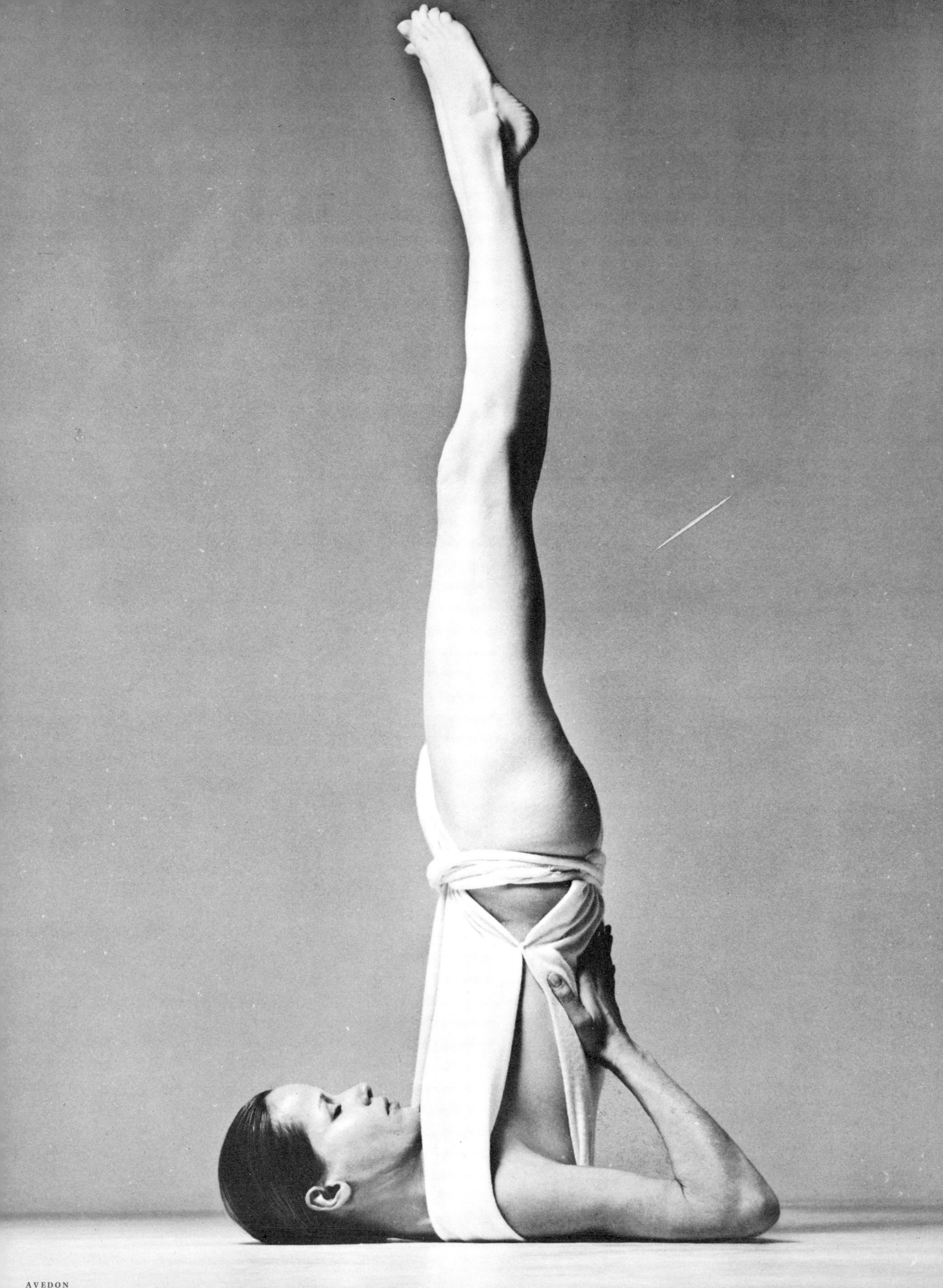

AVEDON

BRONWEN MEREDITH

VOGUE BODY AND BEAUTY BOOK

Guild Publishing, London

For Arabella

This edition published 1978 by Book Club Associates
Reprinted 1979, 1980, 1981, 1982, 1984, 1985
By arrangement with Allen Lane

Designed by Paul Bowden
Drawings by Maria Theresa Barlow
Set in Monophoto Photina by
Oliver Burridge Filmsetting Ltd
Colour separations by Newsele Litho Limited
Printed in Great Britain by Butler & Tanner Ltd
Frome and London

PART I THE BASICS

PART II THE AESTHETICS

PART III THE SCIENCES

One of the pleasures of writing this book was having at my disposal all the knowledge and expertise of all the contributors to *Vogue* since it was first published. It was like having a team of invisible collaborators and I wish to thank them all. *Vogue*, under the editorial direction of Alexander Liberman, has always been the first to introduce new ideas and to recognize the need for change in the health and beauty fields as well as in fashion. I particularly wish to express gratitude to Beatrix Miller, editor of British *Vogue*, who from the start supported my concept of the book; also to Barbara Tims who went through my original manuscript with a discerning eye and skilled pen. Alex Kroll, as editor of Condé Nast Books in London, not only kept track of everything – including me – but chose the illustrations. Maria Theresa Barlow needs special thanks for splendidly interpreting my rough sketches. I also wish to thank all the people at Allen Lane who have helped with this book, especially Eleo Gordon and the many professionals who gave precious time to explain the intricacies of their special expertise. Finally, a word of appreciation to my mother who, during the last frantic month, looked after me like a child leaving me free to worry about nothing but finishing this book.

FOREWORD

The pursuit of beauty is not narcissistic, it is an essential way to build up confidence without which there is little achievement in anything. It gives pleasure, it brings it. Beauty, today, is not a perfect face or a certain look – we have left those attitudes far behind. Beauty now is seen in the way a woman protects, reflects and projects her body power and mental energy. Beauty is individuality. It is glowing health and vitality, it is awareness and action, it is science and technology and of course marvellous looks, a perfect skin, a superb body. We are no longer interested in quick cover-up effects but in long range plans to feel and look better. Within your grasp is the accumulated knowledge of years that can provide you with your ideal health and beauty programme: a straightforward guide to the whole health and beauty spectrum bringing you the basics of body and function, of artifices and aesthetics, of scientific and medical influences . . . all adding up to complete self-awareness. Beauty is a science now. You are responsible for your body; your first move starts here. . . .

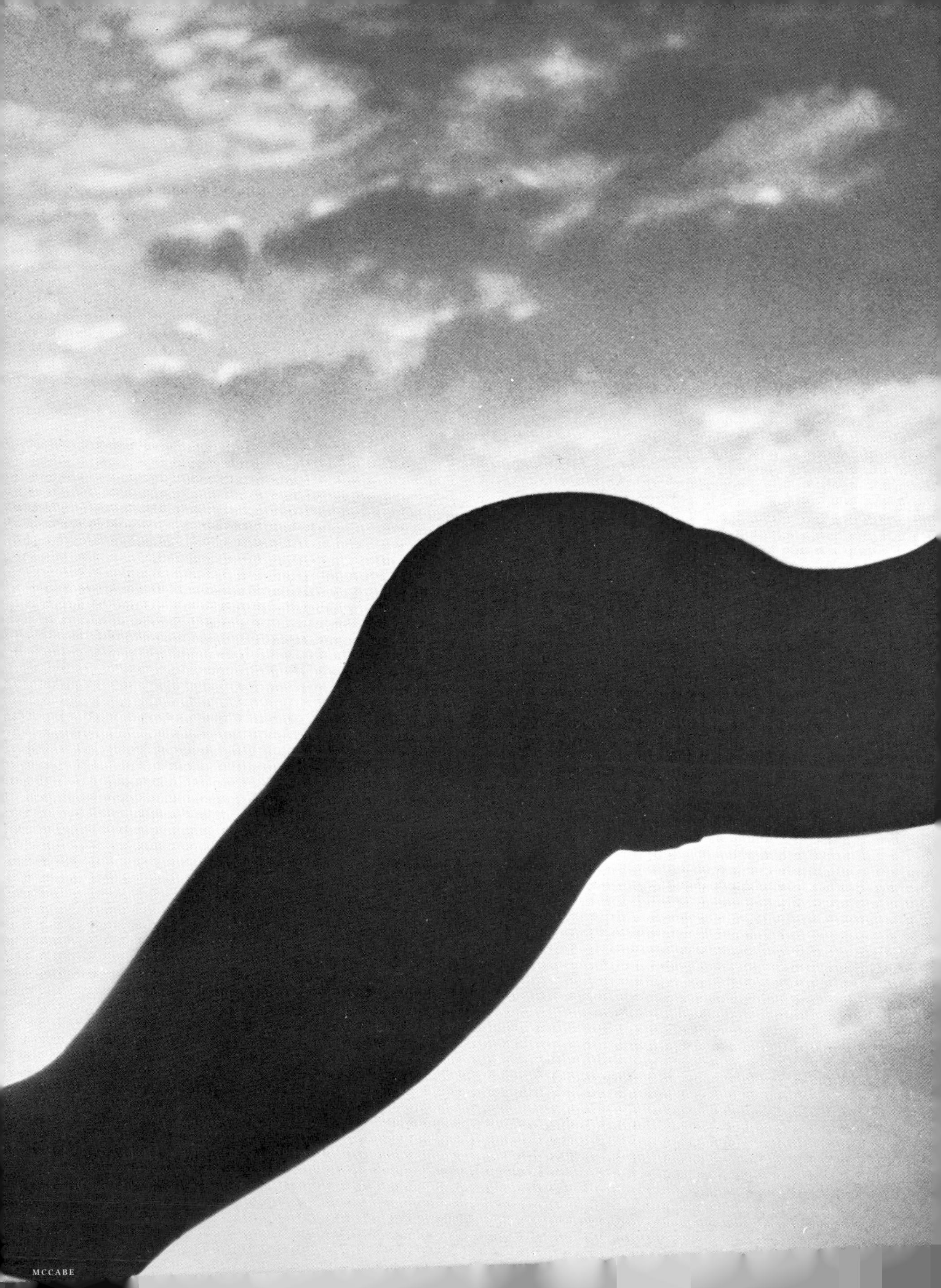

MCCABE

PART I THE BASICS

1

THE BODY

Think of the body as divided into seven systems: bones, brain, nerves, muscles, respiration, circulation, digestion, glands. All are connected and interdependent, though each has a special network of its own.

BONES

The average woman has 206 bones in her body, but not always. She, like Adam, sometimes has an extra pair of ribs. A baby is born with about 350 bones, many of which fuse during the growing years. Bone growth and final size is mostly genetic, but it can be influenced by environment and physical demands. Women usually reach their maximum height at sixteen, but that doesn't mean growth entirely ceases. The vertebral column increases from three to four millimetres between the ages of twenty and thirty. After fifty, stature often diminishes.

The function of bone is diverse. It gives shape and support, it protects certain organs and is an anchor for muscles. Although you may be able to relocate fat and influence muscles nothing can be done to alter this fundamental frame.

The word skeleton comes from a Greek word meaning 'dried bones'. Although one rarely gets an opportunity to see living bones, they are anything but dry. Bones have an outer layer of compact bone tissue that is pinky-white and crowded with tiny openings through which intertwine the network of nerves, arteries, veins and connective tissue. Inside, bones are a deep red with a mesh of spongy material containing that matter vital to life – marrow. Marrow is a combination of fat and tissue which manufactures all the red corpuscles. It also produces other constituents of blood and, most important, is a reservoir of minerals essential not only to the bone itself but to the general health of the body. Calcium and phosphorus are the two main minerals but there are also stores of magnesium, fluoride and chloride. These minerals are not stationary but constantly move on to fortify other areas and need to be replaced. Although rigid, bone is changeable and active.

The skeleton provides both firmness and also extreme flexibility. Some joints move like machinery, others remain locked. Think of what you can do with your thumb and what you can't do with your big toe.

The spinal column is the main bone structure and it supports the whole body. It is very flexible, on the average a little over 2 feet (610 cm.) long and consists of thirty-three vertebrae. These are cylindrical bones with a central canal and strung together. There is a spongy circle of cartilage between each which makes the spine elastic and shock-absorbent. Running down either side are ligaments which help to hold it together.

Attached to the spine is the framework of the chest – twelve pairs of ribs and the breastbone. The ribs are of varying lengths but they all join the spine at the back, curving round to the front where the upper ribs join the breastbone. In this manner they form a protective cage for the heart and lungs, providing ample space for expansion during breathing.

The limbs are attached to the spinal column by special structures – the arms have the shoulder blades, the legs the pelvis. The pelvis is rather like a shell, holding in its strong frame the organs of the abdomen. Freedom of limbs comes from the ball-and-socket joints. The topmost bones of all comprise the skull, where size and placement determine facial features.

BRAIN AND NERVES

The size of the brain has nothing to do with ability. One brain can be twice the size of another without showing any apparent difference in performance. The largest human brains, more than twice normal size, are those of idiots. The brain is a soft lump of 14,000,000 cells and on the surface looks like a jigsaw puzzle fitted together with extreme precision. It usually weighs about 3 pounds (1.5 k.) and is so full of water that it would flop like a jelly if not firmly supported. Anatomically it is symmetrical, but not in performance. Many of its functions are quite one sided. One half of the brain is inclined to be more active and some scientists think this may influence whether one is left- or right-handed.

The forebrain, the cerebrum, is the most important and is over five-sixths of the total. Here is where all higher functions occur – thought, memory and sensory impulses. Brain power is released when a number of factors, physical, mental and social, reinforce one another. The frontal lobe controls muscular movement through a narrow band of cortex which acts as the motor and nerve computer of the body, responding to every single action. An adjacent section receives sensations of warmth, cold and touch; another deals with sound messages. Visual reflexes go through the mid-brain.

The hypothalamus is situated below the cerebrum, mingled with general grey matter. It is an area smaller than a finger joint yet is involved in such diverse operations as balancing, water metabolism, temperature control, appetite, thirst, sleep, fatigue, emotions, weight regulation and sensual responses. Any damage, such as slight pressure from an adjacent tumour, can drastically change body health level, shape and mental attitude. In its control of temperature, the hypothalamus constantly regulates heat loss and gain. Heat is usually gained through metabolic or physical activity and sometimes from the environment, though this is normally cooler than the body. Shivering, which is simply involuntary activity of the skeletal muscles, lowers the temperature. Normal temperature is 98.4 degrees Fahrenheit (36.6 degrees Centigrade). Heat is lost through radiation, convection, conduction and by evaporation through the skin.

The nervous system is closely allied to the brain. The nerve centre of the body runs through the spinal cord. Messages travel as electrical impulses, usually following the quickest route to the spinal cord, and are transmitted from there up to the brain. There are forty-three pairs of nerves; twelve go to and from the brain itself, the rest go to and from the spinal cord. Any disturbance of the spinal cord's balance can have far reaching effects. Nerves go two ways – in and out of the brain. Those passing information to the brain are sensory nerves, those taking messages out are insensory.

MUSCLES

Muscles comprise 36% of female body weight. There are two kinds, voluntary and involuntary, and they perform as the names imply. Involuntary muscles are lighter and function without any indication of their activity. They are hidden away in the body and controlled by the involuntary nervous system. It is impossible to consciously set them in motion or stop them. Their continuous release and contraction is slow and rhythmic; through this action several functions are performed such as pushing food through the digestive channels and pumping the blood.

There are 556 muscles, each consisting of many individual fibres. The longest are 1½ inches (3–4 cm.) and some are less than a millimetre. All muscles exist at birth and grow in size without increasing in number. Strength comes after expansion of each fibre as muscles are made to work. Muscles also have connective tissue which helps to bind the fibres together and secures them to the bones. These take the form of tendons, sinews and bursae – pockets of fluid acting as pulleys at some of the joints. Most muscles are attached by a tendon at just one end, but occasionally at both.

The impulses causing a muscle fibre to twitch are electrical, mechanical or chemical. The time between the arrival of a stimulus at a fibre and the start of contraction is between two and four thousandths of a second.

RESPIRATION

Respiration is more than inhaling and exhaling, it is a very organized method of distributing oxygen around the body. All cells need oxygen to survive. A relaxed person breathes in and out some ten to fourteen times a minute drawing in between 9 and 12 pints (4.5–6 l.) of air. We carry meagre reserves of oxygen so for any physical activity there is an immediate need for more air. Strenuous exercise can require as much as 20 gallons (90 l.) of air a minute with only a second between each breath.

Breathing is controlled by the diaphragm, a large flat muscle separating the chest from the abdomen. It contracts, moving downward – ⅔ of an inch (8 mm.) in quiet breathing, almost 3 inches (7.5 cm.) in deep breathing. This movement increases the capacity of the chest, while at the same time the ribs shift from a sloping position to a more horizontal one. Air rushes in to fill the vacuum in the lungs. For exhalation, the diaphragm relaxes and is pushed upward by abdominal muscles; the ribs return to their former position.

Air is taken in through the nostrils or the mouth or both. It is cleansed by the hairs at the entrance of the nose and by the thin hairs deeper inside. The mucous cells of the nose help to humidify the air, making it less irritating to the delicate structures inside the chest. This is why it is preferable to breathe through the nose rather than the mouth. Air then enters the pharynx, a fibro-muscular passage about 5 inches (13 cm.) long; food also passes down it. Then food and air passages separate, the air going through the larynx at the front of the neck and into the windpipe (trachea), a 5-inch (13-cm.) long elastic tube. Where there's a bump on your breastbone, the windpipe divides into two main bronchi, each subdividing into much smaller bronchioles which in turn divide into many small ducts that lead into the lungs and culminate in alveoli.

The lungs are a pair of large, spongy half cones almost filling the chest area and consisting entirely of air sacs. Together they weigh about two and a half pounds, the right one usually heavier than the left. Architecturally they are rather poor as they have the same entrance as exit. This means there is usually only a partial interchange of gas and about five-sixths of the air present in the lungs is still there when the next breath is taken. Hence recommendations to breathe deeply for good health, as only in this manner is there a chance of exchanging stale air; some molecules can stay in the lungs for life.

It is at the alveoli of the lungs where gaseous diffusion most easily occurs. Each one is covered with a tracery of blood capillaries through which blood cells pass giving off carbon dioxide and taking up the oxygen just breathed in. The two ventricles of the heart are responsible for the blood flow; the right one pumps its blood into the capillary network of the lungs, the left one pumps the oxygenized blood into the capillary network of the body.

Respiration can cause some oddities. Laughter is actually deep breathing followed by spasmodic breathings out. Maybe this way of really cleaning out the lungs is responsible for the belief that if you laugh you are healthy. Yawning is a prolonged deep breath to give the body a reviving and plentiful supply of oxygen. Sighing involves extra breathing-out. Hiccups are spasmodic inhalations which end in a click due to a sudden closing of the vocal cords; either the diaphragm is at fault or the nerves controlling it.

CIRCULATION

On average there are 10 pints (5 l.) of blood in your body constantly being pumped through the circulatory system by the heart. Blood accounts for about 10% of body weight. It is a tissue consisting of red cells, white cells, platelets and plasma, with the plasma occupying a little more than half the volume.

Red corpuscles contain haemoglobin, which picks up oxygen from the lungs and delivers it to the tissues; when carrying oxygen, blood and arteries are bright red. White corpuscles are lighter and fairly transparent; they are less numerous than the red and more varied; they primarily combat infection by their mobility and ability to ingest or absorb bacteria and other foreign elements. Too many white cells, however, can be as disastrous as too few; leukaemia is an overproduction. Blood platelets are smaller than the corpuscles but much more numerous. They influence the clotting of the blood, keeping us from bleeding to death from a nick or cut. They take care of immediate needs at the site of injury. Plasma is not made up of cells; it is 90% water and the balance is proteins, salts and most of the blood cargo such as nutrients, hormones, waste-products and antibodies. Quite often an ill person needs the plasma more than the corpuscles.

Blood's most important job is transportation. During all its travels it carries water, vital to every cell; it takes oxygen from the lungs and carbon dioxide to them; it carries nutrients to the cells and waste products away; it is a distributor of hormones, a circulator of antibodies and it transports heat from the hot to the cool regions. Blood plays a part in every body function and reflects its condition; of all the substances used for testing, blood is by far the most indicative of your health.

The main pumping station, the heart, is the size of a fist and weighs less than a pound ($\frac{1}{2}$ k.). It doesn't lie entirely on the left side of the chest as is often supposed, but is fairly near the centre with about one-third of its bulk over on the right. It has two pumps, each having a similar output; one sends blood through the pulmonary system, the other through the rest of the body. It beats a two-fold sound, roughly seventy times a minute, or four times for each normal breath. With increased physical demand its beat quickens and it pumps blood faster.

Blood pressure is the pressure of blood in the arteries together with a measure of the tension in the arterial wall produced by the blood forced through from the heart. It depends on the output of the heart (systolic pressure) and the resistance to flow by smaller arteries (diastolic pressure). The former is always greater than the latter, and the two are always recorded in that order. An average combination in the twenties would be 120:80. It increases with age and should be frequently checked. Lack of blood pressure can be more rapidly fatal than excess of it. Fainting occurs when there is a short-lived decrease in blood flow to the brain; a stoppage, no matter how brief, would cause brain damage.

A body can lose a quarter of its blood without any apparent severe consequences. One pint (6 dl.) can be given at a transfusion and you can donate a pint (6 dl.) of blood three or four times a year without ill effects.

DIGESTION

Food provides energy and building matter for the body; digestion is the automatic process that converts it into usable units, and storage ones if necessary. The digestive system consists of the alimentary canal through which food passes; it begins at the mouth and ends at the rectum and can be anywhere from 20 to 30 feet (6 to 9 m.) long, twisting and winding to fit in the space provided. Accessory organs are the liver, kidneys, pancreas and spleen.

From the moment food is eaten, it can take from fifteen to twenty-five hours to pass through the body. It is swallowed by automatic contractions in the oesophagus (the foodpipe from mouth to stomach) that propel it onward. The wave of contraction is at the rate of an inch or so per second and is so effective that fluids will get to the stomach even if one is upside down.

On entering the stomach, the proteins, carbohydrates and fats are broken down and changed into smaller particles of protein, glucose, amino acids, fatty acids and glycerine. This is both a chemical and mechanical process; the walls secrete digestive juices and rhythmically contract, causing food units to move into the duodenum, the first part of the small intestine. The stomach's acidity is often a problem, caused by living tissue producing fairly strong hydrochloric acid; this is sometimes diluted and neutralized by food components, but the stomach walls are always protected by alkaline juices.

Practically all digestion is carried out in the small and large intestines and a great proportion of actual absorption of food takes place through the walls. The extraction of valuable food elements is done by enzymes.

LIVER: The largest single organ in the body, it weighs about 4 pounds (2 k.). One cannot live without the liver. It is made of soft, red-brown tissue divided into lobes and covered with a tough fibrous coat. A remarkable feature is that it has a double blood supply: it receives fresh arterial blood and also blood-carrying products of digestion from the intestines. At rest a quarter of the body's blood is in the liver, though a pint or two (6–12 dl.) can leave when exercise is taken. The liver is the central organ of metabolism; its functions are formidable and listed as five hundred. It is capable of replacing its own tissue and its powers of self regeneration are very high.

KIDNEYS: Each kidney is a collection of filter units that absorb virtually everything small from the blood, returning to it what is required. The kidneys eliminate waste products with the formation of urine, regulate salt and liquid intake of the body and maintain the slight alkalinity of body fluids.

PANCREAS AND SPLEEN: Pour crucial digestive juices – 1 to $1\frac{1}{2}$ pints (6 to 9 dl.) daily – into the duodenum. One part of the pancreas is pure gland, secreting insulin.

GLANDS

Some glands, such as those of the skin and digestive tract, produce secretions which have an effect only where they are released; these are called exocrine glands. In contrast, the endocrine glands manufacture substances called hormones which pass directly into the blood stream and affect areas far removed from their place of origin. The secretions are fairly simple compounds many of which are now synthesized. They are effective in very small amounts and are regulators of body processes controlling growth, development, size, weight, sexual activity, reproduction and temperament.

THE PITUITARY: Situated at the base of the brain, it is the master gland. It influences the rest of the endocrine system as well as performing specific functions such as regulating growth, controlling physical and mental development, acting on the sex organs, affecting menstruation, blood pressure and sight.

THE THYROID: Found in the neck, it organizes the body's supply of oxygen. It also secretes an iodine-rich hormone, thyroxine, which works together with one from the pituitary. If the thyroid gland is defective (often due to lack of iodine) metabolism slows down often resulting in overweight and lethargy; it can lead to goitre. Excess secretion causes nervousness, irritability and protruding eyeballs.

THE PARATHYROIDS: Either side of the thyroid, they control levels of calcium and phosphorus.

THE ADRENALS: These affect the nervous system, the emotions and influence the sex glands. They are found above the kidneys. Adrenalin is one hormonal secretion; it stimulates the heart, quickens the pulse and causes a rise in blood sugar. It is released through fear and can cause anger. Cortisone is the other hormone.

THE PANCREAS: Part of the pancreas is used for digestion, the other part is a gland called the Island of Langerhans. This produces the hormone insulin which regulates the sugar level in the blood and the conversion of sugar into energy and heat. Imbalances cause diabetes or hypoglycaemia.

THE GONADS: The sex glands found in the ovaries; they produce oestrogen and progesterone which together regulate the reproductive cycle. A small quantity of male hormones are also produced; if excessive, male characteristics result.

BODY TYPE

Physique varies from person to person and any classification of figure types can only be a general guide. It is important to recognize that there are variations in frame structure, and to acknowledge that you can never change your body type. You have to learn to keep within its range, work within its possibilities. By the early twenties, the dimensions of the skeleton are settled and the appropriate muscle and fat covering is determined. Everything is a matter of proportion, judged three-dimensionally and often in truer perspective from a side view. Height has nothing to do with body type.

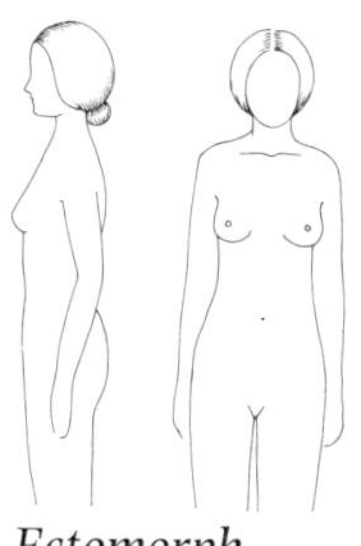

Ectomorph

There are three basic shapes: ectomorph, mesomorph and endomorph and there is a degree of overlapping but no moving from one group to another. A fat ectomorph is a fat person, not an endomorph; while the slimness of a mesomorph in no way resembles the ideal of the endomorph.

ECTOMORPH: Small frame in width and depth, side view slender; narrow shoulders, often still narrower hips; ideally thin with some bust shaping, without much muscle or fat.

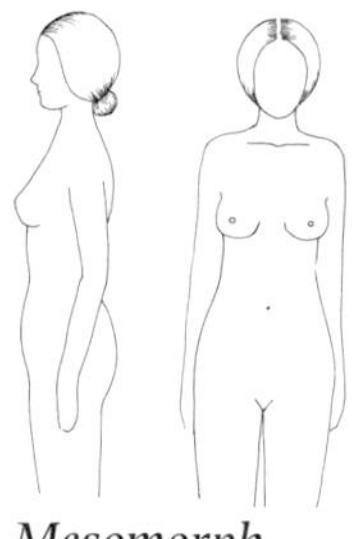

Mesomorph

MESOMORPH: Medium to large frame, ranging from athletic to rounded but always with depth and a certain degree of narrowness through ribcage, waist and hips; sometimes broad-shouldered and a forceful shape; ideally with a lot of muscle and bone, not much fat, controlled hips.

ENDOMORPH: A heavy build but not necessarily a large frame; rounded on all sides with a chunky middle section; shoulders often narrower than hips; ideally well-covered without excess fat and trim muscles.

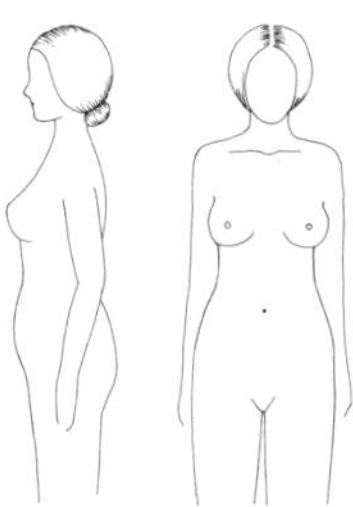

Endomorph

BODY POSTURE

Good posture gives a better figure instantly; it is good exercise and the basis of figure beauty. The way you carry and move your body influences its shape; the effect is slow but steady, and it can work for or against you.

POSTURE EXERCISES

Many figure faults have their origin in faulty posture; aches and body fatigue too. When the spine is carried correctly, it has an easy alignment; when incorrectly held it gives a hollow back, squashes the vertebrae together, sets up friction and tension, and eventually can cause joint thickening and bone displacement.

The habit of good posture can mean a young-looking figure for life; it creates an impression of vitality, confidence and attractiveness.

Standing – Your spine is a long cord; imagine there is a thread running through it and it is being pulled up tautly from above your head. This lifts and stretches straight the whole body; it also makes you feel much lighter and springier. Pull in stomach, tuck buttocks under, chest high, shoulders back but relaxed and pulling the arm sockets downwards, head in alignment with chin parallel to the ground. When picking something up, bend from the knees with one foot slightly in front of the other, bottom tucked under. Good posture strengthens the supportive muscles and through habit they automatically keep firm and in place.

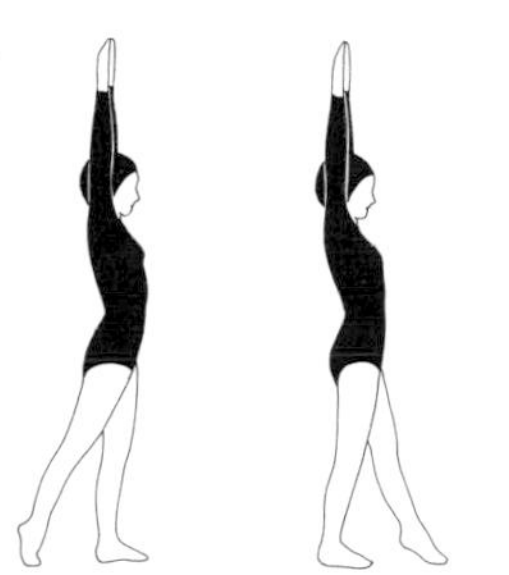

1. *Walking Stretch*

Walking – Check alignment before you start and be sure toes point straight ahead. Relax arms, allowing them to swing, following the body naturally and with ease. Movement should come from the thighs, not the hips; as you walk breathe deeply and slowly to the count of four in, four out. Keep the back straight, up and down hill, up and down steps, lifting and lowering yourself by using thigh muscles. Don't lean forward with buttocks stuck out at the back.

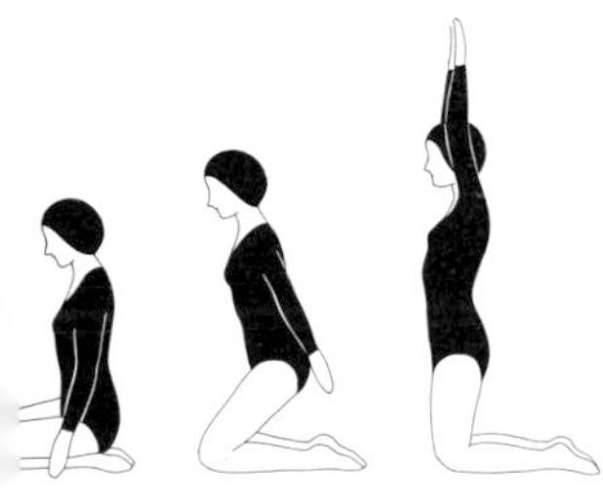

2. *Kneeling Stretch*

Sitting – Before sitting, be sure your back is to the chair and one leg almost touching it, the other a little in front. Keeping the back straight and head aligned, lower yourself by bending the knees. Legs look better together, straight in front or slightly to the side.

1. Align back, hold arms straight above head, thumbs hooked; pull arms back without arching spine. Walk around the room for two minutes, breathing in deeply to the count of four, out to the count of four.

2. Kneel, sitting on heels, back straight, arms at side; using thigh muscles, keeping back straight and bottom under, rise to kneeling position bringing arms up over head; return to heel sitting; never arch back. *10 times.*

3. Lie on stomach, arms stretched out, palms down, shoulders flat, head slightly raised. Bend left leg at knee to a right angle; keeping ribcage firmly on floor, move bent leg across straight one, aiming to touch the floor with the knee; at first it is impossible. *6 times with each leg.*

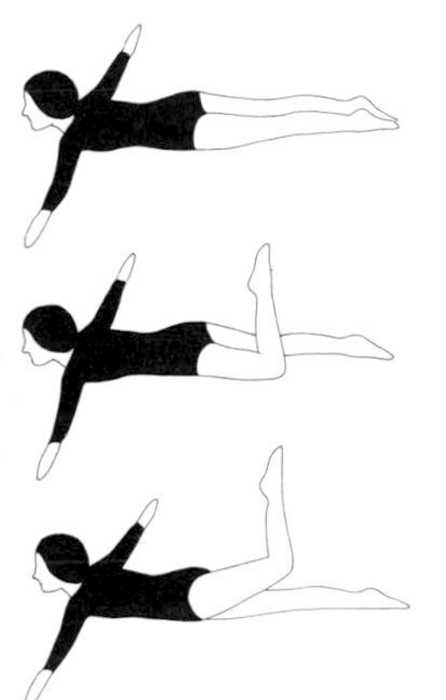

3 *Lying Stretch*

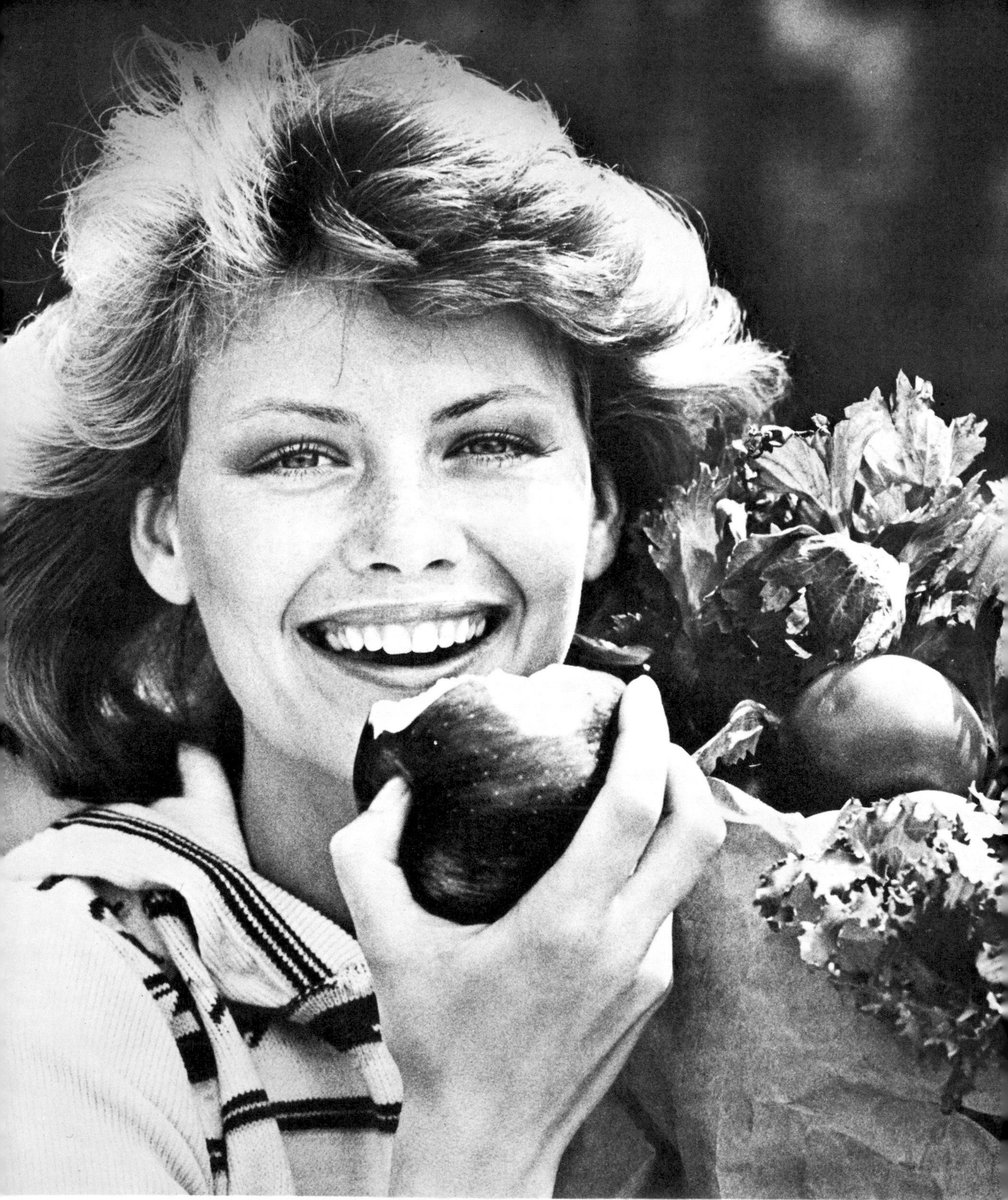

STEMBER

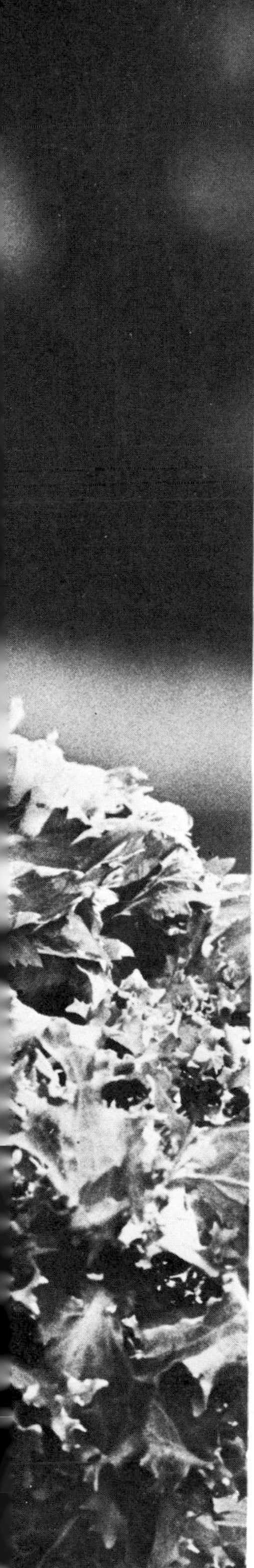

2

NUTRITION

Nutrition is a comparatively new science. We are warned constantly about the adverse effects of refining, processing, of additives and of pollution but there is disagreement on certain points, the main one being health food versus regular food. People eat health food for many reasons: because they like plain good food, because they are worried about chemical additives either in the growing or in the processing of food, or because they feel that food is directly linked to how they look and feel. But there are alternatives to the specialized health shop. There is enough fresh food around to supply all the nutrients anyone normally needs. This is the rational way to nutrition and it takes only a basic knowledge of food constituents, their preservation and utilization, to work out a conscientious diet. It is being aware of food values that matters, so that you do not unconsciously give your body worthless foods – or worse, poisonous ones. A lot is ordinary common sense:

Fresh is best.
Eat plenty of vegetables and fruit, raw when possible.
Certain manufactured, processed or refined food should be avoided.
Sugar and all its derivatives should be cut down to a minimum, preferably cut out.
Eat foods rich in fibre (formerly known as roughage).
Eat less fat.

We should eat as much wholesome, fresh, uncontaminated food as possible. It is the best way to get essential vitamins and minerals. Most of the food we eat has been tampered with in some way; the goodness taken out by refining and processing, chemicals added to prolong shelf life, stabilize, preserve, flavour, colour, sweeten, thicken – all of which may please the eye and the taste, but not the stomach and health.

Be wary of anything white – white flour, bread, pastries, rice, sugar. White means a blank, that most nourishment has been taken out and all sorts of synthetic things put in. Wholegrain cereals, flour, bread and brown rice should replace this fortified white stodge.

Sugar is the number one enemy of good nutrition and sugar supplies about 20 per cent of an average diet in the Western world.

Sugar was unknown to man until 200 years ago, so the body handles it as a foreign substance. In nature sugar is packaged with vitamins and minerals – in fruit as fructose and in vegetables as starch. The refined product is straight sucrose, which the body absorbs much faster than natural sugars, and because it is so similar to blood sugar which has already been metabolized into glucose, it escapes the body's processing action. The body is forced to use its vitamins and minerals and acids to fight the invasion, and this surge of activity can lower blood sugar and body energy levels leaving one tired, mentally slow, irritable, and susceptible to disease. The odd sweet or chocolate bar gives an initial spurt due to acceleration of metabolism, but shortly afterwards you are more depleted than ever. Substitute honey for sugar; brown sugar is next best.

Fruit and vegetables should make up the highest proportion of your diet. They can supply all necessary vitamins and minerals. Wash thoroughly but not overmuch. Eat skins whenever possible, they are often the richest part.

Eat less fat. Evidence is conflicting on this issue but it seems reasonable to keep it to a minimum. This means cutting a lot of fat off meat, restricting butter, using unsaturated fats and vegetable oils. It does not necessarily mean skimmed milk and cottage cheese – that is a personal choice.

The missing ingredient in many diets is fibre. It was once called roughage and considered essential to the proper working of the bowels. Overlooked over the last twenty years, it is now thought to be directly related to the high incidence of colon-rectal cancer, also to the increased prevalence of diabetes, gallstones, appendicitis, varicose veins, haemorrhoids and obesity. Yet fibre passes virtually unchanged through our intestines and is excreted as waste matter.

Fibre is the structural part of a plant, the connective tissue that supports the cells – leaves, stems, seeds, flowers, fruits, bulbs, roots and tubers are all sources of fibre. In itself it doesn't contain nourishment, but it is believed that its bulk is needed to provide a smooth intestinal voyage for other nutrients. What is known is that a high-fibre diet takes longer to consume and you are more likely to reach a point of satiation before you eat too much. Also it takes a lot of chewing, therefore more saliva and gastric juices are produced which aid in the digestion of other nutrients.

Again fruit and vegetables are the main suppliers of fibre, and best eaten raw with their skins, or lightly cooked. Whole grains in cereals and flours are good for fibre and for other reasons; bran, a very good source, can be taken in water, sprinkled on other foods or made into bread.

When working out a nutritious diet think in terms of vegetables, fruits, proteins, grains (the carbohydrate group) and fats in that order of importance.

PROTEINS: Primarily for building and repairing body tissue and helping to counteract daily wear and tear. Essential to life, they satisfy hunger and have so many functions it would be impossible to list them all. A few of the more important are: ability to build hormones and enzymes which aid in energy production; digestion of food and excretion from the tissues and body; the making of haemoglobin within the red corpuscles; maintaining the acid-alkaline balance of the body; assisting in clotting the blood; forming antibodies to fight infection and disease.

Proteins are found in flesh foods, dairy products (eggs and milk are the best source of all), soya beans and nuts, grains (especially wheatgerm) and some vegetables.

CARBOHYDRATES: Provide energy for physical and mental exertion by supplying immediate calories; they assist in the assimilation and digestion of other foods. A deficiency leads to low energy level, poor health and mental depression. There are three forms of carbohydrates — sugars, starches and cellulose. The sugar and starch are converted to glucose for energy; excess not spent as energy is quickly stored as fat. In an effort to burn up this excess, the body uses extra vitamin B, thus depriving other organs. The cellulose carbohydrates (a large part of fruit and vegetables) have no energy value but provide the fibre necessary to regulate the bowels. The best carbohydrates are found in vegetables, fruits, whole grain flours and cereals. Acceptable sugar carbohydrates are honey, blackstrap molasses and dried raisins. Unacceptable sugar and starch carbohydrates are the refined sugars, flours, cereals and breads.

FATS: Provide a delayed source of energy and act as carriers for fat-soluble vitamins. Fats also make calcium available to body tissues, thus promoting growth. They prevent the skin from becoming dry. It is important to have fatty deposits to protect the vital organs and a layer under the skin preserves heat and protects the body against cold. A deficiency of fats can lead to a deficiency of vitamins, and to skin disorders. Excess means obesity and indigestion. There are two types: saturated fats which are hard at room temperature and come mostly from animal sources; and unsaturated fats, usually liquid and from vegetable sources. Some nutritionists say it doesn't matter whether one has animal or vegetable fat, while others point out that hard animal fats create high cholesterol content in the blood. Play safe and limit animal fats like butter and solid unsaturated fats such as margarine and be liberal with the liquid vegetable oils – olive, corn, wheatgerm, sunflower, sesame, avocado and peanut. They all contain linoleic acid which is particularly beneficial to the skin.

There are no wonder foods but there are some foods that contain a particularly concentrated amount of vitamins and minerals. They include honey, brewers' yeast, blackstrap molasses, wheatgerm, yoghourt, powdered skimmed milk and sunflower seeds.

COOKING

A few basic rules are important: no frying in additional fat; meat, poultry and game can be cooked in its own fat or with a little oil (always vegetable oil, avoid butter) or roasted, braised or boiled. When cooking vegetables use a minimum of water and cook for the minimum of time otherwise vitamins and minerals are destroyed. Don't add chemicals such as bicarbonate of soda, use a few drops of lemon juice instead. Learn to bake with wholegrain flours and sugar substitutes.

SELECTION AND SERVINGS

Constantly vary vegetables and fruits, consulting the vitamin and mineral listings to see which are most nutritious. Balance the flesh and dairy products – eggs for breakfast, cheese for lunch, meat for dinner, for example. This is not a diet for weight loss but be sensible and keep to moderate portions. Eat raw fibre food first, it fills you up. An average meat serving should be about 20 grammes. A vegetable serving should be about a cup, the same for rice or other grains. One large baked potato or three new boiled ones. Salads and raw vegetables in any quantity but not too much fruit because of its high sugar content: one apple, orange or banana, a small bowl of berries, a slice of melon, half a grapefruit.

THE MAINTENANCE DIET

This is the blueprint for a daily eating plan that ensures that all the protein, vitamins and minerals, with the right amount of energy foods, are consumed. It concentrates on healthy, wholesome foods and is not at all meagre. It is a preventive health measure as well as one that provides a high degree of energy and helps to keep weight at a constant level. Count calories if you like but it is really not necessary if you keep to the servings suggested. A day's intake should average 2,300 calories, the number needed to balance energy output.

PROTEIN GROUP – 20% OF TOTAL

meats: beef, veal, lamb, pork, ham, bacon, liver, kidney, heart, brains, sweetbreads, tripe
poultry: chicken, turkey, duck, goose, guinea fowl
game: venison, pheasant, quail, rabbit
fish: fresh and salt water varieties, shellfish
dairy products: eggs, cheese, yoghourt, milk
nuts: almonds, Brazil nuts, peanuts, walnuts, pecans
vegetables: avocados, soya beans, lentils
grains: barley, oatmeal, rice, wheatgerm, wholegrain flours, brewers' yeast

VEGETABLE GROUP – 65% OF TOTAL, TOGETHER WITH FRUIT

leafy vegetables: asparagus, artichokes, broccoli, cabbage, cauliflower, celery, chicory, endive, kale, spinach, lettuce, watercress
root vegetables: onions, radishes, potatoes, beetroot, carrots
fruit vegetables: tomatoes, peppers, aubergines, courgettes, cucumbers, marrows, pumpkins, squashes

FRUIT GROUP

citrus: lemons, oranges, grapefruits, tangerines
orchard: apples, pears, plums, apricots, peaches, cherries, grapes
berry: raspberries, strawberries, bilberries, cranberries, gooseberries
tropical: mangoes, bananas, pineapples, papayas, cantaloups, melons

GRAIN AND CEREAL GROUP – 10% OF TOTAL

Wholegrain flours and breads, oatmeal, barley, brown rice, wheatgerm, bran.

FAT GROUP – 5% OF TOTAL

Unsaturated fats such as margarine, limited butter, all vegetable oils.

DAILY FORMULA

Breakfast:

Generally considered essential, as your blood sugar level is low in the morning and a good breakfast will get you going. Some protein must be eaten.

fresh fruit or unsweetened juice
protein – egg, cheese, fish or meat (not less than 20 grammes)
slice of wholewheat bread or toast with butter, honey or home-made preserves or wholegrain cereal such as oatmeal or muesli
coffee or tea.

Lunch:

This is the time to eat raw foods such as salads combined with some protein, but if it's more convenient to have the main meal at midday, reverse dinner menu – nutritionally it doesn't make any difference.

fresh salad or raw vegetables
protein – egg, cheese, fish or meat
wholewheat bread, toast or roll
dessert – yoghourt or fresh fruit
coffee, tea or glass of wine.

Dinner:

This is the main meal of the day, it should be leisurely and can be many courses. Start with something fresh.

salad or fresh fruit or crudités
home-made soup
protein – meat, fish, game or poultry
cooked vegetables – always include one leafy green variety
choice of potatoes, rice or pasta
dessert – fruit, yoghourt, cheese or gelatine with fruit
2 glasses wine coffee or tea.

FLAVOURINGS: All natural herbs; limited salt, preferably sea salt.

SWEETENERS: No white sugars; use honey, natural brown sugar or molasses.

DRESSINGS: For salads, oil and vinegar with added herbs and mustard, home-made mayonnaise; avoid creamy synthetic dressings.

SAUCES: Limit those containing flour or cornstarch; use no sugar.

SNACKS: Fresh fruits and vegetables or their juice; cheese and other protein titbits. No sweet biscuits or cakes.

BEVERAGES: Four glasses of water a day, and when possible sparkling mineral water. Limited wine and spirits; coffee, tea.

VITAMINS

Vitamins are not forms of energy or builders themselves but they regulate metabolism and help convert fat and carbohydrates into energy. They also help to repair tissues. Though each of the vitamins has specific functions within the body, they work as a team, which means that if one vitamin is deficient, it may well affect the efficiency of the others.

You cannot test for vitamin deficiency. Only when it is at the extreme stage do visible symptoms occur in the blood chemistry. So how much vitamin should be supplemented and on what grounds? A new branch of science called orthomolecular medicine uses large doses of vitamin supplements in the treatment of disease. This megavitamin (the name for huge doses) therapy cites success stories such as vitamin C as a barrier against some virus infections, and vitamin E as an aid in heart ailments and in retarding the ageing process. Megavitamins do not have an overall seal of approval despite reasonable evidence to support the claims. Some nutritionists point out that overdoses of certain vitamins can have bad side effects. However, there are strong indications that vitamins may be our best protection against environmental stress and pollutants.

Vitamins fall into two groups: those soluble in fat (A, D, E and K) which generally are stored in the body and do not require daily replacement, and those soluble in water (C and B complex) which must be supplied each day as excess is excreted in the urine. The fat soluble ones are measured in International Units (a tiny measurement) and the water soluble ones in milligrammes (mg) which is one thousandth of a gramme. Below are itemized the most important vitamins, indicating their best sources and their effect on the body. New vitamins are being discovered and named, e.g. P, Q, U, B-15 and B-17 (laetrile), but their properties and functions are not fully formulated, nor their claims supported (e.g. laetrile in the treatment of cancer). If you take your vitamins from fresh natural sources every day you should receive an adequate supply. It is almost impossible to get an overdose. Vitamin supplements are essential if you are without fresh foods and take care not to destroy vitamin content in processed foods by exposure to toxins, light, etc.

VITAMIN A (RETINOL)

Function: Maintains a healthy complexion and helps keep skin in good condition. Promotes good eye-sight and is essential to the formation of visual purple, a substance which adapts the eye to darkness. Protects surface tissues of the respiratory tract. Helps to repair body tissues and skeletal growth.
Good source: Alfalfa sprouts, apricots, broccoli, butter, carrots, chicken liver, cod liver oil, dandelion greens, eggs, kale, kidneys, lamb's liver, mangoes, papayas, parsley, peppers (hot red), spinach, watercress.
Deficiency results: Inflammation of the eyes and inability to adjust to darkness. Dryness and premature ageing of the skin. Aggravation of the respiratory system that leads to infections.
Overdose results: Loss of appetite, headaches, hair loss and aching bones.
Destroyed by: Exposure to sunlight can cause serious loss of vitamin A, although it is not destroyed by cooking; air pollution and watching T.V. have adverse affects; it is not well absorbed if taken in conjunction with excessive mineral oil.
Daily need: 5,000 International Units. It is stored in the liver so daily intake is not absolutely essential.

VITAMIN B COMPLEX

There are 13 separate vitamins which should be taken together in the correct proportion because a large dose of one may cause a deficiency of the others. It is impossible to work this out for oneself but in a fresh food diet nature does it for you. Synthetic vitamin supplements are accurately balanced. All these vitamins dissolve in water and any excess is excreted so it is essential to replace them daily. This is not always easy as refining flours and cereals removes almost all of them and large amounts are destroyed by light and heat during cooking. Extra B vitamins are required when under stress, by pregnant women and alcoholics. Best sources for the whole complex are: green leafy vegetables, brewers' yeast, whole grains and offal including liver and kidney.

VITAMIN B-1 (THIAMINE)

Function: Necessary for conversion of carbohydrates into glucose for energy. Important for smooth functioning of nervous system, heart, liver.
Good source: Alfalfa sprouts, asparagus, Brazil nuts, brewers' yeast, brown rice (not white), haricot beans, lamb's liver, muesli, rolled oats, sunflower seeds, wheatgerm, wholewheat bread (not white).

Deficiency results: Fatigue, forgetfulness, nerve pain, numbness and tingling. A severe restriction causes beriberi, but this is rarely found outside the tropics.
Overdose results: Has been known to cause low blood pressure and trembling, but it is very difficult to take an overdose.
Destroyed by: Soaking and cooking, alcohol and tobacco.
Daily need: 1.5 mg.

VITAMIN B-2 (RIBOFLAVIN)

Function: Helps to break down all food. Necessary for good vision and clear eyes. Needed for cell respiration.
Good source: Almonds, avocados, brewers' yeast, chicken liver, cottage cheese, kidneys, milk, mushrooms, spinach, turnip greens, wheatgerm, wild rice, yoghourt.
Deficiency results: Bloodshot and itching eyes, sensitivity to bright lights, broken blood vessels, split corners of mouth, dermatitis, dandruff, split finger-nails.
Overdose results: Tingling sensations.
Destroyed by: Light – rapidly.
Daily need: 2 mg.

VITAMIN B-3 (NIACIN)

Function: Assists in breakdown and use of proteins, fats and carbohydrates. Important to mental health. Maintains health of skin, tongue, gums and digestive system. Is most beneficial in conjunction with the other B vitamins.
Good source: Chicken, chicken's liver, halibut, kidneys, lamb's liver, mackerel, peanuts, salmon, sardines, turkey, whole grains and breads.
Deficiency results: Lethargy, bad concentration, bad balance, depression, nervousness, diarrhoea, dental decay, halitosis (bad breath).
Overdose results: Flushes, tingling sensations, activation of peptic ulcer.
Destroyed by: Not established.
Daily need: 15 mg.

VITAMIN B-5 (PANTOTHENIC ACID)

Function: Essential for balanced functioning of the adrenal gland, therefore important to the nervous system; cholesterol and fatty acids cannot be formed without it.
Good source: Bran, brewers' yeast, kidneys, lamb's liver, mushrooms, peanuts, whole grains.

Deficiency results: Malfunction of the adrenal gland which means loss of control against stress, irritability, dizziness, nervous headache, blackouts; numbness and tingling of muscles, sometimes cramps. Can lead to premature grey hair – an adequate amount may prevent it. Lack of it plays a major role in the onset of arthritis.
Overdose results: Not established.
Destroyed by: Acid such as vinegar. More stable in hot liquid (such as boiling) than in dry cooking (such as grilling or roasting).
Daily need: Estimated at 5–10 mg.

VITAMIN B-6 (PYRIDOXINE)

Function: Aids in metabolic breakdown of foods; helps form antibodies and red blood cells. Important in regulation of nervous system.
Good source: Bananas, blackstrap molasses, Brazil nuts, chicken, lamb's liver, mackerel, walnuts, wheatgerm, wholewheat grains and bread.
Deficiency results: Nervousness, irritability, depression, mouth disorders, muscular weakness, anaemia, haemorrhoids, dermatitis.
Overdose results: Not established.
Destroyed by: Oral contraceptives, so supplements may be necessary for women on the Pill. A little is taken away by soaking and cooking food.
Daily need: 2 mg.

VITAMIN B-12 (CYANOCOBALAMIN)

Function: Essential for normal functioning of body cells, particularly those of the bone marrow, nervous system and gastro-intestinal tract. Necessary for formation of red blood cells.
Good source: Cheese, eggs, herrings, kidneys, lamb's liver, milk, oysters, sardines, soya beans.
Deficiency results: Most serious is pernicious anaemia; also bronchial asthma, disturbance of central nervous system, unpleasant body odour.
Overdose results: High haemoglobin count.
Destroyed by: Foods used in conjunction with raw egg white.
Daily need: .005 mg.

BIOTIN (VITAMIN B COMPLEX)

Function: Helps form fatty acids, then burns them up together with carbohydrates for energy.
Good source: Blackcurrants, blackstrap molasses, cauliflower, dried milk, kidneys, lamb's liver, leeks, raw egg yolks (only), rolled oats (dry).

Deficiency results: Unlikely, but absorption problems can occur resulting in fatigue and depression, dermatitis and greyish skin colour.
Overdose results: Not established.
Destroyed by: Exposure to air, baking soda; raw egg white prevents absorption. Unaffected by heat.
Daily need: Very small amount, not established.

CHOLINE (VITAMIN B COMPLEX)

Function: Aids distribution of fats from the liver to the cells. Plays a role in nerve transmission.
Good source: Beans, fish, heart, lecithin granules, lentils, wheatgerm, whole grains.
Deficiency results: Cirrhosis of the liver, hardening of arteries, high blood pressure.
Overdose results: Not established.
Destroyed by: Strong alkali. Not affected by heat or storage.
Daily need: Not established.

FOLIC ACID (VITAMIN B COMPLEX)

Function: Helps form red blood cells and nucleic acids, both essential for reproduction. Carries carbon to form the iron-containing protein in haemoglobin.
Good source: Almonds, cod, comfrey, lamb's liver, oysters, raw cabbage, raw kale, walnuts, watercress.
Deficiency results: Anaemia, low white blood count, depression.
Overdose results: Not established.
Destroyed by: Not established.
Daily need: 1.5 mg – stress and the intake of excess alcohol increase needs.

INOSITOL (VITAMIN B COMPLEX)

Function: Together with choline, necessary for the formation of lecithin, which keeps the liver free of fats.
Good source: Bran, blackstrap molasses, lecithin granules, nuts, oats, sesame seeds, wheatgerm.
Deficiency results: Cirrhosis of the liver, poor appetite, hardening of arteries.
Overdose results: Not established.
Destroyed by: Not established.
Daily need: Not established.

PABA (PARA-AMINOBENZOIC ACID, VITAMIN B COMPLEX)

Function: Enables other vitamin B agents to function properly. Especially important in forming red blood cells. May help prevent onset of grey hair.
Good source: Broccoli, cabbage, kale, kidneys, lamb's liver, rice (brown).
Deficiency results: Fatigue, irritability, depression and digestive disorders.
Overdose results: Not established.
Destroyed by: Not established.
Daily need: Not established.

VITAMIN C (ASCORBIC ACID)

Function: Main use is to maintain level of collagen, a protein necessary for the formation of skin, ligaments and bones; therefore helps to mend fractures, heal wounds, form scars. Helps prevent haemorrhaging. Said to aid and prevent some types of virus and bacterial infections (the common cold, for instance).
Good source: Acerola cherries, alfalfa sprouts, blackcurrants, broccoli, Brussels sprouts, cabbage, cauliflower, grapefruit, lemon juice (diluted), orange juice (including pith and peel), papaya, paprika, parsley, peppers, pineapple, rose-hip powder, strawberries, tangerines, watercress.
Deficiency results: Tooth decay, bleeding gums, aching joints, susceptibility to infections, slow healing, tendency to bruise or bleed, bad vision, low body warmth. Prolonged deficiency can lead to scurvy.
Overdose results: Suspected as a contributing factor to kidney stones; large doses cause diarrhoea, activation of peptic ulcer.
Destroyed by: Light, heat, air, prolonged storage, excess cooking, copper and iron utensils. Most easily destroyed of all vitamins.
Daily need: 50 mg. Body's need is increased when under stress, tired, suffering an infection, injury, surgery. More also needed if you smoke, take aspirin or live in a hot climate.

VITAMIN D (CALCIFEROL)

Function: Encourages the transport of calcium and phosphorus to tissues which build bone.
Good source: Cod liver oil, eggs, halibut liver oil, herrings, mackerel, salmon, sardines, sunshine, ultra-violet light (in moderation).
Deficiency results: Weak, brittle bones, spinal curvature, muscle cramp, joint pains, hardening of the arteries, rickets.
Overdose results: Loss of appetite, headache, drowsiness; widespread calcification of non-bony tissues can occur.

Destroyed by: Air pollution inhibits its production via sunlight. Stable when exposed to heat, keeps under storage conditions. Primarily stored in the liver.
Daily need: 400 international units – more if you are on the Pill.

VITAMIN E (TOCOPHEROL)

Function: Not well understood. It unites with oxygen to protect red blood cells and keep them from rupturing. Thought to improve the circulatory system and counteract the process of ageing; used to increase fertility and treat sterility. Externally, used on burns, bruises and wounds to accelerate healing and help alleviate scars.
Good source: Apples, carrots, cabbage, celery, eggs, muesli, olive oil, rolled oats, sunflower seeds, sunflower seed oil, wheatgerm, wholemeal bread, wholemeal flour.
Deficiency results: Degeneration of reproductive tissues, sexual frigidity, early onset of old age, sluggish circulation, varicose veins, liver problems, muscle weakness.
Overdose results: Elevated blood pressure.
Destroyed by: Cooking, storage, iron utensils.
Daily need: 20 International Units – more when under stress.

VITAMIN K

Function: Prevents haemorrhaging, stimulates production of substances involved in the normal clotting process.
Good source: Broccoli, Brussels sprouts, cabbage, cauliflower, eggs, oats, potatoes, strawberries, wheatgerm, wholewheat grains.
Deficiency results: Haemorrhaging deficiencies, but very rare as this vitamin is manufactured by bacteria in intestines.
Overdose results: Fast clotting – thrombosis.
Destroyed by: Alcohol, light and rancidity. Sulphur drugs and antibiotics interfere with its absorption (eating yoghourt can restore it).
Daily need: Widely available, only supplemented in disease conditions.

MINERALS

Minerals occur in minute quantities in the human body and are essential to certain metabolic processes; they help draw chemical substances in and out of the cells; they control the amount of water necessary to the life process; they influence the secretion of glands; they affect muscle responses; and they are important in transmitting messages through the nervous system.

We obtain our minerals through food, but unlike vitamins, which plants manufacture, minerals have to be extracted from the earth by plants. Once in the body, when their work is done, they are excreted in the urine and sweat, so must be regularly replaced.

The problem is that with chemical interference in the soil and atmosphere we are getting too little of some minerals and too much of others; and because the amounts are so minuscule, even a speck of mineral matter can upset metabolism. Reading about deficiencies and their results may inspire you to take capsule supplements. Don't; the borderline between under- and over-doses is too fine. Supplement your diet with natural foods rich in minerals so that the positive and negative electrical charges that minerals carry will be neutrally balanced for proper absorption.

CALCIUM

Functions: To build and maintain bones and teeth; also important in regulation of heart muscles and nerve transmission.
Good source: Almonds, blackstrap molasses, broccoli, cheese (hard varieties such as Parmesan, Swiss, Cheddar), clams, haricot beans, kelp and other seaweeds, milk, powdered milk, olives, sardines, sesame seeds, shrimps, yoghourt.
Deficiency results: Deterioration of bones; weakened tooth structure; muscle cramps, numbness and tingling in arms and legs; blood clotting.
Overdose results: Excess calcium is normally excreted by the body; if not there is a chance of widespread calcification.
Daily need: 600 mg.

CHLORINE

Function: Important in cell metabolism; helps regulate the balance of acid and alkali in the blood.
Good source: Celery, kelp, lettuce, salt (and other sodium-containing foods), spinach, tomatoes.
Deficiency results: Weak water retention, atherosclerosis.
Overdose results: Not established; excess chlorine is usually excreted.
Daily need: Joined to sodium, so provided that intake is sufficient, level is usually correct.

CHROMIUM

Function: Helps regulate blood-sugar levels and improves body's utilization of glucose. Thought to be instrumental in keeping cholesterol low.
Good source: Blackstrap molasses, bran, brewers' yeast, chicken, condiments, fruits, green vegetables, honey, nuts, shellfish, wholegrain cereals.
Deficiency results: Affects tolerance of glucose; hardening of the arteries.
Overdose results: Not established.
Daily need: A trace.

COBALT

Function: Necessary for the proper functioning of vitamin B-12 and for red blood cells.
Good source: Fruits, green vegetables, meat, wholegrain cereals.
Deficiency results: Pernicious anaemia; dry, scaly skin.
Overdose results: Could cause enlargement of thyroid gland but unlikely; toxic in large quantities.
Daily need: A trace.

COPPER

Function: Associated with iron in production of red blood cells; aids in forming hair pigment; a catalyst for body-building enzymes connected with muscle and nerve fibres.
Good source: Almonds, bran, Brazil nuts, chicken's liver, lamb's liver, shellfish, wheatgerm, wholegrain cereals.
Deficiency results: Very rare, but can lead to anaemia, greying or loss of hair, heart troubles and nervousness. Women need more copper during menstruation and pregnancy.
Overdose results: Toxic in large quantities, but body usually discards excess. Schizophrenics have been shown to have a high level of copper.
Daily need: 2.5 mg.

FLUORINE

Function: Improves tooth development and strengthens bones by helping to deposit calcium. Hinders tooth decay by fighting acid-forming bacteria.
Good source: Seafood, tea, fluorinated water.
Deficiency results: Poor bone and teeth formation; tooth decay.
Overdose results: Discoloured and brittle teeth, muscle stiffness, arthritis; toxic reactions.
Daily need: 1 mg.

IODINE

Function: Necessary for the production of the thyroid hormone.
Good source: Kelp, seafood, sea salt, seaweeds, shellfish.
Deficiency results: Abnormal swelling in the throat leading to a goitre; thyroid disturbances that lead to weight gain, nervous tension and lethargy; drying of skin, loss of hair.
Overdose results: Interferes with the thyroid's synthesis of hormones, reducing them to an unsatisfactorily low level.
Daily need: A trace.

IRON

Function: The most important mineral involved in the transportation of oxygen to the cells and in the formation of haemoglobin. Most beneficial when taken in conjunction with vitamin C.
Good source: Blackstrap molasses, bran, dried apricots, egg yolks, haricot beans, kidneys, lamb's liver, shellfish, soya flour, sunflower seeds, watercress, wheatgerm.
Deficiency results: Anaemia, pallid skin, loss of energy, general listlessness and restlessness; brittle nails, premature grey hair; palpitations and breathlessness. Menstruation and pregnancy use up the iron supply and it needs to be replenished.
Overdose results: Usually excreted, but poor performance of the liver or pancreas can result in excessive deposits which are toxic; skin can become pigmented.
Daily need: 15 mg.

MAGNESIUM

Function: Important in cell metabolism; it actuates more enzymes in the body than any other mineral acting as an agent in the utilization of other minerals and vitamins – calcium needs it, vitamin C useless without it. Necessary for nerve and muscle function.
Good source: Almonds, avocado, bananas, barley, blackstrap molasses, Brazil nuts, haricot beans, honey, muesli, peanuts, seafood, whole grains.
Deficiency results: Muscular weakness, heart and circulatory diseases, nervousness and depression, dizziness, diarrhoea, liability to convulsions. Alcoholics and diabetics are often short of magnesium.
Overdose results: Not likely, but could lead to sleepiness and general weakness.
Daily need: 300 mg.

MANGANESE

Function: Activates enzymes; closely related to blood-sugar levels and helps maintain reproductive processes.
Good source: Almonds, apricots, bran, kidneys, lentils, parsley, walnuts, watercress, wheatgerm.
Deficiency results: Poor equilibrium and bad co-ordination; sterility, reduction of sexual drive, abnormal body growth, still births. Deficiency extremely unlikely.
Overdose results: Not established.
Daily need: A trace.

PHOSPHORUS

Function: Found in every cell in the body and the busiest of all minerals; important for growth, maintenance and repair of cells; significant in energy and nerve transmissions; passes on genetic hereditary patterns.
Good source: Brewers' yeast, cheese, chicken, eggs, fish, liver, skimmed milk, wheatgerm.
Deficiency results: Disturbances in cell regulation; poor quality of teeth and bones; stunted growth. Older people need more phosphorus because their systems don't absorb it well.
Overdose results: The body stores phosphorus well with no known toxic results.
Daily need: 1 gramme.

POTASSIUM

Function: Often in partnership with sodium. An important mineral in muscle control including that of the heart and in the stimulation of nerve impulses; helps regulate osmosis and water balance.
Good source: Bananas, butter beans, dried apricots, figs, haricot beans, jacket potatoes, lentils, peanuts, seafood, soya beans, spinach.
Deficiency results: Muscular weakness, irritability, disturbances of the heart; deficiency unlikely.
Overdose results: Affects heart beat, slowing it down and eventually arresting action; weakness and numbness of limbs.
Daily need: 4 grammes.

SELIUM

Function: Not specifically known, but appears to be an anti-oxidant; closely related to vitamin E and may prevent certain types of cancer.

Present in the retina of the eye in fairly high concentration, indicating that it may be important in vision.
Good source: Kidney, lamb's liver, nuts, seafood, wholegrain cereals.
Deficiency results: Difficulty in absorbing and utilizing vitamin E.
Overdose results: Toxicity; brittle bones and tooth decay.
Daily need: A trace.

SODIUM

Function: Important in cellular metabolism; protects the body against excess fluid loss, balances acid-alkali levels, influences muscular activity.
Good source: Chicken, green vegetables, kelp, salt, seafood, water and wheatgerm.
Deficiency results: Rare, but in hot climates excessive perspiration may deplete the body's salt, resulting in headaches, nausea, diarrhoea and muscular cramps of legs and abdomen.
Overdose results: Swelling of body tissues (oedema); unduly aggravates high blood pressure.
Daily need: 2–5 grammes, but for those with high blood pressure, 1 gramme is the limit.

SULPHUR

Function: Present in cells to help in formation of body tissues; necessary for proper function of vitamins thiamine and biotin; acts as a detoxant.
Good source: Cheese, chicken, eggs, fish, haricot beans, meats, milk, nuts, soya beans.
Deficiency results: Rare, but associated with protein lack and its effects.
Overdose results: Toxicity, if excess comes from synthetic supplements.
Daily need: No exact amount, but widely available through protein.

ZINC

Function: Helps in the formation of enzymes and proteins, in digestion, in elimination of carbon dioxide.
Good source: Bran, eggs, lamb's liver, nuts, onions, shellfish, sunflower seeds, wheatgerm, wholewheat flour.
Deficiency results: Retarded growth, delayed sexual maturity. Pregnant women, those on the Pill and older women frequently need extra.
Overdose results: Loss of iron and copper, particularly in the liver.
Daily need: A trace.

VEGETARIANISM

This means eating no meat or fish products. Some vegetarians will eat animal by-products such as butter, cheese and eggs provided the animal isn't killed for them. Others, known as lacto-vegetarians, cut out eggs as well as meat because they are potentially living creatures. The most extreme, the vegans, eat nothing of animal origin.

Vegetarians have a reputation for being slim, healthy and energetic but their claim that their diet provides a healthier and longer life cannot be medically substantiated. Undoubtedly they are more conscious of what they eat. They are well able to get adequate protein, vitamins and minerals from meatless sources though the diet requires some variety. In cooking there is never a question of using harmful animal fats.

A vegetarian regime follows this general scheme:

Breakfast: Choice of: fruit or fruit juice, muesli, oats, wholegrain cereal, dried fruits, honey, wholewheat bread, eggs, tomatoes.
Lunch/Dinner: Salad always, protein ingredient such as nuts, cheese, egg, lentils, haricot beans, avocado, soya beans; carbohydrate ingredient such as potato, brown rice, wholegrain bread; fruit or a dessert made from it.

LIQUIDS

A daily intake of water is essential, a pint if possible, and when on a slimming diet much more. There are basically four kinds of drinking water:
hard water – contains calcium, magnesium and other salts
soft water – contains sodium (which replaces the calcium and magnesium), often some copper, iron and zinc
distilled water – has had all the minerals removed by a steam process
mineral water – natural, untreated water, bottled with nothing added, nothing removed. There are many varieties with reputations for uniform quality and stability of beneficial mineral content. They are still or sparkling and have combinations of minerals that are both good to taste and reputedly good for health. Bottled still waters have considerably less sodium content, which affects water retention, than tap water.

Most community water has been fortified with chlorine for purification and fluorine to help prevent tooth decay but evidence of the toxic effect of sodium fluoride is causing concern.

SOFT DRINKS: Many have chemicals, colourings and flavourings added. It is more nutritious to make your own juices and add sparkling water, soda or tonic mixers. The high sugar content in most soft drinks provides the body with an unnecessary overload of sugar carbohydrates.

WINES, SPIRITS AND LIQUEURS: Very pleasant in moderation; a drink or two before dinner is relaxing, wine complements food, while an after-dinner drink is often a digestive. Most doctors agree that a controlled amount of alcohol won't harm; excess does and can get to the point of being beyond the bounds of self limitation. External signs of puffiness, blotchiness, impeded speech and actions, only indicate what's going on inside. Alcohol is speedily assimilated and quickly dilates the blood vessels which explains why it is sometimes prescribed in moderate amounts for people with circulatory troubles. Within a very few minutes about 50 per cent will have passed into the blood stream and on to the liver. The liver can absorb about one-third of an ounce of alcohol an hour. Feeling 'high' starts the minute you are drinking more than that amount during that time. If you take more than the liver can handle, the surplus is pumped around the body waiting its turn to get into the liver. It literally goes to the head, acting as a sort of anaesthetic. It affects the highest centre of the brain first, the part that controls amongst other things the inhibitions. As a rule effects are quicker and more drastic in a person who doesn't drink much. Regular drinkers develop a medically unexplained slow-down in the rate at which alcohol is absorbed.

Some days one can stand more alcohol than on others. Fatigue, stress, emotional upset, depression or anger can all accelerate alcohol's anaesthetizing action, although in small doses it relieves tension. One's resistance to alcohol is roughly in direct proportion to the fullness of the stomach. This has led to the practice of drinking something creamy (even milk) or oily before setting off on a drinking evening. This doesn't absorb the alcohol but it does reduce the rate at which it is absorbed.

Wine is the most inoffensive of alcoholic beverages and said to be beneficial to the digestion as it contains enzymes active in the metabolization of food. It provides vitamins B-2, B-6, niacin, pantothenic acid and small quantities of B-1, B-12 and folic acid. Minerals are present, too, and dry red wine is a good source of iron. Wines are carbohydrates, and the sweeter or heavier the wine, the more sugar elements it contains.

Spirits and liqueurs are more concentrated alcohol and can take vitamins from the body because like any sugary carbohydrate they need the vitamin B complex. Dry spirits such as whisky, white rum, vodka, gin have less sugar content than sherry, port, vermouths and the sweet liqueurs.

THE BASIC KITCHEN

Three basic grain recipes, plus one for a soup that is all vegetables and full of vitamins. These four items constantly crop up in health cures.

Basic Muesli

2 tablespoons oats old fashioned
juice of ½ lemon
a little milk, fresh or skimmed
2 tablespoons wheatgerm
4 tablespoons water
2 tablespoons honey

Soak oats overnight in water; in the morning add lemon juice, milk, honey and wheatgerm; mix well. Then add as you wish: any fresh fruit (traditionally shredded apple), raisins, dried apricots, nuts, natural yoghourt.

Basic Wholegrain Bread

1 oz. (30 g.) dry yeast
1½ pints (9 dl.) potato water, or warm milk
1 tablespoon honey
3 lbs (1.5 k.) wholewheat flour
pinch of salt

Into a warm bowl, put the yeast with a little of the potato water (or milk), mix and add honey. Leave for twenty minutes. Into another bowl mix flour and salt, then gradually add the yeast mixture and the remainder of the potato water; blend well and knead. Put into well-oiled tins, only filling half-way. When dough has doubled, bake at 350 for 50 minutes or until the bread sounds hollow.

Basic Potato Cereal

4 cups boiling water
1½ tablespoon wholewheat flour
1½ tablespoon bran
2 raw potatoes
wheatgerm, milk, honey

Into the pan of boiling water (4 cups) add flour and bran, stir and simmer for about 3 minutes; shred raw potatoes into mixture, stir until blended, then take from heat, cover and let stand a few minutes before serving. Add the wheatgerm, milk and honey to taste.

Basic Vegetable Broth

1 cup chopped onions
3 stalks celery, chopped
3 pints (1.5 l.) water
2 large potatoes, chopped small
4 carrots, chopped
pepper and sea salt
1 cup root vegetable
1 cup any leafy vegetable

Put a little vegetable oil into a large stainless steel or ceramic pot, braise onions and celery a little, add the water and then the other vegetables except the leafy one. Season; simmer for 30 mins. and then add the leafy vegetable; cook for 3–5 mins., otherwise vitamins are destroyed.

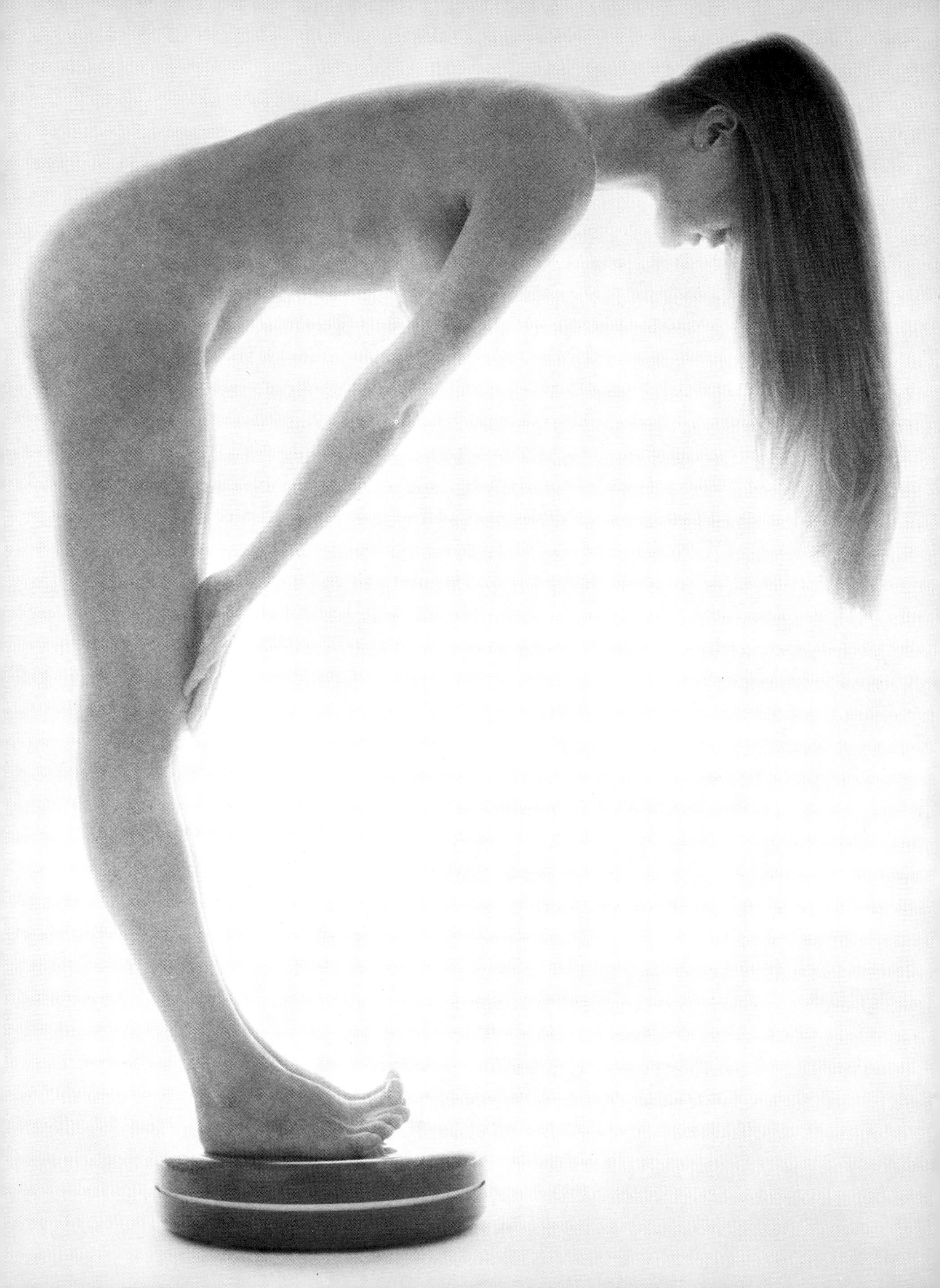

3

SLIMMING

Gradual weight loss is best. To take off pounds is one thing, to do it in a minimum time through drastic means is another. You are probably harming your own health even while you're losing weight. Ideally weight reduction should be planned on a gradual, steady basis resulting in permanent loss and a stabilized weight. For example, by steadfastly following the Maintenance Diet (Nutrition – page 25) in time the body would probably attain and sustain its ideal weight. But that time could be six months or more. Not many have that sort of patience; it is more common for an overweight person to think in terms of taking off x number of pounds for a special purpose (fashion, love, holiday) or initially to lose substantially as an inducement to get going on the long-term haul.

There are ways to quick weight loss, but the question is – which way? There are so many varieties of diet plans that it is easy to be thoroughly confused and it doesn't help to discover that even doctors do not agree about which method is the most satisfactory. Many have their pet theories and so-called recommended diets which appear contradictory.

Dieting is a very individual matter – and reaction to any specific regime varies considerably, be it psychological or chemical. There is no perfect diet that is good for everyone; nor is there any wonder food or formula that will do the trick – despite all the credit given to lemons and grapefruit. But there are several approaches to dieting that work, and it is up to you to decide which suits you best. Here is all the information: the diets summarized into categories to make it clear what theories are behind the various methods together with an assessment of their weight-loss possibilities. However, they all have one thing in common: to be successful they need will power and determined effort. Statistics reveal

LATEGAN

that out of one hundred who slim only twelve lose any substantial amount of weight, and ten are likely to gain back their loss.

What is overweight? What is normal? What is ideal? Apart from measuring in pounds and inches, there have been many ways devised to assess if you are fat or not. Most are a waste of time – can you scoop up thick folds of skin? When you pinch various spots on your body, do you hold more than an inch in your fingers? If you lie on your back can you place a ruler on your side so that it touches both your ribs and hip-bone? Do all this if you like, but the real test is to give yourself an honest look in the mirror. You know if you're carrying around too much fat. You can see it, feel it. Let your eye be the best judge.

Actual weight is not always a true indicator. Weight charts scaled to height should be used as a guide, not as a rule – ten pounds variation up or down could still mean you are at your ideal weight. Most charts record average weights tabulated by insurance companies, and these are usually quite a bit higher than the ideal. Our weight table is worked out from several independent studies and represents a guide to ideal weight for women over twenty. No adding is permitted for additional years; although metabolism and activity slow down as one ages, intake of food should be cut and balanced accordingly to keep weight steady. You usually hit your ideal weight in the mid-twenties. Most women gain roughly a pound a year after the age of thirty, which can add up to an uncomfortable lot over a number of years. Don't allow it to happen. Check the chart to give you a realistic ideal. To determine whether you are small, medium or large frame, refer to figure-type explanation (page 18). Big or small bones don't make as much difference as we would like to think. Bones roughly weigh one-sixth of your weight. They can give you an alibi for about seven pounds at the most.

Weight can fluctuate each day. To keep track of your weight weigh yourself at the same time and under the same conditions each day; weight varies not only daily but during the day as well. It also changes according to the menstrual cycle; most women are heavier and inclined to be bloated just before they menstruate. Weight can also move up and down in a seemingly alarming way – I can gain five pounds overnight after an indulgent dinner but thankfully can lose it just as fast too. Normally one swings within a three to five pound range, and it is only when you find yourself constantly returning to a lower figure that you can be sure you are losing weight on a permanent basis.

IDEAL WEIGHT FOR WOMEN OVER TWENTY

This is to be used as a guide not a rigid rule. To gauge ideal weight accurately you would have to consult a specialist. For a girl from sixteen to twenty, subtract a pound for each year under twenty.

HEIGHT (BAREFOOT)		SMALL FRAME		MEDIUM FRAME		LARGE FRAME	
		kgs.	*lbs.*	*kgs.*	*lbs.*	*kgs.*	*lbs.*
1.42 m	4′8″	39–42	86–92	41–46	90–101	44–51	98–113
1.45 m	4′9″	40–43	88–95	42–47	92–104	45–53	100–116
1.47 m	4′10″	41–44	91–98	44–49	96–107	47–54	104–120
1.50 m	4′11″	43–46	95–102	44–50	98–111	49–56	107–123
1.52 m	5′0″	44–47	96–104	46–52	102–114	50–57	110–126
1.55 m	5′1″	45–49	99–107	48–53	105–117	51–59	113–129
1.57 m	5′2″	46–50	102–110	49–55	108–121	53–60	116–133
1.60 m	5′3″	48–51	105–113	50–57	111–125	54–62	120–137
1.62 m	5′4″	49–53	108–116	52–57	114–128	56–64	123–140
1.65 m	5′5″	50–54	111–119	53–60	116–131	57–65	126–143
1.68 m	5′6″	52–56	114–123	54–62	120–136	59–67	130–147
1.70 m	5′7″	54–58	118–127	57–64	125–140	61–69	134–151
1.73 m	5′8″	56–60	122–131	59–65	129–144	63–70	138–155
1.76 m	5′9″	57–61	126–135	60–68	133–149	65–73	143–160
1.78 m	5′10″	59–64	130–140	62–69	137–152	67–75	147–165
1.81 m	5′11″	61–65	134–144	64–71	141–156	68–77	150–169
1.83 m	6′0″	63–67	138–148	66–73	145–160	70–79	154–174

Excess food is stored as fat. If you are overweight it is because at some time or other you have eaten more food than you need or the wrong food. If your body takes in more than it burns up in energy, the extra becomes a fat reserve. Today to be between twenty and thirty pounds overweight is the norm, though hardly desirable. More than that and you are on the way to obesity, which can easily get out of control. At this stage it is no longer an aesthetic problem, but a serious medical matter and no diet should be undertaken unless supervised by a doctor. It is possible that you are one of those individuals whose bodies for reasons not yet fully understood do not deal in the usual way with food. The advice for everyone who wants to diet is to check with a doctor. Few do. A normal healthy person can embark on limited sensible dieting, but should any adverse effects arise, seek medical advice immediately.

One of the oldest clichés in the diet game is that some people get fat easily no matter how little they eat, while others who constantly overeat stay thin. It's quite true that these two distinct groups exist. Recent research shows that in the case of the constant-weight types, excess food stimulates the body to increase its metabolism, and the food used up for this job exactly balances the additional intake. People who put on fat easily show no increase in metabolism when given extra food, but simply become fatter. This difference is rarely taken into consideration.

Why? No one really knows all the answers. It is impossible to distinguish the two types biologically – those who can very accurately control output and those who are not so good at it. It is a very delicate and sensitive balance; the reason may be metabolic, psychological, glandular or a complex combination of any or all. Scientists have been looking for clues in the fat cells of the body and have found that when fat people lose weight, the cause is shrinkage in the size of the fat cells, while the number of cells is unchanged.

This would seem to indicate that at maturity you have a certain number of fat cells, so that although fatness is difficult to cure, it probably is easier to prevent. It has been suggested that overfeeding in early life may account for the severe weight problem many people have as adults. Heredity may be a factor, not least because a child follows the pattern of over-eating that runs in the family. Each individual acquires an underlying cellular pattern – a sort of blue-print that is established in the early years and carries on. Each person's body has an optimum weight level that it strives to maintain. If weight is lost or gained slowly there is a force returning one to the original weight. With normal people this works in their favour, but with the fat-prone it's yet another battle, as there's a strong tendency for the overload to return. With fat gained over a long period, you must have the will-power to eat smaller quantities and better foods.

Fat cells are all over the body and they behave as an organ, which means they have a rich blood supply which enables them to metabolize. The fat organ is very large indeed, making up from 10% to 25% of body weight in an average person and half the body mass in an obese one. Some fat protects vital organs and for health reasons this fat should never fall below a certain level nor rise too high. However, the majority of cells lie in the layer of adipose tissue just beneath the skin. This layer does many useful things like cushion the body, act as an insulator, conserve heat, metabolize food and burn fat – but above all it stores fat. Here is the main reservoir of fat in the body, and it's usually too ample.

If this fat deposit becomes quite dense – which means there's rather a lot of it – the skin over the fat becomes quite puckered, rather like an orange peel, and this is called cellulite. The French invented the word, implying it was a special sort of fat and had to be treated in a special way but it is ordinary fat that is water-logged, and the best way to get rid of it is through diet accompanied by exercise, and by controlling fluid retention.

Although eating is a neural and muscular activity, it is mostly a brain function. There are certain control centres, primarily – it is thought – in the hypothalamus, from which decisions go out whether to eat, how much, when to stop. Researchers have hopes about a hormone produced by the pituitary, which seems to mobilize fat. It has been isolated but is not yet at the stage of being used. Interestingly enough it is produced by people fasting and those on a mainly fat and protein diet. People on the normal mixed diet don't produce it at all, nor do those on a low calorie intake consisting mainly of carbohydrates. And those with poor pituitary function don't make it either.

What about the glandular system and its effect on weight control? Glands are often unjustly blamed for excess fatty deposits. Glands secrete hormones into the bloodstream, which carries them around the body to act as regulators of various functions. Among other things they control the balance of food metabolism. Take the famous thyroid gland; it can produce too much hormone, thus causing cells to metabolize so fast that food is burnt up speedily as fast as it goes in. Accordingly, high thyroid persons are thin and usually nervous. Too little thyroid production results in slow cell metabolism; the cell cannot keep up with the intake of food, has no time to use it as energy, so stores it as fat. Food requirement for people with a low thyroid production is consequently less, but they frequently exceed the limit and put on weight.

Observations of these effects have led to the use of thyroid hormone for the treatment of overweight but medical opinion is very divided. Some doctors are against it, arguing that when thyroid tablets are given to a person with a normal thyroid, the gland gets lazy and stops making its own hormone. Thyroid extract is useful when there is medical evidence of low thyroid activity. Small doses will speed up metabolism and assist in weight loss, provided effective diet is being taken at the same time.

The pituitary gland has considerable influence on weight control but because it turns out dozens of hormones which stimulate or inhibit other glands, it is not easy to find out how. Under certain circumstances it produces the fat-mobilizing hormone mentioned above; this is under further experimentation. The adrenal gland, together with the reproductive system, produces a special hormone during pregnancy, which is the basis of a controversial weight shifting method used by a number of doctors (see page 65).

Some overweight people retain more water than they need. When on a diet it is necessary to differentiate between loss of weight and loss of water. Usually the latter goes first, and it can mean a magical loss of pounds overnight. In most cases this water loss is frequently recovered. There is a lot of water in the body, some in blood, some in cells, some in connecting tissue. The proportions are very carefully regulated, and one of the chief things that controls the balance is salt. You need an exact amount – no more, no less. If too much salt is taken, water accumulates with it, the tissues swell up and you weigh too much. We need about one gramme of salt a day to keep a healthy water supply. Most people consume ten to twenty times that, which means carrying an extra four pints of water. Most fresh foods naturally contain salt. It is very rare for anyone to take too little salt, and only in very hot climates is it sometimes necessary to supplement it.

If you drink a lot of water it doesn't mean you are going to retain it, in fact quite the reverse. One should have at least three pints a day when on a diet. It is good for the kidneys, and scientific approval is now being given to the old wives' tale that water can also wash off weight. Water is an important part of many slimming regimes. Many thin people drink a great deal of water with meals – something that was considered bad a few years ago – while fat people often drink less and choose more concentrated foods.

Weight loss is directly connected with energy output no matter what the metabolic speed of assimilating food. Each of us has a unique body, but one fact remains the same: if you take in more than you burn off, you will put on weight. Nutritionists calculate the amount of heat or energy released by burning food as a calorie. It is a very small unit, and when we refer to a Calorie, it is a thousand times as big as the original unit. Protein has a caloric value of approximately 4 Calories per gramme, carbohydrate 4 Calories per gramme and fat 9 Calories per gramme. An average woman uses about 2,300 Calories a day.

The principle of all diets is based on the balance of food intake with energy output. But it is not always a strict equation. New thinking is along the lines that it is not only the number of calories you take in, but also the type that helps to balance the energy output. The three groups of food – protein, carbohydrates and fat – react differently. Excess fat, not burned off, is stored as fat. Excess carbohydrate is also stored as fat, while protein has the peculiar ability of making the body burn its fuel more quickly – sometimes to such an extent that it is essential to turn some of the body fat into energy to cope with the breaking down of the protein. This is why many diets are very high in protein. Strange as it may seem, fat – though not healthy in large quantities – is inclined to metabolize quicker than carbohydrates. It is the sugar and starch that are likely to end up as stored fat.

There are certain foods to be stopped no matter what system you follow, some you can take with caution, and others you can eat without a care. Check the tables and use this as a basis for any diet menu. You will notice that it hardly varies from our Maintenance Diet and is a sound plan for healthy eating as well as for slimming.

STOP:

SUGAR CARBOHYDRATES

sugars: all types, glucose, sweets, chocolate, spreads, sweet sauces, confectionery decorations
pastries: biscuits, cakes, pies, tarts
preserves: jams, marmalade, jellies
fruit: tinned, candied or preserved in any way

STARCH CARBOHYDRATES

breads: all white breads, rolls, buns, breadcrumbs
cereals: white flour, refined grains and cereals (wheat, oats, barley, rye), packaged cereals, rice, pasta, flour, puddings, blancmange, flour sauces
vegetables: dried peas, beans and lentils, tinned root and pod vegetables, cream soups

FATS

sauces: all cream ones like mayonnaise, unless freshly made with oil, bottled sauces and relishes
nuts: peanuts, walnuts
delicatessen foods: processed meats, pâtés, sausages
no fat for frying

CAUTION:

STARCH CARBOHYDRATES

bread: wholewheat varieties, any made from unrefined grains
cereals: natural oats, unprocessed rice, wholegrain flour

CELLULOSE CARBOHYDRATES

root vegetables: potatoes, carrots, parsnips, turnips, white onions, beetroot
pod vegetables: peas, beans
fruits: some tropical varieties – bananas, water melons, avocado pears

FATS

dairy produce: butter, margarine, milk, cream

PROTEIN

dairy produce: cheese made from cows' milk, eggs
poultry: goose, duck

GO AHEAD:

PROTEINS

fish: fresh and salt water, shell varieties
meat: beef, veal, lamb, pork, ham, bacon, liver, kidney, heart, brains, sweetbreads, tripe
poultry: chicken, turkey
game: venison, pheasant, quail, guinea fowl, rabbit
cheese: made from goats' milk, mozzarella, feta, cottage cheese

CELLULOSE CARBOHYDRATES

leaf vegetables: artichokes, asparagus, broccoli, cabbage, cauliflower, celery, chicory, endive, kale, lettuce, all salad greens, spinach, watercress
root vegetables: spring onions, radishes
fruit vegetables: tomatoes, peppers, aubergines, courgettes, cucumbers, marrows
fruits: citrus – lemons, oranges, grapefruit, tangerines; berry – raspberries, strawberries, bilberries, cranberries, gooseberries; orchard – apples, pears, plums, apricots, peaches, cherries, grapes; tropical – mangoes, papaya, pineapples, cantaloupes, figs

FATS

vegetable oils: olive, soya, unsaturated fats

Herbs and seasoning are allowed, but use little salt. Never, never, fry in fat. Meat and game can be braised in a non-stick pan, on an iron griddle or on a barbecue rack. Otherwise roast, grill or boil. Fish should be roasted, steamed or grilled. Vegetables and fruit should be eaten raw whenever possible, but when cooked boil in a minimum amount of water or braise in the oven with a little oil. Sugar is forbidden in all diets; if absolutely necessary use a minimum amount of honey to sweeten a beverage.

I've already mentioned the value of water – three pints a day minimum. Coffee and tea are allowed in any quantity – without sugar and in most diets preferably without milk. Some diets permit a lot of milk, others a little, some only skimmed milk, some not at all. I'm inclined to go for skimmed milk with cautious use of whole milk and cream.

Commercial soft drinks are definitely not allowed, and that includes all tonics, sodas, and ginger ales. Some of the diet varieties can be taken in moderation, but it is best to make your own lemon drink from fresh lemons and a sparkling mineral water. This helps to take away excess fluid in the body and is a recognized regenerator of the liver.

The rule concerning alcohol is not as strict as might be supposed. It does not necessarily put on fat. If you normally drink a fair amount you should probably carry on but to a much lesser degree as the tension derived from being without may make you eat more food – with a worse result.

For the purpose of dieting think of alcohol as being equivalent to carbohydrate (roughly 1 gramme of alcohol equals 1¾ grammes of carbohydrate). Alcohol carbohydrate burns at a rather slow rate. Quite a number of alcoholic drinks contain sugar and consequently have to be avoided: beers, ales, ciders, liqueurs, sherries, ports, sweet and heavy wines. Light red and white wines are all right; so are dry spirits such as gin, vodka, rum and whisky.

Again doctors are not in agreement over alcohol. Some say that it checks the combustion of fat, others that it dilates the blood vessels and makes the body work harder, stepping up metabolism to an extent which may more than compensate for the extra calories.

Vitamins as such have no influence on weight, nor can one live on vitamins alone. Even when fasting only supplements of vitamin B and C should be taken; other additions could be dangerous. On a sensible reducing diet extra vitamins should not be required. However there are doctors who recommend taking multi-vitamin capsules, stepping up the intake of vitamin E, C and particularly the full spectrum of the vitamin B complex. This is fine but it is most important to remember that one cannot safely exceed the normal daily requirements of either vitamin A or vitamin D. As for the other vitamins, overdoses are simply washed away by the kidneys if you are drinking adequate water.

Everyone looks for a short-cut to dieting. It would seem logical that one way to eat less would be to curb the appetite. Appetite suppressants, such as the amphetamines, act on the central nervous system, and apart from getting to the centres of appetite control, they also stimulate mental and physical activity – thus increasing energy output. There are snags: some doctors consider them appetite postponers not suppressants and people have sometimes found that they quickly put on weight after stopping the drug. Amphetamines are effective for only a few weeks and can be addictive which causes a withdrawal problem. Because of this the prescription of many has been stopped.

If you look carefully at the formulae for slimming pills you will find that their active ingredient is nearly always a laxative (such as phenolphtalein). Laxatives are one of the oldest ways to lose weight, the most common being Epsom Salts (magnesium sulphate). They will get weight off temporarily due to loss of water and malabsorption of food, but the ensuing thirst usually puts back weight in the form of water desperately needed by the dehydrated body. In any case, you are not losing fat. Constant use of diuretics and purgatives can seriously harm the body.

The 'magic' foods – biscuits, package meals – are low calorie but contain a large amount of stomach filler such as methyl cellulose. This is harmless but it expands and fills up the stomach, so that you feel you have had a reasonable meal. Manufacturers put in protein and vitamins so that undernourishment is unlikely but these foods often lack essential nutrients. They are also expensive and a most monotonous way to diet.

The best and only way to go on a diet is to choose one you can stick to. Yo-yo dieting is hopeless and not worth the effort of the dieting days. The best bodies have worked out a plan of eating that is really a diet for life. They have learned to eat thin without starving and without discomfort. Plan a diet around the way you eat, one that fits into your life-style and temperament. Sometimes dieting is a matter of forcing yourself out of certain bad habits. Judge the pros and cons of each diet, balancing them against your preferences, your schedule, your finances. Then stick to what you have chosen.

There are two main schools of thought on diet. Those who believe that the clue to losing weight is simply to control the quantity you eat. These are the calorie counters who believe that food-in must always be less than energy-out when measured in calories. This is the PORTION CONTROL theory.

Then there are those who argue that it is the type of food you eat that matters and the restriction of food from certain groups. Some are all-protein diets, others contain no fat, others a lot of fat, others a few carbohydrates. These are the PROPORTION CONTROL theories and are deliberately unbalanced.

There are convincing arguments for both sides. Individual metabolism is the deciding factor.

PROPORTION CONTROL DIETS

All these restrict one or two of the food groups. It is claimed that such methods shift fat more quickly than a calorie control system and without the feeling of hunger. They can cause quite dramatic weight loss, though it is preferable to take it off slowly. Because these diets allow more food, often unlimited eating of certain things, they are more appealing to people who don't have the patience to keep track of calories or quantities.

All Protein

meat
poultry
fish
eggs
cottage cheese
3 pints water
no alcohol

FORMULA: No carbohydrates, no fats, 100% protein. Only these foods, but quantity unlimited: lean beef, veal, lamb, chicken, turkey, fatless fish and shellfish, eggs – preferably hard-boiled – cottage cheese. All fat must be cut off meat. No fat for cooking. Food must be boiled, baked, grilled or roasted. Drink at least 3 pints of water daily. As much coffee and tea as you like. Salt, pepper, herbs. Non-caloric beverages allowed. No alcohol. Supplementary vitamin tablets if necessary.

THEORY: Protein makes the body burn its fuel quickly and since in this diet there is lack of immediate fat and carbohydrate it is essential for the body to turn some of its stored fat into energy to break down the protein. Thus fatty deposits are slowly depleted. It is generally accepted that fat cannot be completely broken down in the body unless carbohydrates are present (in this case they are not). This means that during metabolism chemical compounds called ketones accumulate in the blood; they are present in the urine and also cause bad breath. The condition is called ketosis, but healthy people who chose this diet are unlikely to stick to it long enough for ketosis to reach an unsafe level. Long-termers should be under medical supervision; it can be harmful for pregnant women, as well as those with kidney problems.

Low Carbohydrate

meat
poultry
game
fish
eggs
cheese
oil
butter
salad
leaf vegetables
fruit vegetables
citrus fruit
berries
3 pints water
dry wines
dry spirits

FORMULA: Unlimited protein, caution for fats, carbohydrate limited to 250 Calories per day (about 60 grammes).

No quantity control on –

Meat: beef, lamb, veal, pork, ham, bacon, liver, kidney
Poultry: chicken, turkey, duck
Game: venison, pheasant, rabbit
Fish: all varieties
Cheese: hard varieties, cottage cheese, mozzarella and goat cheeses
Beverages: tea, coffee, a lot of water, non-calorific drinks

Limited amounts –

Eggs: any way
Fats: butter, margarine, oils, cream, milk

Control to under 250 Carbohydrate Calories (60 grammes) – total from the following:

Salads: green varieties
Vegetables: confine to leaf and fruit vegetables
Fruit: citrus fruit and berries only
Alcohol: dry wines – white or red, dry spirits – gin, vodka, whisky
Breads: wholewheat – never more than a slice a day

THEORY: This is the compromise between the Proportion and Portion theories. It is not counting calories for everything, but because it acknowledges carbohydrates in any form as a cause of weight gain, it cuts them down, though not out.

It is a slower way of losing weight than the all-protein or the protein-fat regimes. A fair amount of water is lost first and you stay on a plateau before getting really under way. The joy is that there is more to eat and something to drink, so it is considerably easier to live with over a longer period of time. At this 60 gramme a day level of carbohydrate intake there is usually no trace of ketosis. If you are not losing weight, you may cut down further on the carbohydrates. Alcohol is allowed because it is treated as a carbohydrate and comes within the controlled proportion. This diet also comes very close to our general diet rules and is not far off from the Maintenance Diet. When desired weight has been reached, it is relatively easy to make the transition to normal healthy eating, thus avoiding an immediate weight gain which happens after most diets. This low-carbohydrate scheme is not a new principle. It was originally prescribed for a rotund Victorian English gentleman, William Banting, who became famous after he published his 'Letter on Corpulence' showing how he lost 50 pounds in one year and was still going down.

Low Carbohydrate – The Grapefruit Diet

The Grapefruit Diet is based on the low-carbohydrate principle. There is no magic in the grapefruit but this fruit is used because it is very low in carbohydrates and provides necessary vitamins. It becomes most effective after five days.

Breakfast:

Half grapefruit or 4 oz. (120 g.) unsweetened grapefruit juice
2 eggs – any way
2 slices bacon
Coffee or tea

Lunch and Dinner:

Half grapefruit
Moderate portion of meat, poultry or fish
Salad with lemon juice/or portion of leafy green vegetables
Coffee or tea

Protein and Fat

meat
poultry
fish
game
eggs
cheese – hard
oil
butter
cream
salad
lemon
3 pints water
no alcohol

FORMULA: Primarily a protein and fat diet, with a small salad allowed with meals – if you must – providing such an infinitesimal amount of carbohydrate that it hardly counts. No quantity control; eat what you like at any meal.

Meat: beef, lamb, veal, pork, ham, bacon, liver, kidney
Poultry: chicken, turkey, duck
Game: venison, pheasant, rabbit
Fish: all varieties including fatty kinds like tuna and salmon
Eggs: any way, no limitations
Cheese: hard varieties, no processed ones, cottage cheese, mozzarella
Fats: butter, margarine, oils, cream (no milk)
Salads: green salad, limited to a small one each meal
Fruit: juice of one lemon a day

Food can be boiled, baked, grilled, roasted and can be cooked in a pan on the stove in its own fat – in the case of eggs, with a little fat. Drink the usual 3 pints of water daily; as much tea and coffee as desired. Salt, pepper, seasonings. Non-caloric drinks, no alcohol. Supplementary vitamin tablets if you like.

THEORY: This is basically the same principle as the all-protein diet in that, in the absence of carbohydrate, the body is forced into using stored fat for energy. Tests have shown that obese patients lose weight on comparatively high caloric diets so long as food consists mainly of protein and fat with carbohydrates kept to a minimum. Dieting is certainly made more palatable with the addition of fat, though weight loss is usually less rapid. Some people who take little or no fat find they are irritable, tired and inclined to lack concentration. Fat goes through the stomach quite slowly, so you do not feel hungry quickly after a meal and are able to stay on this diet for quite a while. We are constantly reminded about the dangers to health of too much saturated fat so although fat is permitted, it is hardly sensible to consume huge portions, nor is there usually the inclination. Again there is the problem of ketosis, but as explained above, there is no need to worry unduly about a low degree of this.

PORTION CONTROL DIETS

This is the mathematical approach to dieting, where the calorie equation rules: energy out must exceed food in, otherwise it is fat on. There's nothing wrong with it if healthily balanced.

For calorie counting you need a strong will. It is a slow, steady way of reducing weight. In theory it is simple: proteins give 4 Calories of energy per gramme, carbohydrates 4 Calories and fat 9 Calories.

The average woman needs about 2,300 Calories a day to balance energy output. For weight loss, calorie intake should be a maximum of 1,400 Calories a day. 1 pound of body fat represents 3,500 Calories. Therefore, in practice, calorie-counting diets amount to, on the average, 2 pounds loss a week on the basis of a long-term 1,200–1,400 Calories a day diet. This requires will-power.

In theory it doesn't matter how you take your calories, but it does matter nutritionally. If you follow the basic diet charts (page 57) you are on a good nutritional level.

Crash diets follow the calorie principle though they are reduced to survival level and therefore diets cannot be followed for more than a limited period. Crash diets are either for those who are only a few pounds beyond ideal and want to lose it fast, or for those who need encouragement to continue on a permanent weight-loss plan. The minimum is 800

Calories a day, less is a potential danger to health – unless completely fasting which has a different effect on metabolism.

Once ideal weight has been achieved, the calorie principle can be continued within the 2,300 Calorie limit to balance energy output. Choose foods from the 'Go-Ahead' and 'Caution' tables and you will see it is easy to keep within the caloric limit – and within the Maintenance Diet too.

CALORIE CONTROL / *1,400 a day / loss: 2 lbs (1 k.) weekly*

Breakfast: 1 glass unsweetened juice or half grapefruit
1 egg, any way but fried
1 slice wholewheat bread
1 pat butter or margarine
Coffee or tea, no sugar

Lunch: 3 oz. (90 g.) lean meat, poultry or fish
1 portion fresh vegetable or salad
1 slice wholewheat bread
1 portion fresh fruit
Coffee or tea, no sugar

Dinner: 3 oz. (90 g.) lean meat, poultry or fish
1 portion green salad
1 portion vegetable
1 slice cheese – no more than 2 oz. (60 g.)
1 portion fresh fruit
Coffee or tea, no sugar

CALORIE CONTROL / *1,200 a day / loss: 2–3 lbs (1–1.5 k.) weekly*

Breakfast: 1 glass unsweetened grapefruit juice
1 egg, any way but fried
1 slice wholewheat bread
Coffee or tea, no sugar

Lunch: 2 oz. (60 g.) lean meat, poultry or fish
1 portion green vegetable or salad
1 slice wholewheat bread
1 portion fresh fruit – not banana
Coffee or tea, no sugar

Dinner: 2 oz. (60 g.) lean meat, poultry or fish
1 portion green vegetable
1 portion salad
1 oz. (30 g.) cheese
Coffee or tea, no sugar

WEIGHT WATCHERS' PLAN / *very long term / loss: 2 lbs (1 k.) weekly*

A group therapy programme that involves a weekly meeting plus rigid adherence to a very detailed diet regime. It is portion control but through weight not calories – food is weighed on a postage scale. You must eat three meals a day, a minimum of five fish dishes a week, four to seven eggs a week, liver once, beef not more than three times. Many vegetables are unlimited. Off the list completely are the sugar carbohydrates. There are some strange rules – like eggs only for breakfast and lunch, limited vegetables for dinner only. They have no dietary or nutritional purpose, they're supposed to discipline the dieter. A typical day's menu:

Breakfast:	1 egg or 1 oz. (30 g.) hard cheese or 2 oz. (60 g.) fish 1 slice wholewheat bread Coffee or tea, no sugar
Lunch:	4 oz. (120 g.) fish, beef or poultry or 2 oz. (60 g.) hard cheese Unlimited vegetables (from a long list, mostly leafy green) 1 slice wholewheat bread
Dinner:	6 oz. (180 g.) fish, meat or poultry ½ cup limited vegetables (tomato, carrots, egg plant, peas) Unlimited vegetables in any quantity
Include each day:	three fruits – one must be a grapefruit or orange; two cups skimmed milk

CRASH DIETS

These are the drastic reducing regimes that most women resort to as an emergency measure. Over the years many fad diets have gone the rounds; here the most effective are summarized. It is important to limit diet days as indicated because of minimum nutritional value. Diets are of course monotonous, but it is this very repetition of certain foods that has proved easier to follow. Weight loss varies from one person to another, usually related to the amount you are overweight – the greater the excess the greater the loss. Average weight losses are indicated, but you could shed more or less. Do not extend the number of days; it could impair your health and also it is not always worth it as the speed of loss usually diminishes after the initial period. A crash diet can be used as an encouraging preliminary course before a long term dietary plan.

MILK AND BANANA / *5 days / loss: 5 lbs (2.5 k.)*

6 bananas
3 glasses of skimmed milk

This is the entire consumption for the day – eat at intervals when you feel like it. If necessary, add 2 cups of black unsweetened coffee.

COTTAGE CHEESE AND BANANA / *4 days / loss: 6 lbs (3 k.)*

First Day

Breakfast: 4 oz. (120 g.) cottage cheese
1 grapefruit
Black coffee or lemon tea

Lunch: 4 oz. (120 g.) cottage cheese
1 slice melon
Black coffee or lemon tea

Dinner: 4 oz. (120 g.) cottage cheese
1 grapefruit
Black coffee or lemon tea

Second Day

Breakfast: 1 banana
1 cup skimmed milk, black coffee or lemon tea

Lunch: 1 banana
1 boiled egg
Black coffee or lemon tea

Dinner: 6 oz. (180 g.) steak, grilled
2 bananas – grilled with steak if preferred
Black coffee or lemon tea

One cup of coffee or tea is allowed between meals. Repeat the routine of the two days.

BANANA DRINK / *2 days / loss: 6 lbs (3 k.)*

Recipe for drink: Juice of 2 large oranges
1 teaspoon liquid honey
Juice of 1 lemon
Mix these together well, add 1 banana very finely sliced
Mix well together

Take the drink four times a day in place of regular meals – add one cup of coffee or tea.

HONEY AND EGGS / *2 days / loss: 3 lbs (1.5 k.)*

First Day

Breakfast: Honey and egg cup: 2 egg yolks, 1 teaspoon honey and a dash of ground black pepper; beat until thoroughly blended
Black coffee or lemon tea

Lunch: Honey and egg cup
3 oz. (90 g.) hard cheese
Black coffee or lemon tea

Dinner: 1 cup clear soup
1 slice wholewheat bread
Honey and egg cup
1 portion fresh fruit
Black coffee or lemon tea

Second day

Breakfast: Honey and egg cup
1 slice wholewheat bread, bit of butter
Black coffee or lemon tea

Lunch: Honey and egg cup
5 oz. (150 g.) fish, poultry or meat
3 tablespoons boiled cabbage, spinach or courgettes
Black coffee or lemon tea

Dinner: Honey and egg cup
3 oz. (90 g.) hard cheese
1 slice wholewheat bread, bit of butter
Black coffee or lemon tea

WINE AND EGGS / *3 days / loss: 5 lbs (2.5 k.)*

Breakfast: 1 egg, hard-boiled
1 glass white wine (dry, preferably Chablis)
Black coffee

Lunch: 2 eggs, hard-boiled is best, but poached if necessary
2 glasses white wine
Black coffee

Dinner: 5 oz. (150 g.) steak, grilled with black pepper, lemon juice
Remainder of white wine (one bottle allowed per day)
Black coffee

Opposite: Benito, 1926
Overleaf left: Benito, 1926
Overleaf right: Benito, 1927

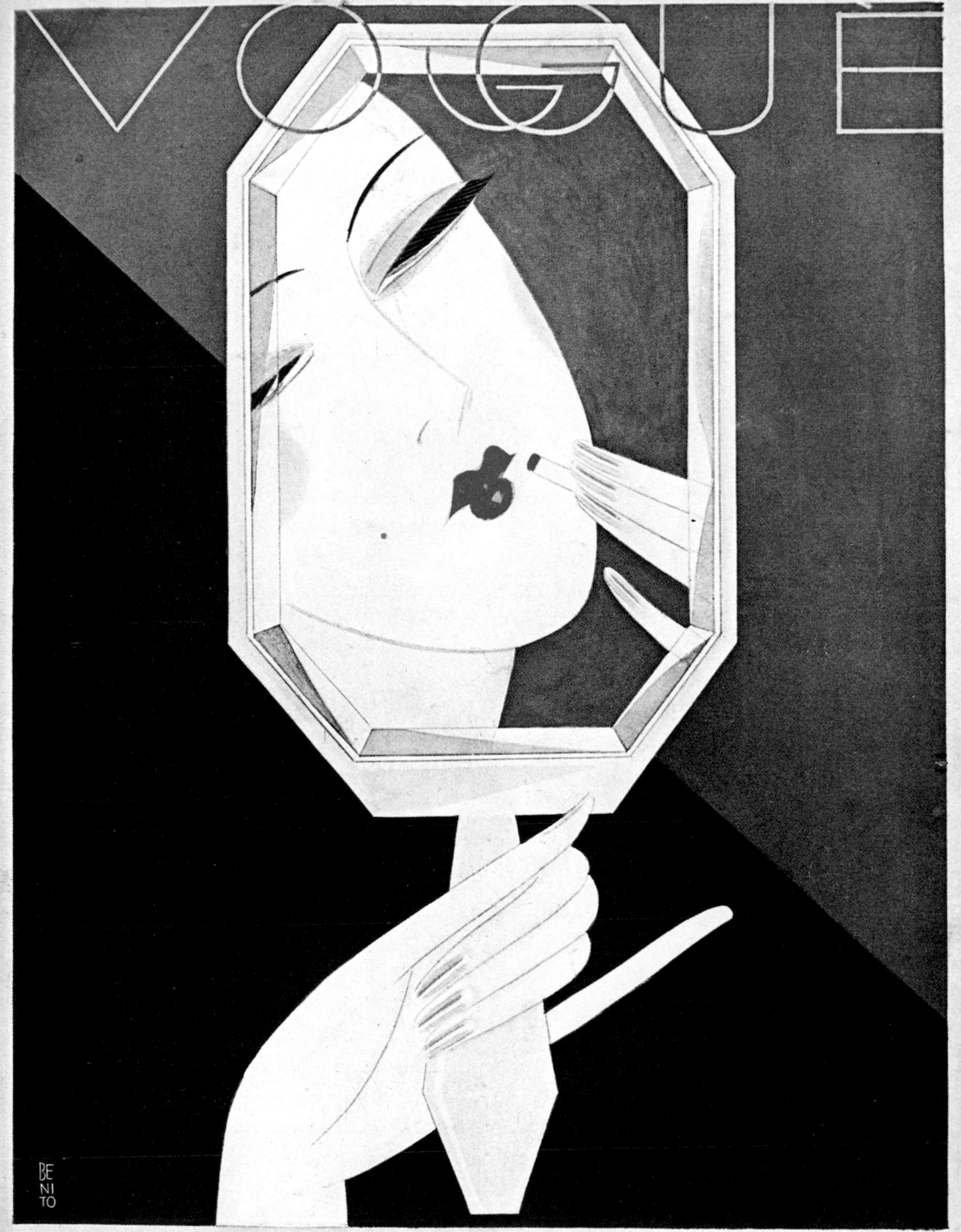

VOGUE

VOGUE

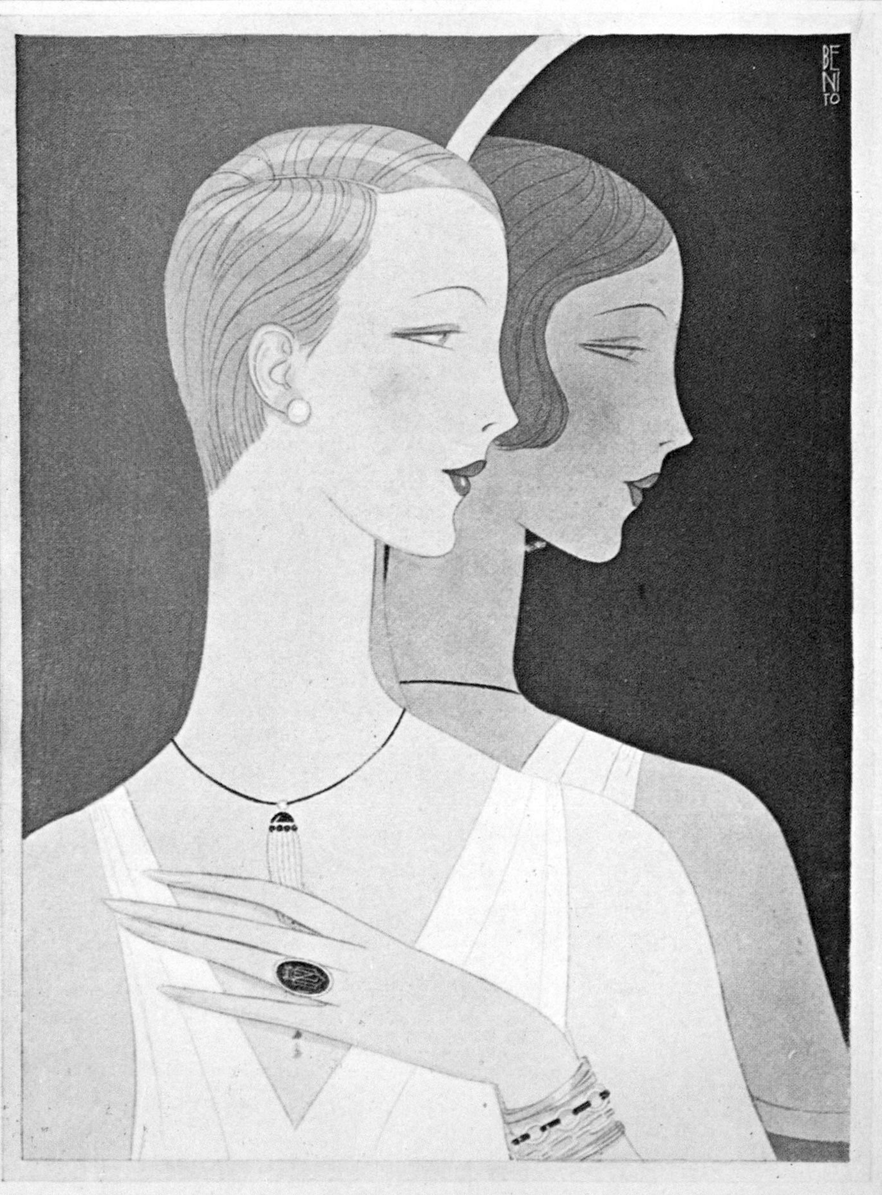

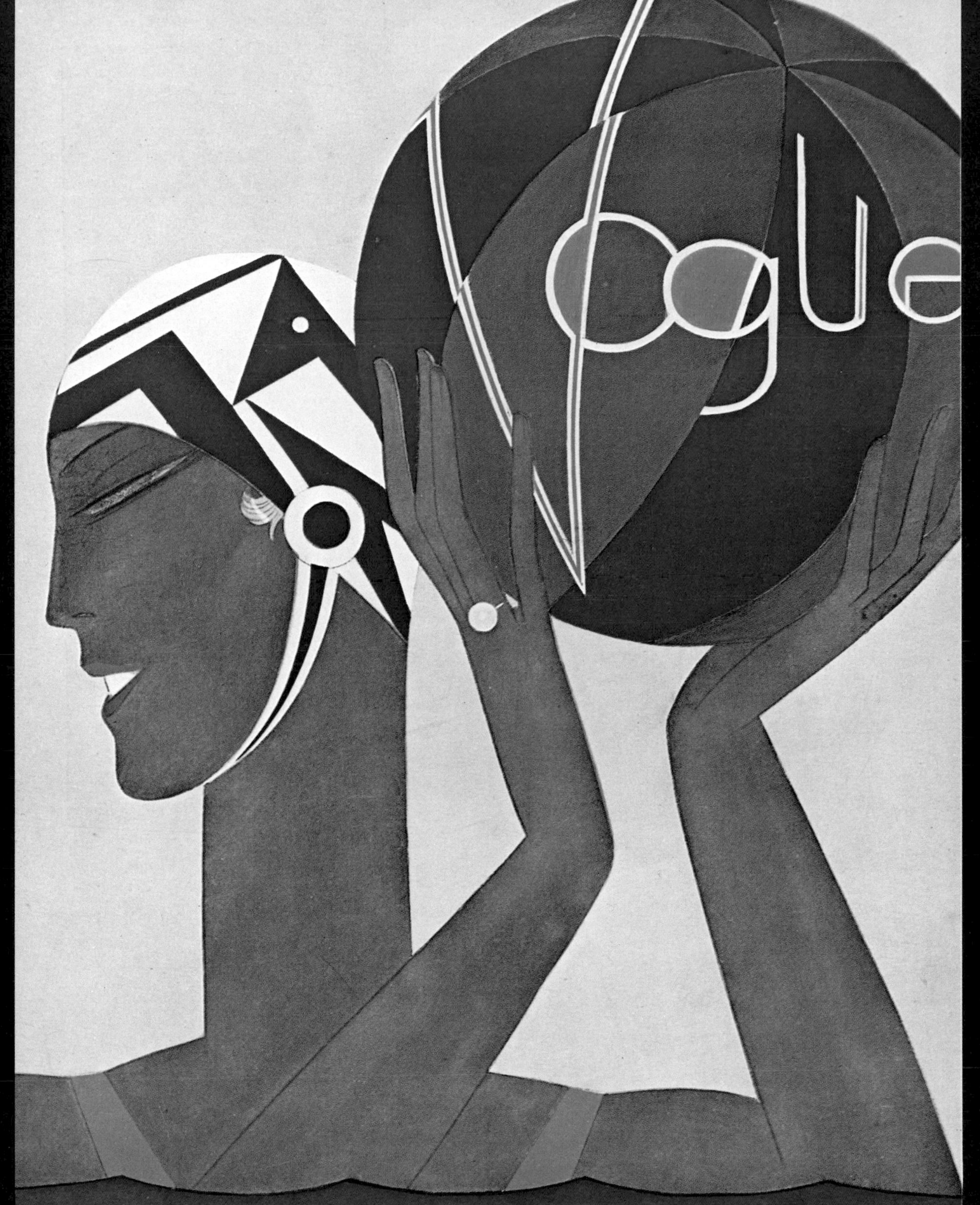
Vogue

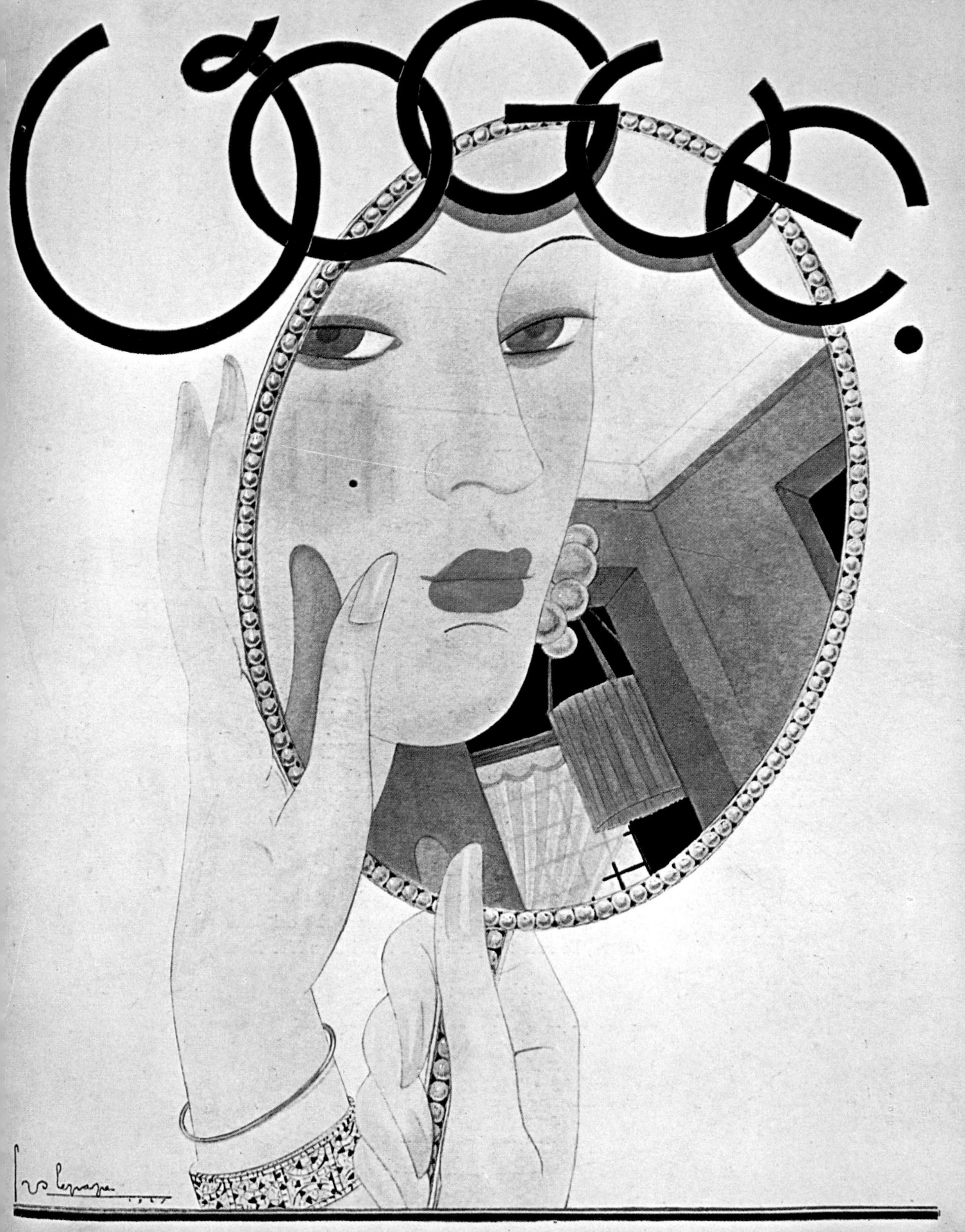

WINE AND STEAK *5 days / loss: 5 lbs (2.5 k.)*

Breakfast: 2 hard-boiled eggs or 4 oz. (120 g.) grilled steak

Lunch: 4 oz. (120 g.) grilled steak
1 glass red wine

Dinner: 4 oz. (120 g.) grilled steak
1 glass red wine

Black coffee or lemon tea allowed as you like, no sugar though. Seasonings and herbs for steak, but no salt.

WINE AND CHEESE / *3 days / loss: 4 lbs (2 k.)*

Breakfast: 4 oz. (120 g.) hard cheese
1 slice wholewheat bread, toasted

Lunch/Dinner: 4 oz. (120 g.) cheese – any kind
2 slices wholewheat bread
1 glass white wine
Black coffee or lemon tea as you like

EGG AND TOMATO / *4 days / loss: 3 lbs (1.5 k.)*

Breakfast: 1 glass tomato juice
1 egg, poached or boiled
3 grilled tomatoes
1 slice wholewheat bread

Lunch: 2-egg tomato omelette or tomato and egg salad using hard-boiled egg, 2 tomatoes and adding a small sliced onion with chopped parsley

Dinner: Tomato omelette or tomato and egg salad or 2 scrambled eggs and parsley
Black coffee or lemon tea

EGG AND GRAPEFRUIT / *3 days / loss: 3 lbs (1.5 k.)*

Breakfast: ½ grapefruit
1 hard-boiled egg
1 slice wholewheat bread
Black coffee or lemon tea

Lunch: ½ grapefruit
2 eggs, any way but not fried, best if hard-boiled
Black coffee or lemon tea

Dinner: ½ grapefruit
2 eggs any way but not fried
Black coffee or lemon tea

Opposite: Lepape, 1927

EGG AND POTATO / *4 days / loss: 3 lbs (1.5 k.)*

Breakfast: 1 glass grapefruit juice
1 boiled egg
Black coffee or lemon tea

Lunch: 1 medium sized potato – baked, boiled or mashed with a little milk
1 apple
Black coffee or lemon tea

Dinner: 1 glass tomato juice
½ grapefruit
1 boiled egg
Black coffee or lemon tea

EGG AND HAMBURGER / *7 days / loss: 5 lbs (2.5 k.)*

Breakfast: 1 glass grapefruit juice
1 hard-boiled egg
Black coffee or lemon tea

Lunch: 3 oz. (90 g.) grilled hamburger, rare
1 apple
Black coffee or lemon tea

Dinner: 3 oz. (90 g.) hamburger, rare
Small green salad
Black coffee or lemon tea

AVOCADO / *3 days / loss: 3 lbs (1.5 k.)*

Breakfast: ½ avocado filled with cottage cheese
Black coffee or lemon tea

Lunch: ½ avocado sliced and mixed with sliced hard-boiled egg, 6 slices cucumber and onion to taste
Black coffee or lemon tea

Dinner: 3 oz. (90 g.) beef steak or hamburger, rare
½ avocado with cottage cheese
Black coffee or lemon tea

VEGETABLE AND FRUIT / *7 days / loss: 6 lbs (3k.)*

Vegetable Day

Breakfast: 1 glass vegetable juice
4 grilled tomatoes
Black coffee or lemon tea

Lunch: Green salad – lettuce, cucumber, celery, watercress, green peppers and onion to taste
Black coffee or lemon tea

Dinner: 1 hot green vegetable – cabbage, spinach, cauliflower, broccoli – boil and flavour with garlic and a little lemon juice
Black coffee or lemon tea

Fruit Day

Breakfast: Small fruit salad – grapefruit, orange, lemon and apple
Black coffee or lemon tea

Lunch: ½ melon
Small fruit salad as for breakfast
Black coffee or lemon tea

Dinner: Same as lunch

Alternate vegetable and fruit days, beginning and ending with a vegetable day.

RICE / *7 days / loss: 6 lbs (3 k.)*

Breakfast: 1 hard-boiled egg
2 oz. (60 g.) boiled rice (preferably brown and weigh after cooking not before)
Black coffee or lemon tea

Lunch: 3 oz. (90 g.) boiled rice (weigh after cooking not before)
3 oz. (90 g.) white fish or chicken
1 raw tomato
Black coffee or lemon tea

Dinner: Same as lunch

ONE MEAL AND LEMON / *5 days / loss: 5 lbs (2.5 k.)*

Lunch or Dinner: 8 oz. (240 g.) beef, veal or chicken grilled or roasted with no additional fat
1 portion fresh green vegetable or salad
1 orange or apple or ½ grapefruit

During the day: Juice of a fresh lemon in a wine glass of hot water – maximum of 6 times
Black coffee or lemon tea

VEGETABLE JUICES / *1 day / loss: 2 lbs (1 k.)*

Breakfast: Glass of tomato juice mixed with one raw egg and a little lemon juice
Black coffee or lemon tea

Lunch: Glass of vegetable juice – any mixture
1 slice wholewheat toast
Black coffee or lemon tea

Dinner: Glass of tomato juice with a raw egg
Black coffee or lemon tea

FRUIT ONLY / *5 days / loss: 5 lbs (2.5 k.)*

Breakfast: 1 orange or ½ grapefruit
Black coffee or lemon tea

Lunch: Fruit salad – orange, lemon, grapefruit, apple and melon
Black coffee or lemon tea

Dinner: Same as lunch – add a little cinnamon to liven the taste

STEAK TARTARE / *3 days / loss: 5 lbs (2.5 k.)*

Breakfast: Steak tartare made from 3 oz. (90 g.) fresh ground beef, 1 egg, peppers and capers
1 slice wholewheat toast
Black coffee or lemon tea

Lunch: Small green salad (eat first)
3 oz. (90 g.) steak tartare
Black coffee or lemon tea

Dinner: Same as lunch

DRINKER'S DIET / *7 days / loss 5 lbs (2.5 k.)*

Breakfast: 1 hard-boiled egg
1 portion of cottage cheese
Black coffee or lemon tea

Lunch: Up to 5 oz. (150 g.) white fish – not fried
1 small green salad or 1 portion green vegetable
2 drinks – whisky, gin or vodka or white wine

Dinner: Up to 5 oz. (150 g.) lean beef or chicken
1 small green salad
1 oz. (30 g.) hard cheese
2 drinks – whisky, gin or vodka or white wine
Black coffee or lemon tea

DIET BOOSTER:
LECITHIN, VITAMIN B-6, CIDER VINEGAR, KELP

The addition of these four to any type of diet is claimed to give it a spurt and provide a higher energy level. Tests are not conclusive on this point but personal recommendations from those who've done it, indicate that it is worth a try. The formula is: 2 tablespoons of lecithin a day, a fifty-milligramme tablet of B-6 vitamin a day, 1 teaspoon of cider vinegar after each meal and 3 tablets of kelp after each meal. The theory is that lecithin helps mobilize fat, the vitamin B-6 helps metabolize it, the cider vinegar contains potassium which helps to keep nerves on an even keel, while the kelp is rich in iodine which speeds up metabolism.

HCG DIET PLAN

This is based on daily injections of HCG (Human Chorionic Gonadotropin, a compound obtained from pregnant women's urine) together with strict adherence to a fat-free 500 Calorie a day diet; a number of medical authorities do not approve it, but many women say it is one of the few ways to not only lose weight but to shift it from the most stubborn places – such as thighs and legs – that other diets do not achieve. Treatment is for a minimum of 21 days and a maximum of 40 under the daily supervision of a doctor; weight loss is usually fairly consistent between half a pound to a pound a day. Never are you allowed to lose more than 34 pounds at a time. It is argued that the same amount of weight can be lost by forgetting the injections and just existing on the miserly diet; maybe, but the injections mobilize the fat and once in the bloodstream make you feel as though you have eaten so there are no hunger pangs. Also, the fat is encouraged into more even distribution. No cosmetics containing grease can be used during treatment.

Breakfast:	Tea or coffee in any quantity without sugar – only 1 tablespoonful of milk allowed in 24 hours
Lunch or Dinner:	3½ oz. (105 g.) of veal, beef, chicken breast (skinned raw), fresh white fish, shrimp, lobster or crab 4 oz. (120 g.) of only one of the following vegetables: cabbage, onions, beet greens, spinach, Brussels sprouts, chicory, tomatoes, celery, cucumber, fennel, lettuce, watercress, radishes 1 breadstick or 1 piece of Melba toast 1 apple or orange, or ten cherries, 2 oz. (60 g.) strawberries or half a grapefruit Black coffee or tea with lemon is allowed

FASTING

The ultimate diet. If you wish to lose between 2–10 pounds (1–5 k.) over a period of two to four days, there is a very good chance you can do it this way. It is possible to lose up to 4 or 5 pounds (2–2½ k.) on a one-day fast, up to 10 pounds (5 k.) on a weekend regime and up to 20 pounds (10 k.) on a week-long abstinence. If you are in general good health, fasting within limits is not dangerous; in fact the contrary for it gives body metabolism a much needed rest and revitalizes the digestive system. Fasting on one's own should have a limit of four days, but under medical supervision and preferably in a clinic, most women can safely fast for several weeks.

A fast means eating absolutely nothing. You can drink, indeed you have to, the medical recommendation of a minimum of 2 quarts (2 l.) of water a day. Some fasts suggest drinking natural vegetable or fruit juices, others allow black coffee or lemon tea, but it is generally accepted that when fasting for weight loss rather than health, it is best to drink only water – mineral water, if possible, but not distilled water. There is no limit to the amount of water you may drink, nor is there any reason for concern if you don't seem to be eliminating as much as you take in; much of it evaporates through the pores.

Hunger amazingly disappears during a fast. After eighteen hours of no solid food, one usually loses hunger pangs and the desperate desire to eat. There is no need to take any vitamin supplements, but if you must, only take vitamin B and C as the others could cause complications.

The rate at which you lose weight is generally in proportion to the degree you are overweight – the more, the faster. It is also said that after fasting, chances are much better for permanent weight control than after other diets. A few pounds may come back at the beginning; this doesn't mean you are eating too much but that the sodium content in food causes the body once again to retain a certain amount of fluid. After an initial fast and weight loss, you should be able to lose an additional two pounds a week on a daily diet of not more than 1,400 Calories (see page 57).

You can fast for one or two days a week, but the total in any one month should not be more than 10 days. A fast should be gradually broken. At first add orange juice to the water, then take some yoghourt, later melba toast and honey. Eat a little every three hours until your body gets back again into the rhythm of regular meals. You will probably find that after a fast, it takes less food to satisfy you, also frequently the taste for sweet and fatty foods is less.

SLIMMING DISEASE

Anorexia nervosa is a psychiatric illness usually caused by compulsive dieting. There is such a thing as too much dieting. It doesn't happen often and it is a relatively small problem compared with troubles caused by overweight. Even the keenest slimmers find that hunger eventually overcomes intentions and any target weight is reached with relief. Not so for a small proportion of women who find that once started they are unable to stop slimming even when they are thinner than is normal. It becomes an obsession. Only prolonged medical attention can reverse it and unless checked this diet mania can lead to starvation.

The prevalence of the disease is on the increase. It usually starts with a desire to be extremely thin or alternatively with a morbid fear of fatness. In the early stages it looks like crash dieting of an extreme kind, but there the similarity ends. Any degree of thinness is not thin enough, and the next step is a refusal to eat almost any solid food and to take a minimum amount of fluids. It is a vicious circle for as the anorexia victim eats less and less she develops an aversion to food. At this point she really cannot eat and cannot be persuaded to try. If she does indulge in a bout of eating she will force herself to be sick. By this time she is usually rather pleased with her emaciated state.

One of the first metabolic symptoms is a specific endocrine disorder that causes periods to stop; other signs are dry skin and often swollen ankles. Medical attention should be sought right away, for it has gone far beyond the point of being a 'diet mad' matter – and beyond self control. Serious cases are immediately hospitalized and treatment starts with several weeks in bed using drugs to overcome resistance to eating and to stimulate the appetite. Psychiatric help is used and in some cases sleep therapy. Most patients leave within two to three months, but often the patient goes back to the old starvation habits, sometimes triggered by an emotional crisis. It can take years to cure and repeated relapses are not unusual. It mostly affects teenage girls. There are many theories as to the cause, but little is specific. Sometimes when a girl is fat and teased about it during childhood she develops an obsession to be thin in puberty. Others are said to wish to retain the shape of a child in order to avoid the sexual implications of growing to womanhood. In a mature woman a hypothalamic dysfunction is cited, or desire to get attention by subconsciously gambling with death.

SLIMMING AIDS:

Most salons use electrical machines that provide passive exercise. They are based on a system of electrical impulses invented 150 years ago by Faraday. Two pads – one negatively charged, the other positive – force body muscles to expand and contract between thirty-five to forty times a minute, thus exercising them. When the available energy these muscles need for exercise is used up, fatty deposits are converted into additional energy. The art lies in the correct placement of the pads so they tighten the appropriate muscles to reshape the figure. Another electrically induced way of slimming employs glass vacuum cups for massage; these stimulate the muscles by suction.

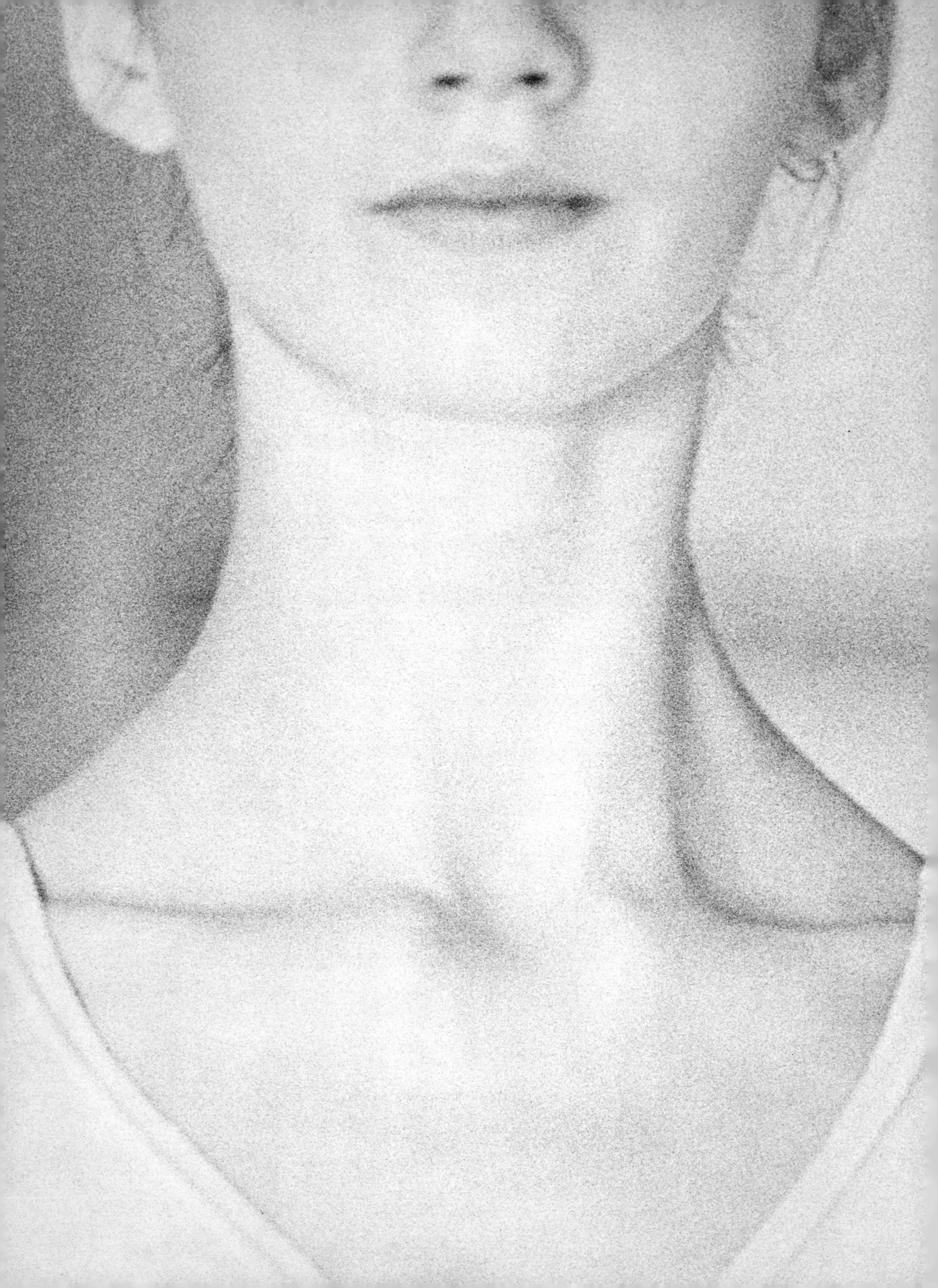

4

EXERCISES

Exercise is vital to overall health. It promotes good circulation and increases oxygen intake and flow. It firms muscles, moves joints, gives flexibility and suppleness; it can help to dispel nervous tension and delay some ageing symptoms. The reason we do not devote more time to it is because of laziness and boredom.

Most physical jerks are thoroughly boring, and it is essential to find the kind of exercise that fits your figure, age, temperament, skills and preferences. There are dozens of systems to choose from; all good ways of getting you into shape and building up energy reserves. One of the surprises for the beginner is the enjoyment that exercise brings. There is pleasure in motion and once you discover this you will find exercise indispensable.

To be effective, exercise must be part of your daily schedule. A burst of activity followed by a few days off just doesn't work. And there is no point in torturing your body with a crash programme: you might jeopardize your health, particularly if you are used to a sedentary life. Slow but sure is the only way. Gradually the body will respond and become capable of doing every movement at its own steady pace.

Exercise cannot alter your weight to any appreciable degree, but it can alter your figure by toning and tightening the body's outer layer of muscles thus helping to restore firmness. It can take inches off upper arms, midriff, waist, hips, thighs and buttocks – but it takes them off slowly.

Exercises are individual and on the following pages are the blueprints for the most effective systems. Each group incorporates a series of eight movements which together exercise the entire body. They are paced so that you can gear them to your own rhythm and timing. They can be

HEUMANN

done in 15 minutes a day – though there's no restriction if you want to do more. Each system has a different approach, different techniques of balance, movement and muscle control. The end result is the same: better health, energy, vitality. You don't have to stick to one routine; change weekly or do two different ones in a day if you wish – variety will retain your interest and keep you exercising.

Before you start, a little preparation and attention to basics:

Decide where and when; make a definite time and be firm and punctual.

If there's no convenient carpet area, get an exercise mat, large towel or blanket for the floor.

Wear leotards, bathing suit, underwear or nothing.

Exercise barefoot if possible.

Move to music, it keeps you at a certain pace, maintains interest.

Each exercise is a series of integrated movements, go from one to the other with smooth, controlled motions.

Body movements should be balanced by deep rhythmic breathing; exhale when body is bent and chest compressed, inhale as you stretch or straighten.

Work gradually into schedule; five minutes at first.

INFORMAL EXERCISE AND SPORTS

Some sort of exercise each day is so important – walking, jogging, swimming, tennis, bicycling. Informal activities and sports, done regularly and in easy stages, contribute to your general health, fitness and all over firmness. Every activity raises your pulse rate above normal and keeps it there while a fresh supply of oxygen pumps through your system. Each breath revitalizes the heart-lung complex and noticeably improves well-being. An under-exercised heart results in lack of energy. Walking should be a daily constitutional of not less than a mile.

Two of the most effective forms of exercise are swimming and jogging. Almost everyone can do one or the other. In swimming the buoyancy of the water makes movement easier, while the pressure makes it more effective. It uses almost every muscle in the body and physical strength is not necessary.

Take a warm shower first, finishing up with body-temperature water. Then a few arm circles to limber up. Breast stroke helps to firm and shape arms and legs, upper chest muscles. Back crawl is good for the shoulders, shaping the bosom and firming upper thighs. Front crawl uses the muscles of upper and lower arms, upper chest, while the leg action tightens the buttocks and the front of the thighs. In swimming you can measure endurance and progress: if you swim regularly you will be amazed at the degree of improvement in a relatively short time. Try to swim three or four times weekly, for forty-five-minute periods.

Jogging is the simplest form of exercise and uses most muscles in the body, especially those in the legs. The lungs are forced to bring in more oxygen, the heart has to beat faster to supply this to the muscles, so the entire circulatory system is put in peak motion. Begin jogging by combining it with walking for periods of fifteen minutes. It is better to do a few warm-up exercises beforehand, then break into a slow trot for about a quarter of a mile. When you are tired walk until you have recovered your breath, then trot again. Do not over exert yourself at first, but try to build up a steady rhythm, keeping that as your beat and speeding it up as you get fitter.

MASSAGE:

Massage relaxes you, relieves tension through touch and, most important, makes you conscious of your own body and its potential. In massage you are not so much toning muscles as trying to achieve a recovery from muscle fatigue; the blood flow is stimulated, the body becomes supple and energy is restored.

A false assumption is that rubbing and manipulation of tissues break up unwanted fat deposits and wash them away in the bloodstream. Women with cellulite problems who explore the possibilities of massage find that although the fat is broken up to some extent it simply moves from one place to another.

Massage helps exercise and diet take effect sooner and makes you feel slimmer and better. It is best to have massage after exercise or late in the afternoon when tension is at its height. It is the great tranquillizer – far superior to a pill – acting on the autonomic nervous system and nerve endings all over the body.

There are several ways of giving a massage and masseurs normally work out their own techniques which are as individual as handwriting. Stroking and kneading may vary from light to heavy depending on the area, but all movements should be gentle, slow, and rhythmic. Most masseurs use a bland oil or emollient, but you can choose what you want. Certain aromatic oils have particularly beneficial effects.

CLASSIC BEGINNER

These formal movements are an introduction to motion, and prove that simple easy rhythms if done every day can quickly bring about a new suppleness and make you more relaxed. When mastered, go on to the intermediate exercises.

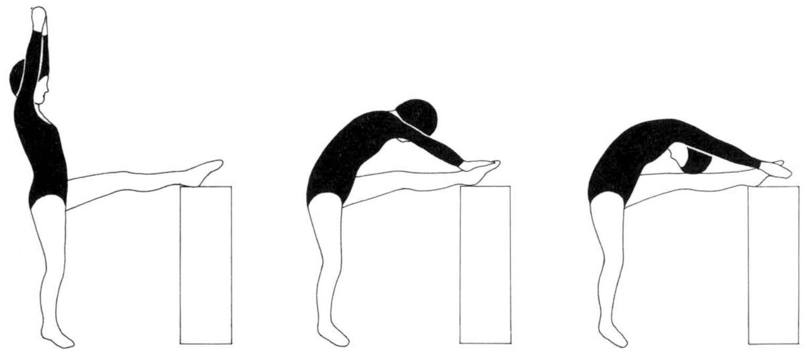

Raised Leg Stretch – Stand a leg's distance away from a support a fraction higher than your leg. Lift leg, rest it there. Stretch hands over head. Bend forward, try to touch feet, head on knee. Keep supporting leg straight. *3 times.* Reverse legs.

Stomach Control – Lie on back, head and shoulders on floor. Bend legs, raise knees to chest, slowly extend legs, lower and hold at 45°. Count 3. Bend legs back to chest. *6 times, work up to 10.*

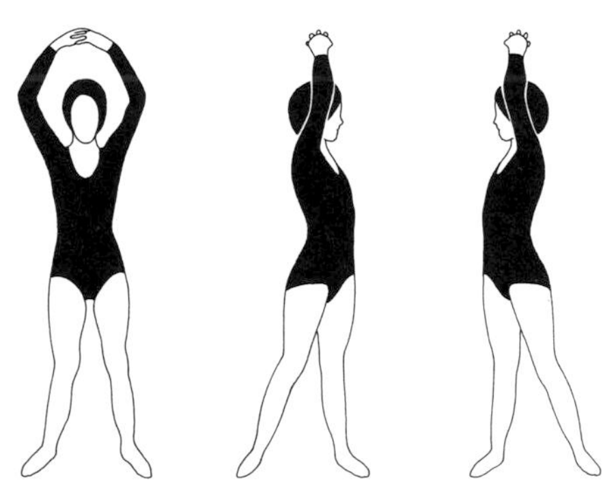

Torso Twist – Stand feet apart, hands over head, fingers linked. Slowly twist the body to left, then right. Move only the torso. *10 times, working up to 20.*

Hip Swing – Lie on back, arms slightly from sides, knees bent. Swing legs down to left, then to right. *20 times.*

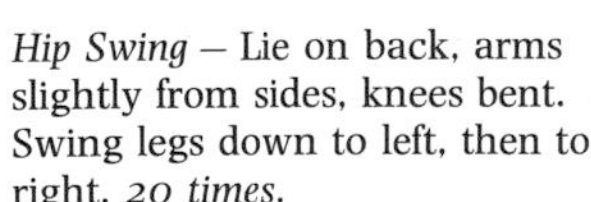

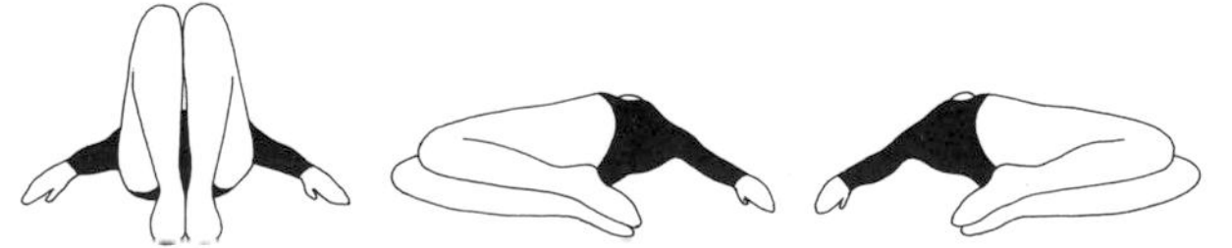

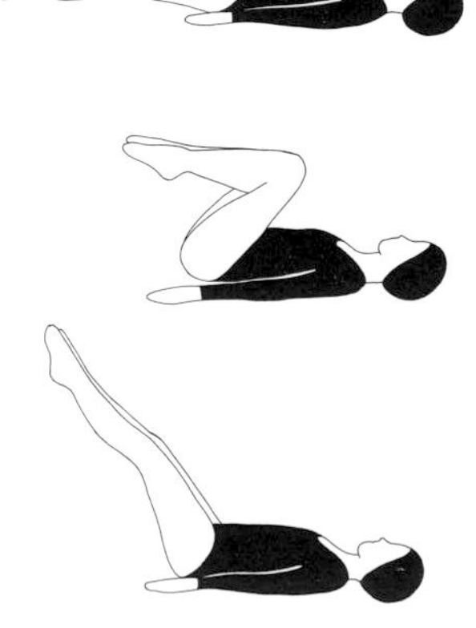

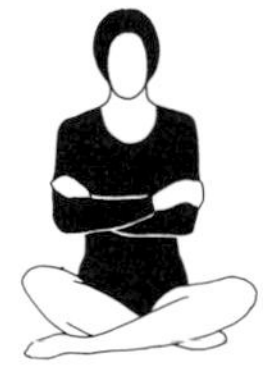
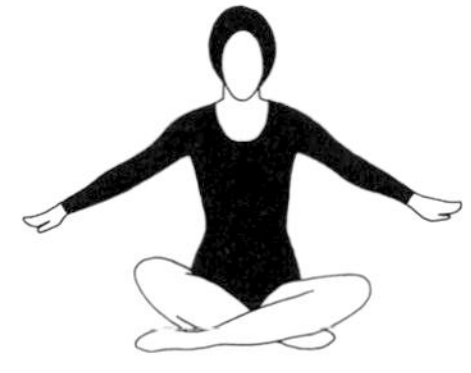
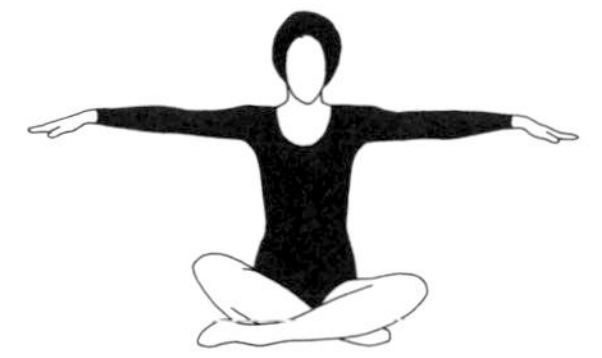

Chest Brace – Sit cross-legged, arms folded. Open arms, gently stretch out and push back. Count 3. Relax. *10 times.*

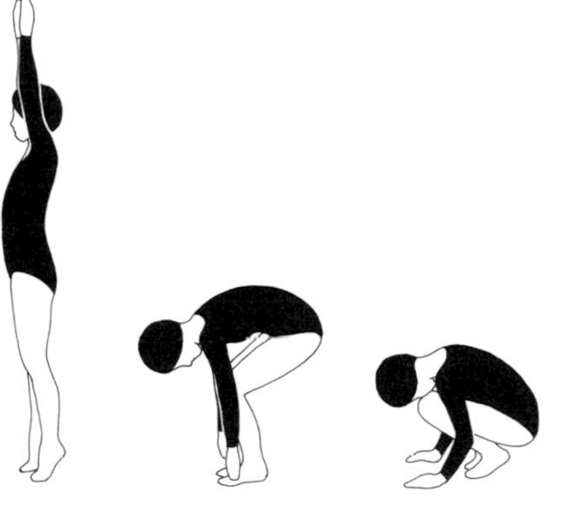

Stretch and Relax – Stand, legs a little apart, arms high. Stand on toes, stretch high. Curve back, relax knees, arms down. Relax completely, unfurl. *6 times.*

Leg Swing – Stand holding a support. Swing outside leg high in front, then way back leaning forward. *20 times*. Reverse legs.

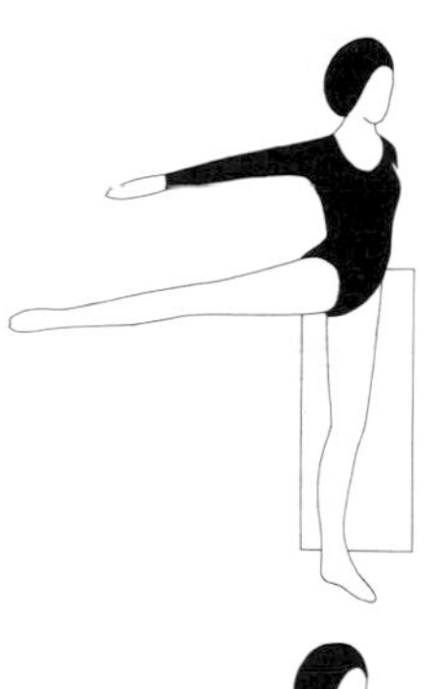
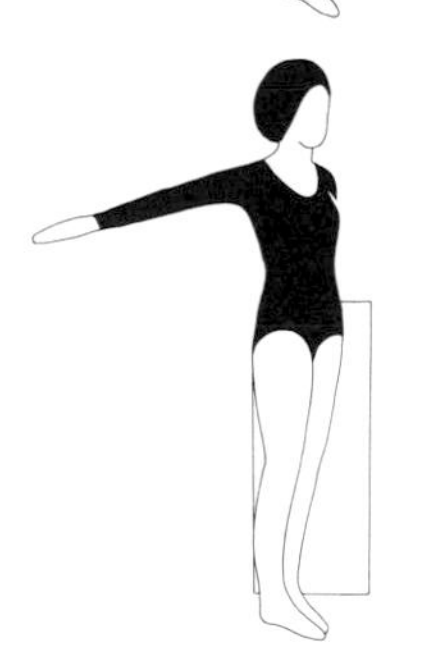
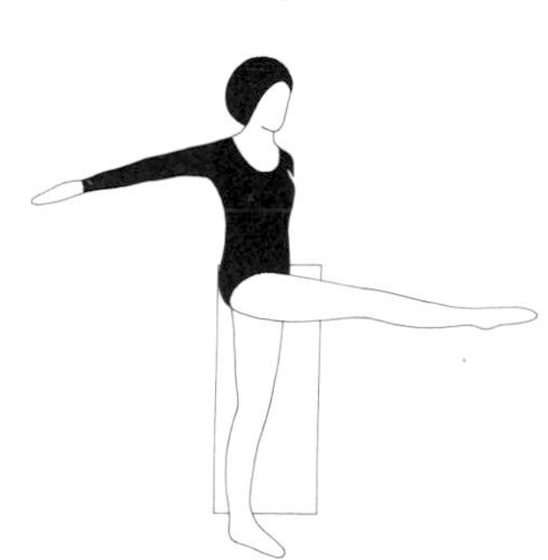

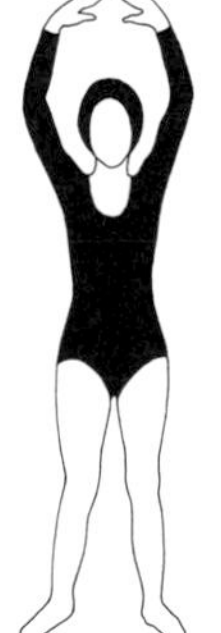
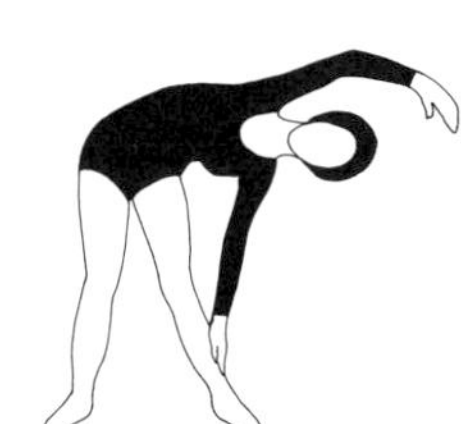
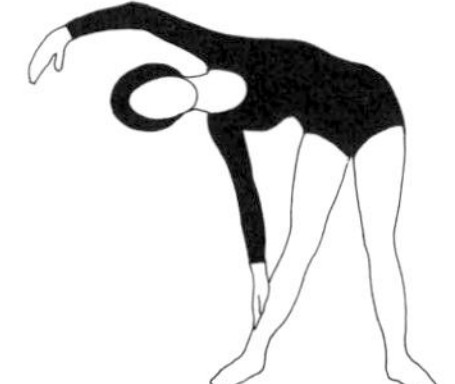

Waist Stretch – Stand feet apart, hands over head. From the waist, bend far to left, then to right. *10 times, working up to 20.*

CLASSIC INTERMEDIATE

For bodies used to a little movement but not really limber, more advanced forms of basic actions already introduced. Now you can be aware of control as well as rhythm. Pay attention to correct breathing. On exertion take deep breaths to fill the lungs; on relaxation, exhale very slowly.

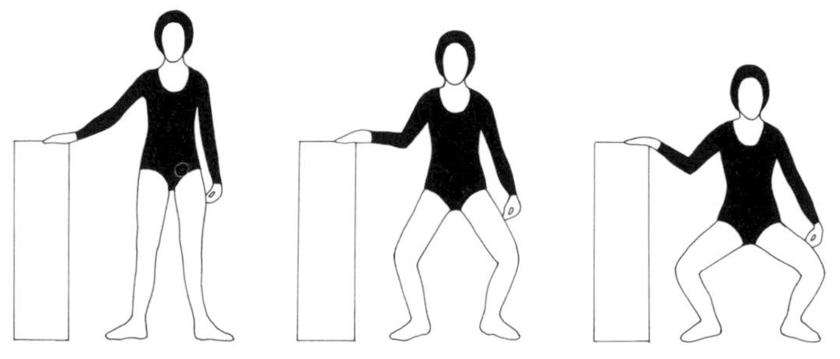

Knee Bends – Stand feet apart, holding on to support if necessary. Keeping back straight, bend both knees outward and down, keeping pelvis forward. *5 times, work up to 10 then 20.*

Kneeling Posture – Kneel, bend keeping back straight, hands clasped behind back. Stretch and curve forward until head is on floor. Return. *10 times, working up to 20.*

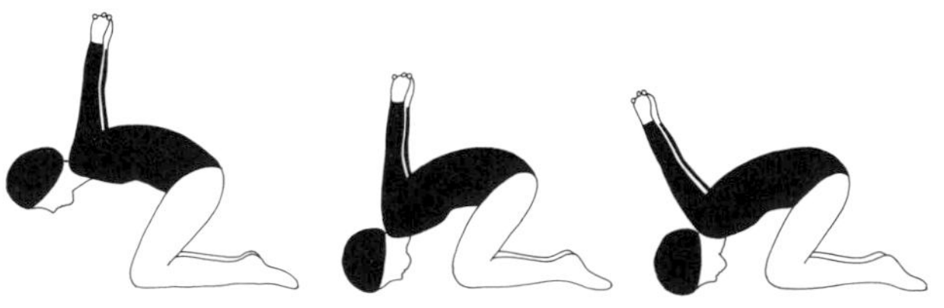

Knee-Tapping – Lie on back with legs well apart, knees bent. Clasp ankles. Bring left knee inwards and down to tap on floor, then right knee. *10 times each knee, working up to 20.*

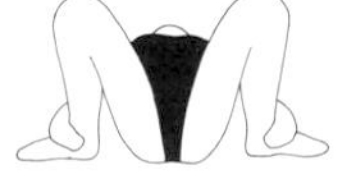

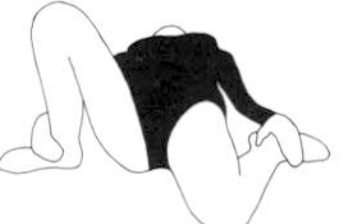

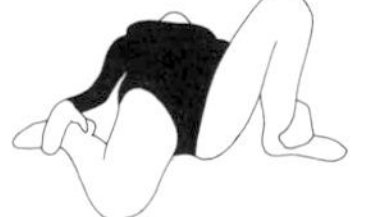

Scissor Raise – Lie on side, head on hand, other hand on floor in front. Keeping torso firm, slowly raise leg high. Lower slowly. *10 times.* Reverse legs.

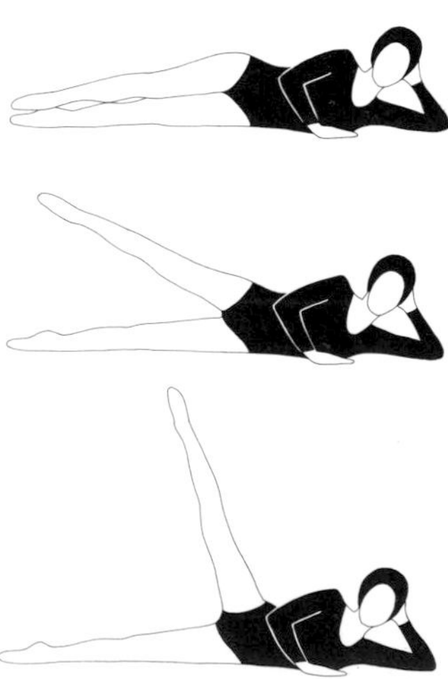

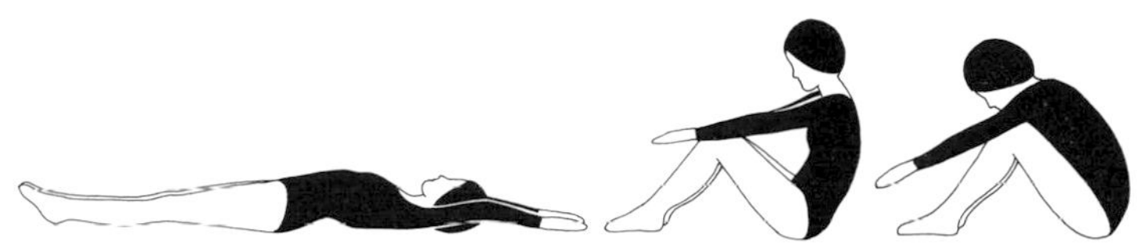

Stomach Control – Lie flat on back, arms over head. Breathe out, pulling up and stretching forward. Breathe in and return. *6 times, working up to 12 and increasing speed.*

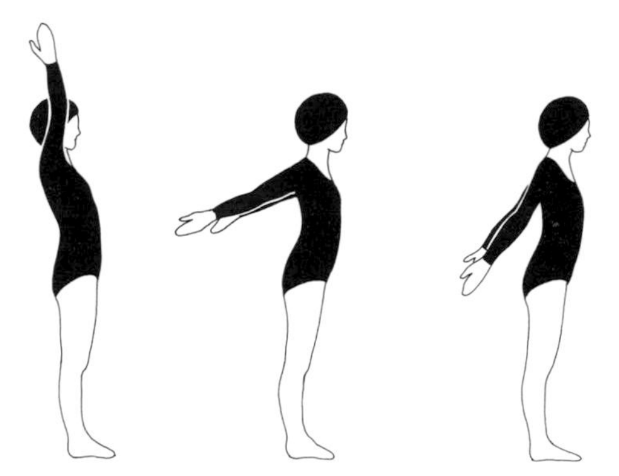

Arm Swing – Stand arms over head, palms together. Bring arms down to sides, push back, pull down and back. Relax. *10 times, working up to 20.*

Waist Bend – Stand feet well apart, link hands over head. Keeping arms and body straight, bend slowly to right, push to the limit. Count 3. Reverse sides. *10 times, working up to 20.*

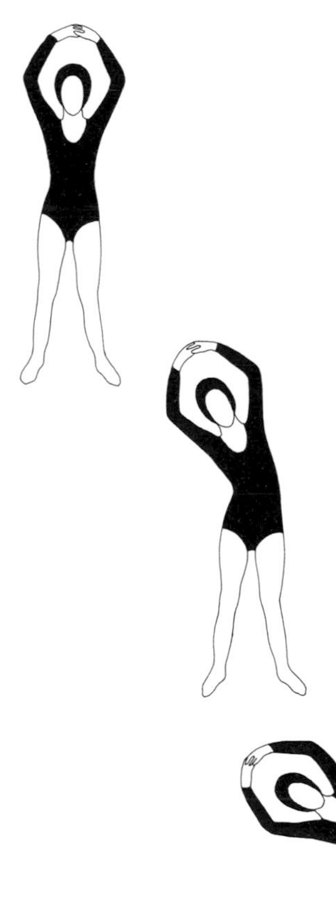

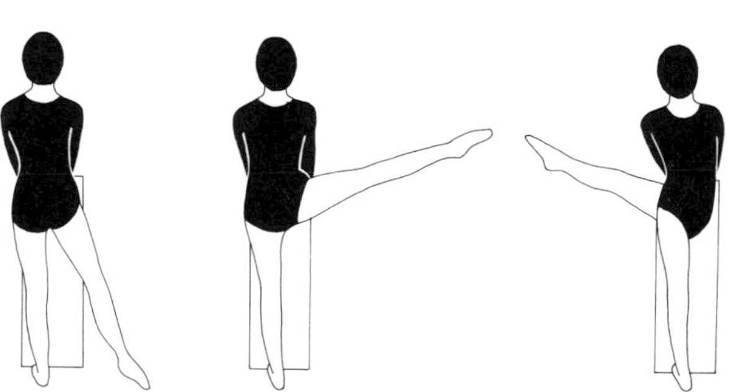

Crossover Swing – Stand about 2 feet away from a support. Keeping legs straight, stretch and lift one leg, swing across body. *20 times.* Reverse legs.

CLASSIC ADVANCED

For these exercises the muscles require more subtle control and should be able to sustain positions longer. Endurance should come with ease. Smooth and clockwork precision is expected. Do beginner series to warm up, activate muscles.

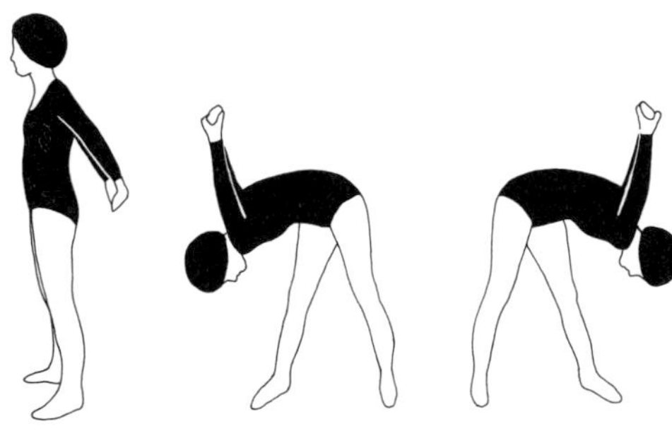

Body Bend – Stand legs apart, hands linked behind hips. Drop upper body forward, with head near knees, move head to right and left. *10 times each side.*

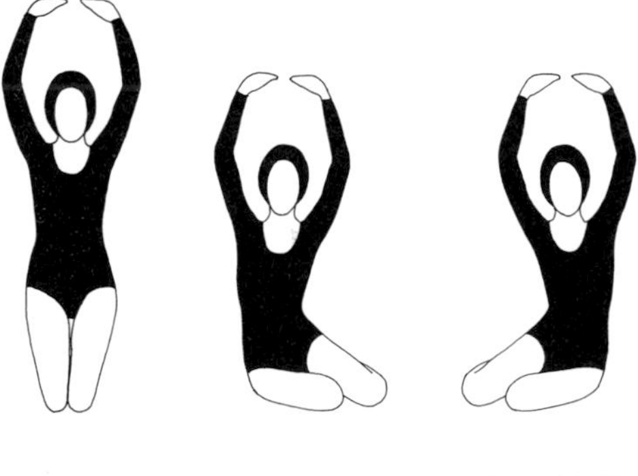

Bottom Bounce – Kneel with hands over head, fingers touching. Keeping body facing forwards, lower buttocks to touch floor on right, then swing to left and down. *5 times each side, working up to 10.*

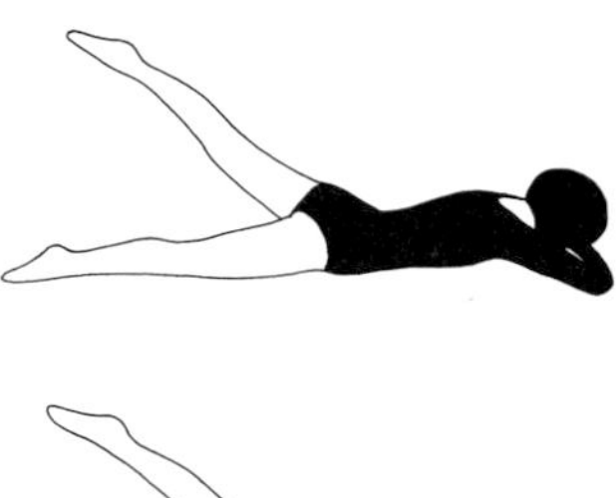

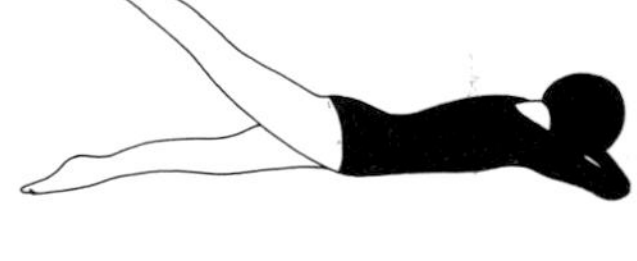

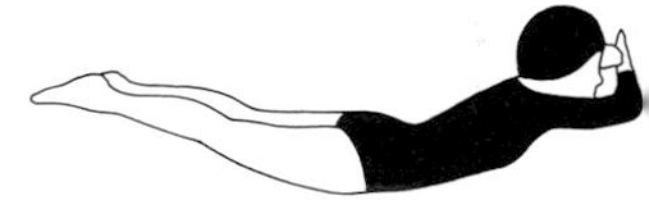

Leg and Head Lift – Lie on front. Raise left leg high. Count 2, lower. Reverse legs. Raise both legs simultaneously, lift shoulders and head with hands on forehead; count 2. *5 times, working up to 10.*

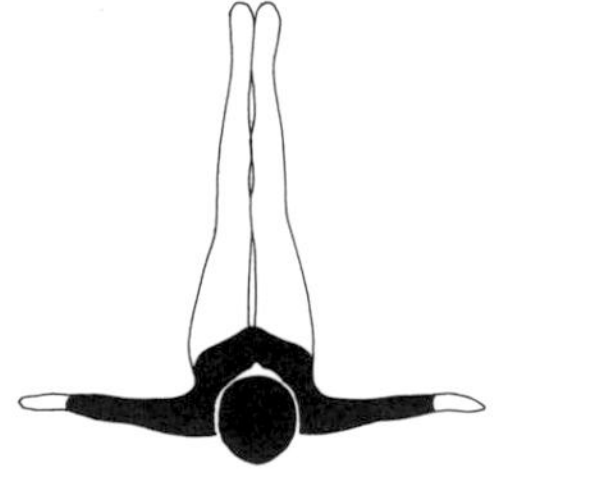

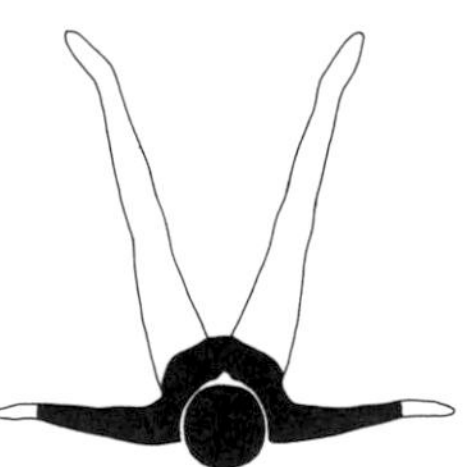

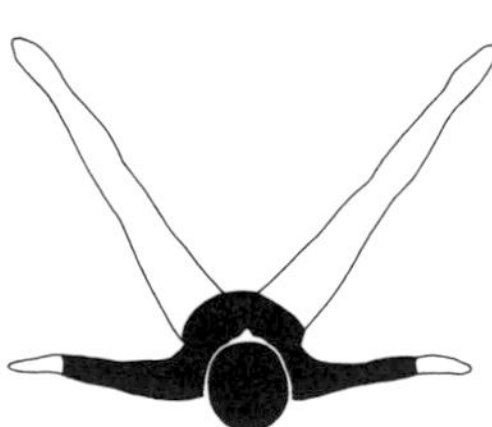

Thigh Control – Lie, arms out at sides, legs at right angles to torso. Spread legs wide, bring together. *Non-stop 20 times.*

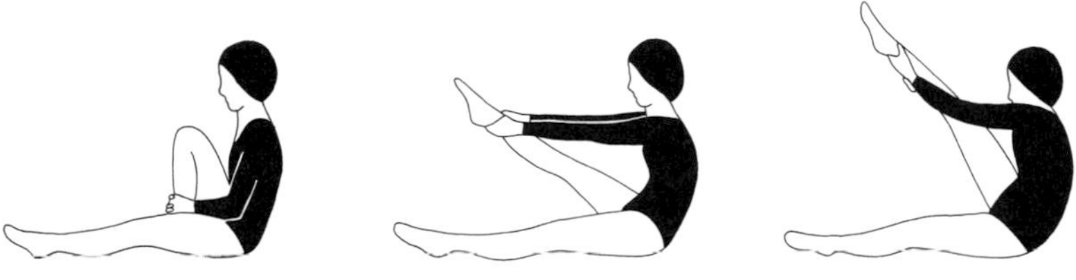

Complete Leg Stretch – Sit, left leg straight, right leg bent. Clasp ankle, bringing heel right against buttocks. Holding firm, straighten leg pulling up high. Count 3, lower leg. *3 times each leg.*

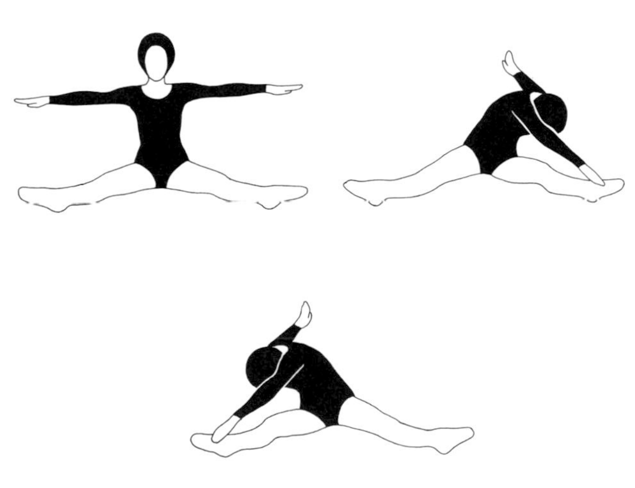

Sitting Stretch – Sit upright, legs wide apart, arms outstretched. Swing forward to touch left foot with right hand, then vice versa. *20 times in rhythm.*

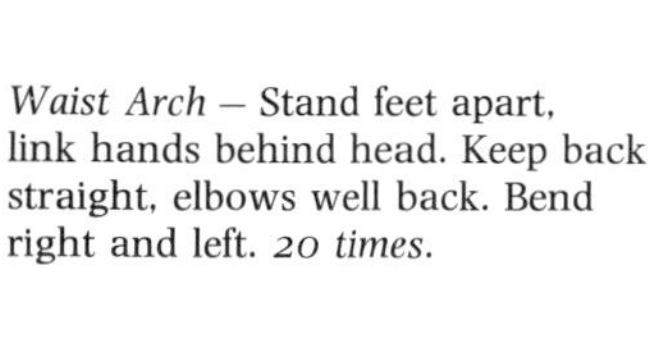

Waist Arch – Stand feet apart, link hands behind head. Keep back straight, elbows well back. Bend right and left. *20 times.*

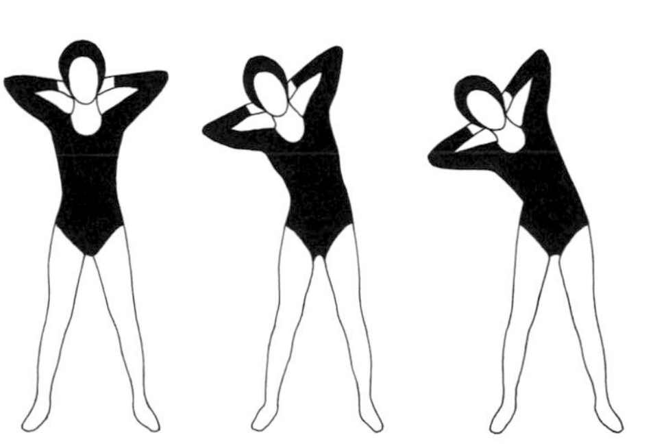

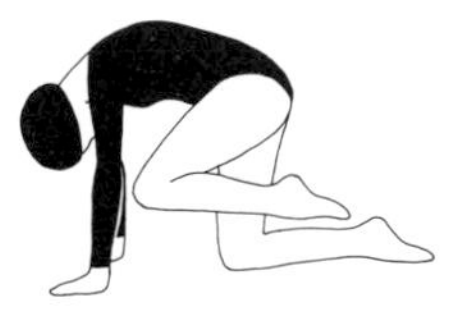

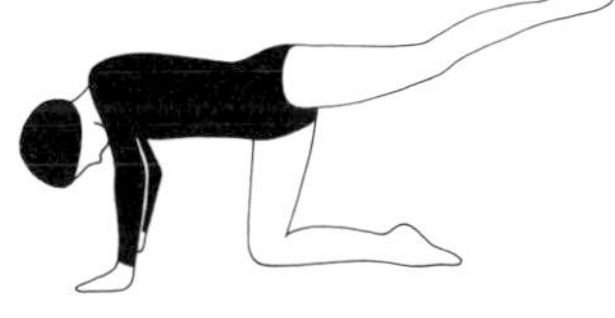

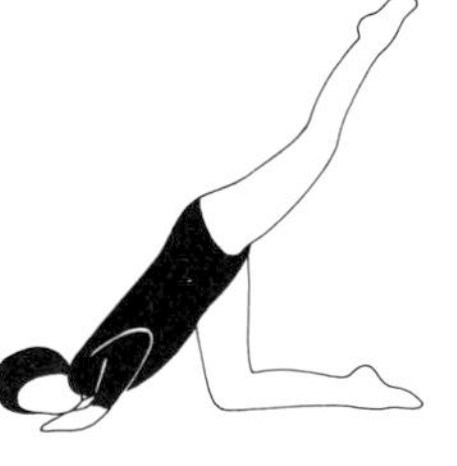

Kneel and Stretch – Kneel, arms straight, head down. Bend left knee to chest, push straight back and up. Count 2. Bend elbows allowing head to rest on floor, holding body in diagonal line from toe to shoulder. Count 2. Relax. Reverse legs. *5 times each leg.*

STICK

These are straightforward classic exercises with a prop to give movements a systematic form. Suggested for women who need some sense of direction for hands; in addition stick controls arm movements, paces distance and provides good balance. Use long pole, broom handle or curtain rod.

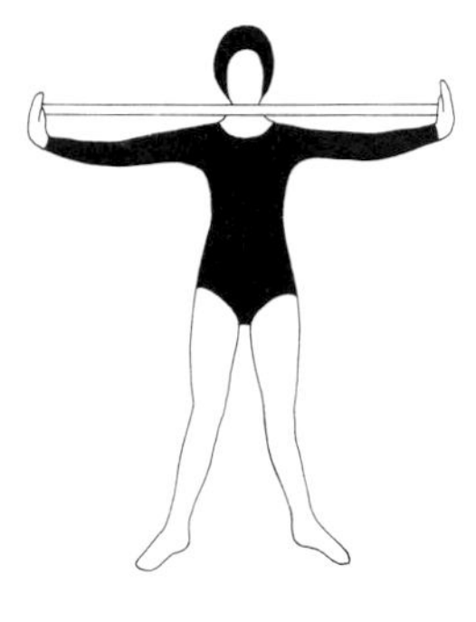

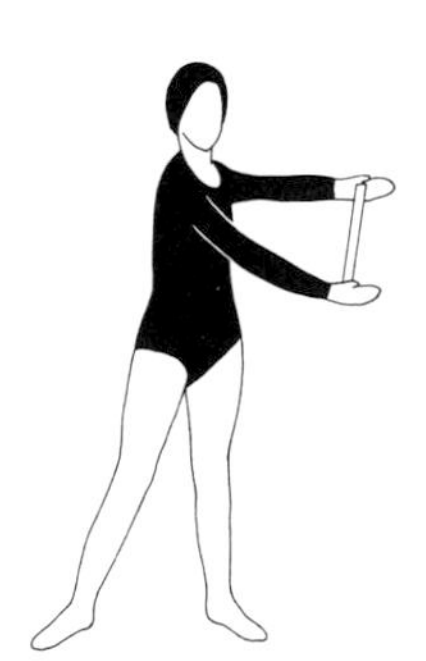

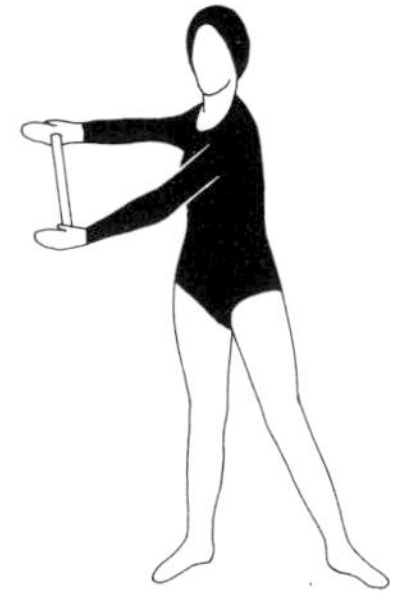

Fore-arm Reach – Feet apart, stick ends held between palms, arms stretched really wide. Swing arms from side to side, holding stick firmly. *20 times.*

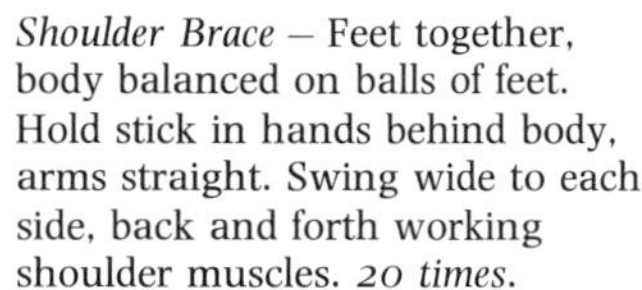

Shoulder Brace – Feet together, body balanced on balls of feet. Hold stick in hands behind body, arms straight. Swing wide to each side, back and forth working shoulder muscles. *20 times.*

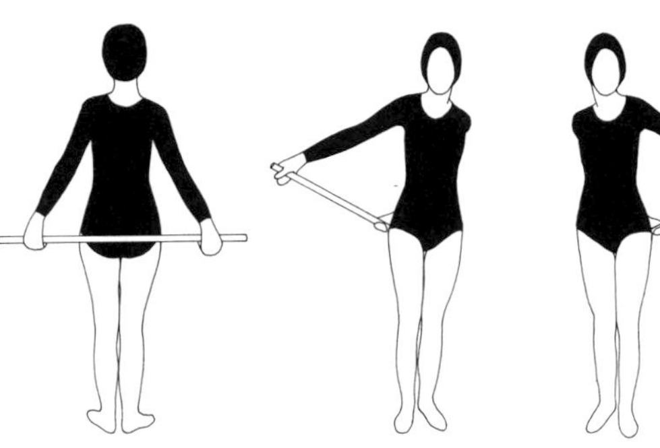

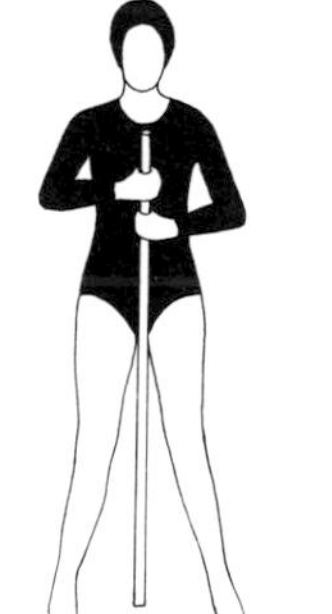

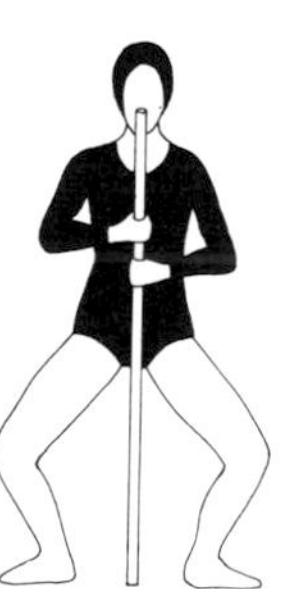

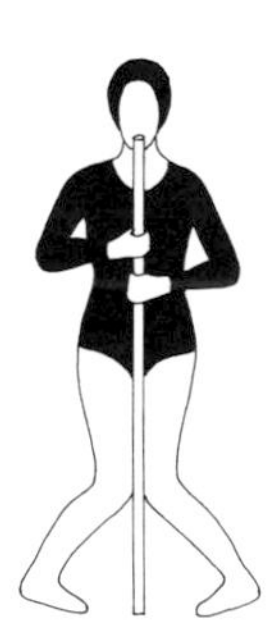

Foot Switch – Stand feet a few inches apart, stick held vertically. Bend knees, turn toes out, straighten up. Bend knees, turn toes in, straighten up. *In-out quickly 20 times.*

Leg Swing – Stand upright, stick vertical. Hold with both hands, balance it. Swing one leg forward and back as far as possible, holding stick firm. *30 times each leg.*

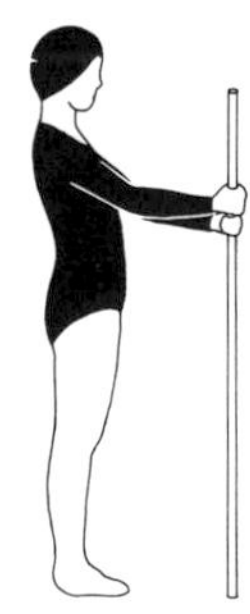

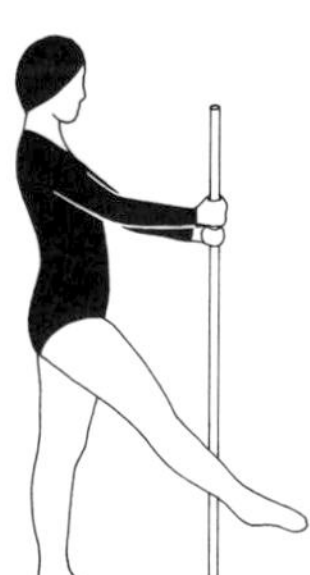

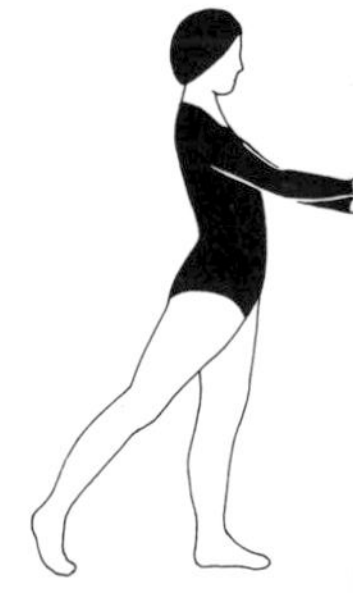

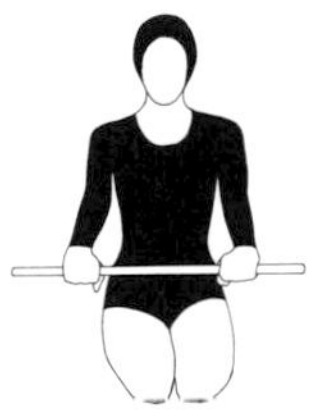

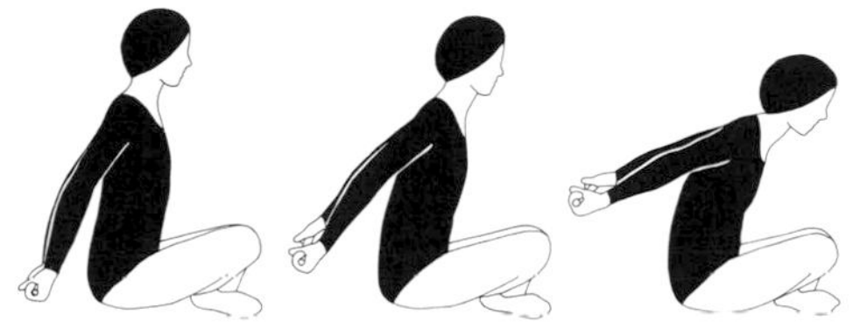

Behind the Back – Sit cross-legged, hold stick behind back, palms upward. Push stick up and down very slowly, keeping arms straight. *30 times.*

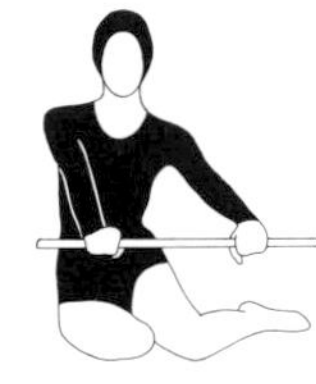

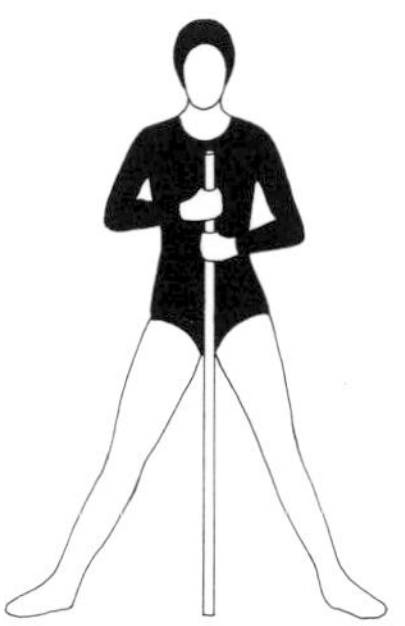

Side Dip – Stand legs apart, holding stick with both hands. Keeping back straight and buttocks tucked under, dip left then right knee in rhythm. *20 times.*

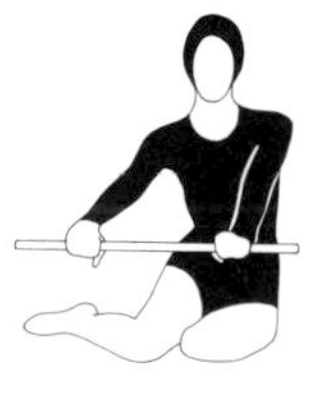

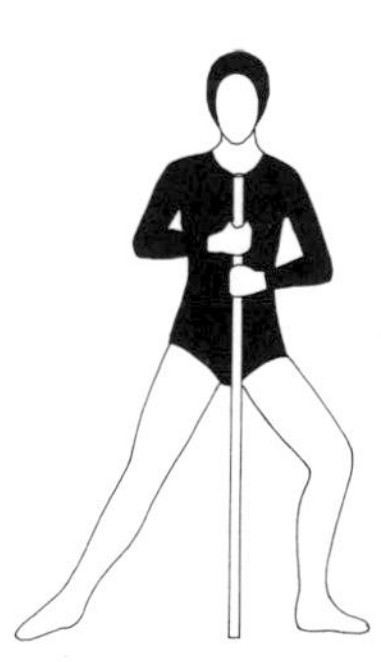

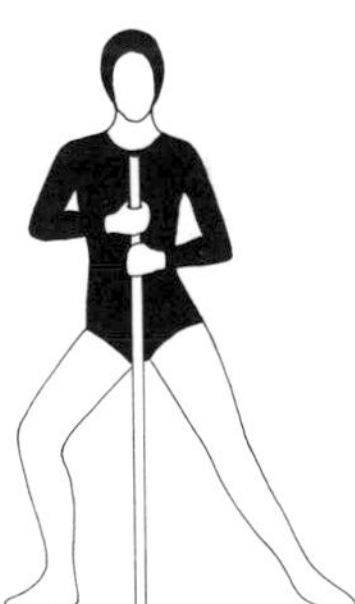

Kneel and Rock – Kneel on heels, stick in front. Move body weight to one side until buttock touches floor. Rock to other side. Try to keep stick steady and level. *20 times.*

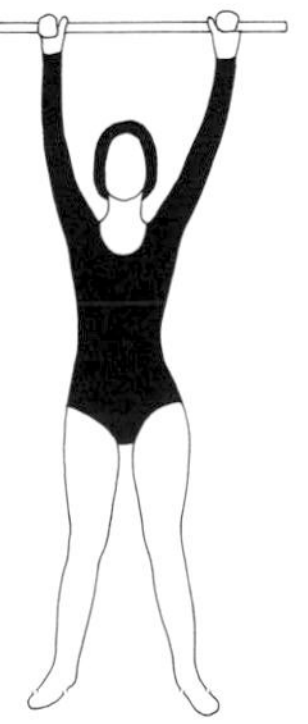

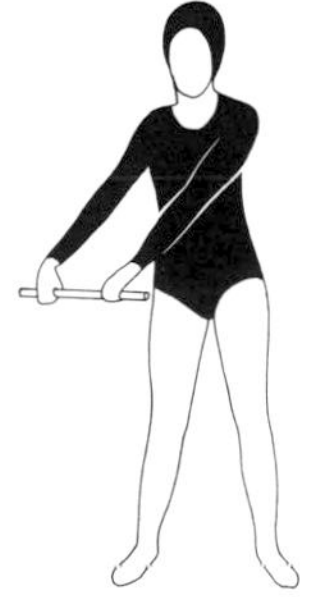

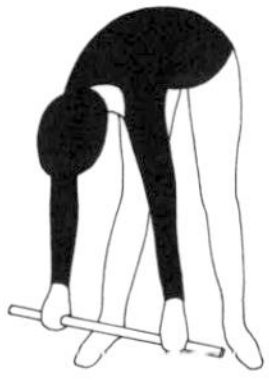

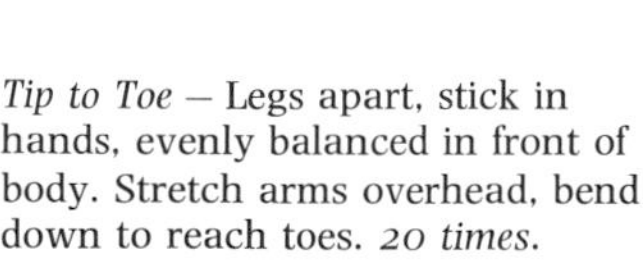

Tip to Toe – Legs apart, stick in hands, evenly balanced in front of body. Stretch arms overhead, bend down to reach toes. *20 times.*

WEIGHTS

Excellent for those with stamina and anxious for quick reshaping. Extra pounds make muscles work harder. Start with 3 pounds (1.5 k.), work up to 5 (2.5 k.), finally to 10 (5 k.). There are weights to hold, tie or slip on. Or make your own sacks. Warning: too much for too long can develop ugly muscles.

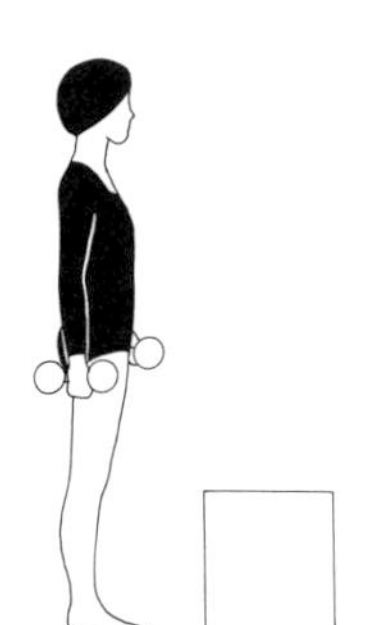

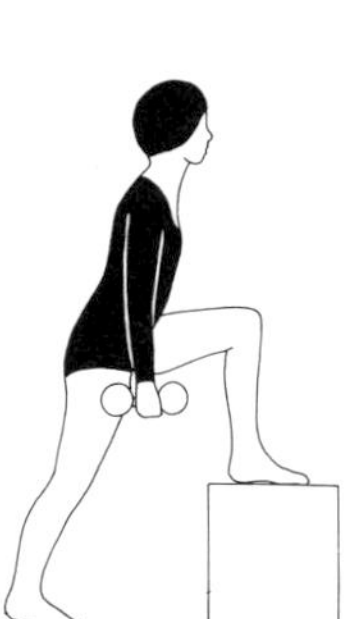

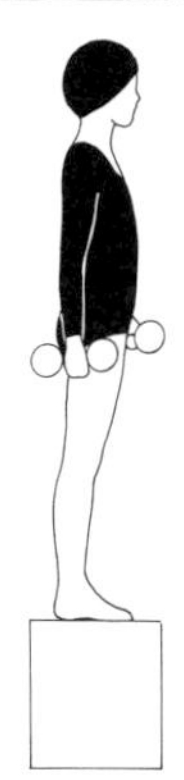

Step-Up – Stand in front of chair, or high step, weight in each hand. Put one foot on chair, draw other leg up to it. Step down same way. *10 times each leg.*

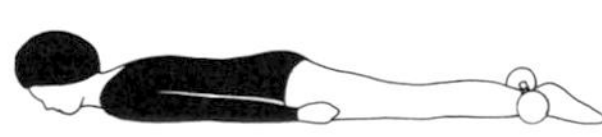

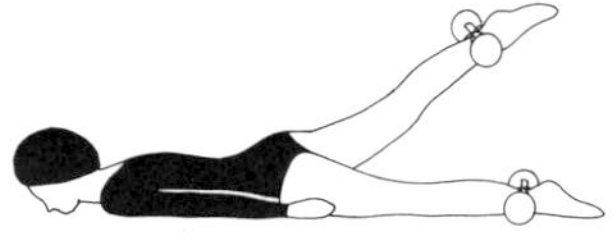

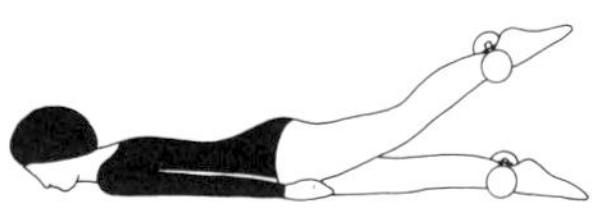

Horizontal Lift – Lie on floor, weights tied on each ankle. Raise one leg as high as possible, count 6, lower slowly. Reverse legs. *6 times each leg.*

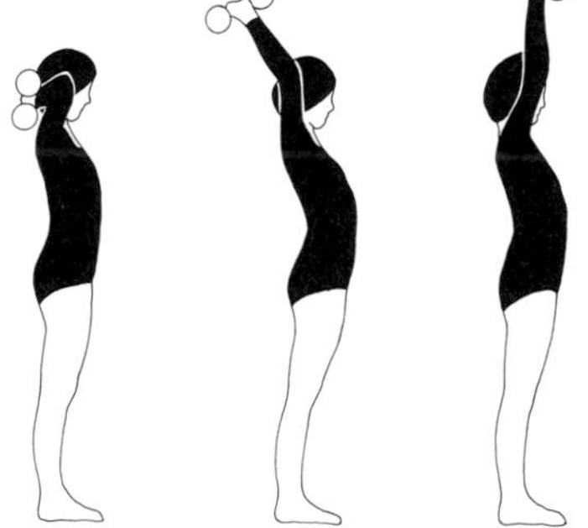

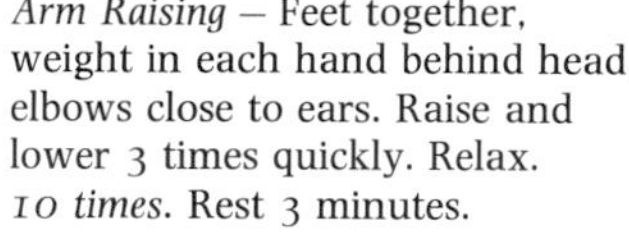

Arm Raising – Feet together, weight in each hand behind head, elbows close to ears. Raise and lower 3 times quickly. Relax. *10 times.* Rest 3 minutes.

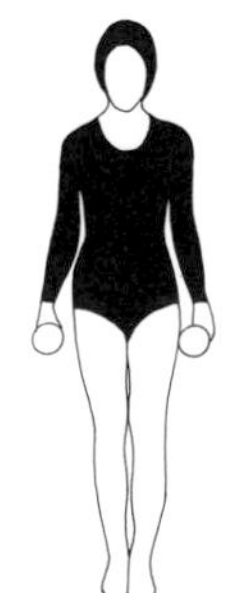

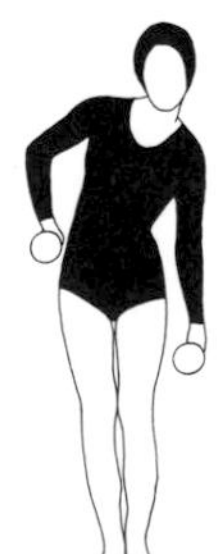

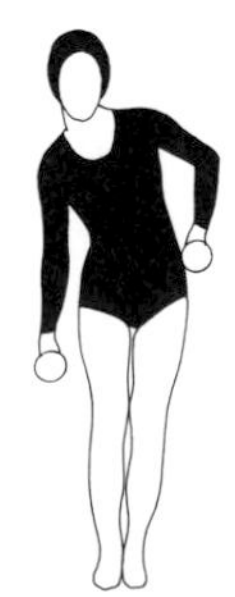

Body Bend – Stand feet together, knees slightly flexed, weight in each hand. Pull right arm up, bend body to left, then vice versa. *10 times.* Rest 3 minutes.

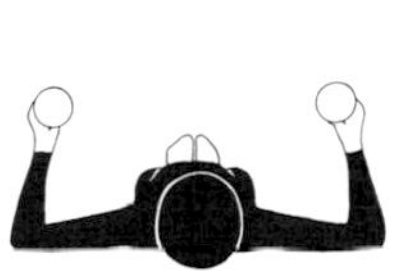
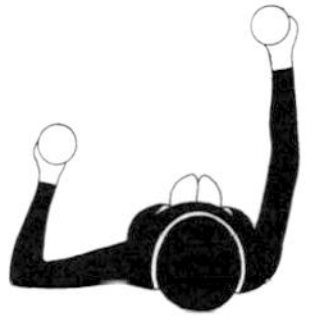
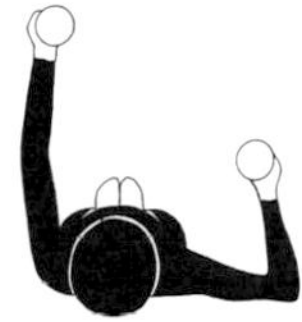

Arm Push – Lie on back, weight in each hand. Elbows bent, upper arms flat on floor. Push alternate arms towards ceiling. *6 times each arm.*

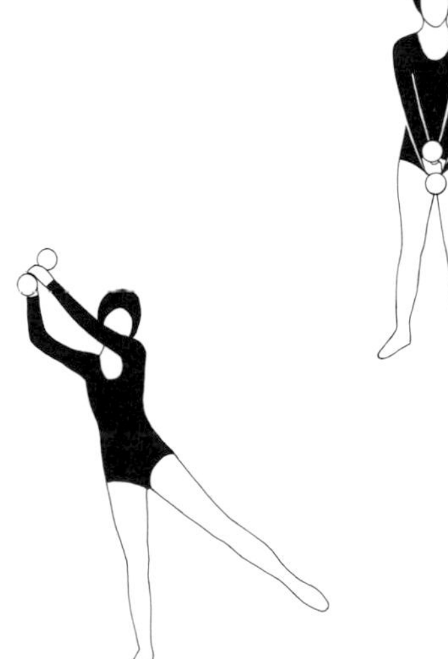
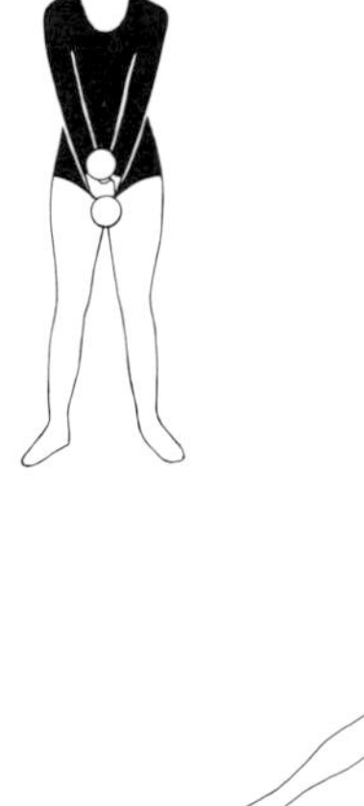
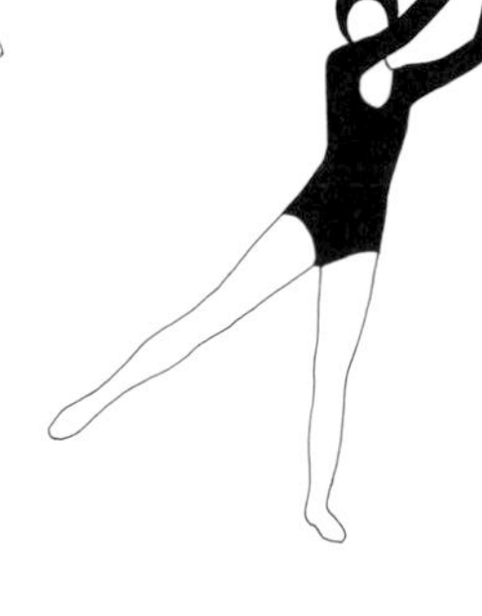

Angle Swing – Stand legs apart, holding one weight in both hands. Swing arms up and out way over to the right. At height of swing, lift left foot for balance. *10 times each side.*

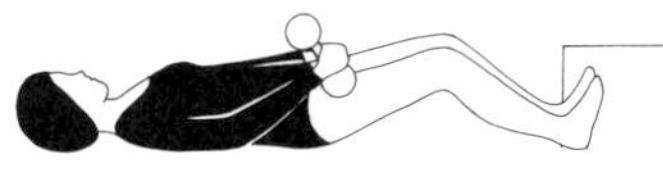
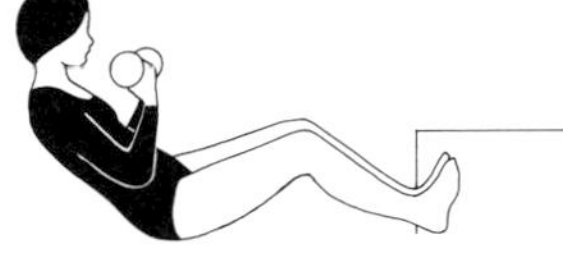
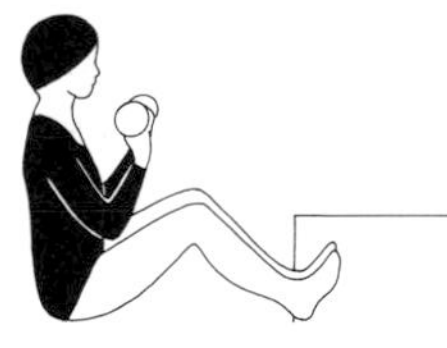

Stomach Pull – Lie on floor with feet on underside of couch, one weight in both hands. Slowly raise body up and down 3 times, knees and feet firm. Relax. *6 times.*

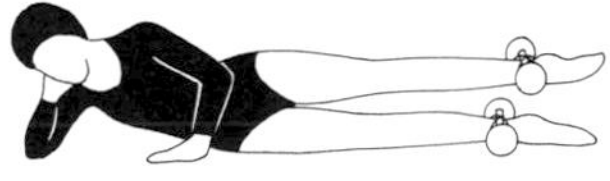
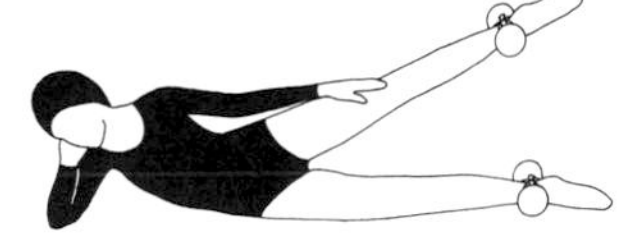
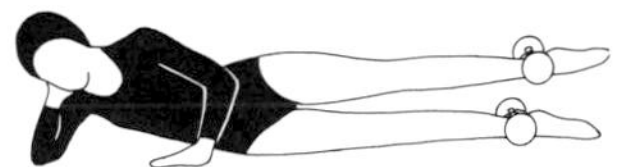

Side Lift – Weights on each ankle, lie on side, supported by one elbow and hand. Lift leg, help with hand near knee, lower slowly. *6 times each leg.*

WATER

Callisthenics in the water is one of the most pleasant and easiest ways to exercise. The buoyant nature of the body gives the illusion of little effort, yet it's the pressure of water that makes movements so effective. Perfect for beginners and older women. Water at shoulder height; best in pool.

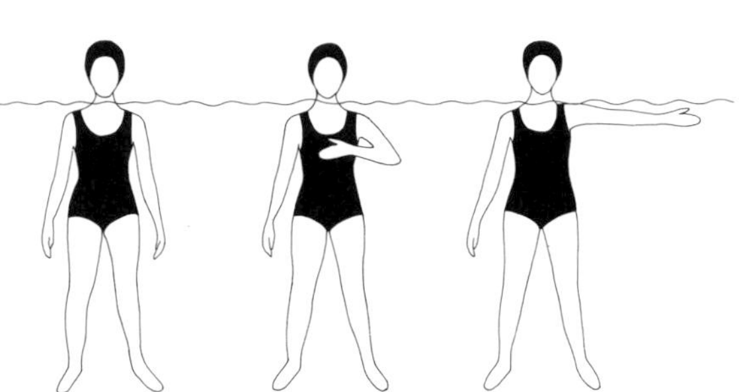

Arm Push – Stand feet apart, arms at sides. Bend arm across in front of bosom, palm facing body. Straighten elbow then push arm back hard against water. Relax to side. *20 times each arm.*

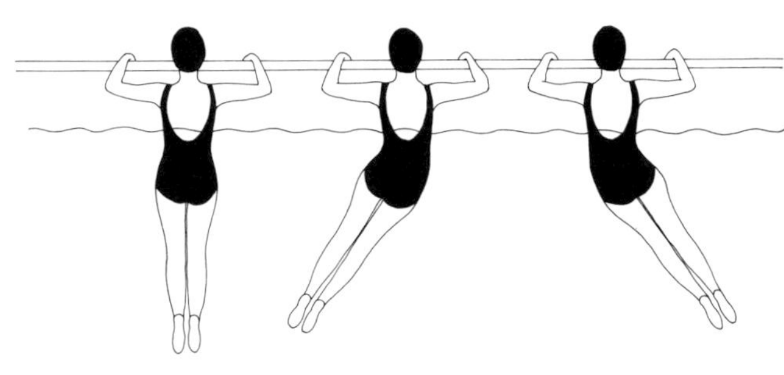

Waist Swing – Hold rail, keeping legs straight and toes pointed, swing each side from the waist, torso firm, for 2 minutes.

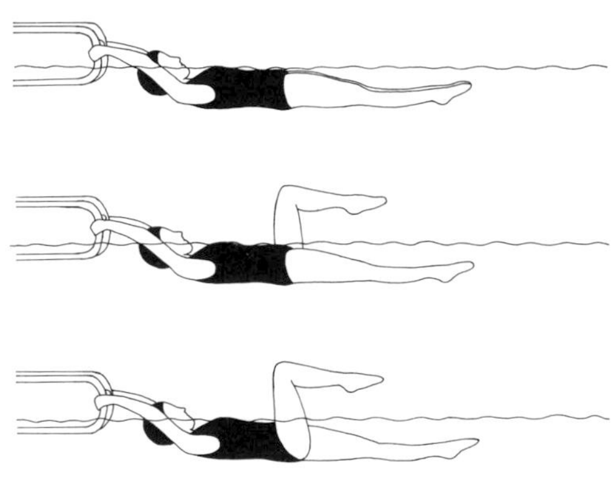

Bicycle Kick – Lie on back, hold ladder or edge. Bicycle kick lifting feet out of water, knees high and push hard on downward kick. *30 kicks or more.*

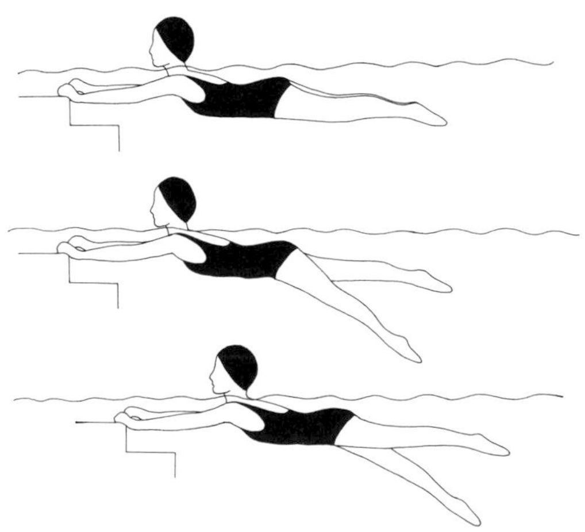

Leg Kicks – Hands on ladder or edge. Float in a horizontal position. Holding knees straight, kick legs fast and hard for 2 minutes. Rest. *4 times.*

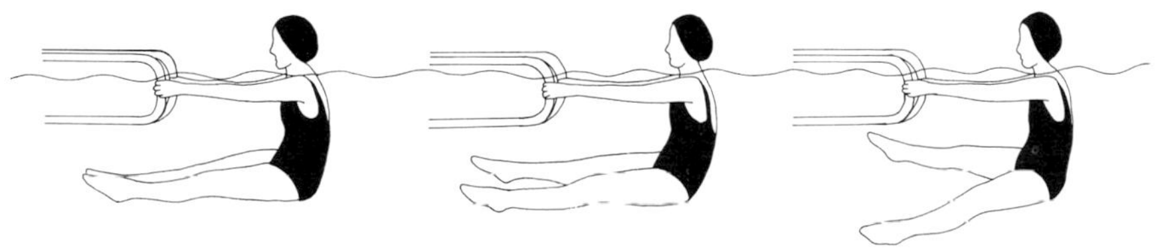

Water Scissors – Grasp ladder, sit in water, arms straight, legs together. With a jump of the body, open legs wide to a scissor, hold, draw together. *Quickly 30 times.*

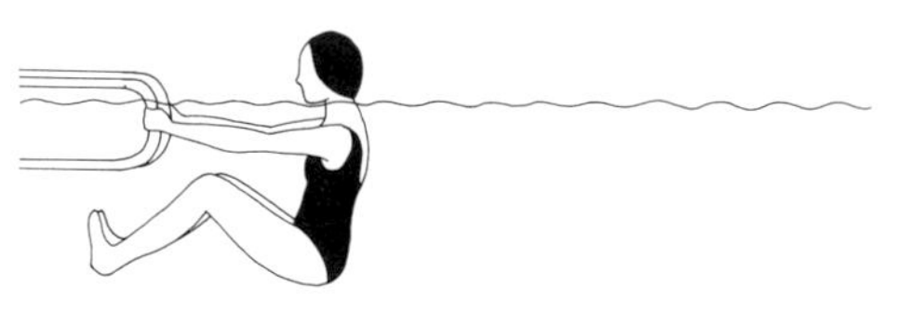

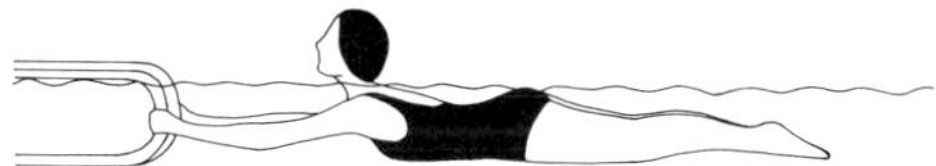

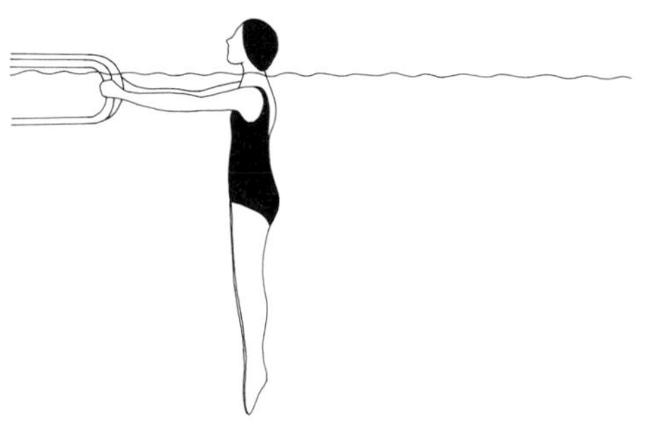

Leg Thrust – Face ladder or edge, hold. Sit in water, bend knees, feet slightly apart. Thrust legs back to prone position. Balance a few seconds; slowly return. *25 times.*

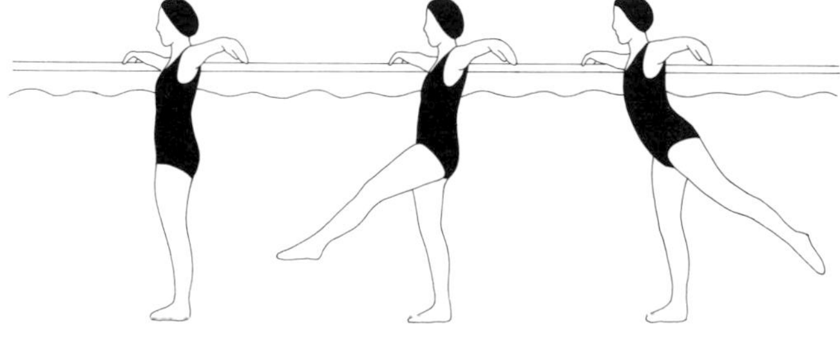

Leg Swing – Stand with one hand holding rail, other arm straight. Swing one leg up high in front, then back really stretching. *20 swings.* Reverse sides.

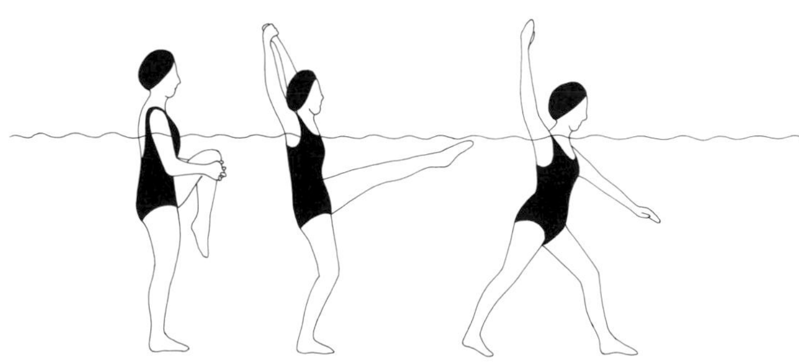

Giant Walk – Bring a knee to chest, clasp with arms. Stretch leg high in front, arms clasped overhead. Take a giant step forward swinging one arm down over front leg, other arm back to balance. Repeat with other leg. Walk for 3 minutes.

BED

If you have trouble getting up in the morning, these exercises are for you. Prime requisite is a firm mattress. Although most exercises are performed lying down, they require more muscle effort than you would think. They build up energy for the day but are also good relaxers after work.

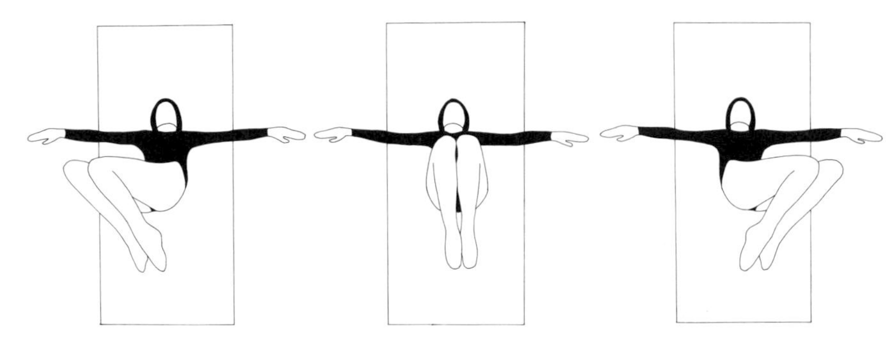

Waist Turn – On back, arms stretched out. Bend knees, lift feet. Keeping knees firmly together, swing legs from left to right aiming to touch bed. *20 times.*

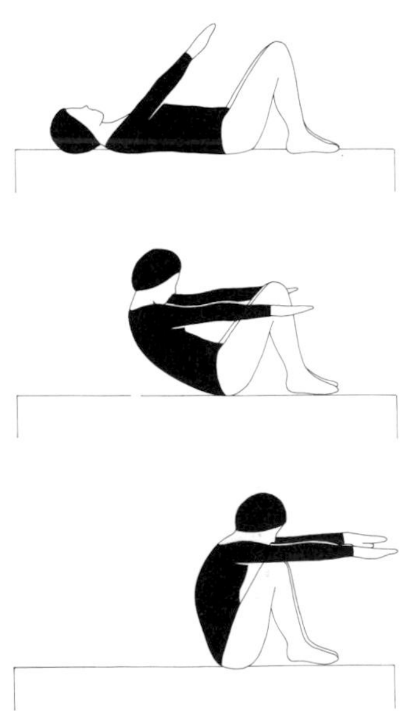

Stomach Tug – Lie on back, knees bent, feet flat, arms out in front, a little apart. Pull up body so chest touches thighs. Lower slowly. *10 times.*

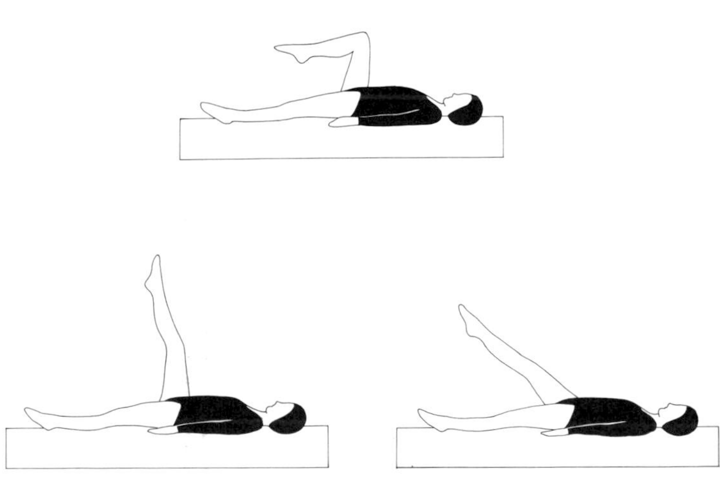

Leg Control – Lie on back, arms at sides, palms down. Bend one knee at right angles, count 3. Stretch to ceiling, count 3. Lower to bed, keeping straight. *6 times each leg.*

Bed Scissors – Lie on side, head supported by elbow. Raise upper leg as high as possible, hold, lower slowly. *10 times*. Reverse sides.

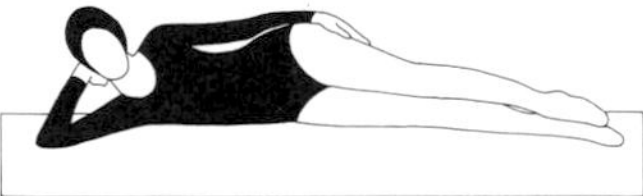

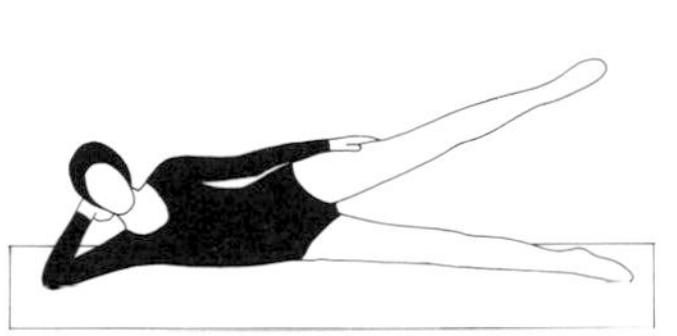

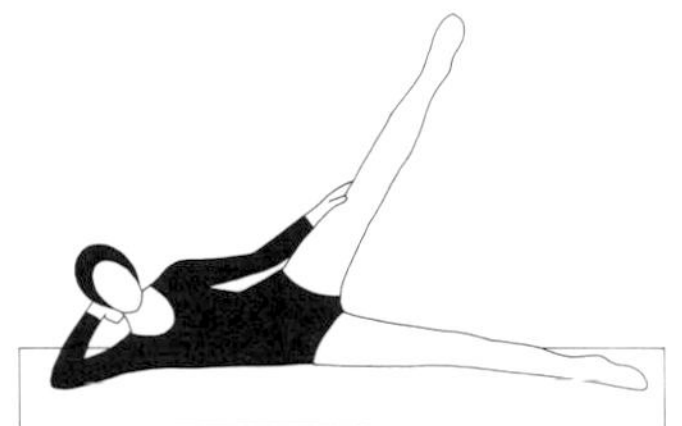

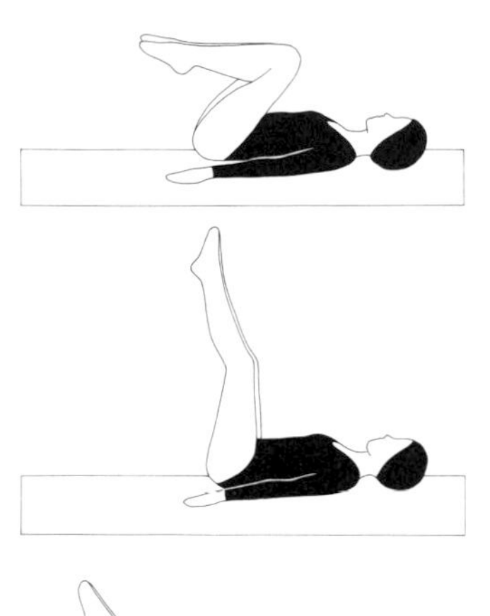

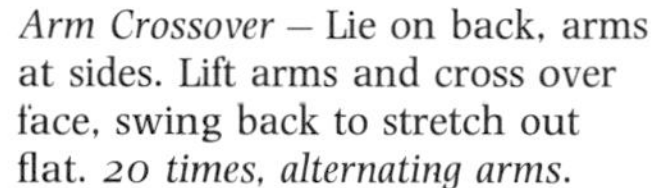

Leg Stretch – Lie flat, arms by sides, palms down. Bend knees against chest. Stretch legs high and straight, lower slowly without bending knees. *10 times*.

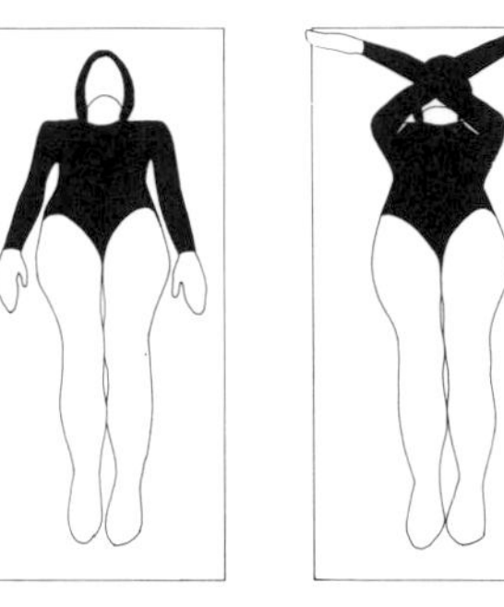

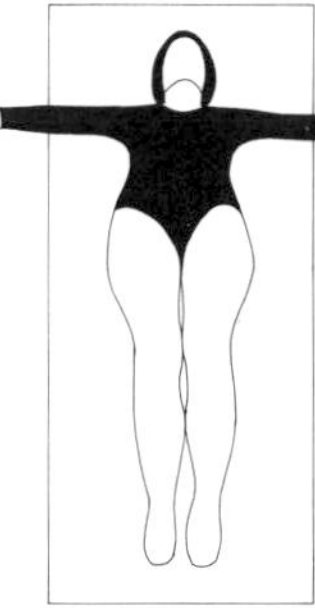

Arm Crossover – Lie on back, arms at sides. Lift arms and cross over face, swing back to stretch out flat. *20 times, alternating arms*.

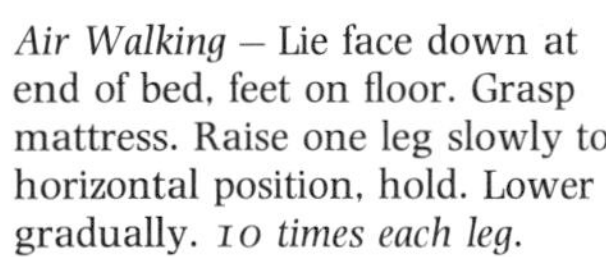

Air Walking – Lie face down at end of bed, feet on floor. Grasp mattress. Raise one leg slowly to horizontal position, hold. Lower gradually. *10 times each leg*.

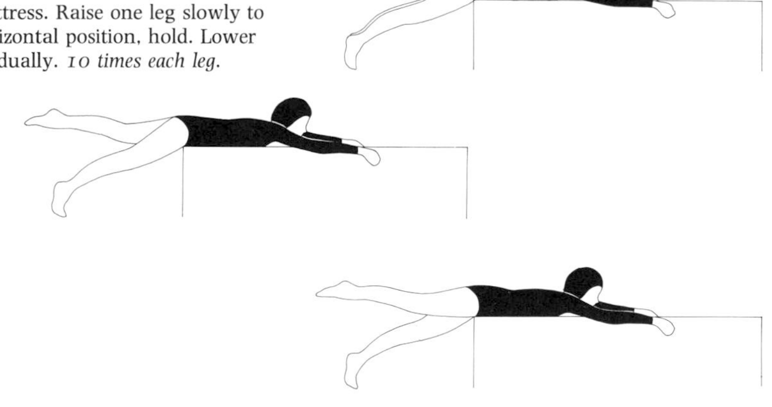

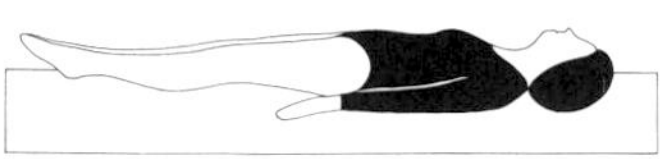

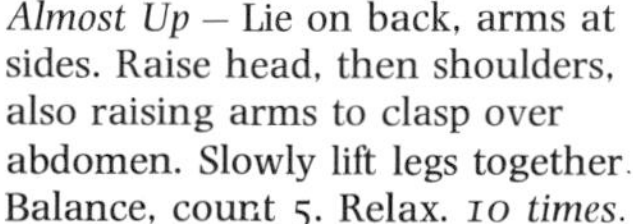

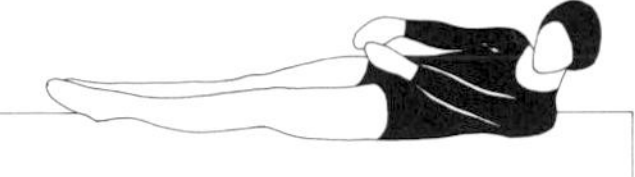

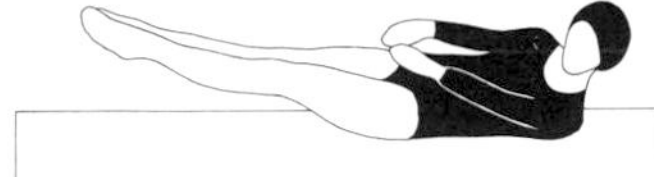

Almost Up – Lie on back, arms at sides. Raise head, then shoulders, also raising arms to clasp over abdomen. Slowly lift legs together. Balance, count 5. Relax. *10 times*.

SCULPTURE

Pioneered by Dr Bess Mensendieck, this is based on the simple premise that by learning to do everyday movements in the proper way one can reshape the body within limits of frame. Movements do not require outward exertion but are muscle controlling schemes motivated by mental concentration. At times limbs are used, but slowly. All ages and figures can benefit from this type of reshaping programme.

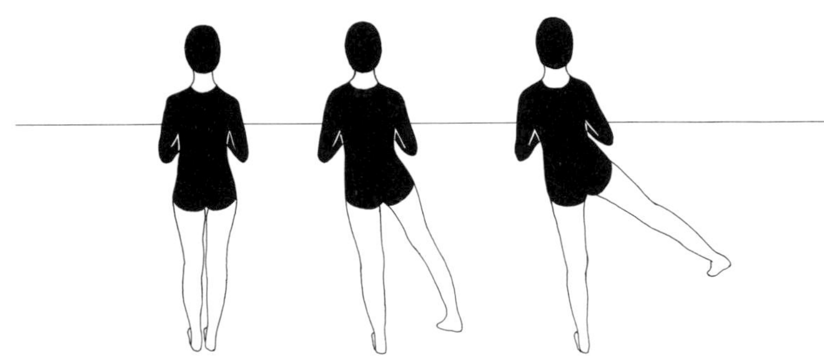

Leg Pendulum – Stand balanced, hold support if necessary. Slowly draw up right leg from hip, draw in stomach. Using right buttock muscle, move right leg backward then up, keeping leg straight. Release buttock muscle slowly lowering leg; then release muscle of right lumbar region, lowering foot. Relax. *3 times each leg.*

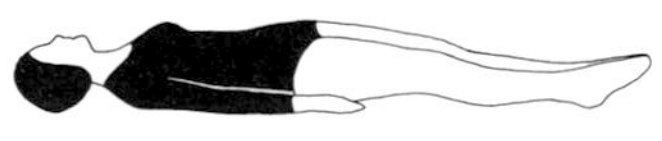

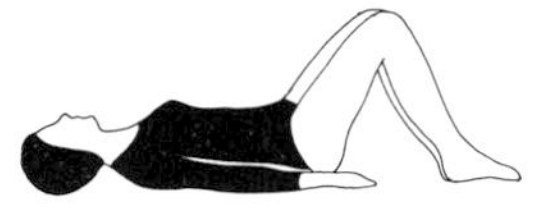

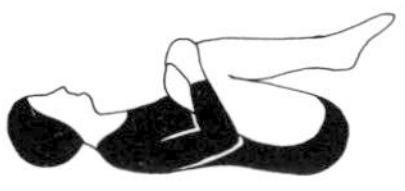

Body Fold – Lie at rest, body supported at all parts on floor. Bend knees so feet are close to buttocks. Bring knees up to the chest, folding body through muscle contraction in back and stomach. Clasp hands around knees if necessary, count 6. Relax. *5 times.*

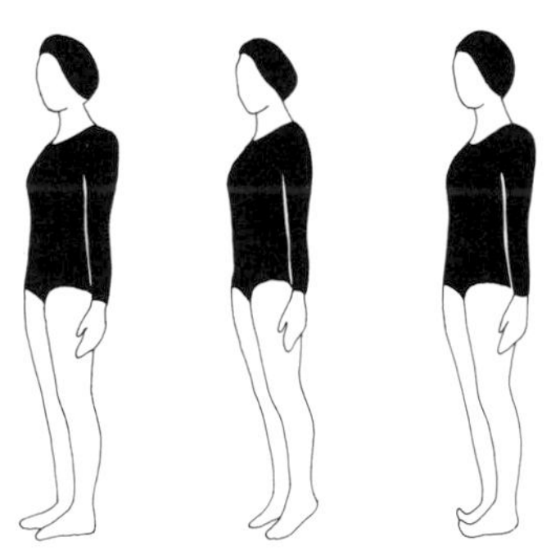

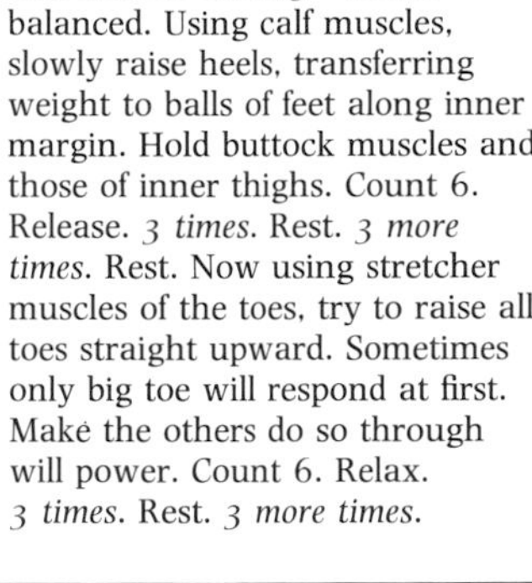

Heel and Toe Raising – Stand balanced. Using calf muscles, slowly raise heels, transferring weight to balls of feet along inner margin. Hold buttock muscles and those of inner thighs. Count 6. Release. *3 times.* Rest. *3 more times.* Rest. Now using stretcher muscles of the toes, try to raise all toes straight upward. Sometimes only big toe will respond at first. Make the others do so through will power. Count 6. Relax. *3 times.* Rest. *3 more times.*

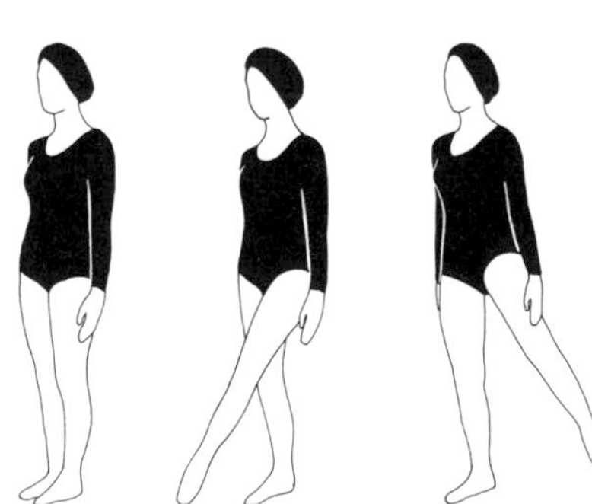

Leg Arcs – Stand balanced. Using muscle in lumbar region, draw left leg up so heel is off floor. Use left buttock muscle to slowly move leg backwards, at same time drawing in the abdomen. Make an arc to the side. With thigh muscle bring leg back to original position. *3 times each leg.*

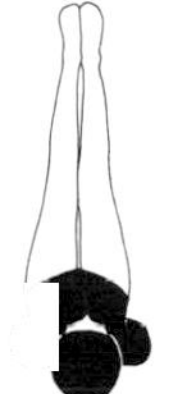
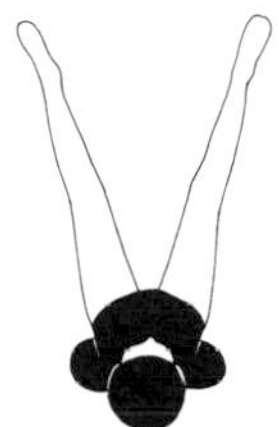
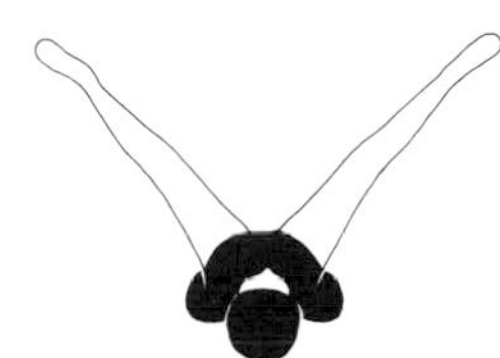

Leg Spread – Lie at rest, arms by sides. With knees straight, lift legs holding close together until at right angles to torso. Slowly open legs wide as possible. Count 6. Return together, relax. *5 times.*

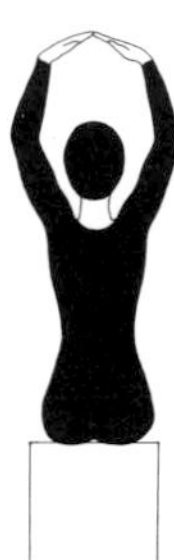

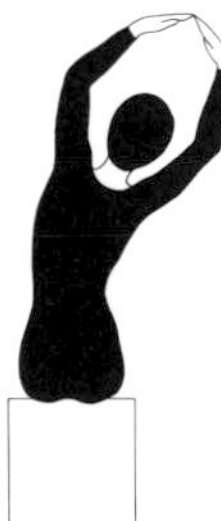

Trunk Bend – Sit balanced, make this posture a habit: sit near front edge of chair on sitting bone, feet flat, parallel and slightly apart. Arms loosely by side. Draw abdomen in and up, beginning near groin and continuing up to chest; use ball of each foot and sitting bone for support.

Now raise both arms overhead, palms facing; stretch elbows as much as possible. Slowly bend over by stretching opposite side of trunk; consciously stretch up before bending. Count to 6 at limit. Return to upright position. *3 times.* Relax. Reverse sides.

Buttock Control – Assume correct balance, which you must consciously adjust to whenever standing: feet parallel, a tiny bit apart, pressing forwards on ball of each foot, weight evenly distributed. Using muscles in front of thighs, pull up knee caps. From small of back, slowly stretch spine upwards, lifting head straight as though a thread were pulling from the top. Shoulder blades back and down. Arms loose at sides – with inside of elbows and palms facing body.

Place palms over buttocks. Slowly draw buttocks towards each other, when as tight as possible count 6. Release. *3 times.* Rest. *3 more times.* Sometimes one muscle pulls faster and better. Consciously make both sides work evenly. Check in rear mirror in the nude.

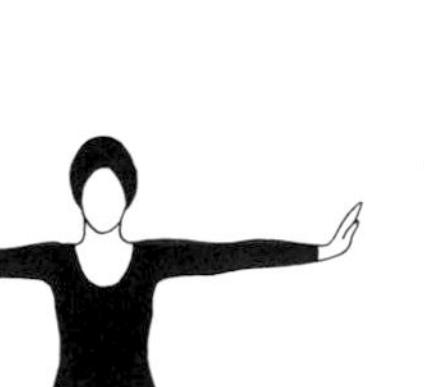
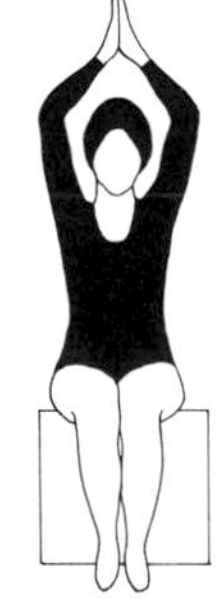
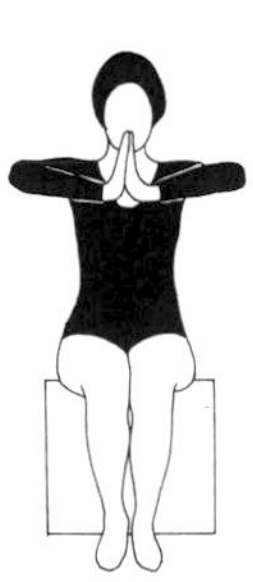

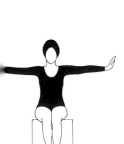

Bosom Lift – Sit balanced. Lift arms slowly to side, then up and over head, elbows as straight as possible, palms together. Using muscles to lower shoulders and arms, push elbows out until shoulder level. Count 6. Relax. *3 times.* Rest. *3 more times.*

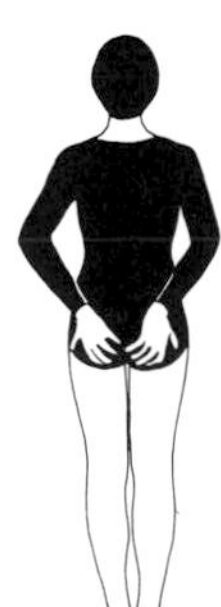
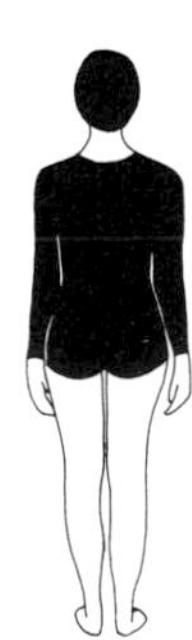

ISOMETRIC

There is very little movement to these exercises and anyone can do them anywhere. The principle is that muscle can be toned by setting one strength against another. Consider these as bonus exercises, to be done at odd moments during the day; at work, on the bus, in bed, and after the bath.

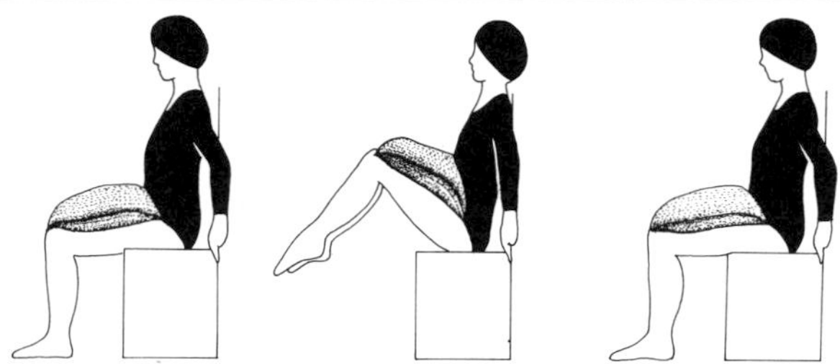

Cushion Squeeze – Sit with cushion on lap. Grip sides of chair. Bend knees, raise thighs trying to squeeze cushion against stomach. Count 10. Relax to count of 3. *3 times.*

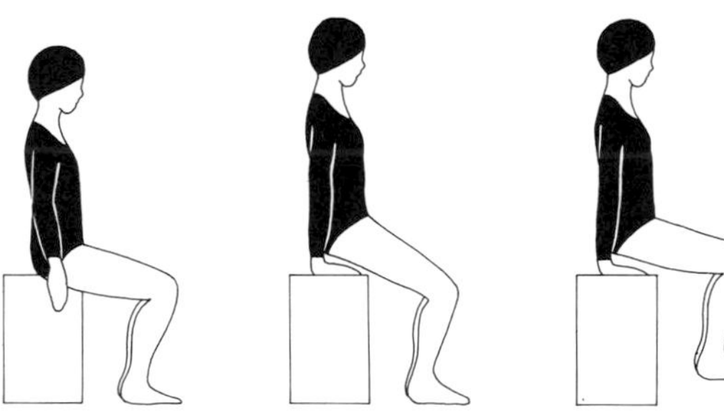

Chair Lift – Sit on armless chair, palms flat on seat, arms straight. Lift buttocks and thighs off chair, feet off floor. Count 6. Relax to count of 3. *10 times.*

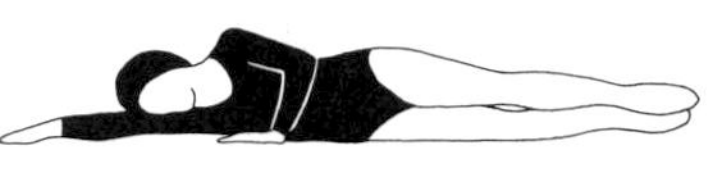

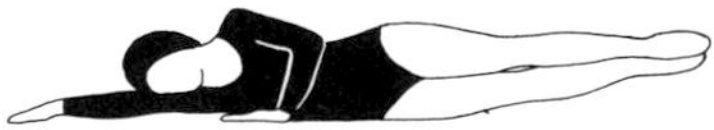

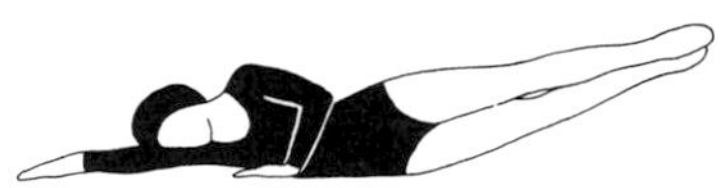

Bed Support – Lie on one side with feet tucked under bed edge. Stretch one arm under head, lift legs to touch underside of bed, keeping them rigid. Count 6. Relax to count of 3. *5 times each side.*

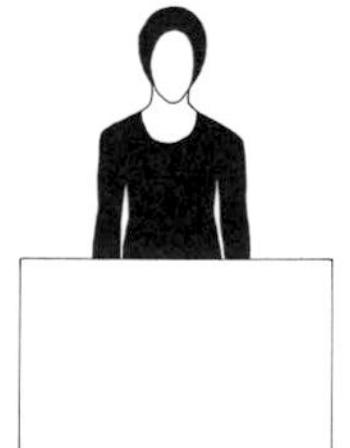

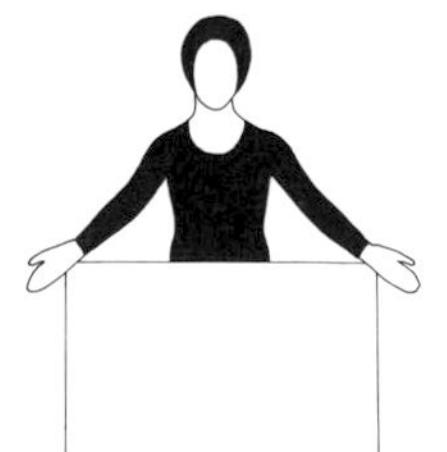

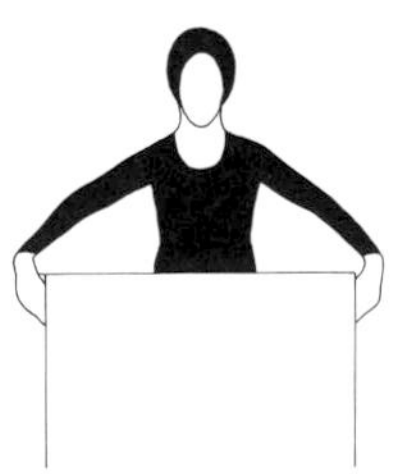

Desk Work – Sit, arms at sides. Lift arms to clutch edges of table and squash together. Count 6. Relax to count of 3. *10 times.*

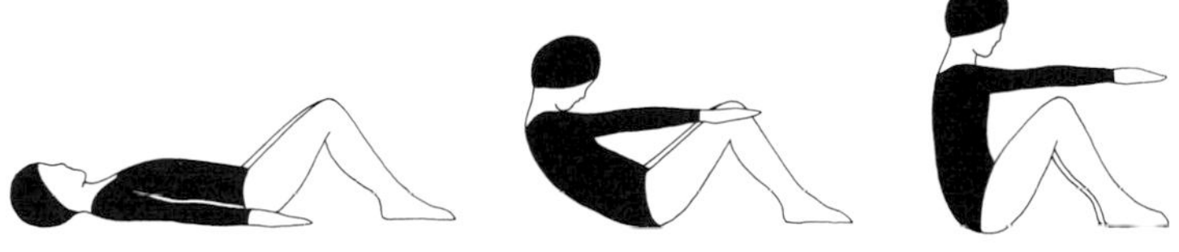

Floor Contact – Lie, knees bent, feet firm. Pushing floor away with feet, raise body bringing arms to knees then beyond. Count 6. Relax to count of 3. *10 times.*

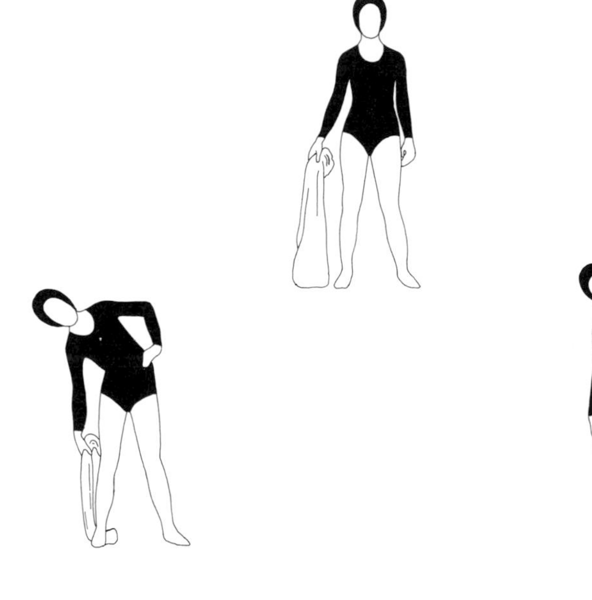

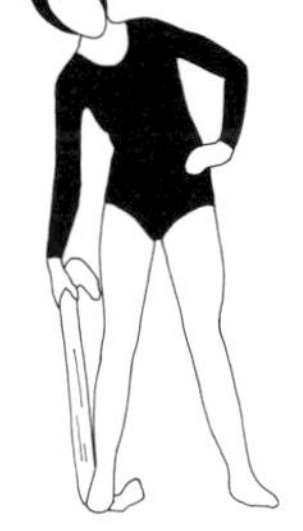

After the Bath – Stand feet apart, put one end of towel under heel, gripping other end near knee. With other hand on hip, keeping body straight, try to stretch towel. At limit count 6. Relax to count of 3. *4 times each side.*

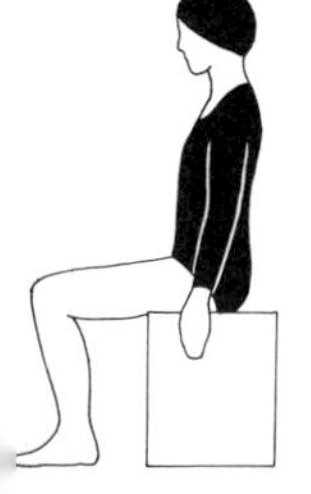

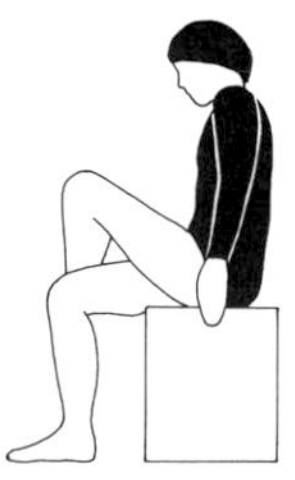

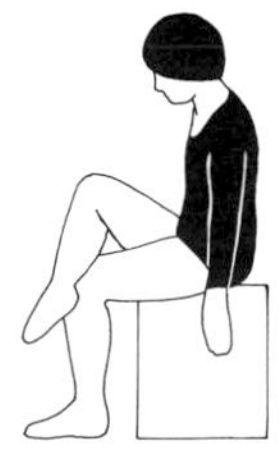

The Cross-over – Sit, hands gripping chair. Cross one leg high over thigh and lean in that direction as though pushing chair away. Count 6. Relax to count of 3. *6 times each leg.*

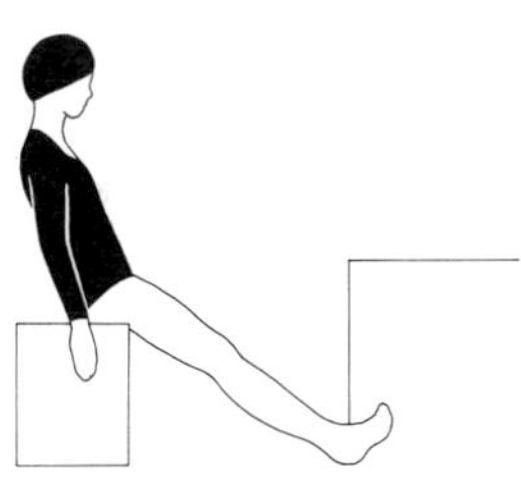

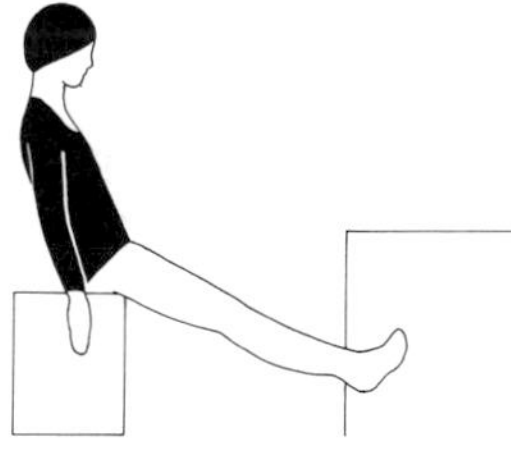

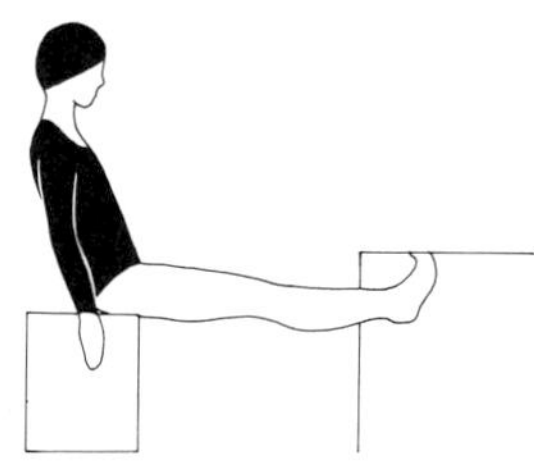

Table Push – Sit a little away from table. Stretch legs under it, toes touching. Press feet upward as if to lift table. Count 6. Relax to count of 3. *6 times.*

YOGA

Yoga benefits both mind and body. Technique depends on breathing, posture, relaxation. Never strain to accomplish an exercise; with each repetition you'll get better. And as you get better try to hold positions longer. This is modified yoga, adapted as daily exercises for figure streamlining.

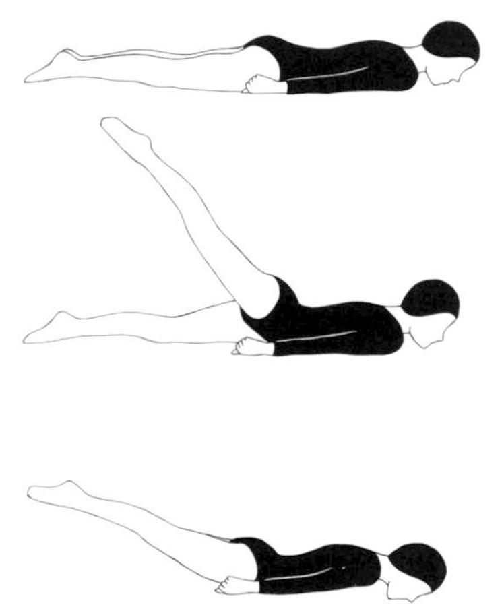

Leg Control – Lie flat, arms by sides, hands making fists. Slowly raise one leg, knee straight, pushing fists against floor to help. Hold 10 seconds. Relax. Starting from same position, legs together, knees straight, raise both legs. This is the locust position. Hold 10 seconds. Relax. *Each movement 3 times, alternating legs.*

Shoulder Stand – Lie flat, slowly raise legs over torso. Tighten stomach muscles, raise legs high, supporting body on hands. Push up; slowly lower knees to forehead. Return torso, legs to floor. Hold 1 minute, work up to 3.

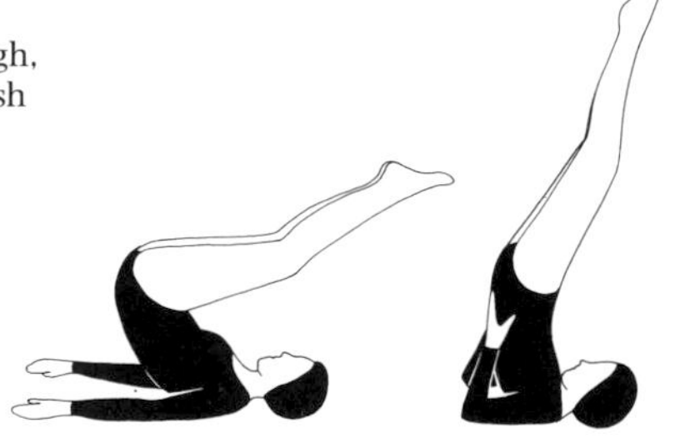

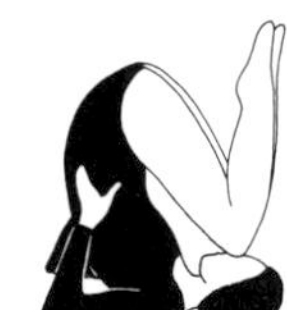

Chest Expansion – Stand straight, arms in front, keeping elbows straight move arms behind back, clasping hands, lean back. Let neck go limp, drop head forward, hold arms high. Hold 5 seconds. Bend forward, hands still clasped. Relax. *3 times.*

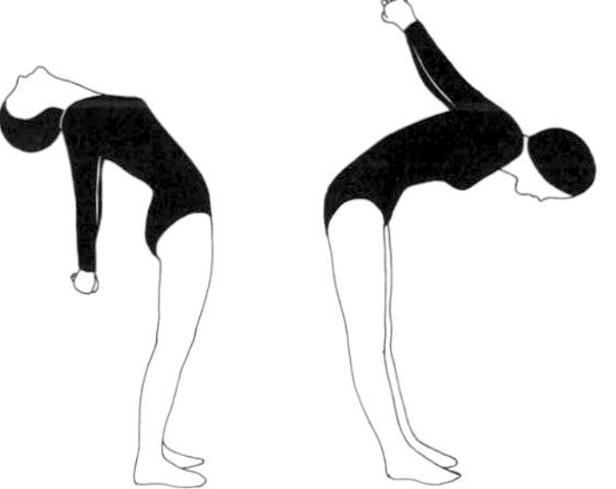

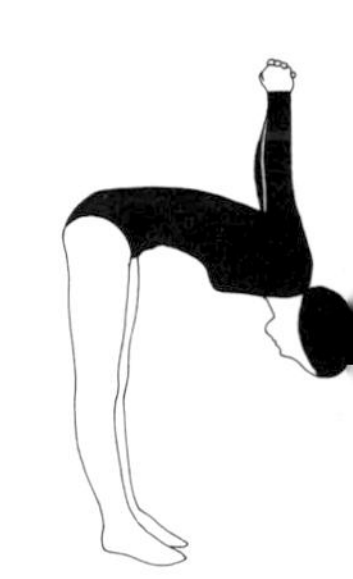

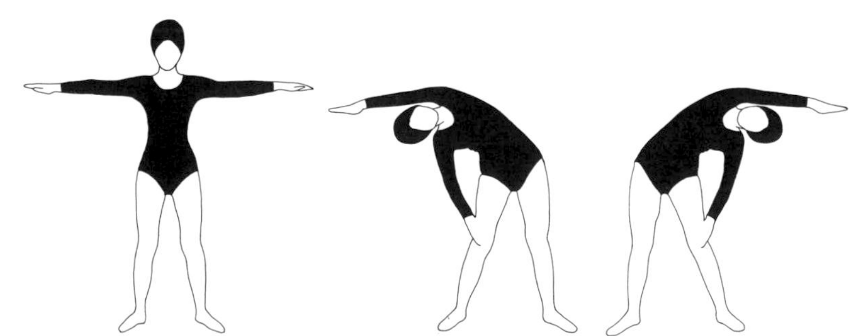

Triangle Bend – Stand erect, feet apart, arms extended. Bend slowly to one side, bringing one arm high over head; slide other arm down corresponding leg. Hold 10 seconds. Relax. *3 times on each side.*

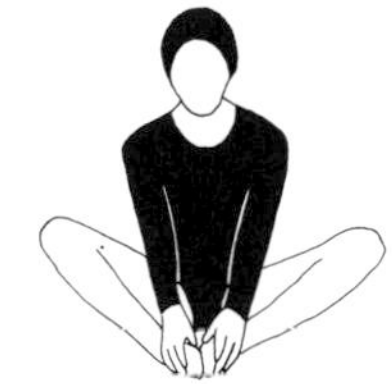
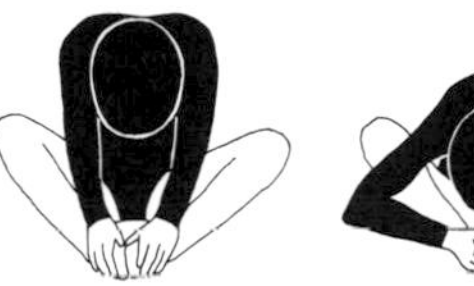
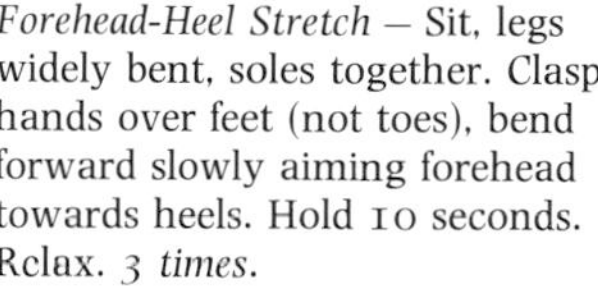

Forehead-Heel Stretch – Sit, legs widely bent, soles together. Clasp hands over feet (not toes), bend forward slowly aiming forehead towards heels. Hold 10 seconds. Relax. *3 times*.

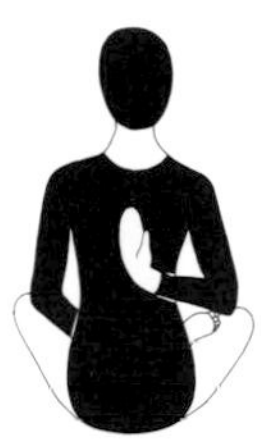
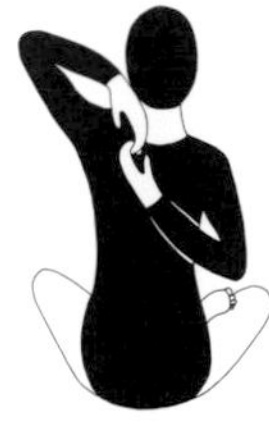
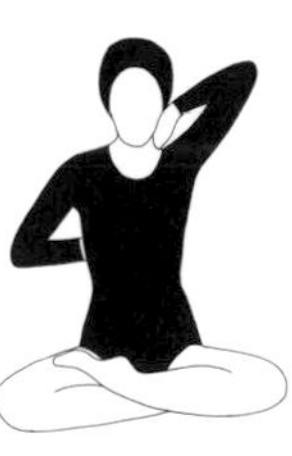

Backward Handclasp – Sit cross-legged, one foot on opposite thigh. Bend right elbow so hand touches spine. Raise left arm, bend back. Inch hands towards each other, clasp fingers. Hold 10 seconds. Relax, reverse hands. *3 times*.

Stretching Spread – Sit, legs spread wide, knees outward, palms on inside of knees. Raise arms, bend forward, sliding hands down outerside of legs, try to clasp ankles. Hold 10 seconds. Relax. *3 times*.

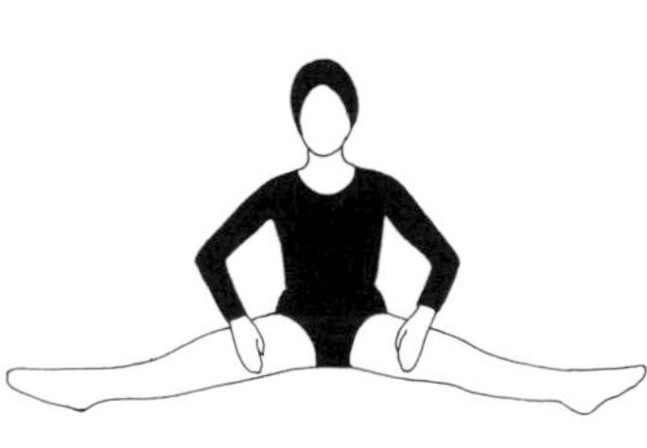
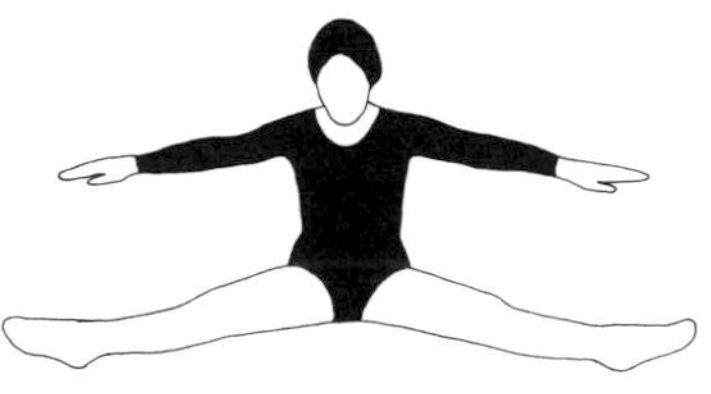
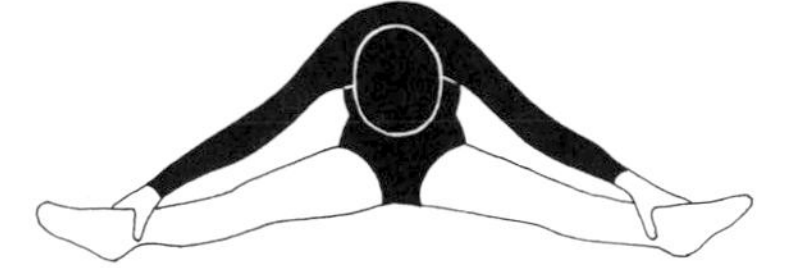

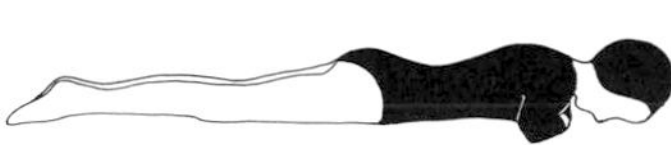
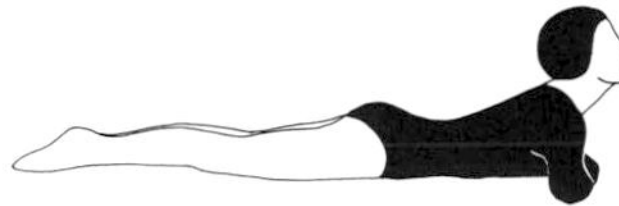
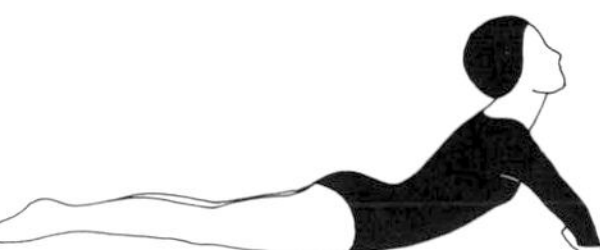

Cobra Arch – Lie face downwards with chin on floor, elbows bent but raised a little, palms flat. Slowly raise head then shoulders, pushing on palms, raise chest and upper abdomen. Head far back. Hold 10 seconds. Relax. *3 times*.

MODERN

At first an endurance test, as controls and concentration are equal for these exacting movements. Developed by Lotte Berk, this system emerges as the most contemporary, well geared to modern thinking and agile bodies. Based on Hatha yoga, ballet and orthopaedics, most routines are done with the pelvis rolled in, accent on lower torso and thighs.

Warming Up – Stand legs apart, hands above head, bend over and down pushing bottom out. Return, down again, curling further, pushing arms through legs. *10 times, work up to more.*

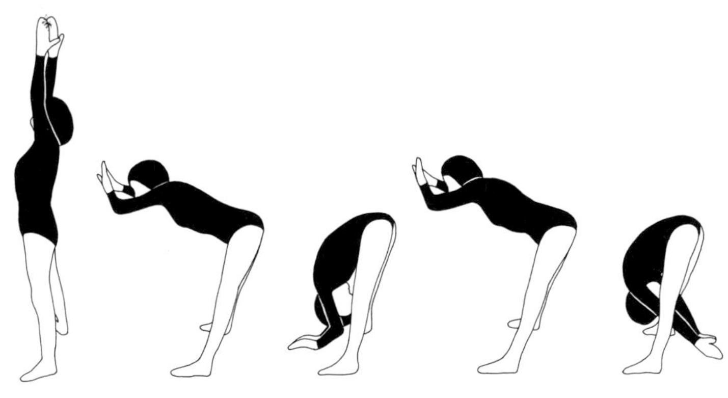

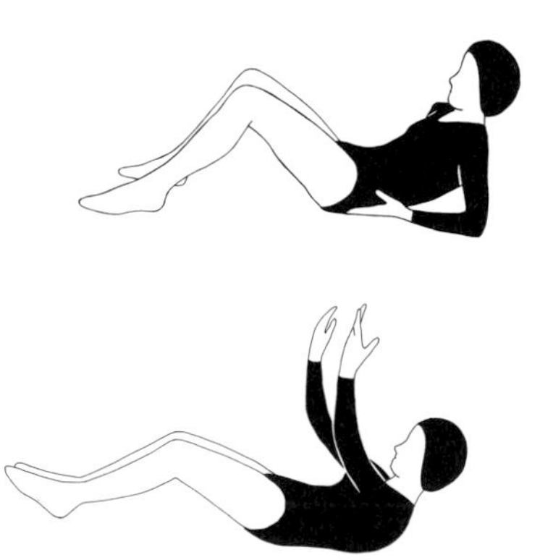

Central Control – Half lie knees bent, elbows supporting. Roll pelvis in, bring arms in front clicking fingers, one, two, three, at the same time raising feet a little off floor. Return. *6 times, work up to more.*

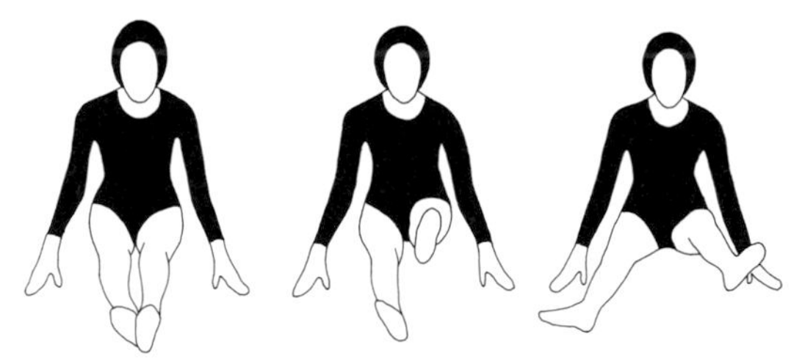

Foot Circles – Sit, legs stretched out, pelvis rolled in, rest on hand Lift leg, twist foot in wide circle around ankle. Make 20 circles. Reverse feet.

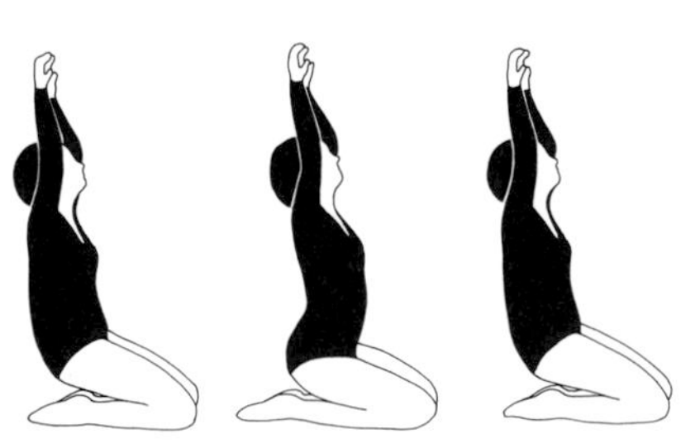

Pelvis Roll – Kneel, knees a little apart, hands linked over head. Roll pelvis in, then with hips and shoulders in a straight line, lean slowly backwards, lifting a little heels. Roll the pelvis forward, once, twice, hold. Relax. *5 times, work up to more.*

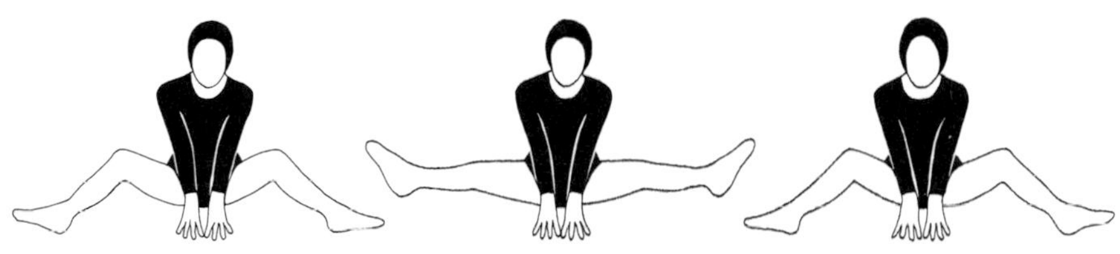

In the Air Stretch – Sit, legs wide apart, arms between legs, palms flat. With weight on hands, lift legs a fraction off floor. Bend legs, stretch, bend, stretch. *10 times rhythmically*. Relax. Repeat.

Crouch Bounce – Stand sideways by a support, crouch low, heels together, pelvis rolled in, back straight. Hold, bounce up and down lifting buttocks from heels. *10 times, work up to more.*

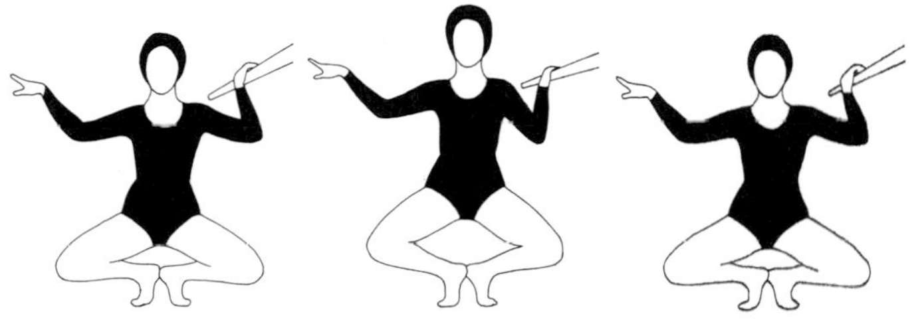

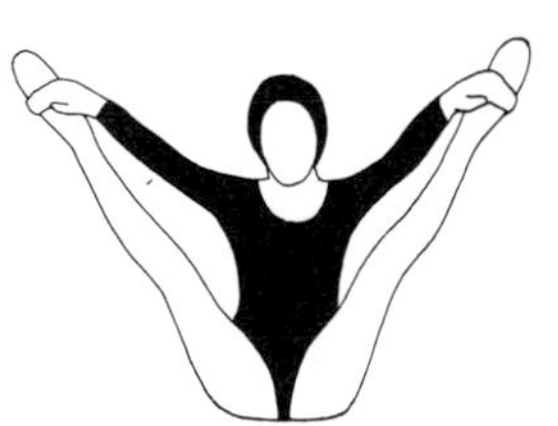

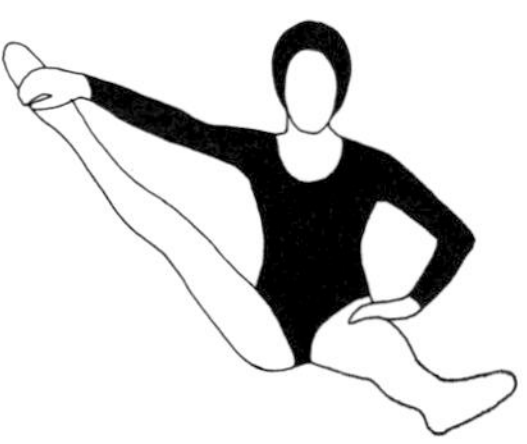

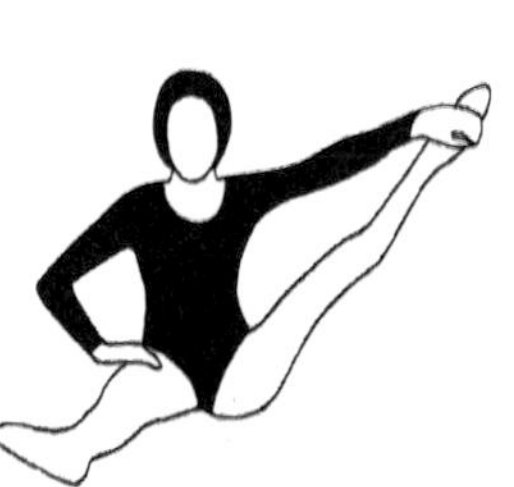

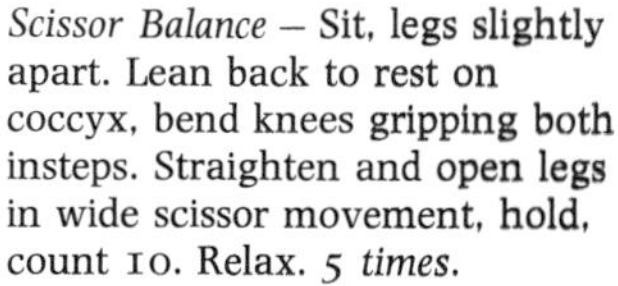

Scissor Balance – Sit, legs slightly apart. Lean back to rest on coccyx, bend knees gripping both insteps. Straighten and open legs in wide scissor movement, hold, count 10. Relax. *5 times.*

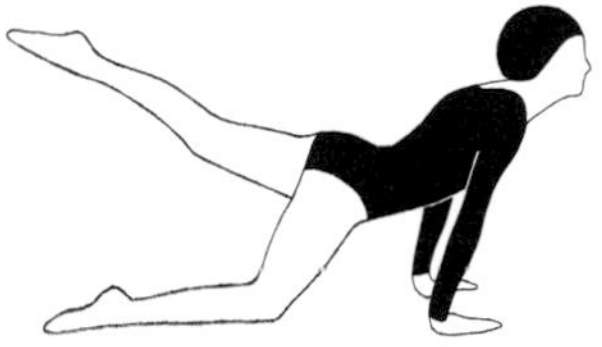

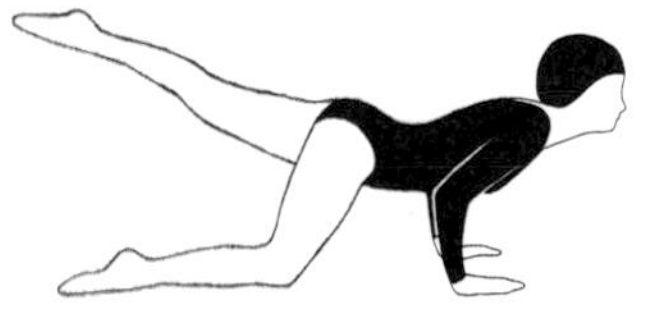

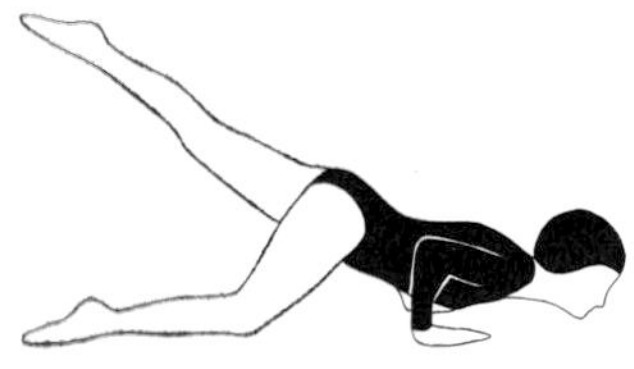

Kneeling Seesaw – Kneel on all fours, arms apart, palms flat. Control pelvis, arch back, lift a leg. Seesaw body by bending and straightening elbows. *10 times, work up to more*. Reverse legs.

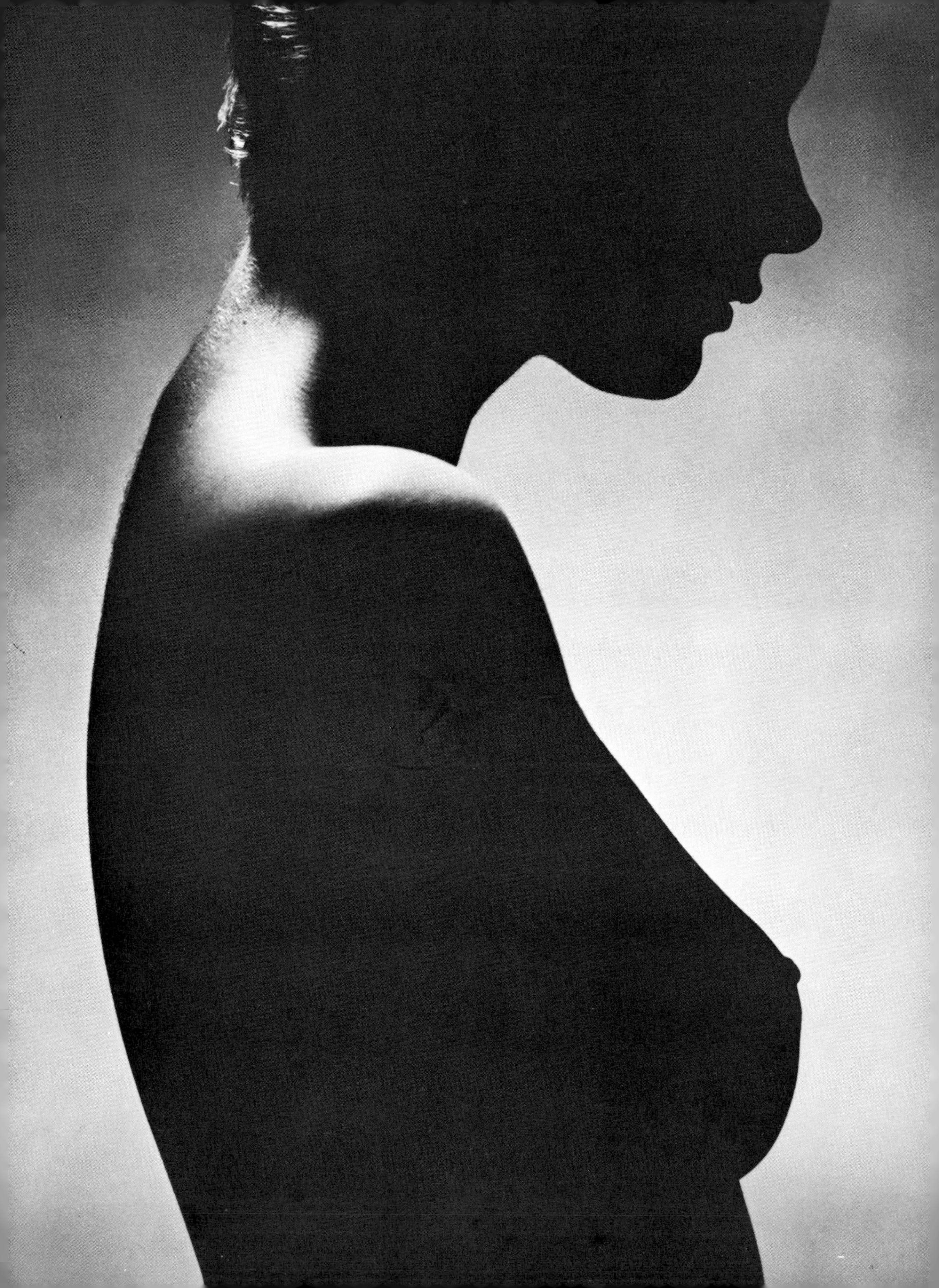

5

SEXUALITY

Sexuality is intrinsically linked with health and beauty. It should describe one's whole being as a woman, but it has come to be thought of as the degree of ability in direct sex functions. Orgasm is still to many women an achievement but it is part of the all-encompassing sex cycle that is a powerful tonic to looks and health. If you make love you will glow and look more beautiful. If you make love you are more aware of your body. Sexuality is knowing your body, liking it, taking care of it. Most women know every pore on their face and what to do about it, but have no idea of the shape of their bosom nor how to take care of it.

We are no longer governed by our reproductive system: the physical and emotional implications of periods, cramps, unwanted pregnancy, premenstrual moods and the menopause can all be handled with confidence and knowledge. The stress effects produced by ovulation are real and biochemical in origin. Knowledge of hormones has changed life for all of us and in this connection the life and beauty of a woman can be divided into three eras. As a girl approaches eleven or twelve, oestrogen and progesterone surge from the ovaries; during the mature years production is steady; as she nears fifty and the menopause production gradually slows down. These hormones are responsible for sexual characteristics: development of the breasts, shaping of the hips, the appearance of pubic hair and the onset of menstruation. For the whole of a woman's reproductive life hormones are produced in a cyclical pattern, usually within a four-week period. They affect looks, skin, hair, vitality, the health of the ovaries and uterus, the menstrual cycle, the state of the vaginal tissue and the structure of the breasts. They have a stabilizing influence on the emotions. Hormones control what is visible and invisible, adding up to the sum total of individual sexuality.

THE BOSOM

More women are concerned about the health, shape and size of their breasts than any other part of their anatomy. If a woman feels they are larger or smaller or rounder or more pear-shaped than others, she can become concerned and the self-consciousness may remain throughout life. Some women feel so strongly that their whole life is affected and under these circumstances, plastic surgery should be considered. Many doctors are sympathetic to the idea, particularly in the case of the flat-chested woman who thinks this is the cause of much of her emotional unhappiness.

The breasts are fundamentally two mammary glands meant for suckling the young. They usually extend from the second to the sixth rib on either side of the breast bone and over the chest muscles. They are contained in fatty tissue, which determines the shape and size. The fine covering of skin is connected by fibrous tissue which decides your bosom type as bouncy or firm. Internally the bosom can be affected by several factors. As it is controlled by hormones, breasts change during the menstrual cycle; they may appear larger or fuller just before menstruation, they may also be a little sore. Crash diets and overeating can also alter their shape; and so can gravity if the pull of the breasts is allowed to go unchecked. Going bra-less is not a health hazard unless your breasts are very heavy, in which case a posture problem may develop. Some women claim their muscles are forced to work harder and so breasts actually take on a better, firmer shape. However unless you are watchful about exercise or conscious about muscle control during the day you can preserve the shape of your breasts better if you use some support.

Apart from plastic surgery, there is little one can do to noticeably change size and shape but it is possible to improve the way breasts hang, their texture and resiliency, with improved posture, exercise, water therapy and oil massage.

Posture – slouched shoulders and hunched backs produce sagging breasts. Improved posture can make the biggest improvement; this does not mean shoulders back and bosom obviously thrust forward. It involves lifting the bosom up from the diaphragm, stretching the vertebrae from the pelvic muscles, and lifting the head as though it were being tugged skywards with a string.

Exercise – the pectoral muscles at the sides and curving underneath the breasts cradle, control and uphold a good bosom but only as long as they are firm and well-toned. Do a couple of exercises a day; these are simple and effective and although the bosom will not show immediate improvement, muscles will slowly strengthen to give the breasts a better placement on the chest cage.

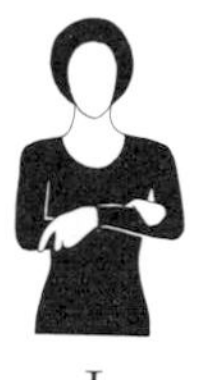

1

1. Forearm Push: fold arms, grasping each forearm below the elbow with the opposite hand. Push hard towards the elbows without moving the hand up the arm. Feel a pull in the pectoral muscles. Do 20 times.

2. Arm Stretch: stand with elbows bent at shoulder level, the backs of the hands facing the body. Push arms back unbending to slowly stretch straight, keeping arms at shoulder level. Back and forth 10 times.

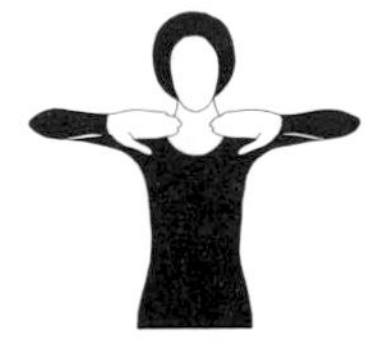

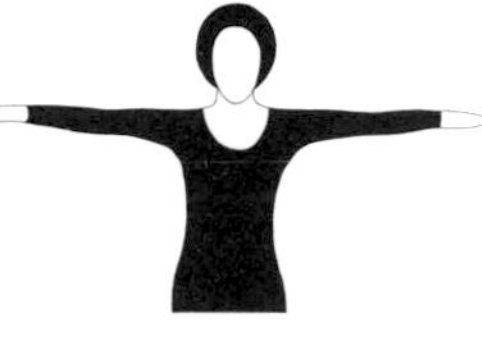

2

3. Swimming Stroke: stand legs apart, don't bend knees, lean forward as far as possible with one arm stretched out. Now bring the other arm up in the crawl swimming stroke movement. Continue, building up to 10 strokes per arm.

Water therapy – cold water stimulation can tone the breasts. After bathing, turn the shower on cold, full force, and spray directly on each breast, two minutes each side. If you don't have a shower, splash with cold water. When bathing, keep the warm water below breast level.

Massage – for improved texture, massage body moisturizer, lotion or oil into the breasts; always apply a liberal coat of sunscreen lotion before tanning.

Make-up – to create the illusion of depth and curves, brush blusher down your cleavage; a frosted blush for evenings.

Irregularities in the breasts are a cause for concern. Breasts are often sore and painful, particularly prior to menstruation, and to touch appear to be full of undulations. Doctors emphasize that if a lump is painful it is rarely malignant and is probably due to one of the following conditions:

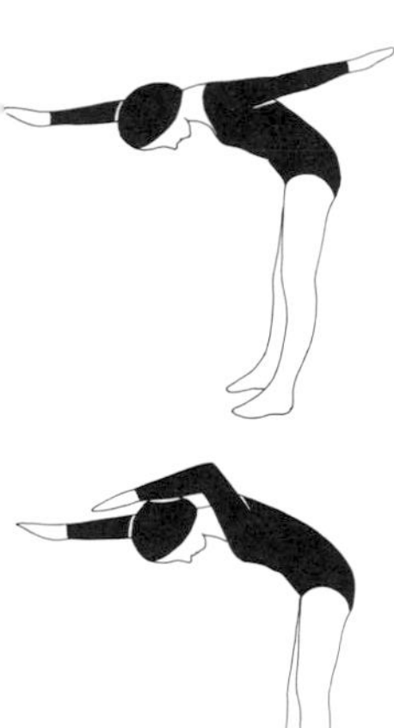

3

CYSTS AND FIBROADENOMAS: These are definitely non-cancerous, but cause obvious breast lumps and swellings. Cysts occur because the liquid that is secreted by glands in the breasts has not properly drained through the breast ducts. They are usually regular in shape, mobile when handled – move under the skin. They frequently crop up just before menstruation and disappear by themselves after bleeding has started. They can be removed by draining them under local anaesthetic, which is considered less of a physical or psychological trauma than surgery – which is also sometimes used.

Fibroadenomas are growths of the fibrous tissue that holds the breast together. They may occur in just one part of the breast or in several spots on both breasts. They should be reported to a doctor who will remove them if they are uncomfortable. Some women suffer from chronic cysts or fibrous growths. These should be constantly checked even though neither condition becomes cancerous.

CANCER: This is the big fear – cancer is now the leading cause of female deaths in the 40 to 44 age groups and the primary cause of cancer deaths among women of all ages. All women can develop breast cancer but some seem more susceptible: those in the mid to late forties who never had children or did not begin having them until after 30, whose mother or sister has had the disease, who are overweight. There are indications that women who are married have a slightly lower breast cancer rate than those who are single, also those who have breast-fed several children have fewer breast malignancies than those who have not. The evidence is statistical only and there is no certainty of developing cancer even if you fit into all the risk categories. One thing is certain: if left untreated, breast tumours can spread rapidly invading lungs, skeleton, liver or brain.

Despite years of research, the cause of breast cancer remains unknown. Reports indicate that there is no correlation between cancer and the Pill. Diet has been cited as a factor, based on statistical evidence showing breast cancer's greater prevalence in countries where people eat large quantities of animal fat. Injuries – bumps and bangs on the bosom – do not initiate the disease.

Early detection is vital; when malignancies are small they are completely curable. It is a woman's responsibility to keep watch over herself. Breast lumps are sometimes found by doctors during routine examinations but most changes of tissue are spotted by accident or during self-examination. Finding them in the early stage can be a problem because cancerous growths rarely cause pain or feel sensitive to the touch.

Three techniques are used, often in combination to ensure detection: physical examination, thermography, which is a method of measuring heat given off by a tumour, and mammography, an X-ray technique which can spot very small tumours before they can be felt even by an experienced examiner. One of the best methods is a type of mammography known as xeroradiography, which reveals tiny dots of calcium that are commonly present in breast cancer.

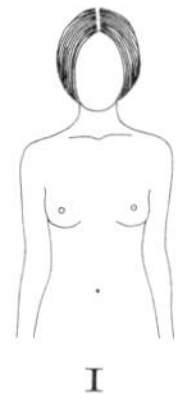

1

SELF-EXAMINATION OF THE BREASTS: The importance of monthly self-examination of the breasts cannot be over-emphasized. Many women know they should examine themselves but do not because they are scared of what they might find. Don't worry if, on first examination when you are not familiar with the feel of your breasts, they appear to be full of irregularities, bumps and nodes.

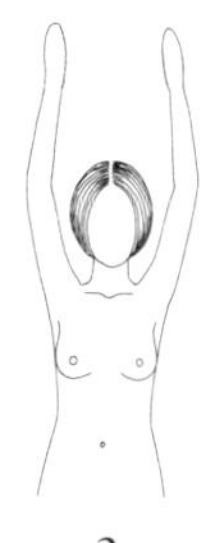

2

The earlier you start examining your breasts the better. Sixteen is not too young; this does not mean that a young woman should start worrying about cancer; it simply helps her become familiar with the feel of her breasts and establishes a habit of self-examination.

Examination should be done in the week following menstruation and continued for six days. It is a ten-minute procedure. A woman who is familiar with the feel of her breasts in their normal state should be able to detect any thickening. Do it after a bath, as this is relaxing and allows the superficial blood vessels of the breasts to dilate and thus become easier to observe. If you do find anything, see a doctor without delay.

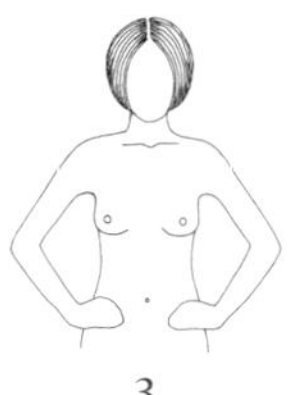

3

1. Sitting or standing in front of a mirror, take a good look at your breasts, get to know their shape, the tracery of the blood vessels. Be alert to any unusual puckering or dimpling, any change in the look of the nipple, or the appearance of bigger or more vessels.
2. Stretch arms above the head, observe any changes.
3. Place hands on hips, check the shape and fall of the breasts.

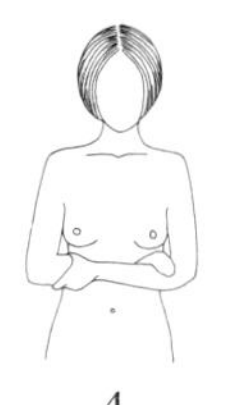

4

4. Fold arms, push hands against the area between wrist and elbow so that the pectoral muscles flex under the breasts; observe.
5. Lie down, place one hand behind the head, then with the fingers of the other hand, flattened, gently feel the breast, starting at the nipple and working outwards in concentric circles; be careful not to miss any spots; be very aware of any swellings. Repeat with other breast.
6. Check the armpits by raising one arm over your head. Insert the fingers of your other hand well into the armpit and with flattened fingers press it against the chest wall, checking for irregularities. Do the same on both sides. Armpits are as important as the breast area because they contain both the lymph glands and the tail of the breast.

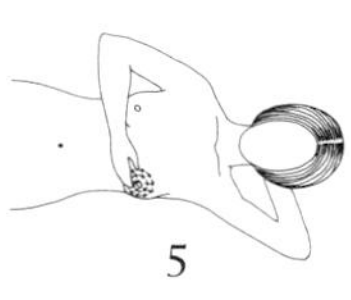

5

When a lump is found some women try to ignore it in the hope it will miraculously disappear. Frightened women often wait as long as a year: don't, it could be fatal. And remember that statistics indicate that 65% to 80% of all breast lumps are not cancerous.

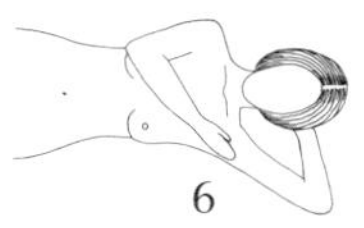

6

On examination doctors can often determine the type of growth. If it hurts it is unlikely to be malignant, also if it appears to be unanchored it is usually all right. A needle biopsy can be used – a needle is inserted and fluid or cells withdrawn for examination. However some growths are too small or too hidden to be checked by these methods and so a surgical procedure is necessary. The lump is cut out and immediately checked; within minutes the surgeon can tell if cells are cancerous.

If the result is positive, something has to be done as soon as possible. Many surgeons feel that the only prudent method is immediate surgery and frequently take the precaution of asking permission from the patient to perform a mastectomy (removal of the breast) if cancer is present. This, they say, reduces both the risk and the expense of two operations. Even so, most women would rather know beforehand; a few days doesn't make any appreciable difference in growth, though a few weeks can.

A woman with breast cancer should know what options she has. The size of the lump is the determining factor. The choices are: radiation only, lumpectomy (the cutting away of only the lump), simple mastectomy (the removal of only the breast), radical mastectomy (the removal of one breast and the nearby regions) or double radical mastectomy (the removal of both breasts and their regions). It is usual for mastectomies to be followed by radiation treatment, which can be painful and irritating.

Efforts are being made to improve the ways in which radiation alone can be used on a cancerous spot to avoid mutilation, but this therapy is still debatable. Ultra-sonic treatments are being investigated, but are still in the exploratory stage. The current choice is a decision about the extent of surgery. Many doctors feel that complete amputation is not always necessary. Research has shown that where lumpectomy (removal of the lump only) was performed, cancers have not spread to the lymph nodes. In this respect it is considered as effective as more radical operations and less damaging psychologically. Other doctors point out that these were lucky cases. Partial mastectomy is also possible which, while more extensive than lumpectomy, still spares most of the breast. The arguments against these procedures is that most cancers have been growing from six to eight years before they are discovered. By that time invariably they may have spread in microscopic clusters elsewhere in the breast.

THE SEX ORGANS

The two ovaries are the source of female germ cells (ova) and the female hormones oestrogen and progesterone. They are each the size of a bean, supported by ligaments and touched by the fallopian tubes, the ducts for the passage of ova to the uterus (or womb). The uterus has a narrow neck, the cervix, dipping down into the top end of the vagina, which is about three to four inches long, opening at the vulva, the surface sex organs where the clitoris is the most sexually receptive area. The whole system is T-shaped, the bar of the T being the fallopian tubes, the stroke being the uterus and vagina.

This area controls general health patterns and emotions. We are very dependent on the hormone production and any lack or excess can have far reaching effects. Our reproductive capacity depends on the menstrual cycle; our sexual responses on its stimuli. Regular gynaecological check-ups are important and should not be reserved only for when obvious symptoms appear. Most women are bothered by varying degrees of vaginal discharge or vulva irritation, some are harmless secretions, common and normal, others need attention.

VAGINAL INFECTIONS: A group of low-grade infections are prevalent but neither dangerous nor likely to spread; they should be controlled and cleared up by medication if they persist. They are not necessarily contacted through sexual activity but produced by the body's own flora. Many women have one or more of them on different occasions and they may occur simultaneously in what is called a mixed infection. Self-help involves avoiding hot baths as the fungus thrives on warmth; keeping the body as cool and dry as possible. Cotton underwear or no underwear helps prevent infections by allowing air to circulate more freely to the outer vaginal area. Constant douching can also destroy the beneficial flora and upset natural balance. The occasional use of mild douche powders, or a little salt in warm water, is acceptable.

Moniliasis – also known as leucorrhoea, vaginal fungus, yeast infection or 'whites'. Discharge is white and thick; can provoke vaginal and vulva itching, areas may become reddened, the vagina sometimes has white patches. Local vaginal creams or suppositories are effective.

Trichomoniasis – produces an abundant malodorous, yellow or greenish-white discharge. Can cause inflammation, itching, soreness and bleeding of the vagina. It is passed back and forth between sexual partners although the male usually does not have symptoms. Treatment involves oral medication to be taken by both partners.

Bacterial infection – discharge is white or yellow, heavy and viscous. It covers the vaginal walls and may cause burning or frequent urination. Can be cleared easily with medication.

Cervicitis – inflammation of the cervix, often associated with a vaginal infection. Symptom is painful and frequent urination. It can be treated with oral antibiotics. Drink lots of water, especially after intercourse.

GONORRHOEA AND SYPHILIS: Both are sexually transmitted and can be extremely harmful if not treated in the early stages. The incidence of gonorrhoea has trebled in the last ten years, and the problem for women is that they have no obvious symptoms until the disease is quite far advanced. If there is any possibility you may have been exposed to it have a test every six months. A sample of discharge from around the cervix is taken to the laboratory for culture.

The early symptoms of gonorrhoea usually include an inflammation of the urethral lining, causing a discharge and frequent burning urination. These are usually mild, and invariably passed as a transient bladder irritation. Later on, infection induces an abundant yellow discharge. The real trouble begins when the virus invades the fallopian tubes causing inflammation and the development of pus within the ducts. At this stage there is often copious discharge, fever, lower abdominal tenderness following the menstrual period and pelvic pain during intercourse. This invasion of the fallopian tubes must be treated within 36 hours after the onset of pain, otherwise the result might be scarring and blocking of tubes finally to cause permanent sterility. Penicillin remains the most effective drug for treatment, and is also used for checking the progress of syphilis.

Syphilis is considered a three-stage disease that spreads over many years. It starts with the intrusion of an infectious organism into the skin or mocosal tissue. The area becomes red and swollen, then ulcerates turning into a painless sore; the adjacent lymphatic glands usually become swollen and hard. This is the primary stage of the disease and at this point it is highly contagious. The sore heals within six to ten weeks and although a skin rash erupts, it often goes by unnoticed.

Syphilis can be detected early, within weeks of contact by a blood serology test. If not treated during the first phase of development, the infection makes its way into the bloodstream. This stage can last from ten to fifteen years but is no longer contagious and presents few overt symptoms. In the third and final stage, the virus attacks vital organs.

VAGINAL WARTS AND HERPES: Warts often occur between the vagina and rectum, beginning as little grains of tissue. They can be treated in a doctor's surgery by the application of a solution that causes them to fall off within two or three days. If they are allowed to develop surgical procedures may be necessary. The herpes group of viruses is responsible for cold sores and fever blisters, but when they appear in the vaginal area they are of a different genre and are linked with the possibility of cancer of the cervix, so should be thoroughly checked.

OVARIAN CYSTS: These are growths on the ovaries which occur frequently. The most common type is soft and 3 to 4 centimetres large, and will often regress within two or three menstrual cycles. Ovarian cysts that are larger and persistent require surgical intervention. In rare cases, cysts will rupture, bleed or cause problems. Surgery gives immediate relief. Young women are frequently afflicted. While they usually cause no problems, they may lead to emergency situations if left undetected. Fertility is not affected.

CANCER: Cervical cancer is 100% curable if found early. It is practical to have a smear every six months. For this, cells are gently scraped from the cervix with a wooden spatula and are sent to a laboratory for examination. Results are available in about a week. If positive, it is usually considered necessary to have a hysterectomy, which is the removal of the uterus and fallopian tubes together with the ovaries. Because the cancer is usually localized within this area, there is rarely a chance of it having spread. A hysterectomy is also performed for some infections that cannot be helped in ways other than surgery. Hormonal substitutes are given to compensate for loss of natural production.

D AND C (DILATION AND CURETTAGE) OPERATION: This is one of the most common operations performed on the female sex organs and can be used in the diagnosis of many different conditions as well as part of treatment. It is sometimes known as scraping.

In a D and C, a fine metal rod is first inserted into the opening of the cervix, to measure how far in it is possible to put the dilators – a series of curved metal rods of progressive thickness which the surgeon uses one after the other until the cervix is open enough to provide a passageway into the uterus. This part of the operation is called dilation.

The curettage involves the introduction of an instrument called the curette, which is passed across the lining of the uterus to scrape away sections of it. This does no harm because it does not remove any tissue that is not normally shed automatically. The lining of the uterus is naturally lost every month in a period. There is no incision, no stitches.

The operation is done to check on the health of the uterus should any infection or fibroid build-up be suspected. It is often used as a treatment after a miscarriage, to ensure that all the debris is cleared away. In the same way it is used to terminate pregnancy. Often the first period after a D and C is a specially heavy one.

MENSTRUATION

A 28-day cycle is average; longer and shorter cycles within a year are perfectly normal, while many women never have a cycle longer than three weeks or shorter than 30 days. Duration and quantity of blood loss also varies, but it should be more or less the same each month. The cycle is controlled from the hypothalamus which responds to nervous stimuli and nudges the pituitary gland into the action of sending out appropriate hormones at the appropriate time of the month. The first one is released into the bloodstream at the beginning of menstruation, going straight to one of the ovaries to ripen an egg. Simultaneously the ovary produces oestrogen which goes to the uterus to prepare the endometrium (the inner lining) for the arrival of the mature egg.

About 14 days after the start of menstruation, the mature egg moves from the ovary through the fallopian tube to the uterus. This is known as ovulation and is the time of possible conception. Meanwhile in the follicle that held the egg in the ovary, another hormone is being produced, progesterone, which also goes to the uterus to assist in making it the perfect environment for a fertilized egg. If the egg is fertilized new hormones are summoned by the pituitary to aid in pregnancy. If it is not the unwanted lining disintegrates and is shed together with the unfertilized egg as the menstrual flow. Then the whole process starts again.

It is a highly complicated, sensitive and responsive activity, based on interrelated endocrinal activity. Because it is controlled by the hypothalamus where emotional stress is also registered, any upset readily disturbs the cycle – enough either to bring on or delay menstruation. Persistent excess bleeding or pain should be medically checked.

DYSMENORRHOEA (PAINFUL PERIODS): The most common cause of menstrual distress is hormonal imbalance. There are two types of period pains: spasmodic and congestive dysmenorrhoea. Spasmodic sufferers get sharp uterine cramps as the periods start. This often afflicts young women and may be eliminated after having a baby, as one cause is believed to stem from pain when the egg and menstrual blood pass through a tight cervix. If it continues, it can be helped by introducing oestrogen, at times in the form of the Pill.

Congestive dysmenorrhoea often intensifies with age and successive pregnancies. Symptoms heralding menstruation include depression, lethargy, water retention, head or backache, tender breasts and constipation. Hormone therapy is indicated, probably progesterone which can be given in pessaries or suppositories. Treating with the Pill does not always work out in this case, as the Pill contains progestogen, which is a synthetic substance and does not necessarily act like progesterone.

AMENORRHOEA: This is the absence of periods and thought to depend on psychological elements due to some kind of response to stress in the hypothalamus. A drastic change in life patterns can cause it, some medications such as tranquillizers, while a few women have it after stopping the Pill. Sudden weight gain or loss are other causes, particularly anorexia. It always requires medical attention; currently hormone therapy is considered the best treatment.

MOOD CHANGES: Researchers report that from 25% to 95% of all women suffer mood changes prior to having a period, mostly depression, irritability, anxiety and low self-esteem. Usually this occurs 4 days before and during the first 4 days of menstruation. Moods are predictable through the whole cycle and are due to hormone levels. During the first half of the menstrual cycle, most women feel alert, happy, out-going and competent. These feelings reach their peak at the time of ovulation, which is also when libido is at its height. During the second half women feel more passive and self-centred, while just before the period begins they become tense, anxious and sometimes aggressively bad tempered. The emotional changes parallel hormone changes; oestrogen production increases up to ovulation, afterwards progesterone levels begin to rise and both hormones circulate; then a few days before menstruation, both levels drop.

CONTRACEPTION

Today women have reliable and hygienic control over the number of children they have. There is a choice of contraceptive alternatives:

THE PILL: The most reliable form of reversible contraception. Used correctly it gives 100% protection against pregnancy; it does not interfere in any way with the sexual act. It alters the body's hormonal mechanism by combining progestogen with relatively small doses of oestrogen and inhibiting ovulation. The early pills had a high oestrogen content but this has been greatly reduced because it was considered responsible for some side-effects. Progestogen pills are often misleadingly referred to as mini-pills. These work by bringing changes in cervical mucus making it hostile to sperm penetration.

The Pill has had a bad reputation for causing weight increase, but the low-level oestrogen varieties limit this. Should weight go up by over seven pounds, check with a doctor. The most troublesome occurrence when the Pill is first taken may be break-through bleeding. It should cease, but if it continues after two months, a change of preparation is advisable. The Pill should not be self-prescribed; a clinic or a doctor can decide which type of pill is best for your particular metabolism.

All the pills are taken in the same way: one each day for 21 days then dropped for 7. Some packs contain dummy pills so that one is taken every day. It is important to take the pills in correct sequence. During the fourth week, light menstrual-type bleeding occurs, but this is not a true period. The progestogen pills have to be taken throughout the cycle and timing needs to be precise because coverage is of limited duration.

The biggest fear is side effects. A few hypersensitive women may experience a rise in blood pressure but the incidence of thrombo-embolic trouble has decreased since the withdrawal of high-oestrogen pills. However, there is a definite risk and the Pill should not be taken by any woman with a known predisposition to thrombosis. Pill taking should also stop for six weeks before surgery. It is also advisable to terminate three months prior to an anticipated pregnancy.

IUD (INTRA-UTERINE DEVICE): This is a small device in the shape of a loop or coil, usually plastic or plastic and copper, inserted into the uterus. How it prevents conception is not fully understood but it permits intercourse at any time. It is specially fitted and can be left in place for several years with regular medical check ups. Many women expel them and some suffer heavy periods. Coils can come out unnoticed during the first few months especially during a period. Conception can take place with the IUD still in position in which case it must be removed immediately otherwise it may harm the foetus. Most coils are not given to childless women because they can be painful to insert and more likely to be ejected, but the copper IUD usually known as the Copper-7 is an exception as it is smaller, easier to insert, and less likely to be expelled.

DIAPHRAGMS AND CAPS: Mechanical devices, effective if used properly. They should be left in for at least six hours after intercourse. They are dome-shaped rubber preventives, fitted after examination at a clinic or by a doctor. Instruction is given on how to insert and remove, which can be messy. Diaphragms should be checked once a year for fit and impermeability. They should preferably be used with a spermicide.

CONDOMS: An ancient method and effective if condoms are properly manufactured. They are made of rubber and simply collect the semen. Apart from possible rubber allergies, they have the drawback that the rhythm of love-making has to be interrupted to put them on, and there is the possibility of leakage, particularly if the penis is not withdrawn immediately after climax. For maximum reliability use with a spermicide.

RHYTHM METHOD: This relies on restraint in not having intercourse during ovulation which lasts about a week in between the cessation of the last cycle and the beginning of the next. It is difficult to estimate, as it varies so much. Timing by temperature is not always reliable.

COITUS INTERRUPTUS: This means withdrawal of the penis just before ejaculation and is not for the sensitive. It is also messy and can be a strain on sex and relationships.

SPERMICIDE CHEMICALS: These include creams, pastes, jellies, foaming tablets and pessaries, which have to be put into the vagina just before intercourse. They are not very satisfactory if used on their own.

STERILIZATION: An operation on fallopian tubes which stops eggs passing from ovaries to the womb. The normal menstrual cycle continues, but the operation is hardly ever reversible. It is a more serious operation than that for men (vasectomy) which involves a minor procedure on ducts leading from the testicles which prevent ejaculation of sperm with seminal fluid.

PREGNANCY

The best age for a woman to have a child is between 20 and 35. In younger mothers there is a much bigger chance of premature birth, while older mothers risk chromosomal errors including Down's Syndrome and mongolism. In this respect, the breakthrough is a process called amniocentesis – a technique of examining the chromosomes of the unborn foetus. A needle is inserted through the abdominal wall of the mother to draw off a sample of the amniotic fluid surrounding the baby. This enables such abnormalities as mongolism to be diagnosed. The sex of the unborn child can also be determined, which is important for families with sex-linked disorders.

Preferably a man should beget children before he is 45.

Ideally there should be an interval of at least two years between children, otherwise the younger one may be of lower intelligence.

Don't take drugs during pregnancy. That includes aspirin, nose drops, even supplementary vitamins, unless medically prescribed.

Don't smoke; studies indicate that smokers tend to have smaller babies, which means they are more susceptible to disease.

Avoid X-rays during pregnancy, including dental ones; make sure teeth are attended to early in pregnancy.

Every woman should see a doctor as soon as she feels reasonably sure she is pregnant. Regular check-ups will be arranged, the date of confinement estimated, and then it is up to you to take good care of your body.

Diet – a diet rich in protein, vitamins and minerals is important to the infant's health as well as your own. Pregnancy is never the time to lose weight though sometimes the more solid areas will slim down due to the fact that deposited fat is mobilized during pregnancy and put at the disposal of the growing foetus. Try to stay within a 2,000 Calorie a day regime, concentrating on meat, fish, poultry, fruit, fresh vegetables, cheese and wholegrain breads and cereals. No fried food, few fats. There is no need to drink extra milk, sufficient calcium is found in the other foods. Avoid sugar, white grains and breads; no alcohol. One of the early symptoms of pregnancy is an aversion or craving for certain foods. Control any desire for sweets, ice-cream or sugary confections. Don't eat raw, rare or undercooked red meat; it can adversely affect the foetus.

Exercise – swimming and walking are the best forms; add to that, housework, if necessary. Wear low or medium heeled shoes, and put your feet up should they be inclined to swell. If there is a tendency to varicose veins, wear a supporting stocking. Do one or two foot exercises a day. Keep breast muscles strong by wearing a fully supporting brassiere and during the last few months at night as well as during the day. Bathe the bosom with cold water night and morning. Do a simple exercise to strengthen pectoral muscles.

Rest – plan two rest periods a day, one before the midday meal and a longer one before dinner. Put your feet up, completely relax if you can.

Skin – this is twice as active which means it can improve more quickly and often does. It usually needs more cleansing, more frequently. Pigmentation marks sometimes appear but vanish when the baby is born. Some doctors advise patients to take vitamin D.

Stretch marks – they are less likely to occur if you don't get overweight and keep active. Rub in olive oil or lanolin cream. Weight should not increase more than ½ pound (240 g.) a week.

Nails – can prove difficult, need regular hot soakings in oil and nightly massage with a rich cream.

Hair – it will probably look marvellous during pregnancy but may fall out after the birth. This is usual beginning around the third month and not later than the seventh after confinement. If it is an excess amount or appears to be getting progressively worse, consult a trichologist.

Fifty per cent of conceptions are achieved within six months of trying and 80% within a year. If you have trouble conceiving, don't wait too long before seeking medical advice. Factors preventing pregnancy can be complex but many are straightforward and can be put right easily. Subfertility requires checking of both partners for mechanical or physical blockage of either sperm or ovum availability or effectiveness.

Spontaneous abortion occurs in 10–20% of all pregnancies. The majority should not be averted, particularly if they occur once or even twice during the first three months. The reason may be that the foetus is not perfectly normal. If miscarriage is repeated, especially after the initial three month period, the reasons should be medically ascertained.

ABORTION

Clinical abortion is available in almost all the major nations of the world. It is a relatively riskless procedure if done under the proper conditions; termination is technically simple and unlikely to lead to damage of the uterus which might affect later pregnancies. Up to three months and sometimes a little beyond an abortion is performed by doing a D and C operation and scraping the womb of the early foetal growth; it involves overnight hospitalization. More advanced pregnancies can be aborted by inducement and generally a salt solution is injected into the uterus bringing on contractions and abortion; several days are required. The decision to have an abortion is not a matter of medical uncertainty but one of morality. However, emotional upset is proving not to be nearly as high as was either expected or women were led to believe; it is more likely to bring relief.

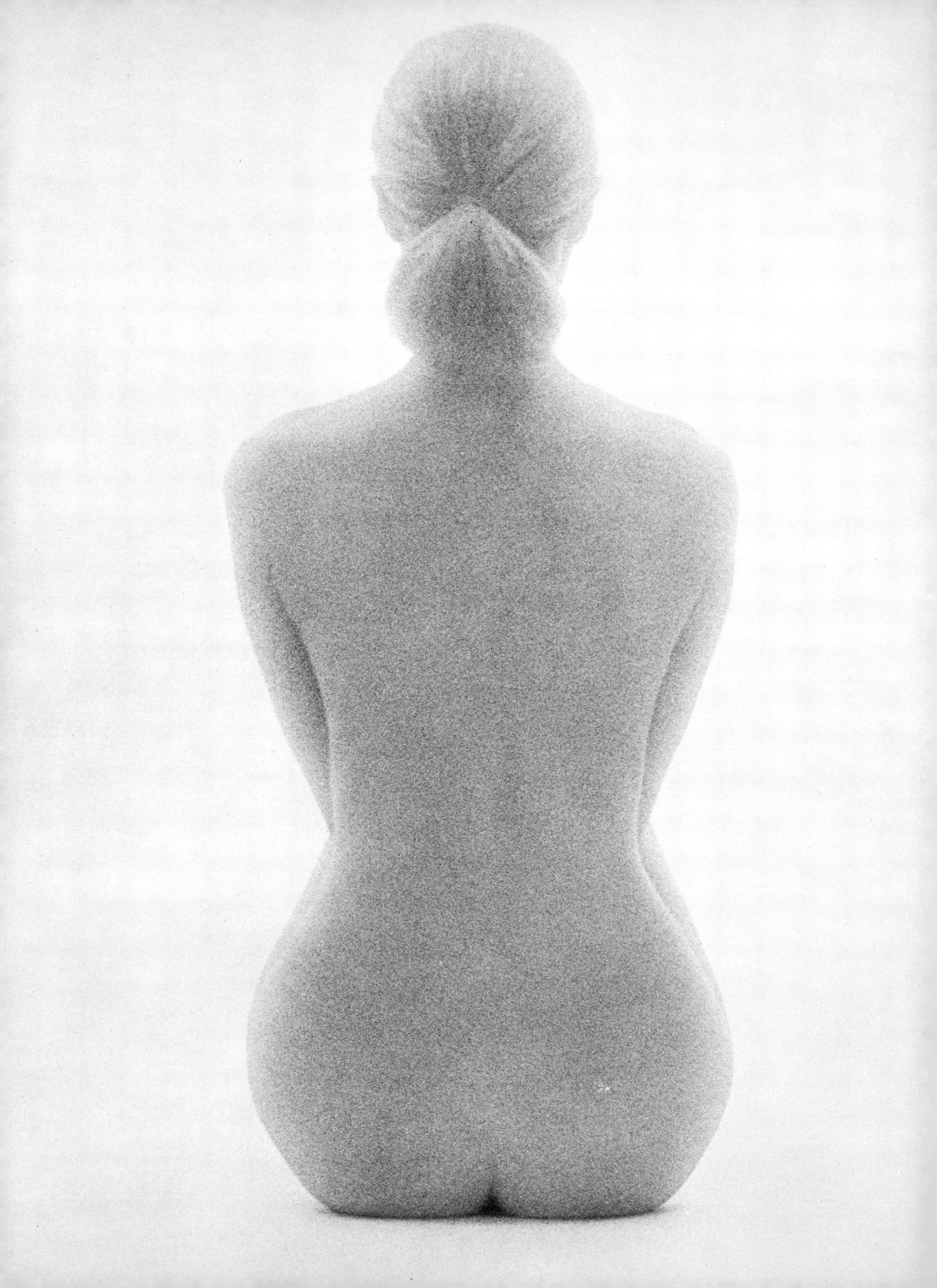

6

SKIN

The skin is a very complex structure. Four things affect it: genetics, environment, age and attention. Skin renews itself with biochemical efficiency and invariably responds well to treatment. A good skin is unblemished and uniform in colour, whether dark or light. It is firm, smooth and resilient. We are apt to think of skin in terms of the face only, but all body skin (except that of palms and soles which is hairless, thicker and tougher) is the same and will react in the same way. Every woman can have a great skin at any age, it's just knowing how to care for it.

Skin is the body's largest organ, 2 millimetres thick, weighing approxmately 6 lbs (3 k.) with a hardworking life of its own. It is a protective covering, guarding the body against bacteria, chemicals and foreign objects. It breathes, contains blood vessels, sebaceous gland ducts, nerves and hair follicles. It acts as a thermostat, retaining heat or cooling the body with its sweat glands. It absorbs the shock of blows to the body and through its receptive sensory organs, keeps you in touch with the world.

It is made up of two main layers: the epidermis which you see, and the dermis. The outer layer protects by sealing in all the body's fluids and keeping out potentially harmful things. The inner layer supports, nourishes and supplies it with that most essential commodity – moisture. In structure the two layers are dissimilar. The epidermis consists of several rows of living cells covered by compact sheets of dead cells (sometimes referred to as the keratin layer). It is constantly growing and about every twenty days new cells are born at its base. They quickly die and the dead cells are then pushed to the surface by the arrival of the new ones underneath and are continuously shed. Every new top layer is another chance to have a beautiful skin. Even if you remove a portion of the outer layer it will grow back as good as new. The living reproductive cells are nourished through the blood vessels, but the dead cells have

ATEGAN

only one requirement: water. It will plump, soften or smooth. The amount of water the outer layer holds determines the skin's texture and to some extent its contour. It receives a steady supply of water from the dermis, but this is limited and frequently not enough.

The epidermis also holds the skin's pigment; the darker the skin, the greater the pigmentation. Oil and sweat glands belong to this layer, though they are actually situated below, communicating through ducts that end on the surface. Oil glands greatly influence the skin's condition.

The inner layer helps determine contour and is responsible for tone and resiliency. It is all living, though it cannot replace itself and only grows until maturity. Damage to this layer results in permanent degeneration or scarring. It consists of bundles of tough supporting tissue (collagen) interlaced with elastic fibres and blood vessels that transport water and nutrients, and set complexion tone. The emotions often affect these vessels. Embarrassment can cause them to flood resulting in a blush; panic can cause them to empty, leaving the skin dead white. If you feel bilious, you can turn green as the yellowish bile from the liver is transported to the surface.

Care of the skin requires a nutritious diet, plenty of water, fresh air, exercise, sleep and minimum stress. The skin needs to be protected against the environment – sun, wind, cold – by using barrier creams. Poor health habits, too many fats and sugars, too many stimulants like coffee, are bad for the skin; so is excess smoking, excess alcohol. Weight fluctuations should be avoided as, after sun, they are the prime cause of wrinkled skin. When you gain weight the skin has to stretch and this puts strain on the elastic fibres of the inner layer. When you lose weight the skin does not always spring back to its original shape, particularly if the loss has been quick and drastic. Apart from wrinkles, visible scars remain – stretch marks – and they are seen mostly on upper thighs and stomach. (They can sometimes be alleviated by rubbing in pure coconut oil or cocoa butter, particularly as a preventive measure during pregnancy.) Fat pads are extremely important to the skin's appearance; they lie directly beneath the skin and separate it from the deeper muscle and bone. Their function is to cushion and support the skin, to supply the sebaceous glands and to act as a vehicle for the oil-soluble skin vitamins A, D and E. Loss of almost all fatty tissue through extreme dieting or disease can alter the appearance and quality of skin very quickly.

A wholesome diet is essential. It is important to get enough proteins, vitamins and minerals; lean meat, fish, poultry, eggs, fresh vegetables and fruits; avocado, cucumber and cabbage are particularly recommended. Vitamin A is the skin's most needed vitamin, but it is widely available in everyday foods and excess can be detrimental. A supplement of C and E can do no harm. It is generally accepted that vitamins A, D, E and K can be absorbed through the skin, though how much, under what circumstances and to what value, varies with the source. The case for vitamin E is debatable. Dermatologists are dubious about its supposed skin-regenerating claims, but some people burst a 200 mg. vitamin E tablet and squeeze oil directly on the skin, saying it thickens it, dries up whiteheads and helps erase wrinkles.

Hormones play a tremendous part in the condition of the skin. The hormonal balance is responsible for the coarsening of pores at puberty: the sex hormones stimulate the sebaceous glands; these enlarge and so do the ducts and the pores. Over-stimulation can lead to acne. The hormones involved are oestrogen and progesterone, the female ones that make the skin finer, less oily, less porous, and androgen the male hormone that makes the skin coarse, oily and porous. We have a mixture of all but in varying proportions. Large doses of oestrogen can provide a smoother, better skin, but are not advisable in adolescence or during child-bearing years. The Pill has a high oestrogen content, but its effect on the skin is individual; most women report there is no noted change, some say skins improve, others that it worsens. There is no evidence to support the idea that sexual activity affects the skin for the better. Skin changes are often apparent during or after pregnancy, but that's the change within you and nothing to do with your sex life.

The ageing of skin is a gradual process, but it can be slowed down and reversed within limits. Regardless of how much care is given, minor structural changes will eventually occur, but the more serious skin problems are caused by neglect and abuse. The most important structural changes are cellular build-up, dryness and pigment increase; they cause problems in texture, contour and colour. Older skin produces a different type of epidermis cell that tends not to shed so easily when dead. Because of this, the sheets of dead cells mount up, giving the skin a coarse, leathery look. These older cells do not hold water so well and unless moisture supply is constant and increased they can become dry and shrivelled. In addition there is a decrease in oil gland function which further aggravates the moisture problem. Pigmentation increases with age. This is not noticeable in black, brown or even dark olive skins, but fair skins darken a shade or two and not always evenly. Discoloration may appear as blotches or as freckle-like areas on hands and face commonly called liver-spots, although nothing to do with the liver – the sun is the culprit, for it dries and discolours.

Ageing changes the inner layer. As the supporting tissue degenerates, the elastic fibres lose their effectiveness and the skin is unable to maintain its normal resiliency. Wrinkles, lines and creases appear; the skin of the eyes and neck is the most vulnerable. Finally the blood vessels respond to age by expanding, sometimes causing the complexion to take on a ruddy look, sometimes breaking to form red spider lines and spots.

SKIN TYPES

What your skin needs in the way of treatment and preparations depends upon its type – and that depends upon texture, colour and condition. There are three textures – oily, dry and balanced (often known as normal); many skins are a combination of oily and dry. Colour influences texture while any skin can have a sensitive or blemished condition. To determine skin type, cleanse skin thoroughly and using a magnifying glass in strong light, examine it closely.

TEXTURE:

Oily – Caused by overproduction of sebum by the oil glands. Affects darker skins mostly; but even a light skin is inclined to go sallow. Skin shines constantly, is coarse and has enlarged pores. It is often plagued with blackheads, occasional break-outs and is the skin most prone to acne. It stays younger-looking longer, has few wrinkles and usually improves with age. Trying to remove all oils from the skin only encourages greater gland activity. It is important to remove only excess oil from the surface, leaving a sufficient amount to ward off any over-activity. Too enthusiastic a treatment with harsh soap or cleansing lotion will often dehydrate the epidermis, leaving skin in a flaky condition.

Dry – Three different things cause dry skin: dehydration, insufficient amount of oil secretion and ageing. It affects 85% of all light-skinned women. Skin is generally of a fine texture, but looks and feels tight and drawn. It chaps, flakes and peels easily, and even at an early age may show wrinkles and lines, particularly around the eyes and mouth. Contributory factors to this condition are: use of wrong cosmetics, strong soaps, exposure to sun and wind, indoor heating and air-conditioning. One of the most important steps in dealing with a dry skin is to try and avoid further dehydration by sealing in moisture. The lack of natural oils must be compensated by rich external lubrication.

Balanced – Exists when oil, moisture and acidity are harmonious. It is ideal but rare. Skin is fine textured with no visible pores, smooth to touch, neither wet nor greasy. It has a tendency to become more dry with time, so it needs assistance to retain the status quo.

Combination – This is really skin in transition between dry and oily state. It gives off too much oil in the T-area of forehead, nose and chin; the rest is dry particularly around eyes and on cheeks. The dry and oily areas have to be treated separately.

COLOUR: The colour of the skin depends on the degree of pigmentation. Light skin tones are graded from pale to pink, beige to rosy; dark skin tones go from olive to caramel, brown to black. The general term 'black' covers a much wider range than does 'white'. One dermatologist differentiates 35 variations of basic shading for black skins, 10 for white. There is no basic difference in structure and quality – therefore no difference in skin-care regimes. Black skin is usually more oily and has more sweat glands. However it still suffers the effects of dryness, which shows in its ashen cast in cold weather. In general the darker the skin, the slower the ageing process. The reason is a combination of heredity and habitat. The sun is the great enemy of light skins which usually have dry tendencies so lines are created faster. The evenly distributed pigment in dark skins acts like a sun filter and its more oily surface acts as a shield keeping moisture in. Dark skins, even black skins, can tan and burn, but they do so less drastically and more evenly than light ones. Dermatologists say that black skins are less likely to develop acne or skin cancer.

CONDITION: *Sensitive* – Usually dry skin plus. Fine textured often with a transparent look, the upper layer being particularly thin and sensitive and likely to develop broken capillaries. Reacts quickly to both external and internal influences – sun, wind, emotions, food, drink. Needs usual dry-skin care plus extra protective lubrication. Watch for any allergies.

Blemished – Usually oily skin plus. Troubled with pimples, sometimes to the intensity of acne. Needs usual oily skin care plus attention from medicated preparations that dry and heal – and professional advice.

BASIC CARE

Body skin usually can be taken care of by retaining moisture through a body lotion, using oil in the bath if skin is dry and by rubbing away the flaking skin. Facial skin is more vulnerable but consistent care can give lasting results. It need not take more than three minutes morning and evening but is vital. The key to good skin is activity; you must keep the renewal rate of skin cells as high as possible. The only way to do this is by regularly keeping the skin clean, moist and thinned of its dead-cell build-up. It's easy to get into the habit, and once attained it is hard to break. The preparations only influence the epidermis, but that's enough. The steps to good skin are: cleansing, freshening, moisturizing, conditioning, exfoliating (thinning) and stimulating. The first four are daily procedures, the other two are weekly unless you have a special problem – then more often. Check this chart for treatment necessary for each skin texture; check below for complete details. Warning: corrective skin care is minimal. If you try to do more you can possibly harm the skin.

SKIN TREATMENT SCHEDULE

	OILY SKIN	DRY SKIN	BALANCED SKIN
Twice daily (morning and evening)	cleanse with soap or rinsable cleanser – and water astringent light moisturizer	cleanse with mild soap, rinsable cleanser, cream or lotion – and water diluted toner rich moisturizer	cleanse with soap or rinsable cleanser – and water toner light moisturizer
Daily	eye cream emollient for throat area	eye cream rich emollient conditioner	eye cream light emollient conditioner
Weekly	exfoliation treatment (twice a week is better)	exfoliation treatment (more if dry skin builds-up)	exfoliation treatment
Weekly	stimulation and clearing masque (twice a week is better)	stimulation and clearing masque	stimulation and clearing masque

CLEANSING

It is necessary to remove stale make-up, pore-deep grime as well as some natural secretions which can cause skin problems. How you do it is important: cleansing incorrectly is worse than not cleansing at all, as the skin's natural moisturizers and oil protectors can be removed in the process. Cleanse twice a day, always in the morning and at some time in the evening, not necessarily just before going to bed.

There are four types of cleansers: oils and greases, creams, soaps and rinsable cleansers (creams and lotions). The greases and creams dissolve make-up but are not so adept at removing dirt or themselves. Tissuing off is not enough, a freshener is always needed. There is no substitute for soap and water. Even if you're fair skinned and fragile, cleansing creams and oils do not provide the kind of cleansing soap can and there are many mild soaps suitable for the face. Rinsable cleansers are the next best solution for older and particularly dry skins, and although these may be creams and lotions, they should be rinsed, not wiped, off.

Many women never use water in the belief that it is bad for the skin. It is not true. Frequent and excessive contact with water can cause dry and chapped skin, because in time it will remove most of the skin's moisturizers, but you are hardly likely to soak your face that long. The entire cleansing routine should not take more than two minutes and should be done no more than twice a day.

Procedure:

Use cream or oil for make-up removal, particularly for eyes; tissue off.
Wet skin with lukewarm water.
Using soap or rinsable cleanser, work up a quick lather for 30 seconds.
Rinse with warm water till soapy traces have gone; three times is usual.
Pat with towel to absorb residue water, don't rub.

FRESHENING

Fresheners do the important job of rinsing off all traces of cleanser and pore dirt and restoring the skin's acid mantle. They also help stimulate local circulation and refine skin texture. Freshener, toner and astringent are the three names for the preparations used and are basically the same product in graded strengths depending on the alcoholic content. Astringents are the strongest and are recommended for oily skins; fresheners and toners for dry and balanced skins. Medicated lotions are astringents with more alcohol and the addition of anti-bacterial agents.

Procedure:

Apply straight after cleansing; saturate cotton pad with freshener, wipe over skin thoroughly.

A between-cleansing clean-up can be done by wiping face with a freshener; recommended for very oily skins.

Natural Aids:

A teaspoon of cider vinegar added to $1\frac{1}{2}$ cups of water. Use as liquid toner.

Rub skin with a slice of raw potato.

Rub with a slice of lemon, or splash with lemon juice and water.

Cucumber freshener: squeeze juice of 2 cucumbers, heat to boiling point, skim away froth, bottle and refrigerate.

Sprinkle a few drops of camphor in the last cleansing rinsing water.

MOISTURIZING

Helps to offset the evaporating effects of the environment. Moisture is not actually fed to the skin, but preparations form a protective film holding in the skin's moisture. Moisture is the single most important ingredient in skin chemistry. Dry and older skins which don't have as much moisture as they need, are additionally helped by an emollient that attracts moisture from the atmosphere, holds and feeds water to the skin. A moisturizer smoothes and plumps skin surface, improves the feel and fills in the gaps giving a good base for make-up. If used without make-up a heavier type is best. Most creams and lotions moisturize, as they trap water.

Procedure:

Best time to apply is directly after a bath or face-washing; even after drying with a towel, skin is damp and retains some moisture – that is the time to seal it in.

Dot on forehead, nose, cheeks and chin; smooth emulsion all over face and throat, using upward strokes and finger-patting around the eyes.

Wait for moisturizer to be absorbed before applying make-up.

If weather is harsh, reapply to driest and most vulnerable areas.

Natural Aid:

Milk of almonds: skin 1 oz. (30 g.) almonds by dipping alternately in boiling and cold water. Grind until a powder, add drop by drop $\frac{1}{2}$ pint (3 dl.) of distilled water, continuing to blend until liquid is milky; strain.

CONDITIONING

Its purpose is to keep skin soft and supple as well as smooth; most effectively done when you are sleeping or resting and the skin is relaxed. Dry skins need a deep lubricating cream that stays on overnight or for several hours during the day. Balanced to dry skins require a lighter emollient; oily skins are better with just a moisturizer. Combination skins should have each area treated separately. Ideally conditioning should include the use of an eye cream since the area around the eyes lacks natural oil and is very prone to dryness and wrinkling. A light-weight emollient is as effective as a special cream.

Skin needs to be conditioned every day. It is impossible to correct a neglected or damaged skin overnight by applying a thick layer of emollient. A thin film adheres and is adequate; the rest is waste. All preparations of similar consistency give much the same results; the important difference is the concentration, which determines whether a product is light or heavy. An emollient can be used as a daytime barrier cream against inclement weather.

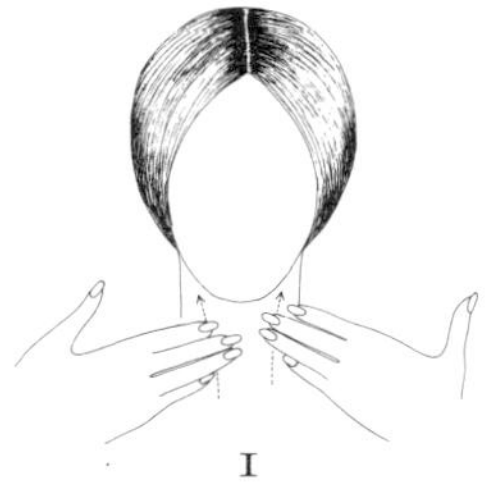

1

Procedure:

Apply after cleansing and freshening.

Pre-wet skin by covering with a wet facecloth; this increases effectiveness of conditioner.

Finger-pat eye cream around eye area.

Gently massage conditioner into skin. This is an opportunity to firm and contour the face and throat. Too much manipulating of facial skin is not good so do it quickly. Use both hands, fingertips only, many strokes.

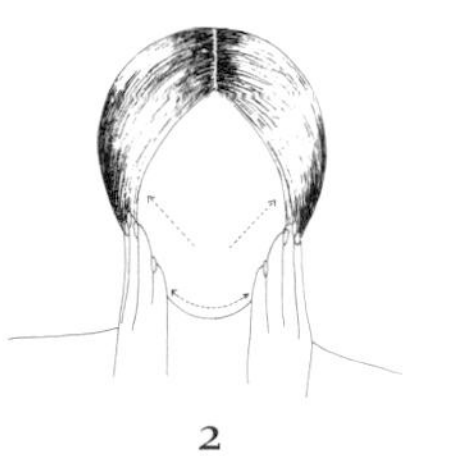

2

Skin Contouring – the same movements should be used for all skin care.

1. Neck: use long alternating strokes from collar bone to jawline.
2. Cheeks: from centre line, smooth upward and outward from chin to ears, nose to temples; stroke the nose bridge downwards, sides outwards.
3. Forehead: stroke upward, in high arcs to the hairline.
4. Eyes: using one tip, finger pat, starting in the centre between eyes, making a semi-circle going outward both above and below eye.

Leave conditioner on a few hours or overnight.

Before applying make-up, cleanse, freshen and moisturize.

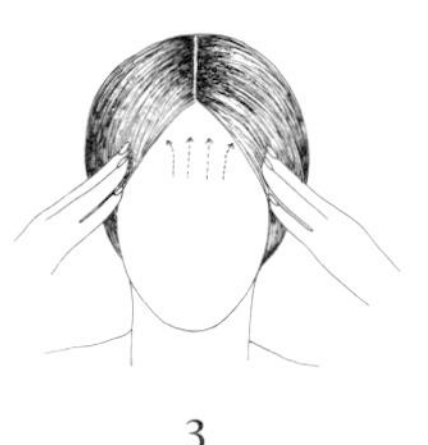

3

Natural Aids:

For extremely dry skin, melt a teaspoon of butter and beat in 2 tablespoons of milk; apply liberally and leave a few hours.

Apply a thin film of petroleum jelly for dry and balanced skins.

Any vegetable shortening makes an effective weather barrier.

20-minute honey conditioner: moisten face, massage in raw honey; rinse away with warm water.

Honey-and-cream: mix 1 teaspoon honey with 2 tablespoons light cream; beat together, apply, leave for 20 minutes, rinse away.

For dry skin – oil of avocado, almond, wheatgerm or olives.

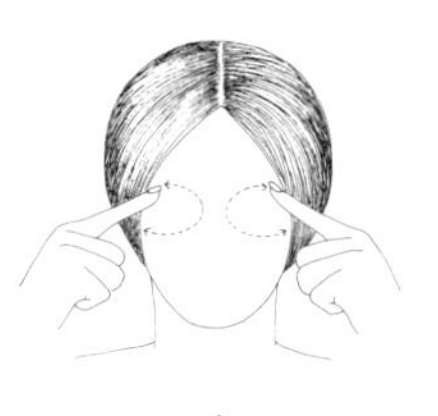

4

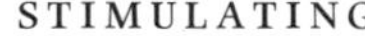

STIMULATING

This is the way to give the skin a quick pick-up, to exercise it by activating circulation and bringing nutrients and oxygen to the surface. It is usually done through masques, sometimes through steam facials. Nearly all masques contain a high percentage of water; the rapid evaporation that follows application causes them to be cooling, soothing and contracting. This is often reinforced by the addition of sharp aromatics and alcohol. When the masque is taken off, the blood vessels expand and the skin looks rosier; fluid from the enlarged vessels plumps up the inner layer, smoothing the skin and compressing the pores. There is a definite improvement in the appearance of the skin, and although this 'masque effect' is transitory, the skin is exercised and stimulated.

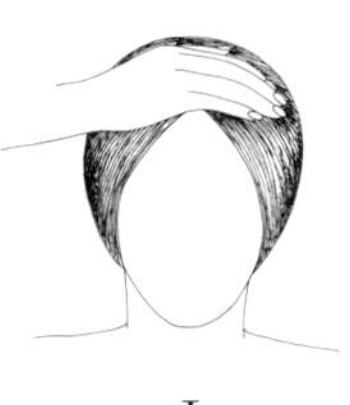

1

In addition, masques may have one or more corrective effects on the skin. They usually contain materials that act as cleansers and purifiers, drawing out dirt, toxins and grease. All masques rely on a drying process; they are divided into rinse-off and peel-off types. The rinse-off ones are the better cleansers; many contain clay or silicas (forms of sand) with the ability to suck out oil and dirt. Some masques contain gums and proteins. Peel-off preparations usually contain rubber, wax or some type of plastic. They work like a sticky piece of Scotch tape removing surface dirt and a few dead cells; they are not such good cleaners as the rinse-off ones, but equally good stimulators. Oily skins need a masque twice a week, dry and balanced skins, once.

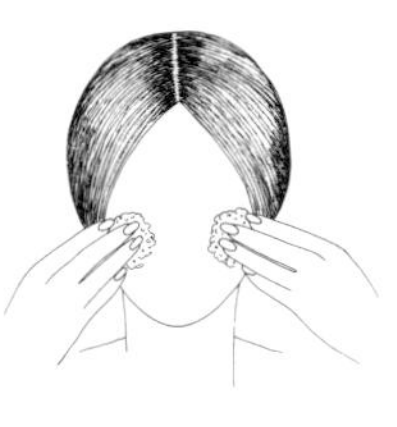

2

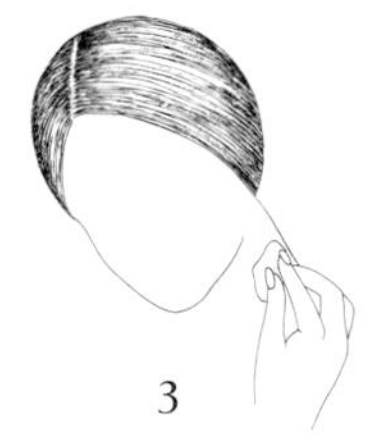

3

Procedure:

This is a facial: here are the professional steps. It takes about half an hour.

1. Smooth hair away from face and tie back.
2. Apply a cleanser using motions illustrated for skin contouring (page 119). Tissue or rinse off depending on cleanser.
3. With cottonwool pad, apply freshener to remove last traces of cleanser.
4. Dot light moisturizer on forehead, cheeks and chin; blend in.
5. Rinse with clear lukewarm water.
6. Apply masque all over face and throat; leave a free circle around the tender eye area.
7. Cover eyes with cottonwool pads soaked in milk or a non-alcoholic freshener. Leave masque on and relax lying down for 20 minutes.

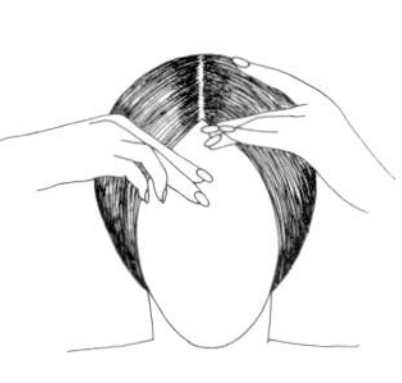

4

8. Remove all traces of masque, blot face and throat with towel; finish with a thin film of moisturizer.

Natural Aids:

The following facial applications should be left on for a minimum of 20 minutes, then thoroughly rinsed off with water.

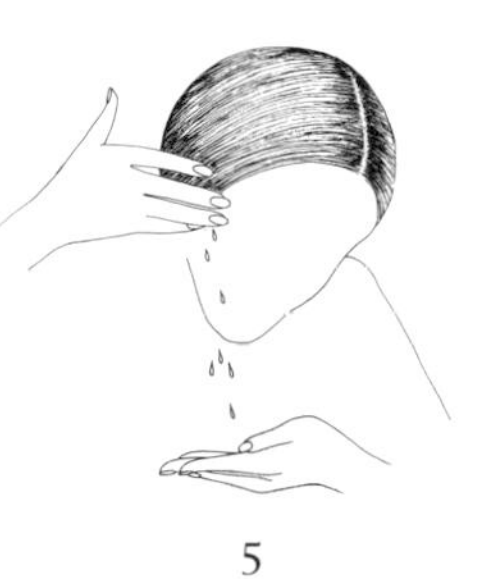

5

Crushed strawberries used alone or mixed with oatmeal.

Ripened pears give an astringent action to oily skin.

Apply juice from a few green cabbage leaves.

Cucumber masque: grind or mash enough to cover face; refreshing.

Brewers' yeast facial: 1 teaspoon of powdered yeast and 2 teaspoons warm water; adjust consistency so it spreads like a paste.

The beaten white of an egg – with the optional addition of $\frac{1}{4}$ teaspoon lemon juice or cider vinegar; good for oily or balanced skin.

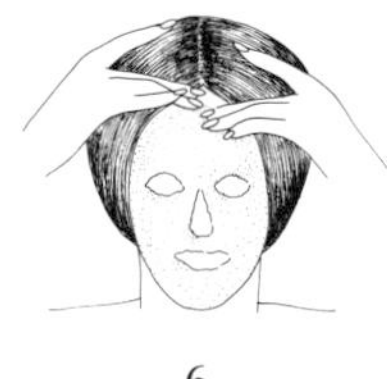

6

Another version of an egg-white facial is to beat it with a tablespoon of skimmed milk.

An egg yolk, a few drops of cider vinegar and a little vegetable oil; good for dry skin.

Honey masque: 2 tablespoons honey and $\frac{1}{2}$ teaspoon of lemon juice or cider vinegar.

Steam Facial

This is a method of stimulation; steam encourages the pores to push out dirt and impurities, it promotes perspiration and stimulates circulation. Sensitive skins or those with broken veins must not be treated.

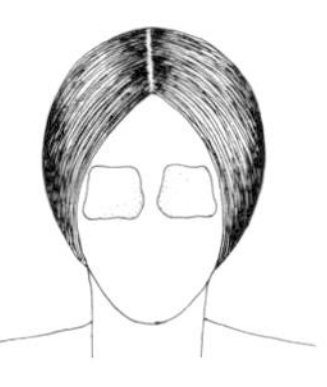

7

Steaming with a herb infusion is most beneficial. Pour boiling water over herbs in a bowl; make a towel into a head tent and steam face over bowl for 10 minutes. Blot dry, freshen, then moisturize. The following can be used individually or combined.

For cleansing, soothing: camomile, lady's mantle, nettle, rosemary, thyme.

For tightening: peppermint, elderflower, tincture of benzoin, gum arabic.

For drying: yarrow.

For healing: leek, comfrey, fennel.

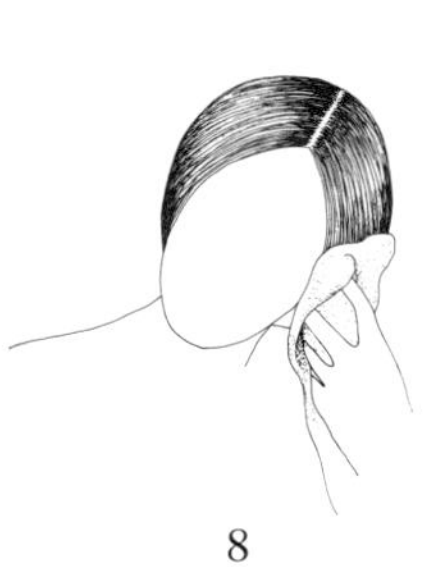

8

EXFOLIATING

This takes cleansing a step further and is the removal of dead surface cells (flakes) from the skin. It is one of the most important skin-care procedures and one of the least known. The skin's texture and contour are both improved; the thinned skin feels smoother, appears more translucent and has a lighter and more uniform colour tone. Pores look smaller and an additional benefit is that the outer layer is more easily moisturized after the dry hard surface cells are removed. Slough-off products can be lotions, gels or creams, sometimes with visible abrasive ingredients like grains. Some astringents act as very mild exfoliators. Young skin may be thinned simply by rubbing with a rough facecloth wrung out in lukewarm water. Older skin requires heavier thinning, using a preparation and a complexion brush, sponge or textured cloth. It is really a mild peel and should be done once a week, sometimes twice if skin looks scaly. Deep peels are drastic remedies to get rid of lines and blemishes; they are done by physicians or specialized cosmetologists.

Procedure:

Thinning is done immediately after cleansing.

Apply preparation according to instructions.

Remove by wiping or brushing off, using circular movements for forehead, chin and cheeks, vertical movements for nose, facial borders and neck; use water if necessary to clear skin.

Moisturize immediately.

Guard against early sun exposure.

Natural Aids:

Sprinkle ordinary salt on a wet facecloth; rub face lightly, rinse away; not for delicate skin.

Papaya mint tea removes skin debris; pour 2 cups boiling water on 2 tea bags, steep for a few minutes; soak a facecloth in the tea, wring out, apply to the face holding cloth against skin. The tea must be hot to be effective; keep heating, and renewing cloth. Continue for 15 minutes.

SUNTANNING

The right amount of sun can help you to look wonderful – tawny, glowing, healthy. Too much sun and you will be doing your skin irreparable damage and depleting your body of vitamin B. Prolonged exposure, year after year, is responsible for both premature ageing of the skin and many skin cancers. The damage is cumulative. It is only about one per cent of the sun's radiation that affects the skin and all the burning and tanning is caused by the invisible short-wave ultra-violet rays.

Activity takes place on two different levels in the epidermis. First, the pigment-bearing cells, tucked away on the underside of the epidermis, are activated by the ultra-violet rays – only the shortest of these rays are strong enough to penetrate the cells making them produce melanin (the brownish pigment). The effect cannot be seen for about two days, but it is this action that produces a long-lasting tan. Meanwhile the longer-wave rays work on the melanin granules that already exist in the upper layers of the epidermis, turning them a dark brown. The reason why the long-lasting tan is slow in coming is that the lower melanin granules gradually work their way to the surface. Tan disappears not because it 'fades' but because the pigmented cells flake off. To preserve a tan, involves controlling the natural shedding of cells. This can be done by using oil in your bath and a body lotion afterwards.

A suntan is a defence mechanism. The granules of melanin act as a screen on the surface, filtering out harmful rays and protecting the delicate underlayers. If this were the only effect of the ultra-violet waves, there would be few problems, but they also release a chemical that penetrates the skin's inner layer. It is this that causes the blood vessels to dilate, accounting for a lobster red colour. Some hours later the dilated vessels allow serum to enter the tissues. This leads to swelling, pressure and irritation on nerve endings; peeling follows and in severe cases, blisters. Damaged cells work their way to the surface, become harder and thicker, forming a tough layer. This is the second line of defence for the skin, as it reflects and scatters light, but also makes the skin look leathery and dry.

Whether you live under the sun all the time, or whether it is a transient exposure, protection is essential. If you want to acquire a tan, you also need patience. Sunburn protectors come in varying strengths, the most effective being the opaque sunblocks. These reduce the likelihood of damage, but also reduce the likelihood of tanning. Some sun lotions are only moisturizers or greases which attract the rays and prevent drying. Be cautious, read labels. Quick natural protectors are cocoa butter, or a mixture of salad oil and cider vinegar.

A protective screen should be used all over exposed areas. The most vulnerable parts are the face, nose, shoulders, upper chest, midriff, backs of knees and backs of hands. If you are in the sun for the first time for several months, take it slowly. The first day sunbathe for only half an hour in the morning, keep in the shade until the late afternoon, then take a little more sun. Increase your time in the sun each day; avoid midday rays, strong reflection from the water and the combination of sun and wind.

Some skins burn and dry, others tan. Generally the colour of skin and eyes determines the effect of the sun on the skin. The lighter, the more cautious you need to be. The very fair skinned with little melanin can't expect a deep tan ever; redheads who sit in the sun often go freckled. Both types should use a strong sunblock. It has been reported that some people susceptible to sunburn have been able to take more exposure by supplementing the B vitamin of PABA (see Vitamin Chart, page 32) to the degree of 1,000 milligrams a day; also by applying it as an ointment, delicate skins can tan.

Olive to caramel skins need a sunscreen only, a stronger one if you don't want to deepen the tone. Brown to black skins require a mild sunscreening lotion, one that simply moisturizes and lubricates with emollients. It is true that dark skin does not burn as easily as fair skin, and can take more exposure, but this does not mean that it should not be helped. Any skin dries out in the sun without lubrication.

Artificial tanning by means of a sun-lamp is a practical way to build up a tan slowly, or to keep a healthy colour. It is preferable to go to a clinic where lamps are used under supervision. The temptation at home is to take an extra minute, which can be very harmful indeed. Half a minute is ample for fair skins with a gradual increase in time according to skin colour. Goggles are essential as concentrated ultra-violet rays can harm the eyes. There is no need to use any protective cream, but apply an emollient or oil afterwards to alleviate drying.

If you get a sunburn and it is red and painful, try these remedies: equal parts of baking soda and water, patted onto sunburn and left on for half an hour, rinsed off with tepid water. Beat the white of an egg with 1 teaspoon of castor oil, smooth over skin as a lotion. Cover with a mashed pulp of cucumber. Soothe with a strong solution of ordinary tea or sage tea. A diluted solution of vinegar and water brings relief. Mix $\frac{1}{4}$ cup buttermilk with 2 tablespoons rose water, splash over skin and wait until it dries, rinse off.

SKIN BLEMISHES

Skin is subjected to various growths and infections which look ugly and can develop into serious disorders. Here are the most common problems:

ACNE: One of the most distressing skin disorders, and primarily affects young skin. If neglected it can cause extensive inner-layer scarring. Acne is caused by sex hormones. Diet, once thought to be so important, is only a minor consideration – though too fat a diet can aggravate the condition. The male hormone, testosterone, is mainly responsible, because its production is apt to be inconsistent at puberty. The sex hormones stimulate the skin's sebaceous glands and regulate oil output. Overactivity results in excess oil secretion and thickening of the pore openings. The pore becomes blocked and in addition fatty acids are produced by enzyme action. The result is a pimple, a whitehead (a waxy point with no surface outlet) or a blackhead. At this point infection often sets in and pus ruptures the wall of the oil gland, the infection spreading to the inner layer. This inevitably results in a permanent scar.

Since one cannot eliminate the cause of acne, treatment is limited to measures that suppress infection and keep it from breaking out in the oil gland. Although a healthy diet, good skin hygiene and medical preparations are of some help, antibiotics are now considered the basis of therapy. These remove the bacteria that cause infection; cortisone is used but sometimes this has undesirable side effects. Oestrogen, the female hormone, can be given to balance the excessive output of testosterone, but caution is necessary particularly in young women. Natural sunlight and ultra-violet treatments often help, so does superficial X-ray therapy.

BLACKHEADS: These are oil plugs in the pores that blacken on exposure to air – the colour has nothing to do with dirt, it reflects oxidization. They are the most common form of skin blemish, sometimes become infected and turn to acne. Regular, proper cleansing helps prevent them and alleviate mild ones. Removing the firmly entrenched plugs is often better done by a professional. The procedure is to open the pores first through steaming or hot compresses. Pressure around the opening is applied either with a special instrument or clean fingertips (never nails). This forces out the blackhead. Some cosmetologists use a suction technique. Afterwards skin must be dabbed with alcohol, then wiped with an astringent to close the pores. At home use hot compresses soaked in a mixture of 1 teaspoon of sodium bicarbonate in 1 cup hot water.

BROKEN VEINS: The legs and face are usually affected. The faintest tracery is the most difficult to get rid of. There are technical ways of draining veins with a special needle and a chemical fluid. It often requires a series of treatment sessions over a period of time.

DERMATITIS: This is a general term that covers inflammation of the skin caused by physical or emotional means. Eczema and psoriasis come into this category and are said to have emotional or nervous origins.

Medical treatment can control them during flare-ups, but cannot control the source. The conditions often come and go, but do not leave scars.

MOLES: These patches of dark pigment can look unattractive particularly when raised or sprouting isolated hairs. They can be removed quickly and painlessly. Don't pluck or pull at hairs, if necessary cut them close to the skin. The slightly raised mole, particularly if it has been there from childhood, is usually harmless. But if a flat mole suddenly becomes darker or larger or more raised, or if it bleeds, go to your doctor at once.

PIGMENT BLOTCHES: If you have been careless about the sun, you have probably acquired a few brown spots varying in size. Removing them is not easy, and many bleach creams are too harsh for safety. They can be removed by planing or deep peeling. Should any pigmentation appear in the form of rough red spots, professional advice is absolutely necessary, as they can become malignant. Skin cancer is every bit as serious as any other kind; certain types stay localized but others spread rapidly to the lymph nodes and on throughout the body. Red patches can be treated in the early stages by cutting, burning, scraping, freezing, acids or X-ray.

WARTS: When they are small, warty growths can be removed easily by scraping them off the surface; this usually leaves no scar. The larger ones must be cut or burned off and sometimes a scar results.

WHITEHEADS: These appear as tiny white beads of waxy matter just under the skin and have no way out to the surface unless helped. A tiny opening has to be made and the application of oil helps to force them out.

SKIN PEELING

There comes a point where certain old skins or blemished skins cannot be helped except by literally getting rid of the old skin and growing a new one. This is a drastic measure, but it can be done. It is entirely different to plastic surgery which corrects contour problems. Peeling is aimed at improving the skin's texture. There are two methods: chemopeel, which involves the use of chemicals to burn off the outer layer, and dermabrasion which planes it down. Both are medical procedures.

CHEMOPEEL: Sometimes called chemical surgery. It is used to treat skin scarred by acne and other blemishes, but the results with ageing skin can be dramatic. A caustic is used to destroy all the epidermis and part of the inner layer. This not only gets rid of the old surface skin which is thickened, large-pored and wrinkled, but also all the things attached to it such as warts, rough spots, pigment blotches. The removal of a portion of the inner layer stimulates growth of new tissue and helps to rebuild the skin effectively. It is a very delicate operation with success depending on precision control and timing. The whole face, usually together with neck area, is treated at the same time to avoid tide marks. Localized touch-ups can be done later if necessary. The degree of penetration of the chemical determines the depth of peeling.

It is not as painful nor as uncomfortable as you might expect, but the caustic does cause intense inflammation. This looks horrific and is often combined with swelling. Understandable when you consider that at the end of the peel there is no outer layer of skin and only two-thirds of the inner one. A new epidermis grows gradually and completely; initial protection from all outside elements is essential. The final covering is smooth, unblemished and fine-textured. The inner layer is a little thicker than before, firmer and more resilient; it has the effect of plumping up the skin.

It takes about three to six months to see the complete visual improvement. There is one drawback: the new skin often has an artificial look about it. This is primarily because the inner layer consists entirely of scar tissue, lacking the tone and depth of the original skin. It is also less durable and can relapse within one to ten years depending on how well you treat it. The operation can be repeated to maintain the effect.

Some complications can occur; the most common is the formation of more pigment than before. This may be due to a strong reaction to the caustic or to early exposure to the sun. The reverse can happen – no pigment and the skin is left ruddy.

DERMABRASION: This is often the preferred method to reduce scars, or acne, remove surface blemishes and reduce fine wrinkles. The upper layer of skin tissue is removed by an electrically operated rotating wire brush or steel burr. The depth of planing depends on the severity of the case; it can also be done in isolated areas. A scab forms very quickly, which is first softened by a prescribed ointment, then with lukewarm water. It usually comes off within a month and at first the face looks badly burned, but in time the redness diminishes. Protection from sunlight is essential for six months. Fine dermabrasion is often used in conjunction with a face lift.

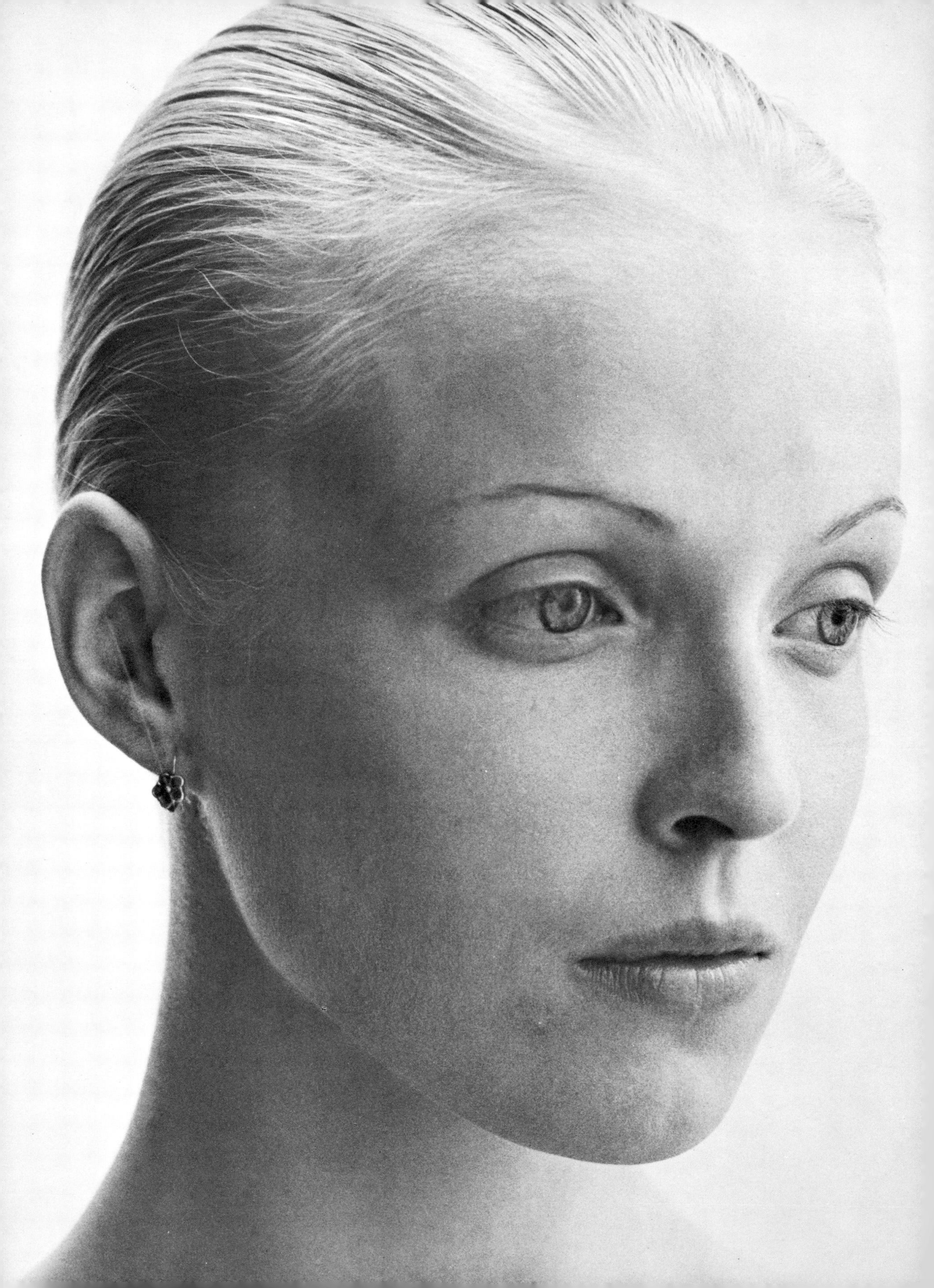

7

THE FACE

The most important bone of the face is the frontal bone. It forms the forehead, eye sockets and bridge of the nose. The size and angle vary tremendously and primarily contribute to the individuality of each face. The cheek bones form a flat area below the eye sockets and determine the moulding and planes of the face. The other bones are the nose bones – two small ones which link with the frontal bone – and the upper and lower jaw bones which hinge together close to the ears and hold the teeth. The ear has no bone structure and is made up of cartilage and muscle.

The eyes are delicate and intricate, depending for effectiveness not only on the condition of the eyeball but on muscles and nerves.

The muscles of the face are very intricate, giving mobility to every single inch of it. The most important, from the beauty point of view, are the zygomaticus muscles which extend across the cheeks from the temples to the corners of the mouth, keeping the contours of the face firm. All these muscles determine the expression of the features. Chewing exercises the face. Smiling and laughing, although they may add a few lines around nose, eyes and mouth, also exercise cheek muscles and pull the corners of the mouth in an upward direction, preventing the face from sagging.

The face will age long before the body. Its muscles react negatively to stress, emotion and tension. It is easy to get into the habit of grimacing, frowning and raising eyebrows and this leads to lines and wrinkles that become more definite each year.

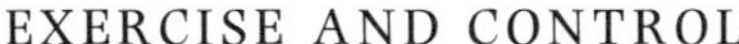

EXERCISE AND CONTROL

Like any other part of the body, the face and interrelated neck structure needs exercise and muscle control to keep it in good shape and condition. Control is primarily awareness. It does not mean immobility but being more conscious of the changing movements of your face when you are talking and listening; try not to exaggerate expressions.

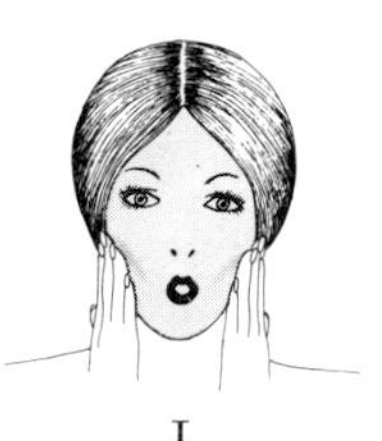

1

FACIAL EXERCISES: To improve and maintain the characteristics of a youthful contour and covering. They may look weird, for they are face-pulling gymnastics that manoeuvre the face to correct it, but you will quickly see that when you do them, certain lines and wrinkles are momentarily ironed out. Done with regularity, they are very effective. Do them in the bath or in front of the mirror before making up.

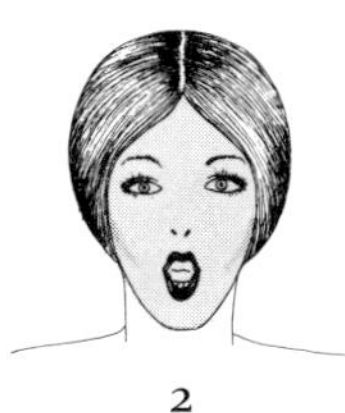

2

1. *Mouth and Cheeks* – Purse lips and at the same time fill cheeks with air. Place the 3 middle fingers of each hand on each cheek, either side of the mouth. Press fingers in against the blown-out surface, but don't let the air out. Count 10. Relax. Repeat 10 times. Work up to holding to the count of 30.

2. *Mouth, Cheeks and Eye Area* – Open mouth wide as if screaming, open eyes wide and staring at the same time. Count 3. Repeat 10 times. Then repeat, turning face first to the left, then to the right – 5 times each side.

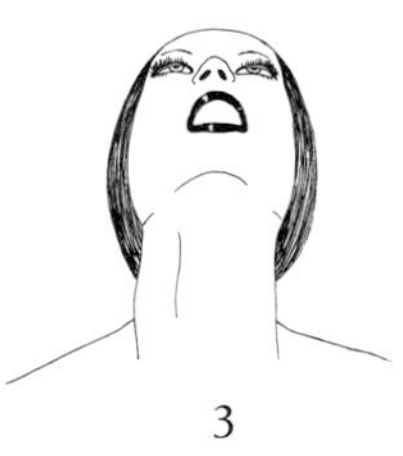

3

3. *Mouth and Jaws* – Open mouth wide, fling head back. Open and close mouth moving the back teeth. Open and close 10 times.

4. *Forehead* – Using palm of hand, push scalp back from the hairline smoothing out any furrows. Count 3. Repeat 10 times.

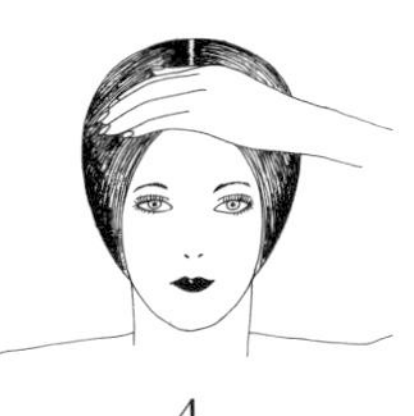

4

NECK EXERCISES: Bad muscle habits in the neck cause crêpiness and lines. When neck muscles are properly toned, the skin is held smooth and taut. When they are not, the horizontal lines crease and the contours sag. The neck is not an isolated area, but part of good posture, vital in keeping the throat area smooth and agile. Most women do not realize how little control they have over the set of their heads, or in moving from side to side. These exercises help to give you control by freeing the neck from tension, loosening and lowering the shoulders, elongating the neck muscles. It is important to be aware of what the neck is doing, how it is being held. Feel it; feel the distance between neck and ears; feel the shoulders hanging freely without knotted-up tension.

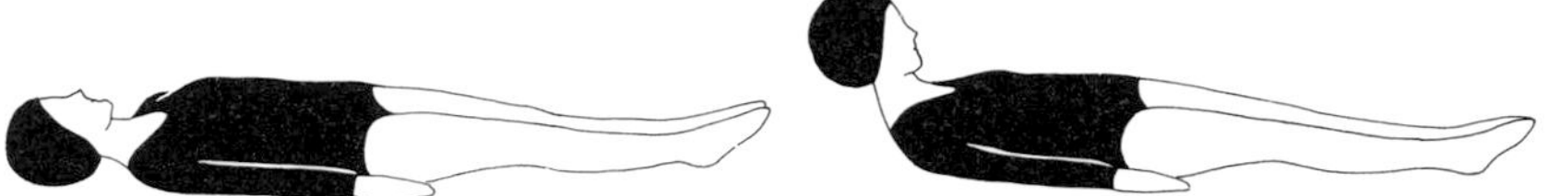

1. *Neck Stretch* – Lie down (on the bed), arms by sides, legs straight and together; slowly raise head and neck, stretching the neck as you raise it. Lower slowly. Do 5 times, work up to 20.

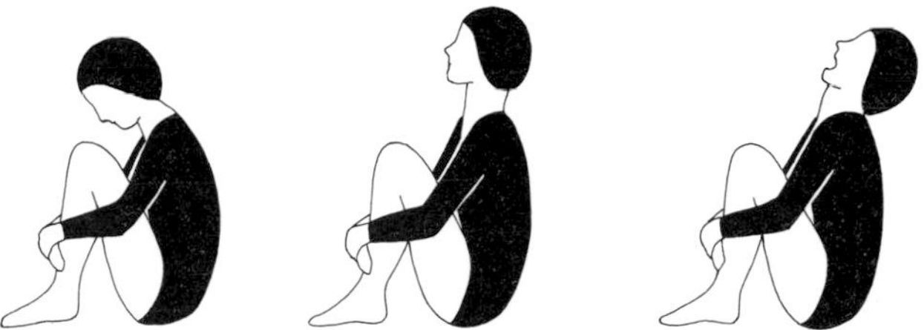

2. *Muscle Toner* – Sit (can be done on the bed also) with knees up to chest. Stretch neck up, shoulders down. Now tilt head forward; slowly pull head back as far as possible, open and close mouth slowly, 3 times. With mouth closed, bring head forward. Repeat 5 times.

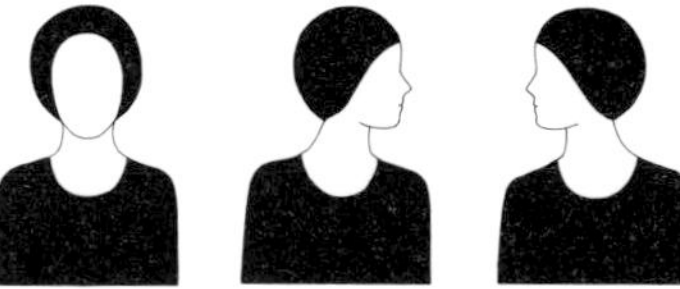

3. *Neck Control* – Sit (on the bed) cross-legged, palms flat just behind buttocks; shoulders down, back straight. Without moving the torso at all, turn chin slowly over each shoulder, keeping neck stretched high. Repeat 5 times each side.

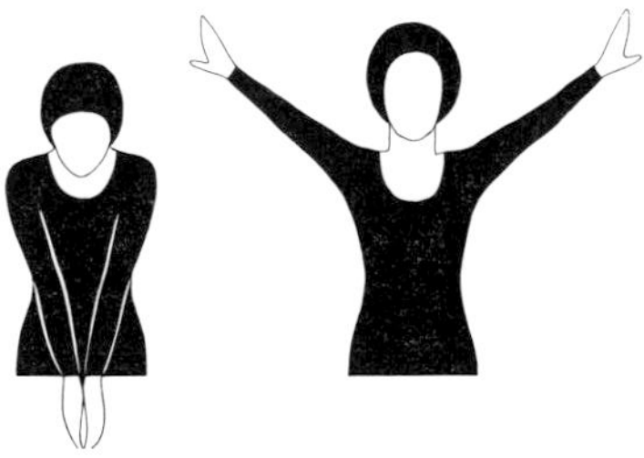

4. *Shoulders Free* – Stand with feet a little apart, arms in front with backs of hands touching, head lowered. Slowly lift head, stretch arms up and back, fingers apart, palms facing back, neck stretched. Repeat 10 times.

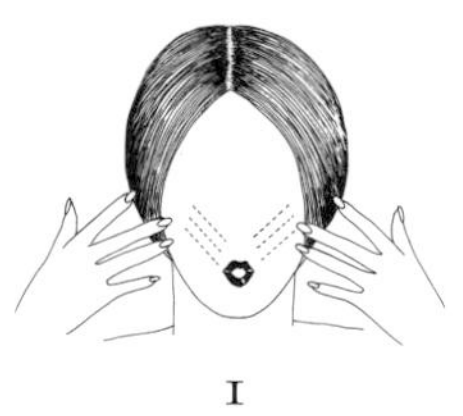

1

FACIAL AND NECK STROKING: This is much lighter than massage and is done with the tips of the third, fourth and fifth fingers; glide them across the skin with the lightest touch. This gentle stroking directs the skin into smoothness, no pulling or pushing. Heavy massage can be destructive, and these almost undetectable movements get better results if done consistently. Aim for 8 to 20 minutes a day. Best place: in the bath, in bed, watching television.

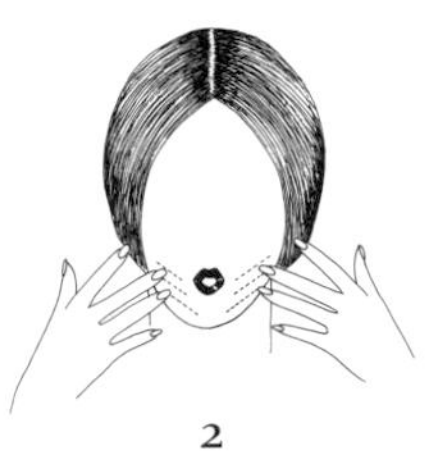

2

1. *Cheeks and Mouth* – Purse lips in an O-shape, breathe normally. With three fingers (first, second and third) stroke upwards from the outer corners of the mouth, making a V-shape up across the cheeks. Stroke slowly, 6 times.

2. *Chin and Mouth* – Purse lips; with the tips of the three end fingers stroke upward from the centre of the chin out to the hollow cheeks. Do 6 times.

3. *Forehead* – Mouth normal, lips together. Starting at the centre, stroke outwards in a circular movement, back in at the top. Repeat 6 times.

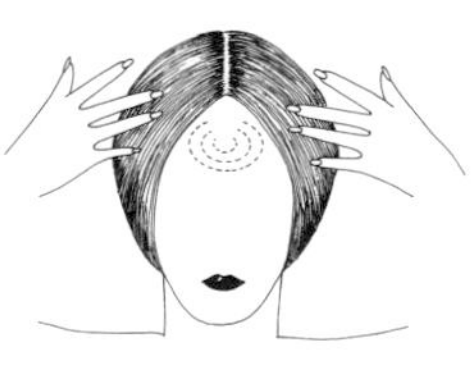

3

4. *Throat and Underchin* – Mouth together, trace fingers up from collar bone brushing off the edge of the chin; movement should be slightly outwards, fingers starting at the bottom, palms down. Repeat 6 times.

EYES

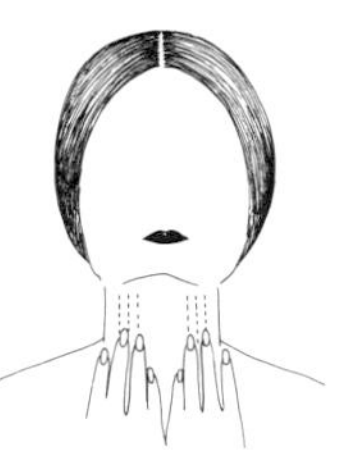

4

The eyeball is circular, roughly one inch in diameter, but only about one-twelfth of it shows. The part you see through is the black pupil, where light passes through to the back of the eye. Pupils appear small in daylight and wider at night because the surrounding coloured iris contracts and expands; it shrinks when it is dark allowing the pupils to expand and let in more light. The cornea is the eye's transparent surface and is a kind of lens that enables it to focus. Further back is a lens that refines what the cornea absorbs. This is slim and relaxed when eyes look into the distance, and thicker when viewing something close up. Eventually an image reaches the retina at the back of the eye which in turn passes it to the brain. All of this happens in a split second.

An eye is functionally mature at ten years of age and usually no serious changes occur in it until after forty. A healthy eye can focus easily at its nearest point as well as adjusting to distance. The focusing power depends on the anatomical arrangement of the cornea and lens, and refractive errors are usually genetically determined. Dysfunctions such as short and long sightedness and astigmatism usually occur because the lens is the wrong proportion for the eyeball. No permanent damage

Opposite: Guy Bourdin, 1973
Overleaf: Norman Parkinson, 1972

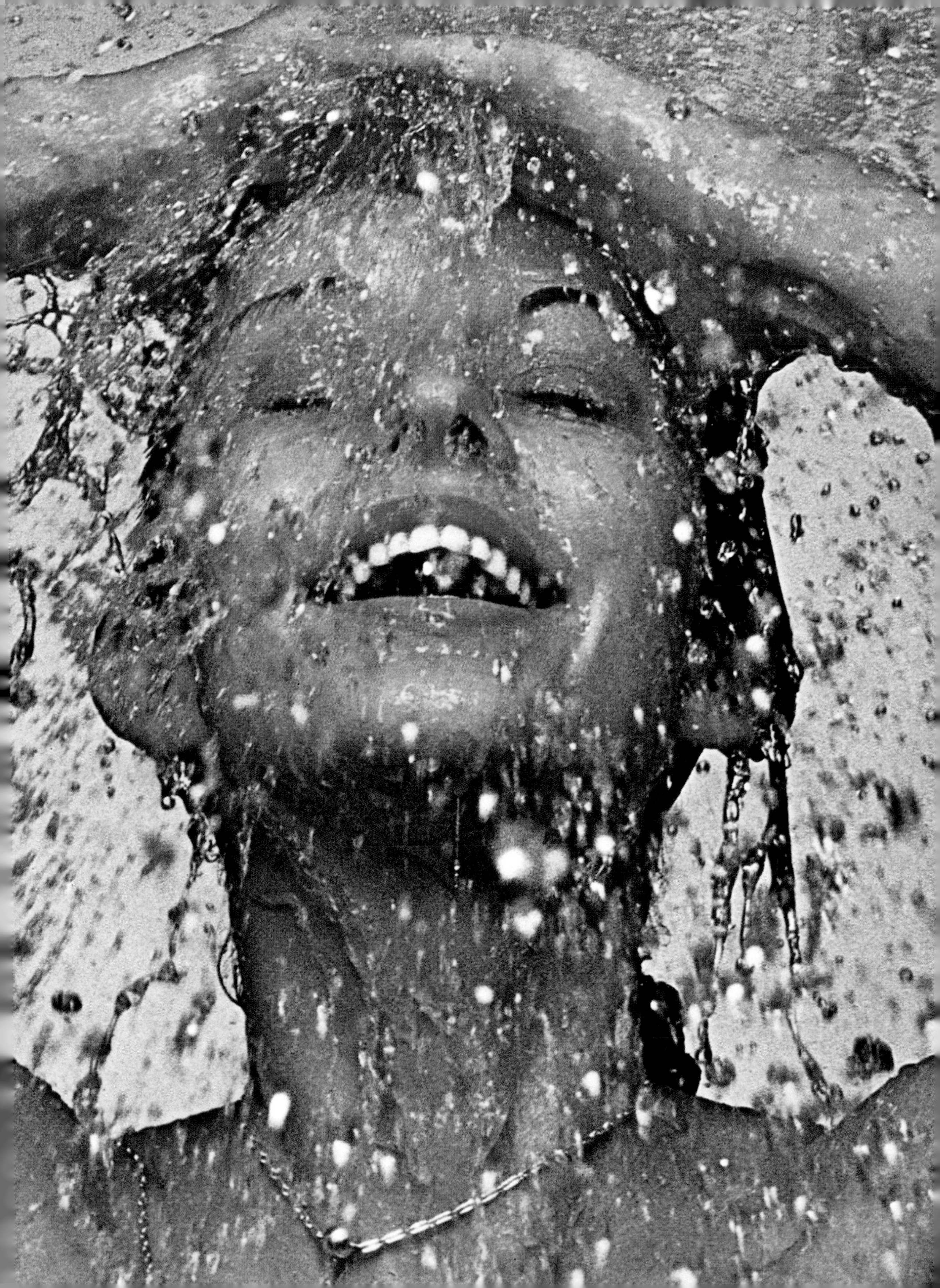

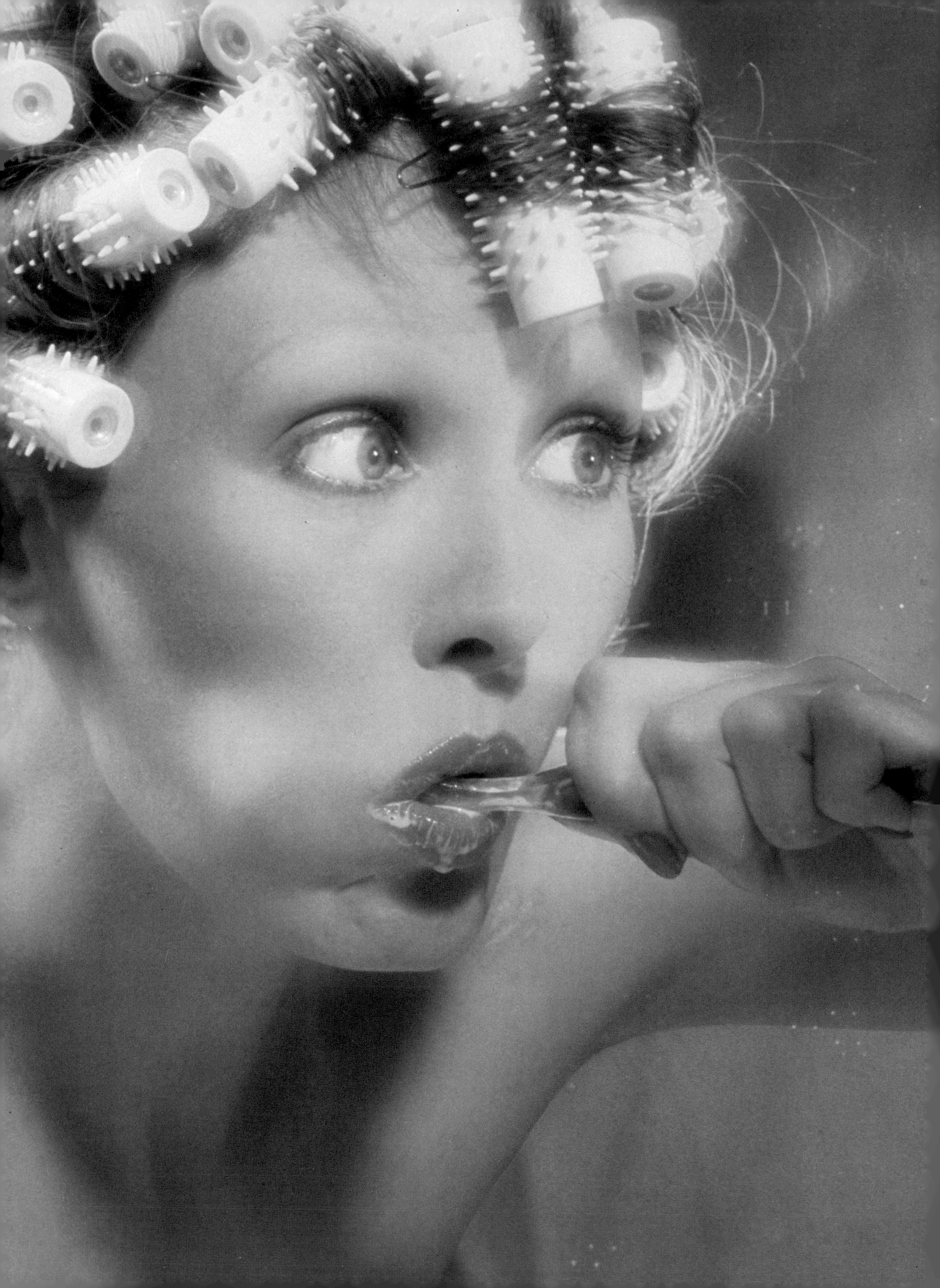

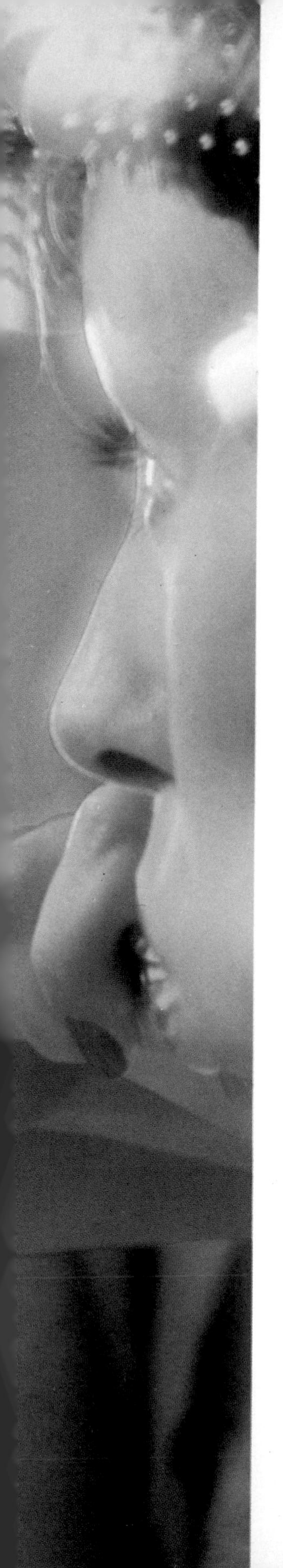

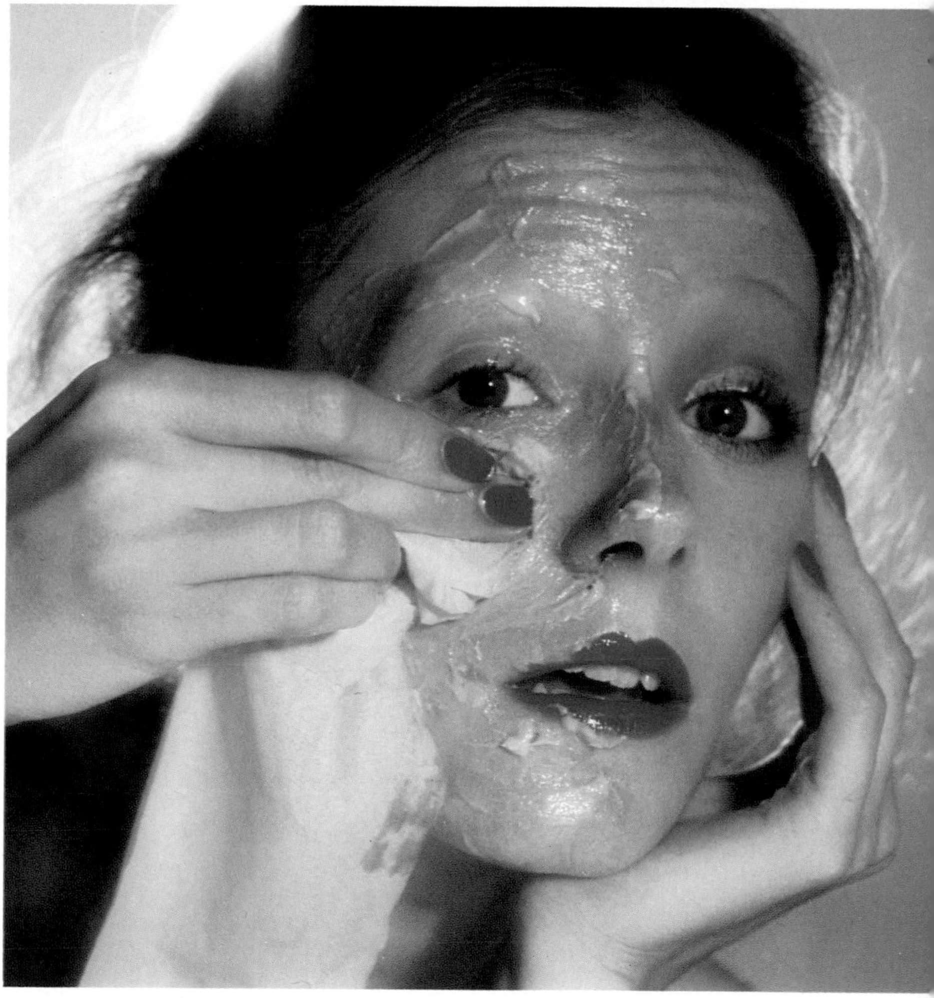

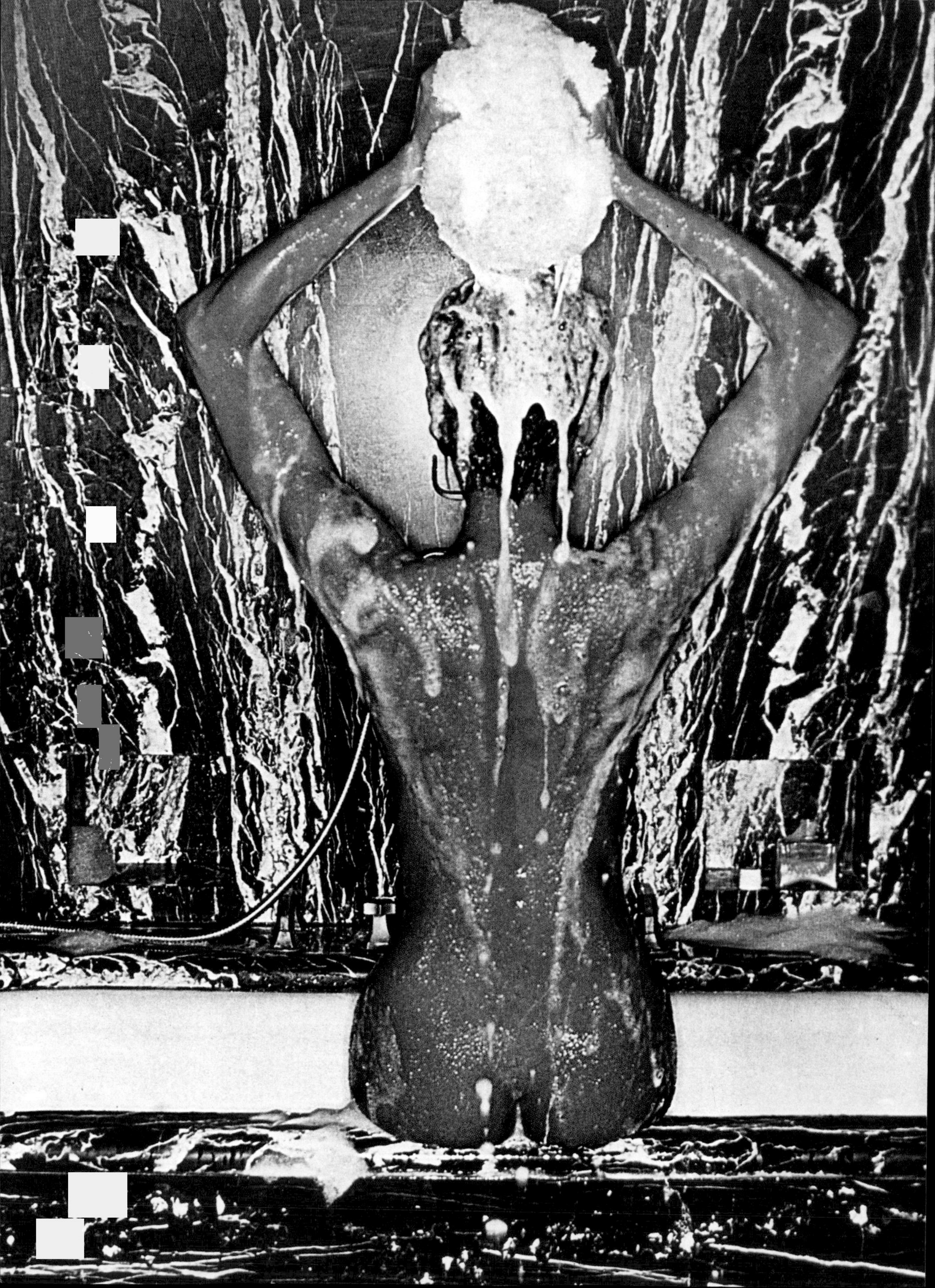

can come through eye strain or incorrect spectacles, or watching too much television.

The basic measurement of good eyesight is that one should be able to see clearly into the distance as well as close up. An optician classifies normal sight as 6/6 which means that you can see at 6 metres (20 feet) what has been precisely gauged to be visible at that distance. For example you should be able to read a car's number plate at 23 metres (80 feet). If your eyesight is 6/8 that means you only see clearly at 6 metres what you should be seeing clearly at 8.

Short sight: Known as myopia. The short sighted eye tends to be longer, so light has further to travel from the eye's own lens to a point on the retina at the back of the eye, which relays the image to the brain. Sometimes the light does not get there, and an unclear picture results.
Long Sight: Known as hypermetropia. The eye is shorter, so the image-carrying light rays go beyond the retina instead of focusing on it. This means that eyes are more comfortable looking into the distance than at close objects.
Astigmatism: This is when part of your vision is blurred, usually because the cornea is misshapen.
Squinting: Usually due to a lazy eye, where the muscle lacks pulling power. When the good eye focuses the other can't, so instead turns inwards, outwards, up or down. Sometimes eyes can harmonize in one direction but not in another. Squints usually show up very early in life and should be corrected before twelve otherwise it may be too late. Sometimes an eye requires a minor operation; exercises often help; or lenses to strengthen the lazy eye.
Colour Blindness: This is not actual blindness, but inability to recognize a few colours only, usually green and red.

INFECTIOUS DISORDERS: Conjunctivitis is inflammation of the thin protective layer over the eye together with a sticky discharge. It usually occurs with an allergy or as a symptom of a nervous disease. It attracts bacteria and sets up an infection, making it possible to infect others too. There are various lotions and ointments which soothe and lubricate the rough areas but the only quick cure is the use of antibiotics.

Blepharitis is inflammation at the roots of the eyelashes, and is inclined to appear if there is a tendency towards dry skin, dandruff or acne. All make-up has some potential allergy problem and unless well cleaned off can produce this sort of inflammation. It is easily treated.

Opposite: Barry Lategan, 1976

AGEING DISORDERS: In old age, the lens of the eye tends to become more opaque and when sight is seriously impaired by this clouding over, it is called a cataract. Cataracts develop slowly and the only treatment when they become severe is surgical removal of the lens which is replaced by strong glasses.

Also with age, pressure within the eye area increases, causing headaches and radiating pain, also coloured haloes around lights. This is known as glaucoma and is often hereditary. Treatment usually comprises keeping open the drainage channels between the iris and lens by contracting the pupil. A small operation may be necessary to increase the channels.

CARE

Conservation of eyesight involves using eyes, not abusing them. Watch for fatigue and if your eyes are constantly tired see a specialist. Try not to read in moving vehicles. Make sure you are living with adequate light: the light should come from behind or above rather than in front. When reading, stop after an hour to give your eyes fifteen minutes' rest.

Vitamin A is important for eyesight and is readily available in vegetables including carrots, celery and tomatoes. Vitamin B-2, vitamin C and vitamin D are also necessary. When there is a lack of B-2, eyes often become bloodshot, itchy and watery.

Eyes need rest and exercise. During the day rest your eyes by simply putting the palms of your hands over them, cutting out the light for five minutes. Another way: sit in front of a picture, look at it. Now gently close your eyes and cover them with the palms. Relax for three minutes or more. You will notice that eyes will see first grey-black, then deep black. Open your eyes and look at the picture again. An additional way to relax tired eyes is to look far into the distance, just gazing.

Eye exercises are simple, quick and efficient. Roll eyes to the right, then to the left in complete circles; 20 times each way. Also look at the tip of your finger, held quite close to the face, then look at a very distant object, then back at your finger. Repeat a few times.

Dark circles and puffiness can be due to lack of sleep or a sluggish kidney. Otherwise it is normal relaxation of tissue which comes with the passing years. Applications of iced water or milk often reduce swollen or puffy eyes. Witch-hazel is helpful – pour a trace over cottonwool pads:

it is best if the witch-hazel is ice cold. Grated potato left under the eyes helps to reduce swelling, as do rosehip tea, fresh figs or strawberries.

For inflamed eyes, squeeze in fresh cucumber juice, or place slices over the eye and leave for 15 minutes. Compresses of an infusion of eyebright or camomile are good natural aids for the eyes.

Bloodshot eyes could be caused by blood vessels congenitally dilated or by some sensitivity. Often alcohol is the cause. Eyedrops are safe but over a long period are not a good idea.

CONTACT LENSES

For aesthetic reasons many women use contact lenses to correct defective sight. Decide with your optician which type most suits your needs.

Corneal lenses, the tiny ones, sometimes only 8 millimetres in diameter, fit only over the cornea. The larger haptic lenses fit over the whole eye, and because of the type of protection they give, are excellent for sports. Hydrophilic lenses, made of extremely soft and flexible plastic, are micro-corneal covering only the iris. These can be worn by those who find the heavier lenses irritating.

Lenses come in many colours. The plastic is patinated. Most people choose light grey to filter the light, or blue or green shades slightly deeper than their own eye to accentuate the colour. The first time you try contact lenses tears will probably stream down your face, but as you get used to the feeling, your vision adjusts. To start with lenses are usually worn for only two hours at a time, twice a day for three days. Then the wearing time is increased by fifteen minutes each session.

The new soft lenses, really flexible flakes of plastic, require less adjustment time. You can wear them for several hours immediately, and finally sleep in them too. Tolerance is no problem, but there is sometimes difficulty in getting exact vision in cases of high astigmatism. They move with the movements of the eye, floating on a cushion of natural eye fluid. They must be expertly fitted and for this a special machine is used to measure the curvature of the eye. There are about fifty-six different kinds of curves and most lenses are made not in one continuous curve, but in a series of three, four or five. If you wear contact lenses, avoid greasy eye make-up because it can work its way into the eyes and even the smallest speck between the lens and the eye can cause blurred vision. Particles of face powder and sparkling eye shadows can cause watering; mascara must be waterproof.

GLASSES

Choosing glasses is not easy. Here are some guidelines:

Always stand in front of a full-length mirror when trying on frames; it is the only way to get the correct sense of proportion.

Make sure glasses fit, sit securely on your nose, don't clamp your head, and that the tops of the frames line up with your eyebrows otherwise you get two sets of parallel lines close together.

Square faces look best in large square or rectangular shapes with the lower corners wider than cheekbones. Round faces need wide but short frames. Long faces need long, deep frames that cover a lot of the face. Short faces are helped by short, narrow, rectangular frames or enormous round ones that sit up on the nose.

Colour is ruled by hair colour, but it is better to keep to neutral tones of beige, browns and greys or light steel rims.

Tinted lenses can be attractive: for indoor wear choose a light tint, darker for sunny or bright artificially lit rooms, while grey is often the best in sunshine.

Eye make-up often needs to be altered when glasses are worn: a little more colour and extra lashes or mascara. Glasses for short sight tend to make the eye appear smaller, so use a darker liner under top lashes for emphasis. Lenses for long sight can magnify eyes, so use light lines and paler colours. Dark frames require a stronger tone of lipstick. Blushing colour should not disappear under frames, so keep it low and use as a contour rather than a highlight.

SUNGLASSES

Tinted glasses are convenient wherever there is a glare and can be very flattering but to wear them consistently is not advisable. The sun is beneficial for it forces the eye into constant activity adjusting from shade to bright light. Good sunglasses help absorb both the infra-red and ultra-violet rays while less expensive ones absorb one or the other or a little of both. Photochromatic lenses are those that change colour depending on the exposure to light – they are very pale in reduced light and darken immediately in the sun.

EARS

Most of us are born with more acute hearing than we ever need and keep it throughout life. If in later years the ability to hear high tones lessens there is nothing to worry about. Constant city and industrial noise can aggravate the ears considerably; loud noises can injure them and affect the general nervous system producing tension.

The ear works this way: sound waves can only exist by a vibration of some material – water or solid matter, but in most cases, air. It is a vibration of the air that we pick up. This is multiplied in pressure many times by the mechanical arrangement of little bones behind the ear drum; then it is taken up within a fluid-filled cavity, which in turn activates the auditory nerves and registers in the brain. It is possible for sound of great intensity to damage this mechanism while some sounds can be beneficial. Music, for instance: no one understands why it can be calming or stimulating or why certain sound patterns can have rejuvenating effects.

Hearing impairment can be congenital, the result of an infectious disease, an obstruction due to dirt, wax, an abscess or congestion, a slight blow on the ear, or a nerve disorder. Over-zealous blowing of the nose can cause damage. Infections of mouth, nose and throat can attack the ear. High levels of cholesterol often coincide with diminishing hearing.

Professional advice should be sought immediately there is any disorder or noticeable change in hearing. More than regular cleaning is not advisable on your own. Even poking around to dislodge impacted wax can be harmful. There is often reluctance to admit to hearing disability yet many surgical and mechanical correction procedures ensure help and minimum inconvenience. In many cases, deafness is due to a hardening of the middle bones; this is called otosclerosis and can almost always be reversed by the manipulation of a tiny bone, the stapes, within the middle ear. Another cause is pressure on the Eustachian tubes which responds well to delicate finger surgery. Finally, artificial eardrums can be inserted.

Modern technology provides amazing miniature units for amplifying hearing. Some are small enough to fit in the ear, others go behind it with a transparent tube leading into the ear's cavity, others are fitted to glasses.

Ear Piercing: Done correctly it is a painless and harmless process. A local anaesthetic should be applied, then the ear lobe punctured by diathermy; afterwards a tiny silk thread is inserted through the hole and acts as a dressing. A few days later, the thread is replaced by a gold ring or rod-and-stud pin which must be worn continually for three months after piercing.

TEETH

It is widely known that teeth need calcium. They are composed of the hardest substance in the body, calcium phosphate. What is not so well known is that a lack of vitamin D restricts the absorption and use of calcium. Vitamin C is also important to strengthen the connective tissue. Fluorine protects teeth and is added to some municipal waters and can be painted on or applied through a toothpaste. Bone meal supplement is said to help fight decay, as it is rich in calcium, phosphorus and fluorine. It is made from finely ground veal and young beef bones and sold as a powder or in tablet form. Apples, celery and carrots clean as well as strengthen teeth. The enemies of good teeth are sugar and white flour. Bacteria thrive on them and decay can start almost at once unless food particles are cleaned away.

The colour of teeth can be deceptive. Very white teeth are not necessarily the healthiest. The whiteness may indicate that they are covered with soft porous enamel, which is thick and transparent. Usually hard enamel is thin and clear showing the yellowish-white dentine underneath. It is impossible to get teeth with this hard enamel coating completely white; all abrasive tooth powders do is to scratch the enamel surface and cause cavities.

DECAY AND DISEASE: Before the age of thirty-five the greatest cause of tooth loss is decay and resulting cavities. After thirty-five the chief culprit is periodontal disease which infects the gums and erodes the supportive tissue and bone structures. Infection can also be carried to other parts of the body and cause trouble. In most cases, periodontal disease can be stopped and prevented. It is a question of controlling plaque, the main cause of both decay and gum disease. Plaque is a mixture of bacteria, saliva and food residue which adheres to the tooth. It is colourless, transparent, invisible. Even very white teeth can be coated with plaque. It settles in the spaces between teeth and around the necks of teeth along the gum line. After twenty-four hours it produces acids which attack the enamel, initiating decay and also providing the perfect environment for the formation of tartar – a rough, hard formation which requires professional treatment for removal.

Unless plaque is removed daily through brushing and flossing it can cause inflammation of the gum tissues, known as gingivitis. The build-up is progressive – gums become inflamed, they bleed, ulcers flare up and the gums begin to recede. At this stage, it can be cured, but if left untreated, it can progress to pyorrhoea (or periodontitis). The teeth become loose as the gums shrink and infection spreads to the underlying bones. This is very serious but surgical procedures by a periodontist may help if the disease is not too far advanced.

Mouth and gums give clear warnings of the disease and the main symptoms are: red, swollen and itchy gums that often bleed, bad breath, pain and pressure between teeth after eating.

HOME-CARE: Normal routine brushing misses 80% of the plaque. If you don't believe it, check by using a disclosing tablet: after you've brushed put one in your mouth and wait until it has dissolved completely. Then look closely in the mirror – the areas where plaque and food debris still remain will show up bright red or purple. There is also a disclosing solution that can be applied to the mouth before brushing. This stains the plaque and so you know where to brush, taking the colour away at the same time. When brushing check these points:

Toothbrushes – should have soft thin bristles with flexible filaments, rounded at the ends, not jagged. Nylon is good because you can change the texture by putting the brush into cold water to make it firmer, into hot to make it softer. A toothbrush should be replaced every three or four months. Electric toothbrushes do not necessarily do a better job. When brushing, angle bristles towards gums, brushing in the direction the tooth grows, downwards for the upper teeth, upwards for the lower teeth, and wiggle the brush around the gum line. A good way is to loosen up plaque first with just the brush, then add toothpaste for polishing. It should take between two and five minutes.

Dental floss – designed to clean between the teeth and under the gums where a toothbrush cannot reach. It should be done once a day, preferably at night and before brushing. It requires a degree of manual dexterity: take a good length, at least a foot (300 mm.), wrap it around the index finger of both hands, winding it from one finger to the other as you need a fresh section, keeping the floss taut. After gently working between teeth, slide it under the gums and scrape the side of the tooth towards the biting surface. Unwaxed floss is usually better.

Watersprays – useful in mouths where bands or extensive fixed bridgework are secured, they clean out debris and help to flush away plaque.

Mouthwashes – dentists warn of overuse of commercial ones, particularly those to freshen breath, as they can disturb the natural flora. An oxidant such as hydrogen peroxide can be used regularly: it kills bacteria and strengthens gums. A good natural mouthwash is a peppermint tea infusion or a mixture of equal proportions of rosemary, anise and mint leaves steeped for half an hour. Parsley and watercress alleviate the bad breath caused by eating over-spiced food.

PROFESSIONAL CARE: Dentistry is now subdivided: a regular dentist does the repair work and cosmetic alterations. The endodontist treats root canal problems. The orthodontist is a dentist who has been trained to consider the good function, balance and alignment of the teeth; he may never do a filling, but his work may eliminate the need for cosmetic dentistry later on. He is concerned with the health of the mouth, gum and bone condition. The hygienist does routine cleaning and scaling: an ultrasonic cleaning device is used with vibrations so fast you don't feel a thing. By gently stroking beneath the gum edge and down the tooth, every particle of plaque is removed.

Everyone should have a clean and a check-up every six months. Cavities should be filled as early as possible but often you cannot see or feel early cavities on your own. Drilling and filling should not hurt at all. Most dentists apply a topical anaesthetic (sometimes a tranquillizing injection beforehand) and then inject a novocain-like liquid into the gum. If enough time is left between the local pain killer and the injection you should not even feel the needle.

Some cavities need root canal work: infection is cleaned out and the area sterilized, then filled with silver or rubber-like materials. Sometimes a post is inserted in the root so a porcelain cap can be attached on the top. There are many filling preparations so like natural enamel that they no longer show. Silver amalgams are still used for back teeth for resistance reasons and there is nothing better than gold for a really big filling.

COSMETIC DENTISTRY: A denture is an unsatisfactory substitute for teeth and cosmetic dentistry can radically change what nature or neglect created. Permanent crowns and bridges look like natural teeth, including the slight imperfections and variations of colour. Porcelain is usually more effective than plastic and is fused onto a strengthening metal, normally a mixture of an amalgam and gold.

Having a tooth capped means first grinding it down to a pointed peg and a temporary plastic jacket being cemented over it. An impression is made, and the permanent crown is cemented in place on the following visit. If teeth are missing, a fixed bridge can be made, attached to neighbouring teeth which either have to be capped or pinned with metal points to base the bridge. The life of the crown or bridgework cannot be guaranteed as the tendency of the gum is to recede as you get older, necessitating additional work at a later date. A minimum of four to five years can be expected, ten is reasonable, and many caps have been known to last much longer.

An alternative to capping a chipped, cracked or broken tooth is to adhere a special malleable resin to the damaged spot; this blends in with the colour and texture of the natural tooth. These resins are also used as a protective coating for eroded areas near the gum line.

Sometimes removable bridges need to be constructed and these have precision attachments as fine as jewellery. They don't look like false teeth and only need to be taken out for cleaning.

Implants are not always one hundred per cent successful. Natural ones, such as resetting a tooth knocked out but still intact in itself, last only about five years as the jawbone usually invades the weakened root area and kills the tooth. Artificial implants involve securing a steel base or post to the jawbone, then capping it with porcelain or plastic. Individual reaction determines their lasting power.

Another cosmetic technique is contouring where teeth are shaped to give the illusion of regularity without altering the basic structure. Bonding is the process that puts a white veneer over teeth to mask any discoloration and pitting. It also helps to prevent decay.

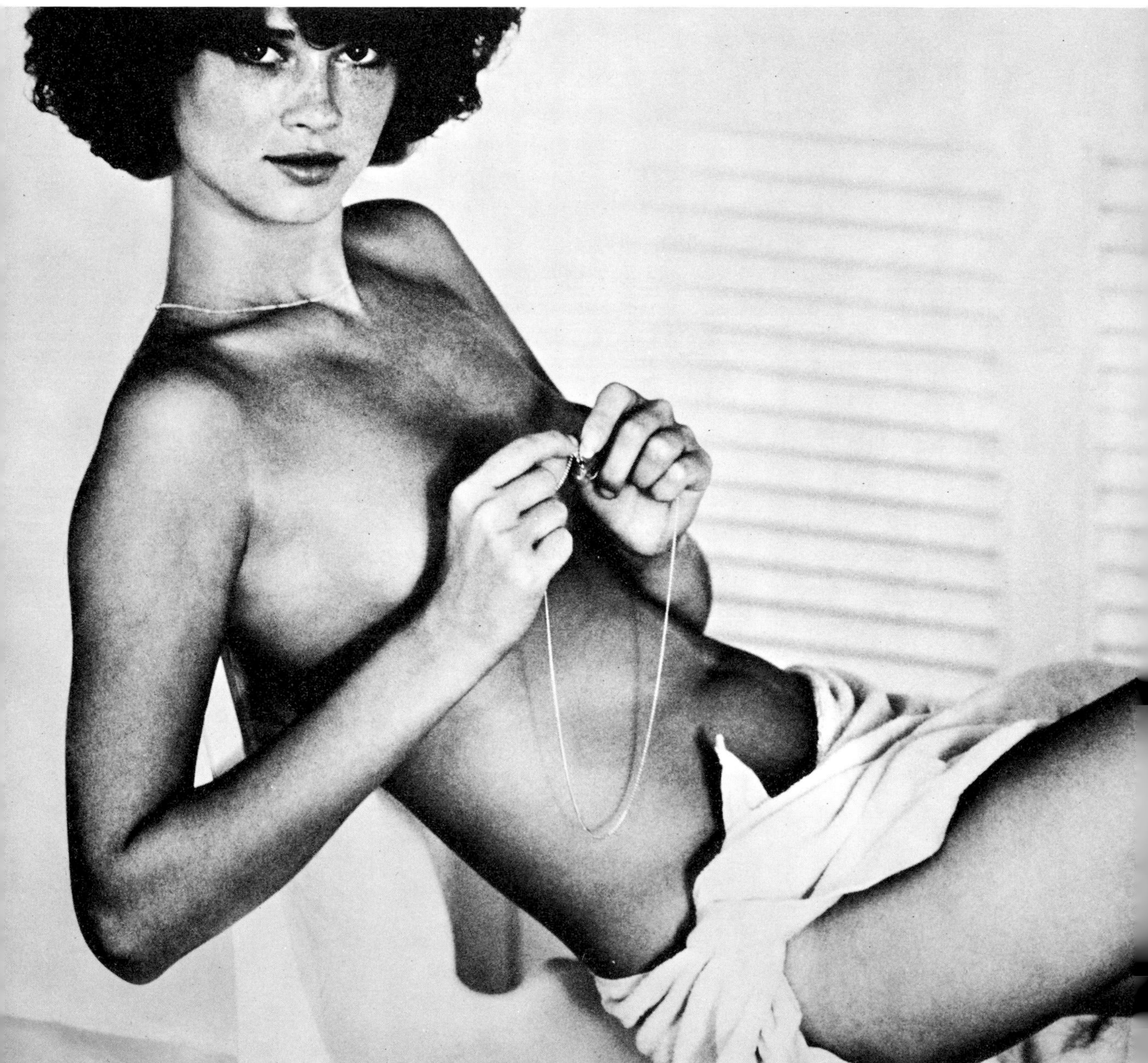

MCCABE

8

LIMBS

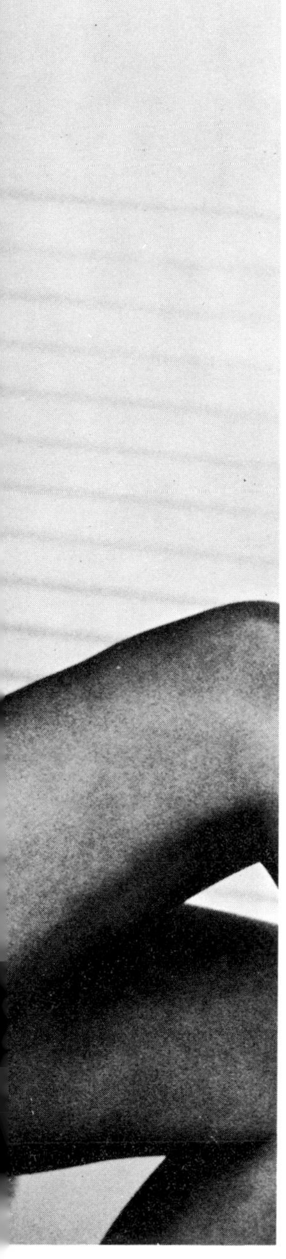

ARMS

Changing the shape of arms is very difficult. Though slender arms are desirable, skinny ones are not – but to put flesh on the arm is almost impossible unless combined with an overall weight increase. There is a tendency for the upper arm to be flabby, particularly noticeable as one gets older, and this is usually due to poor muscle tone. Also upper arms can get a mottled look because of sluggish circulation. Daily exercises can help both conditions – see below for illustrated details. If upper-arm flab is really excessive and hangs down, in some cases it can be corrected by plastic surgery. This is often necessary when considerable weight loss results in loose skin, as there is no other way to eliminate it.

Arms need moisturizing and massaging just like any other part of the body. When applying lotion, use the entire palm with strong upward motions that start at the wrist and go all the way to the shoulder. Don't forget the elbows and try not to lean on them as this causes a rough and bumpy surface – rub the lotion in with circular movements. If elbows are badly ingrained with dirt, use a deep cleansing cream or rub with lemon; if rough, try first kneading in an oatmeal-and-water paste, which is also a marvellous cleanser. All arms have hair; unless it is particularly heavy, it is best to leave it. If it is very dark, bleach first before thinking of removal. If it really bothers you, never shave – use other methods of depilation.

ARM EXERCISES

Four good exercises to help improve muscle tone and circulation of the upper arm. They should be done daily; a little constant exercise produces better results than a lot once a week. It is not necessary to do all, choose just two, if you prefer.

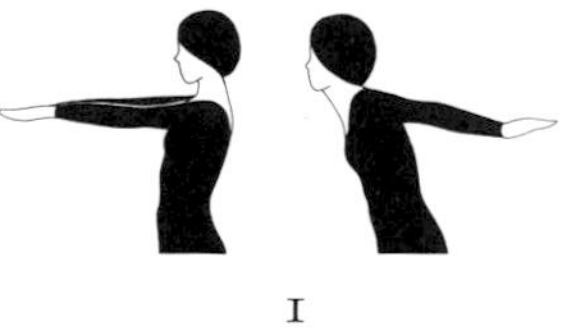
1

1. *Arm circle:* Stand with feet a little apart, stretch both arms out in front, holding them at shoulder level with palms turned down. Swing arms backwards trying to keep them high all the time, and at the back push hard until fingertips touch. Repeat a minimum of 6 times.

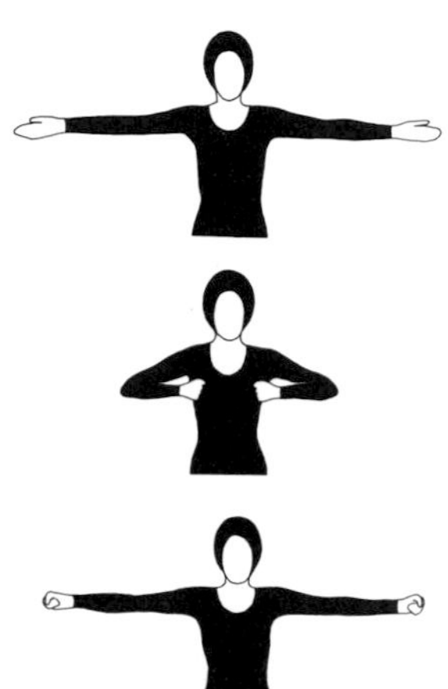
2

2. *Shoulder bounce:* Stand, feet apart, raise arms straight out at sides to shoulder height, palms facing front. Clench fists. Draw fists to touch shoulders above bosom, imagining you have a force resisting this movement. Push hard as though you were squeezing the sides of the bust together. Bounce fists twice in this position; extend arms slowly to starting position. Repeat a minimum of 6 times.

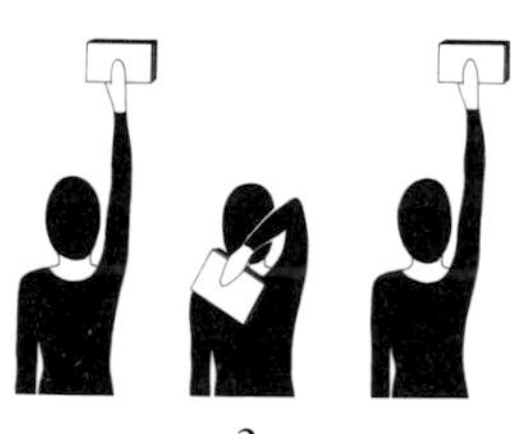
3

3. *Weight lift:* Use a weight of about 3 lbs – dumb-bell, weight-sack, book – grasp firmly in hand and raise arm above the head, keeping it straight with elbow close to head; keep back straight too. Bend elbow and lower weight backwards to touch back of opposite shoulder. Raise arm up again. Repeat 10 times for each arm, slowly, firmly. Work up to 20 times.

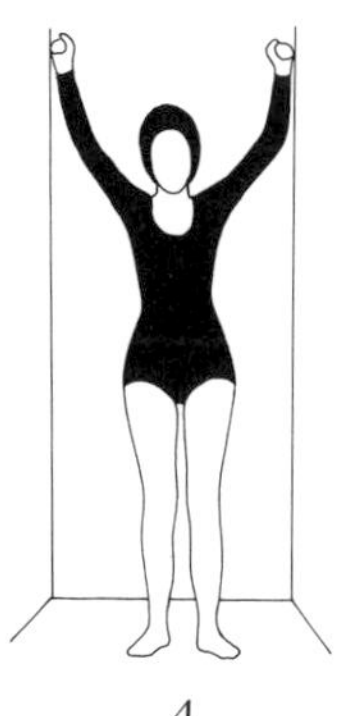
4

4. This is an isometric exercise, where action presents resistance to movement. Stand in a doorway, feet a little apart; make fists of hands and raise arms in a triangular position to rest fists against door-frame – palms facing forwards. Breathe in deeply and try to push out the door-frame. Push, counting to 3, relax. Start with 3 pushes and work up to 5.

HANDS

There are twenty-eight bones in the hand and the wrist, all finely balanced to give remarkable mobility. The skin on the back of the hand is fine and soft, with numerous sebaceous glands (those that produce oily sebum to protect the skin) and sweat gland openings. The palm of the hand is coarser and tougher: well supplied with sweat glands, but unlike most other parts of the body, it has no sebaceous glands. This means that it is one of the dryest parts of the body.

A hand can show age faster than any other area – a face can be lifted, a hand can not. Liquid silicone has been tried for 'plumping up' hands, but its transient properties proved dangerous. Therefore, prevention through care is essential. First, water is fatal to hands; detergents and household cleaning agents are destructive. Exposure to elements – sun, cold, wet, sea, earth – takes its toll. Protection and care are a daily concern.

Some points to remember:

Wear rubber gloves for all wet work; cotton-lined are the best to absorb excess moisture. Wear heavy fabric gloves for gardening, cotton gloves for housework, gloves outdoors when it is cold or raining – or snowing.

Every time your hands get wet, dry them well and smooth on hand lotion.

Wash hands thoroughly several times a day with a mild soap, run clean water over them before patting dry, cream; at least once daily scrub fingers and nails with a firm brush.

A smooth pumice stone used with soap and water removes stains and rough skin.

Once a week massage (twice if time) with a rich lubricating cream; begin at finger tips and work firmly down each finger, then over the palms and backs; a good time to do this is before going to bed.

When you can, wear cotton gloves overnight – put on over a layer of hand cream or petroleum jelly.

First aid treatment: a sheath of warm paraffin wax which opens pores, removes toxins, and cleanses.

A lemon will clean and bleach fingers; cream afterwards, as the juice is drying.

A masque – the same as the one you use on your face – will cleanse and tone hands.

Warmed oil – preferably olive or almond – is the best handbath for dryness; soak once a week for half an hour – marvellous for nails too.

Rinsing in a mild vinegar-water solution after washing will protect hands against drying, chapping, and other irritations.

There are certain conditions that need special care:

Brown spots: The development of these so-called 'age-spots' can be retarded and in many cases prevented by the use of a suncream. Existing spots can be partially bleached out with a de-pigmenting cream, or hidden with a waterproof cover-up make-up (good for hiding veins too); dermatologists can professionally lighten these spots and remove scaly bumps by therapies including cryotherapy and electrodesication.

Chilblains: Usually due to lack of finger activity and inadequate protection from the cold and damp. Exercise to stimulate circulation, massage fingers frequently and check you have enough calcium in your diet. Wear warm gloves.

Rough skin and cracks: Caused by cold weather, hard work and handling drying things. Remove dirt from cracks with lemon, then rub olive oil into cracks with absorbent cotton. Wash hands in warm soapy water, rinse with clear water. Follow with a massage using a really rich emollient hand cream. Do this daily. If cracks are bad, you must not allow air to get to them: seal by covering with adhesive tape or plaster, and only remove for cleansing and creaming. Even the most stubborn cracks will vanish this way.

Swollen knuckles: Could be due to a rheumatic or arthritic condition, in which case check your diet and see your doctor; can also be aggravated by over-exertion. Important to do finger and hand exercises and give hands a daily massage.

Tobacco and fruit stains: The most reliable stain removers are peroxide or lemon juice. Pressure is needed to remove the more stubborn marks, so use a pumice stone. Afterwards cream well, as both peroxide and lemon juice are very drying.

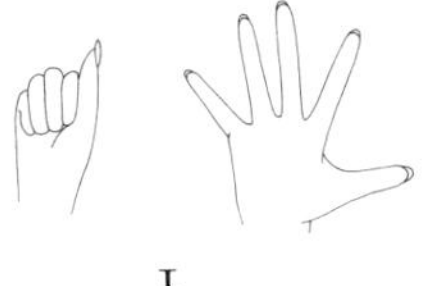

1

HAND AND FINGER EXERCISES

Exercises for hands to make them more flexible and graceful – and to aid circulation.

1. *Fist fling:* Clench the fist tightly, hold a second, throw open the fingers, forward and as wide as possible. Both hands at the same time, repeat 6 times.

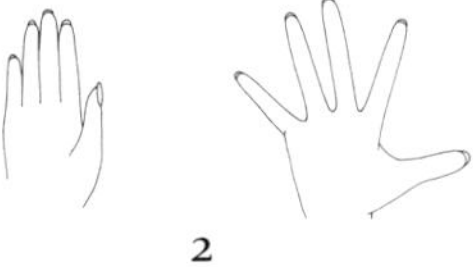

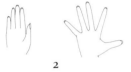

2

2. *Finger spread:* Put hands straight in front of you, palms down, fingers pressed tightly against each other; thrust fingers apart, opening to as wide a separation as possible. Repeat 6 times.

3. *Hand circles:* Be sure hands are limp and relaxed, then rotate them from the wrist in circles, first in one direction, then another – 10 in each direction.

4. *Vertical lift:* Holding hands gracefully, palms down, lift up slowly from the wrist, then move down. Keep the hand very relaxed, but not absolutely limp; 10 times.

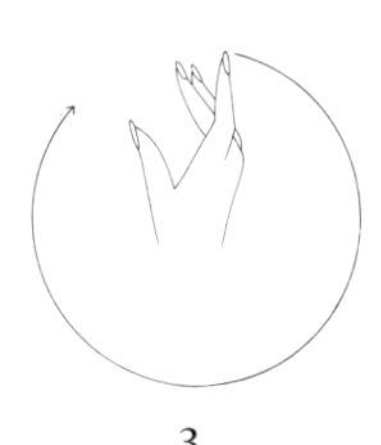

3

NAILS

Nails are horny extensions of the skin. The visible nail, that hard plate, is only about half. The other half is the matrix, invisible except for the uppermost tip which we recognize as the half-moon or lunula. The rest of the matrix is oval, rather like the nail itself, and extends down to the first joint. This is where the nail is formed, where the body turns protein plus a few trace elements into fingernails. Nails are composed of horizontal layers of keratin and how strong or brittle your nails are is partly a

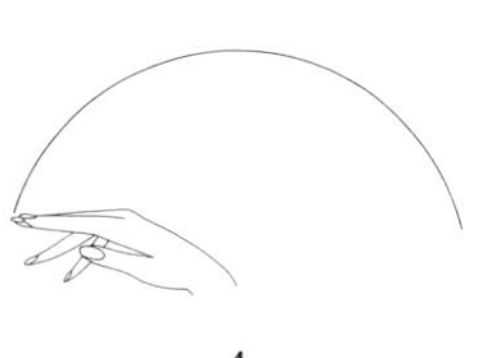

4

matter of inheritance, but nutrition is also important. A protein-high diet rich in iron, calcium, potassium, vitamin B, and iodine will help keep nails healthy. Foods such as yoghourt, celery, carrots, soya, eggs, and seafood are particularly good. Nails are good indicators of circulation: if you put pressure on the nail, watch how quickly the blood returns.

What causes irregularities? From time to time we all get a few ruts, bumps, and marks. Horizontal ridges, regular on all nails, denote a past illness – though if only on one nail, it means you've given it some rough treatment and possibly damaged the cuticle by using a sharp instrument. Good nail care will eliminate most horizontal ridges. Vertical lines tend to be hereditary and the older you get, the more they show; sometimes they indicate dryness. White spots can be a sign of disease or stress or caused by air pockets forming in the nail as it grows in which case they eventually grow out. Yellowing of the nails comes from smoking or medicines or because of nail polish pigment – that is why it is important to apply a base coat. Lack of care causes split or broken nails.

Nails grow at the rate of a quarter of an inch a month, so a new nail takes about four months to reach the tip from the cuticle. If you start helping your nails now, you can soon see the results. Nail growth varies with the individual: fastest in youth, decreasing with age. Pregnancy increases nail growth, so does warm weather, any activity of the fingers (like typing, piano-playing), and massage of the fingers towards the tips. Middle fingers grow fastest, and nails on the right hand (if you are right-handed), which indicates the greater the activity, the faster the growth.

Nails become brittle if they are exposed to extreme cold, too much sun, chlorine or cleaning chemicals. They become soft if you use too much soap and water. Cutting with scissors encourages splits and fractures. Nail polish is not harmful, it protects and strengthens as well as beautifies. A few women are allergic to nail enamel; for them there are formulas free of irritants. Nail polish remover, however, is very drying. To use neat acetone is false economy; even an oily remover should be used sparingly just once a week when you manicure. It is better to touch up polish when there's a chip rather than remove it every time. Cutting the cuticle is generally bad since it protects the nail base from infection – cuts in the cuticle, if too deep, can cause infection.

Basic rules for nail care:

Shape by filing with an emery board, safer and easier than a metal file.

File to an oval; filing to a point is asking for breakage. Don't file too deeply down the sides.

Keep cuticles soft by keeping them well moisturized; after applying hand lotion, gently push back softened cuticles with a towel or tissue as often as you can.

Problem nails need special care, but if you stick to the following guide lines, you may be amazed at the good results:

Keep hands out of water as much as possible; wear gloves; cream-clean hands instead of washing them several times a day.

Use cuticle cream at bedtime; get it to the root of the nail using an orange stick to gently lift the cuticle and put the cream underneath.

Once a week soak nails in olive oil, leave some on; wear gloves in bed.

When manicuring, use warm oil instead of soapy water, but go over nails again with remover before applying enamel or it will slither off.

Before applying polish, buff nails with paste or powder polish; this stimulates circulation and provides a smooth base for the enamel.

Avoid using metal manicure instruments: use emery boards for filing, orange sticks for lifting cuticles and cleansing nail tips.

Paint nails with white iodine before applying polish.

Try the gelatine cure – three level teaspoonfuls in cold fruit juice or dissolved in a cup of hot consommé; taken every day this should improve nails after two months. There is one snag: sometimes when the treatment is discontinued, nails once again become brittle, flake or break.

MANICURE

An expert, professional manicure is not difficult, and done slowly, methodically, and regularly, will result in good-looking, immaculate nails. You need one every week to keep nail shape and cuticles in trim. A professional manicurist spends about half an hour on the job – you will need longer, about forty-five minutes, and if you do it with your legs resting and raised your feet will benefit too.

Equipment:

Basics – towel, absorbent cotton, bristle nail brush, dish of warm soapy water (no detergent, but a shampoo, or a bath product).

Tools – emery board, nail clippers, cuticle clippers, orange sticks, nail buffer.

Creams – hand lotion, cuticle-remover cream or oil, cuticle massage cream or any rich emollient cream, buffing paste – tinted or clear.

Nail Cosmetics – oily polish remover, white nail pencil, base coat, nail enamel, top sealer, nail patch paper and fixative.

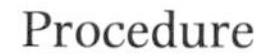

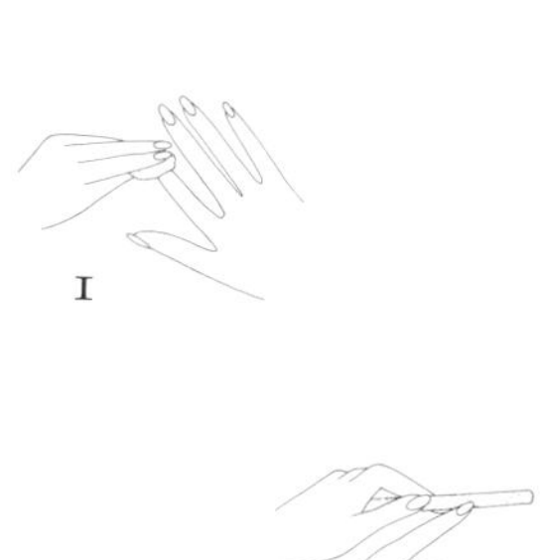

1

2

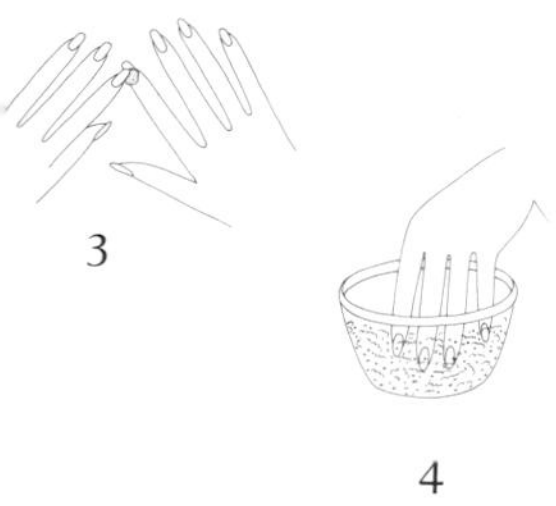

3

4

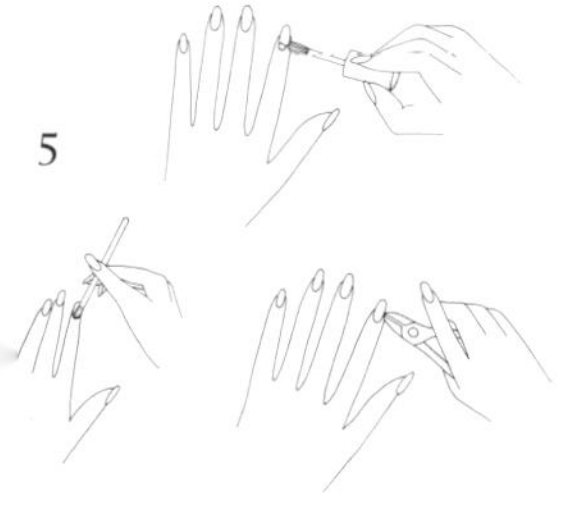

5

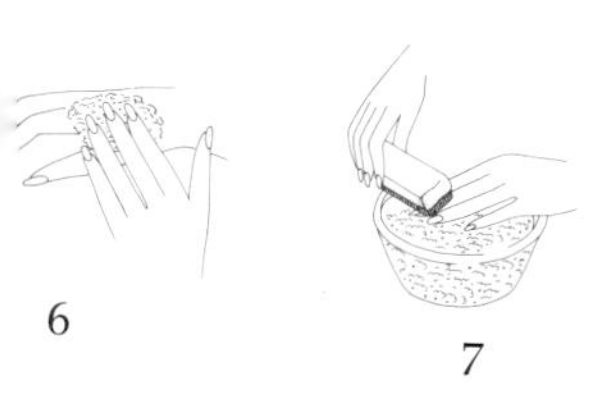

6

7

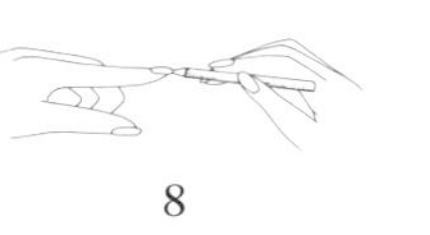

8

Procedure:

1. Remove old nail varnish: wet cotton with oily remover and press it against nail for a second to pre-soften polish, wipe off slowly. A quick swish over is not enough; this press-then-wipe method cleans the varnish from under the cuticles as well.

2. Shape nails into an oval with an emery board, working with long strokes from side to centre. Don't saw, and never cut nails with scissors. If nail is damaged or much too long, use nail clippers to trim it straight across then smooth edge with emery board, leaving tip and sides straight if nail is short. The nail will grow out stronger in this squarish shape and can be rounded later. If nails are brittle, keep them short – just slightly longer than the finger is still long enough for elegance. Don't file too low at the corners; this weakens growth.

3. Massage nails with cuticle massage cream or any rich emollient; this stimulates nail base and helps loosen dry skin.

4. Soak nails in warm soapy water for ten minutes; if grimy and stained scrub gently with a bristle nail brush. After soaking, dry each nail in turn gently with a soft towel.

5. a) Apply cuticle remover or oil around the cuticle.

b) With an orange stick wrapped in cotton wool and kept moist by dipping in the soapy water, push back and carefully lift the cuticle away from the nail. Very gently; if pressure is too great, the matrix of the nail may be dented and the new nail will grow in ridges.

c) If there are still loose pieces of dead skin or cuticle, clip neatly with cuticle shears. Do not clip the entire cuticle; too much trimming should be avoided, as it makes the cuticle tough and encourages it to grow back stronger. If stains have got under, or down the side of, the nail, dip cotton-wrapped orange stick into peroxide and rub them away.

6. Apply hand lotion and massage hands and fingers; during massage give the fingers a good pull from their joints.

7. Dip fingertips back into the water and wash and scrub away the left-over bits of skin. Remove all traces of grease from the nail area.

8. If tips of nails need whitening, run a white nail pencil under them.

9. If you are going to buff your nails, or if you have splits or breaks that need mending (for details see below), now's the time to do it. Buffing is one of the best treatments for nails, either as a pre-polish reviver to stir up blood circulation, or as a polish in itself. Dab buffing paste on nails and buff gently in one direction only with a nail buffer or a soft chamois

cloth. Continue for about one minute a nail. For a pink shine, use a tinted paste. If you are buffing for circulation before applying polish don't use the cream.

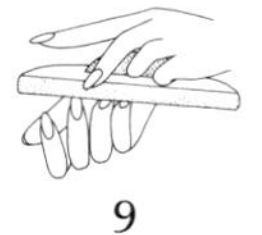
9

10. Apply varnish. With all applications try to do it in three straight strong strokes: one down the middle, one either side. A base coat gives a smoother surface and prevents colour pigment from discolouring the nail. The enamel strengthens as well as colours; the number of coats is up to you – two is a minimum, while top manicurists recommend four. The top coat or sealer helps protect the nail and guards against chipping. In addition to covering the surface of the nail, brush across the top edge and behind it. Colour tricks with polish: minimize the look of large hands by polishing the entire nail; cover all the nail if it is short or small; lengthen short fingers and make wide nails appear narrower by applying polish down the centre only, leaving sides bare; pale shades are best on short nails or stubby hands; dark shades give hands a delicate look; apricot, golden reds, and pink flatter a tan.

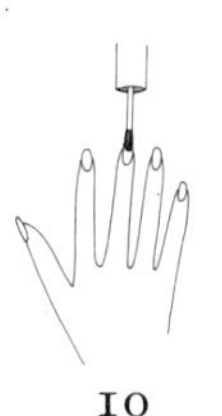
10

11. For a neat finish, run an orange stick tipped with cotton and dampened with polish remover along the outside edge of the cuticle and finger tip, to remove any smudges of polish.

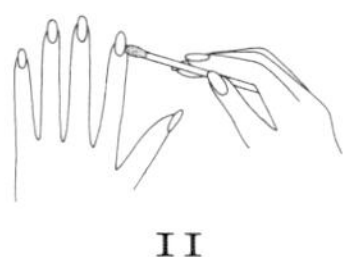
11

Patching:
If a nail splits or tears, it is often not necessary to clip it down – sometimes if the rip is deep, it can be both painful and ugly, as well as inviting infection. It can be temporarily patched until it grows out. There's a knack to doing this and it takes time to learn, but you can make a patch smooth enough to be invisible under any nail enamel:

1. With cotton dampened in remover, take away all traces of polish, oil or cream from nail.
2. Tear off a patch of nail paper – slightly larger than the area to be covered. Don't cut, the ragged edge blends more easily with the nail surface and resists peeling off.
3. Brush over patch with the fixative; lift it with tweezers or brush onto the nail. The jagged edge should face the base of the nail, and there must be a flap-over long enough to fold under the nail tip.
4. Mould the patch to the nail with a cotton-wrapped orange stick dipped in remover. Tuck extension under nail tip; be sure edges blend on the surface and excess glue is removed; check to see there are no air bubbles between patch and nail.
5. Cover first with base coat, then layers of polish and finally sealer. A patch should last through two polish changes, if you treat it with care.

Protective Patching:
The same principle can be applied to problem nails to protect them during regrowth. On each nail apply a tissue patch at the top – a jagged edge at the bottom to mould onto the surface of the nail, an extension at the top to tuck under the tip. You might need a little extra glue under the tip to secure the paper. Cover with base coat, polish layers and sealer.

False Nails:
Only to be used in an emergency. There are two kinds – those you glue on, and those you build up with a kind of cosmetic cement. They can look very effective, but they are drying, not good for the nails, and can be detrimental to new growth.

LEGS

The length and basic shape of the leg is hereditary and cannot be altered . . . fat and cellulite are accumulated, and can be prevented or controlled. Most things that go wrong happen after maturity or because of complete neglect in the teenage years.

The leg is about one-third of body weight, but the ankle has to bear the entire weight of the body and is one of the strongest hinge joints we have. The knee-joint is the largest and has to support the largest, heaviest, strongest bone in the body: the thigh. The look of the thigh depends on the upper and lower sections of muscles and flesh which cover the bone. It is in this area that trouble starts, partly because most of us don't use it enough, and partly because it has a particularly thick layer of adipose tissue, just waiting to be filled out with stored-up fat. Only regular exercise and diet control can prevent, correct and maintain shape. What's wrong with most legs is simply that they are too fat above the knee. Swollen legs are another matter, for they retain too much fluid.

Legs by nature are rather dry – there are not enough active oil glands in the limbs to keep them smooth and gleaming. It is important to lubricate them with a body lotion or cream after every bath; more often in the summer when they are bare and drier because of exposure to sun and sea.

Legs grow hair. Though in some cultures it may be considered erotic to keep it on, from a beauty point of view, it is better off.

CELLULITE

Cellulite is ugly and it tends to accumulate on thighs, around the knees, on hips and buttocks. It is the result of abuse more than age. It can affect women of normal weight, indeed even thin women are often troubled by cellulite. It takes time to appear and a long time to repair. It is caused by bad circulation and retention of fluid, the latter being the reason why the skin looks puffy, dimpled and soggy. It is also a sign of lack of exercise and a diet too full of the sugar and starch carbohydrates. Some doctors believe it is caused by an excessive secretion of oestradiol (female hormone) and it would seem logical that there could be a counter-balancing treatment. But at present cellulite is helped only by physical means – self care and salon treatment. Try the following with daily regularity – the only way to get good results:

Diet: Cut back on fats, sugars and starches; concentrate on high protein meats, green leafy vegetables, salads and fruit. Eat plenty of cucumber, first and foremost a diuretic food which helps to firm tissues. Every day eat cucumber salad – finely sliced complete with skin, a little olive oil, garlic, lemon juice and parsley (to counteract the smell of garlic).

Exercise: Walking and swimming are ideal, so is bicycling whether the real thing or simulating the movement by lying on your back supporting hips with hands and cycling in the air. Walk around the house doing the goose-step – you'll feel the inner thigh muscle working hard to keep the leg in a straight line.

Applications: Anti-cellulite creams can be massaged into the skin (see below for method) but it is usually the movement more than the cream that aids the area. Ivy is an ingredient in many creams and when used on its own it has a noticeable effect on cellulite. Ground ivy can be crushed and rubbed into the skin or applied as a poultice. You can make a solution by steeping ivy in cold water for twenty-four hours and using it as a wash to bathe the dimpled areas repeatedly.

Friction: The idea is to improve circulation, stepping up the metabolism of the fat cells. Pinch flesh through a towel; slap area alternately with hot and cold sponges or cloths; rub with a loofah or a friction glove made of string, nylon, or rubber nodules; put rough kitchen salt on the glove and vibrate the flesh.

Massage: You must be careful not to over-massage and be too rough with your flesh; use an oil, emollient or cellulite cream, and always be sure movements go up in the direction of the heart, never down. Don't just rub; using both hands wring and twist the flab as though you were squeezing out water; then with fists, iron the flesh upwards. For legs, grasp one ankle with both hands, wring and twist up to knee. For inner thighs, knead, then iron out. For buttocks, stand sideways about four inches away from a wall; turning slightly hit first one side then the other.

Water: Any force of water against the flesh is good – a jet in a swimming pool, a strong shower faucet; contrasts of hot and cold water help – take a cold shower followed by a hot bath, or force alternate hot and cold blasts from the hand-shower on special areas; nightly warm baths with Epsom salts are recommended.

Treatments: Beauty specialists offer individual methods to get rid of cellulite – wax, mud, steam, water, electrical and enzyme treatments, usually followed by a massage. Aromatherapy also claims to have good results with cellulite. See also page 289.

THICK ANKLES

Some people have naturally fleshy or sturdy ankles and no amount of attention or exercise can alter them. In these cases the flesh, though ample, is usually firm. However, if flesh is flabby, it is caused by fluid retention on the same principle as the formation of cellulite, and the same rules apply for getting rid of it – diet, exercise, massage, treatments.

SWOLLEN ANKLES

The sort of swelling that is usually temporary and abnormal: to test, press a finger on the swollen area. If it leaves a dimple that slowly disappears, then it is a transient condition. Gravity causes the most simple form: blood and body fluids fighting against gravity to return to the heart from the lower body extremities. When you have been on your feet all day, some of the body fluid can seep into the tissue around the ankles and puff them up. If you are barefoot or wear open sandals the feet swell instead. This can be dealt with easily by resting the feet, raising them higher than the head, to help the fluid back into circulation and upwards. The swelling will go down but it can take more than an hour. The swelling caused by varicose veins is similar; this too can be helped by raising the feet, and support stockings are of value.

Another cause of ankle swelling – and one of the most common – is the shift in hormone balance which occurs in the premenstrual period and in pregnancy. Many women in their thirties and forties complain of swollen ankles the week before their period begins. Artificial increases in hormone levels cause fluid retention and for this reason some women are unable to tolerate birth control pills. Older women who take hormone pills may have the same trouble. To counteract swelling it is essential to minimize fluid retention. First, control salt intake; it is the high hormone level that causes the kidneys to hold salt in the body and retention of salt always causes retention of water. Second, eat foods that are diuretic;

green vegetables, fruits, and herbal teas all have diuretic properties – cucumber and artichoke are of particular value. Third, bathing the feet and ankles in Epsom salts can help, also ivy compresses.

SPIDER VEINS

Little clusters of veins can gather on thighs, behind knees and around the ankles. They may look unattractive but usually have no serious effect. Sometimes thread veins are controlled by hormones, which is why they can appear during pregnancy. You may get them if you take the Pill and other causes include alcoholism and cirrhosis of the liver, but in such cases they are accompanied by other symptoms. Tight girdles, garters, and boots don't cause vein trouble but it is not healthy to wear them all the time, nor constantly to have legs encased in synthetic fibre tights; legs need to breathe. Thread veins are really a cosmetic problem and can be concealed by leg make-up applied in upward strokes. They can be treated by injections of a chemical and although the veins will fade and usually disappear, bruise marks may show for a while. Surface veins can be prevented from spreading by an electrical treatment that coagulates the blood. The time required to clear up blemishes of this type depends on how long you have had them; a series of treatments is usually needed, and the blue-purple veins are easier to eliminate than the reddish spider ones.

VARICOSE VEINS

This is an ugly and potentially dangerous condition. Varicose veins are caused by malfunction of the blood vessels in the legs, and are very common among Western peoples. Great pressure is put on the leg veins, as they have to defy gravity when they take the blood up to the heart. Some veins cannot stand the strain. Veins are long, elastic-walled tubes with a one-way flow of blood controlled by valves. Sometimes the vein walls become flabby or the valves don't work well and instead of closing to prevent backflow, they relax, sag, and let some of the blood seep back where it promptly meets blood going in the other direction. This makes the elastic wall bulge and in time there is a permanent knotty bulge with twisted bluish veins. The causes of valvular inefficiency are not known exactly, but there is a hereditary factor. Overweight puts pressure on the veins, and in pregnancy hormones relax muscular strands in the vessel.

The varicose vein cannot cure itself. The condition is usually progressive and should be treated in the early stages, for it can get so bad that there are medical complications of thrombosis, eczema and ulceration. The most serious type of varicose vein is the post-thrombotic. It usually appears as a group of small veins around the ankles that cause swelling and produce brown pigmentation marks. If not treated, they can lead to ulceration.

Varicose veins can be treated by surgery or injection. The two methods are completely different and it is a personal and medical decision as to which is preferable. The most commonly affected vein is the great saphenous which travels from the foot up the inside of the leg to the groin: the short saphenous may be affected and this shows at the back of the leg. Surgery is successful in 95 per cent of cases. The operation is called 'stripping' and involves removing the whole vein from the leg. It is literally pulled out by a special instrument; incisions are made in two, sometimes four, places. Many surgeons prefer stripping in a downward direction as there is less risk of nerve damage in the ankle area. It is usually necessary to be in hospital for a week. A careful operation means that this particular vein will never cause trouble again but other veins may need treatment later on.

Injections are used for all types of veins, but it is not just a matter of injection. Treatment consists of injections plus bandaging plus exercise plus patience, and the whole procedure involves a minimum of six weeks before legs are cured. A sclerosing fluid is injected into the vein; this acts as an irritant, roughens the surface walls and encourages them to close up. Legs are then tightly bandaged from thigh to ankle. The fluid injected is of far less importance than careful diagnosis and the technique of compression bandaging. The injection simply initiates a chain of events that results in the vein emptying itself and fusing the two surfaces. It is most important that the bandages are not disturbed; you cannot take a bath, only shower with plastic bags protecting the bandages. It is essential to walk a minimum of a mile each day (some doctors say two miles). The injections and bandaging take less than an hour, but the subsequent care is considerable. The method has a high proportion of success; some brown pigmentation marks are often visible after the veins have fibrosed up but these can be covered by make-up.

Prevention, of course, is better than anything. If there is a family history of vulnerable veins, you should rest your legs often, wear support stockings, avoid standing for too long, and walk as much as you can every day. Watch your diet; obesity puts great strain on legs, and even a slim woman is less likely to develop varicose veins if she eats plenty of protein and cuts down on sugar and starches.

SCORCHED LEGS

Scorch marks are caused by sitting too near the fire. Once the skin has been damaged, it takes time for the marks to disappear. This is because the damage is usually below the top layer of skin which has to flake off before the scarred cells come to the surface – and they in turn flake off in the growth cycle. To help bleach the discoloration, try diluted peroxide in water. Keep legs moist by thoroughly creaming after bathing, particularly around the shin bone where there is a minimum of flesh.

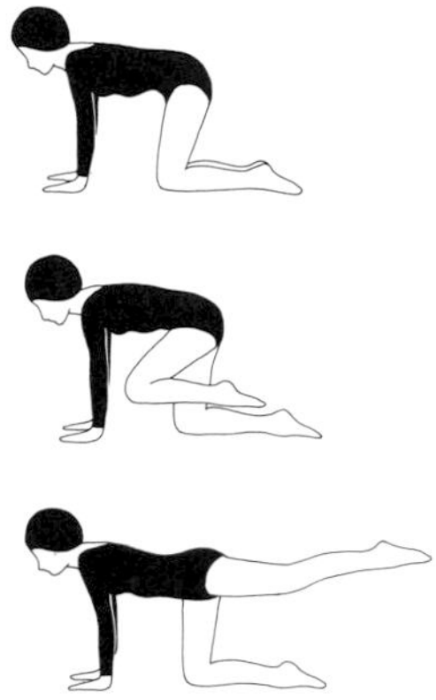

LEG EXERCISES

To keep legs in good shape and condition requires daily exercise. Here are four basic movements designed to trim and firm them. Do each a few times at first, and work up to twenty minutes for the group. This is the sort of attention legs ideally require; not only will shape improve, but health benefits by keeping circulation at an invigorating level.

1

1. *All-fours stretch:* (for thighs and buttocks). Position yourself on hands and knees with back straight, arms rigid; bend left knee forward and up to chest, then extend back, stretching in line with buttocks. Do 10 times without touching floor. Repeat with other leg.

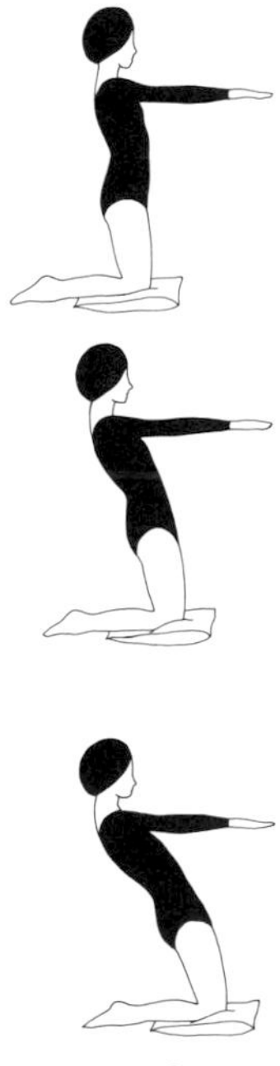

2. *Angled kneeling:* (for thighs and legs). Kneel on floor with back straight, arms at shoulder level; keeping body in a straight line with bottom tucked under and hips forward, slowly lean back as far as possible – without straining thighs, without collapsing. As thighs become stronger, you'll be able to go further back. Return to vertical position. Repeat 8 times.

3. *Knee bends:* (legs and thighs). Stand with feet a little apart, palms on thighs; raise toes, then bend knees pushing them outwards and lower the body to a crouching position, straighten legs, lower heels. Repeat at first 10 times and gradually work up to as many as possible.

4. *Knee bounce:* (for knees and calves). Sit on floor with legs spread in a wide V; bend knees slightly, drawing heels in towards you; stretch legs and bounce backs of knees on floor twice; bring legs together, straight in front, bounce knees on floor twice. Repeat 10 times.

2

FEET

Feet make our vertical posture possible. Much of the strength comes from the big toe, which is attached to a muscle centred across the shin; weight is absorbed by the arch. The true point of balance is in the ball of the foot, the exact position is individual. The way you place your feet and balance your body determines your standing and walking posture. This ideal point of balance can be found by standing barefoot, feet straight ahead about eight inches apart. Relax, hold arms loosely at sides, then keeping heels on the floor, sway gently. If you do not tense your body, it will steady itself at the correct balancing point for you. Concentrate on the spot, remember its exact position on the foot and from that moment on be conscious of using it. You'll be surprised how much lighter you feel.

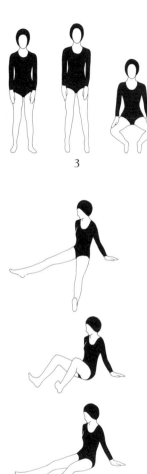

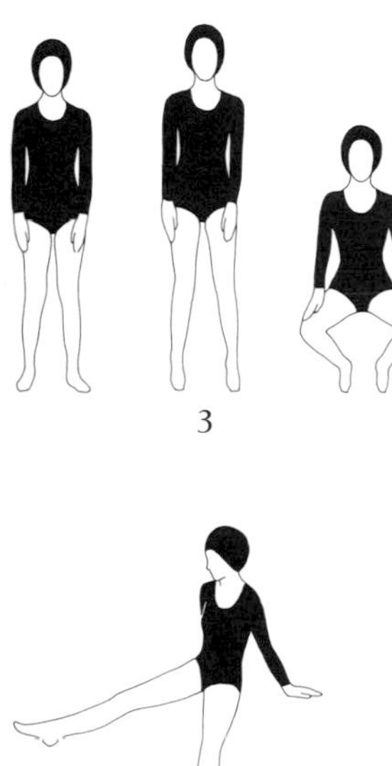

3

In the structure of the foot the order of importance is: muscles, bones, then skin, for it is in this order that feet deteriorate. There are twenty-six small, delicate bones in each foot, the highest concentration of bone in the body. There are also three to four times as many ligaments and muscles which bind the bones into place and give spring and elasticity to the foot. The arch, which has to bear the weight and provide the grace, is strictly not one arch but three, two being in the length of the foot and one across it.

The structure of the foot is very similar to that of the hand, but the toes lack the mobility of thumb and fingers. However, feet should not be so inactive and inert as they generally are. Feet with toes that are practically never used are feet with poor circulation and subsequent problems. Feet that are never exercised permit muscles to slacken so that they can no longer take the weight of the body, nor bind or support the bones as they should. This means that the bones, because they take too much wear and tear, get out of alignment, arches drop, bunions form and the skin gets rubbed so corns and callouses appear.

Ninety per cent of foot trouble is caused by wearing a shoe that is too small, too narrow, too pointed or too high. Limited width causes corns and bunions to build up in defence against pressure; any heel over two inches upsets the shock-absorbing function of the arch, causes headaches and backaches, and adversely affects leg muscles and posture.

Alternate heel heights during the day and from day to day. The lower the heel, the better the legs are exercised naturally, but as each heel height exercises muscles that others don't, vary them. Avoid wearing shoes that have no support, but wear sandals in warm weather – the thong type with low or no heels that permit the feet, particularly the toes, to straighten out without restriction.

4

Make sure shoes really fit. There should be a good pinch of leather between the outer and inner side of the shoe across the ball of the foot (usually the widest part), and no less than a quarter of an inch of space between the end of the big toe and the tip of the shoe. Never buy shoes with the idea of breaking them in. The best time to buy them is in the afternoon; feet are at their smallest in the morning and a shoe that might be fine at nine, is murder at four. Think of shoes like gloves and take them off when you get home.

Footcare: Daily attention goes a long way towards getting feet in better shape and they respond very readily to such consideration:

Scrub feet daily with a stiff bristle brush, toe by toe, arch, sole, heel.

Pumice any callouses or hard spots.

Massage feet often with a hand or body lotion, working around each toe, particularly the heel area.

Push back cuticles when you cream, just as you would for finger nails.

Powder feet, this helps absorb moisture.

Pamper feet with cologne before putting on shoes or stockings.

Give yourself a pedicure every ten days.

For dry sandpaper heels and soles try an overnight treatment of petroleum jelly rubbed well in then sealed in with cotton socks.

Protect sensitive areas by wrapping or covering with absorbent cotton.

For tired feet, give them an Epsom salts bath – two tablespoons of salt to a quart of lukewarm water; then immerse in cool water, rub with alcohol, moisturize with a cream, prop them up for twenty minutes.

Another tired feet remedy – plunge them into hot water softened with bath salts or oil, then put them into very cold water adding a little astringent.

A few drops of lavender oil in a tepid footbath will relieve fatigue.

Lemon juice softens skin and helps tired feet.

For sweaty feet, dab twice a day with surgical spirit, then powder – particularly in hot weather.

A foot soother: stir one teaspoon of malt vinegar into a small carton of natural yoghourt (enough for three applications but keep in fridge); brush on mixture then rub over feet, between toes; leave on for five minutes and rinse away with warm water; the vinegar works on the dead skin and rough patches, the yoghourt softens hard skin and cools it.

Blisters are helped by sprinkling on cornflour.

Go barefoot whenever possible – on sand, grass, carpets; feet need air and freedom.

Check stockings: if they are too tight or too short they can lead to foot problems in the same way as shoes do.

Feet need vitamin D to help maintain bones – and the sun is a good source.

Feet that hurt should be taken to a chiropodist for treatment; even a simple corn should be professionally attended to.

CORNS

Corns are formed because of pressure or friction from footwear. They are really the foot's protection, with the body trying to form a thickened layer of skin to buffer and pad the foot. They are built up of hard dead skin, cone-shaped, with the point facing inwards and known as the eye. When this presses on a nerve, it can be very painful. Corns usually appear on the joints of toes; quite common is a hammer toe, where the second toe (often the longest) becomes bent at its two joints and forms corns over the bends. Corns also appear on the under surface of the foot, caused by unevenness of the sole of the shoe. When corns are between toes, they are moist and are known as soft corns.

The way to get rid of corns is to have them professionally removed. In the meantime, relief may be obtained by bathing your feet in hot salt water for a quarter of an hour, then wearing a ring of felt around the corn to free it from pressure. It is unwise to use a knife, scissors or razor blade to reduce the corn yourself; you could set up an infection.

BUNIONS

A bunion is found over the joint at the base of the big toe; it is a thickening of the skin at the head of the metatarsal bone and forms a painful lump at the side of the foot. It is started in many ways – short shoes, narrow shoes, tight stockings. Particularly significant is the slackening of muscles around the centre of the foot and lack of activity in the big toe joint, which consequently becomes stiff and rigid. At the first sign of a bunion, see a specialist, do foot and toe movements and wear a pad of lint or rubber for protection. If the joint becomes really angled with the built-up bunion, surgery may be the only answer, because although the bunion is hardened skin to an extent, it is basically bone growth. An incision is made along the joint of the big toe to a point just beyond the widest point of the bunion. The part of the bone forming the bunion is removed. The operation requires a week in hospital and the immediate after-effects can be painful, particularly at first attempts to walk. Stitches are removed after two weeks but it is six weeks before normal shoes can be worn.

CALLOUSES

Caused by friction from badly fitting shoes, a callous is an area of flattened hard skin. It is less painful than a corn because it has no pointed root, but it can cause a very unpleasant burning sensation. It is better to have it removed by an expert, but you can help by rubbing the area with a pumice stone or friction pad, afterwards creaming well.

VERRUCAS

These are warts, caused by a virus picked up by bare feet. Because they grow inwards, they can be painful. Sometimes they appear singly, sometimes in clusters. If the spot is relieved by a hollow ring of felt, the infection will often clear up. Otherwise go to a chiropodist who will get rid of the virus as well as removing the verruca. There are four methods of removal: acid pastes or liquids, an electrical treatment, freezing, or surgery if the wart goes very deep.

ATHLETE'S FOOT

This is a fungal infection, so-called because at one time only athletes ran the risk of catching it by going barefoot in gyms and swimming pools. It thrives in warm, damp skin, spreads easily and is highly contagious. A kind of ringworm, it can appear between toes and on the soles of the feet. Symptoms include an itchy rash, splitting and peeling of the skin between the toes, and blisters under the toes.

Prevention is not easy: wash feet after walking around a pool, drying them thoroughly, particularly between the toes. Keep feet as dry as possible at all times, and free them from moisture-holding stockings and shoes. There are a number of preparations in both liquid and powder form for dealing with this problem, but should it persist, get professional help. Treatment is effective within two weeks.

NAIL INFECTION

The most common foot infection is one that attacks the nails. It is called onychomicosis and is caused by a fungus that makes the nail discolour and thicken to such a degree that it is impossible to cut or clip it. It is not necessarily painful, but looks dreadful, and can cause a corn or sore if it presses against an adjoining toe. The big toe nail is most affected. The fungus is infectious and flourishes in warm, damp conditions. Treatment consists of paring and filing away the thickened nail so that a liquid can be painted on the soft surface underneath to kill the fungus. This may have to be done over some weeks, but it only takes a few minutes. Sometimes the whole nail must grow out before it is completely healthy again.

INGROWING TOE NAIL

This can be terribly painful as the sides of the nail are forced into the skin. It is caused either by incorrectly cutting the nail (down the sides instead of straight across) or by wearing shoes that are too tight or shallow. At the beginning seek expert advice; the longer it is left or mismanaged, the more difficult to cure. Some toe nails remain problems for life simply because they were not taken in hand early enough. Feet can be poisoned easily, so don't risk inflammation or the chance of dye from stockings or shoes getting into the bloodstream via a nail cutting into the flesh.

FOOT AND TOE EXERCISES

Feet get little opportunity to exercise freely; here are four exercises that should be a daily routine – to be done barefoot:

1. *Joint stretch:* Stand and take weight on one foot, raise heel of the other foot and bend the toe joints at right angles to the rest of the sole; hold to the count of 2; then balance the foot on tip toe, to the count of 2; return to bent position and finally to floor. Repeat 6 times for each foot.

2. *Muscle toner:* Standing on a book or a step, let toes hang over the edge; then bend them firmly downwards, hold to count of 2; pull them strongly upwards, hold to count of 2. Repeat 10 times.

3. *Toe control:* Sit or lie with legs straight in front, hold feet up and try to spread out toes as you would fingers; then try to work each toe up and down individually. Repeat 10 times. (At first you will find it almost impossible to do this exercise, and it helps at the beginning to hold four toes and let the free one work individually. Start doing it in the bath, when foot circulation is usually at its peak.)

4. *Foot circles:* Sit or lie with legs stretched out in front, knees braced. Make wide circles outward, arching the foot. Do 10 times. Repeat, making inward circles. (Particularly good for strengthening and trimming the ankles, as well as helping to improve the shape of the foot.)

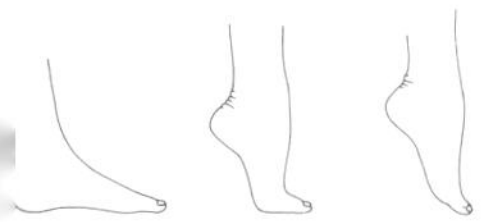

1 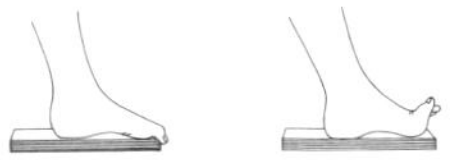 2 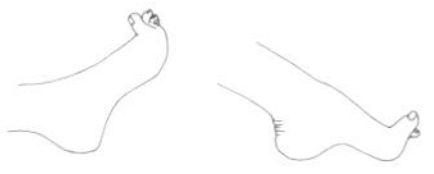 3 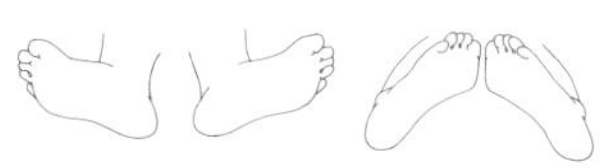 4

PEDICURE

You need a pedicure every ten days and it takes about forty-five minutes.

Equipment:

Basics – towel, absorbent cotton, bristle nail brush, pumice stone or friction block, large bowl of soapy water (bath oil or foam is preferable).

Tools – emery board, nail clippers, cuticle clippers, orange sticks, nail buffer, foot scraper.

Creams – hand or body lotion, cuticle-remover cream or oil, buffing paste, tinted or clear.

Nail cosmetics – oily polish remover, base coat, nail enamel, top sealer.

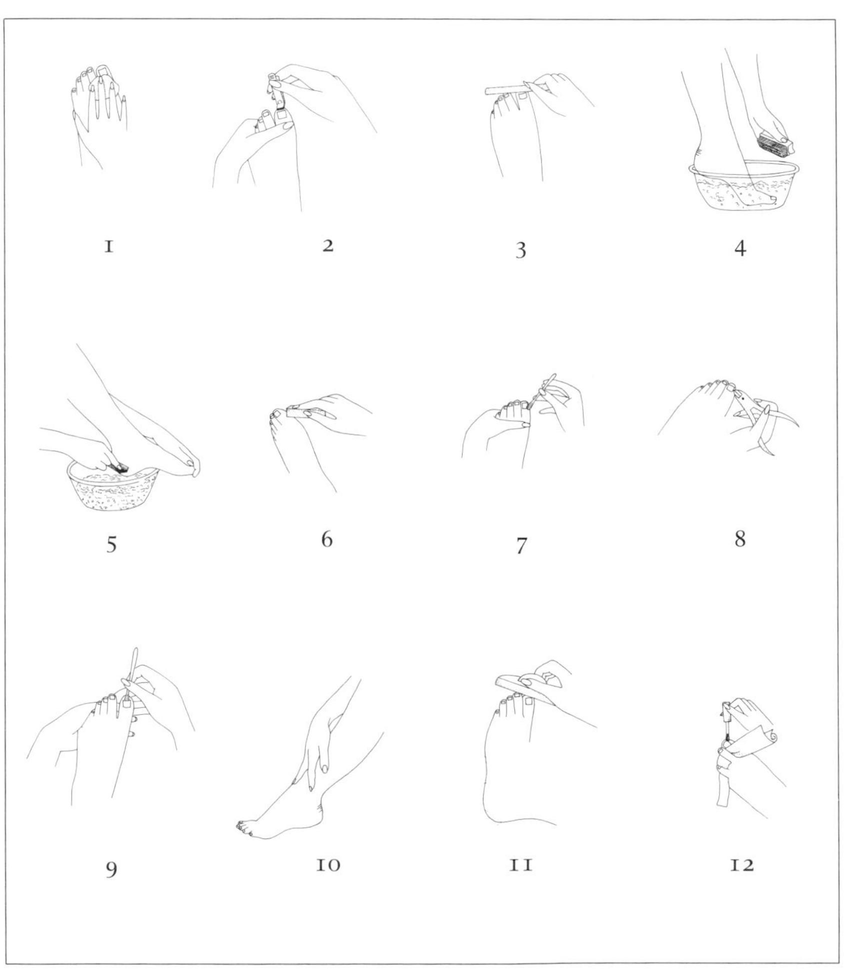

Procedure:

1. Remove old varnish by pressing cotton soaked in oily remover against nail, then wiping off.
2. Clip nails straight across, neat and square, using nail clippers, never scissors. It is particularly important to keep toe nails straight even if long, to prevent the possibility of an ingrowing nail.
3. File nails smooth but not to a shape; keep straight and square line; no sawing back and forth.
4. Soak feet in sudsy water for a good ten minutes; scrub feet with a bristle brush – across the toes, the heel, the underside of the foot.
5. Use a pumice stone or friction pad on the really dry rough spots, on any calloused area too. If there is a lot of flaky dry skin, this can be scraped away with a bladed foot-scraper, but be careful to use this gently. It's easy to nick the skin – short swift movements are the best. Put feet back in the water to brush away remaining shreds of skin.
6. Clean under the nails and down the sides with a cotton-wrapped orange stick dipped in the suds. If nails are stained, dip stick into peroxide and try to rub away. Stains, however, may be due to infection, not dirt.
7. Apply cuticle-remover cream or oil around the cuticles, massage gently and with an orange stick-plus-cotton push gently back.
8. If there are stubborn strands of skin – they often appear at the side of the big toe – that do not break away with the cuticle cream and massaging, clip with cuticle shears to neaten edge. Don't clip the entire cuticle, only the straggly ends.
9. Check toe joints to see if hard skin is beginning to build up, if so gently file down with a pumice stone or a sandpaper stick.
10. After dipping again in the water to get rid of the last bit of skin or dirt, towel dry, then massage in body lotion – over the foot and lower leg with firm upward strokes; massage each toe individually.
11. Buff nails to aid circulation – in one direction only otherwise the nail becomes too heated. One minute a nail is adequate. If you are not going to use polish afterwards, a tinted paste gives a coloured sheen – just cream it on before buffing.
12. Apply polish as for manicure but before doing so, separate toes with wads of cotton or a strip of tissue. This prevents polish smudging from one toe to another. After base coat, apply two colour coats, then a sealer. Clean away any smudge marks with a cotton-tipped orange stick dipped in polish remover.

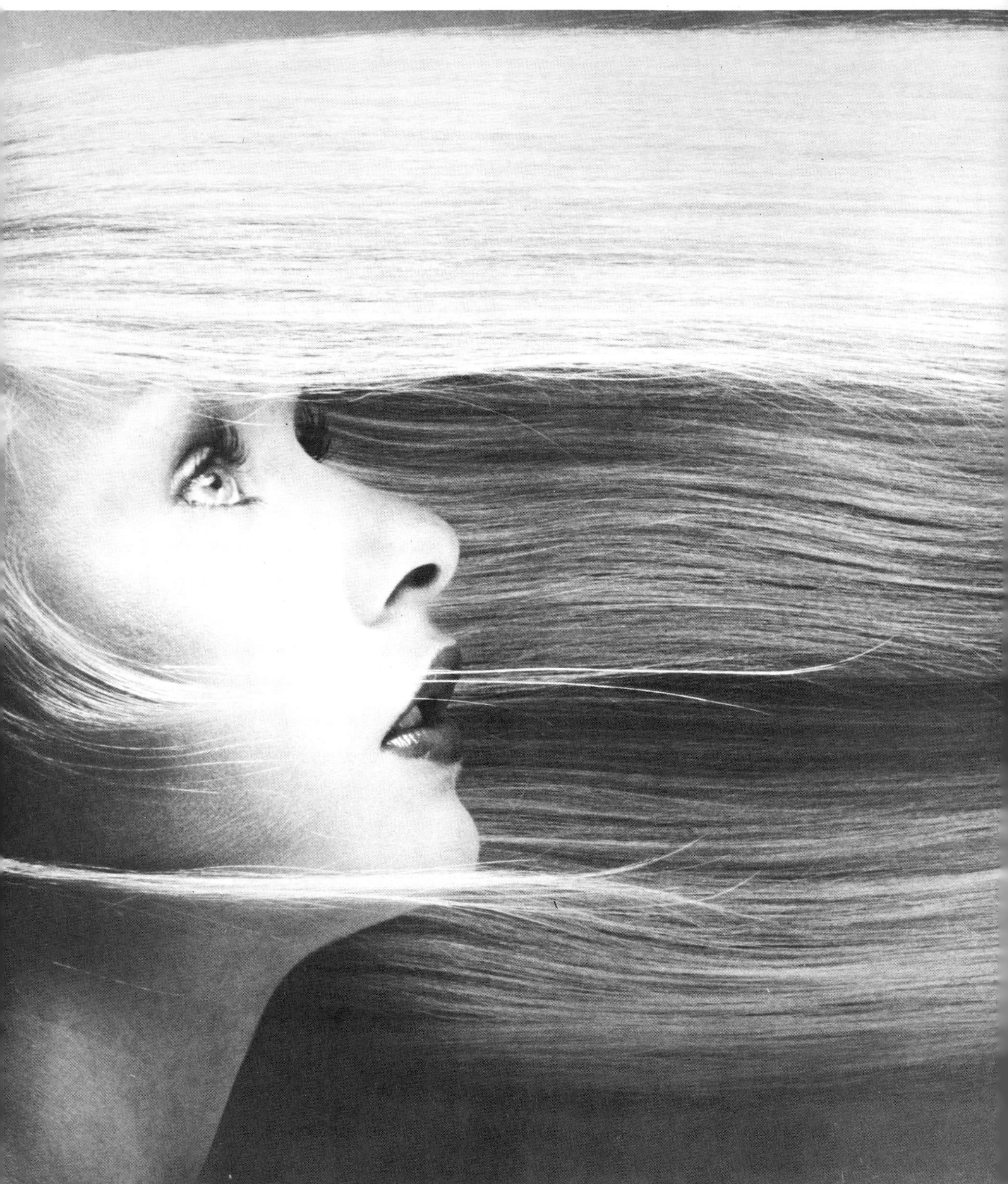

PATRICK HUNT

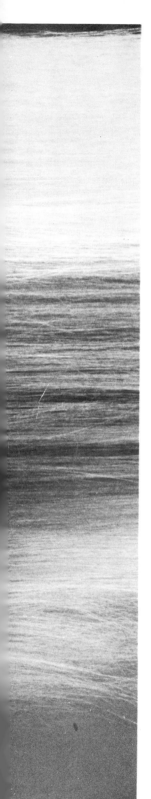

9

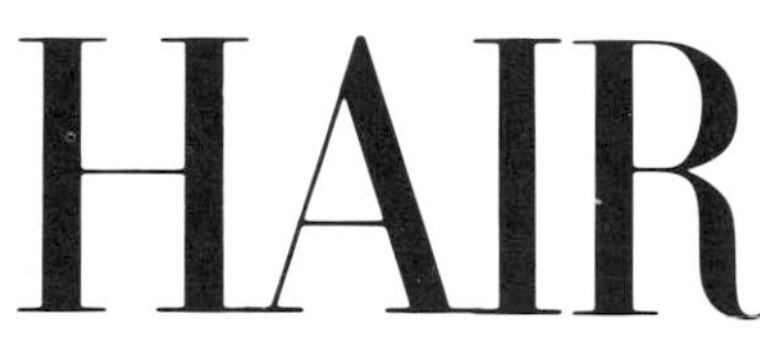

More time, thought, energy and money are spent on hair than on any other aspect of body-beauty. And yet we don't see nearly enough good-looking heads around. Health and beauty are of equal importance and there is no possibility – as in the case of skin and make-up – of covering up lack of one with the other. Texture, condition, type, colour and shape have to be taken into consideration simultaneously. Hair that bounces, shines and has a look of vitality and control is the result of a healthy working body together with a programme of correct care.

ELEMENTS

Hair is a complex cellular structure and varies from one person to another. The structural form is basically the same: each strand, no matter how fine it may look, consists of three layers. The outer layer, or cuticle, is made up of overlapping scales which protect the inner layers. The next layer, or cortex, is made up of long thin cells and is the most important for it gives the hair its elastic resilience and contains the pigment which provides the colouring. The innermost layer, or medulla, is spongy tissue and the cells sometimes contain granules of colour pigment.

The part of the hair that you can see above the skin is the shaft, and the part that lies beneath the scalp is the root. The root is not a single entity, for it is enclosed in a sac known as the hair follicle, and at the base of this is a tiny nodule called the papilla, which is really the store house for nourishment of the hair strand. When you pull hair out 'by the roots', although there is a tiny globule of white at the end of it, you leave behind the papilla which will eventually manufacture and nurture a new hair. This is why plucking is never a permanent way to get rid of unwanted hair, and why hair loss through abuse and breakage can eventually be replaced.

Interlinked to the follicles are sacs containing sebum which lubricates the hair and gives it gloss and suppleness. An underactive or blocked sebaceous gland means dry hair, an overactive one means oily hair.

Each strand of hair grows out straight or curly depending on the inner structure of the root. If the root is smooth, the hair comes out as a perfect cylinder and is straight. If the root is distorted, the hair shaft is more oval, at times quite flat, and emerges as waves or curls. Whatever the texture, you usually have between 90,000 and 140,000 individual hairs on your head. Blondes, because their hair is finer, have the most; then dark-haired people, whilst redheads have the least though their hair is the thickest and therefore appears the most abundant. The life-span of a single hair can vary from a few months to several years. Each strand has its own cycle of growth, then a period of rest which ends in its falling out and being replaced by a new hair. This process is evenly distributed at different stages throughout the head and it is perfectly normal to lose a certain number of hairs every day.

On the average, hair grows at the rate of half an inch (13 mm.) a month, though this slows down as we get older. It grows faster during warm weather, and faster at night. The reason why some women can grow hair to their waists is because they have the combination of a quick growth rate and a relatively long life-span for each hair. It usually happens when you are young and in good health. Nothing can make hair grow faster and most hair, after reaching a length of ten inches (255 mm.), slows down to half the normal rate of growth. It is not true that cutting will encourage the hair to grow. It may seem to simply because, having got rid of split and impoverished ends, the illusion is created of thicker, healthier hair.

Hair colour is determined by three pigments – black, red and yellow. Black and dark brown hair are concentrations of black; red begins to show up in brown hair; light brown hair contains traces of yellow; red hair is mostly red pigment with black or yellow shadings; blonde hair is yellow with traces of red. Hair doesn't really turn grey, but loses its colour. The middle section of the hair shaft stops producing pigment and fills up with colourless air bubbles,.but because the white hairs are intermixed with the coloured ones, the general effect is grey. The age at which hair turns grey is usually hereditary. It cannot turn grey overnight but it can lose its colour quickly due to an illness or emotional shock.

We are inclined to forget that healthy hair is part of a healthy body, and directly affected by physical metabolism and emotional balance. Its texture may be determined by genes but its strength and condition are determined by what it is fed. A high-protein diet with lots of fresh fruit and vegetables is good for hair. Foods containing vitamins of the B complex are essential. Important too are vitamins A and C. Of the minerals, iron, iodine and copper are the most beneficial, and lack of iodine can be most detrimental. A supplement of brewers' yeast tablets is recommended for anyone with a hair problem. In some cases, if premature greyness has been caused by a nutritional deficiency, it can be helped by massive doses of vitamin B.

TYPES AND TREATMENTS

Beautiful hair is immaculately clean and glossy, and the result of a planned programme of care. To work out a routine, it is important to know your hair type. Is it dry, oily or balanced? Has it been tinted, bleached, permed or straightened? That is all you need to know. Texture, thickness and curling ability influence styling and shape, but not basic care. The wonderful washability of hair is one of its main assets, and all hair needs frequent washing. Once a week is average for normal or dry hair, but if you are exposed to city grime or pollution, do it every five days. Oily hair usually requires washing every two or three days. The rule is: wash when hair looks or feels dirty. Some hair requires special rinsing. All hair needs pampering from time to time with a deep conditioning treatment. Check the chart overleaf to work out your general pattern of care, then check for details of each procedure.

THE ROUTINE

The ritual of washing hair was probably the first beauty routine you learned – but it's worth checking to see if you are getting the most out of it. The modern rule is: wash often, wash lightly, use shampoo sparingly; in this way enough lubrication stays in the hair, and the natural fungicides and antiseptics are not removed – they are useful for they protect the scalp from infection. Here are the steps to a perfect wash:

1. Brush hair gently to remove dead hairs and particles of skin that cling to the hair and scalp.
2. Massage scalp with gentle kneading motions; use pads of fingers and do it gently; this helps loosen more dead particles.
3. Deep conditioning treatment is given now, when needed.
4. Wet hair very thoroughly with warm water, lots of it – using a shower

spray is the easiest method. Work a small quantity of shampoo into a mild froth. Rinse hair with warm water. If necessary work in a second limited portion of shampoo – but it shouldn't be necessary.

5. Rinse hair thoroughly until it is squeaky clean. This may take three or four rinsings; let the final one be of cool or cold water to close the pores.

6. Use instant conditioner or cream rinse now if you need one; rinse away if instructions say so.

7. Mop hair with a soft towel to absorb a lot of the wetness; don't rub, simply blot dry.

8. Comb gently into shape for setting or drying; never brush hair when it is wet.

FORM	DRY	OILY	BALANCED
Natural hair not tinted, bleached, permed or straightened	Shampoo for dry hair Cream rinse Deep conditioning treatment every 3 weeks	Shampoo for oily hair Astringent rinse Deep conditioning treatment once a month Dry shampoo when needed	Mild shampoo Natural rinse, avoid very creamy ones Deep conditioning treatment once a month
Tinted, permed or straightened hair; hair overexposed to sun or chlorine; problem split ends	Shampoo for tinted or dry hair Cream rinse Instant conditioner once a week Deep conditioning treatment every 3 weeks	Shampoo for tinted or dry hair Instant conditioner every 2 weeks Deep conditioning treatment once a month Dry shampoo when needed	Shampoo for tinted hair or mild one Instant conditioner every 2 weeks Deep conditioning treatment once a month
Bleached or lightened hair – or hair bleached then coloured with a light shade	Shampoo for lightened hair Cream rinse Instant conditioner once a week Deep conditioning treatment every 3 weeks	Shampoo for lightened hair Instant conditioner once a week Deep conditioning treatment once a month Dry shampoo when needed	Shampoo for lightened hair Instant conditioner once a week Deep conditioning treatment once a month

BRUSHING AND MASSAGING

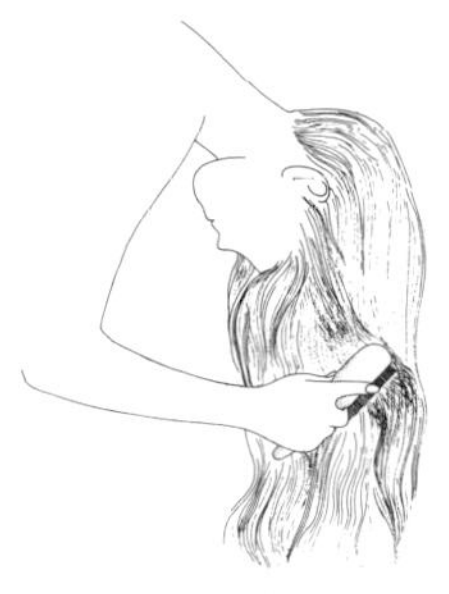

Daily brushing stimulates circulation and gives new body and fullness to the hair. Brushing before a shampoo is essential and the first step in the cleansing routine. Invest in a first class brush. Natural bristles are the best, but if you choose nylon be sure the ends are rounded. Always keep your brush spotlessly clean, otherwise you'll brush dirt back into the hair. A quick dip of the brush in a mild solution of ammonia and water quickly lifts the grime, then swish around in warm soapy water, rinse and dry upside down. Use two brushes if you prefer, one in each hand.

Hair should be brushed firmly but not over zealously – it responds better to a gentle treatment than to an attack. Every time you brush your hair you are going to lose some hairs. It's quite normal; hairfall is estimated at between forty and a hundred hairs a day. Hair should be brushed inside out: stand or sit, bending head forward and down, so that your hair is hanging in front of your face. Start with the brush at the nape of the neck and close to the scalp – though not scraping it – and make long lifting strokes away from the head. If hair is snarled, divide it into sections and work your way piece by piece towards the forehead. Stand up and throw your head back, and when the hair has settled back and down, use your brush to smooth it lightly. If you are not going to shampoo, put a piece of silk over the brush to polish the hair.

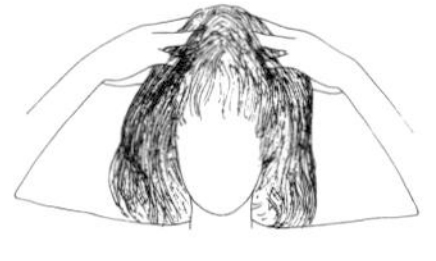

Massaging helps to improve circulation and loosen tense muscles. Do it before a shampoo and whenever you can spare a few moments. Start at the back of the head with fingers rotating slowly and gently; don't scratch, don't push with palms. Work your way in circular movements up the sides, over the crown and to the rim of the forehead. The scalp should move even with the slightest pressure.

SHAMPOOING

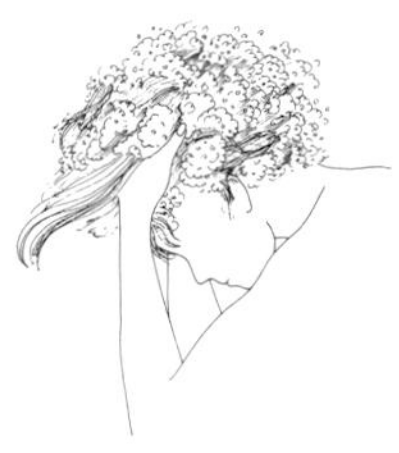

Careless shampooing can be harmful, either because it is the wrong type of shampoo for your hair, or because it is wrongly used. After wetting the hair thoroughly with warm water, use just a teaspoon of shampoo for a mild lathering. No hard rubbing; the hairline can be cleaned with a soft nailbrush, while the ends of long hair should be treated as you would treat fabric. Only if the hair is very dirty should two soapings be necessary. Modern detergent shampoos are very concentrated and if over-used stimulate the oil glands to greater activity.

Commercial shampoos are basically divided into two categories – soap shampoos and detergent ones. Read the labels which provide information as to whether the shampoo is for dry, oily or balanced (normal) hair; whether for tinted or bleached hair; whether enriched and with what; whether medicated or hypo-allergenic, whether based on natural sources or not. Tests have shown that some of the protein molecules from enriched protein shampoos are absorbed by the hair shaft and feed the hair; the remaining molecules coat the strand temporarily and are washed away with the next shampoo. They can make hair more manageable and slightly thicker. Many products make a reference on the label to pH, which means a measure of the acidity or alkalinity. Hair is surrounded by a liquid mantle of moisture (from the atmosphere, perspiration etc.) and it should be slightly acidic. However, certain alterations to hair – including colouring and perming – frequently leave an alkaline residue which makes the hair less resilient and can cause breakage and splitting. So the pH content of a shampoo (or a rinse, or conditioner) can be significant if you need to restore or maintain the natural acid-alkaline balance of the hair. A scale of numbers is used to define the acidity or alkalinity of any solution: 7 is neutral, 7 down to 0 are acidic, 7 up to 14 are alkaline. Most shampoos range from 6 to 8.

To find the right shampoo is a matter of experiment. Judge by seeing how effectively it cleans your hair, how your hair feels and behaves.

There are several shampoos you can make yourself:

Simple Soap Shampoo: For really delicate hair there's nothing better than soap; buy old-fashioned green cream soap and dissolve 4 oz. (120 g.) in a pint (6 dl.) of warm water – it may take a few days to coagulate evenly. Use in small quantities.

Herbal Shampoo: Add a strong infusion of herbs – rosemary or thyme – to a Castile shampoo.

Egg Yolk Shampoo: Beat 2 egg yolks into a cup of warm water; massage into scalp and hair for 5 minutes; leave to saturate for 10 minutes. Rinse off – no other shampooing before or afterwards is necessary.

Egg and Brandy Shampoo: Beat 2 egg yolks into ½ cup brandy and ½ cup warm water; massage into hair, leave to absorb for 10 minutes. Rinse.

Camomile and Egg Shampoo: Make a strong infusion of camomile flowers; for oily or balanced hair add an egg white, beaten to a froth; for dry hair add a beaten egg yolk. This shampoo is for light hair only. For dark hair use the same recipe, but substitute an infusion of sage or rosemary in place of the camomile.

Oily Hair Wash: Beat 4 whole eggs, massage through hair; leave for 15 minutes; wash off well with water; then rinse with a mixture of a cup of rum with a cup of rose water.

DRY SHAMPOOING

If pressed for time or in case of illness, a dry shampoo can be useful. Most come in powder form and the most common error is to use too much. Shake a little into the hair, gently rub in and around, then brush it out, using upward strokes away from the head. It takes about five minutes, and it helps to put a piece of gauze over the brush to absorb dirt and oil. Hair can also be dry cleaned with eau de cologne: cover brush with a piece of gauze or cheesecloth, sprinkle it with eau de cologne and brush through the hair. A natural dry shampoo is powdered orris root: sprinkle a minimum amount in the hair, brush for 5 minutes.

RINSING

Hair that has not been properly rinsed might just as well not have been washed at all. A water rinse is essential after every type of shampoo. Rinse, rinse, rinse – three, four or more times until every particle of soap has gone. The slightest residue of soap will leave hair dull and sticky enough to attract dirt immediately. The final rinse should be cool water, cold if you can stand it, particularly for oily heads as it closes the pores tight. Dark hair can have a little vinegar added to the last rinse; light hair benefits from the addition of lemon juice to the final water. These both help to restore the acid covering of the hair and remove the last vestiges of soap. Natural rinses with special effects are:

To add sheen to hair: boil parsley in water for 20 minutes, strain and use as a final rinse.

To add lustre to dark hair: pour a pint (6 dl.) of water over 2 tablespoons of rosemary, steep for 30 minutes, strain, add to final rinse.

To improve natural hair colouring: simmer a handful of nettles in a pint (6 dl.) of water until soft; strain, add to final rinse. It also gives the hair body.

To restore light tones to blonde hair: simmer a cup of dried camomile flowers in a pint (6 dl.) of water, after 30 minutes strain and use as a final rinse; catch the liquid in a basin and repeat the rinsing several times.

To lighten hair: simmer 4 tablespoons of ground rhubarb root in 1½ pints (9 dl.) water for 30 minutes, steep for several hours, strain; rinse through hair several times.

There are also cream rinses which act like fabric softeners. They make the hair silky and easy to comb after shampooing, reducing the pulling and tangling that causes breakage and split ends. They add sheen and also help control the hair by minimizing static electricity. It is important to control the quantity used, otherwise the hair becomes too slithery. They should not be used on oily hair.

Here's a natural recipe that adds sheen and softness: pour 1 pint (6 dl.) of boiling water over 2 tablespoons of rosemary (for dark hair) or camomile (for light hair), steep for 30 minutes, strain; add 3 oz. (90 g.) oil of sweet almonds and 20 drops of lavender essence.

CONDITIONING

Regular conditioning is a protective measure for all hair. It is essential for hair that shows signs of dryness, dullness or breakage. It is necessary to counteract the alteration treatments of tinting, dyeing, perming, straightening and bleaching. The purpose of conditioning is to restore hair to its natural condition, to make it manageable, to prevent breakage, to reduce split ends and to smooth out rough straw-like texture.

There are two types of conditioner – instant and deep. An instant conditioner is usually an enriched liquid (more likely than not containing protein) that is combed through freshly washed hair. It softens, adds resilience and bounce. Some have to be lightly rinsed away; others stay on to also serve as a setting lotion.

Deep conditioning involves products or home treatments rich in creams and oils. They are massaged into the hair and left on for anything from 10 to 30 minutes in order to allow the rich ingredients to penetrate the hair shaft. They are extremely valuable for dry hair and hair that has been abused or damaged. They are sometimes applied before the shampoo and sometimes afterwards – read instructions carefully. If hair is in very bad condition, a weekly deep conditioning is recommended until there is an obvious improvement. Usually a treatment every three weeks is adequate to preserve and maintain it.

Deep conditioning treatments can be made from household items:

Hot Oil Treatment – warm 2 tablespoons of olive oil, gently massage into every part of the scalp. Wring out a towel in hot water and wind it turban-style around the head. As it cools, repeat the process 2 or 3 times to ensure total saturation. Afterwards shampoo hair and rinse thoroughly. Good for brittle, dry hair.

Procedure

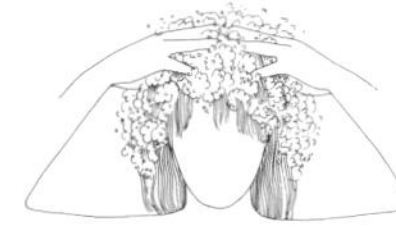

1. Shampoo hair and rinse until absolutely clean – till it squeaks.

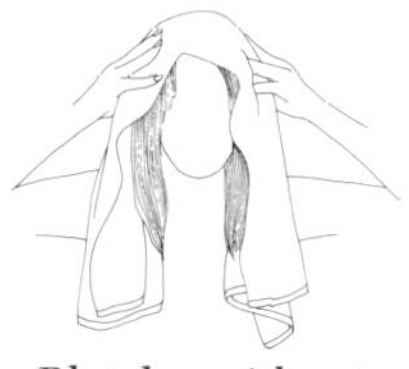

2. Blot dry with a towel, gently comb until smooth without tangles.

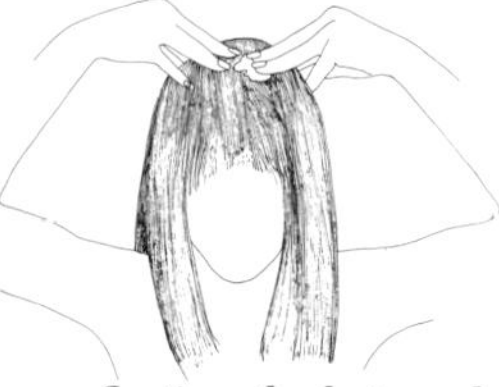

3. Section the hair and apply treatment product; massage into scalp.

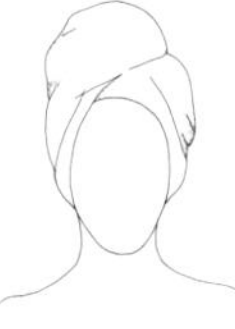

4. Dip towel in hot water, wring out, wrap around head; leave 15 to 30 minutes.

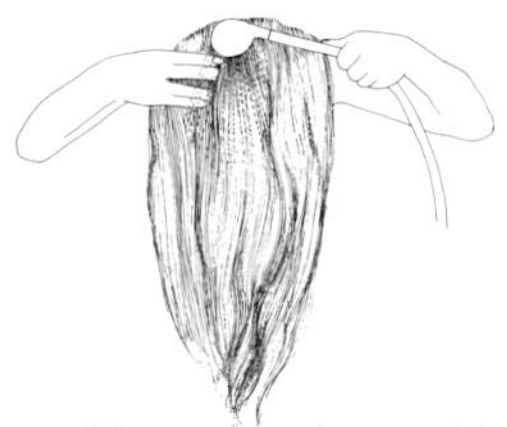

5. Rinse very thoroughly, 3 or more rinses preferably with shower.

Castor Oil Treatment – warm ½ cup of castor oil, massage into scalp and gently comb it through hair; wind a steaming hot towel around the head; wait 30 minutes before shampooing. Good for fragile hair.

Olive Oil and Honey Treatment – stir together ½ cup of green olive oil and 1 cup of liquid honey; shake vigorously; allow mixture to steep for a day or two. Massage into scalp, comb through, but don't let teeth scrape the scalp. Cover with a plastic bag, make airtight to permit the heat of the head to aid penetration. Leave for 30 minutes. Then shampoo and rinse. Keeps dark hair shining and lustrous.

Protein Treatment – beat 2 eggs, continue beating and slowly add 1 tablespoon of olive oil, 1 tablespoon glycerine and 1 teaspoon cider vinegar. Apply after initial shampoo and rinse; leave on for 15–30 minutes. Rinse well. A restorer for all types of hair.

Cocoa Butter Treatment – in the top of a double boiler, melt ½ cup safflower oil, 1 tablespoon cocoa butter and 1 tablespoon anhydrous lanolin; when completely dissolved and blended, take off heat and beat. Then take 3 tablespoons of the mixture and add 1 tablespoon of water, mix thoroughly. Massage into hair, leave on for 15–30 minutes. Then shampoo, rinse. Gives new life and lustre to dark hair.

Salad Dressing Treatment – beat together 1 egg, 1 tablespoon vinegar, 2 tablespoons vegetable oil just before using. Massage well into scalp and comb evenly through hair; leave on for 15 minutes. Shampoo and rinse. Helps to moisturize the scalp and provide lubrication for dry hair.

PROBLEMS

If hair is treated well it is easy to keep in good condition. It is by nature both elastic and plastic: elastic because it can be stretched and pulled around without breaking; plastic because it can be moulded temporarily or permanently into any shape you please. Yet resilient as it is problems crop up time and time again. Home treatment is often effective but any persistent or serious disorder should be treated by a trichologist.

ENVIRONMENT

It is not only air pollution that is bad for the hair. Day in day out, whatever the climate, hair is constantly exposed to heat, humidity, wind, cold, sun, water, central heating or air-conditioning.

Industrial pollution – particles of soot, grime and smog attach themselves to the hair, particularly if it is oily or sprayed. This makes hair dirtier and it is thought that it can affect the colour of tinted or bleached hair.

Sun – a little is good for the hair, but too much can be its worst enemy. It dries out hair, often causing breakage and split ends. It lightens natural-coloured hair, but seriously changes the shade of tinted or lightened hair, making it dull or brassy – it always brings out the reddish tints. If exposed to a lot of sun, keep the head covered and have a deep conditioning treatment every three or four weeks. Hair often acclimatizes to sun so that women from the tropics find their hair deteriorates in a northern climate and of course the reverse is also true.

Heat – intensifies the natural condition of hair: if it is dry it will become drier, if it is oily, oilier. It usually makes hair dirtier due to the head perspiring and dirt adhering to the moisture. Normal balanced hair will need washing more frequently and deep conditioning once a month. Dry hair will require an instant conditioner after every wash and a deep one every three weeks. Oily hair requires more shampooing than usual, and a long conditioning treatment every three or four weeks.

Humidity – adversely affects all hair. Curly hair becomes curlier, straight hair, straighter and even balanced hair will lose its shape more quickly. Choose simple styles and a stronger setting lotion. A deep-conditioner for all types of hair is a great help.

Water – rainwater is harmless – unless in polluted areas – but sea and swimming pool water can harm. The chlorine in pools dries and bleaches normal and tinted hair; it is always better to wear a cap, and if you can't, wash hair immediately on coming out of the water, adding an instant conditioner if possible. Sea water dries and bleaches hair, often because the hair is also exposed to the sun and the salt content accelerates both the drying and the bleaching processes. Always rinse hair in fresh water after swimming in the sea, again adding an instant conditioner if your hair is naturally dry or chemically altered.

DANDRUFF

The most common of all scalp disorders. It forms noticeable white flakes near the roots of the hair and is really dead tissue from the scalp and not in itself an infection although it can lead to one. It is an unhealthy condition and early and mild cases should be dealt with by a vigilant programme of home care. A very irritated scalp should be treated by a trichologist. Hard brushing, combing or scratching can precipitate a condition called seborrhoea by removing partially attached scales leaving exposed sore areas in which bacteria flourish. There are two forms of this condition: dry and oily. In the dry type, the scales are constantly visible; it is not only unsightly but can lead to eye trouble. The oily type is common in adolescence and is often accompanied by acne.

The causes of dandruff are many but difficult to pinpoint. Not enough fresh air in the hair is one reason, so is sleeping in rollers, never brushing the hair, fatigue, emotional upset and climatic conditions – people who live in cold areas tend to have more dandruff than those living in tropical climates. Doctors suggest hereditary factors and hormone imbalance – but nothing has been proved.

If you suffer from dandruff first look to your diet. Too much sugar and starch can lead to acidity and skin eruptions while a diet too high in fats can stimulate overactive oil glands and aggravate the condition. Stick to lean meats, vegetables, salads and fresh fruit.

It is essential to keep the scalp clean. Dandruffy heads need constant washing with a medicated shampoo, and this applies to dry as well as oily hair. A teaspoon of antiseptic in the rinsing water is helpful. A treatment is to make a liquid of 1 part apple juice to 3 parts water – to be rubbed into the scalp 2 or 3 times a week.

ABUSE

Tinting, bleaching, perming and straightening all damage hair to some extent, but the two treatments that cause the most trouble are bleaching and straightening. Strong bleaching should be avoided: it can weaken the hair and the scalp. If you are dark don't bleach year after year but try to be content to lighten it just a few tones. Straightening can stretch the hair dangerously: it is far worse than permanent waving. Other things that destroy hair are: constant use of brush rollers, heated rollers, hot irons, pulling the hair when blowing dry, elastic bands and any constant restriction.

Damaged hair results in broken strands, split ends and dryness. The way to counter-balance these problems is constant use of a conditioning treatment. The only remedy for split ends is to have them cut off, if not they will continue to split up the entire hair shaft. Even long hair should be cut regularly so that the ends are healthy. Some hairdressers singe the strands to remove split ends: a section of hair is twisted tightly so that the broken or split ends pop out and are carefully singed off with a flame. It is a time-consuming job, and only for an expert.

HAIR FALLOUT

Alopecia areata can mean loss of hair in patches or a diffused hair fall all over the head. It is causing concern because an increasing number of women are beginning to lose their hair. As women assume more responsibilities and tensions, it is thought that they are also producing more of the male hormone androgen. The normal ratio of hormones in a woman's body is eight parts oestrogen (female hormone) to one part androgen. The oestrogen affects skin texture and hair resilience. If the balance is disturbed, trichologists believe that regrowth of hair is affected.

Traditionally women have often suffered excessive hair loss a few months after giving birth because after a very high oestrogen level during pregnancy a sudden reduction adversely affects hair. The Pill keeps female hormone levels high and it has been found that women who stop taking it are often subject to the same post-natal symptoms of hair loss.

Anxiety, worry, lack of sleep and bad teeth all contribute to alopecia areata. Mistreatment through indiscriminate colouring or heating can go further than breakage and produce permanent hair loss.

Pulling the hair tightly back into a pony tail can cause inflammation on the scalp's surface or below the outer layer. This disturbs normal growth and the intolerable strain on the hair when repeatedly stretched can make it give up growing at all. The papilla sometimes shrinks and dries up and either a straggly hair emerges or there's stoppage.

Hair loss can often be reversed by finding the source of trouble. Extreme and sudden loss is a medical problem not an aesthetic one. An examination of the body and not just the head, is necessary including a thyroid test, kidney, calcium, enzyme and liver studies. The latest test is to establish if the body is manufacturing enough oestrogen.

UNWANTED HAIR

Everyone has body hair and except in a few cultures it is considered attractive to get rid of it. Dark-haired women usually have more of a problem than fair, because the hair shows more and is coarser. Haphazard hair growth is normal in every woman past puberty. Hormonal changes are a prime influence which is why growth becomes more profuse after the menopause and sometimes during pregnancy. There are many hair-removing methods and the choice depends on personal preference and place of removal:

Abrasion: Use a pumice stone or sandpapery glove. First cut hairs level with the skin, lather with soap and water, then rub away hairs using circular movements. For arms and legs.

Bleaching: For dark hair that is only a soft down. If you use a commercially prepared bleaching preparation, follow instructions carefully. You can make one yourself by mixing 30 per cent peroxide with a little ammonia and water. It is wise to make a skin-patch test 24 hours before the first bleaching. Swab on where needed; hair must be completely stripped of colour, not just to its reddish tones, and this may require two bleachings – done 24 hours apart. For facial hair, forearms and body.

Depilation: The application of chemical depilatories in powder, gel, cream or spray form. They soften and dissolve the hair shaft but do not disturb the root, therefore do not prevent regrowth. They take from 10 to 15 minutes to work on some areas and longer if you have previously shaved. Use of depilatories over a period of time tends to weaken hair growth so new hair is slower to appear and often less noticeable. If you are using one for the first time, make a trial test on a small patch of hair. For legs, arms, underarms – avoid using on the face unless definitely specified for such application.

Electrolysis: This is the only technique that offers reasonable assurance of permanent removal of superfluous hair. A fine wire needle – of platinum or stainless steel – is introduced into the opening of the hair follicle. An electric current of low voltage, lasting up to 40 seconds, is transmitted down the needle to destroy the papilla. The hair shaft is automatically loosened for instant removal. When it is done properly there is a slight burning sensation, though the intensity of feeling varies from person to person. Some women can sleep through a treatment, others find it really hurts. There are no ensuing scars and the hair from that particular papilla should never grow again. The operator needs skill, patience and good eyesight – plus good co-ordination. It takes time because only a certain number of hairs can be removed during one session. Multiple treatments are usually necessary. The alternative to destroying the papilla is to use the same electronic treatment to cauterize the blood vessel and hence stop growth; this is called diathermy. Electrolysis is expensive, but for those with a chronic problem it is worth it. For facial hair primarily, where the area to treat is quite small and doesn't take long, provided you haven't used other methods before. It is often used for hairs around the nipple.

Shaving: The quickest, easiest and cheapest method – and it does not cause hair to grow faster, coarser or darker. What happens is only that the new hair from the shaved pore emerges blunt-cut rather than tapered, so it seems – and indeed feels – more bristly. Use a safety or an electric razor. Watch out for, and try to prevent, dryness and nicking or scraping the skin. The nicks are prevented by always using a clean, sharp blade; for dryness use a special shaving soap or cream which lubricates the skin and stops moisture evaporating. Never shave dry. Wiping a blade can dull its shaving edge, so to clean loosen razor and rinse with hot water, shake, drain. Shave legs upward in long even strokes. Regrowth is rapid because the root is neither removed or damaged but this is a normal rate of growth. For legs and underarms. Don't shave the face, forearms or sensitive body areas. Pubic hair that extends to the upper thighs can be eliminated this way.

Tweezing: Plucking with tweezers is the only practical way to get rid of isolated hairs on the face and chest; it is the one method for trimming eyebrows too. Before tweezing, swab area with an astringent-soaked cotton pad to remove any oily covering and help you to grip the smallest hairs. Re-plucking is required after two to twelve weeks.

For scattered facial hairs – but don't pluck if hair is coming from a mole or wart, check with a dermatologist first. For hairs around the nipples, pluck in the direction of growth while holding skin taut with the other hand. It can hurt.

Waxing: One of the oldest methods of temporary hair removal – a thin layer of melted wax is applied to the skin, allowed to cool, then quickly stripped off tearing the hair out with it but not destroying the roots. The hairs are pulled out from just below the surface of the skin (though the papilla is left intact) which means new hairs are only visible after quite some time, even months. There is no regrowth stubble and in time waxing retards and weakens regrowth. It can hurt enormously depending on the part of the body and your pain endurance level. It can be done in a salon or with a commercial product at home. A home-made recipe is to mix 5 tablespoons of sugar into 5 tablespoons of water, add the juice of half a lemon; cook slowly or in a double boiler, stirring and waiting until it turns a caramel colour. Pour onto a plate and work into little balls. Press the ball firmly onto the skin, hold, pull it up sharply extracting excess hair with it. It takes a long, long time.

THE FACE

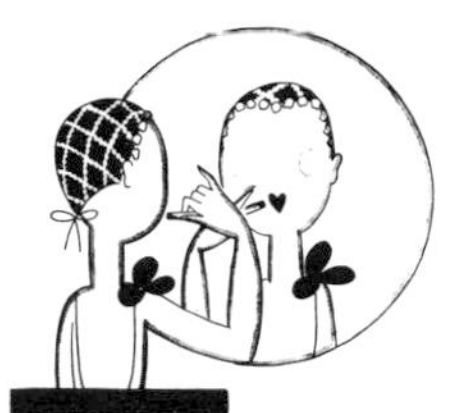
Groundwork

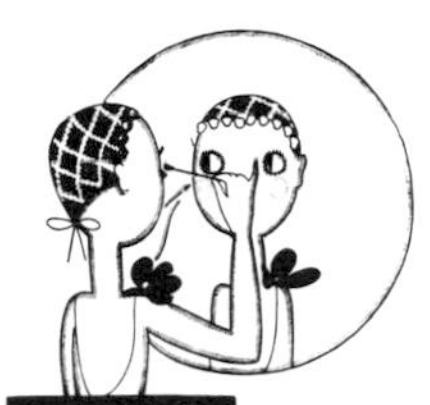
Chiaroscuro

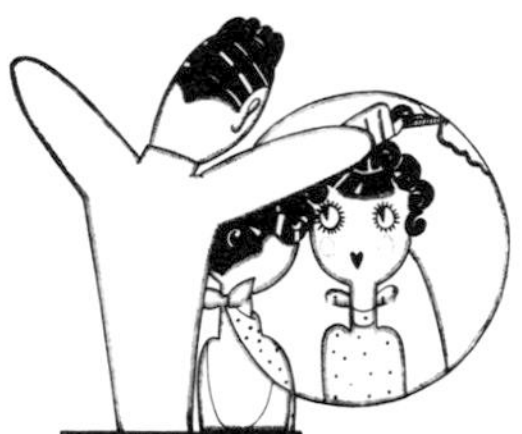
Expert Assistance

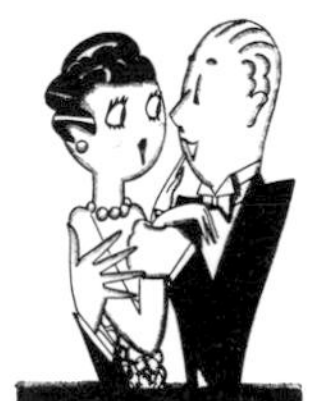
The Kill

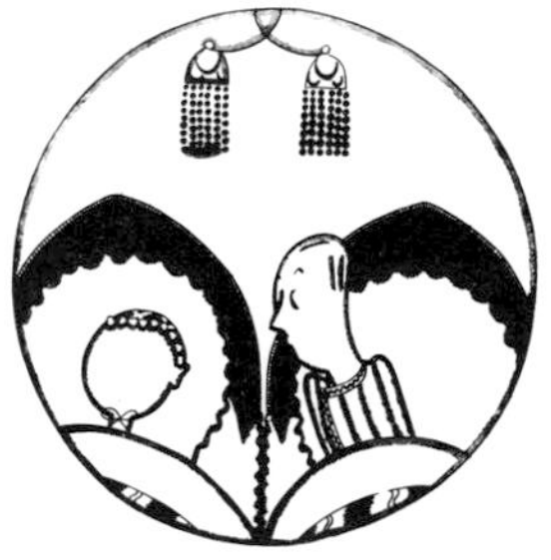
Disillusion

An Artistic Adventure
With A Catastrophic Climax
Drawn by Fish

In 1921 Vogue *said: 'The face that can render a song without words has a lasting charm, for expression is the better part of beauty, being much more than skin deep.' Obvious make-up was in 'disrepute' and cosmetics designed to 'reproduce natural tints to perfection'. But by the end of the decade beauty meant more than 'a pink and white doll's face' and it could 'cost as much in upkeep as a Rolls Royce'. In the 1930s the movies were 'the most perfect visual medium for the exploitation of fashion and beauty'. Everyone wanted Joan Crawford's bow-tie mouth, Dietrich's plucked eyebrows, Vivien Leigh's gypsy colouring.* Vogue *said: 'It is your job to spend gallantly, dress decoratively, be groomed immaculately – in short to be a sight for sore eyes.' Cyclax promised to transform 'jaded Lady into glamorous Jade' and Tattoo lipstick offered 'soft, inviting, youthful lips . . . luscious alluring colour that does not smear but stays on . . . through cocktails, cigarettes . . . everything!' With the war cosmetics disappeared from the counters but ladies were reassured: 'Four fundamental cosmetics you need are unrestricted – sleep, diet, exercise, rest for 20 minutes a day after lunch.' But in 1947 Dior's New Look gave women a new outlook on beauty and 'natural' make-up was considered rather 'mawkish'. Skin care was all important in the 1950s with the 'famous three' steps – cleansing, stimulating and nourishing. With a 'Magic Iron' you could make 'fine lines disappear . . . crepiness give way to smoothness . . . and formant tissues wake up to fresh activity'. With Helena Rubinstein's Estrogenci Oil you could even make 'time stand still'. Eyes became 'doe eyes' and eye make-up even more important than lipstick.* Vogue *suggested: 'Eyes made mysterious with eyebrow pencil and a dusky shadow, and strip eyelashes of nylon.' The 1960s saw the beginning of the back to nature trend while the cosmetic industry still promised 'miracles' . . . 'revelation in nail polish chemistry' . . . 'revolutionary creams and preparations'. The London Look of the mid-1960s was copied throughout the world and Jean Shrimpton's was the look; Elizabeth Taylor the last of the world-famous movie stars. With the 1970s your face, like fashion could be as you like it . . . spectacular like Bianca Jagger . . . naturally sophisticated like Twiggy . . . naturally beautiful like Marisa Berenson. A last suggestion: 'Try looking like a lady.'*

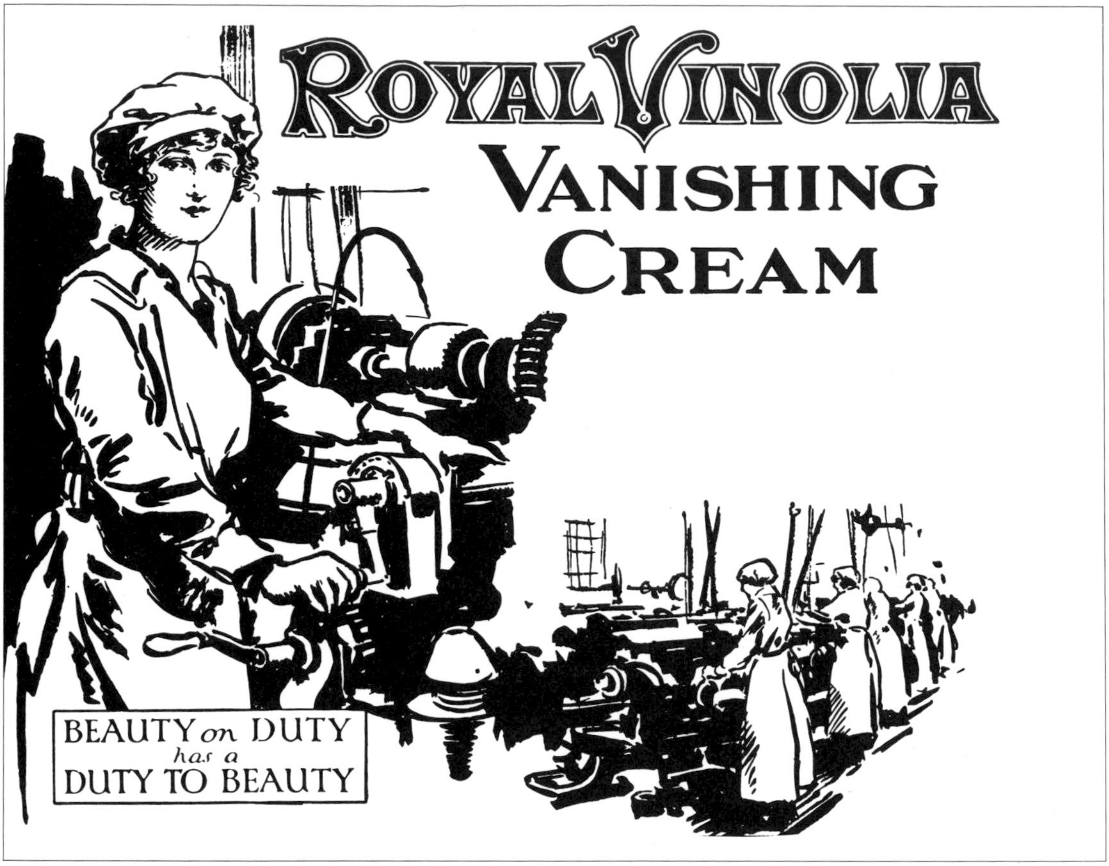

ROYAL VINOLIA
VANISHING
CREAM

BEAUTY *on* DUTY
has a
DUTY TO BEAUTY

1918

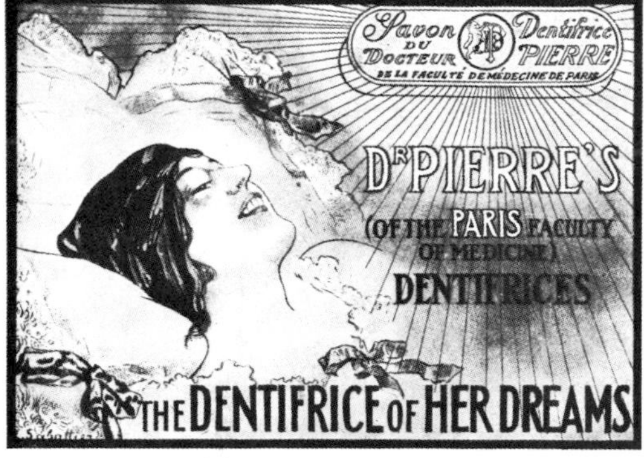

1919

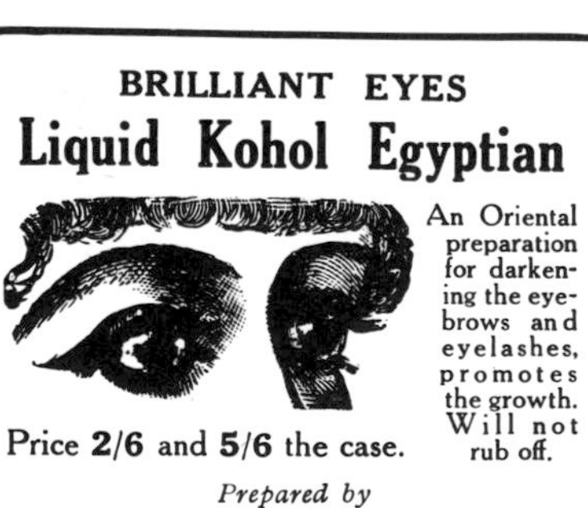

1916

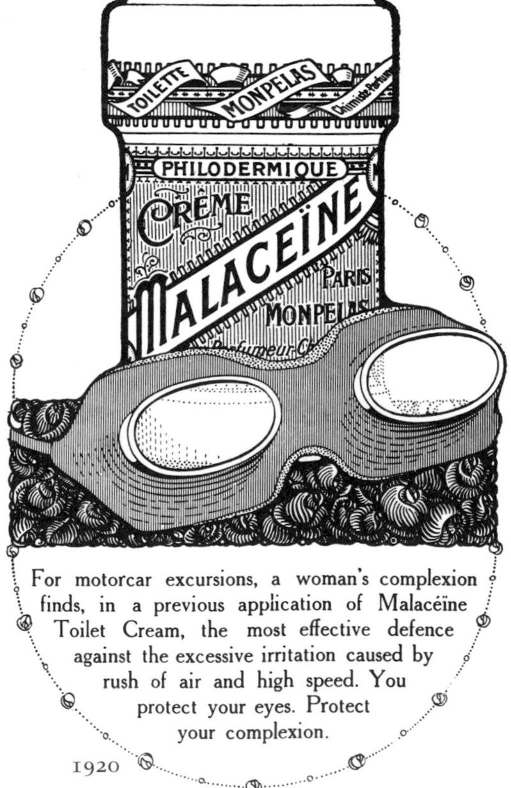

TOILETTE
MONPELAS
PHILODERMIQUE
CRÈME
MALACEÏNE
PARIS
MONPELAS
For motorcar excursions, a woman's complexion finds, in a previous application of Malacëine Toilet Cream, the most effective defence against the excessive irritation caused by rush of air and high speed. You protect your eyes. Protect your complexion.

1920

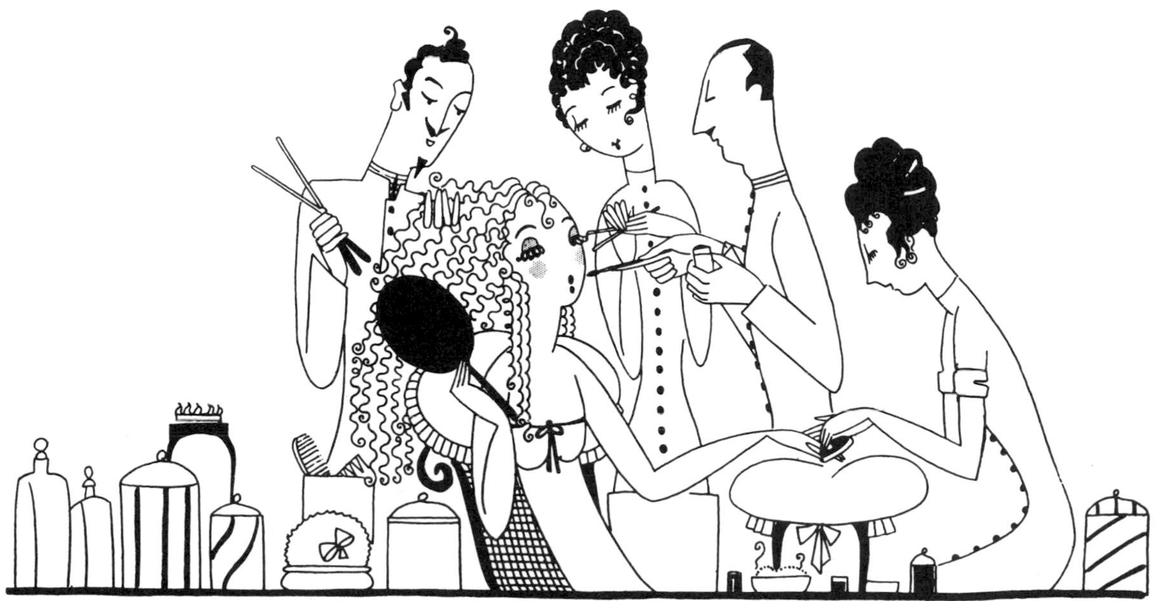

FISH 1923

'A woman who is a beauty has no need – and no time – to be anything else. Courage, patience and perseverance must be among her virtues, but the end justifies the means. Success in her chosen career brings everything that is most dear to the heart of woman – a jealous husband, envious women friends and admiring grand-grandchildren. Besides which she gives pleasure to connoisseurs and employment to many amiable and deserving people.'

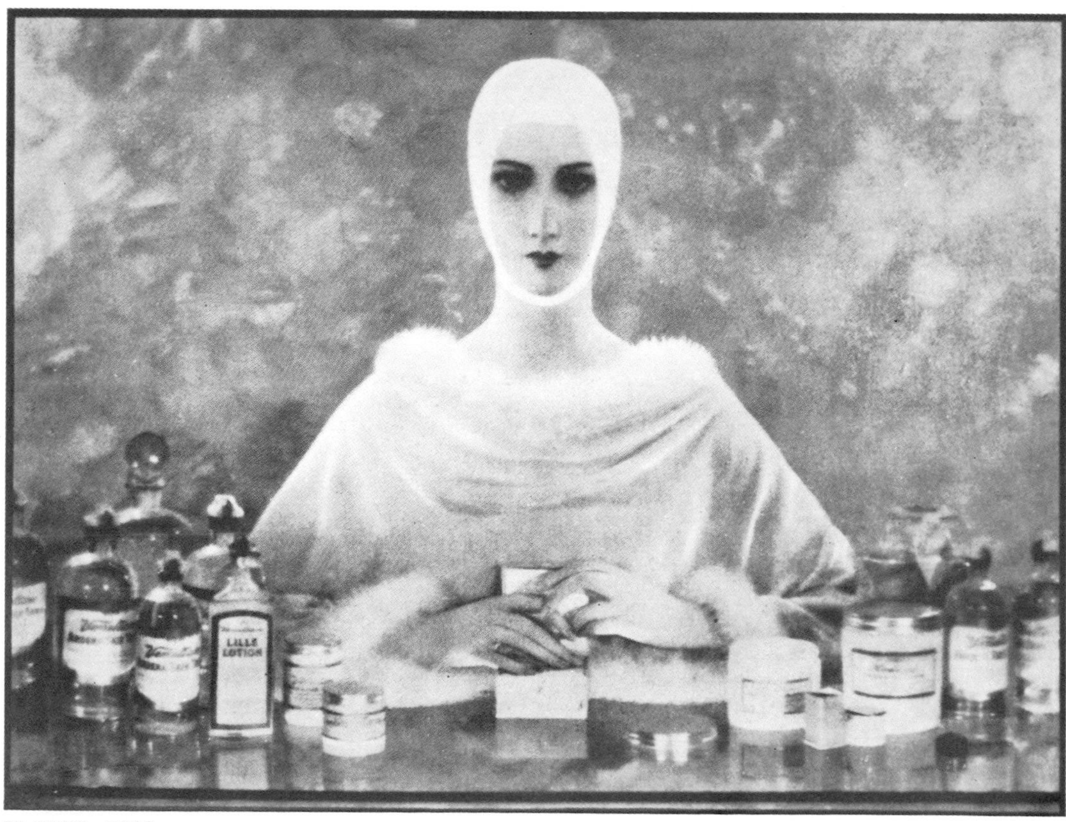

DE MEYER 1932

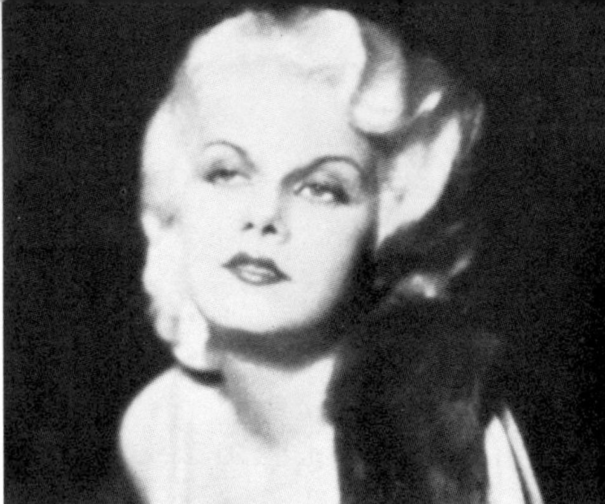

Jean Harlow

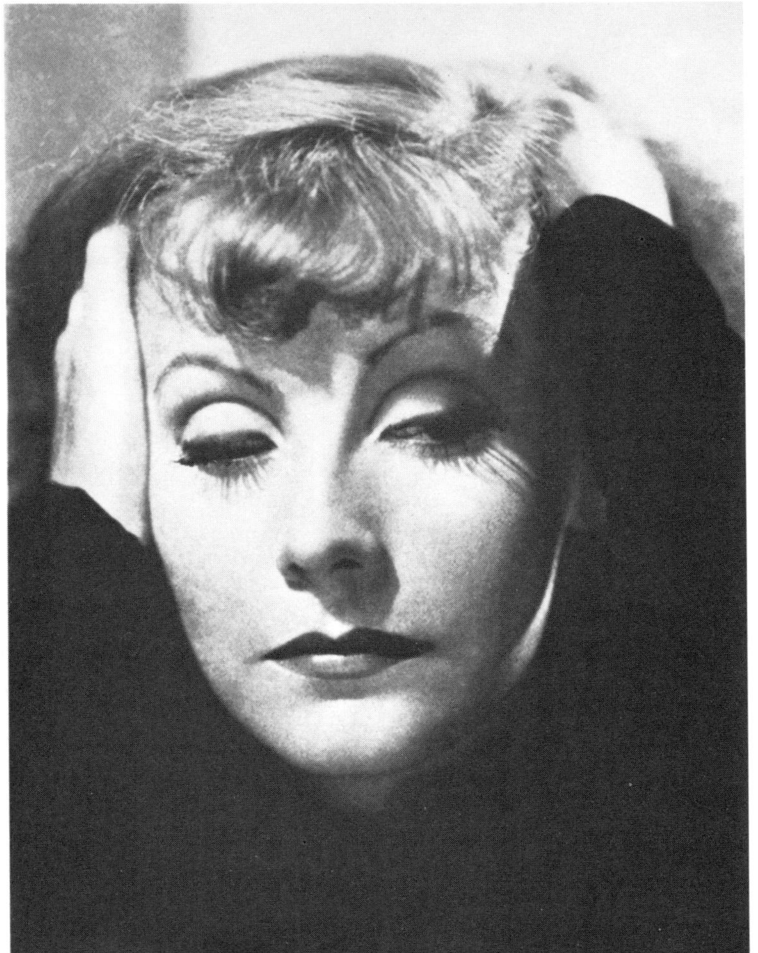

Garbo STEICHEN

'Anthropologists of the future, when bending their beards over cinema archives, will unearth a perplexing phenomenon. They will discover that whereas early in the twentieth century the female citizens of Hollywood were various in type, about 1931–32 they suddenly all began to look alike. The chief points of this resemblance are blondish hair, worn untidily in a long bob, narrow eyebrows arching skywards, and incredibly long eyelashes. These are augmented by a sullen lower lip and a gaunt look which will doubtless cause the inference that all actresses at this era were the victims of an unpleasant internal disorder. Of course, this is not true. What has really happened is demonstrated in the photographs (below). The upper row depicts them in the sunny days of their pre-Nordic innocency. Then came Garbo. Below are shown the ensuing metamorphoses.'

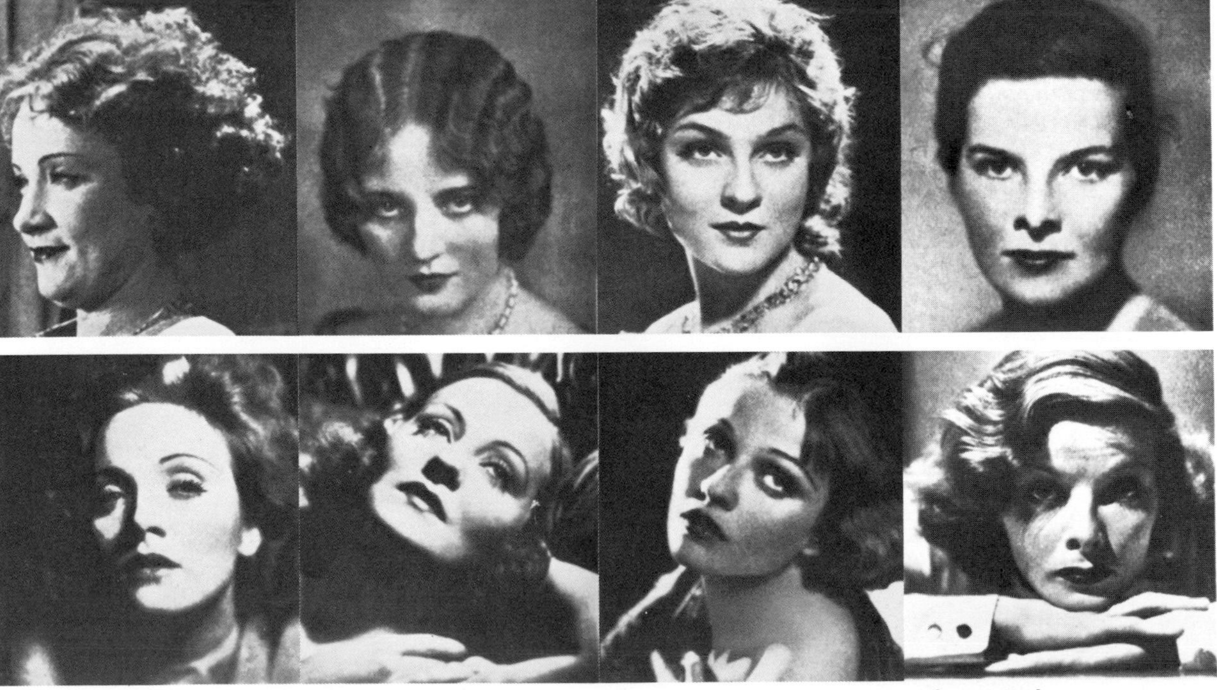

Marlene Dietrich   Tallulah Bankhead   Anna Sten   Katharine Hepburn

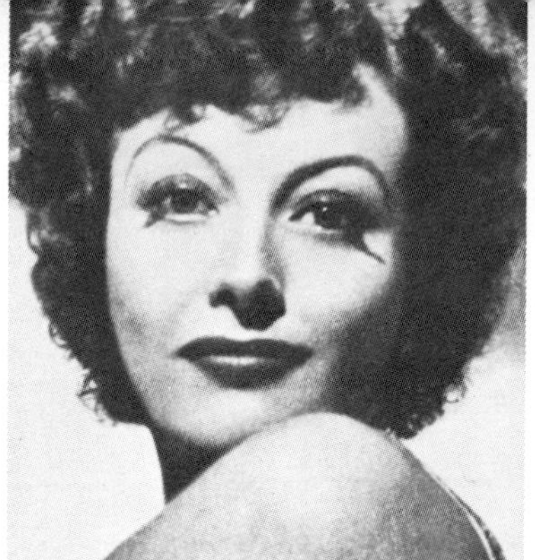

Joan Crawford

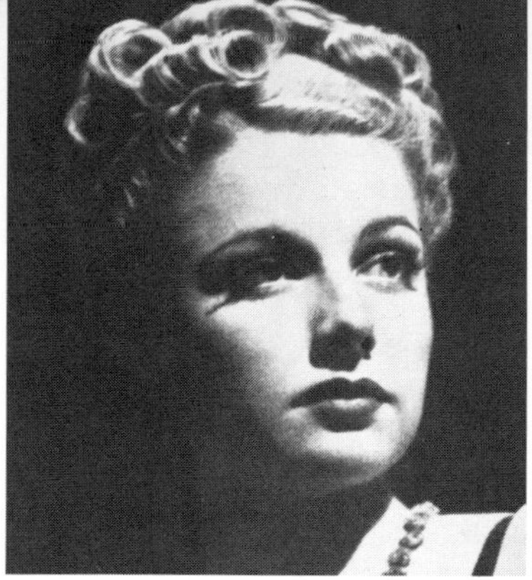

Ann Sheridan

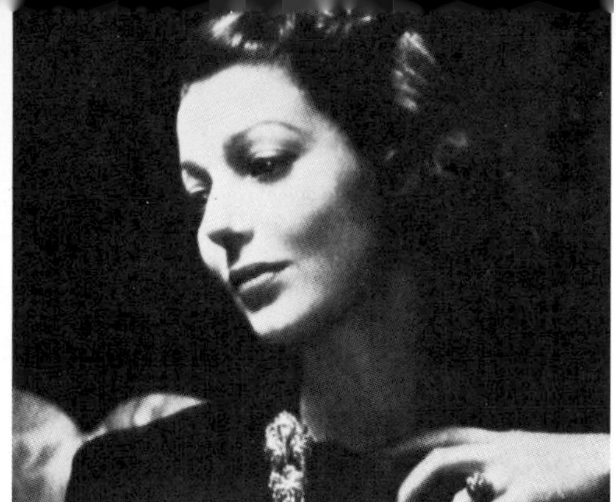

Loretta Young

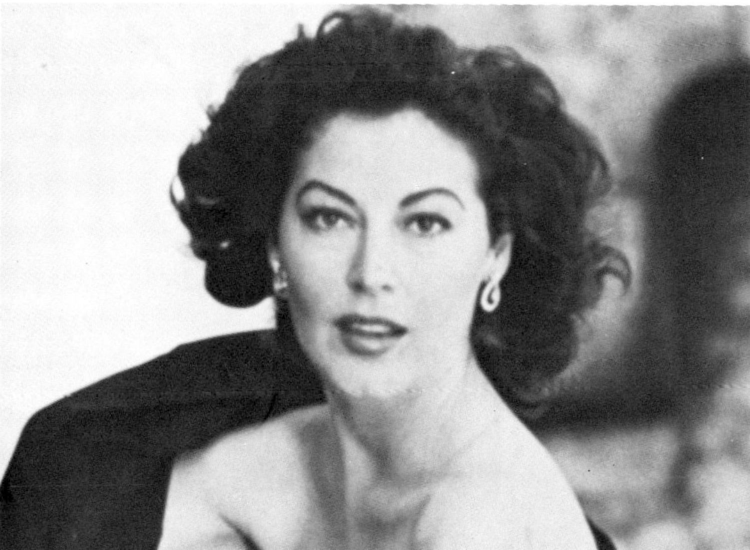

Ava Gardner

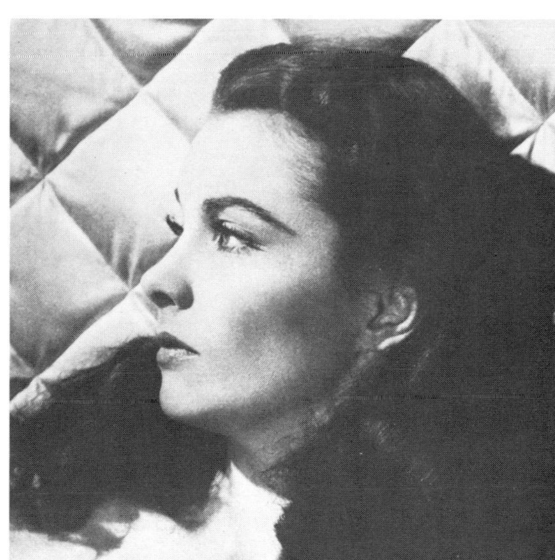

Vivien Leigh

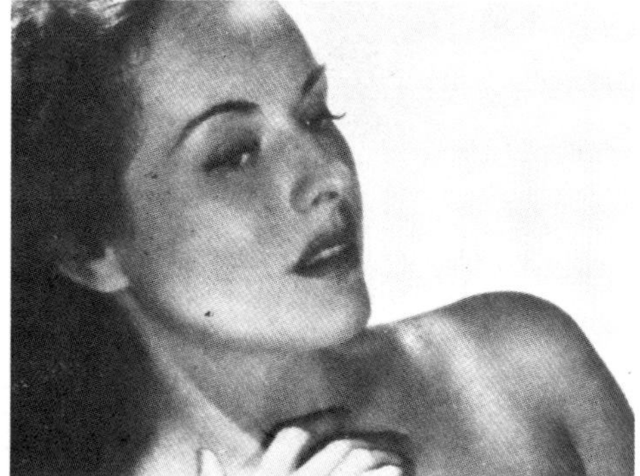

Paulette Goddard

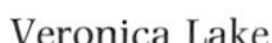

Veronica Lake

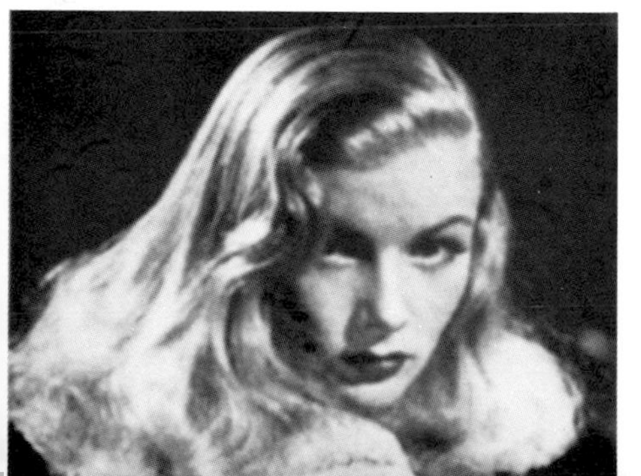

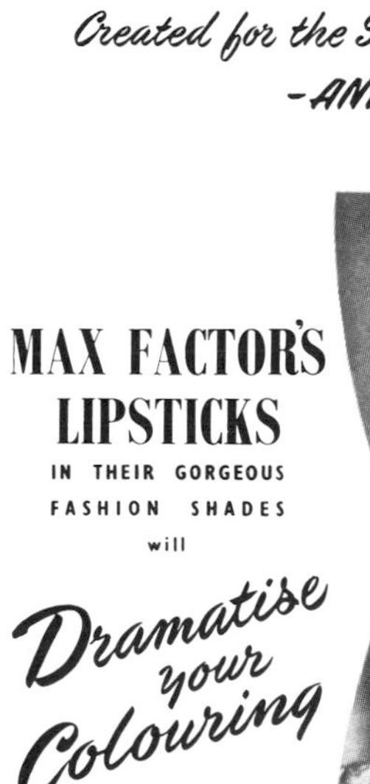

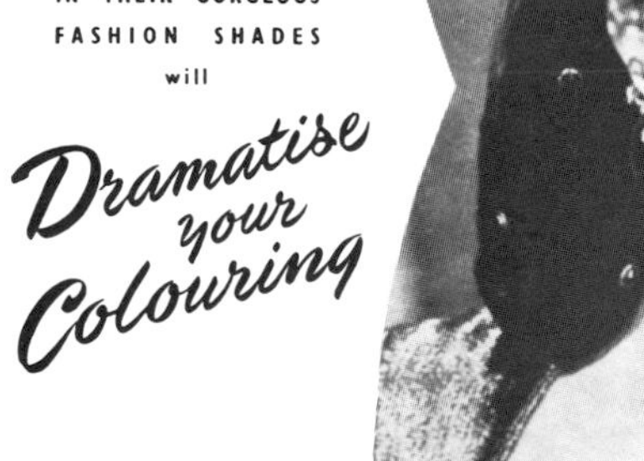

Hedy Lamarr

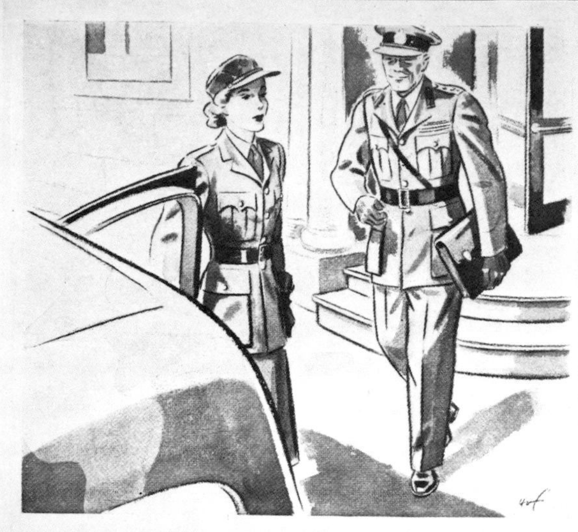

CHARACTER

A WOMAN'S LIPS are a key to her character, and to-day lips have a firmer and more resolute line, for they shape words of command, laugh at danger, and with a smile suppress weariness and pain. A little lipstick gives added character to the mouth and added self-confidence to the wearer. It is for this reason that the makers of Gala continue to manufacture this famous lipstick and suggest that its use in moderation is an asset to our wartime morale.

The Liveliest Lipstick in Town Gala

Gala Lipstick, 4/6. Refills (fit almost any case), 2/6. Gala Powder, 4/6. Gala Cream, 4/6.

1943

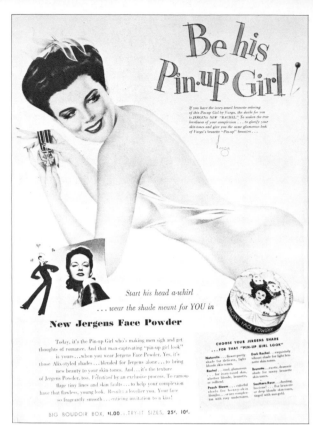

Be his Pin-up Girl!

If you have the ivory-toned brunette coloring of this Pin-up Girl by Vargo, the shade for you is JERGENS NEW "RACHEL." To waken the true loveliness of your complexion . . . to glorify your skin-tones and give you the same glamorous look of Vargo's brunette "Pin-up" beauties . . .

Start his head a-whirl

. . . wear the shade meant for YOU in

New Jergens Face Powder

Today, it's the Pin-up Girl who's making men sigh and get thoughts of romance. And that man-captivating "pin-up girl look" is yours . . . when you wear Jergens Face Powder. Yes, it's those Alix-styled shades . . . blended for Jergens alone . . . to bring new beauty to your skin-tones. And . . . it's the texture of Jergens Powder, too. *Velvetized* by an exclusive process. To camouflage tiny lines and skin faults . . . to help your complexion have that flawless, young look. Result: a lovelier you. Your face so fragrantly smooth . . . enticing invitation to a kiss!

CHOOSE YOUR JERGENS SHADE . . . FOR THAT "PIN-UP GIRL LOOK"

Naturelle . . . flower-pretty shade for delicate, light blonde skin-tones.

Rachel . . . cool, glamorous . . . for ivory-toned skin, whether blonde, brunette, or redhead.

Peach Bloom . . . colorful shade for honey-skin blondes . . . or any complexion with rosy undertones.

Dark Rachel . . . exquisitely vibrant shade for light brunette skin-tones.

Brunette . . . exotic, dramatic shade for tawny brunette skin-tones.

Southern Rose . . . dazzling, luscious! . . . For brunette or deep blonde skin-tones, tinged with sun-gold.

BIG BOUDOIR BOX, $1.00 . . . TRY-IT SIZES, 25¢, 10¢.

1943

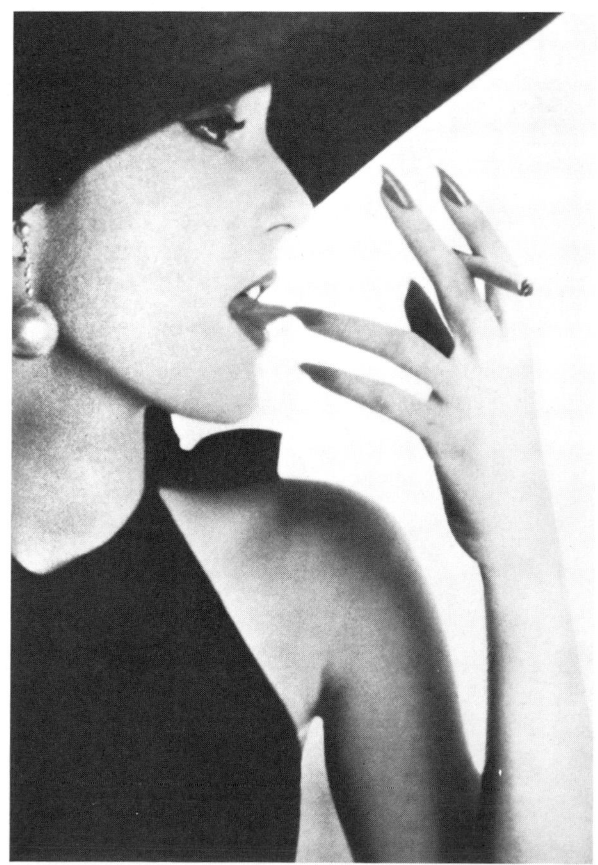

PENN 1951

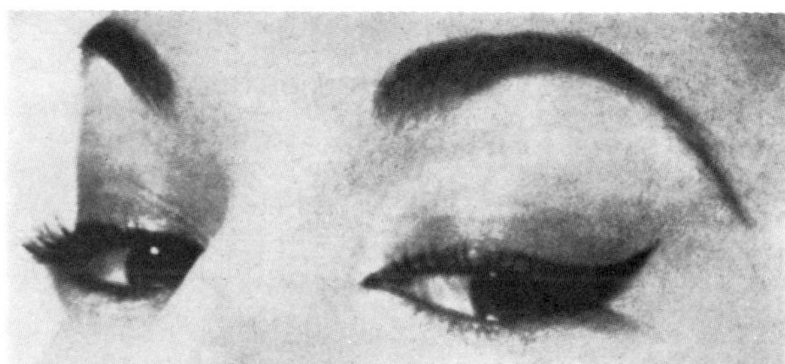

BLUMENFELD 1950

'The 1950 look is the "doe-eyed" look introduced by Piguet in Paris. It could become, we think, as generally and excitingly new as the use of lipstick was in the twenties.'

'With summer and the prevalence of black and white comes a new silhouette-sharpness of make-up. The eyes, lips and nails – often the only colour in the ensemble – are emphasised with bold strokes. Strengthen the browline, sharpen the outline of your lips. This is the moment to use your eye and lip liners, your battery of brushes, and – new too this season – to file your longer nails to an accentuated point, as those of the girl in the picture.'

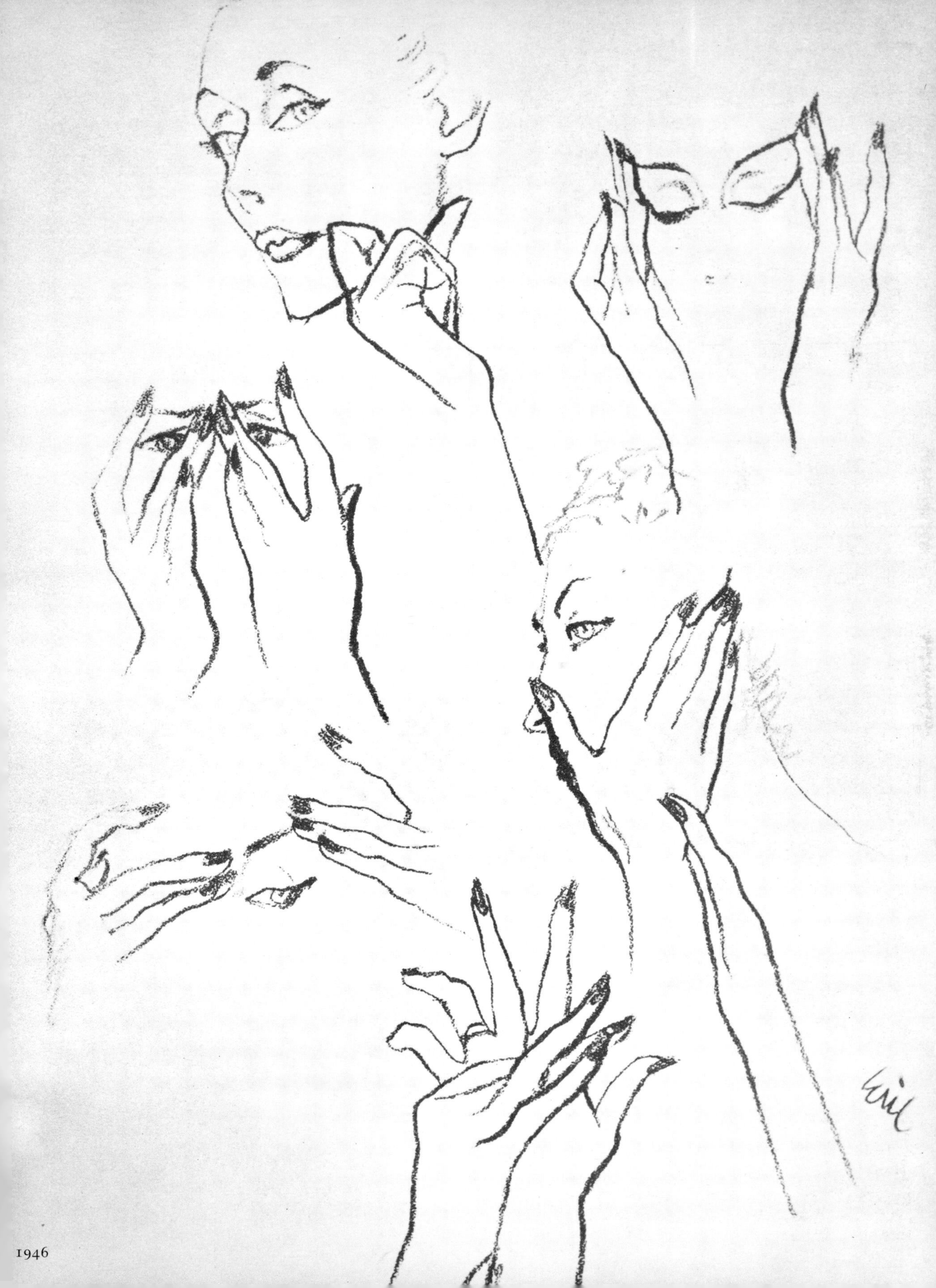

1946

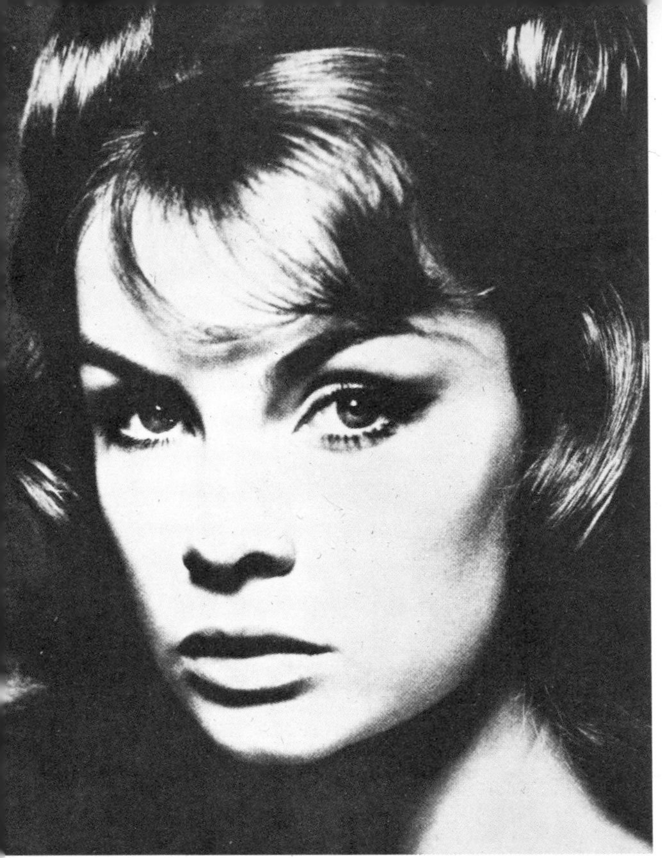

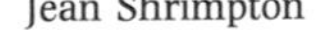 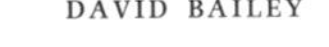

Jean Shrimpton DAVID BAILEY

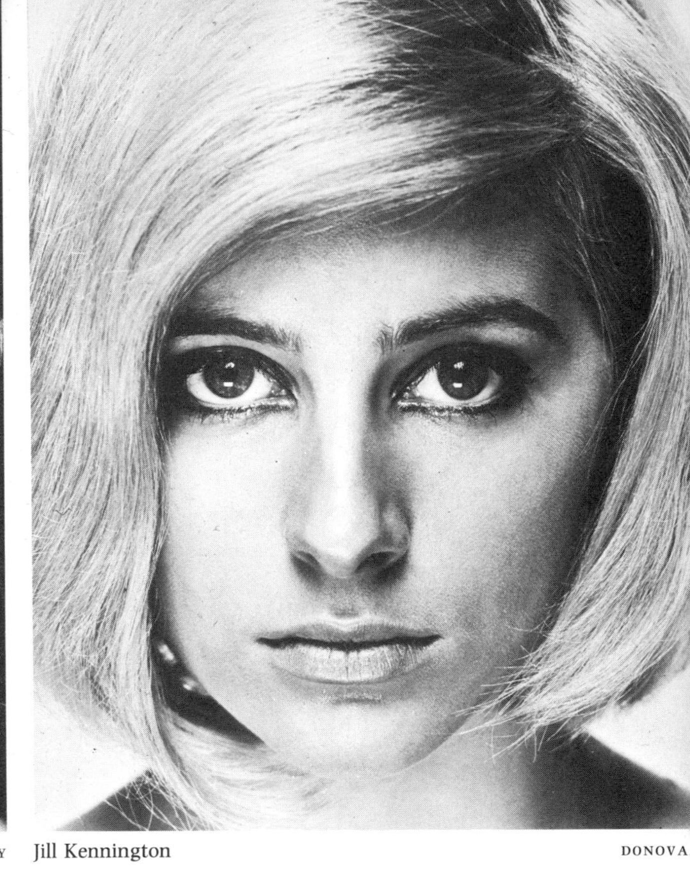

Jill Kennington DONOVA

Twiggy NORMAN PARKINSON

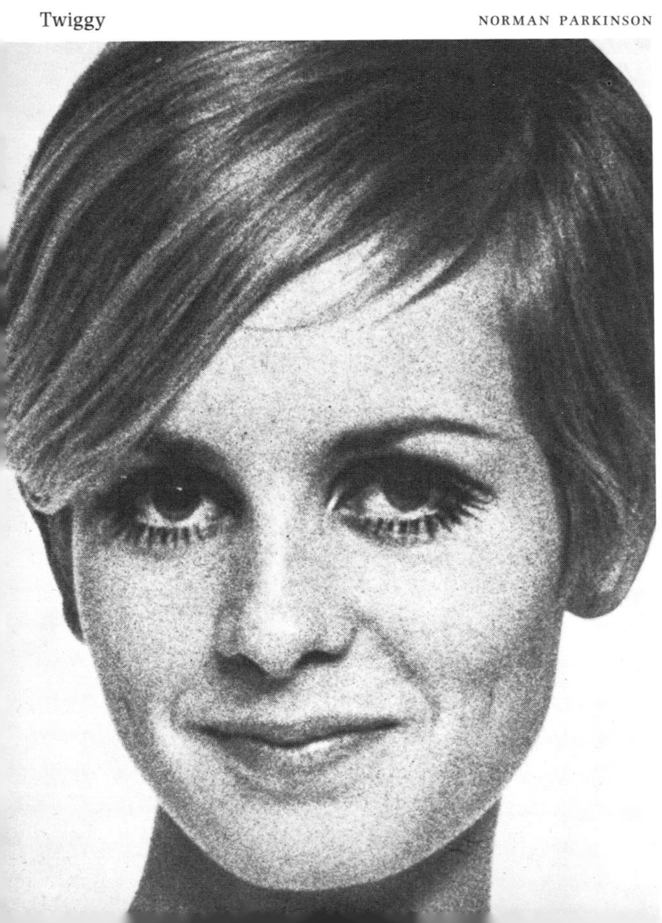

Françoise Hardy ROBERTA BOOT

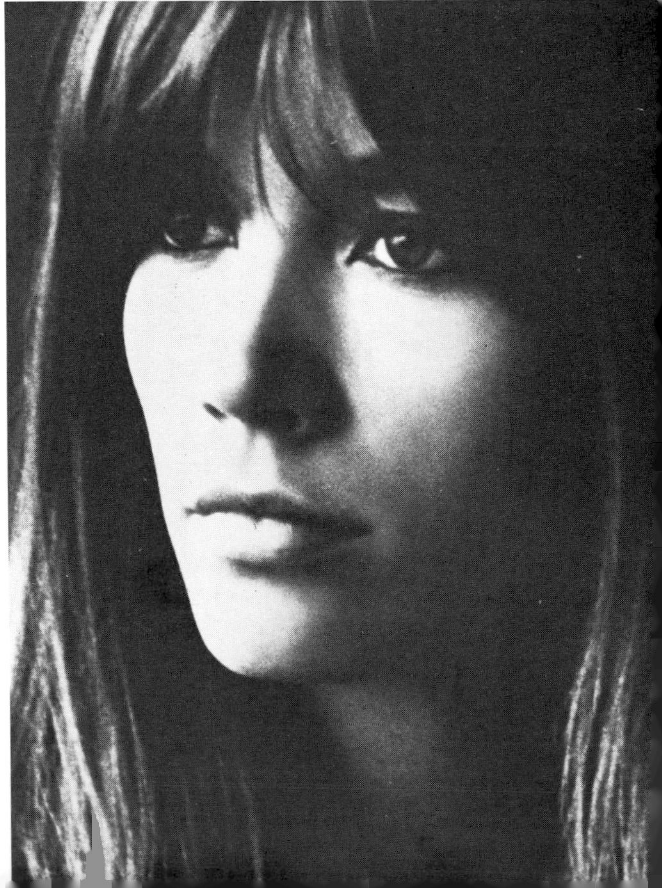

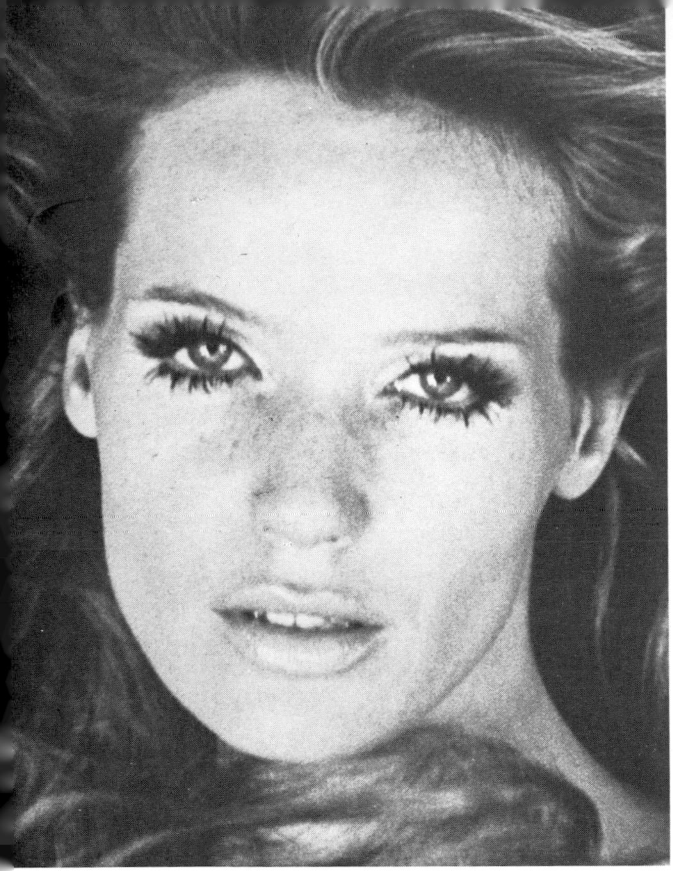

'erushka RUBARTELLI

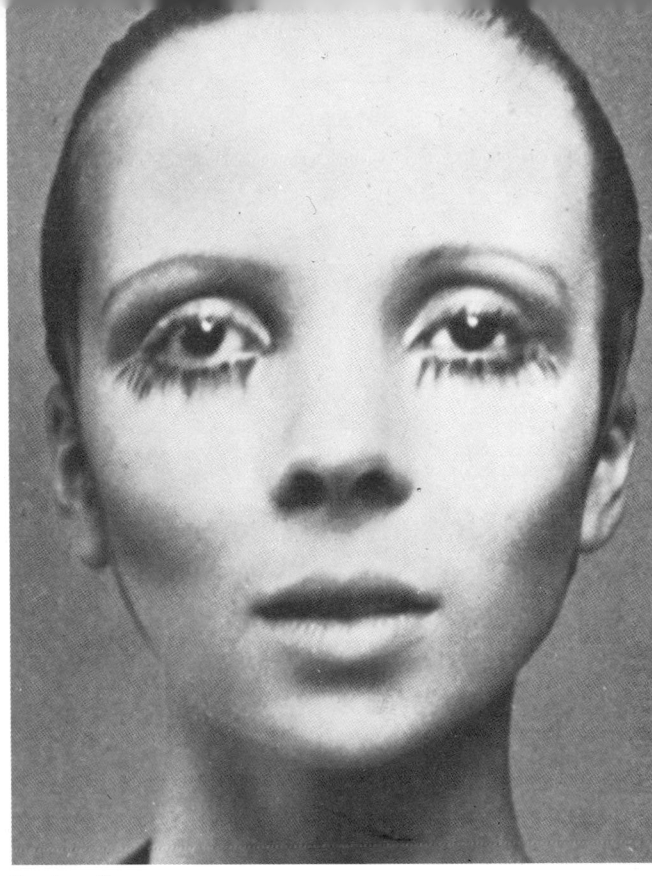

Penelope Tree AVEDON

aren Graham KOURKEN PAKCHANIAN

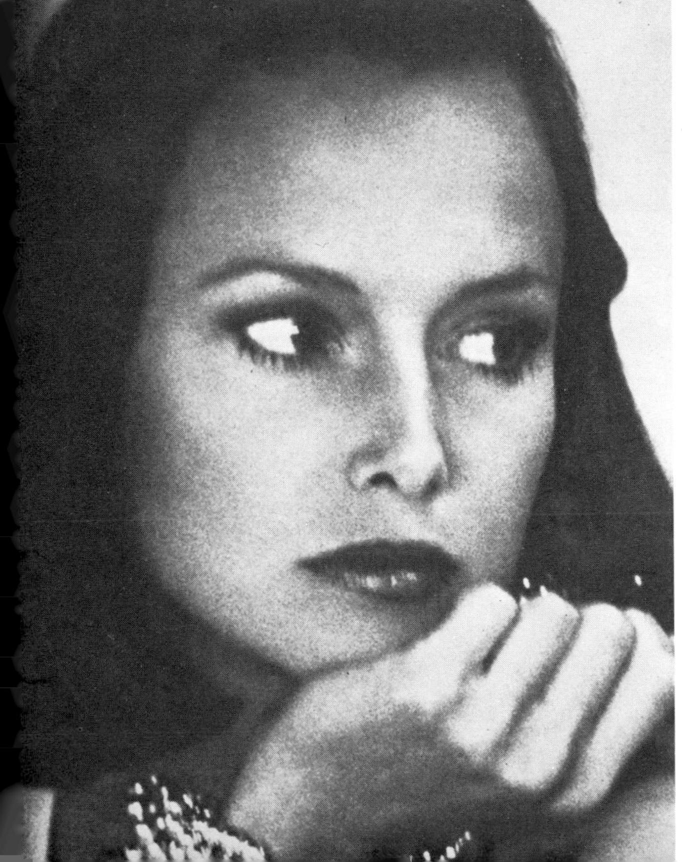

Maudie James DAVID BAILEY

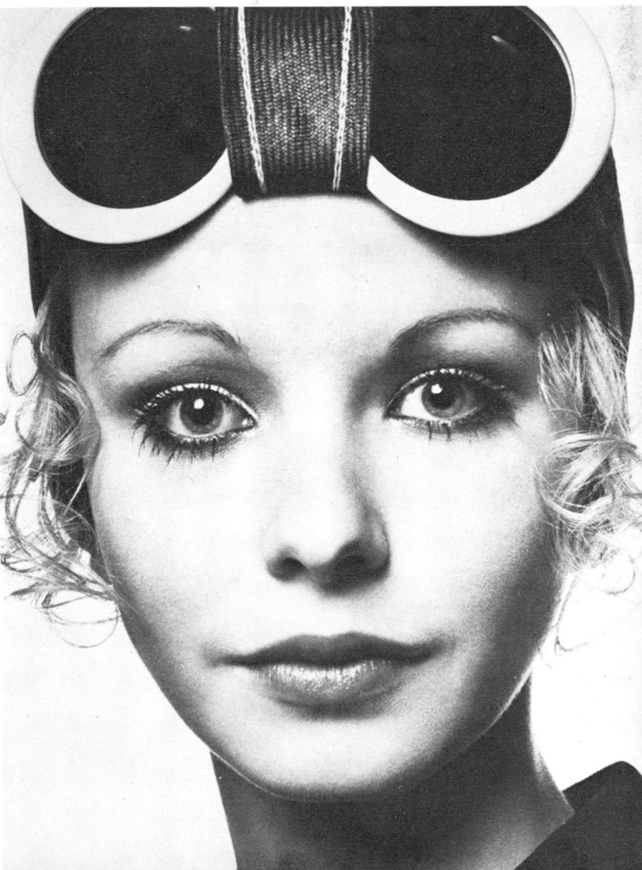

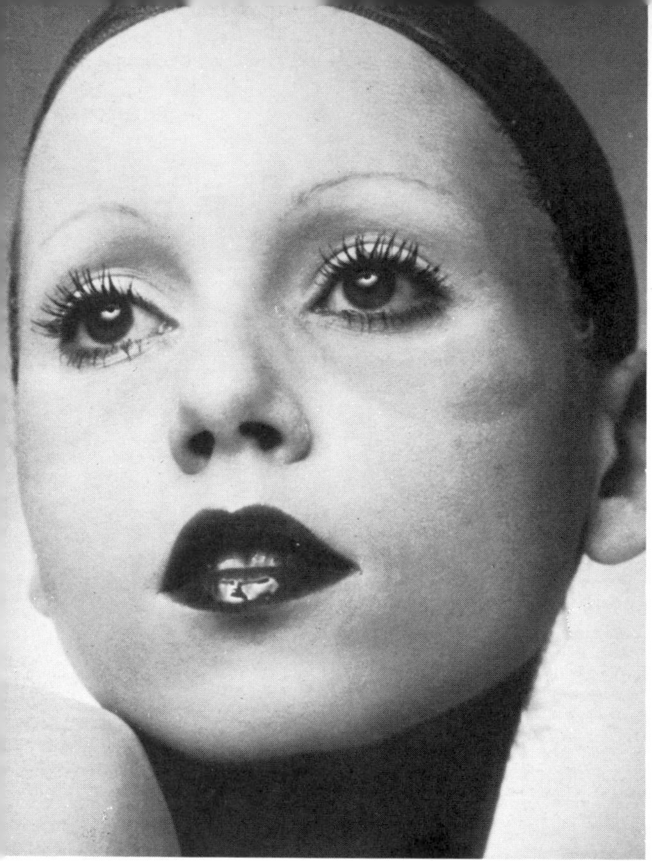

Annie Shaffus ARROWSMITH

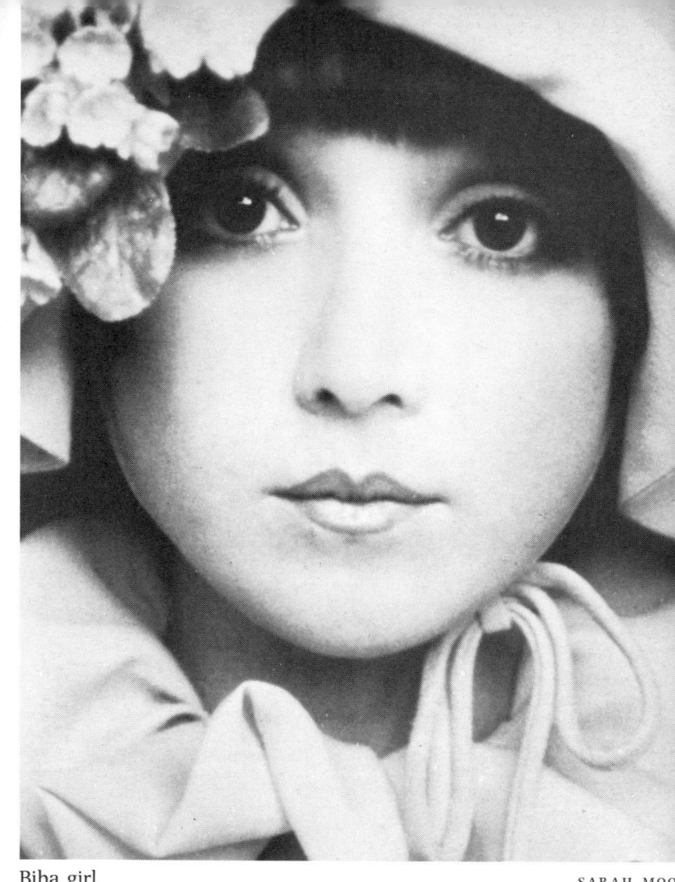

Biba girl SARAH MOO

Grace Coddington BARRY LATEGAN

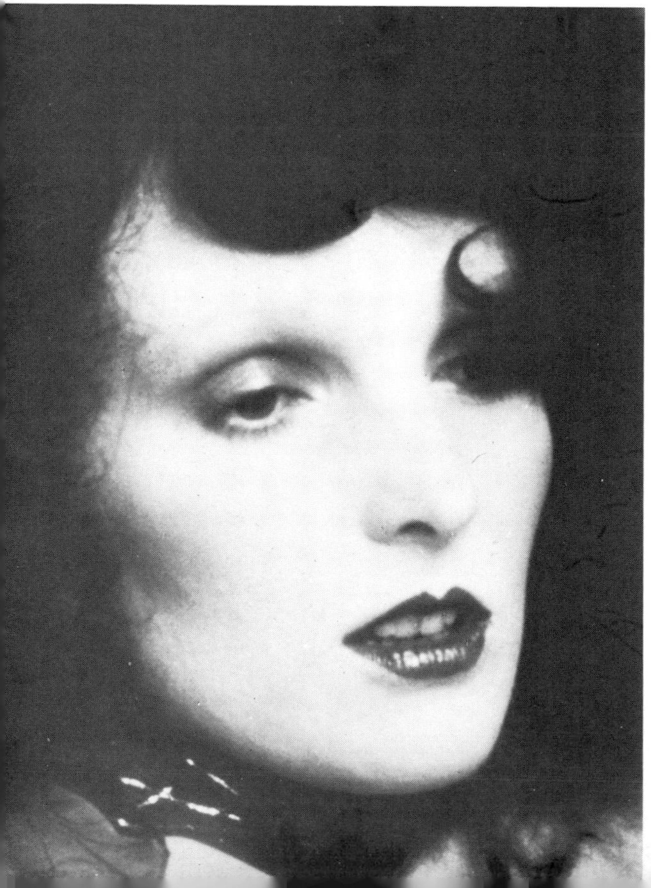

Lauren Hutton EVA SEREN

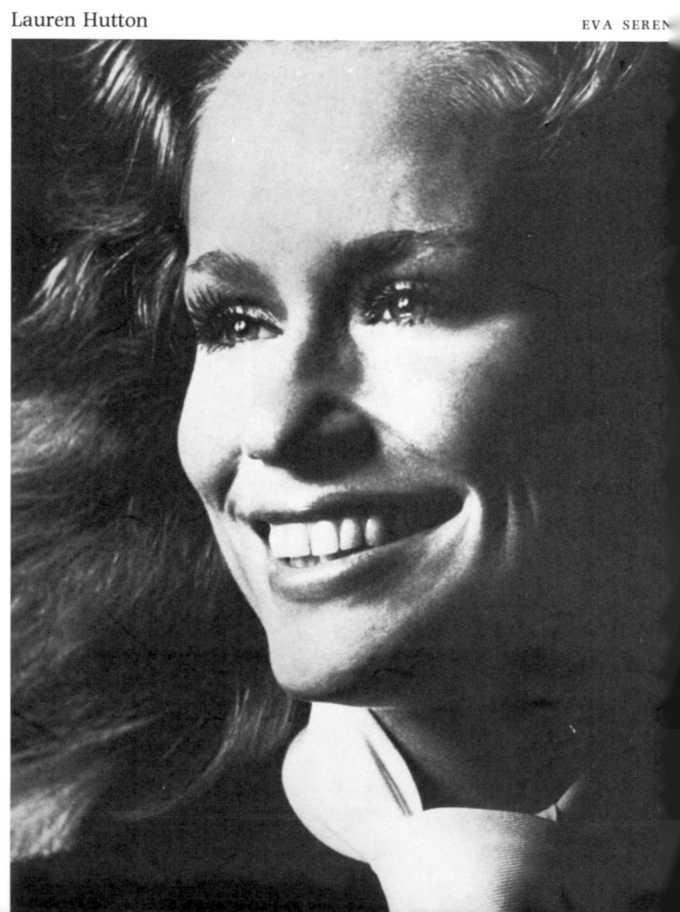

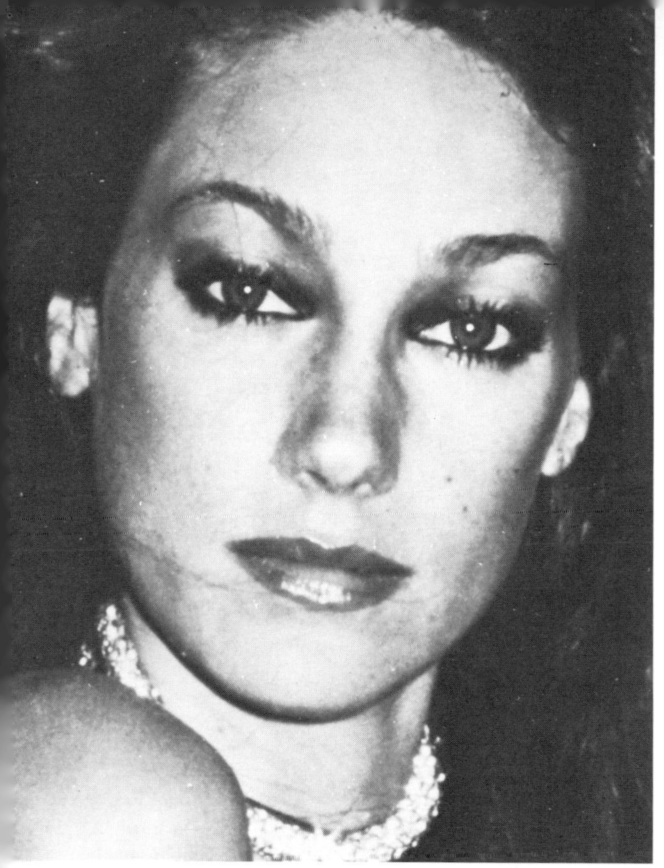

arisa Berenson HELMUT NEWTON

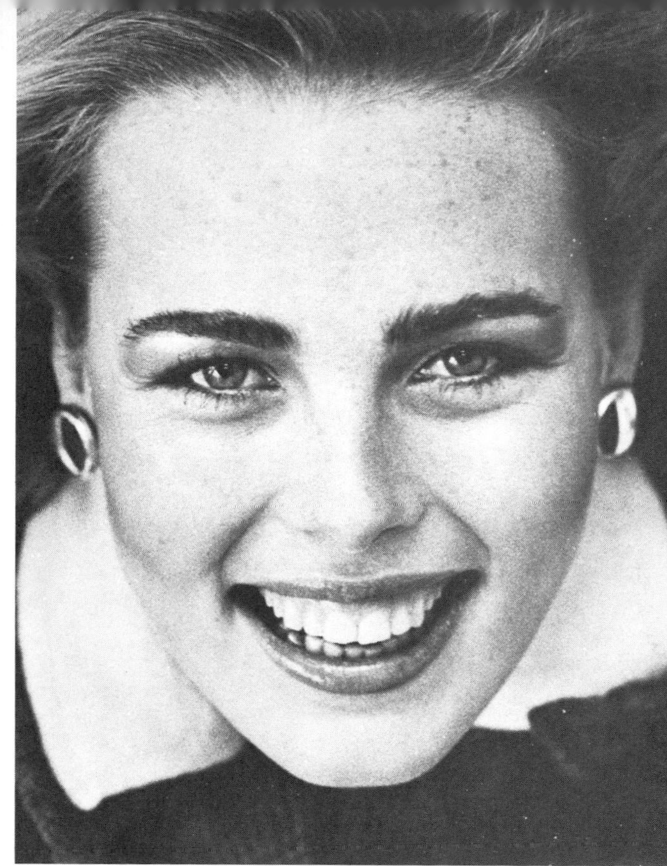

Margaux Hemingway TOSCANI

anca Jagger DAVID BAILEY

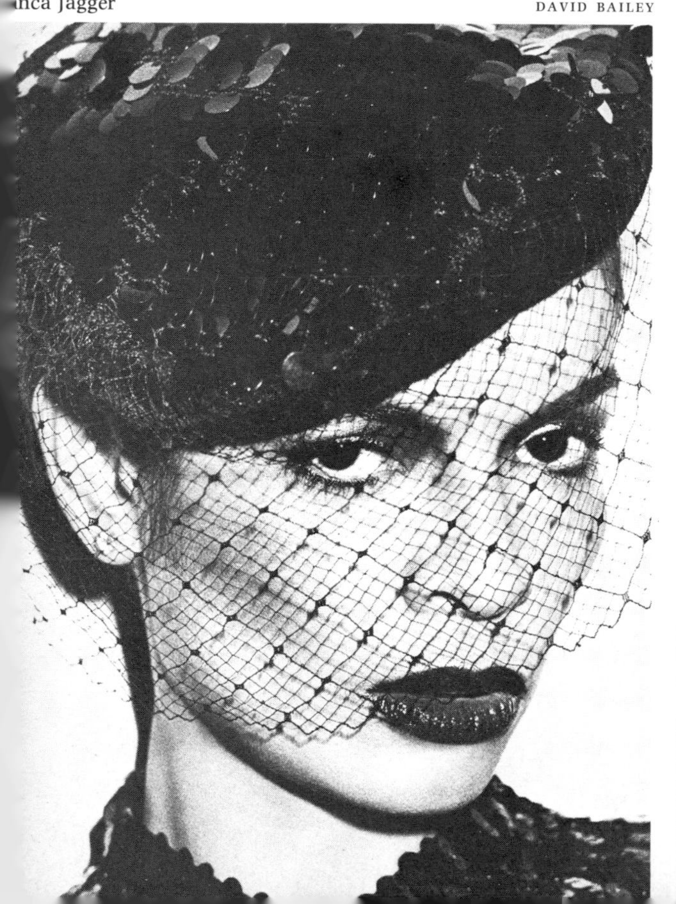

Marie Helvin DAVID BAILEY

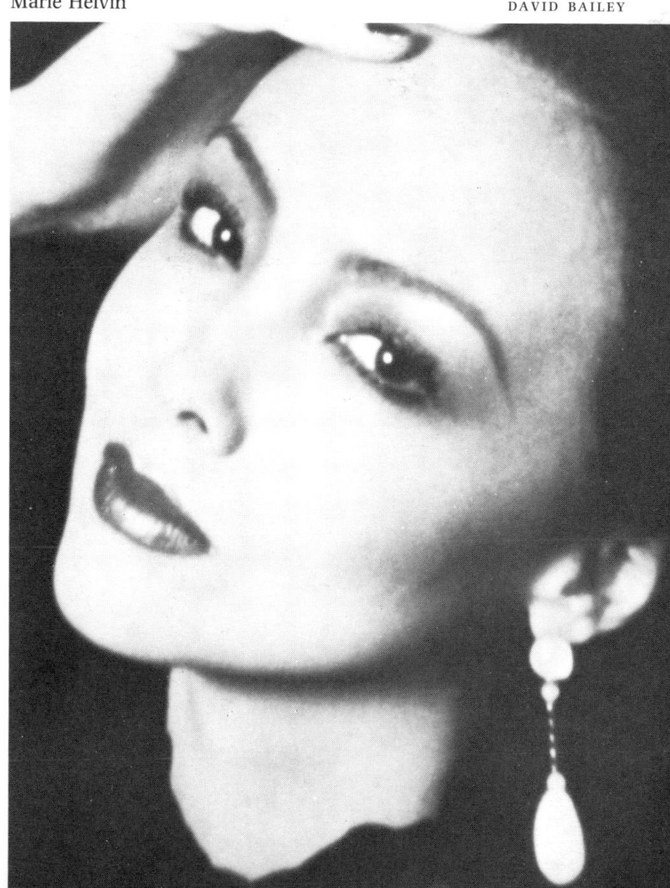

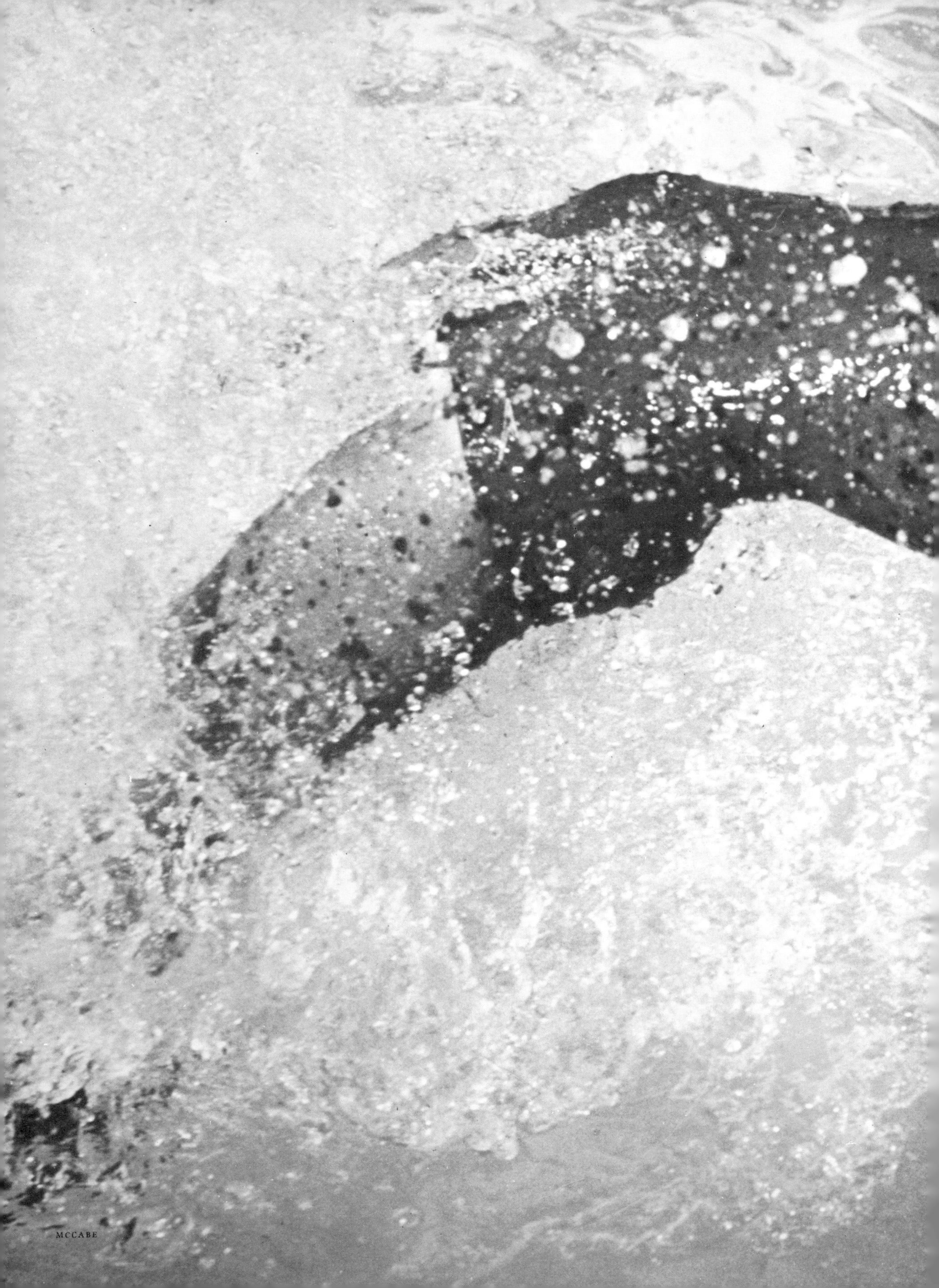

MCCABE

PART II THE AESTHETICS

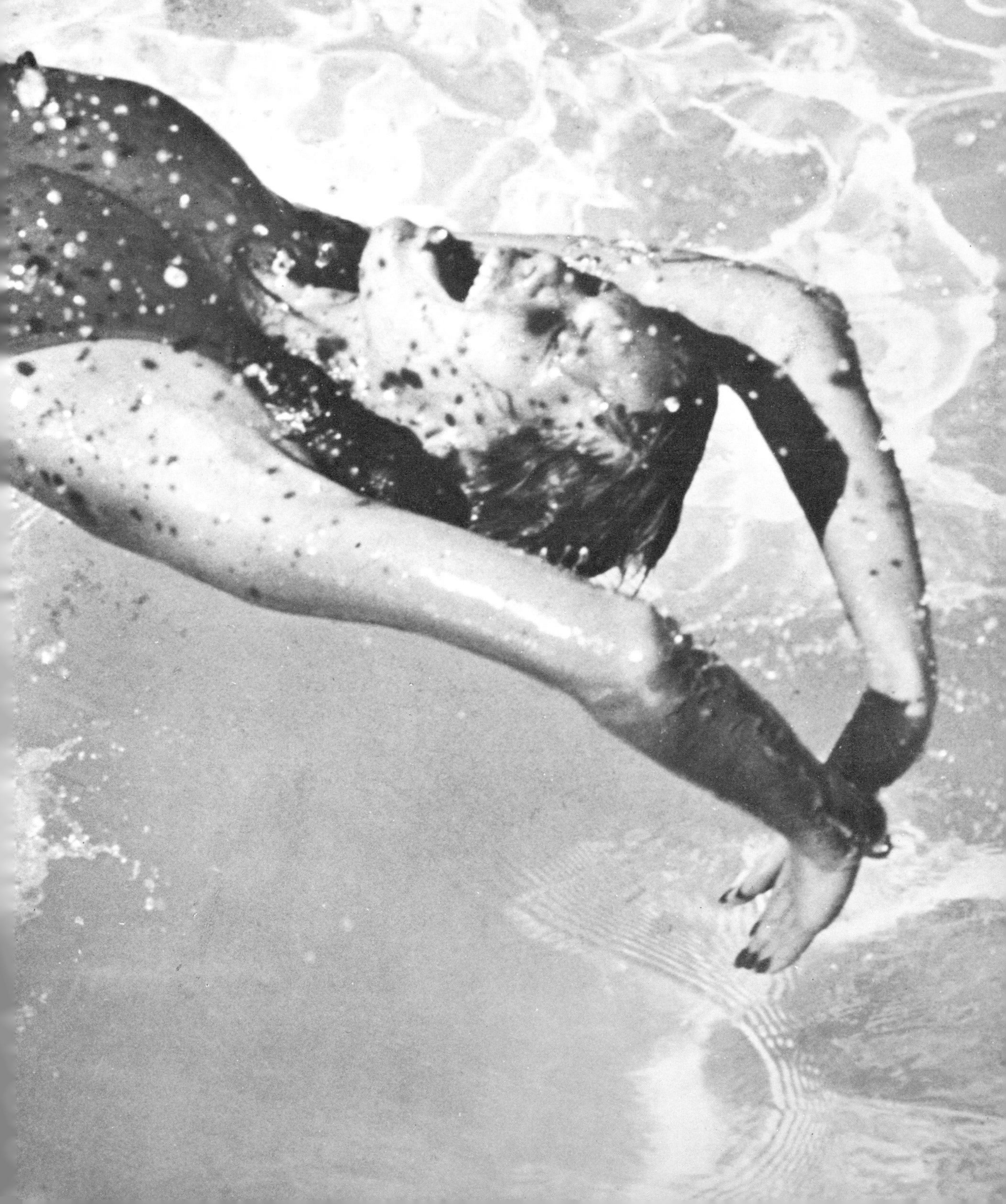

1

NATURAL PREPARATIONS

Some of the most satisfactory beauty products – facials, cleansers, conditioners, tonics – are those you can make yourself with familiar ingredients from formulas handed down, added to and improved upon over the years. It will take time to determine which are the best formulas for your particular skin. Not every recipe will be right or bring exceptional results. You need to learn to adjust the ingredients, to meet your own specific requirements; climate conditions often alter textures.

Home made skin preparations lack the usual preservatives of chemical additives, so will not last long. Make small quantities, and keep chilled any recipe containing perishable food, such as milk, eggs, wheatgerm.

The following recipes are classified according to their function. They are limited to the more simple preparations requiring the minimum effort in the making and in the search for ingredients.

CLEANSERS

Almond Cleansing Cream

4 oz. (120 g.) oil of sweet almonds
1 oz. (30 g.) hydrous lanolin
1 oz. (30 g.) petroleum jelly

Melt the fats slowly in a double boiler; remove from heat; beat until cool.

Lotion for Dry Skin

1 oz. (30 g.) mineral oil
$2\frac{1}{2}$ oz. (75 g.) glycerine
4 oz. (120 g.) milk of magnesia
4 oz. (120 g.) witch hazel

Stir slowly together all the ingredients; keep in a tightly covered glass bottle and shake before use.

Lotion for Oily Skin

1 oz. (30 g.) spirits of camphor
2½ oz. (75 g.) glycerine
4 oz. (120 g.) eau-de-Cologne
2 oz. (60 g.) distilled water

Mix together, adding the water last. Shake before using.

Apricot Cleansing Cream

4 tablespoons apricot oil
2 tablespoons sesame seed oil
2 tablespoons butter
1 tablespoon distilled water

Beat the ingredients, by hand or in a blender, until completely smooth and creamy. Keep in refrigerator.

Olive Cleansing Cream

4 tablespoons green olive oil
2 tablespoons sesame seed oil
2 tablespoons lard (vegetable fat)
2 drops of any essence

Beat the ingredients together until creamy. Keep in refrigerator.

Almond Meal Cleanser

½ cup oil of sweet almonds
½ cup corn or powdered oatmeal
½ cup grated Castile soap

Mix ingredients together without any liquid. Keep in jar and on use add just enough water to the handful necessary for cleansing.

CONDITIONERS

Night Cream

3 tablespoons almond oil
2 tablespoons hydrous lanolin
2 tablespoons cocoa butter
2 teaspoons rose water
½ teaspoon honey

In a glass bowl placed in a pan of boiling water, melt and smooth the almond oil, lanolin and cocoa butter. Remove from heat and add the rose water and honey; cool, then beat until blended.

Strawberry Conditioner

½ cup fresh or frozen strawberry juice
1 dessertspoon lanolin
1 dessertspoon powdered oatmeal

Melt lanolin in a bowl over water, add the oatmeal and when mixture is smooth stir in the strawberry juice, beating until creamy.

Lettuce Cream

1 cup chopped lettuce
½ cup lanolin
2 drops rose geranium oil

Heat lanolin over water in a small bowl. When it has liquidized add lettuce and beat until blended. Remove from heat and perfume with rose geranium oil. Strain.

Elder Flower Cream

(Freshly picked flowers
give the best results)

1 tablespoon lanolin
6 oz. (180 g.) sweet almond oil
1 cup elder flowers

Melt lanolin in a bowl in boiling water, add almond oil, blend well. Put in the elder flowers and simmer for 30 minutes; cool and strain.

Lily Cream

1 cup distilled water
2 tablespoons powdered lily roots
1 tablespoon honey
1 oz. (30 g.) lanolin
½ teaspoon rose water

Simmer the lily root powder in the water for 30 minutes. Strain, add the honey. Meanwhile, melt lanolin in a glass bowl in boiling water, remove from heat; add the lily, then the rose water.

Cucumber Cream

½ oz. (15 g.) white wax
2 oz. (60 g.) oil of sweet almonds
1 cucumber

Melt the wax in a glass jar standing in boiling water; add the almond oil. Peel and chop the cucumber very finely, and add just enough to the jar so that it is covered by the wax. Cover with foil and leave simmering for one hour. Remove from heat and stir thoroughly. Strain.

Enriched Avocado Cream

2 eggs
1 teaspoon glycerine
½ teaspoon lemon juice
2 teaspoons avocado oil
½ teaspoon cider vinegar
2 egg yolks, beaten
2 tablespoons distilled water

Blend the eggs, glycerine and lemon juice; slowly add enough avocado oil to thicken the mixture to a heavy cream, then stir in the vinegar. Add the beaten egg yolks and water – slowly, blending all the time. Keep refrigerated.

Honey and Almond Cream

4 oz. (120 g.) natural honey
8 oz. (240 g.) hydrous lanolin
½ cup oil of sweet almonds

In a double boiler warm the honey, blend in the lanolin, and as it melts add the almond oil. Stir well; remove from heat and beat until thoroughly creamed. Refrigerate.

RESTORERS

Mayonnaise Facial Masque

1 egg
½ teaspoon sea salt
2 tablespoons lemon juice
1 cup olive oil

Blend half a cup of the oil with the remaining ingredients; whip until thick, pour in the remaining oil very slowly. Keep refrigerated. After applying to face, allow 15 to 30 minutes before rinsing off.

Oatmeal Masque

½ cup milk
2 tablespoons unprocessed oatmeal
2 teaspoons elder flower water

Cook the oatmeal and milk as though it were porridge, until soft. Take off the heat, add elder flower water. Beat together and when just warm, spread over the face. Leave for 20 minutes.

Cucumber Masque

1 cucumber
¼ teaspoon lemon juice
1 teaspoon witch hazel
1 teaspoon alcohol
1 egg white, whipped

Peel the cucumber and extract the juice, add lemon juice, witch hazel and alcohol. Stir well; then blend in the whipped egg. Allow to dry on face for a minimum of 15 minutes. Rinse.

Wheat Germ Facial

1 egg yolk
½ teaspoon wheatgerm
¾ cup oil of sweet almonds
1 teaspoon distilled water

Beat the first three ingredients together, add the water, beat again. Brush on the face, leave 20 minutes.

Honey Masque

1 tablespoon honey
1 egg yolk
1 teaspoon olive oil

Beat the egg yolk into the oil, then blend in the honey. Apply to the face and leave for 15 minutes before rinsing away.

Parsley Facial

2 handfuls parsley
1 cup distilled water
1 tablespoon honey
1 egg yolk

Boil the parsley in the water for 15 minutes; strain. Stir in the honey and beaten egg yolk when liquid has cooled. Brush on face, leave for 15 minutes.

Honey and Oatmeal Paste

1 oz. (30 g.) honey
1 teaspoon lemon juice
2 unbeaten egg whites
½ teaspoon oil of sweet almonds
2 tablespoons powdered oatmeal

Mix everything together except the oatmeal. When smooth slowly add sufficient oatmeal to make a paste moist, but not sloppy. Apply to face and neck for 20 minutes before rinsing off.

Apricot Wrinkle Cream

2 tablespoons lanolin
1 tablespoon apricot oil
1 teaspoon lemon juice
3 drops tincture of benzoin

Melt lanolin in a glass bowl in a pan of simmering water; stir in the apricot oil and lemon juice; blend very well and finally add the benzoin; beat again.

Almond Refining Paste

4 oz. (120 g.) blanched almonds
1 egg white
1–2 tablespoons rose water

Pound the almonds into a smooth paste; add the egg white, unbeaten, and enough rose water to make a malleable paste. Leave on the skin for about 10 minutes.

Pimple Clearing Cream

2 pints (1 l.) rose water
2 sliced apples
2 tablespoons chopped fennel
2 tablespoons chopped celery
¼ oz. (7½ g.) barley meal
3 egg whites
1 teaspoon lanolin

In a double boiler simmer in the rose water, the apples, fennel, celery, and barley meal; when mushy, add beaten egg whites and lanolin. Strain; beat until smooth. Keep in refrigerator.

Basic Pimple Cream

1 tablespoon castor oil
1 tablespoon glycerine
1 tablespoon lanolin

Melt all ingredients together in a glass bowl placed in simmering water. Cool and keep in glass jar.

French Freckle Cream

1 oz. (30 g.) grated Castile soap
3 tablespoons distilled water
3 teaspoons lemon juice
$\frac{1}{4}$ oz. ($7\frac{1}{2}$ g.) oil of bitter almonds
$\frac{1}{4}$ teaspoon cream of tartar
4 drops olive oil

Put the grated soap and water in a double boiler, melt over low heat; when all water has evaporated, blend in thoroughly the rest of the ingredients. Rub over freckles, leave for 30 minutes.

Paste for Blackheads

8 oz. (240 g.) powdered oatmeal
4 oz. (120 g.) ground almonds
2 oz. (60 g.) powdered orris root
$\frac{1}{2}$ oz. (15 g.) grated Castile soap
2 tablespoons water

Mix dry ingredients well together, then add 2 tablespoons boiled water to make a paste. Rub into blackheads and leave 1 hour.

Lotion for Blackheads

1 tablespoon Epsom salts
3 drops white iodine
1 cup boiling water

Dissolve Epsom salts and iodine in the boiling water. Apply hot.

Freckle Removing Cream

$\frac{1}{4}$ cup of sour milk
$\frac{1}{2}$ teaspoon of grated horseradish
1 tablespoon of cornmeal or powdered oatmeal

Mix all ingredients together into a paste; put between two layers of gauze, then apply to freckled areas. Don't let it get too near the eyes. Leave for 30 minutes.

STIMULATORS

Raspberry Vinegar

2 cups raspberries
1 cup rose petals
1 teaspoon honey
2 pints (1 l.) cider vinegar

Steep the first three ingredients in the vinegar for one month – in a covered earthenware pot. Strain, dilute with an equal part of distilled water. Use as a toner.

Oily Skin Astringent

$\frac{1}{4}$ teaspoon boric acid powder
1 dessertspoon witch hazel
2 oz. (60 g.) glycerine
2 oz. (60 g.) alcohol
$1\frac{1}{2}$ oz. (45 g.) rose water
$\frac{1}{4}$ teaspoon friar's balsam (benzoin)

Dissolve the boric acid powder in the witch hazel, add other ingredients. Mix thoroughly.

Lavender Water

2 cups lavender flowers
1 oz. (30 g.) powdered orris root
1 pint (6 dl.) vinegar

Steep the dry ingredients in the vinegar for three to four weeks; strain, dilute with the same amount of distilled water. Use as a toner.

Rose Vinegar

4 cups dried red roses
½ cup essence of rose
1 pint (6 dl.) vinegar

Put all ingredients in a lidded glass jar; allow to stand for three weeks, often shaking it. Strain, dilute with equal parts of distilled water. Use as a toner.

Cucumber Toner

1 peeled cucumber
1 teaspoon witch hazel
1 teaspoon rose water
egg white

Mash the cucumber, add witch hazel and rose water; beat the egg white to a froth; mix very well. Refrigerate. Strain before use.

Elder Flower Rinse

1 cup elder flowers (fresh or dried)
1 pint (6 dl.) boiling water

Pour boiling water over the flowers and allow to steep for a minimum of eight hours. Strain. Use as a toner.

Peppermint Vinegar

1 pint (6 dl.) cider vinegar
1 pint (6 dl.) distilled water
1 cup mint leaves

Bring all ingredients to the boil, remove and place in a glass container. Allow to steep for five days; strain. Use as an astringent.

Sage Astringent

½ cup dried sage
½ cup alcohol
1 teaspoon glycerine
3 tablespoons witch hazel
¼ teaspoon friar's balsam (benzoin)
¼ teaspoon boric acid powder

Steep the sage in the alcohol for a week; strain. Dissolve boric acid powder in the witch hazel, add this and all other ingredients to the sage extract.

PROTECTORS

Sesame Tanning Lotion

¼ cup lanolin
¼ cup sesame oil
¾ cup distilled water

In a double boiler, melt the lanolin; take off the heat and blend with sesame oil and water. Keep in refrigerator.

Sun Protection Lotion

1 peeled cucumber
½ teaspoon glycerine
½ teaspoon rose water

Extract the juice from the cucumber and mix the liquid with glycerine and rose water. Refrigerate.

Anti-Sunburn Cream

1 egg white, beaten
1 teaspoon honey
½ teaspoon witch hazel

Blend all ingredients together until even. Smooth over bad sunburn. Always refrigerate.

Iodine Bronzing Lotion

1 cup olive oil
10 drops iodine
juice of a lemon

Blend all ingredients together very well and always shake before using.

FRAGRANCES

Lavender Toilet Water

½ oz. (15 g.) oil of lavender
2 pints (1 l.) ethyl alcohol

Mix the lavender essence with just a little of the alcohol until thoroughly blended; then slowly add the rest of the alcohol. Keep in sealed jars – mature for a minimum of 6 weeks before using.

Cologne Water

1 pint (6 dl.) ethyl alcohol
1 teaspoon orange water
1 teaspoon lemon essence
1½ teaspoons oil of lavender
1 teaspoon bergamot

Blend all the oils and essences, then gradually mix in the alcohol. Allow to mature for 6–8 weeks; keep in firmly lidded bottles.

Rose Essence

3 handfuls of dried rose petals
sweet almond oil as needed

In a glass bowl or jar, put dried rose petals and cover with the oil. Put the pot in a pan of simmering water, heat until the oil has removed all the colour of the petals. Strain; keep tightly lidded.

Herb and Flower Cologne

¼ oz. (7½ g.) bergamot
¼ oz. (7½ g.) orange oil
¼ oz. (7½ g.) balsam of Peru
¼ oz. (7½ g.) essence of cloves
¼ oz. (7½ g.) thyme
¼ pint (1·5 dl.) orange flower water
2 pints (1 l.) ethyl alcohol

Put all herbs and essences into a glass jar, pour over the alcohol very slowly and stirring all the time. Allow mixture to mature for two weeks before using – jar must be tightly lidded.

After-bath Splash

1 cup fresh rose petals
½ cup alcohol
1½ tablespoons lemon peel
1½ tablespoons orange peel
½ tablespoon dried basil
1 tablespoon dried peppermint
1 cup boiling water

Steep rose petals in alcohol for 1 week; strain. Steep lemon peel, orange peel, basil and peppermint in the boiling water – make as tea – for 12 hours; strain. Combine two liquids, cover tightly, always shake before use.

Fresh Floral Cologne

1 oz. (30 g.) rose water
3½ teaspoons oil of lavender
½ oz. (15 g.) oil of cloves
6 oz. (180 g.) ethyl alcohol

Blend the two oils with a little alcohol until thoroughly united; beat in the remaining alcohol. Add the rose water. Bottle tightly and mature for 6–8 weeks.

Spicy Toilet Water

2 cups rose water
2 cups wine or cider vinegar
2 bay leaves
½ tablespoon crushed cloves

Boil all ingredients together, but add a little extra water all the time to keep the liquid at the original volume. Allow to mature for a month.

FOR THE HANDS

Protective Cream

(to be worn under gloves)

1 dessertspoon fuller's earth
1 dessertspoon almond oil
2 egg yolks

Mix all three ingredients together into an even blend; keep chilled until use. Keep on during work, then rinse off.

Cuticle Softener

2 tablespoons fresh or frozen pineapple juice
2 tablespoons egg yolk
½ teaspoon cider vinegar

Mix together – a very sloppy texture in which nails should be soaked for 30 minutes. It can be preserved for a while in the refrigerator.

Chapped Skin Cream

½ oz. (15 g.) white wax
6 tablespoons sweet almond oil
2 oz. (60 g.) rose water
1 teaspoon cod liver oil

In a double boiler melt wax and oils; add the rose water drop by drop, slowly beating all the time.

Honey Hand Cream

¼ oz. (7½ g.) white wax
¼ oz. (7½ g.) spermaceti
½ oz. (15 g.) sweet almond oil
4 oz. (120 g.) honey
few drops perfumed oil

In a glass bowl over hot water dissolve the wax and spermaceti; stir in almond oil and honey. Blend well, cool and then beat in perfumed oil.

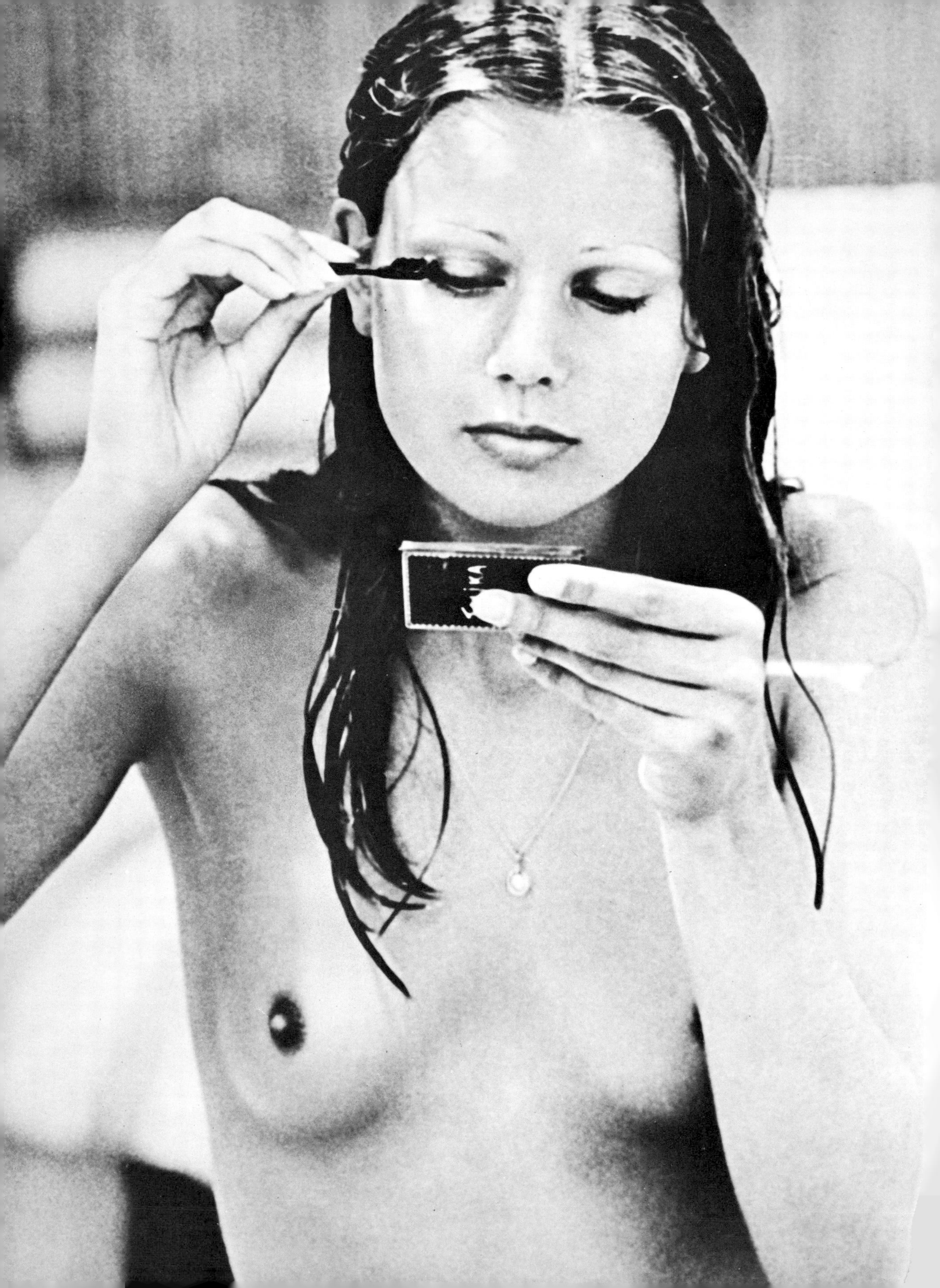

2

MAKE-UP

Make-up is any formulated preparation used for cleansing, treating, embellishing or altering the appearance. All contain a variety of ingredients, both natural and synthetic. The selection is vast, yet within the categories, compounds are basically the same. Differences are in the finer points – texture, colour, perfume, or in the addition of a special nutrient. Is there much difference between expensive and inexpensive brands? Performance does not vary a lot; it is usually how you use a product not what you use that determines the effect. It is true that more research goes into the more expensive items. Also the higher the price, the more attractive the containers, the better the depth and choice of colour, and sometimes ingredients are finer and perfumes rarer. But the real difference is psychological. If you think a certain product is more effective, it invariably is. The look, the feel, the smell, the image of a cosmetic – all contribute equally.

The make-up you use depends on what suits you. Some products are in agreement with your skin, others are not. There are also several ranges of hypo-allergenic cosmetics and manufacturers are increasingly concerned with purity. Cosmetics containing no chemicals whatsoever are likely to be more expensive because not only are natural ingredients often rarer, but the life of the preparation is usually limited.

SKIN PREPARATIONS

CLEANSERS: These contain oil to dissolve the grease of make-up and an emulsifying agent to make removal easier.

Creams – very good at removing make-up and dirt, but apt to cling to the skin. Generally better for dry and normal skins. Remove with tissue.

Cold Creams – more fluffy and can be used on oily skins too. Remove with tissue.

Liquids – contain more water than creams and come as lotions of varying creaminess. For all types of skin. Remove with tissue.

Rinsable Cleaners – light creams or liquids that can be rinsed off with water. Fine for all skins.

Pad Cleaners – thick wads of absorbent material saturated with a liquid cleanser. Good for special areas like eyes and for touch-up cleansing.

FRESHENERS: Remove last traces of cleanser, refresh and refine skin texture, sometimes acting as thinners of dead cells. They come in three strengths according to alcohol content. Apply with cottonwool wads.

Fresheners – the simplest, consisting of an aromatic substance dissolved in water, sometimes with a little alcohol. Soothe and cool the skin.

Toners – slightly more bracing because of higher alcohol content. Good for dry and normal skins.

Astringents – the strongest with highest percentage of alcohol. Tingle on skin and have a temporary pore-tightening effect. Good for oily skin.

MOISTURIZERS: A misnomer, as these products do not give moisture themselves, but promote moisturization by sealing in the available water. They do so by filming the skin with the thinnest invisible layer of oil or grease. The most essential of all skin preparations, they come in different formulas for different skins, so read the labels. Apply with finger tips.

Creams – the heaviest, also act as lubricants and protectors in extreme climates. Good for dry skin, ageing skin and for use overnight.

Lotions – lighter but still mild lubricants. Go well under make-up as they fill in surface irregularities, thus allowing foundation to adhere more smoothly and evenly.

CONDITIONERS – Also called: emollients, lubricants, nourishing, treatment, enriched or night creams. Eye creams and throat creams also come into this category, as do body and hand lotions. All are heavy duty preparations aimed to help skin that needs oil or moisture or both. They do three jobs – lubricate, moisturize and protect.

Creams – all contain oils or greases or both; the main difference between the many types is the concentration and proportion of the two. All oils and greases, whether of animal, vegetable or mineral origin, will act in much the same way.

They are tenacious, forming a protective barrier while the skin absorbs the fatty molecules; they smooth the surface and provide an anchor for moisture. They are applied with fingertips and massaged gently into the skin. They should not disappear, but be visible on the surface. The effectiveness of these heavier creams is increased by pre-wetting the skin. Leave on for a minimum of an hour. Tissue off, then cleanse the face.

Many creams contain extra ingredients claiming special properties. Most are intended to encourage the skin into increased cell renewal. Skin is capable of absorbing certain outside elements, but which and to what degree is controversial. Some of the more common additions are:

Hormones – satisfy the skin's need for oestrogen during and after the menopause. The hormone content of creams is too small to affect the whole system, and there is a legal limit as to how much is permitted in an ounce (30 g.). They do improve skin condition to an extent as they change metabolism of cells, causing them to expand, thus plumping and smoothing the surface.

Tissue extracts – include tissues from the embryo, placenta and ovaries of young animals. Their action is to increase capillary circulation and stimulate metabolism. Their content in cream is limited, but they can help to hydrate and nourish ageing skin, also remedy excessive dryness and oily problems.

Collagen – in its natural state is an important part of connective tissue and responsible for smoothness and resilience of the skin. It is used in creams to improve elasticity and help skin retain natural fluids.

Eye Creams – particularly concentrated conditioners with a high percentage of a finer oil. To be patted around the eye area.

Throat Creams – not very different from regular conditioners, but sometimes a little richer in oils. Apply with fingertips, massaging with upward strokes.

Body Lotions – water-based emulsions that are really diluted creams, but often containing additional aromatics and sometimes a freshener to give a cool feeling. They perform the same service as any other conditioner – smooth, lubricate, moisturize and protect. Apply by hand.

Hand Lotions – water-based emulsions of varying degrees of thickness. The same basic formula as a body lotion but often of a heavier consistency. Some hand creams are glycerine based, formed into a jelly substance by gum tragacanth. Protection properties are important; they also lubricate and moisturize. Apply by hand.

SUNSCREENS: These consist of a chemical screen plus a base which may be a water-alcohol mixture, a lotion, a cream, an oil or a grease. The type of base makes little difference, though the oily and greasy ones are more water resistant, and many women prefer creams because they also soften the skin. However the criterion for a sunscreen should be its efficiency at protecting the skin against sun and light. They work by selectively blocking out the ultra violet rays that are responsible for skin damage.

They fall into three groups; the names of the chemicals are impossibly difficult but to be selective you must read labels and recognize them.

The best – para-aminobenzoic acid, but with the disadvantage of being poorly soluble, so alcohol is needed to keep it in solution. This means that sunscreens containing it may be drying to some skins. It also tends to stain fabrics.

Pretty good – para-aminobenzoic derivatives such as iso-amyl and glyceryl, also benzophenone derivatives. These are available in all bases, but beware of a heavy application of benzophenone as it will almost eliminate tanning completely.

Fine – menthyl anthranilate, homomenthyl salicylate, triethanolamine salicylate, cinoxate, digalloyl trioleate. Found in all bases, don't stain and approved for limited amounts of sun. Apply liberally everywhere including lips.

Fake Tanning Creams – emulsions containing a chemical agent that darkens the skin. On the whole they work well, but some skins are inclined to go orangey instead of brown. Colour is temporary.

MAKE-UP PREPARATIONS

FOUNDATIONS: Their purpose is to provide the look of better skin colour and texture. They leave a film on the skin covering minor imperfections and unify colour. Generally made from a water-in-oil formula, the basic idea is that each drop of water is surrounded with drops of oil. The proportion of each varies to produce different textures and effects, but all give an even tint. They range in colour from flat white to the deepest mahogany. Some can be used without powder.

Liquids – provide a light protective film, can be of the creamy moisturized kind ideal for dry and normal skins, or oil-free formulas for greasy skins. They do not cover well, therefore are not good for camouflaging blemished skin. Sometimes difficult to control, and more efficient when applied with a sponge.

Creams – thicker and heavier with consistency varying from milky to whipped cream. Give the glossiest look, and easy to apply with fingertips or sponge. Usually waterproof.

Opposite: Guy Bourdin, 1974
Overleaf right: Norman Parkinson, 1972

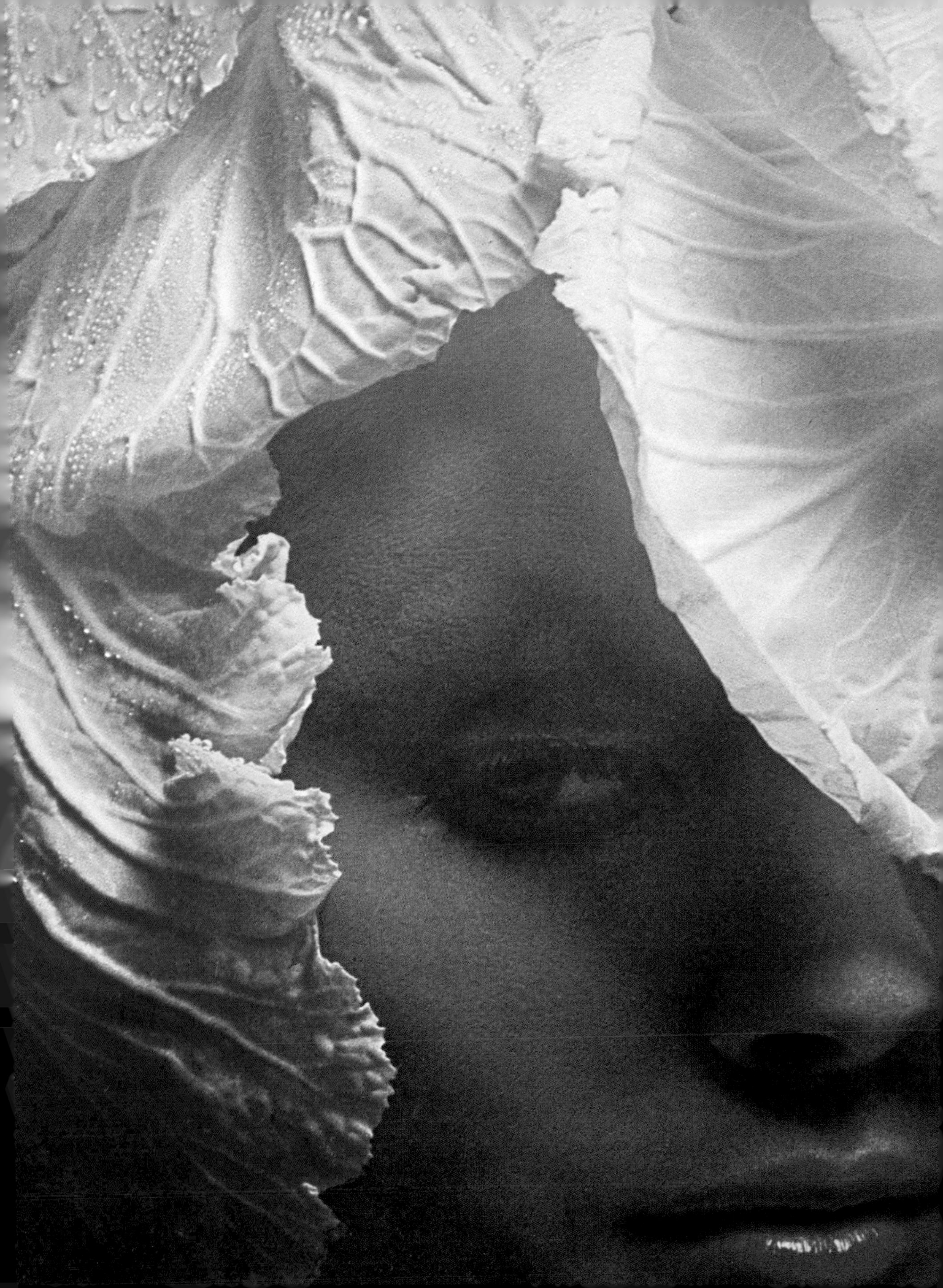

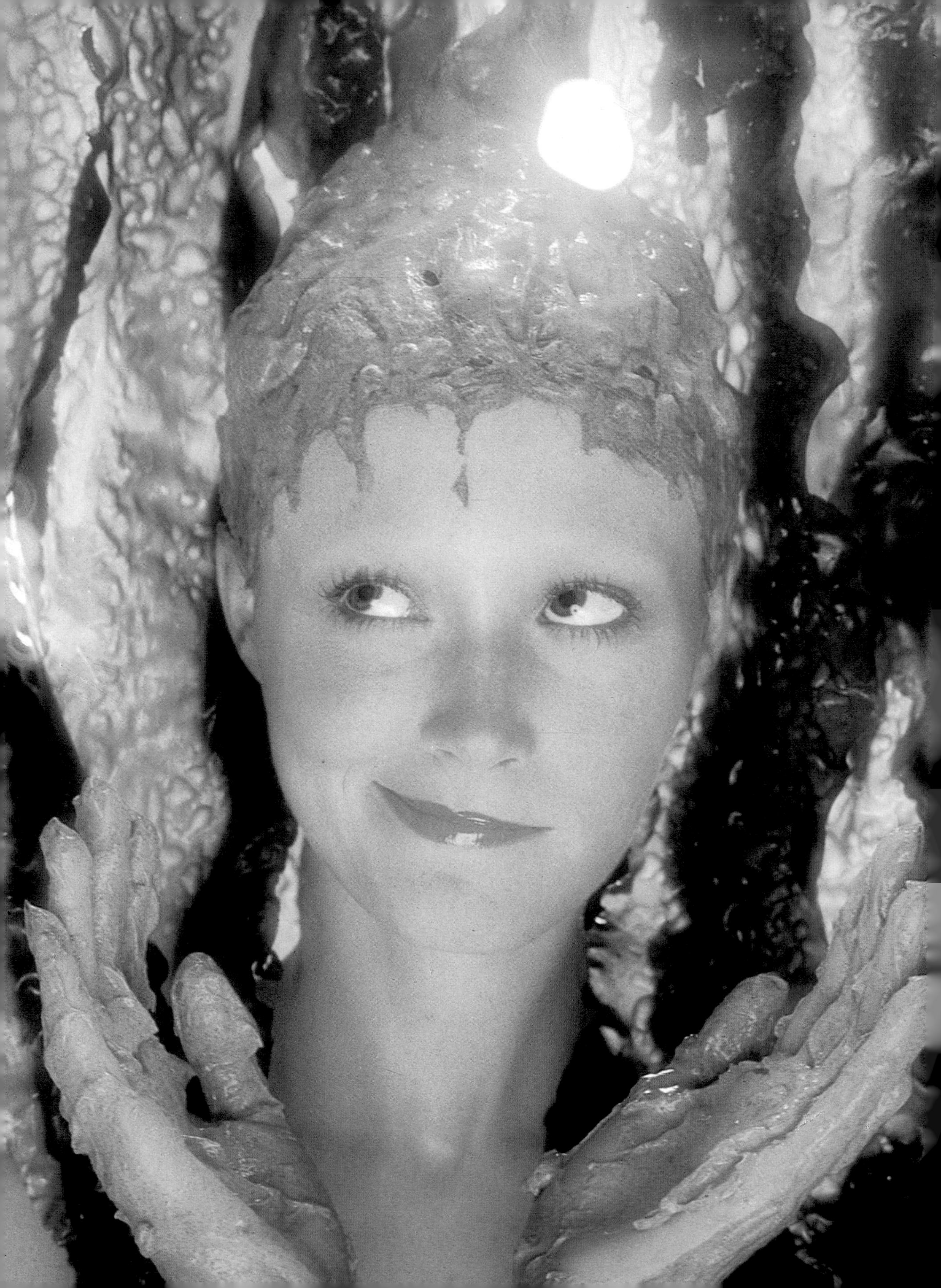

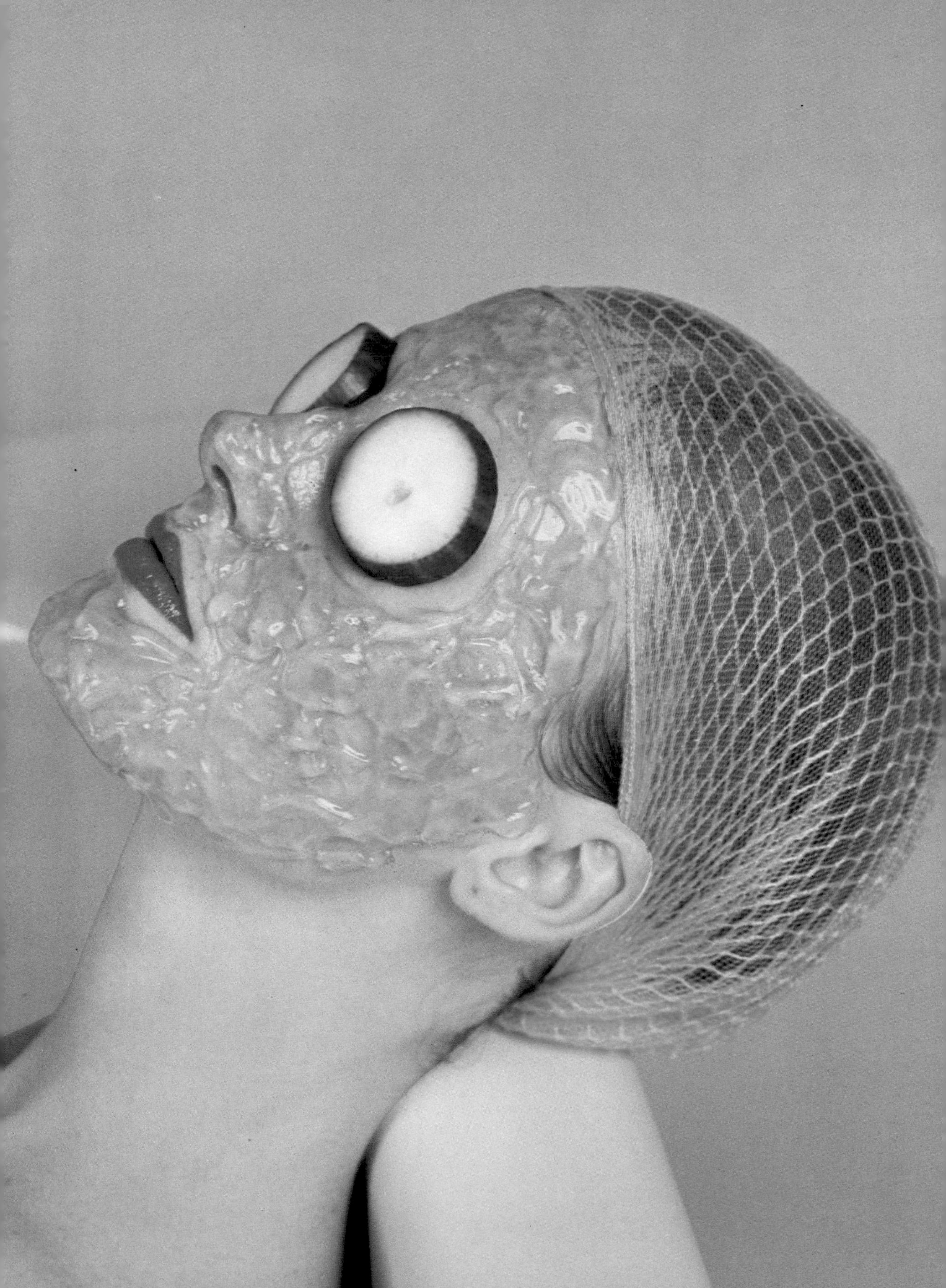

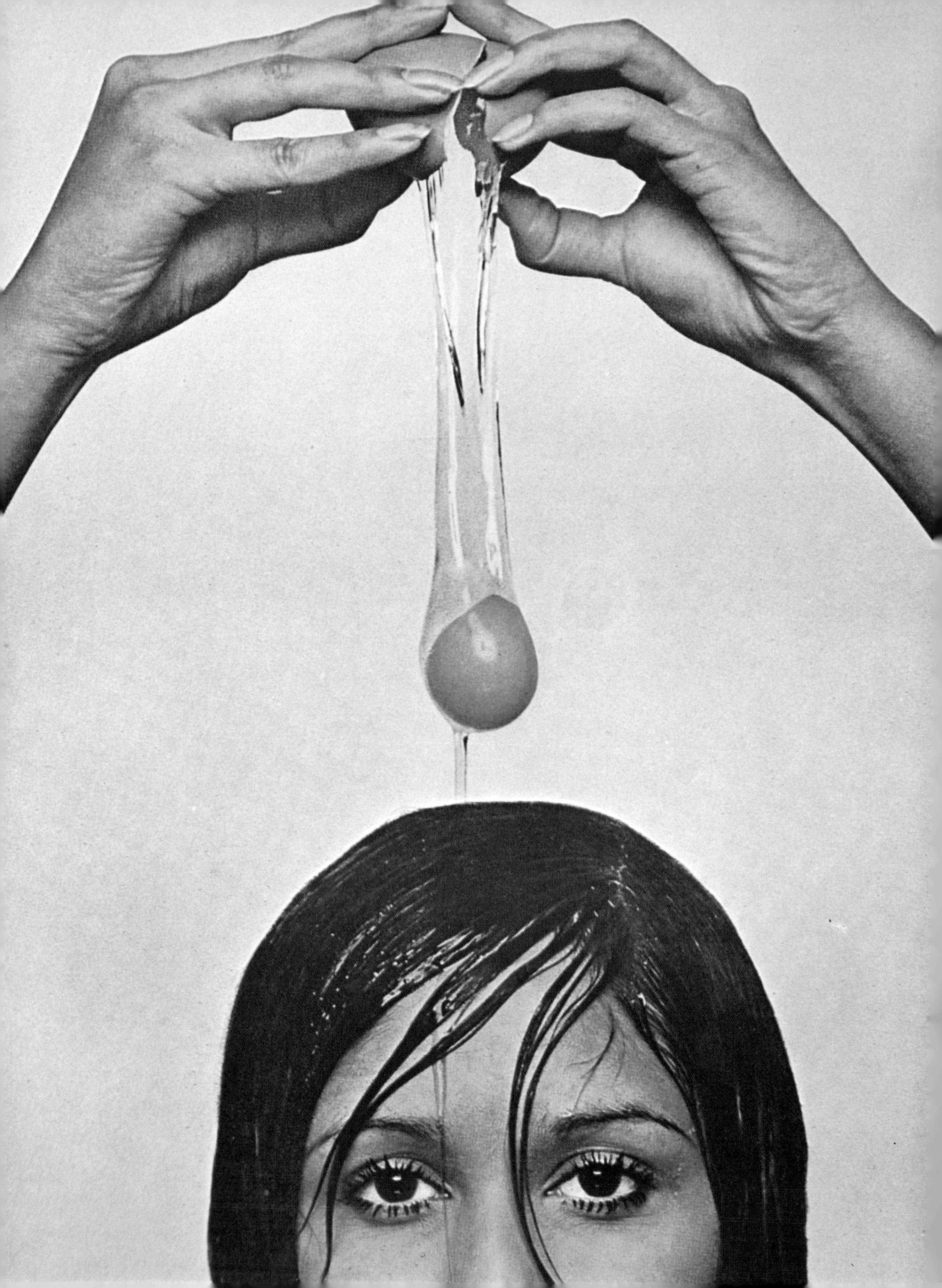

All-in-One Bases – a mixture of cream and powder, often more difficult to apply as they tend to drag the skin; a damp sponge eases application. Not suggested for dry skins. Do not require fixing with powder, but finish is drier.

Cover-Ups – very dense creams that feel like putty and often in stick form. Used to cover skin blemishes and alleviate dark circles under the eyes. Pat on with fingertips. All cover-ups require extensive blending afterwards.

Solid Cream Sticks – very thick formula, add the most colour, hide blemishes, dark circles, freckles. Stroke on directly, then blend with fingers.

Gels and Glossies – like a more fluid petroleum jelly, but coloured and scented; easy to smooth on with fingertips, provide a transparent shine, good for adding colour and a healthy looking gloss.

Cakes and Blocks – dense dehydrated formulas, add a lot of colour, good for covering blemishes. They can be drying so are not advisable for dry skins – but a great help to oily ones. Apply with a damp sponge.

POWDERS: Set make-up with a sheen or matt look. Translucent powders are usually preferred as they do not affect other make-up colours. Otherwise the colour spectrum is in four groups: the neutrals, the pinks, the goldens, the browns. If you use a colour, the general rule is to choose one shade lighter than the foundation.

Loose Powders – best for the final finish to make-up; apply with a puff or cottonwool wad.

Pressed Powders – usually in compacts and convenient for touch-ups, but do not apply layer upon layer, it will cake.

BLUSHERS: Used to be known as rouge. Now also known as shaders, contourers or, when light, as highlighters. Function is to add colour, warmth, shading or luminosity. Rosy, peach and tawny colours tone the cheeks; the deep tawny and brown shades are used to give the illusion of fading out undesirable features and hollowing cheeks. Apply powders with a brush, others with fingertips.

Creams – add moisture as well as colour. Blend in with fingertips; use over foundation but under powder.

Powders – brushed on face after powder; translucent varieties reflect more light and appear to glow.

Gels – transparent colours for a glossy look; apply over foundation, but don't cover with powder.

Opposite: Barry Lategan, 1969

EYE-SHADOWS: Add colour and dimension to the eyes, the look of which can be dramatically improved by intelligent shading. Often known as highlighters in the white and creamy tones. Full spectrum of colour.

Creams – oil based, soft spreading and easy to blend on skin. Should be set with powder – translucent or talcum – to prevent crease lines. Apply with fingertips or brush.

Sticks – more solid creams with oils dispersed in a waxy base. Like lipsticks, apt to go soggy in hot weather and hard to spread in cold. Apply stick directly to lids, then blend in with fingertips. Set with powder.

Liquids – usually provided with a built-in brush or wand applicator. Contain more water than creams and sticks, long-lasting when dry but difficult to apply as they're inclined to run.

Gels – easy to apply but often more gloss than depth of colour, so a couple of coats are required. Apply with fingertips.

Powders – based on compressed powder with a moisturizer added to give cling. Staying power is good, sometimes feel taut on dry skins. Apply with brush or sponge applicator.

Water-Colours – cake-like shadows applied with a wet brush. Long-lasting and painting-on property facilitates artistic effects. Some powders can be used in this way, but once water has been added there's no returning to using it as a simple powder.

Crayons and Pencils – waxier and softer than for brows, so easy to apply without pulling or dragging over the skin. Colour is drawn on with strokes or curves, blended with fingertips.

EYEBROW COLOURINGS:

Pencils – waxy narrow leads that have to be sharp to be effective. Draw on colour with tiny diagonal strokes.

Powders – like compressed powder, moisturized a little. Apply with slant-edged brush.

EYE LINERS: Define outline of eye by colouring all or part of the rim.

Liquids – oil-based in water; difficult to control unless applied with a fine sable brush.

Cakes – block of water-colour powder; one of the best ways to draw eye lines. Use fine brush, dampen powder.

Wands – contain a creamy fluid and built-in brush. Can be a bit gooey; allow time to dry otherwise they smudge.

MASCARAS: Generally oil-in-water formulas, giving colour and thickness to lashes.

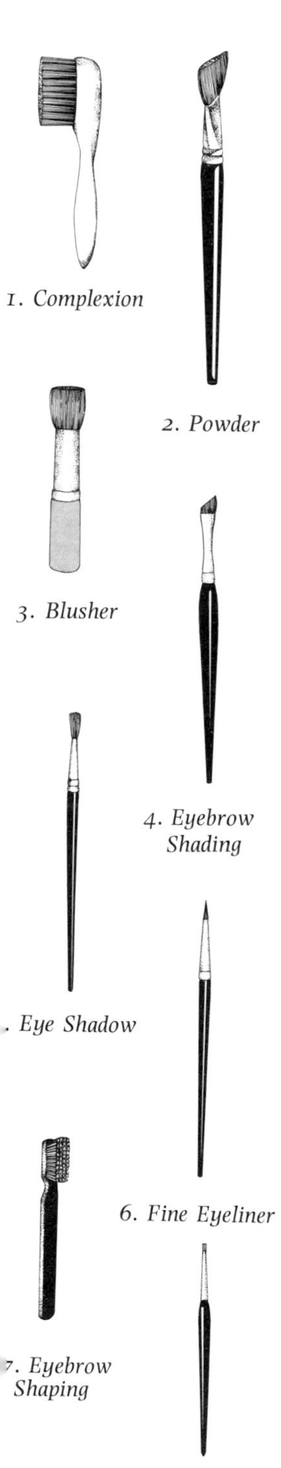
1. Complexion
2. Powder
3. Blusher
4. Eyebrow Shading
. Eye Shadow
6. Fine Eyeliner
7. Eyebrow Shaping
8. Lipbrush

Cakes and Blocks – one of the oldest kinds and still one of the most efficient. Apply with a wet brush. Build it up slowly and gradually allowing to dry between coats. Long lasting, and lashes usually separate well.

Creams – thick, oil-based, waterproof. Messy to apply so use a brush.

Wands – contain creams that are rolled on either with a spiral brush or screw-like rod; some have teeth applicators and creams are combed on. Several have additions of fibres or filaments to build up lash length and thickness.

LIP COLOURINGS:

Sticks – basically colours and oils dispersed in a wax base, many colours combined to make one shade; lanolin is added for softness and pliancy. The creamy, lustrous looking lipstick doesn't stay on very long, but is good for the lips and prevents drying. Some shades slightly stain the lips. Application can be direct, but better with a brush.

Gels and Gloss – with glycerine or petroleum-jelly bases, they give lots of gleam but usually not much colour. Clear colourless gels are often used over lipsticks. Apply with brush or fingertips.

Pencils – soft, wax-base crayons used to outline lips.

APPLICATION

Think of features: look in the mirror, forget overall shape. What is your best feature, the most attractive, the most unusual?

Think of emphasis: eyes, mouth or cheeks; decide which. Avoid the pitfall of trying to play up everything.

Think of skin tone: is it right for you? Would you look better a little paler, beiger, darker, browner, blacker? Think of the best blushing tone to go with it – pink, peach, amber, tawny, plum.

Think of change: a common fault is to go on believing in one particular look too long. Slight alterations can give the face a new contemporary look without losing its basic image.

The art of contemporary make-up lies in putting together all the separate parts to give an overall impression. It is not difficult but it takes know-how. Decide what to emphasize, then work on the background. The art is in the blending – textures, tones, shadings, colours, lines, features. A lot of make-up blended well looks more natural than a little make-up slapped on. Blend mostly with your fingertips, but also with brushes. It is easier, more accurate and more effective to apply make-up with brushes, and there are special ones for each application.

THE BASIS: COLOUR TONES

Skin tones can be altered only within a shade or two. Lighter skins have the advantage over dark, as the range of going deeper through make-up is far greater than that of going lighter. Skin tone controls other colour areas too: the cheeks and lips always, the eyes sometimes.

The choice and blending of colour tones is the most important part of make-up and various tints can be mixed together before application. Use the palm of the hand as a palette and work with fingers or brush. If the consistency is a little too thick, thin it by adding a drop of moisturizer or non-alcoholic freshener.

Generally the foundation shade closest to your natural skin tone is best and the darker the skin the more transparent looking it should be.

Pale – needs a delicate touch, a film of creamy ivory for the foundation; a blush of pink or amber; pastel lip tone.

Creamy – often an oriental skin, needs a bisque or golden beige make-up base; peach or rose tints for cheeks and lips.

Beige – a medium-tone skin that can take many shades – beige, golden and suntan tones; coral, rose-reds, bright pinks and tawny shades to balance.

Olive – golden colours with a touch of rose in the foundation; cheeks and lips need warm corals, deep rose tints or tawny shades.

Brown – the darker the skin, the less make-up base it usually needs, often the shine of a gel is the best. Dusky tones can be covered with cool brown or earthy shades of foundation; amber, cinnamon and grape tints for blushing, for lips.

Black – gels give glow and bronzing sticks are good for the darkest skins. Cheeks can be buffed with amber or plum shades, the same for lips which can often take a vivid rose too.

FOUNDATION

Use sparingly, two thin coats are preferable to one heavy layer. Creams, liquids and gels can be broken down on the palm of the hand first to give a smoother and finer application. Then dot on nose, each cheek, chin, forehead. If you are using a cream stick, put a stroke in each place. Blend very well with fingertips – upward and outward across the chin, outward over the cheeks, across the forehead, down the nose, under the tip and very lightly around the eyes and on the lids. Continue foundation just under the chin. There is no need to cover the neck area, but make sure there are no demarcation lines. Cake foundation is applied with a damp sponge. Sponging over all make-up bases evens out the film.

CORRECTING

Blemishes and dark shadows can be concealed; facial planes and dimensions can be corrected by light and dark shading.

Blemishes – use an opaque cover-up product. If flaw does not contrast too much with the skin – broken veins for example – use a shade that matches foundation. To cover a reddish scar or dark birthmark, use one shade lighter. To cover a lightened area, such as a white scar or pigment loss, use one shade darker. Apply concealer to the exact spot, gently stroke and blend the edges in with the foundation. If necessary cover with a thin film of foundation.

Shadows – usually under-eye circles which can be camouflaged by lightening. It is better to do this with a very light foundation or with a thick white crayon stroked on, then blended with the fingers. Blend until the whitened area merges with the make-up base.

Contouring – emphasize the best and diminish the least using light and dark shadings interspersed with a red tone: moving down from the eyes, the rule is – white first, red in the centre (see make-up for cheeks) and the beige-browns underneath. It is easy to make a mistake, as the inclination is to do too much. Concentrate on the highlights: automatically the rest of the face will recede. Use a white base (on the palm first) or a soft greasy crayon. Lighten the ridge of the nose, the upper edge of the cheekbones (out from under the eye up to the hairline), put a stroke in the crease by each nostril, a dot centred under the bottom lip. Blend. Be cautious with shading. Use one shade deeper than foundation: narrow a broad nose by shading the sides from eyebrows to nostrils; subtract from prominent jaw or chin by shading the outer edges. And blend.

CHEEKS

This is quite a large area and it is more practical to consider it two levels – upper and lower. The upper is a small oval area high on the cheekbone and slanting outwards from under the eye; the lower is a larger oval starting in the hollow of the cheek at nostril level and going up and out towards the hairline. The upper cheek is for highlighting, to give radiance during the day and luminosity on an evening face. The lower area is for contouring the face, using a muted tint to give dimension. The one smoothly flows into the other, remembering that the upper cheek colour has to be blended into the previously lightened area under the eye.

Creams and gels – are preferable for the upper cheek as they reflect more light. Put a little on the palm, mix with an equal part of foundation and blend. Apply to the cheek, blending up and out towards the temple. Don't let colour stray, but let it merge. The same substance can be applied to the larger lower area, but make the colour a little deeper. Don't go below the nostril level, blend off the face into the hairline. For evening use, luminous and frosted tones can be applied.

Powders – effective for lower cheek shading, but not always for the upper area. They are brushed on after face powder. Suck in cheeks to indicate natural hollow, brush up and out from there. If cream colour is used for the lower cheek, it is often advisable to brush on extra shading at the end of complete make-up to adjust depth and dimension.

FACE POWDER

This sets make-up, giving it a finished look and staying power. Translucent powders (with talcum and baby powder as alternatives) are more reliable as tinted powder can change colour according to skin chemistry.

The puff is a matter of preference – swansdown, velour, cottonwool, sponge or brush. Take a generous amount of powder and starting at the chin apply upward with gentle press-and-turn motions. Cover the entire face, eyelids too. Now with the other side of the puff or a fresh one, dust across forehead, down cheeks and nose, across the chin. Brush or whisk away any excess. Powder should be an all but invisible film.

EYES

Eyes give your face much of its personality and most women emphasize their eyes above other features. The general idea is to shade down the minuses and shine up the pluses. It is done with shadow, lightener, liner, mascara and additional lashes. It is up to you to decide which and to what degree.

First Degree – the casual eye: smudge shadow on the lid, blend up and out towards the brow until it fades away; carry a touch of shadow round the corner to tuck just under the bottom lashes. A suggestion of eyeliner, mascara.

Second Degree – the contoured eye: achieve extra dimension by intensifying shadow colour and adding a deeper tone in the crease of the eye, following the natural curve of the socket. Lighten under the brow line; give a smudgy outline to the eye; mascara and scattered extra lashes.

Third Degree – the evening eye: planned to shine under artificial light. More vivid, stronger colour for shadow, a very definite line in the crease of the eye; luminous highlight under the brow; eyeliner and much fuller lashes with a false section added if necessary.

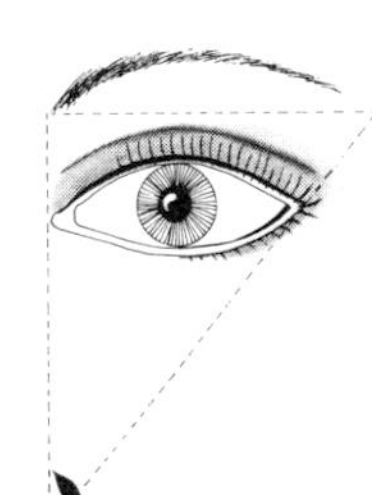

Eyebrow Proportions

EYEBROWS: Eyebrows give expression and balance to a face. They require grooming and definition but try not to alter their basic form. Some eyebrow hairs are temperamental and once plucked don't grow back again. The brow should start at a point above the inside corner of the eye; the highest part of the curve above the outer rim of the iris. The arch should be gentle with the end of the brow never lower than the beginning. It should terminate at the extension of the diagonal from nostril to outer eye.

Brush eyebrows into shape, up first, then across; pluck out hairs between and underneath the brow lines, never above. Tweeze with a quick, firm tug, always from underneath. Apply cream first, then astringent.

Define brows with a pencil or brush-on powder. The pencil must be sharp; apply in short diagonal strokes. The brush for powder application has a special slanted edge; make short feathery strokes. Colour looks darker on the brow, so select a shade lighter than your own colour. Dark brown is better than black; light brown for fair hair.

EYE SHADOW: This gives the eye its shape and shine. Bear in mind the colour-contour rules: deeper tones de-emphasize and brighter, pale ones emphasize eye features. All contouring is more effective with neutral and pink tones. If you can not resist blues and greens, keep them pale, so they are almost grey or tinged white. Any texture of shadow can be used, but blend and blend; strips of colour are most unattractive. Cover the eyelid, blend colour up and out. Define the crease, the curve of the eye socket with a thick crayon, smudge and blend. Lift the eyebrow and reflect light to the whole eye area by blending a highlighter under the brow, either at the outer or inner edge depending on the shape of the eye. White, creamy or pinky tones are best, or a transparent gel. For evening, dark colours can go deeper, light ones more luminous or pearly, and the crease definition stronger. Here are the best ways to make-up eyes.

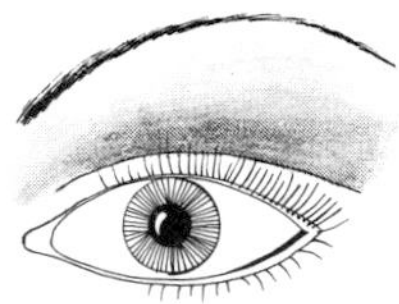

Deep-set

Deep Set

Eyes can be brought forward by applying pale shadow over the lid, carrying it to just above the hollow. On the bone between lid and brow put a little brown, taupe or grey shading; highlighter under the brow and a dot on the centre of lid. A smudged socket line above the natural crease. A light eyeliner in a fine line under upper lashes.

Prominent

The lid must be pushed back by covering with a deep tone of matt eye shadow, blending into lower brow area and curving around just under the bottom corner of the eye. Use a fleshy or pink tone on the underbrow section. Define a dark crease line, smudge it. Eyeliner helps minimize lid; emphasize top lashes, first by curling, then adding many coats of mascara.

Small

To give more importance to the eye you have to lighten part of the lid and recede the area around it. Begin by applying dark shadow around eye leaving inside top corner free; build shadow out at the sides, but only a small rim underneath. A pale tone should go in the corner, taken up and across the lid. Lots of lashes – false ones help; highlight under brow.

Round

Shading gives the eye width, but should be kept light. Cover the entire upper lid with a pale shade then, in a deeper tone in the same colour range, fill in the socket area, extending at corners parallel to the brow line. Outline the eye extending both top and bottom lines; add lashes from centre of lid outwards. Lengthen and darken the crease definition.

Heavy lids

Here you need to reduce the emphasis on the lid and increase focus on the eye. Use a matt colour in medium tone; make a triangle starting at inside corner, going up near inside of brow and angling back down to outside of eye. Put a small highlight at centre of lid. Define socket crease, make darker and smudge towards end of lid. Mascara the top lashes only.

Close-set

The accent has to be shifted to the outer part of the eyes. Pluck a bit more between the brows; blend cover-up between inner corners and bridge of

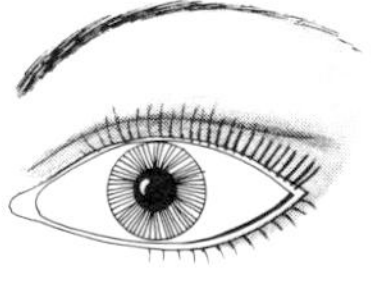
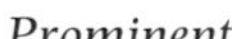

Prominent

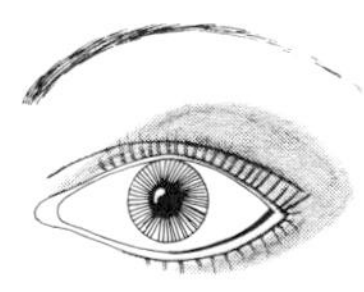

Small

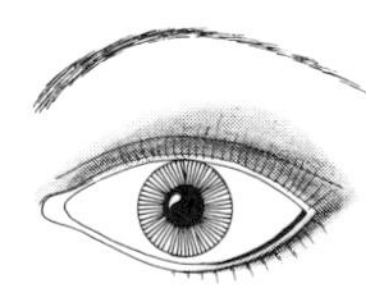

Round

nose. Start shadow towards the centre of the eye and blend outwards. Begin lid crease line at the same place and extend. Begin eyeliner half an inch in from the inner corner and extend. Add lashes to outer corners.

Wide-set
To bring eyes closer, use dark shading between eyes and the bridge of the nose, filling upwards to brow line; arch down, tapering to outer corner. Highlight a deep area under outside edge of the eybrow. Emphasize socket crease near nose, thicken eyeliner there but smudge to avoid harshness. Add extra lashes or heavy mascara towards centre of eye.

Droopy
Uplift is needed at the outer corners; it is more effective and less obvious to do it with shadow and a suggestion of eyeliner. Wing shadow out and upwards, almost touching brow line. Draw in a false socket line, raised at the outer edge, smudge. Feather an upswept eyeliner from centre of upper lashes; blend pale shadow at outer corner; curl up lashes, mascara.

EYELINER: Liner helps define shape and opens the eye, but it should be done with a delicate line. Black eyeliner is only for those with dark hair and dark skin, otherwise dark brown is deep enough. For fair skins, soft brown, taupe and grey tones. For evening, a coloured eyeliner can be effective when it tones with eyeshadow.

Apply with a very fine-tipped brush. Look down, and with one finger holding the eye taut, draw a fine line along the upper lid and as close to the lashes as possible; end at the outer corner, do not extend. Most women should use liner on the upper lid only; just dot or feather strokes on the bottom if you have no definition at all. Sometimes a line under the upper lashes is better, but keep it thin and even. Eyeliners often look better when smudged a little to blend in with lashes and shadow. Liquid and cake liners give a sharper line, pencil is more subtle.

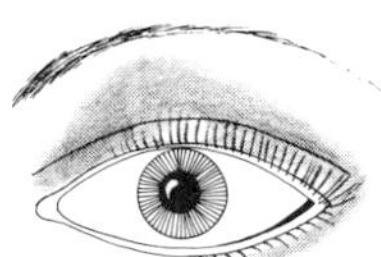

Heavy lids

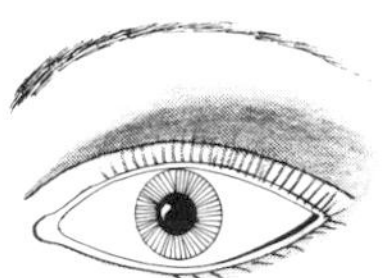

Close-set

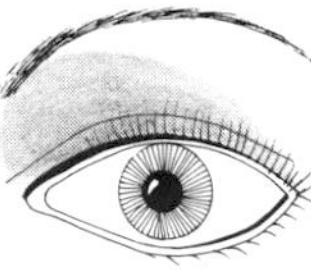

Wide-set

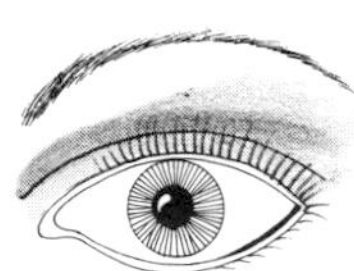

Droopy

MASCARA: Lashes need to be obvious, not spiky or thick, but long and feathery. Natural lashes are rarely long enough or dark enough to frame the eyes well. Mascara can be dark, and you can often take black even when your hair is brown; always use a shade much darker than your hair colour, in the brown, taupe or grey range.

Brush and lightly powder lashes providing a built-up surface for the mascara. It is often better to curl them first for a more fluttery look. Build up mascara in layers; many thin coats are better than a heavy one. Start by applying to the tips of the lashes, and working down to the base. Brush upper lashes downwards from the top, then brush up from below. This ensures both sides of the hairs are coated, and sweeps the lashes upwards. For the lower rim, brush up first, then down. Allow each layer to dry before applying another; you may need several coats depending on the fullness you want. It is important to keep lashes separated; should they cake and stick together, separate them with a fine, clean comb.

FALSE EYELASHES: Extremely effective and often more natural looking than layers of mascara. They can change a face considerably and make it more youthful. Use the same rule for colour as for mascara. The object is to supplement your own lashes, so they look thicker and longer, not stuck-on; put them on upper lids only.

There are three ways to supplement eyelashes:

A full strip: Check the length; lashes should begin a little in from the inside corner and not extend beyond the outside one. Cut with a razor if necessary.

If new, soak lashes 3 to 4 minutes in warm water to remove sizing that makes them stiff.

Flex base lightly to shape it to the contour of your eye.

Taking a wooden toothpick, dip in surgical glue and trail a streak of it along the lash strip. Let it get a little gummy. Pick up lash, hold as close as possible to natural lash line; using toothpick or emery board, press lashes downward in gentle vertical strokes until both lash lines meet.

Draw a thin eyeliner to fill-in any gap and cover up any excess glue. A very little mascara over the real and extra lashes blends them together.

Remove by peeling off gently beginning at outside corner. Pick off the adhesive. Lashes can be washed in clear warm water or a special liquid. To dry, roll in a tissue around a pencil.

Strip section: Cut off desired length from long strip with a razor.

Flex lashes around a finger so that they will follow the curve of the eye when applied.

Apply and remove as for full strip.

Lash by lash: Patience is required for this method. They are not attached to the skin but to your own lashes. The idea is to double the thickness of natural lashes not their number. Takes a minimum of half an hour for both eyes.

From a strip, select lashes – smaller ones for the inside of the eye.

Start from the inside and build outwards: with tweezers pick up lash, dip in surgical glue and using the hair base like a brush, stroke adhesive all the way down your own lash. Then press false lash base against natural lash base; hold a second.

Lashes should last a week, but do not use oily eye make-up. Mascara is not necessary nor advisable as it cannot be cleaned off without taking the lashes with it. To remove, apply an oily make-up remover.

LIPS

Lips need shine, colour, and careful shaping. Learn to outline lips, using a pencil or brush and a darker or lighter tone than that of the overall colour. It gives a cleaner, neater, fresher look than a stick alone. For greater control, rest elbow on the table using the hand like a lever. Outline bottom lip first, from centre to right corner, from centre to left corner. Extend slightly at the corners to give the mouth an upward lift. Outline the upper lip, again from the centre to the corners. Fill in with colour either with a brush or the lipstick. Don't run over the outline. For extra shine use gloss over the lipstick.

Making lip corrections is not always successful as alterations can be very obvious, particularly when lipstick starts to wear off. Never attempt to reshape the whole mouth; keep the colour subdued: These are subtle corrections:

Too big: outline just inside the natural line, using a light shade, fill in with a deeper but still lightish tone.

Too full: avoid bright, shiny or heavy colours, keep lipstick just inside natural lip line; outline in almost-matching shade.

Too thin: outline in a light shade just outside the natural lip line, stopping a little short at the corners; fill in with a deeper tone.

Uneven: when lips don't match in thickness, use two different shades – a darker one for the thickest lip, a lighter one for the other.

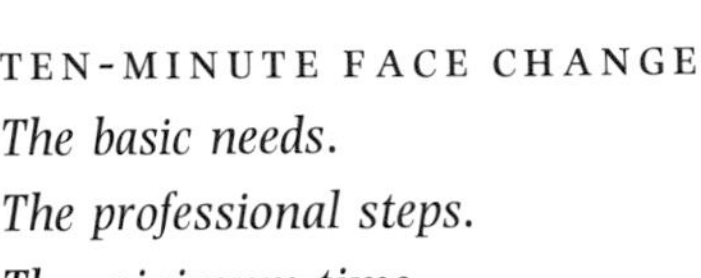

TEN-MINUTE FACE CHANGE

The basic needs.
The professional steps.
The minimum time.

Success depends on technique and that is only acquired through practice. The correct sequence of making up is of the utmost importance. Emphasize one area only – eyes, mouth or cheeks – keep the rest in subdued tones. The professional plan: a clean, well moisturized face, a simple range of cosmetics.

Equipment: tweezers, tinted foundation, pale cover-up or crayon, darker shading, cream blusher, translucent or baby powder, eye shadow, eye crayon, eyeliner, eyelash curler, mascara, eyebrow pencil, powder blusher, lip pencil, lipstick, gloss or petroleum jelly.

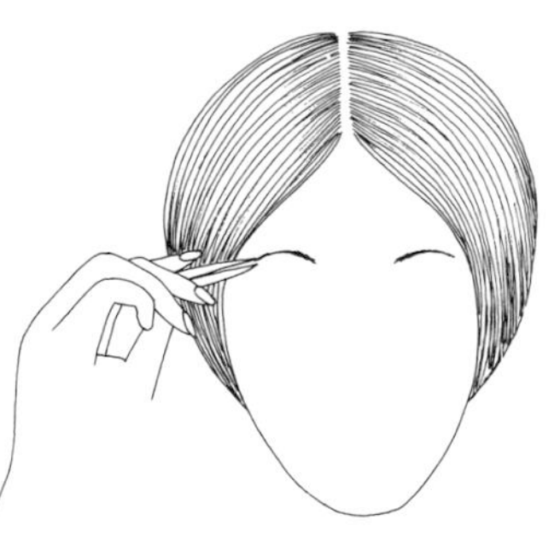

1. *Check brows* first to see if they are properly shaped, no stray hairs. Open up the arch, pluck only from underneath. The curve of the brow is important for the balance of the entire face; can be extended and colour defined later.

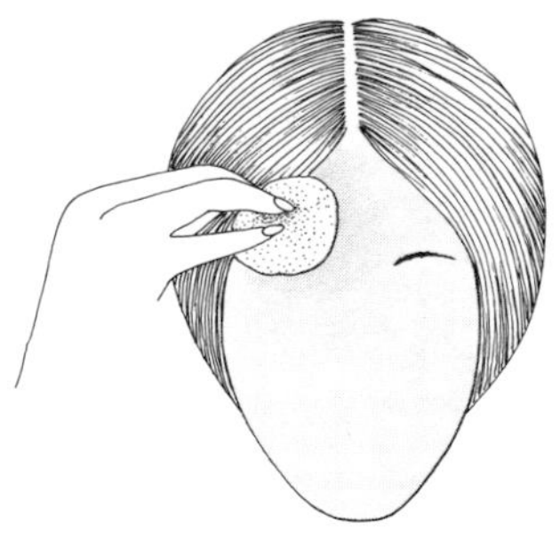

2. *Cover skin* with foundation smoothed evenly over face and under chin, blend well, no tide marks. Two thin applications better than one thick; use palm as palette to make consistency more malleable. Sponge for evenness.

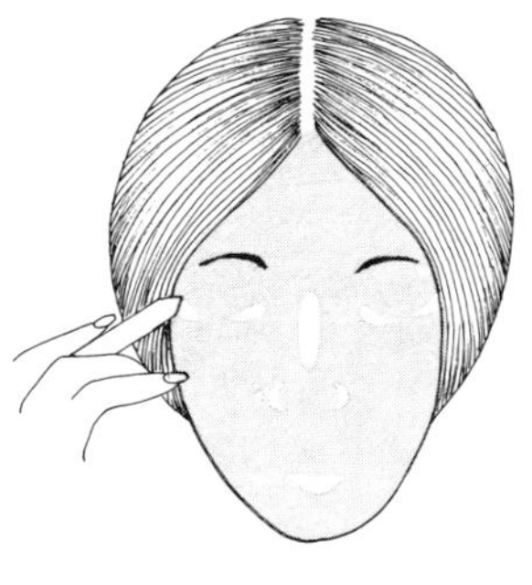

3. *Lighten up* dark areas under eyes, around nostrils, under lips, with light cover-up or white crayon. Also apply to high plateaux: ridge of nose, upper edges of cheekbones. Blend well until only a light shine remains.

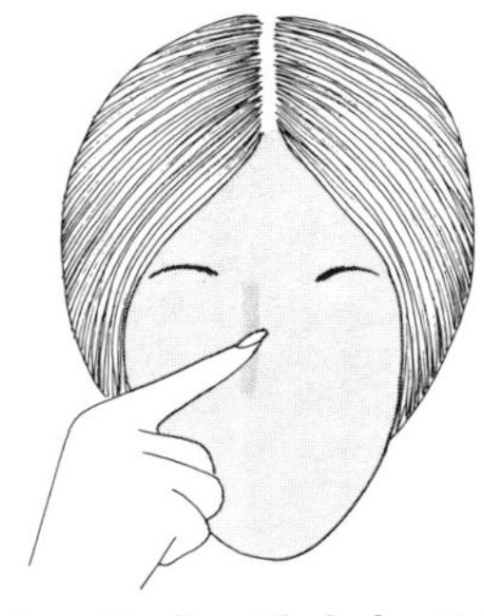

4. *Fade out* faults with darker tint, but very slightly as worse errors can result from doing this incorrectly. Sides of nose and heavy jaw lines can be eased away. Blend to almost nothing, mere shadows.

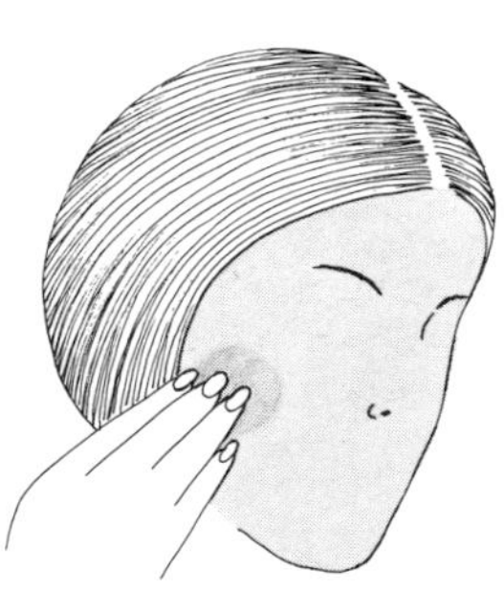

5. *Colour cheeks* with a cream blusher, applying in a diagonal sweep upward and outward towards the top of the ears along the top of the hollow. Blend so you can only see a radiance and no lines suggesting colour stops or starts.

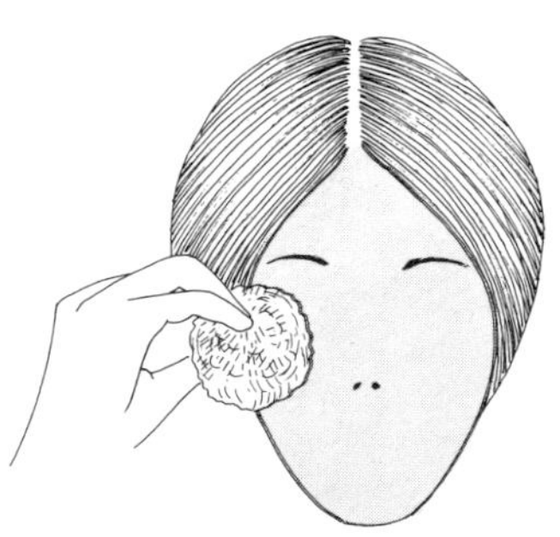

6. *Powder lightly* with a translucent or baby powder. Use cottonwool, puff, brush or dry sponge. Gently pat powder on with lots of tiny, circular press-in motions to ensure setting. Flick down to remove excess. Brush for lightest look.

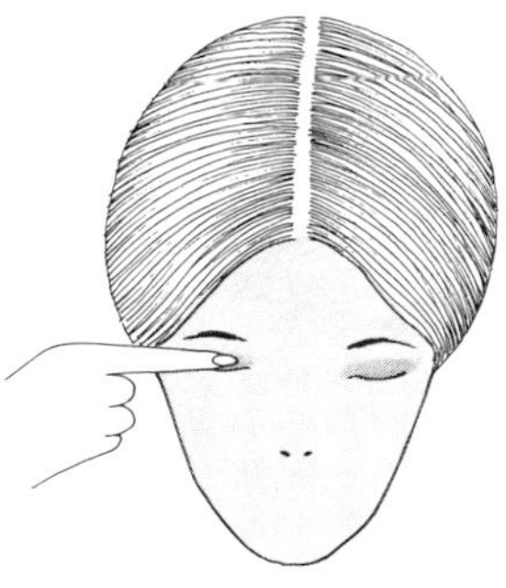

7. *Shade eyes* according to pattern decided. First apply colour to entire lid, then blend in swiftly with fingertips, adding and subtracting as you go. Look downward to prevent smudging. If cream, set with powder.

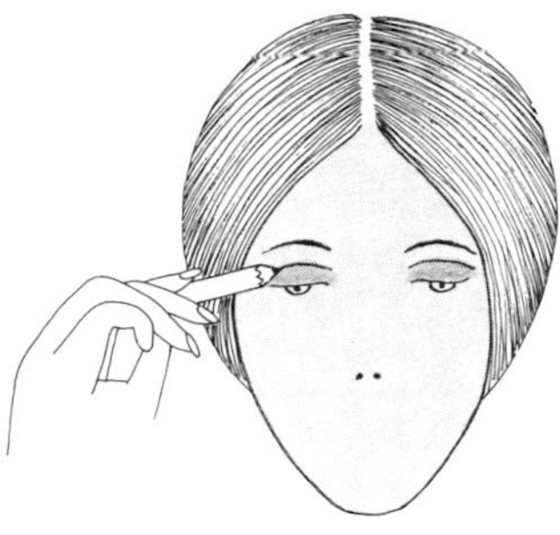

8. *Contour crease* of eye socket area to give dimension. Draw arc with thick eye crayon, using deeper shade than eye colour. Blend with fingertips or cottonwool swab. To emphasize eyes for evening, make line darker and definite.

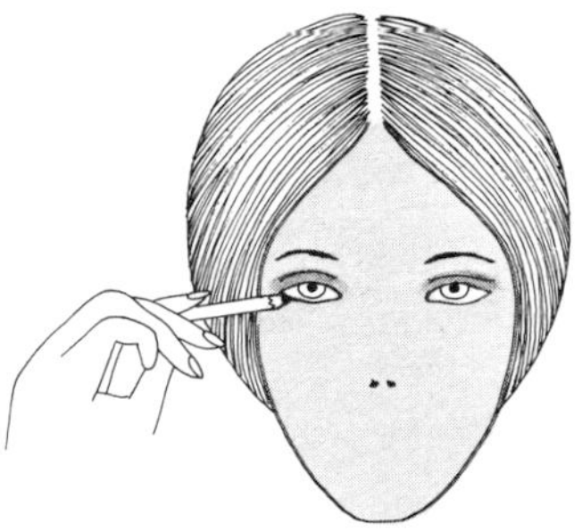

9. *Outline eyes* to define shape and make lashes look even thicker. Avoid hardness; softer lines are more effective. Consider it like shadow; dot and blend into smudgy line becoming darker and thicker towards outer corner of eyes.

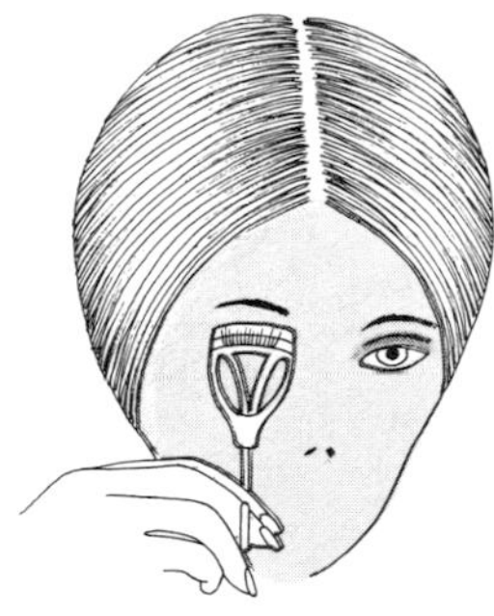

10. *Curl lashes* with special curling instrument. Eyes can be opened up, giving the illusion of more lash too; makes mascara application easier. Lightly powder.

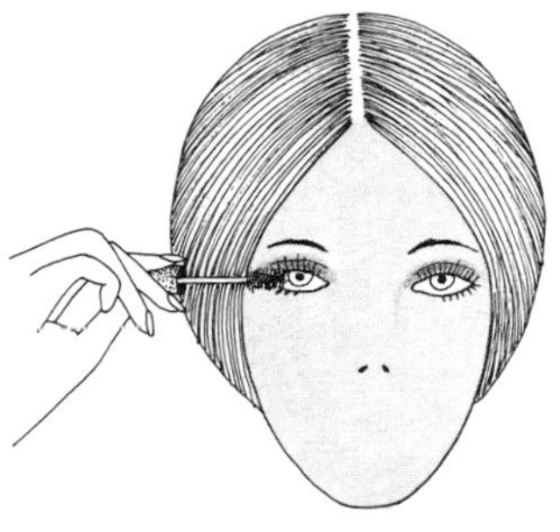

11. *Apply mascara* starting with tips of lashes and working to base for a feathery line. Brush upper lashes downwards from the top first, dry, then brush up from below. Lower lashes up first, then down. Use plenty but in thin layers.

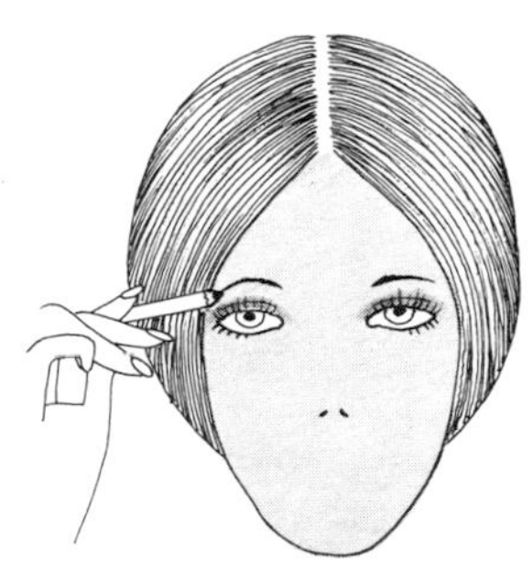

12. *Define eyebrows* after brushing to remove any trace of powder, up then across to smooth hairs in place. Apply eye pencil in light tiny diagonal strokes simulating a hair. Extend slightly at the end; brush to blend and soften line.

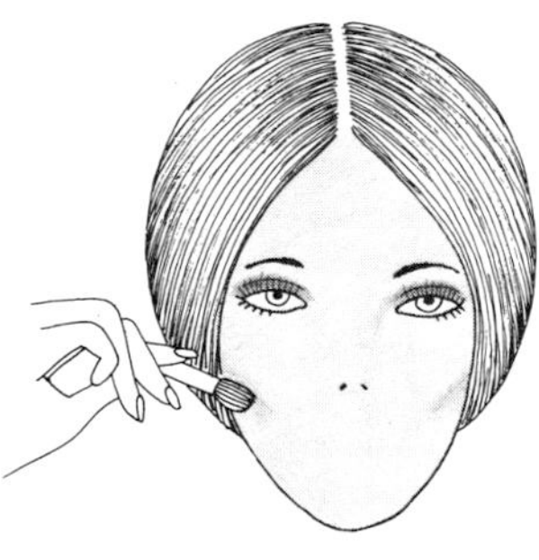

13. *Brush blusher* powder lightly over cheeks to stabilize colour and add a luminous touch. Suck in cheeks and flick the brush across the top of the indent, in upward strokes. Shade choice here can determine whether day or evening face.

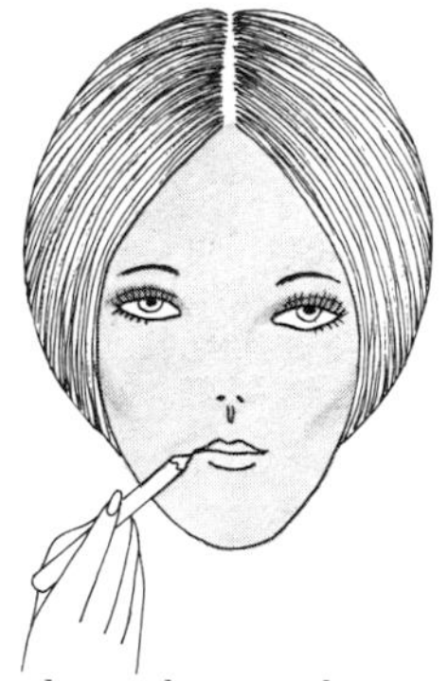

14. *Outline lips* with a pencil to establish shape, whether natural or not; the colour a little darker than lipstick. Draw in bottom line first, extending slightly at corners. Or do this with a brush using a deeper lipstick like paint.

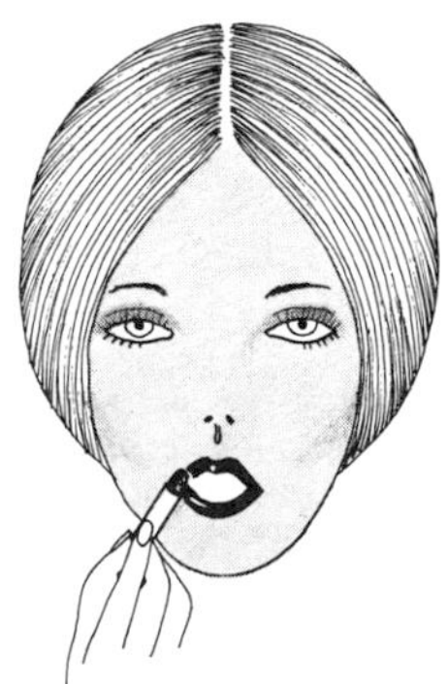

15. *Colour and gloss* lips, first filling in with the lipstick applied directly or with brush, blend into the outline but don't completely cover it. Blot. Apply another light coat. For extra shine, smear on a lip gloss or petroleum jelly.

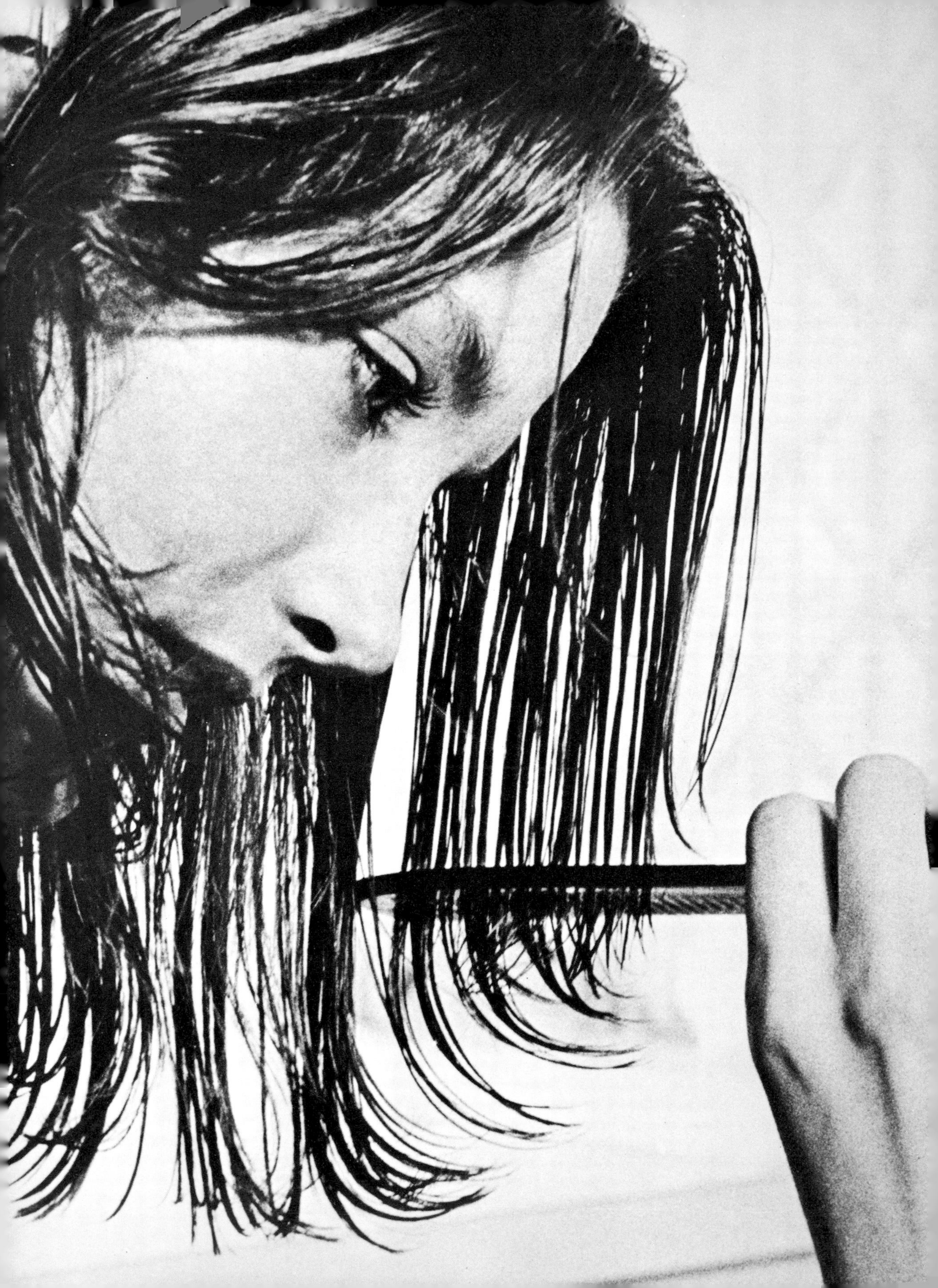

3

HAIRSTYLE

Before any decision can be made on style or colour, the first thing to establish is what type of hair you have. Three aspects have to be considered: texture, body and pattern.

TEXTURE – FINE OR COARSE

Fine hair is narrow in diameter, inclined to be weak, limp and lacking in body. It is usually thin and looks fullest and best when it is blunt cut and not much longer than chin length. Styling depends on how curly it is. Anglo-Saxons and Nordic people often have this sort of hair.

Coarse hair is fat, generally strong and sometimes wiry. It can be hard to manage and style depends on thickness and curliness. Women in hot climates – Mediterranean, African and Eastern areas – often have strong coarse hair. It can respond well to a longish cut, unless wiry and very curly. When straight or wavy, too short a cut will make hair stand out.

Medium hair is somewhere between the two extremes and combined with medium body has the fewest limitations of style.

BODY – THICK OR THIN

Thick hair means there's a lot of it. If it is coarse, it is easy to tell, but fine hair can be deceptive. Warm climates and thick hair usually go together. Straight thick hair can look marvellous cut to one length, but generally thick hair is better cut in different lengths to reduce bulk and give shape. If it is curly and thick, beware of cutting it too short – unless it is cropped Afro hair – because it is difficult to control.

Thin hair is usually best kept to short to medium length and cut evenly to give the illusion of bulk. Curls can also give the impression of body.

PATTERN – CURLY, WAVY, STRAIGHT

The more you take advantage of the natural tendencies of hair, the easier it is to take care of it.

EDWARD OLEKSAK

Curly hair, cut in layers, can work at most lengths, but don't let it grow beyond the shoulders, particularly if it is thick.

Wavy hair usually reverts to its natural state very quickly after being persuaded into a contrary style. It can be cut straight or tapered; looks best medium length. Hair with only a suggestion of wave has a certain fall and it is important to follow that in styling. When hair is wet, after being combed back from the forehead, push forward with hands – it usually falls into its natural parting, and it is advisable to keep to it.

Straight hair can be coaxed into turning up or under and if necessary will take to permanent waves and curls. When straight and fine, blunt cutting gives it body and fullness; short to medium lengths are best. Straight coarse hair can look very attractive long, it swings at medium length, but can be a problem when short.

PATTERN CHANGE

The body and texture of hair cannot be altered, but the pattern can. It is done through a combination of chemicals and heat. The more drastic the change, the more severe the procedure and the more care is needed to compensate the altered hair.

BODY WAVE

This gives a loose wave 1 to 2 inches (25–50 mm.) in depth; it doesn't give a curl and doesn't change the overall shape of the hair. It is done on large rollers.

PERMANENT WAVE

This gives a tighter wave; it is done on small bone-shaped rods and the curl pattern is every ½ to 1½ inches (12–35 mm.). The idea is not to provide rigid rows of waves, but to offer texture and a base for certain styles, particularly the short ones. It often helps fine, straight hair.

AT-HOME PERMING

A simple procedure if you follow the directions: most disasters stem from failure to do this. Read labels and instructions very carefully; don't take short cuts and don't omit any steps. Each product has its own specific directions, but follow these general rules:

Do a test curl; this is important to help judge timing for the strength of curl. Try one section on a narrow rod, another on a roller, to decide if you want a curly perm or just body.

Home permanents usually come in three strengths: for fine, medium or coarse hair – check. Some are done in two steps: a waving solution first, then a neutralizer to stop the action and stabilize the degree of wave. Others are one-step procedures, where a timing element is built in; the snag is, there's no individual control.

If hair structure has been previously altered in any way – tinted, bleached, waved – it is porous and more susceptible to the wave solution.

The coarser your hair the more it will take the curl; the finer, the less.

The bigger the rollers, the looser the curl. If hair is short you are forced into using the small rods. Long hair is easier to handle on large rollers. Avoid putting too much hair on the rods. The pattern for rollers is the same as for setting (see page 232).

Hair must be washed before perming, dirt and grease can affect action.

Try not to perm more than three times a year, and twice is better.

STRAIGHTENING

This is a permanent wave in reverse. The chemical method is by far the most successful, though waxes and gums are sometimes used temporarily to smooth out hair. Coarse hair is the easiest to straighten. It is not obligatory to do the whole head, the more problematic areas around the hairline and temples can be straightened separately. Straightening makes hair less heavy. It shouldn't be done more than once a year; it is preferable to do it at the start of summer, as curly hair is particularly affected by hot weather humidity. Afterwards hair should be protected from sun and sea water, and it can react to the chlorine of swimming pools.

Because it is a more complex and difficult procedure than waving, few women are capable of doing it at home. This is how it is done professionally.

Hair is shampooed, blotted dry and combed; the straightening lotion (mixed 15 minutes beforehand) is put on by brush or with fingers, soaking all surfaces; it is then combed through the hair. Head is wrapped in plastic for 20 minutes. Hair strands are now soft, and the next step – the most important and most arduous – is to continuously comb from 10 to 20 minutes, relaxing or altering the curl pattern. Afterwards hair is rinsed, towelled to remove excess water, combed; then a neutralizer is applied, combed through and takes about 5 minutes to stabilize straightness before being rinsed out. The process takes about 2 hours. Bleached, tinted or toned hair may not react as well as natural hair.

COLOUR CHANGE

No cosmetic can achieve a greater illusion of naturalness than hair colouring – if it is done well and suits your skin. The rule is not to change the colour too much; best is one or two shades lighter and it is rarely recommended to go darker. Very few women can take really drastic changes. Professional colourists prefer to mix at least three tints together which give three or four tones to the hair. This looks much more real than a solid mass – natural hair is always a combination of several shades. When deciding on colour you must consider the tone of your skin and the colour of your eyes. Experiment by trying on a few wigs and hairpieces. There are cool shades, ashen tones, warm shades with bright and reddish hues. If your skin is pale, choose a warm shade, but if your skin is colourful or if you want to lessen a too red or brassy look, try a cool colour. Even if you go to a professional colourist, have an idea of what you want and don't judge a new hair shade immediately. It takes a few days for natural oils to return and they can make quite a difference to the final colour impression.

Most women can handle toning that involves a temporary or semi-permanent colouring. Lightening within a moderate colour range is not difficult either, but a more drastic change should be done at a salon. During lengthy bleaching, hidden tones often come up – brown hair can prove to have a lot of red in it, for instance – and special toners are needed to eliminate brassy tones. If colouring is done correctly it does not harm hair, though it is important to condition it after washing. It often helps fine hair by giving it more body.

There are three basic kinds of hair colouring – temporary, semi-permanent and permanent:

TEMPORARY RINSES

These are the most short-lived of all forms of colouring and last only until the next shampoo. They contain no bleaching agent so do not lighten hair. They contain no penetrating agent so they simply coat the outside of the hair shaft. They make only subtle changes in colour, adding high-lights within the same colour family as your own. On light to medium brown, rinses can highlight, darken, tone down reddishness or add it. They are good for dulling brassiness in over-bleached hair. On darker hair, rinses have less effect but will brighten, darken or add highlights. Rinses won't cover grey, but will blend in adding a little colour. Rinses often have built-in conditioners, some also act as a setting lotion. They are generally hypo-allergenic and unlike other types of hair colouring require no skin patch test.

SEMI-PERMANENT TINTS

These work in the same way as temporary rinses, only more intensely; they also last longer, through four to five shampoos. They have no bleaching agents, so they cannot lighten. They contain a very mild penetrating agent so the hair shaft is diffused with a little colour as well as being coated with it. They substantially alter tones within the same shade range – fading gradually, leaving no appreciable demarcation line between the tinted portion and the new growth of hair. With each shampoo, a little colour is washed away. Finally it goes and you simply repeat the process. Semi-permanent tints can turn a muddy blonde into a golden one, add a sable glow or reddish tint to brown hair; and they can darken. Like temporary rinses, they usually contain a conditioner. There is some build-up colour which gives the hair a heavy unnatural look, but only a professional can spot this or know how to counteract it.

PERMANENT COLOURINGS

These last as long as the hair does, though exposure to sun and certain air pollutants can cause discoloration. They contain both bleaching and penetration agents. They can lighten hair and colour it by duplicating the process of natural pigment distribution. They alter the structure of hair, as the bleach not only strips colour but makes the shaft more porous and therefore more receptive to new additions. Any colour change is possible – lighter, darker and eliminating grey. Partial lightening can be very effective.

For a moderate change, from medium brown to medium blonde for instance, you can use either a shampoo or a cream formula. Shampoos are worked into the hair and they colour as they clean. Although more convenient than creams, they are much less effective. Cream formulas are brushed or swabbed on dry hair section by section. Both processes require mixing of two preparations: the colour, called an oxidation dye, and the bleach (usually 20 volume hydrogen peroxide), called a developer because this is what makes the colour develop in your hair; the chemical reaction takes place within the hair shaft.

To lighten your hair more than a few shades – from darker brown to very blonde – a two-step process is necessary which separates the bleaching and colouring actions. It should be done professionally. Hair is first stripped of all colour – called pre-lightening – and it can take up to an hour. After comes the colour – golden, fawn, red or whatever. If you want a really pale blonde look, a toner is rinsed through the hair after stripping to drab or ashen it, eliminating brassiness. The greater the degree of colour change, the longer it takes. From black to blonde – the extremes and not recommended – might have to be done in two operations with a day's rest in between. Hair suffers from bleaching and must be conditioned constantly to combat brittleness and breakage. There are also special shampoos for lightened and tinted hair.

Darkening hair is much simpler than lightening, and less hard on the hair because pre-bleaching is not necessary.

Any permanent hair colouring needs retouching every 3 to 4 weeks to cover regrowth. Just the roots are treated, then before washing the formula is quickly combed through the entire head of hair to ensure even colour.

PARTIAL COLOURINGS

These are alternative colour possibilities, all permanent, but growing out gradually and without the necessity of frequent touch-ups. They usually involve lightening strands here and there to produce a blend of light and darker shades that look like the natural effects of the sun.

Highlighting – also known as frosting. Hair is lightened in very fine strands beginning approximately one inch away from the parting. It can be done all over the head or just around the face. A perforated rubber cap is put on the head and selected strands pulled through the holes with a crochet hook; the number depends on how much highlighting you want. These strands are bleached then toned – the whole shaft or just the tip.

Streaking – several slender streaks are lightened along the movement edges of the hair, following the line of the cut. The bleach is usually painted on, then toned with an overall rinse.

Framing – just two rows of fine streaks are lightened and toned around the hairline, to frame the face. Of necessity this must be very delicate.

Tortoise-shelling – dark streaks are put in over lightened hair to bring it closer to a natural colour without the shock of a total darkening. It is done the same way as highlighting.

Collage – three shades are blended together in the front and at the sides. First, fine sections of hair are bleached. After shampooing, some of the natural hair is blended with the bleached hairs and treated with a toner. The result – if you start with brown hair – would be a blend of brown, honey blonde and caramel.

AT-HOME COLOURING

Temporary rinses and semi-permanent tints that are shampooed in are no problem; tints that require section application can be mastered with practice; bleaching and its complementary colouring or toning is better done by a professional. Before starting, check these points:

The examples of hair colouring found on many charts and packages show how that particular colour looks on colourless hair. The colour result changes according to the colour of hair it's applied to. Before buying be sure you have the right colour for the right type of hair.

Don't straighten or perm hair for two weeks before colouring.

Read directions carefully, be strict about timing, too many minutes or too few can greatly affect colour depth. After mixing chemicals, they must be used immediately.

Before treating the entire head, it is essential to make two tests:

Patch Test – for allergic reactions. In a salon this is done on the skin behind the ear. If you think this spot is difficult to observe, an alternative is just inside the crease of the underarm. Prepare a small amount of colouring; wash skin, swab on formula, leave for twenty-four hours being careful not to rub or wash it off. If there's no reaction, go ahead. If there's any sign of irritation, don't use that product.

Strand Test – to check colour reaction. Cut off two or three dozen strands near the scalp and using the remainder of the trial mixture prepared for the patch test, follow colouring procedure exactly as instructed. What happens to the strands will happen to your whole head. Look at the results in strong light.

NATURAL VEGETABLE COLOURINGS

Henna is totally vegetable with no chemicals at all; it is non-toxic and can also be used on pubic hair. It does not disturb the molecular structure of hair as it coats the hair shaft, and thus also increases body. It is slightly astringent, so it is a good idea to rub oil on the skin before using. The colour lasts several months.

Henna must be used with caution. It is difficult to stabilize the colour except with experience. Its intensity of colour varies according to individual hair conditions, and amateurs often have been left with strange shades. A strand test is an absolute necessity. It is a long tedious process but by experimenting you can achieve rich auburn, mahogany or red tones. Brown tones can be acquired when henna is mixed with other vegetable dyes. For example, one-quarter henna and three-quarters camomile will bring a warm chestnut to fading brown hair. A half-and-half combination of henna and camomile will give reddish tones.

Hair must be shampooed before using henna. Wear gloves because it can stain hands and fingernails. Mix 2 cups henna powder with 1 cup warm water into a thick paste; add 1 teaspoon of vinegar to help release the dye. Let it stand for an hour. Stir mixture in top of double boiler until well warmed, leave for about half an hour. Brush on hair divided into sections; comb through all strands. Wrap in towel. For a brown colour leave for about 3 hours, longer for reddish tones and keep checking until you get the colour you want. Wash hair and keep rinsing until water is clear, combing all the time.

Sage can give a brown tone to grey hair. Make a strong infusion, preferably combined with black tea; boil half an hour and let it steep for several hours. This liquid must be dabbed into the hair every day until it deepens to the correct shade.

Saffron or Marigold Flowers will give a reddish tint; use a steeped infusion as a rinse, putting it through the hair many times.

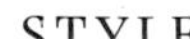

STYLE

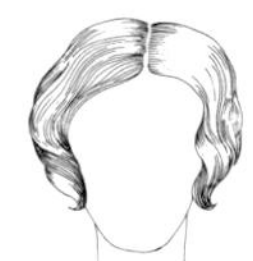

Round Face

Contemporary hair styling stresses individuality rather than fashion. The aim is healthy naturalness. It is how hair swings and moves that matters.

The basis of all modern hairdressing is the cut: when that is done to perfection hair can be styled to swing and curl. The shape of your hair can change the shape of your face, emphasizing best features, minimizing others. This is why body is significant. Move your hair around to see what direction works best for your face. Where features are good, pull hair back to reveal them – eyes, forehead, ears, chin, throat. Where there's a fault of too much or too little, cover with hair – a low forehead, a high one, fat cheeks, strong jaw. Balance a prominent nose, a receding chin with hair so placed that the eye is drawn away from it.

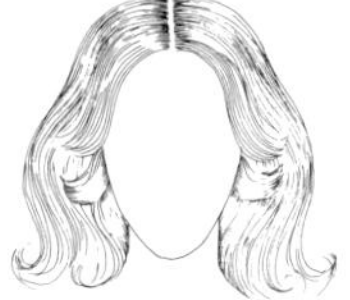

Long Face

Round Face – emphasize the top or cover the cheeks; usually short cuts work better.

Long Face – make width at the sides by fluffing out hair with waves or curls; best with medium-length hair, fullness starting around ear level.

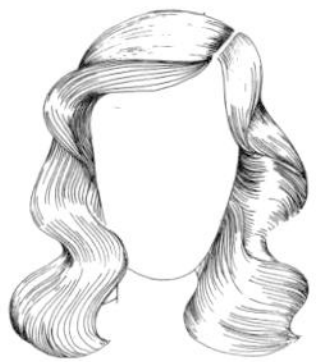

Square Jawed

Square-Jawed – cover the jaw line; straight hair can be cut to hang over the cheeks, wavy hair can break the line; leave forehead clear.

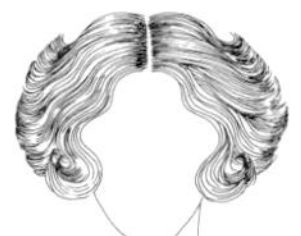
Heart-Shaped

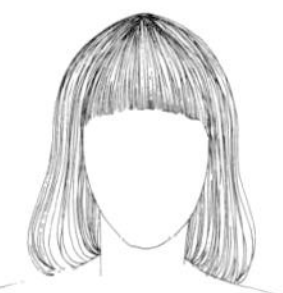
Low Forehead

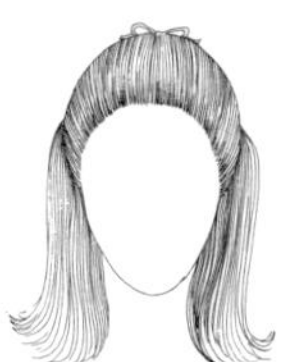
Small Face

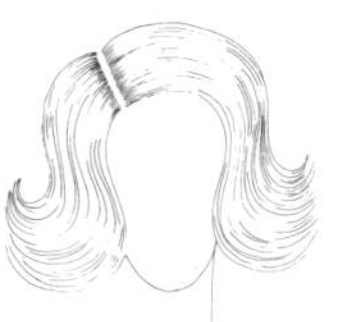
Big Face

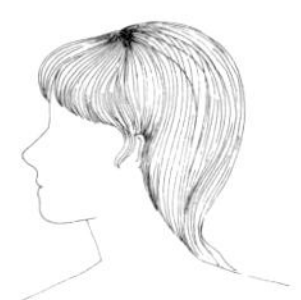
Prominent Nose

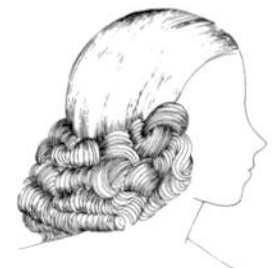
Receding Chin

Heart-Shaped – hair should be given volume over the fullest part of the cheeks; even straight hair can achieve this through good cutting.
Low Forehead – or one that narrows towards the hairline; simple to cover it with a deep fringe that only looks right when it almost reaches the eyes; it should start far back at the crown; the rest can be any length.
Small Face – providing features allow it, take all hair away from face, framing it with height and width.
Big Face – let hair fall over the face, covering part of the cheeks, possibly at an angle over the forehead.
Prominent Nose – balance it by drawing the eye to the other side of the head; emphasize the crown, giving bulk to short hair or arranging long hair into an up-swept style.
Receding Chin – hair must be long enough to arrange fullness along the jaw line.

THE CUT

Whatever the length of hair, it should be cut about every six weeks, more frequently for a very short look. It should never be allowed just to grow long. This produces split ends and a straggly appearance.

Hair should be cut wet, after it has been shampooed. It has to be done with precision. Hair is parted into half-inch horizontal layers and each piece cut in turn following the shape of the partings. Cutting starts at the neckline, the rest of the hair being pinned up and brought down piece by piece. Modern styling calls for scissors and a blunt cut which means hair is clipped straight across even when cut into different layers. This helps discourage split ends and achieves a clean, swinging line.

Hair can be cut all one length, which is good for thin fine hair in need of fullness, and for long straight hair. It can be shorter in certain sections, but in any segment hair is the same length. If hair is to be turned under it is usually cut shorter underneath; if hair is to be flipped up, the upper layer is cut shorter.

A layered cut is when hair is cut to different lengths all over the head. It is usually good for thick hair and encourages waves and curls. Hair is sectioned into layers – the shorter ones can be on top or underneath, depending on the style.

These two basic ways of cutting can be used alone or in combination to create a variety of styles. Look at the sketches on the following pages.

SHORT

The most contemporary cuts are usually short; the best ones are those you can care for yourself. The expertise of the cut is vital; shape is everything and even short hair can look like lots of hair if done right. Curly hair is usually better short, thin hair too. To change the pattern of short hair is, of course, easier than at other lengths, and this is one of the main advantages of keeping hair at a minimum:

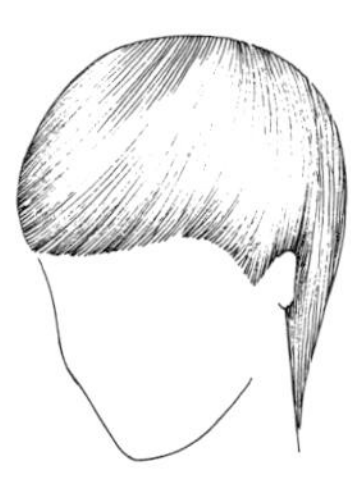

1. Cap cut brushed forward over forehead; good for straight hair whether fine or thick.

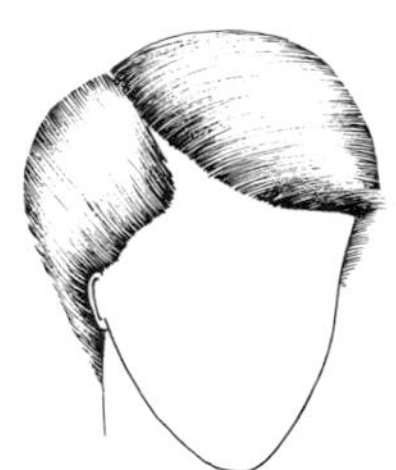

2. Hair brushed back like a boy's, flicked over forehead; hair must have some body.

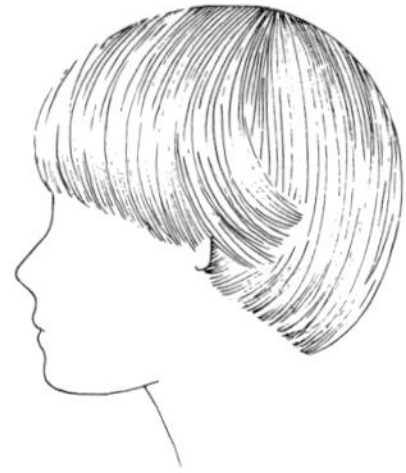

3. Classic fringed bob, hair almost touching eyes; straight hair only, thick or thin.

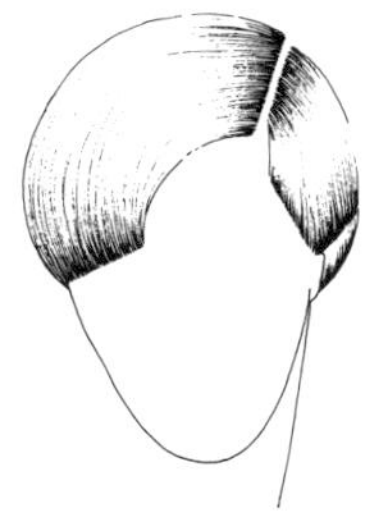

4. Angled cut, side-parted and geometrically shaped; best with straight thick hair.

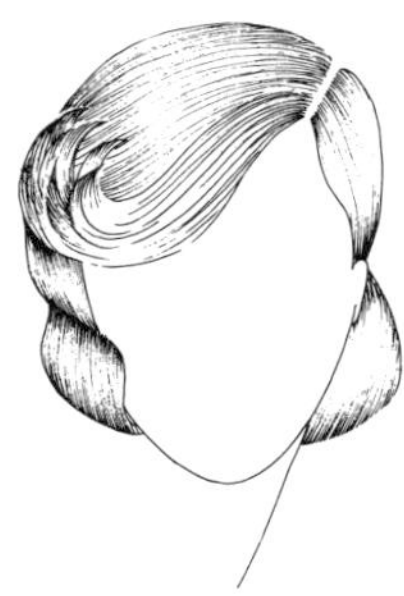

5. Hair is actually blunt cut, but waved with curling iron for layered effect; needs body.

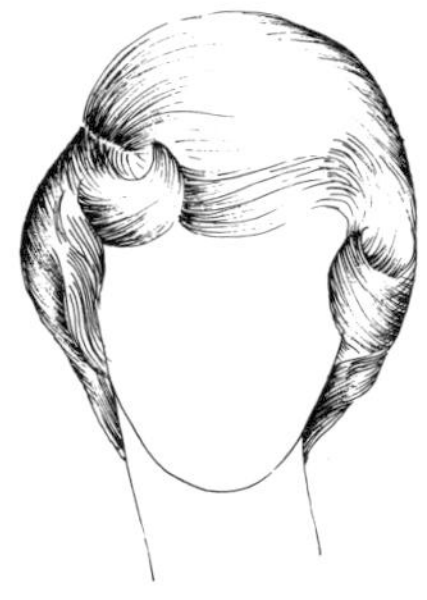

6. A layered cut for wavy hair, good for thin hair to give illusion of more bulk.

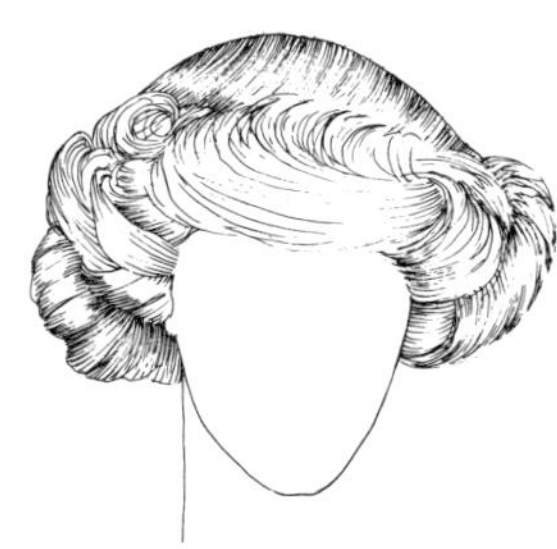

7. For wavy hair with lots of body, cut in sections to give maximum side width.

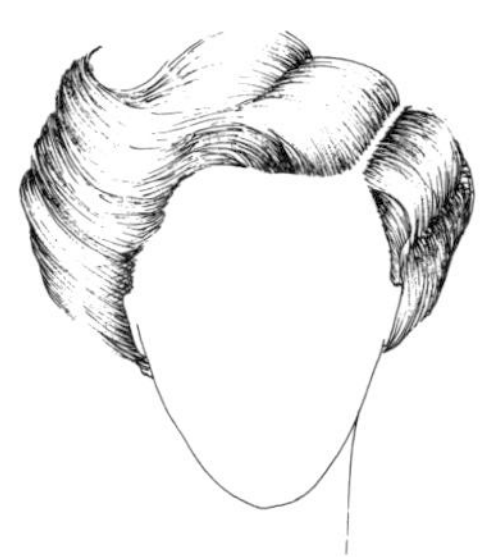

8. Hair blunt cut for a one-sided flick; hair must have body, some wave.

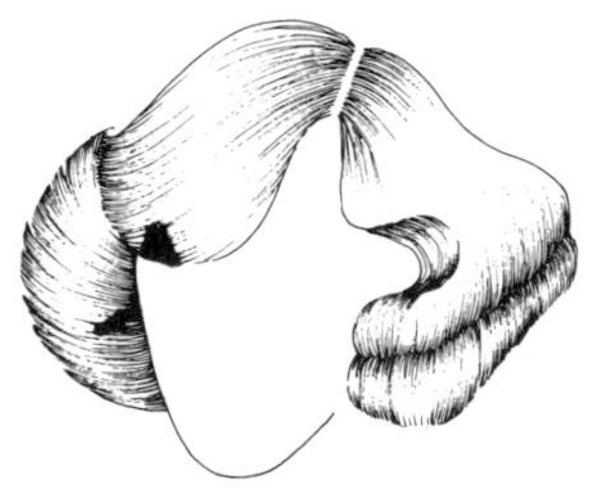

9. Only for thick hair; semi-wavy; blunt cut for side width.

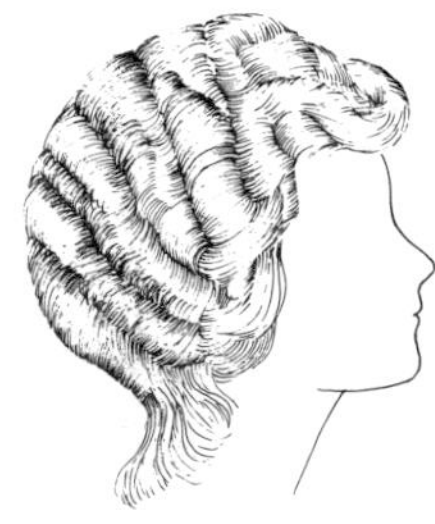

10. Curly or wavy hair cut in layers for wavy curls from forehead to nape.

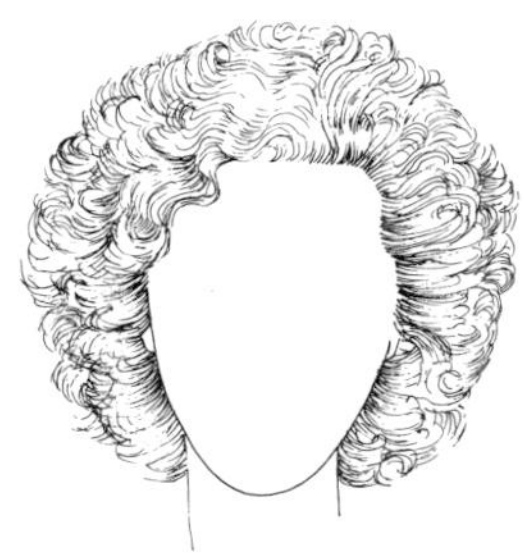

11. For curly or very wavy hair; the cut is the same even length all over, brushed up.

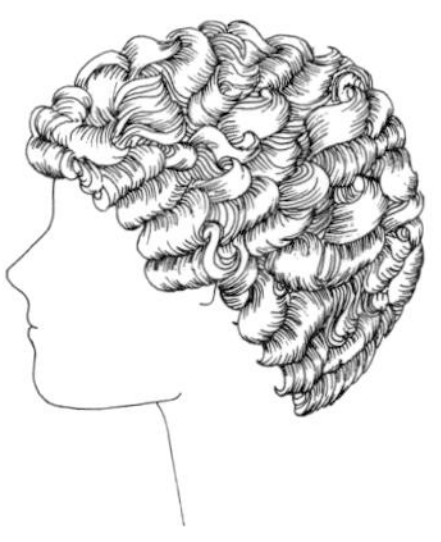

12. The only way to style very curly hair, the Afro cut with short tight curls massed over entire head.

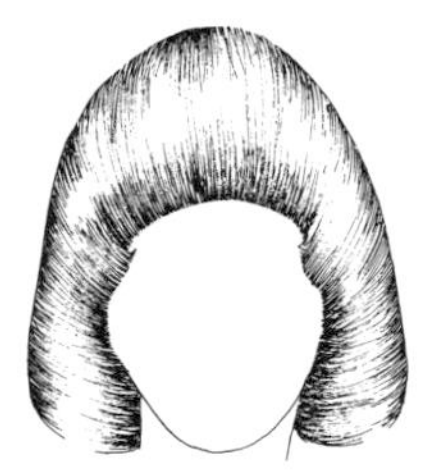

13. A cap page-boy ending just below ears; for thick straight hair with body.

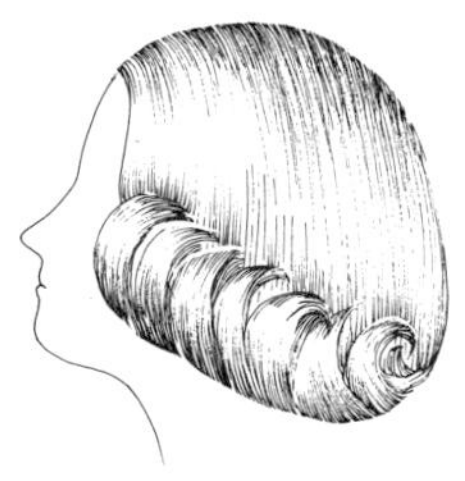

14. Classic flick-up bob looks best when moving over cheek; straight or wavy hair, all textures.

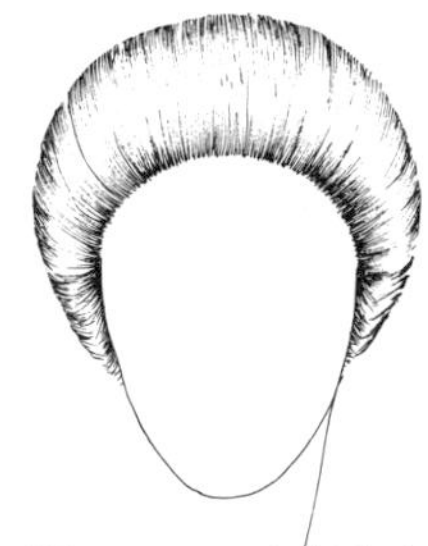

15. Wavy or straight hair can be done this way; hair cut to one short length; brushed up and back.

MEDIUM

In general, this is the most flattering length, but effect and staying power absolutely depend on the right cut for your type of hair. Note that at this length hair is more likely to fall into its natural ways faster, so follow its inclinations; a continual pattern change is not advisable. Cut and style according to texture and pattern; wavy hair is best at this length, so is thick hair. Medium length styles require the most upkeep.

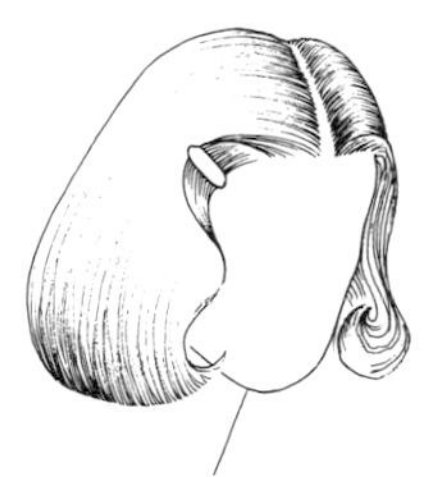

1. Hair blunt cut to same length; straight hair or a slight wave, all textures.

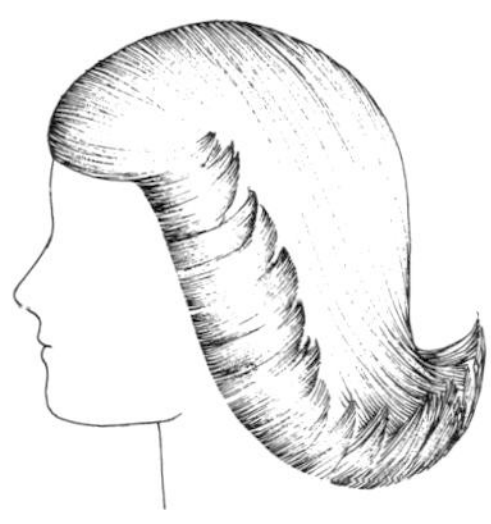

2. Body needed for this style, minimum wave; blunt cut in a graduating curve.

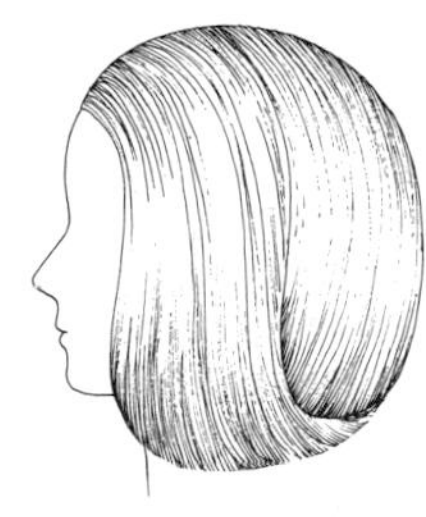

3. Good for straight hair, any texture; even length blunt cut coaxed to turn under and back.

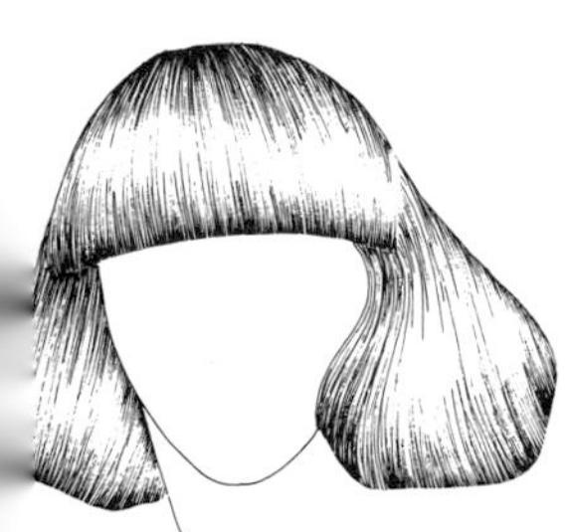

4. Hair must be thick and straight; it's the under layers that provide fullness.

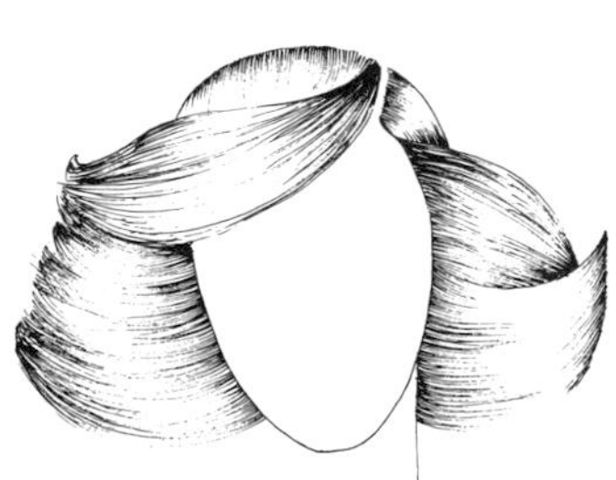

5. Works well on semi-wavy or straight hair, but body is necessary to maintain width.

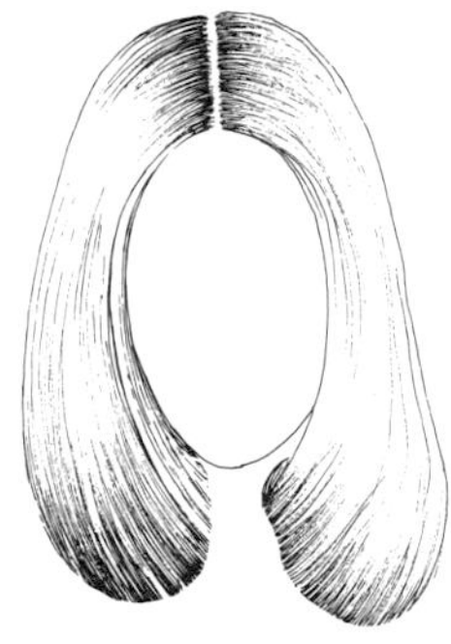

6. For straight hair only, thick or thin as hair is turned under to provide fullness at base.

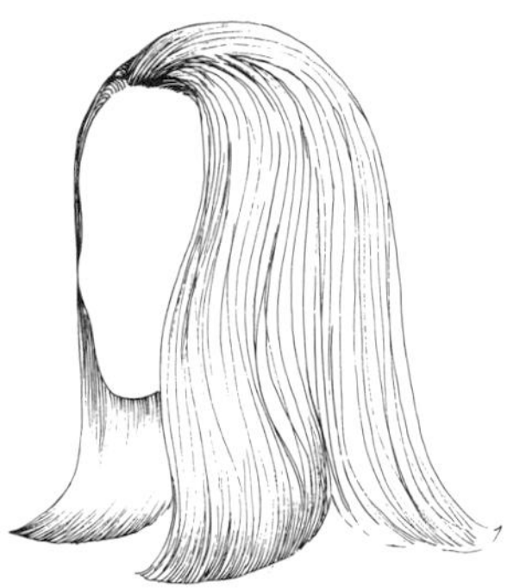

7. Straight or wavy hair of all textures can adapt to this classical fall of hair.

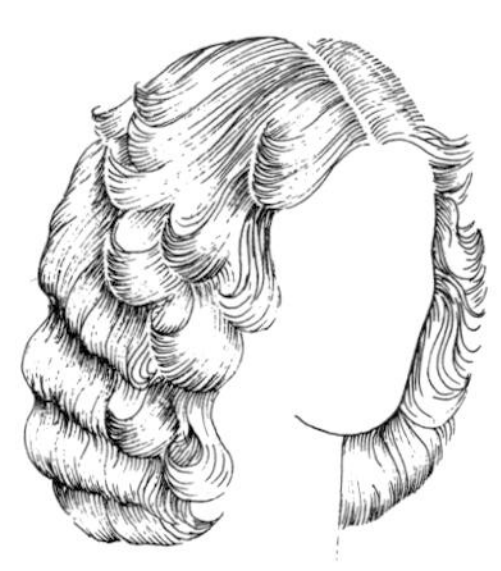

8. A layered cut for curly or wavy hair; centre parting here, but easily adaptable to side combing.

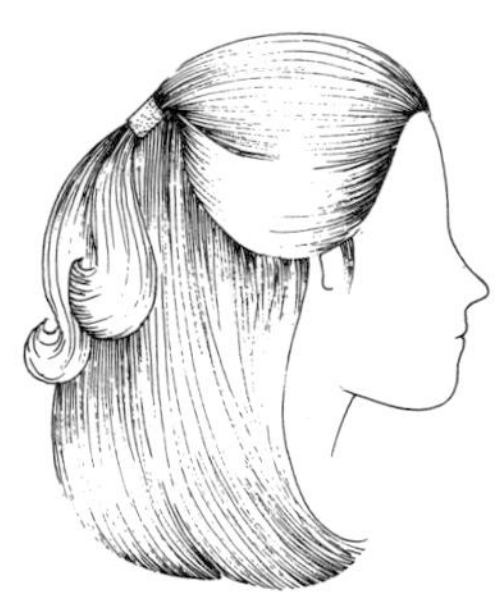

9. Blunt cut to one length, upper section drawn back; for all textures, straight or semi-wavy.

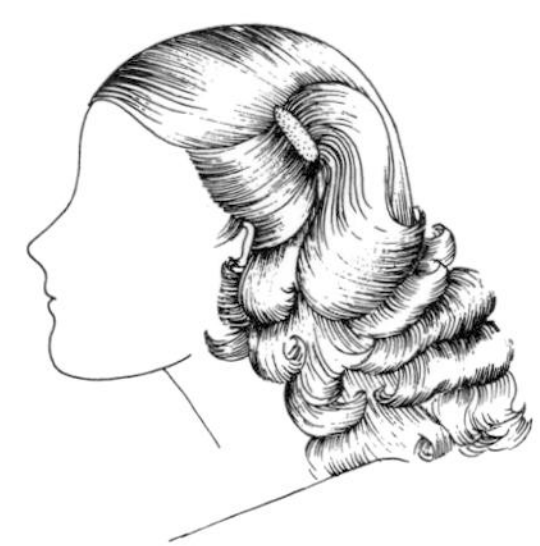

10. Semi-wavy hair cut in layers from the ears down, the crown left smooth; body not necessary.

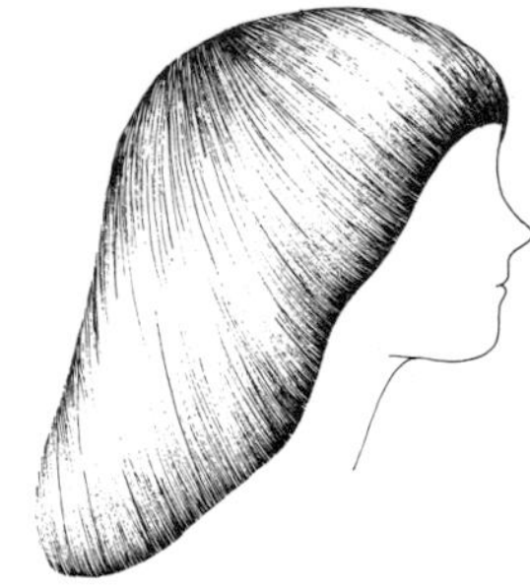

11. Page-boy cap only for straight hair and better if some body; blunt cut in graduation.

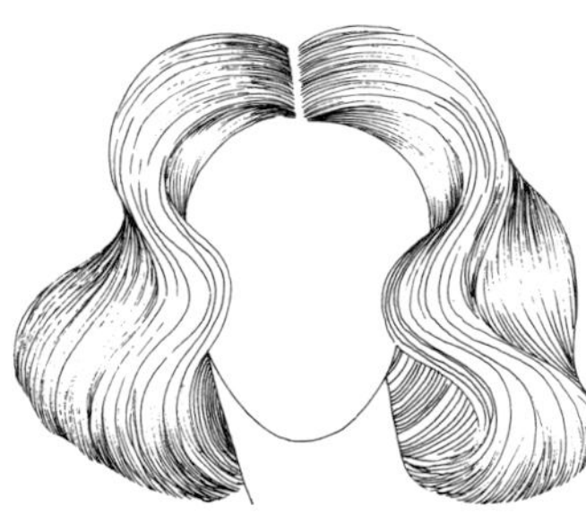

12. Only for thick wavy hair; the basic cut is blunt of even length; parting easily switched.

LONG

Often the easiest to control, long hair can provide the widest range of styles. The trick is knowing how to handle it: manipulate hair in sections, secure the main bulk with pins or covered elastics, use the free pieces to drape for interesting effects. All textures of hair can achieve sculptured effects; straight hair is easier to place, but even curly hair can be coaxed into sleek shapes. Most styles here can also be done with medium length hair plus hair pieces.

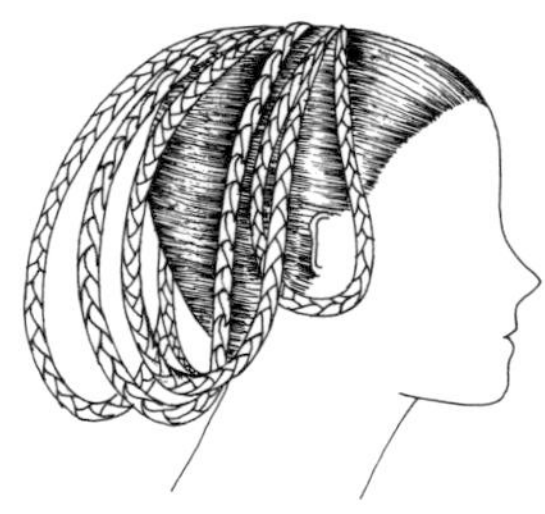

1. Coarse frizzy hair plaited in a series of narrow looped plaits; can remain until next washing.

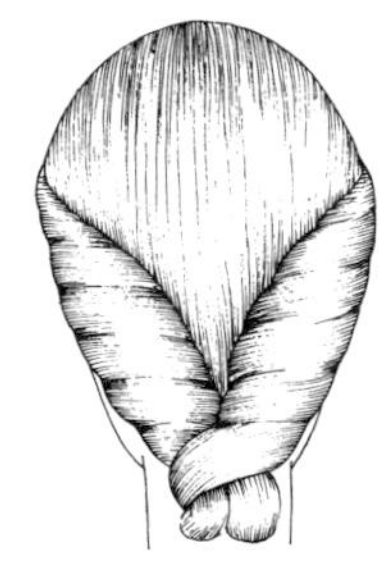

2. Straight hair only, plus addition of hairpieces; centre plait at crown.

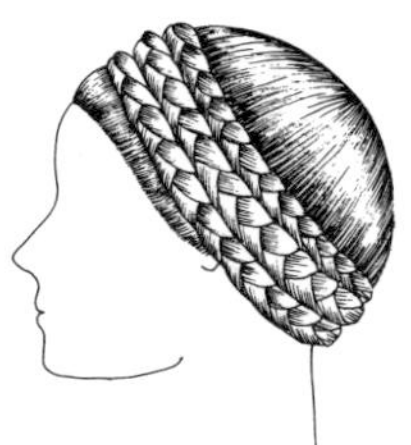

3. Renaissance feeling, plaits true or false are wound around head.

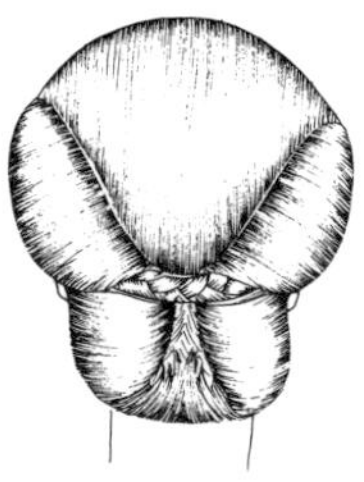

4. False plait pinned in semi-circle is the base for wrapping of hair in rolls.

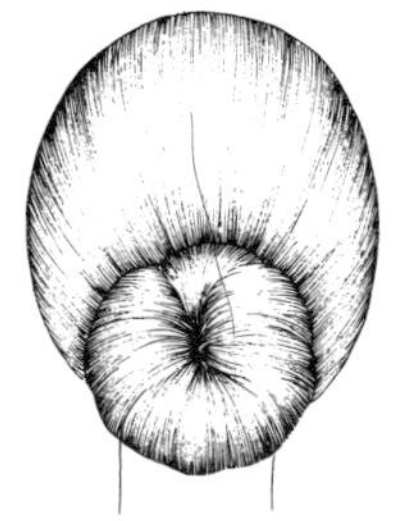

5. Classic bun; hair is drawn back in elastic, back combed and curved under.

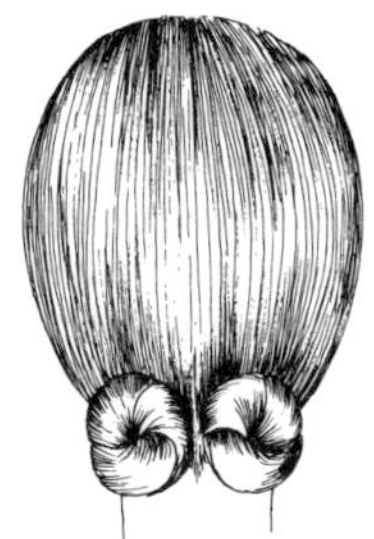

6. Hair secured in two sectio[illegible] at base of neck, back combe[illegible] and pinned in two circles.

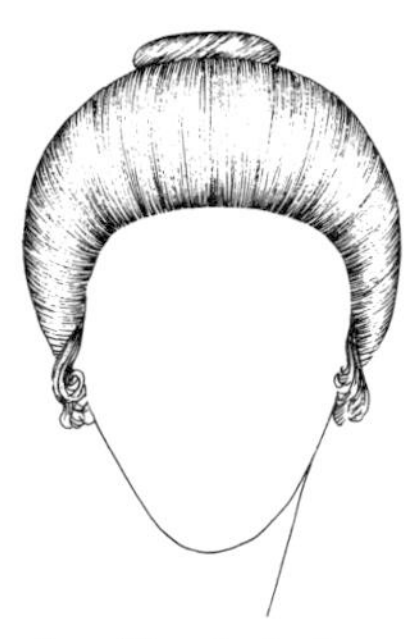

7. Edwardian idea, hair drawn high and evenly from face, a circular top knot on the crown; a few strands over cheeks.

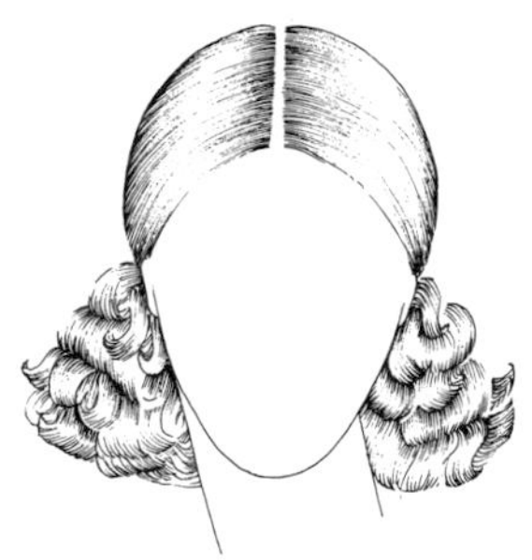

8. Wavy or curly hair can be tautly forced back into a band then curls allowed to spray from there.

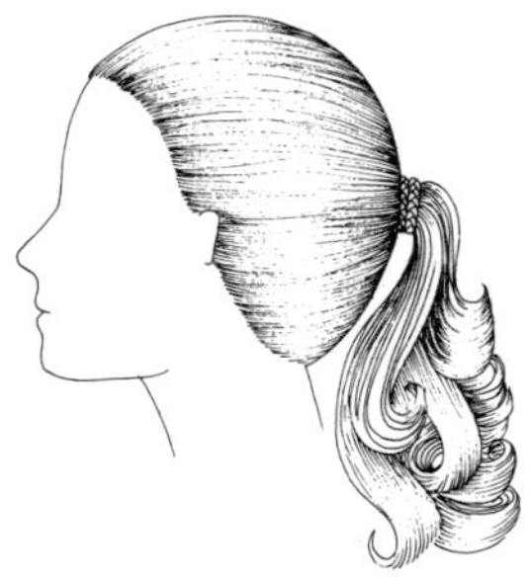

9. A simple pony tail, covered with a fine plait at the knot, the rest curled.

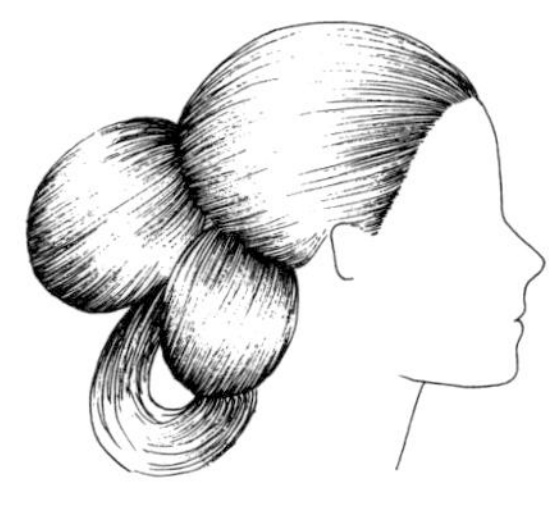

10. Hair is secured with a band at nape of neck; divided into three parts and formed into giant loops.

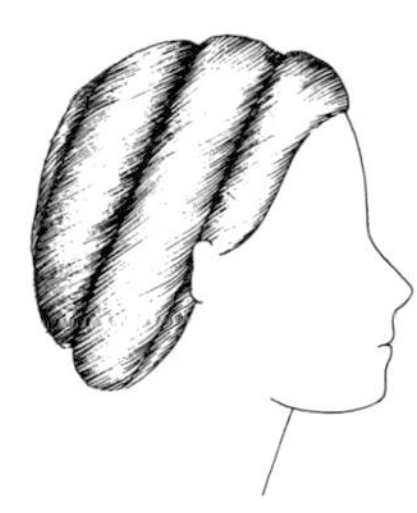

11. Straight or wavy hair can be divided into sections and pinned in parallel rows; strings on crown help control.

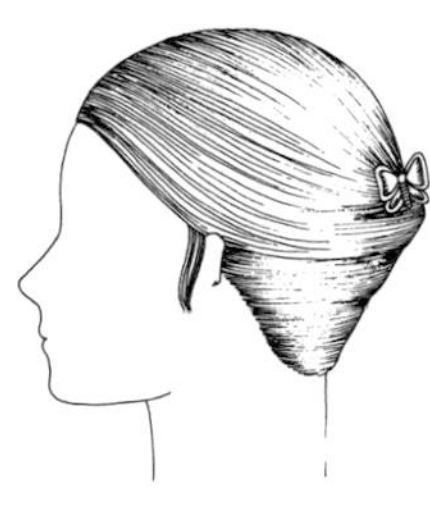

12. The classic French twist softened by cheek strands; for straight or slightly wavy hair.

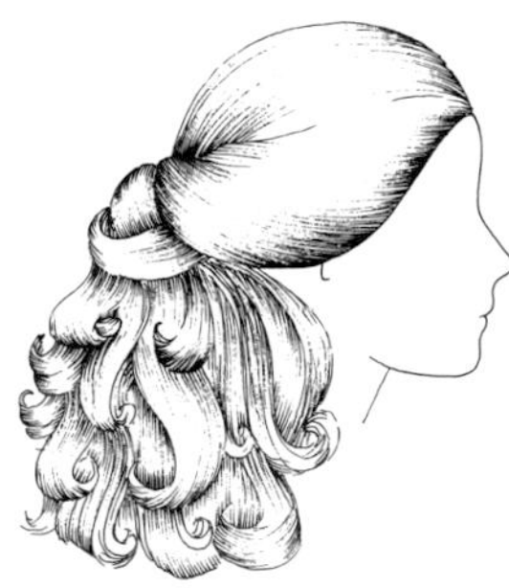

13. Wavy hair caught in a loose knot; side sections are draped over covered elastic band.

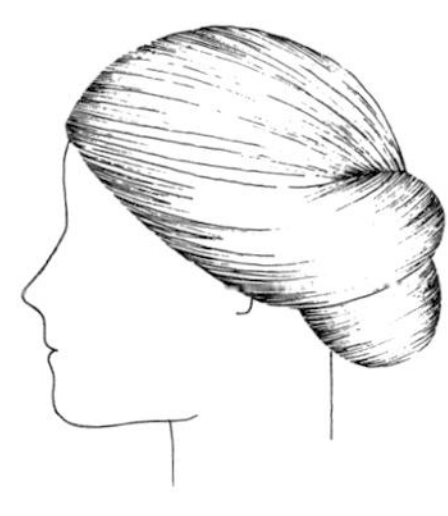

14. Very simple and only achieved with thick straight hair; two side sections and lower one form large rolls.

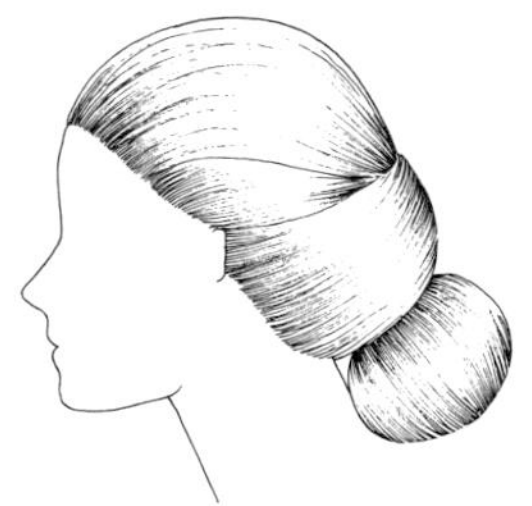

15. Centre section pulled into low pony tail; folded under, side sections swathed over band.

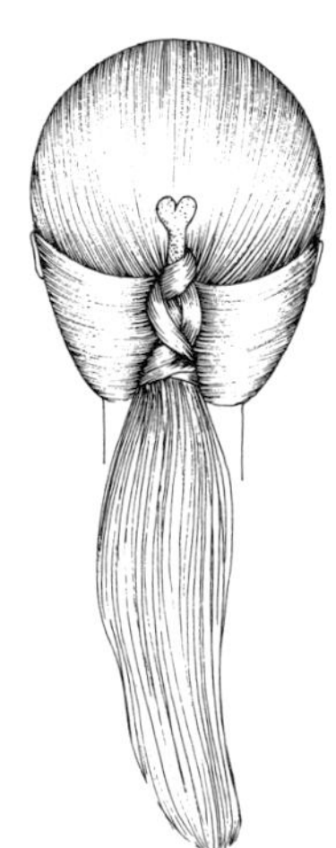

16. Only straight thick hair can be rolled like this; side sections are twisted across each other at nape.

17. False pony tail added to sectioned hair; natural hair draped over pin conceals attachment.

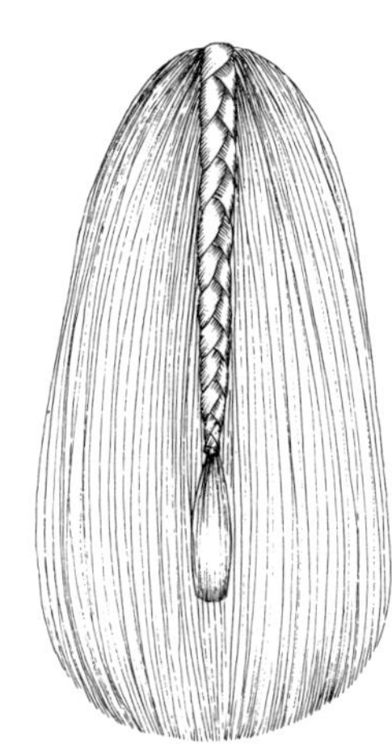

THE SET

There are two ways to transform your wet cut into a living manageable style – by setting in rollers or blowing dry into shape. Curly, wavy and thick hair is often better controlled through rollers.

1. For no parting or centre division, roll crown hair back from hairline. Six rollers are average to reach nape; four rollers, wound down, in double rows either side. Six flat clip curls at nape, two more at ear level – substitute rollers if hair is long. Fringes can be incorporated in crown rollers; when brushed forward they give a fuller effect.
2. For side division of hair; three diagonal rollers wind downward from side part across crown. Side hair rolls down, top back hair winds down. At nape and sides near ear, clip curls or rollers according to length.

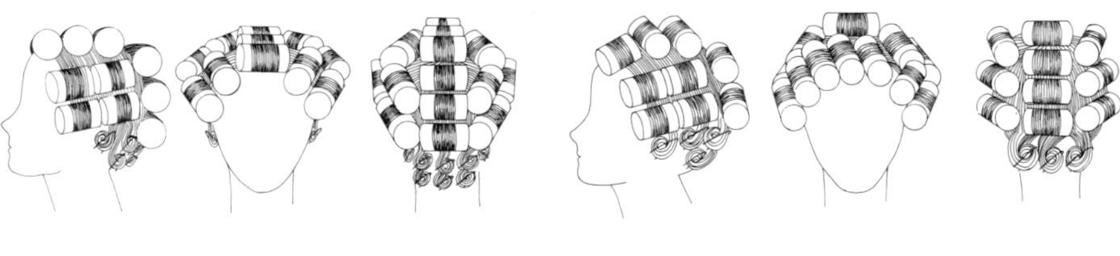

1 2

3. For a flat straight fringe, comb forward while wet, hold in place with tissue or cottonwool secured with clips or transparent sticky tape. Other rollers as for first pattern.
4. For getting long hair as straight as possible, use the head as though it is a huge roller; set two big rollers at crown, hair wound down and back; wrap hair firmly around the head securing it with clips. When almost dry, take down and wrap in the opposite direction; dry completely.

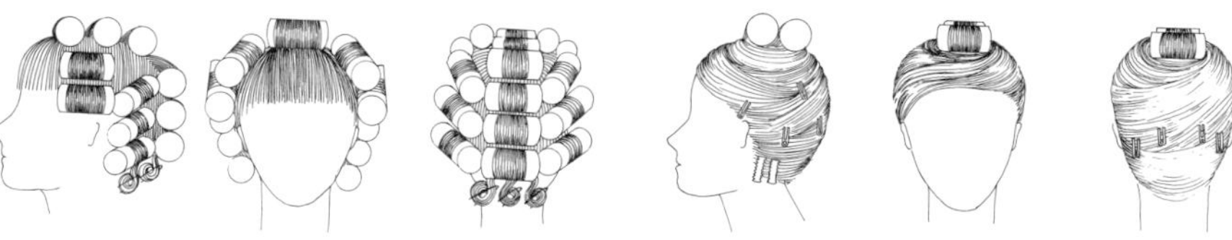

3 4

SOME GENERAL RULES

Setting lotion makes hair more manageable and easier to handle.

Rollers with brushes inside are rough on hair.

End papers help hold ends of hair smoothly and prevent crimping.

Be sure hair is smooth and taut, but not tight on rollers; stretch it a little first by pulling in the opposite direction from which it is to be rolled.

Divide the hair and work with thin sections of one-and-a-half to two inches (40–50 mm.) wide, well combed out.

The bigger the roller, the looser the set; the smaller the roller, the tighter. Most hairdressers use six sizes ranging from three-quarters to two inches (20–50 mm.) in diameter.

The coarser or curlier the hair, the larger the roller you need.

BRUSHING OUT

Before taking hair down, allow hair to cool off at room temperature after a hot dryer. Take the bottom curlers out first. In brushing out, always brush straight back to evenly distribute the curl. Put into final shape with minimum of back combing; use hand dryer and brush, or curling iron for special curling or straightening effects.

BLOW DRYING

A precision haircut is a necessity for a good blow dry result. If straight, time can be saved by towel-drying first; if curly and you want to get hair as straight as possible, you must start to blow dry while it is soaking wet. One very important point – do not pull wet hair too taut in an attempt to smooth and straighten it; this destroys hair and can cause hair fall-out. Don't have the drier near the scalp so hot that it almost scorches. Never concentrate too much heat on too small an area.

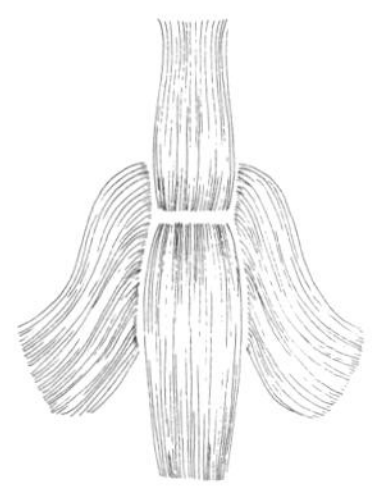

You can style with a circular brush and a hand dryer, though some dryers are equipped with built-in brushes. This is the procedure:

Divide hair into four sections – crown, back and two sides; keep separated with clips.

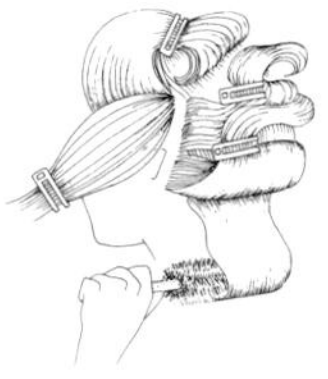

Start blow drying at the back at the nape; place brush under hair at the roots and blow over it. Dry roots first, then middle strands, then ends.

Dry upper back section layer by layer; move to sides and dry in the same way, beginning at neck; finally dry the crown.

For extra bounce, blow hair in opposite direction to the way you want it eventually to go, until almost dry; then switch direction for final minutes.

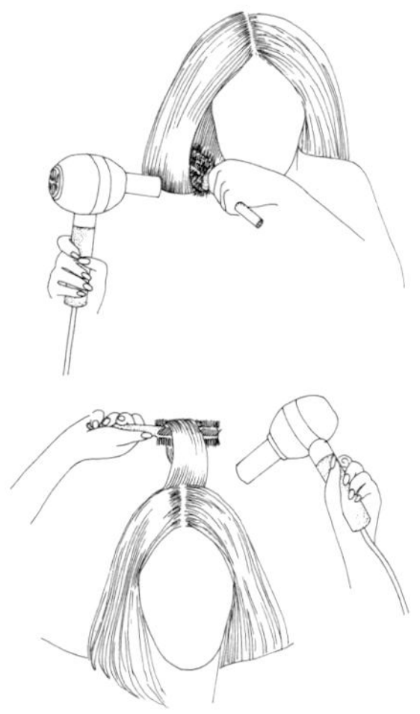

If hair needs to be turned under, wrap dried hair around brush, blow with hot air for a minute, continue to hold brush in place until hair has cooled. To turn hair up, wrap in opposite direction.

If hair is layered, brush all hair over head while drying to give a lift; when hair is not quite dry and you have the necessary height, brush and dry in direction of style.

Short curly hair should be brushed away from scalp.

For fringes – brush backwards first until almost dry, then bring forward twirling around brush, dry and let air cool hair completely before removing brush. For straight fringes, brush flat on forehead.

ELECTRIC ROLLERS

These are used on dry hair to restyle and shape hair between shampoos. They are fast and effective but should not be used every day as they are inclined to dry out the hair, even those with a 'mist'. They can be used for the whole head or certain sections to give curls, a wave or smooth according to the size of the rollers. This is how to get the best results:

In general electric rollers will make curls about twice as large as those with the same size ordinary rollers.

Large rollers make loose, casual waves, medium rollers bouncy waves, small rollers tight waves, curls or ringlets.

The more hair you wrap around each roller, the looser the curl will be.

The use of end papers ensures a smoother set.

Some electric roller units recommend a special conditioner to use while setting – check instructions.

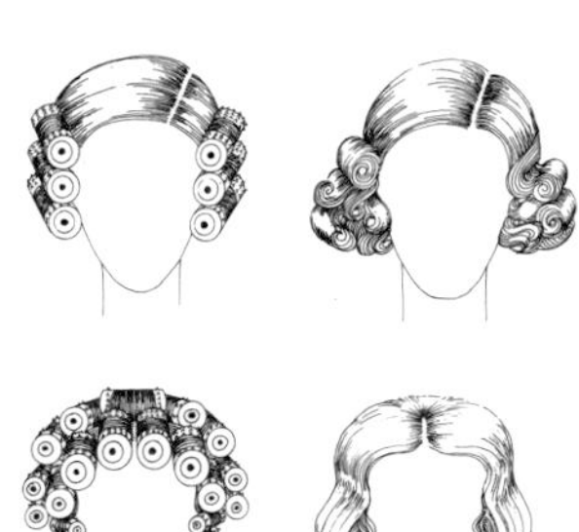

Rollers remain active for about 15 minutes after you have taken them off the heating rods.

When putting in rollers, start at the top of the head, working neckwards; when taking out vice versa.

Allow the hair to cool in curled rolls before brushing them out.

CURLING IRONS

A quick and successful way to pick up a dropping curl, shape fringes, organize ends and lift the hairline. Use with caution as they can easily scorch hair. Plastic or Teflon-coated irons minimize risk. Don't put a metal iron on bleached hair.

Time-test a strand, building up from 2 to 20 seconds to judge how much heat it can tolerate and how quickly it curls. A good idea is to briefly dip iron into diluted setting lotion as this provides protection for the hair. Curl hair in the same direction as you would if it were going in rollers. After curling, clip strands until cool.

WIGS

A wig can either improve the way your hair looks naturally or create a totally different style. The most important thing is that it should look natural, have swing and motion.

Your first wig should be close to your own style and colour. Choose one that is relatively simple to handle. All wigs can have a professional haircut and it is not essential to invest in a human hair wig; some of the synthetic fibres are very convincing, but check colour in daylight and check its springiness. Fibre has the advantage of being more stable than real hair, does not react to the environment and is easy to care for.

Take time selecting a wig; proper fit is crucial – too tight a wig will ride upwards, too big a wig will roam around on the head. A well-fitting wig should not need to be clipped or pinned to your own hair. If you prefer hair away from the face, a more natural look is achieved if an inch of hair at the hairline is combed into the wig; of course colours have to match perfectly. If the colour is different, a wig should have a fringe or be styled in such a way that hairline is invisible. Shape and untangle a wig with a wire brush, there is less fibre loss than with a comb and less static electricity than with a nylon brush. Before putting on a wig, your own hair must be securely pinned back and up; long hair can be wrapped around the head, a net or cap securing it if necessary.

Human hair wigs should be washed and set by a hairdresser, but fibre wigs can be done at home:

Shampoo every month, using a mild shampoo. Follow instructions of the manufacturer.

Dry on a wig block.

If you want more curl, set on conventional rollers, dry under a hair dryer. Follow the original curl and pattern, don't attempt a complete restyle.

HAIRPIECES

These help to add dimension or build up a style, and are particularly useful in creating imaginative up-swept effects. Colour matching must be exact and always checked in natural light. Fibre pieces are invariably as effective as real hair and less expensive. They are washed in the same way as a wig, dried and styled on a wig block.

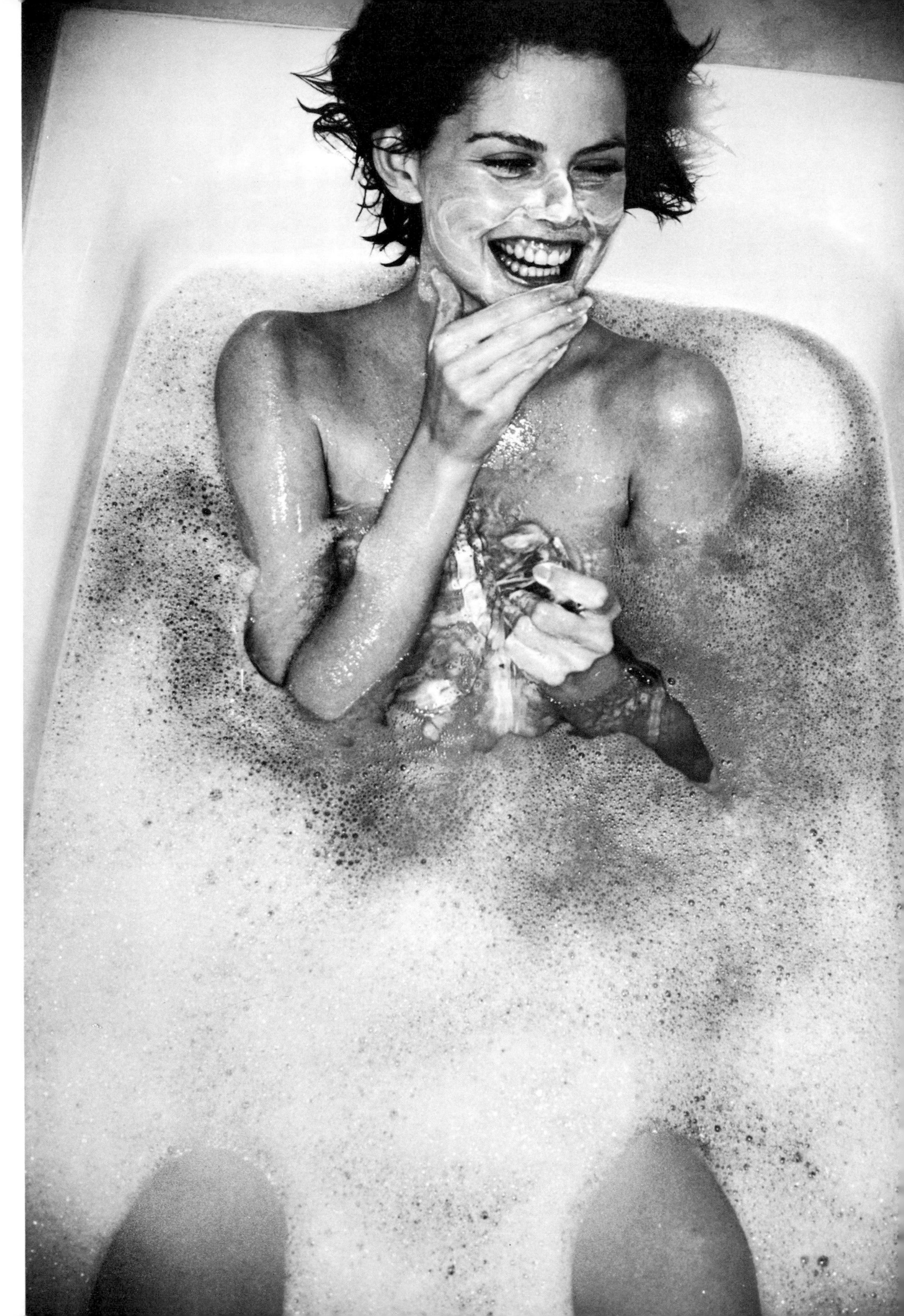

4

BATHING

Bathing is the only way to keep fresh and immaculate; it cleans the skin as nothing else can, it also refreshes and stimulates it. It is the first act of beauty and without it, all preparations and perfumes would be useless. If it is just cleanliness you want all you need is water, a bar of soap and a towel. But there's more to bathing than that.

A bath is therapeutic. It can be used to relax, soothe, stimulate, exercise and perfume your body – as well as clean it. Bathing is one simple daily event that can impart a feeling of luxury. To be a pleasure it must be sensually appealing to the touch, to the eye and to the sense of smell. It must be an exercise in relaxation and tranquillity.

There are times when speed is the criterion. Then it's a quick bath or, better still, a shower. A morning shower wakes you up in a brisk, invigorating manner and takes no time at all. Turn on the water full force to stimulate circulation and to give you a warm glow. It gets you going, it refreshes, it cleanses – but it's quite a different thing from a bath.

Many people think of a luxurious bath or a luxurious bathroom as extravagance – something to feel guilty about. Bathrooms reflect this feeling, and are usually the smallest and most miserable-looking rooms in the house. We are changing though and the message is getting across that a large, comfortable bathroom is an investment in well-being.

So first rethink your bathroom. What can be done to make it more appealing? In these days of washable carpets, protective papers, and treated metals, it is not necessary to make it strictly a tile and chrome set-up. Try cotton or nylon carpets, waterproof paper; instead of an ugly medicine cabinet use interesting cupboards and shelves, framed mirrors – many, not just a functional one above the washbasin; hang prints and paintings, attractive lamps; cover chairs, stools, and hampers; have potted plants, a table for books. Some of the best bathrooms are those that were once bedrooms, porches or terraces; they have space, light, large windows, a view. They are places of beautiful efficiency for cleansing, relaxing, thinking. The true benefits of the bath begin like this:

BATHTUB

Bathtubs should be deep and long enough to stretch the legs, but not so long (as some are) that you have trouble touching the end with your toes. A non-slip mat is a good idea, so is a comfortable foam pillow or folded towel on which to rest your head.

IMPLEMENTS

Body groomers for the bath all have to do with scrubbing and rubbing.

Loofah – a very dry rough-textured vegetable gourd that swells and softens when wet; it is perfect for rubbing off dead skin and leaves the body tingling. Natural loofahs are usually from twelve to fifteen inches long, and able to reach any part of the back.

Friction strap – usually made of hemp, blended with horse hair; long and flat, stringy-looking with strap handles at each end; it is gentler than a loofah but serves the same purpose.

Sponge – an elastic porous mass of interlacing fibres that was once the skeleton of a marine animal; comes in various shapes, sizes and porosity. If a sponge becomes too clogged with old soap, it can be cleansed by soaking overnight in vinegar, then rinsed. There are silk sponges for really delicate skins and nylon sponges in all colours.

Flannel or wash-cloth – a small square of cotton towelling used for rubbing on soap, rubbing away dead skin and rinsing; launder frequently.

Bathmitt – basically two kinds: one has soap in it, or a pocket in which you can slip soap or any cleansing product; the other kind has a rough surface and sometimes contains an abrasive or a stimulant; good for giving skin a rub down.

Body brushes – preferably made of stiff, natural bristles; long-handled ones for the back, smaller ones for arms, legs, fingers, toes, nails.

Pumice stone – a piece of ultra-porous volcanic lava; rubs away skin on elbows and particularly on heels and soles of feet, also sides of fingers that may get work stained; modern substitutes are synthetic friction blocks, as effective but not so sturdy.

ROUTINE

Drink a glass of water to encourage perspiration before you step into a steaming bathtub. Set your hair, cover it with a cap and it will be fresh and bouncy when you comb it out. Take off make-up, apply any treatment that is necessary (masque, lubricant – see page 121). If it's a morning bath, or pre-going-out bath, put on make-up beforehand; it will set in the bath, look more natural and oddly enough, fresher; it will also last longer. Lower yourself into the bath slowly; allow your body to drift in the water with spine immersed, head on pillow. Soak first, and exercise at the same time if you wish to take this good opportunity to work-out muscles (see Bath Exercises – page 250). Then wash, working up a fine lather with soap, stroke limbs with a loofah underwater, this helps firm flab as well as getting rid of dry flaky skin. Brush and pumice where needed. Rinse well, with a hand shower of fresh water if possible. The soaking time varies depending on the type of bath and the temperature.

VERSATILITY

A bath can be relaxing and intoxicating, or energizing and circulation building. With the addition of oils and softeners, it can help prevent the skin from getting rough, replacing moisture, oil, and acidity. With the addition of herbs, it can be soothing, healing, calming or reviving. Bath-time is a treatment for skin and muscles. The heat urges pores to open, making them more receptive to skin lubricants and cleansers; the warmth and humidity relax muscles, relieve tension and increase the stretch and contract capabilities of muscles. Warm water calms because it temporarily lowers blood pressure; cold water quickens circulation and gives you an extra spurt of energy.

TEMPERATURE

Depending on the temperature, water can be a great relaxer or a great revitalizer. Meticulous bathers use a thermometer; the rest rely on the elbow test or how it feels to the hands. Anyone with circulatory complaints should never expose themselves to extremes of temperature.

Hot (100° to 110°F, 38° to 43°C) – this is de-energizing and drying; it can bring out the little surface veins on legs and thighs, and if your bosom is covered, hot water can soften it and encourage sagging.

Warm (85° to 100°F, 29° to 38°C) – this is the best temperature for relaxing and perfect for treatment baths – herb, mineral, oil and aromatic additions. It's the bath to soak in, to read in for up to twenty minutes but not too much longer, otherwise the skin begins to crinkle. Keep water at an even temperature by replenishing it often. Choose which temperature you prefer; the exact body temperature, 98.6°F (37°C), is recommended. At its warmest, this range is fine for unstiffening muscles, or warming you when you are chilled to the bone.

Tepid (75° to 85°F, 24° to 29°C) – relaxes, revives, and refreshes in hot weather; prolonged for 10 to 15 minutes it gives the circulatory system the chance to expand and release internal heat through the skin. Such a bath can keep you cool, or at least cooler, for five to six hours; a colder one may cool you only temporarily.

Cool (65° to 75°F, 18° to 24°C) – a quick pick-up after a day's work, or if you feel sluggish in the morning and can't stand a cold bath or shower. Don't stay in for more than 10 minutes.

Cold (less than 65°F, 18°C) – really stimulating; should be an in-out plunge with quick soaping and rinsing. It's better as a bracing shower with the shower power turned on at its fullest – the high water pressure exercises muscles, gives circulation a real boost.

TIME

Convenience and your way of life dictate bathtime. Whether you are a night or morning bather is a matter of taste, but make it a daily routine.

Morning: If you like a morning bath – and it is a gentle easing into a heavy daily schedule – use an oil or milky powder, or if you prefer a brisker start, try a salt or seaweed bath. Soak, exercise if you like, wash, scrub and finish with a lukewarm splash followed by a quick colder one.

End of day: After a day's work, many women find it ideal to unwind in a soothing bath, to ease tension for a quiet evening at home, or to recuperate for an evening out. Have a mineral, herb or aromatic bath; exercise first, then relax for 10 minutes. A cooler rinse will give you extra energy.

Night-time: To encourage a good night's sleep, laze in a milky, foamy or protein-enriched bath (oatmeal, for instance); if it's perfumed, choose a drowsy, sweetish one. Rinse with water of the same temperature; dab dry, don't rub vigorously.

TYPE

There are four basic baths – nourishing, toning, lubricating or restoring. All are more rewarding when perfumed. Some general rules are: mint and rosemary for energy, sandalwood for tranquillity, cedar and pine for meditation, jasmine for soothing nerves, and rose for calming – carnation is said to be an aphrodisiac. Over the ages, there have been dozens of stories about famous beauties and their special use of herbs and aromatics in the bath to maintain their beauty. It is simple to work out your own formula from kitchen items and everyday herbs. Below are several recipes which may be made up as stated or with an addition of a favourite herb or fragrance.

Nourishing: Usually protein-based baths that soften and enrich the skin and combat dryness. These are soothing baths, good for morning and evening.

MILK:

A cup of powdered skimmed milk in a bath of warm water – the modern version of the ancient milk bath.

OATMEAL:

Stir 1 lb (½ k.) of oatmeal into a deep bath. It contains oils that smooth and nourish. Rinse well afterwards.

OATMEAL BATHMITT:

1 lb (½ k.) oatmeal
¼ lb (120 g.) bran flour
¼ lb (120 g.) powdered Castile soap (finely shredded will do)
¼ lb (120 g.) powdered orris root

Mix thoroughly and put into a muslin or cheesecloth bag, then into a towelling bag or mitt.

This can either be used as a bathmitt and directly rubbed on to the skin, or soaked in the bath itself.

OATMEAL, ALMOND, OR BRAN BAG:

Make a muslin bag, and fill it with oatmeal, almond meal or bran, and let soak in the bath the way tea bags soak in water. Put the bag on a long string hanging from the tap and use for two or three baths.

MILK AND HONEY:

This is probably the most expensive home-made bath, but has become a weekly ritual with several well-known beauties.

1¾ oz. (55 g.) bicarbonate of soda	1 lb (½ k.) honey
3 pints (1·5 l.) dried milk	4 oz. (120 g.) salt

Dissolve soda and salt in a pint (6 dl.) of lukewarm water. Make 3 pints (1·5 l.) of milk from dried milk, following proportions indicated on the package; warm it, and dissolve in it the honey. First put the salt-and-soda mixture in a warm bath, then stir in the milk and honey.

STARCH:

Hard water can be softened with the addition of a couple of teaspoons of ordinary laundry starch, which also gives a milky, softening texture to the water and in turn smooths skin.

Toning: Mineral salts help stimulate circulation, making the skin tingle; they are invigorating and recommended as a start to the day; they are especially reviving during bleak winter months when one cannot get to the sea. They aid in the removal of toxins, and often help get rid of liquid weight.

SEAWEED:

Fill a muslin bag with seaweed (preserved from summer or found at a health shop) and let soak for 10 minutes in a warm bath before getting in.

SEA SALT:

Rub handfuls of coarse salt over body – everywhere except face and genital area. Salt can be contained in a mitt, if preferred. Rinse salt off with warm water, then wash in bath with lubricating additions.

EPSOM SALTS:

Use ½ lb (240 g.) in a warm bath; this is additionally therapeutic if you add mint, pine or eucalyptus extract or oil.

TEA:

A colour toner this, for it tans the skin and keeps up the shine of summer; make a strong tea (just ordinary tea) with four dessertspoons to a quart of boiling water; let it steep for 10 minutes, then pour into warm bath – not too deep, otherwise tea becomes too diluted and less effective.

Lubricating: Oil in the daily bath is the easiest way to counteract skin dryness; it gives the body a silken feeling, and helps restore moisture. Oils that disperse in water are few (though there are now many commercial combinations) but it doesn't matter, as floating oil will cling to the skin and lubricate it equally well. Just a few drops of oil are effective.

AROMATIC OIL:

Mix ¾ cup castor oil or almond oil or avocado oil with ¼ cup any aromatic oil. Suitable fragrances are: rose, jasmine, lavender, mint, pine, lemon flowers, citron. Use only a few drops in each bath.

KITCHEN OIL:

1 cup corn, sesame or olive oil
1 tablespoon liquid detergent shampoo
½ teaspoon aromatic oil

Pour all into a bottle, shake well; use a couple of tablespoons for each bath, remembering to shake again before use.

SHAMPOO OIL:
Oil-base shampoos are as beneficial to the skin as to the hair; it's a quick and inexpensive way to lubricate the skin; a couple of dessertspoons are enough for a deep bath.

Restoring: Herbs and other natural botanical sources are the bases of the restorative bath. These are treatment baths in the tradition of the spa. They are always warm baths, which draw out the beneficial elements. Some are relaxing, some reviving; they are ideal for recuperation after a day's work or for soothing before going to bed.

HERBALS:
There are many herb baths, simple or compound ones, the recipes of which have been handed down over the generations. Don't throw herbs into the bath; they will stick to your body and play havoc with drainage. There are two ways to use herbs in the bath:

1. Pouchette – put herbs in a bag of porous fabric such as cheesecloth; to please the eye more, put this in a patterned silk or muslin sack and hang over the tap for several consecutive baths.

2. Infusion – crush or break-up herbs and make an infusion as you would tea; a pint (6 dl.) of boiling water to 2 tablespoons of leaves or flowers. Never boil the herbs themselves – pour the water over them and let them steep for a minimum of 15 minutes. The longer you allow a herb to steep the more effective it will be but 3 hours is the maximum. Keep pot covered; use ceramic or glass pots, never enamel-lined pans.

LAVENDER MIX:
Dried lavender flowers mixed with smaller amounts of mint leaves, rosemary, comfrey root. Put in a muslin bag and pour on boiling water. Steep for 15 minutes, pour liquid into bath and also hang pouchette from tap into bath.

ROSEMARY MIX:
Rosemary, fennel, sage and yarrow; make an infusion or pouchette.

CAMOMILE:
This mild yellow-white flower contains azulene which is very soothing and restoring to the skin. Use fresh or dried flowers. For an extra zing, add dash of rosemary and pine needles (infusion or extract). Camomile also protects you from insect bites.

ELDER:
Restores nerves and calms, as well as healing and stimulating the skin; either an infusion or pouchette.

COMFREY:
Good for healing scars – make an infusion from the leaves.

LADY'S MANTLE:
An infusion in the bath is said to help menstrual difficulties.

BLACKBERRY:
Spring tonic to restore a dull skin, use several nights in a row. Make a strong infusion, add to warm bath.

PINE:
Boil pine needles for 20 minutes and allow to steep for 12 hours.

Or – put needles in a vacuum flask, add boiling water and leave for 24 hours.

Strain and use a cupful per bath; add to basic lubricating bath.

LEMON:
Add slices of lemon to a lemon-scented bath oil (either commercial or your own concoction); use slices to rub over skin.

CIDER VINEGAR:
Restores the acid mantle to the skin and can be very important in keeping this balance. Add one cup to a bath; the water takes on a velvety quality, but the skin does not retain the smell of vinegar afterwards.

SOAP

Soap is the best way to cleanse the skin. Facial skin may need special care but rarely is a woman so sensitive to soap and water that she must use only cleansing oils or creams for her body. Soaps are made from fats and oils, combined with an alkali. This alkalinity is neutralized on contact with most skins. Talk about soap being too drying and the cause of flakiness is exaggerated, as this condition is usually brought about because of over-use or abuse and not because of the soap itself. Too much soaping is definitely bad and quite unnecessary. Every soaping must always be followed by a thorough water rinsing, and in the case of dry skins by an application of cream or a moisture-preserving lotion. Soap is neither old fashioned nor ineffective.

Conventional soaps are reasonably mild and there is a wide range of products to choose from. Choice is a matter of experiment; if one soap tends to make your skin taut, change to another. There are soaps based on olive oil as were the first soaps made in Castile, soaps using natural botanical sources, soaps rich in lanolin, soaps superfatted with cream. The fattier soaps are midway between regular soaps and a rinsable cleanser. They don't clean as well as regular soaps, but are milder. The rules to follow are: for an oily skin, use a drying soap; for a dry skin a superfatted one; for a normal skin, any good mild soap.

Cleansing detergents are not to be thought of as meagre substitutes for soap because they're synthetic. They come as bars, liquids, lotions and gels – and clean exactly the way soap does; they must be very well rinsed away. They are very effective in hard water, and also lather in sea water. For oily skin, use an alkaline detergent to strip away excess oils; for dry skin, a detergent with built-in moisturizer is best.

Home-made soaps are complicated to produce and frankly not worth the effort, but here is a recipe for liquid herbal soap that's simple to make, soothing and nourishing to sensitive skins:

HERBAL LIQUID SOAP:

2 tablespoons dried camomile flowers
12 tablespoons milk (fresh or made from powder)
1 egg
1 teaspoon honey
1 tablespoon almond oil
2 tablespoons herbal shampoo with oily base
2 tablespoons rubbing alcohol

Steep camomile flowers in the cold milk for three hours – covered with a cloth. Beat egg into almond oil, add shampoo, then honey and finally alcohol, beating all the time. Blend in the milked camomile. Put in a tightly sealed jar; shake always before use. If you want a more perfumed soap, substitute part of the almond oil with an aromatic oil.

PREPARATIONS

Bath products cleanse, soften and revive the skin and soothe the senses. Here are the general types, for bath and afterwards.

In the Bath:

Bubbles – soften and scent water; often not necessary to use soap.

Crystals – mineral salts, coloured and perfumed to soften water.

Gels – transparent cleansers that can be used as an alternative to soap, gentle and good for dry and tender skin; pour into bath to give a foam or squirt straight onto body before shower.

Milks – essentially water-conditioners, rich in fats and oils; soften water and smooth skin.

Oils – some float on the water, some mix with it; all lubricate well, leaving a film on the skin that acts as a conditioner and moisturizer.

Salts – those made from Epsom salts, perfume and colour water; some from sodium derivatives, soften water; some are carbonated and make water effervescent. Special herbal salts indicate therapeutic benefits.

After the Bath:

Bath oil spray – softens and scents skin, less drying than a perfume or cologne, therefore good for dry skins, or special dry areas.

Body lotion – a moisturizing creamy fragrance, important to help keep skin supple; smooth on all over when you are still a little damp as pores are clean, open and ready to soak up extra moisture.

Dusting powder – lighter version of talcum powder; to be shaken, sprayed or patted on; it cools and smooths, helps absorb moisture and enables you to slip more easily into clothes.

Splash and friction waters – tangy colognes and toilet waters that brace, cool, and stimulate the body.

Talcum powder – a smooth mineral powder, sometimes with antiseptic properties due to the addition of boric acid.

After-bath lotion to make at home:

$3\frac{1}{2}$ oz. (100 g.) of red rose petals steeped in 2 pints (1 l.) of white vinegar for fifteen days. Make in a ceramic jar, covered with gauze.

The same lotion can be made with lavender, orange blossom, mint.

DRY FRICTION BATH

This is said to be conducive to sleep and a cure for insomnia. Using a friction glove – made from hemp, horsehair, heavy cotton or plastic – massage the body gently in upward sweeping motions. Switch glove from right to left hand to reach all parts of the body. There is no need to massage roughly as the glove does most of the work with its heavy texture. Accumulated dead cells and surface dirt are brushed off; skin is given a chance to breathe, blood circulation is increased and consequently toxins lying on the surface are disposed of more quickly. Over a period of time, this can really cleanse and refine the pores. Done once a week, it's a real tonic for the skin.

SPIRIT SPONGE BATH

2 oz. (60 g.) spirit of ammonia
2 oz. (60 g.) of camphor
1 cup sea salt
2 cups ethyl alcohol
Put all ingredients into a quart bottle, fill to brim with boiling water. Allow to cool slightly.

Shake lotion before using, then with a cloth or sponge, rub the spirit all over the body, but do it gently as the liquid itself invigorates as it cleanses. Afterwards just dry with a towel, don't rinse or sponge over with water.

PERSPIRATION AND ODOUR

If you ask most people what causes body odour, they will answer perspiration or sweat. It's not true. Moisture excretion, which is the body's air conditioning system, is not to blame. Sweat is colourless and practically odourless when it appears on the surface of the skin. It consists for the most part of pure water and a few salts, which are responsible for giving a faintly salty smell that's rather attractive and considered aphrodisiac. What causes body odour is a group of bacteria that turns the innocuous moisture into stale smells through decomposition. This only happens if moisture cannot evaporate fast enough.

Areas exposed to air have no problem getting rid of surface moisture, but when perspiration is trapped next to the skin, body odour begins. The underarms, feet and outer vaginal areas are the usual problem spots. Synthetic materials hinder evaporation – tights, underwear, shirts, and sweaters shut off air circulation more when not of natural fibres.

Perspiration is caused by the activities of two different types of glands. They both secrete moisture through tubular ducts. They are:

Eccrine glands – these are evenly distributed all over the body, between 2 to 3 million of them. Their secretion is 99% clear water with a few salts. They act as the main temperature control and through thermal sweating endeavour to hold the body at an even normal temperature. Interfering with this process in any major way can be fatal.

Apocrine glands – these are less common and are concentrated in specific areas: underarms, groin, buttocks and the nipples. Their secretions are also mostly water, but they are cloudy and contain some protein and fatty substances which attract the bacteria. These glands are larger than the eccrine ones, and commonly associated with hair follicles; they usually develop during puberty. Apocrine glands take care of a certain amount of thermal regulation through sweat, but their activity is mainly due to nervous and emotional reactions: a slight argument, a tense conversation, a moment of agitation, is enough to get them going. Environment temperature doesn't make any difference to the apocrine glands. Whether it's 110°F (43°C) or below freezing, their secretion is the same.

All-over perspiration is adequately dealt with by regular bathing. Underarms need particular control for the problem here is not only odour but visible wetness. Extra precautions are usually necessary and this is one reason for shaving under arms though in many cultures it is considered a de-sexing procedure and therefore not done.

The problems of wetness and dryness have two basic solutions in the underarm area.

Deodorants and deodorant soaps which control odour by impeding bacterial action.

Anti-perspirants which limit both odour and wetness by reducing the volume of perspiration as well as fighting bacteria.

The safety of deodorant soaps has not been definitely established. They contain antiseptics which, when exposed to sunlight, sometimes cause an adverse reaction in the form of blisters and swelling.

Deodorants and anti-perspirants come in cream and liquid form and allergic reactions are extremely rare. They must be used regularly and are most effective when applied to a thoroughly clean area. It is helpful to remove hair, as this traps sweat and makes it harder for the controlling agents to reach the skin. Apply when the body is cool and at rest – not directly after a shower because the skin is hydrated and perspiration ducts are not sufficiently open; fifteen minutes later is better. One application a day is sufficient for most women, while an additional one gives complete 24-hour protection. For excessive sweating it is advisable to apply before going to bed with another application in the morning.

How well deodorants and anti-perspirants work depends on many factors – temperature, clothes, exertion, stress, tension, and whether you naturally perspire lightly or heavily. Odour is more easily brought under control than wetness, and no anti-perspirant is 100% effective. Nor should it be. 50% is a more realistic level, but it is quite enough for aesthetic reasons. Even if it were possible, it wouldn't be desirable to block completely the flow of perspiration. A deodorant or anti-perspirant does not last until washed off; its durability is limited.

Why use a deodorant instead of an anti-perspirant when the latter does two jobs instead of one? Some women are irritated by the additional chemicals that go into an anti-perspirant. A deodorant is simply a germicide (a very small amount, 1% or less), a fragrance and a mixer that makes it easy to apply. Anti-perspirants contain aluminium or zinc salts which penetrate the sweat duct openings, and it is this activity that prevents the delivery of a lot of the sweat to the surface. However these salts can sting sensitive skins. Allergic reaction to anti-perspirants is rare.

Irritations

Underarm irritation is not necessarily directly caused by a deodorant or anti-perspirant. It could be from a chemical finish or dye in fabric, from sensitivity to your own perspiration, from cutting or grazing your skin when shaving or because of a more serious disease. If irritation doesn't clear up or shows signs of spreading, it is important to check with a doctor right away. To help prevent irritation, the first thing is to make sure you shave correctly. A blade must be sharp, otherwise you drag off layers of skin. It is a sensible precaution to delay using a deodorant or anti-perspirant for 24 hours after shaving. If you have an acid skin condition, you are likely to get an irritation from deodorants – try many, as some are less acid than others. The cause of irritation may also be a particular perfume in a deodorant.

Natural deodorants

These help counteract odour, but cannot control wetness.

Chlorophyll has a marked effect on the bacteria that cause body odour, so eat foods rich in this substance, i.e. green leafy vegetables.

Rub underarms with leaves of parsley, watercress, outer dark lettuce leaves, tops of beets or radish.

Use an infusion of sage under arms or in bath.

Lovage in a hot bath acts as a deodorant and purifier; put shredded leaves in a muslin bag.

Lavender oil is effective though too strong to use as it is; make a lavender water to dab on or smooth over particular problem areas.

3 drops lavender oil
1 lump sugar (or 1 tablespoon)
1 pint (6 dl.) distilled water
Leave for two weeks before use; always shake beforehand.

Other herbs that help control body odour are: cloves, leaves of chrysanthemum, camphor and patchouli. Make infusions or pouchettes either for body application or for adding to the bath.

BATH EXERCISES

The time spent enjoying the benefits of a bath, can be usefully and easily employed for a few basic exercises that will tone muscles and keep the main trouble areas in trim.

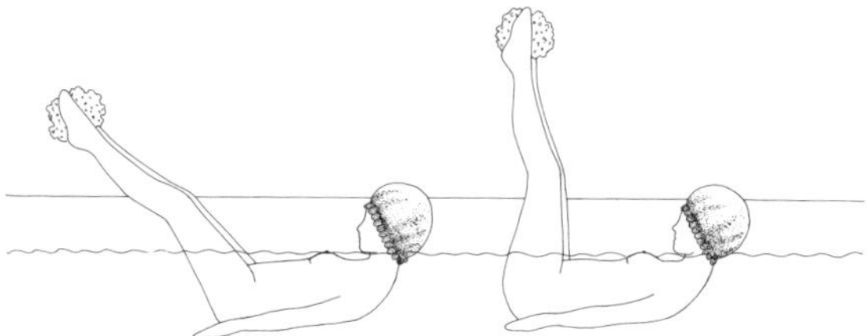

1. *Sponge grip:* Lie almost supine in bath, grip sponge between feet and slowly raise legs as high as possible; hold at zenith to count of three, lower slowly. Repeat six times. Good for the hips.

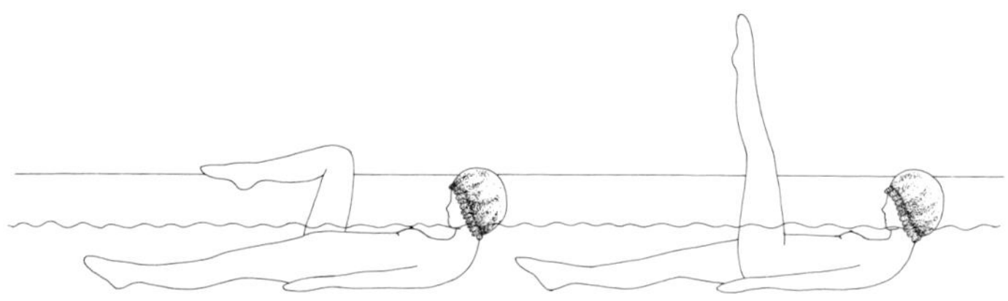

2. *Leg kick:* Lying in bath, put legs up, bent at right-angles at the knees; kick one leg up straight, toes pointed, foot arched; alternate with other leg. Do twenty kicks. Helps shape legs.

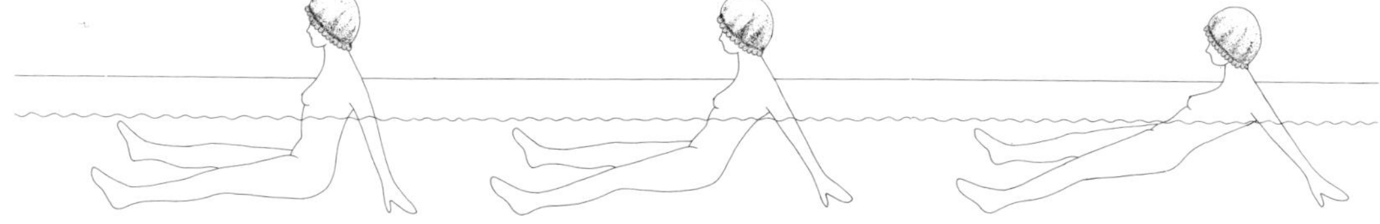

3. *Stomach pull:* Sit with legs straight out in front, a little apart, supporting body with arms behind torso; move torso slowly to a backward slant, using stomach muscles and shifting arm support backwards too; return equally slowly. Do six times.

4. *Shoulder circle:* Using sponge, make wide circles with hand in the centre shoulder area. Do six circles with each hand, going from left to right with right hand, right to left with left hand; for breast and upper arm muscles.

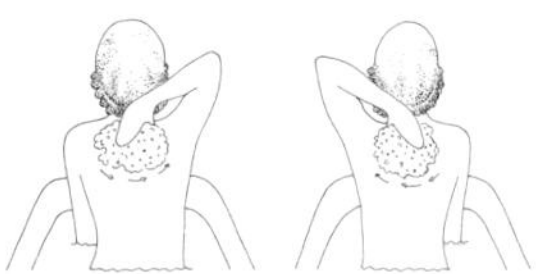

SALON BATH TREATMENTS

Sauna – A special type of dry heat. A sauna is taken in a small room built entirely of pine logs with slatted timber platforms at different levels. A central stove, sometimes wood-burning, sometimes electric, is covered with heat-resisting stones. The temperature is high – around 200° F (93°C) and if water is ladled onto the hot stones it produces a sudden burst of heat. The object is to perspire and through perspiration lose weight, open the pores, clear the skin, stimulate circulation and relieve aching muscles. Tension is helped too. To stimulate sweating, the real enthusiast hits the body with birch brooms. At first it is not advisable to stay in for more than 10 minutes; then 5 minutes or so outside – a quick cold shower is suggested – then back in the sauna for another 10 minutes. In many salons a sauna cabinet is used, an encasement where only your head is exposed – with dry or steam heat inside.

Wax – Paraffin wax is particularly good for the treatment of stiffness; it also helps get rid of excess fluid and improves skin texture and colour. The wax is solid and cloudy white; it has a low melting point and when heated becomes clear and completely fluid. It is painted onto the body and forms a second skin of wax. The body is usually wrapped with towels or linen. Heat is built up inducing perspiration; afterwards the wax is sponged off. The treatment usually takes about an hour and is often followed by a massage.

Mud – Volcanic mud contains therapeutic minerals and when it covers the body it induces perspiration, drawing out impurities. You can either soak in a mud-filled tub for about 15 minutes or be layered with the mud.

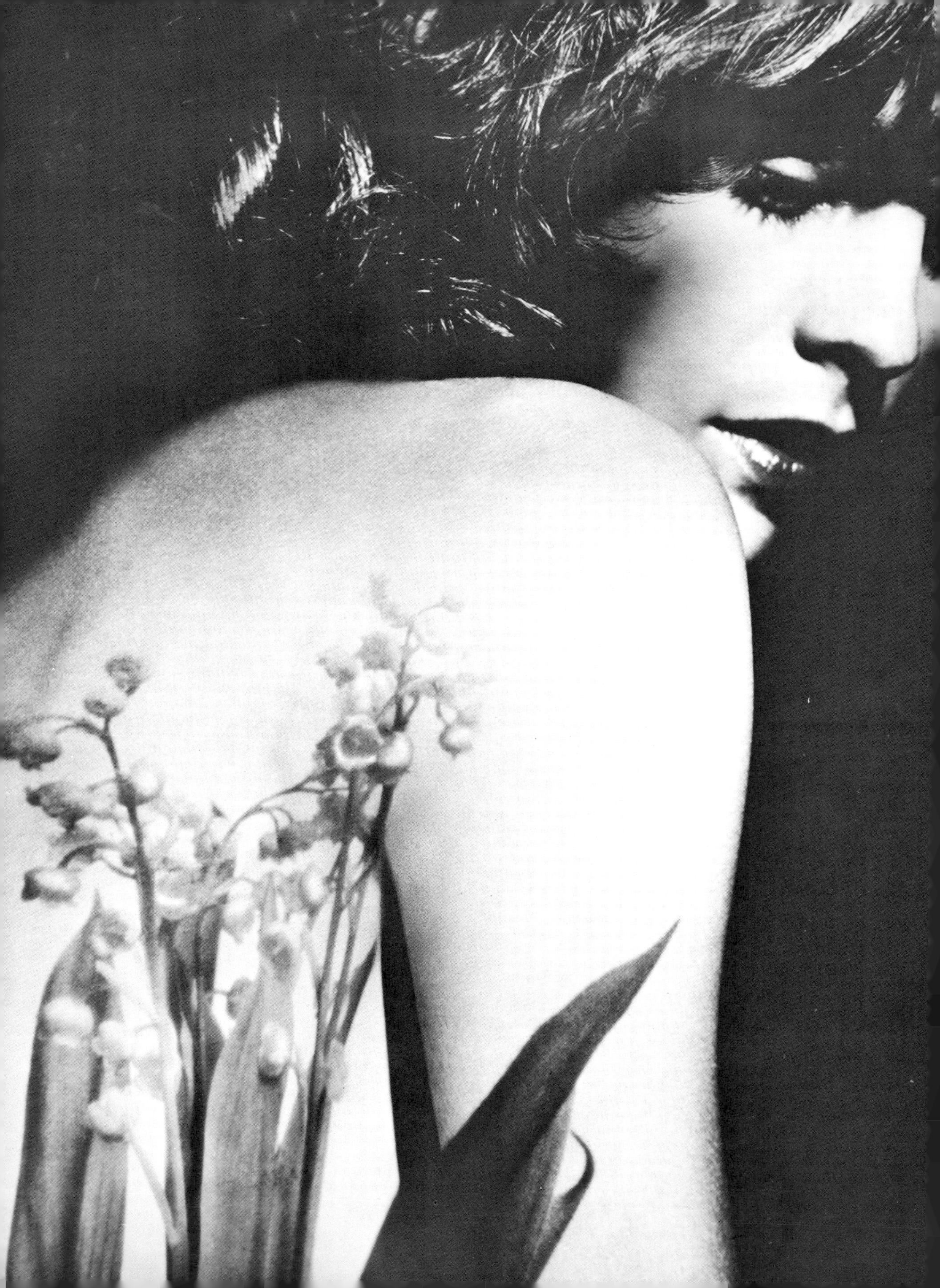

5

PERFUME

Scents trigger emotions in all animal life, and though our primary sense of smell may be less acute than that of animals, it is now believed to be a great deal keener than we have supposed. We have all but suppressed any natural odour instincts and we have little practical use for smelling, but odour is still very much part of our instinctive lives and memories.

Scientists are puzzled by our sense of smell and particularly by body odours that could affect behaviour. These are called pheromones, and are clearly evident in the animal world where they attract, repel, warn or reassure. Do they function in people? There is no evidence that they do not, and some indication that they do, particularly in sexual situations. We produce pheromones in abundance, but are very busy suppressing them or covering them up. And yet perfume can act like a pheromone, as the habitual use of the same fragrance registers on the subconscious and is immediately associated with a particular place or individual. This emphasizes the unique property of perfume: under its influence we recall and relive.

The brain transmits thoughts and memories, but the olfactory cells are responsible for our sense of smell. These are assembled in a membranous tissue high in the nose and receive the odour messages through the nose or through the rear of the mouth (during eating taste and smell are closely related). From here, via the olfactory nerves, information is directed to the brain. Natural odours produce instinctive reactions; perfume aromas stimulate the senses in a more excessive, more varied and more subtle way.

It is impossible to give a scientific analysis of the sense of smell. What smells nice is tied to the psychology of association which varies from person to person.

RICHARD DAVIS

Perfumes did not originate in France, though they have been perfected there, and now the world centre of the industry is at Grasse, a hillside town just inland from the Côte d'Azur. Perfumes were already used more than three thousand years ago in Egypt as aphrodisiacs, medicines, and cosmetics. The name comes from the Latin *per fumam* (through smoke) which indicates its extensive use as incense at that time. Perfumery is an art as well as a science; the master perfumier is known as a 'nose' because although he may be mostly chemist, he is an artist too and with one whiff he can discern if a perfume will be successful or not. No computer has been found to replace him. The language of perfume is artistic too; perfumiers use analogies of other arts, notably music, and borrow acoustic terms to register effect. So we hear of 'high or top notes', 'low or base notes' and middle notes. A perfumier's 'top note' is the first heady fleeting impression received as the bottle is opened. It lingers briefly to give way to the 'middle note' which is the heart of the perfume portraying its character and richness. This can last several hours and the better the perfume, the longer the time. Finally comes the 'base note' composed of the longest lasting elements usually known as 'fixatives'. These are the odours of low volatility that cling and could be unpleasant if used alone, but as part of a total composition add a warm, permanent glow to a fragrance.

Most perfumes are complex intertwinings in which each accent sets off another. There can be dozens, even hundreds, of ingredients artfully blended to produce one distinct smell. Each component has its separate identity, but loses it as it is blended. A professional 'nose' can identify most aromas in turn, but the end result depends on two autonomous things: the touch of a particular perfumier and the woman who wears the perfume. The same ingredients with slight adjustment can result in something quite different, and no two 'noses' are alike. Also, perfumes react differently on different skins, so one can never say that any perfume always has exactly the same odour.

The art of the perfumier as we know it is about 200 years old. Today's perfumiers have inherited the techniques and methods invented by the French in the 18th century. It can take many years to create a new scent, and it takes a rare power of discrimination to balance the formula. There are three stages in the making of a perfume: the selection of raw materials, their preparation and blending, then the formulation. Raw materials are in two categories – natural and synthetic. The natural components come from all over the world. They have been the traditional sources of perfume since earliest times and are both botanical and animal in origin. Synthetic ingredients – called aldehydes – have been developed over the last thirty years. They have strong characteristic odours reminiscent of natural essences; sometimes they are more real than the real thing. They lend force and character to a perfume, but rarely contribute subtlety. As a rule, the higher the price of perfume, the more expensive its raw materials and the more effective the aroma.

'Enfleurage' is the French term for the old and tedious method of extracting the scent from flowers. Enormous quantities of the natural source are required to produce a fraction of concentrated oil. To obtain 1 pound (½ k.) of concentrated jasmine oil, about 300 lb (150 k.) of flowers (or 2½ million flowers) are needed. These are soaked and softened in purified cold fat. In time the flowers will yield their essential fragrant oils to the fat, then an alcohol wash is used to remove the scent. In turn the scent is separated from the alcohol by distillation. It is these floral essences that provide the top and middle notes of a perfume. The low notes are established by a 'fixative' which adds staying power. This is a misnomer as such ingredients (often animal in origin or from green or bark sources) don't 'fix' the components. They are more the tenacious lasting notes of a perfume.

Animal ingredients are as expensive as floral ones. In their concentrated state, they smell pretty awful, but in minute quantities they are an enticing and humanizing element. No good perfume can do without them; they give a distinguished air to a fragrance, but because they have an aphrodisiac quality, they must not be overdone. Can a perfume be an aphrodisiac? Technically the answer is 'no', but any good perfume is sexy and any skin smelling of jasmine, Bulgarian rose or whatever is infinitely more erotic than the same skin smelling of nothing in particular. For the practical, there is this information: it has been established that in a person who is unable to smell, sex interest is less pronounced.

The effect of a perfume depends upon its category, and fragrances are divided into groups. The type of fragrance not only indicates its components, but also its impression. For example, light floral perfumes refresh, citrus, greens and moderns revive and stimulate, spicy, sweet florals and oriental musky perfumes lull. There are general categories, but nothing is straightforward about fragrance: just as no one scent is made up of a single essence, sometimes no one overall sensation comes through. Underlying notes of sweetness can penetrate a sharp perfume, or tangy overtones give clarity to a warm sweet scent. The following categories are a guide:

Floral

Single florals are one-note perfumes that give the essence of a single blossom. This does not necessarily mean that the essential oil used is only from that particular flower. Usually when the perfumier wants to copy a natural flower fragrance, he blends together a number of different essences which produce the effect of the flower.

Then there are the floral bouquets where various flowers, often represented by aromatic or synthetic essences, are harmoniously blended. Sometimes one note predominates, but there are other notes as well. Usually specific flowers are not readily recognizable. Floral perfumes are frequently light and refreshing; some however can be very sweet (see category below) though not as overpowering as the orientals.

Citrus

These are perfumes dominated by lemon, orange and bergamot notes. They are particularly sharp, fresh, and stimulating to others as well as to the wearer. They are ideal for 'cooling' the body and perfect for those who turn perfume very sweet – people with oily skins for instance.

Green

As the name implies these fragrances are essentially fresh and woody, crisp, clean, and dry. Aromatic sharp woods from temperate climates – such as pine and cedar – are blended with mosses, ferns, grasses, and flower stems.

Modern

These have been developed over the last thirty years and primarily use synthetic oils. They are highly complex products of the chemical laboratory and the professional 'nose'. Individualistic and distinctive creations rather than duplications of nature, they are characterized by brilliant top notes, a rich middle section, and often provide a depth and emphasis that natural perfumes alone cannot achieve. Many contain notes from several fragrance categories, but on the whole they are bright, cheery, and cool, ideally suited to an active modern life, pleasant and uncomplicated. This modern group has been the most popular category in recent years, and has had the most additions. Modern florals are sparkling with specific flower notes not easily identifiable. Modern green and woody florals are drier blends – grassy and fresh, but not as dry as the modern greens which are noticeably tangy with the zest of the outdoors. Modern mossy and herbal blends are sharp and run from light to resinous. They are very bracing and said to have a 'sexy dry-out' which in the language of the perfumier means that once the distinct high notes have evaporated, you are left with a clean fleshy scent which is more human than botanical. This green-moss-herb group is cited as the trend of the future.

Spicy

These are heavier in character than the florals and can be quite pungent. The blends combine essences of cinnamon, cloves, vanilla – and sometimes ginger – with the more exotic flowers.

Sweet

Mostly floral combinations made from the more penetrating of the fragrant blossoms – jasmine, tuberose, and gardenia. They can be very sweet and need to be used carefully as they are likely to become overpowering after a very short while, particularly if the metabolism of one's skin is such that it turns a perfume sweeter. Many skins react this way and another person is usually more aware of it than the wearer.

Oriental

Very rich and full-bodied fragrances, based on the more aromatic of the eastern woods and grasses (like sandalwood) and heavy with the scent of musk, ambergris and civet. The most sultry perfumes, their appeal is very much an individual reaction. They may be exotic to one person, and too much for another.

Whatever category a perfume may fall in, most come in three strengths: perfume, toilet water, and cologne. Today the terms toilet water and cologne have become interchangeable, though the former is considered a little stronger. Both are diluted perfumes containing a higher percentage of alcohol which accounts for their cooling and refreshing quality: the result of the rapid evaporation of spirit. The fragrance lingers on though not as potently as that of the concentrated perfume. This lasting power is particularly true of modern blends, where the synthetic aromatics provide a forceful middle note. Scent permeates all beauty products and frequently the same one is found in a series of preparations: soap, bath oils, and foams, body lotions and powders, hand lotions, towelettes, solid perfume sticks and cream sachets. All are soothing and economical ways to extend fragrance enjoyment.

How do you set about selecting a perfume? There is really only one way: with authority, tenacity, and leisure. Perfume is expensive; perfume is an investment in personality and mood; perfume is complex and individual; perfume is hundreds of different fragrances. You have to sniff, to sample, to sniff again. It is a matter of trial, error and eventual success. You are not expected to buy the whole bottle to find out if you like a perfume or if it likes you. Tester bottles are there for testing. Use them; the more you try, the more discriminating you become.

Scent must reflect mood and occasion as well as personality. Women are experimenting with different fragrances more than before. The idea of finding one perfect perfume and sticking with it forever is now considered too restricting. Some women find two and stop there – one fresh scent for day, a more brilliant one for evening. Others use several and choose the one that strikes the right note at the right time. No perfume evokes the same mental image to any two women. Find the one that makes you feel fresh and lively, the one that stimulates your mind, evokes your sensuality.

Professional noses evaluate perfume by testing it in its most diluted state – as a cologne or toilet water. A drop of perfume is a potent thing, and it can overstimulate the nose to a state of numbness. The best way is to spray a cologne on your left wrist and another on your right. Sniff it right away to get the impression of the top notes, but don't make a decision for about an hour. Within that time it will have reached the final drying out stage, when the top note has given away to the main body of the perfume. Keep checking your reaction throughout the day, but don't try any new scents. You could sample a third fragrance on the back of one hand at the same time as spraying your wrists but usually more than two is confusing, particularly for beginners. Another point: it has been shown that your sense of smell is least acute in the morning and early afternoon, so it is better to test later in the day.

What affects fragrance? The chemistry of the skin can change a perfume. For instance, a woman with fair skin will get better results with a delicate fragrance than a woman with darker skin because of her type of sebum (oily substances). Perfume lasts longer on an oily skin but tends to become sweeter. If you smoke you lessen the effectiveness of fragrance, not only because the smell of tobacco pervades body and clothing, but also because the nicotine is apt to alter the chemistry of the skin, reducing the staying power of a perfume. Medications, including the Pill, can affect your fragrance as they intentionally interfere with the body's metabolism and consequently change the skin's reaction to a scent. This can also happen if one's diet is suddenly switched from its usual pattern. If perfume is subject to even a minor odour deviation the end result will be different. During menstruation natural body odour doesn't alter but your perception of smell is not the same. This explains why a woman may think her perfume is going 'off' – but to others she smells the same. Climate and environment can also affect fragrance: in a warm climate perfume evaporates quicker and tends to bring out the base notes earlier, which explains why so many perfumes seem sweeter and heavier in tropical conditions. In cities air pollution seems to strangle some perfumes, which means you have to re-apply scent more often than in the country.

The ultimate effect of perfume is in the way you use it. Don't think of it as the last thing you put on before leaving the house. That is the wrong method and the wrong psychology. Perfume should put you in a certain mood. It is for your benefit first, so apply fragrance directly after a bath or shower, before getting dressed. Learn to layer it. Begin with scented soap, bath oil, and powder. Splash on a cologne or toilet water – all over and generously. Then follow with dabs and strokes of perfume essence, used sparingly. The best way is to emphasize the pulse points from the toes up; these warm spots of the body bring out the true note of the perfume and accent the general impression given by the cologne. The spots for dabbing are: ankles, behind the knees, between thighs, bosom, throat, back of neck, wrists, and crook of the elbow. Behind the ears is not such a good place as the oil secretions there are often different from the rest of the body.

Whether to put perfume on clothes is mainly a matter of taste. Perfume does stain, so it should be sprayed under hems, under collars etc. and remember that essence not in contact with your skin doesn't take on its individual character. Don't use perfume as an antidote for sweat – the chemical reaction is invariably fatal. Perfume must be refreshed during the day. When the heart of the perfume gives way to the base notes, it is time to renew it, not only because the best part of the perfume has gone, but also because the last lingering tones can be unpleasant. A good perfume lasts from four to six hours.

Once a bottle of perfume is open, it is uneconomical not to use it. Keep it in the cool and dark because it oxidizes when exposed to heat and light. Once the seal is broken, slow evaporation means a less perfect, less balanced perfume. For travelling, a spray container is best, or a small securely sealed bottle. Avoid plastic, scent tends to evaporate through it.

What finally ends up in a bottle has taken years of judgement and preparation. This is one reason why perfume is expensive. The perfumier puts his heart, his expertise, his nose, endless time and different kinds of flowers, grasses, barks, roots, leaves, and fixatives into a single creation. Listed below are the more important of these ingredients – all from natural sources. The synthetic aromatics (with formulas and names only a chemist can digest) follow parallel lines in smell and use. But here are the more important and most commonly used basics, the elements that have gone into perfume making over the centuries.

Botanical Sources

BERGAMOT: Small, fragrant member of the citrus family that looks like a green orange; it is inedible but filled with an oil that has a clean, tangy scent. It grows only in Calabria in Southern Italy. In some countries natural bergamot is no longer used in perfume as it can cause dark splotching of the skin but the chemical synthesis is extremely good.

CEDARWOOD: This tree gives an oil which provides a woody undertone to a perfume; it is also valuable as a fixative. The best cedars are found in Morocco.

CLOVE: Best known as a spice, but the buds provide attar of cloves, a useful component in the spicy and oriental scents.

CYPRINUM: An essence that comes from the flower of the henna; heavy and long-lasting, particularly sweet scented.

JASMINE: Possibly the most precious of floral ingredients. White jasmine provides the fragrance and reaches its peak of intense perfume at dawn. Almost every perfume contains some jasmine and although chemists have been able to isolate all the essentials of the essence, no one has been able to synthesize its fragrance – very close, but not its equal. The flower is a native of Persia and Kashmir, but today is grown commercially in Mediterranean countries, particularly around Grasse in France.

LAVENDER: Used when a delicate fresh fragrance is required; grown mostly in the hills behind the Côte d'Azur, at times the scent is so strong that it permeates the whole area.

ORANGE FLOWER: Often added to a floral bouquet to give fullness and a tinge of intoxication; if too much is used, the effect can be rather sweet.

PATCHOULI: A member of the lavender family and a native of Bengal; the essence is obtained from the leaves and stem of the herb, and because of its wild, haunting odour it is used mainly for the musky and oriental perfumes.

ROSE: First of the natural perfume oils, the most pleasantly fragrant of blossoms and the most versatile. It can be used alone or incorporated into fragrances. The species used for perfume is *Rosa Centifolia*, and vast fields are cultivated near Grasse. Flowers are hand-picked at night when their scent is at its zenith. A more opulent version is the Bulgarian rose which has a more voluptuous scent and is also a favourite with perfumiers.

SANDALWOOD: Comes from the white wood of *Santalum Album*, a parasitic tree found in India and Australia. It is a seasoned, exotic scent and because of its density and capacity to provide long-lasting base notes it is used as a fixative.

VETIVER: This is extracted from the roots of a grass that grows in the Far East and parts of Central and South America. Eastern in quality, it provides a heavy aroma and is used mostly as a fixative.

VIOLET: One of the enigmas of perfumery, this flower which would seem such an obvious choice for an essence inhibits our sense of smell. When we sniff a violet for more than a certain length of time, the flower seemingly loses its fragrance – in fact we lose our ability to smell it. Perfumiers have discovered that the root of the Italian iris produces the best approximation to the fragrance of violets.

YLANG YLANG: The blossom this essence comes from is pale green. It is oriental and the fragrance wildly sweet, yet when woven into musky blends it makes them subtle and rich.

Animal Sources

AMBERGRIS: The most unlikely of all perfume ingredients, this grey, odourless, porous, fatty substance is the spew of the sperm whale. It is found floating on the sea (it dissolves in alcohol but not in water) and is a perfume fixative of the highest order. A perfume infused with ambergris is sexy as it gives a fragrance of an erogenous animal note. It is rare and expensive simply because it is difficult to find, and likely to become rarer and more costly as whales are an endangered species.

CASTOREUM: An oily brown substance produced by the lymph glands of the Canadian beaver – like all animal derivatives, it is used to give a sexual, lasting quality to perfume. It is the strongest of all animal fixatives, and so blatant is its scent that it is used sparingly and, in modern fragrances, hardly at all.

CIVET: The secretion from a gland under the tail of a civet cat. It is useful as a fixative, but rather strong, so must be used discreetly.

MUSK: A glandular secretion of the male musk deer whose habitat is the Himalayas. As with all animal elements in perfume, it is strongly erotic and used as a fixative. At one time, it was used on its own as a one-tone natural aphrodisiac. Now, on a more restrained level, it is added to floral blends. The musk deer is in danger of becoming extinct, so rather than forgo the obvious advantages and appeal of musk, chemists are now producing synthetic versions which are considered as effective.

Despite the various basic natures of ingredients, perfume is the most intangible of beauty sources. It will not help looks in any way but it can uncannily provide an aura, change an attitude, create a mood and stir up emotions to a remarkable degree. Perfume is not necessarily a mere beauty agent, but is a way of soothing one's own physical and emotional state. The heavier perfumes, those with more animal elements or with a heavy scented floral base, have a drowsy effect that puts the mind at rest and so chases away mental distraction. This mysterious curative power is also seen in the way a fresh sharp scent can stimulate our sense of smell; we breathe in deeply, nasal passages are cleared, the head is relieved of tension and we feel refreshed. Such a scent is the classic eau-de-cologne. And surely, the fact that for centuries perfume has been closely associated with seduction must be based on more than hearsay. Indeed, because of this, perfume is often regarded with suspicion. Perfume is certainly complex as much is unknown and much is contradictory. But there are facts that establish its realities and possibilities and facts that help define the human reaction.

THE HAIR

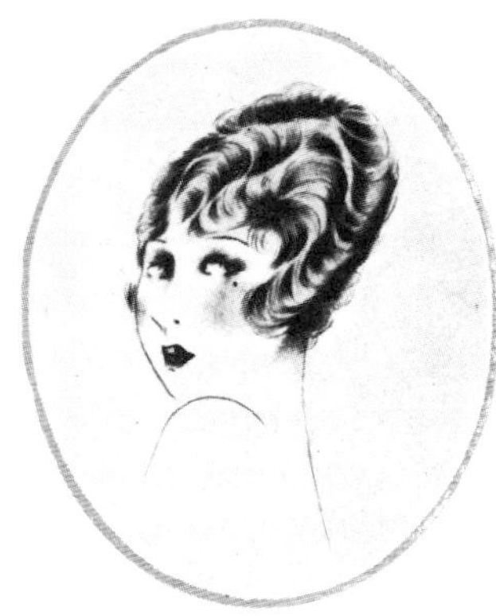

Nestlé's wonder machine for 'perming', although invented in 1906, only really hit the masses in the 1920s, changing the manes of nations. In London Eugène claimed to be the 'ablest and most renowned permanent Hair Waver of Paris & London' . . . the Mason Pearson hairbrush was 'enjoyed by all' . . . and Inecto-Rapid was 'used by ROYALTY, endorsed by 5,000 leading hairdressers' and 'permanently restored colour to Grey Hair in 15 minutes. Vogue *warned: 'Ill-kept hair spoils all possibilities of good looks and smartness.' By 1929 the shingle had succeeded the bob and the Eton crop was soon to come. With the 1930s came a 'new sense of individuality'. 'Curls must never appear untidy and so, to hold them in perfect control, some of the smartest women are adding to their coiffures decorative details that are practical, smart and becoming.' You could keep your hair in 'perfect order' with a Lady Jayne Slumbernet and 'science' discovered a way to bring back colour and gloss to faded hair 'by natural methods' – the only method 'endorsed by the Press'. But just in case that didn't work you could buy a bobbed head-dress for eighteen guineas. There was increasing interest in hair care and* Vogue *advised 'a good shampoo every two, or perhaps three weeks'. In the 1940s hair fashion was dictated by the war: girls working in factories had to wear turbans and snoods to stop their long hair getting into the machinery and servicewomen had to wear their hair above the collar.* Vogue *asked: 'Why does that shoulder-mane seem so out of date?' With the 1950s the teenagers took over, first with the ponytail, later with the loose hair cult and the Carita sisters in Paris made the first fashion wigs – to match Givenchy dresses. The accent was on* <u>you</u>*. André Bernard's 'creations moulded to suit your individual charms'; French's creations 'for you alone'; Riché's 'short-styled softly waving coiffure – the fashion follows you'. The wig boom began in 1960, Harrods – like other big stores – opened a wig counter and by the end of the decade the State was supplying human hair on the N.H.S. In 1963 Vidal Sassoon created his revolutionary new haircut – hard, architectural, thick chopped bob – and later came Jean Shrimpton's 'tiger mane', pre-Raphaelite 'ripple waves' and the first 'afro' styles. With the 1970s hair health became a fetish; henna brightened the colour, added shine and weight. 'With less backcombing, less lacquer, more brushing, more shine, there's a new deal in hair health.'*

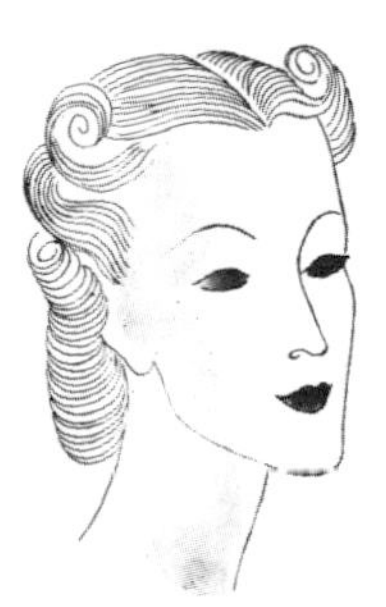

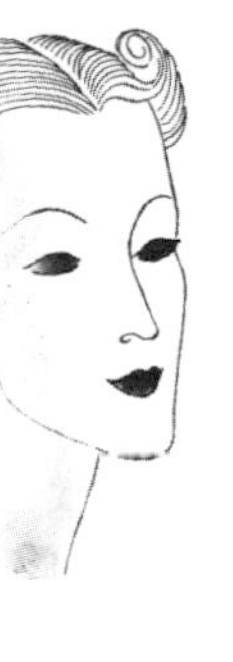

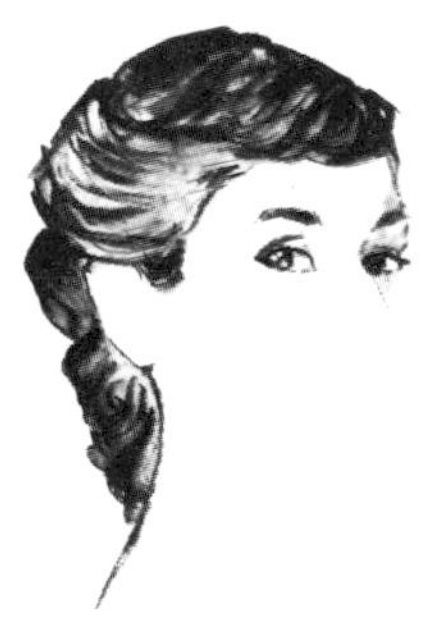

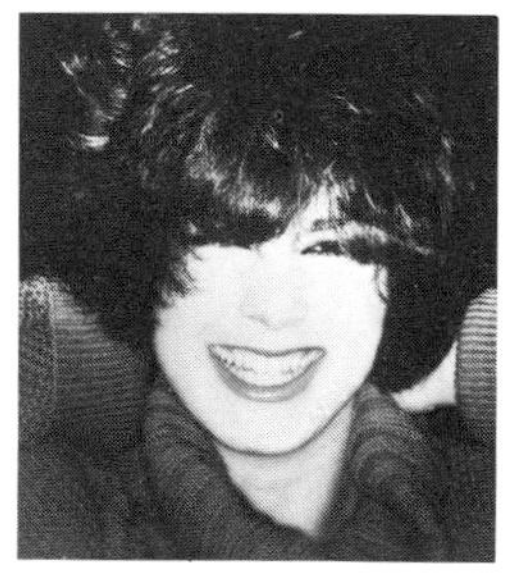

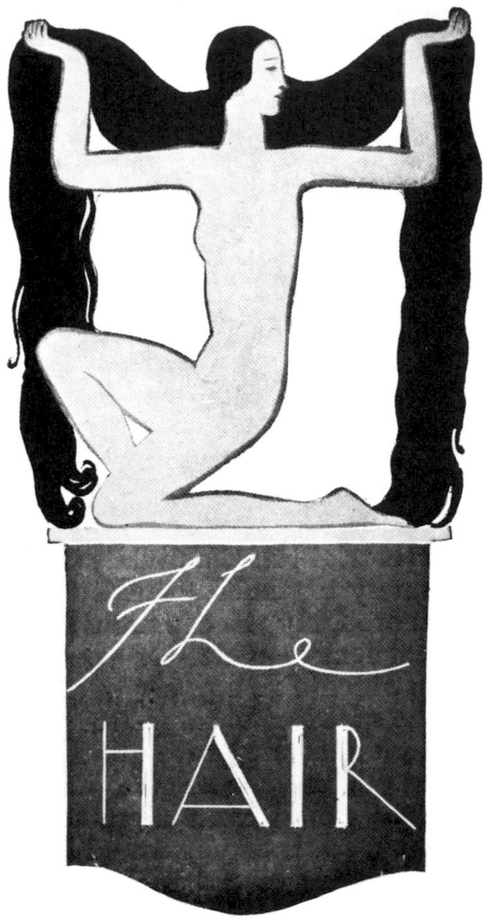

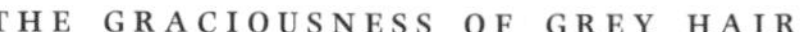

THE GRACIOUSNESS OF GREY HAIR

By a Sophisticated Charm, a Fitting Choice of Costume, and Exquisite Grooming, the Wearer of Grey Locks Becomes a Personage.

'Alas, poor might-have-been, who mourned her raven hair and failed to see that grey was vastly more distinctive. Too soon, the dye-pot did its work – and robbed her.'

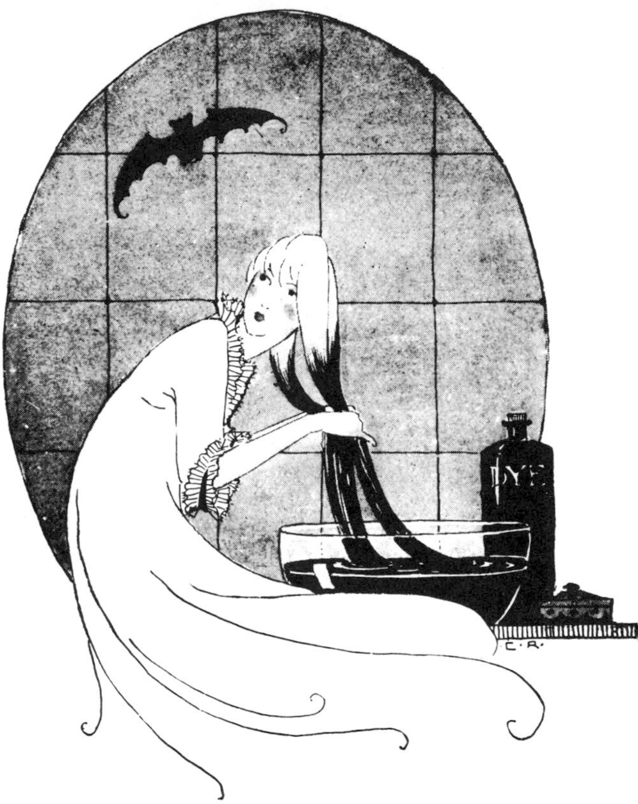

PARIS MAKES AMAZING EXPERIMENTS IN COIFFURES

No Two Heads – No Head on Two Days – May be Coifed the Same

'The return of the gowns of the Princesse de Clèves is, naturally, the occasion for the return of her coiffure, and this, too, makes novel and striking use of braids.'

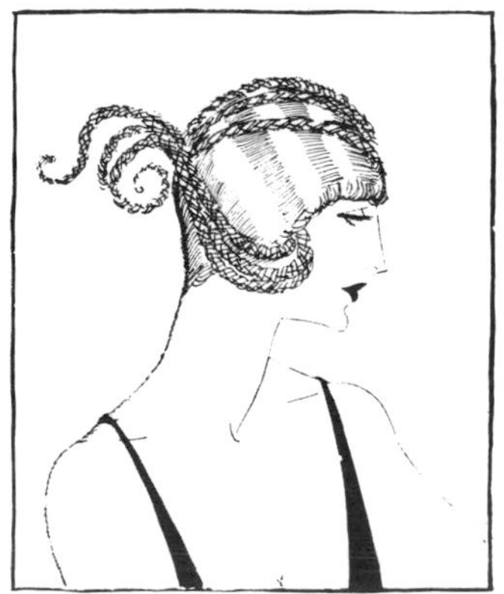

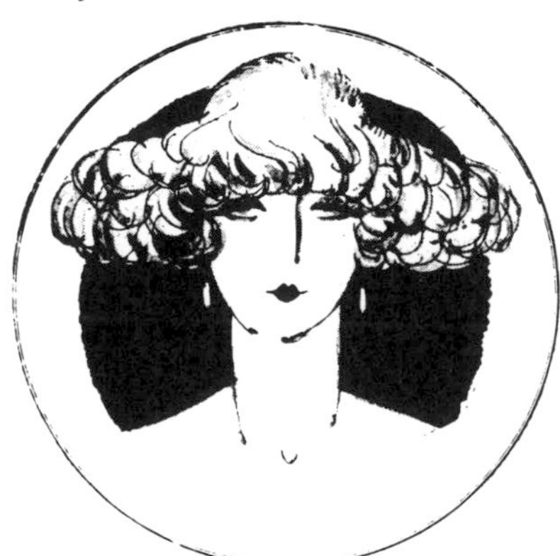

'So great an aid to the toilette is that newest invention, the electric wave, that even the woman of soft and silky hair occasionally attains such coiffures as this, although, in time, she will doubtless decide not to.'

'With the high collar, one may expect the high coiffure which lifts the hair away from the neck. Less readily will woman part from the puffs about the ear.'

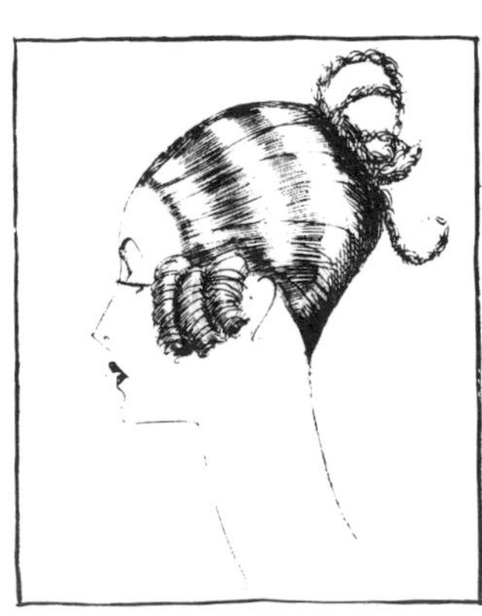

Mr. Eugène has personally given, in his Paris Salons, a demonstration of his famous Patented Appliances to the well-known film producers, Messrs. Gaumont. This series of cinema demonstrations may be seen throughout Great Britain during September, and show how Eugène's wonderful process can transform the lankiest hair into soft becoming waves.

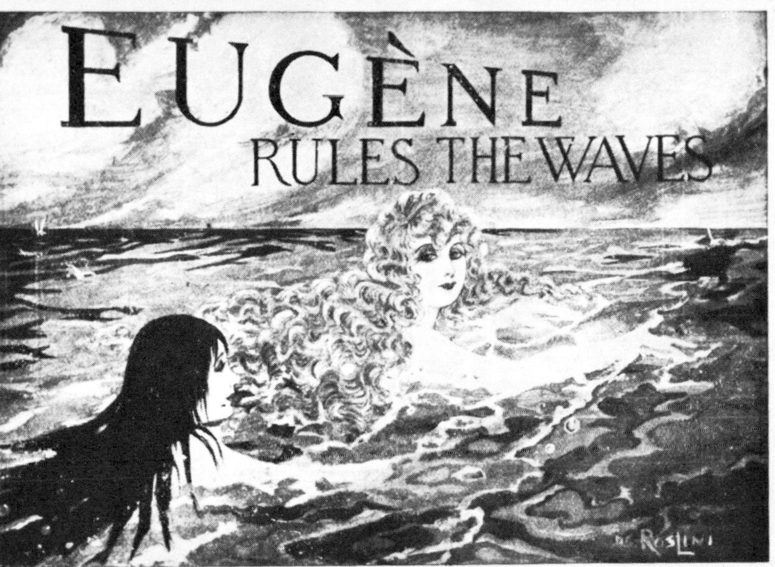

Inventors and Patentees of the world renowned EUGÈNE APPLIANCES for Permanent Hairwaving

Eugène Ltd.

LONDON
23 GRAFTON ST. W.1
Telephone: Gerrard 4607
178 New Bond St. W.1.

MANCHESTER
2 St. Anne's Place
Telephone: Central 2803

PARIS: 265 Rue St. Honoré

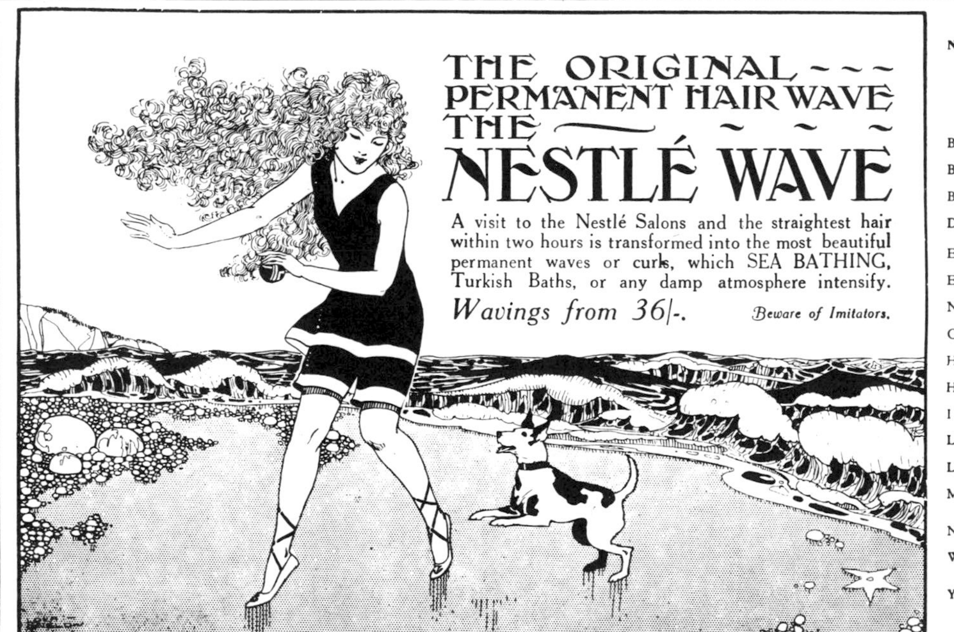

NESTLÉ LICENSEES
THE PROVINCES

The following firms are licensed to carry out the Nestlé Wave:

BATH.—Mills & Watkins, 3 Georg Street.
BEDFORD.—W. J. Wilkinson, 41, Tavistock Street.
BOURNEMOUTH.—S. A. Thomson, 92, Poole Road.
DUNDEE.—Miss Hill Rennie, 7 Union Street.
EDINBURGH.—John King, 52 Princes Street.
EXETER.—D. Theuwissen & Co., The Arcade.
N. FINCHLEY.—Mrs. H. Norris, 79a, High Street, N.
GLASGOW.—Maison Lewis 140, Douglas Street.
HARROGATE.—J. Kasper, 19, Parliament Street.
HULL.—Swallow & Barry, 24, George Street.
ILFORD.—Madame Seabrook, Cranbrook Buildings.
LEEDS.—Miss Manning, 27 County Arcade.
LEICESTER.—Alfred E. Bird, 77, Queen's Road.
MANCHESTER.—Maison Taylor, 26-28 King Street; 131, Oxford Road, All Saints.
NEWCASTLE.—Marguerite Joyce, 1, St. Mary's Place.
WOLVERHAMPTON—Madame Elizabeth Hewart, 152, Tettenhall Road.
YORK.—Swallow & Barry, 26 Stone Gate.

THERE IS NO DIFFERENCE BETWEEN NATURE'S WAVE AND THE NESTLÉ WAVE.

WRITE FOR NEW ILLUSTRATED BOOKLET.

C. NESTLÉ & CO., LTD.
Directors: Alfred Harris, George Aldworth.
Telegrams: "Kantist, Wesdo, London."

48, South Molton Street
Phone: Mayfair 2986.
43, Dover Street, Piccadilly
Phone: Regent 1/34

LONDON, W.1

1920

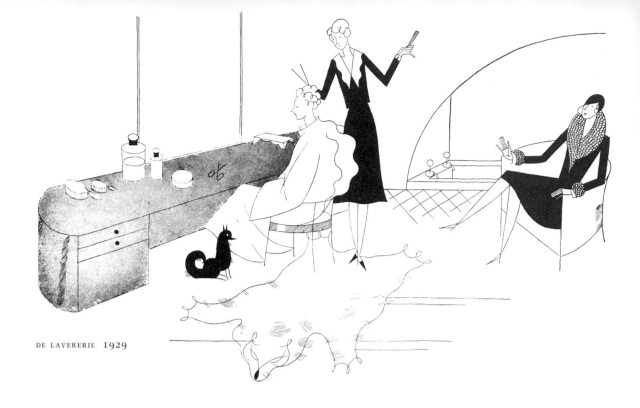

DE LAVERERIE 1929

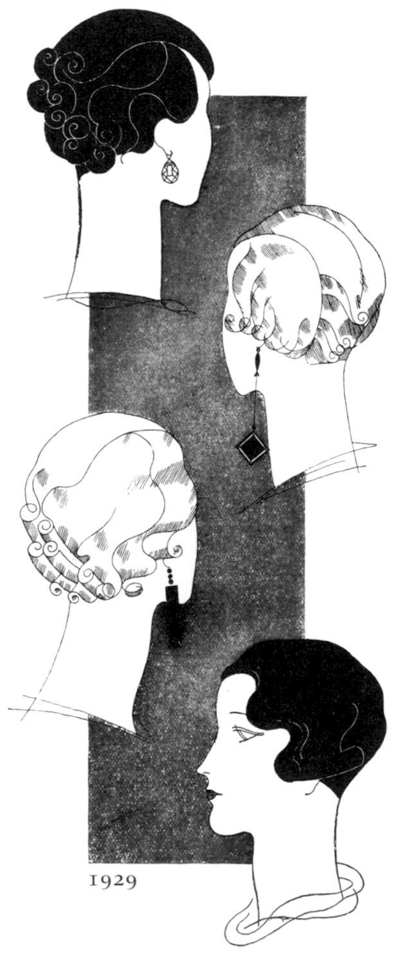

1929

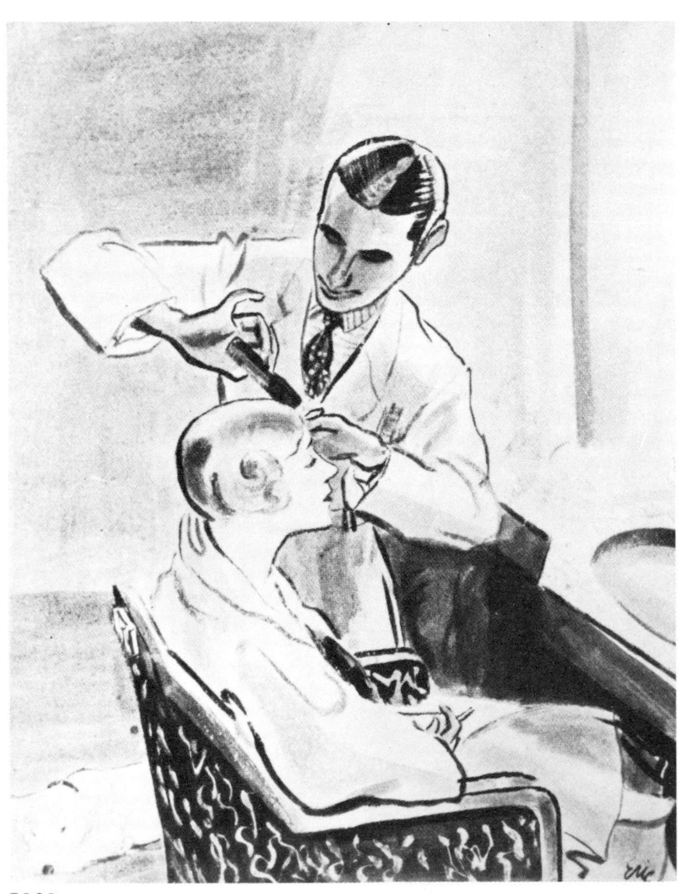

1930

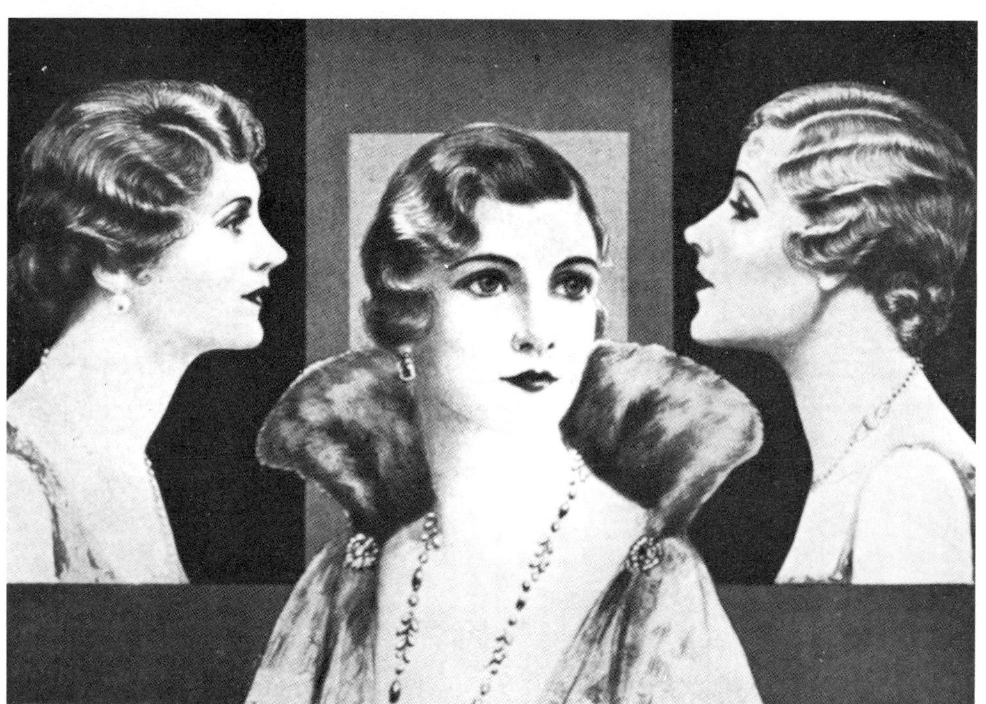

The Triumph of Maison Georges 1930

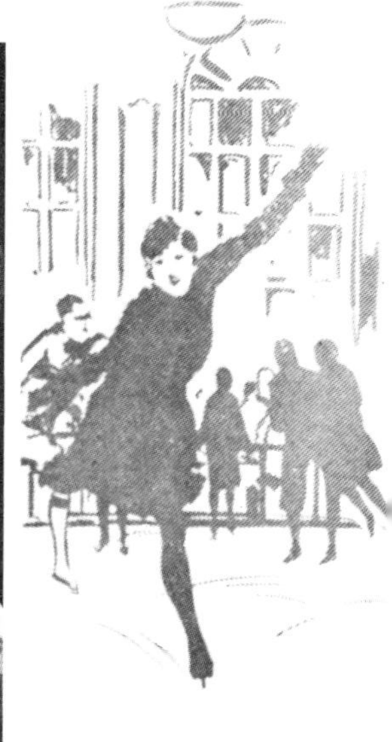

'Your choice will provide you with the PERFECT COIFFURE.'

'Up aloft does Guillaume dress their hair: the Princesse Jean Poniatowski and Madame Pol Roger. Ear-revealing, forehead-revealing, nape-revealing – these two coiffures call for a good natural hairline and clear-cut features. But if you can't boast these assets, there are many modified versions of the up-and-up line, including at least one which is sure to suit you: study the sketches given here.'

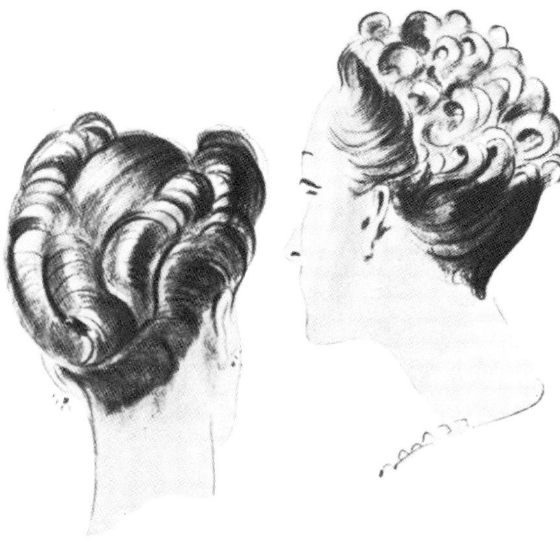

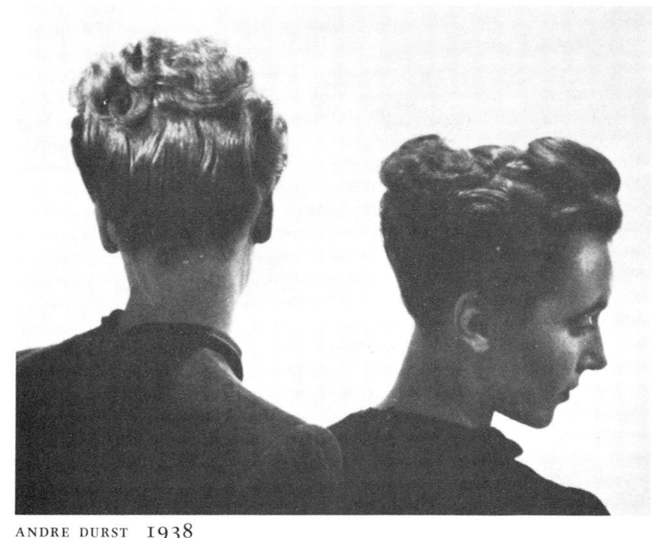

ANDRE DURST 1938

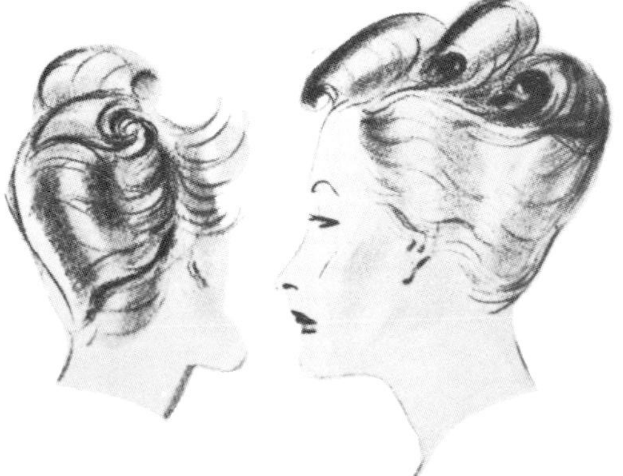

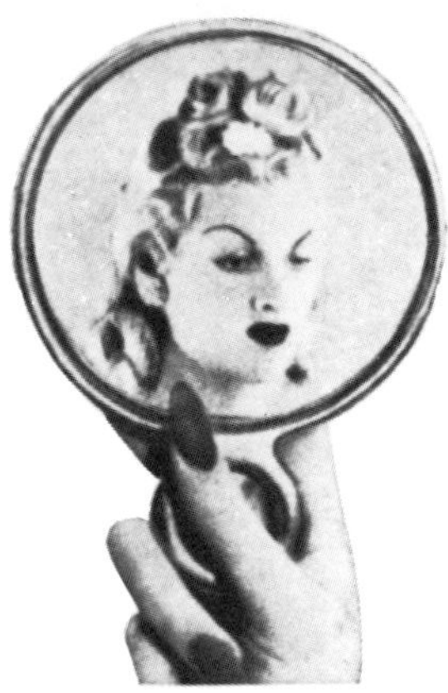

1939: Plucked eyebrows

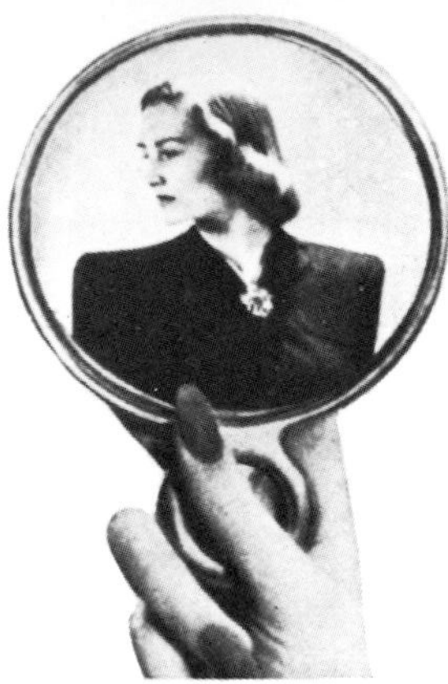

1943: Page-boy cut

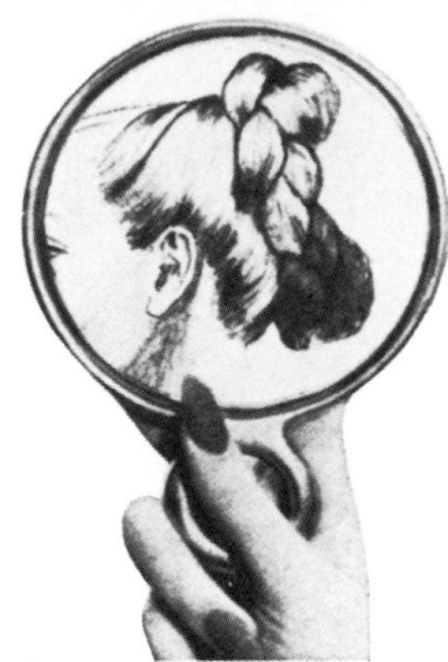

1946: Pinned-on plaits

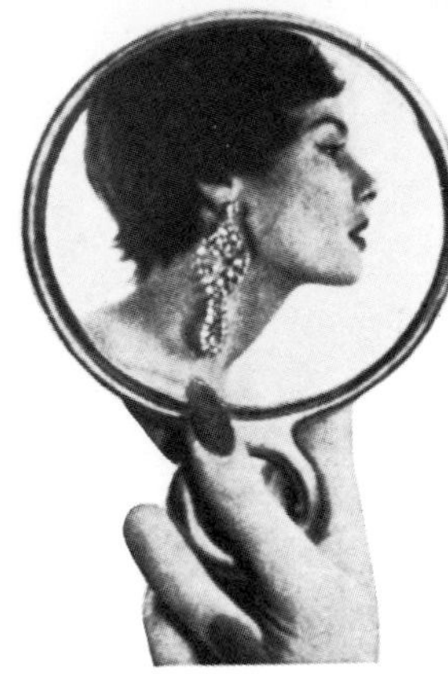

1949: Gamine style

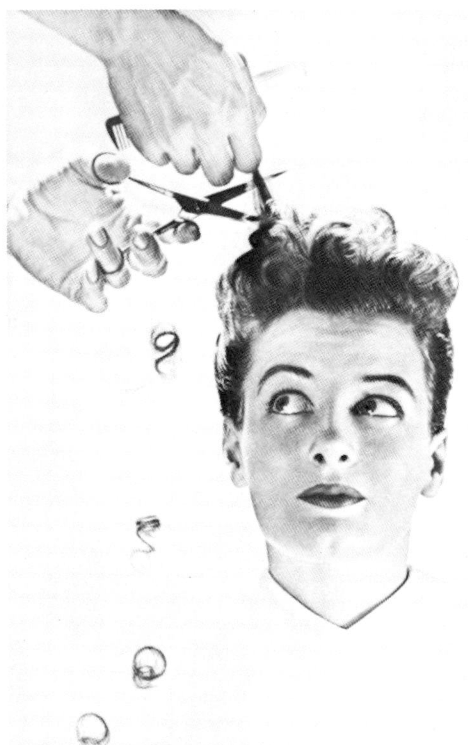

'SNIP, SNIP . . . go the shears, nibbling away at long locks, lank locks, Lorelei locks. Officially – the Government's all for it, because short hair can't get in the way of war work, takes little precious time.

RAWLINGS 1943

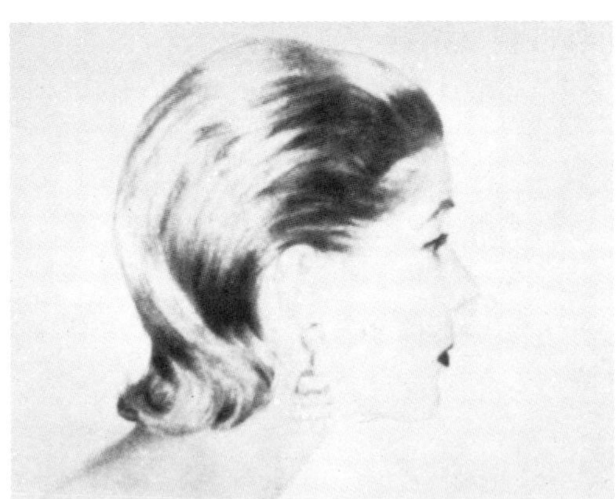

New York

KLEIN 1955

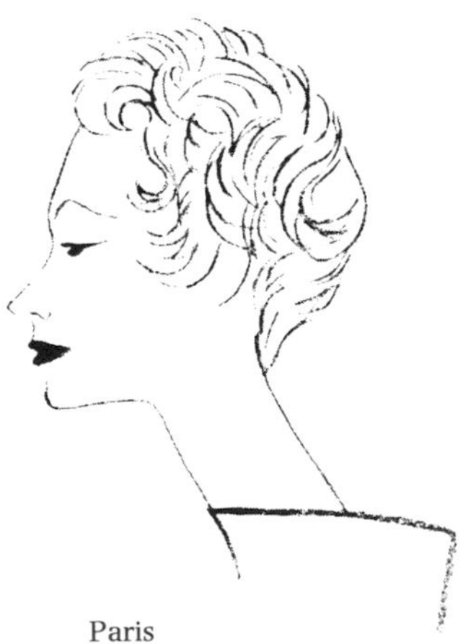

Paris

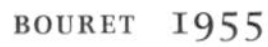

BOURET 1955

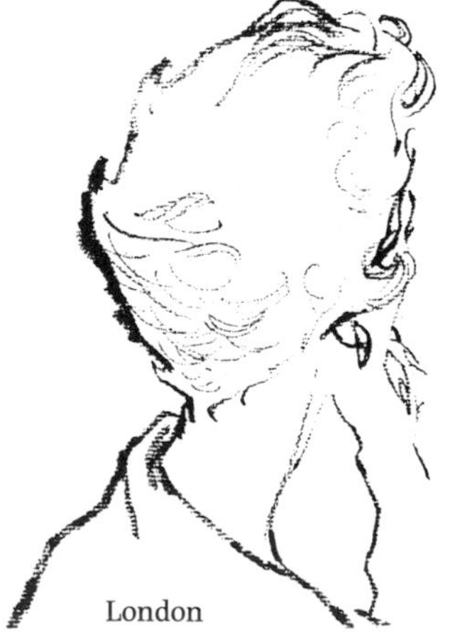

London

STEMP 1955

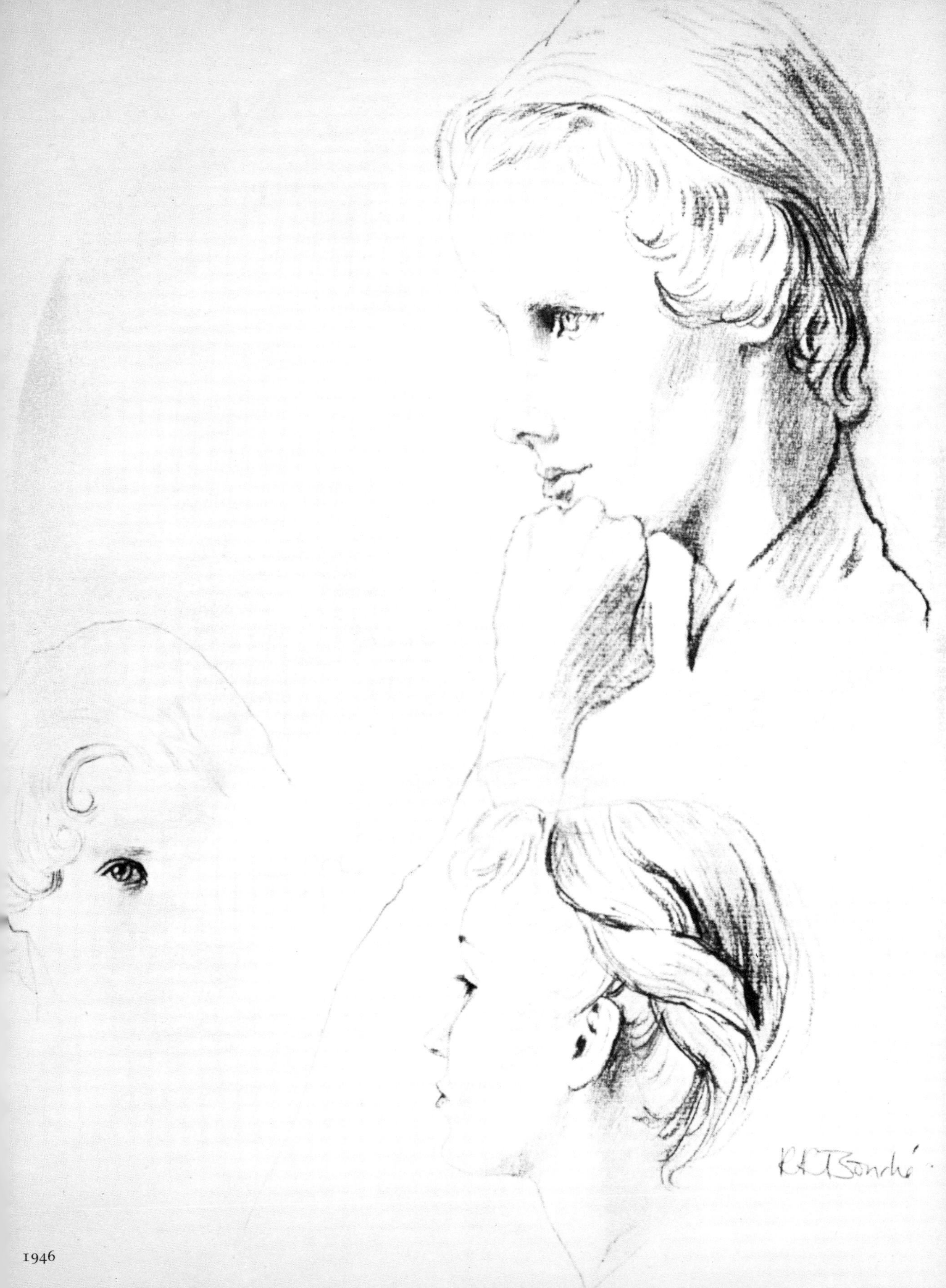

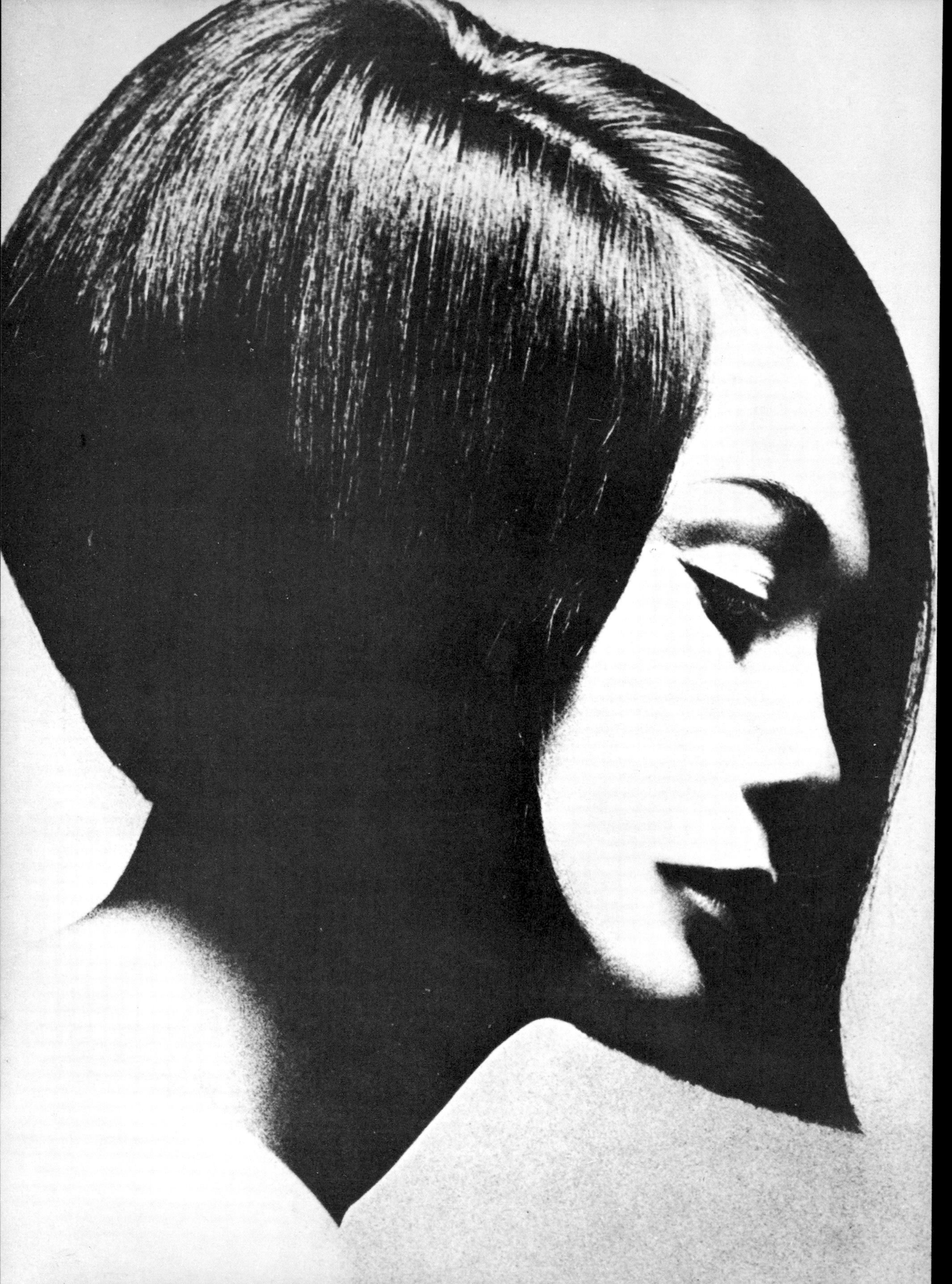

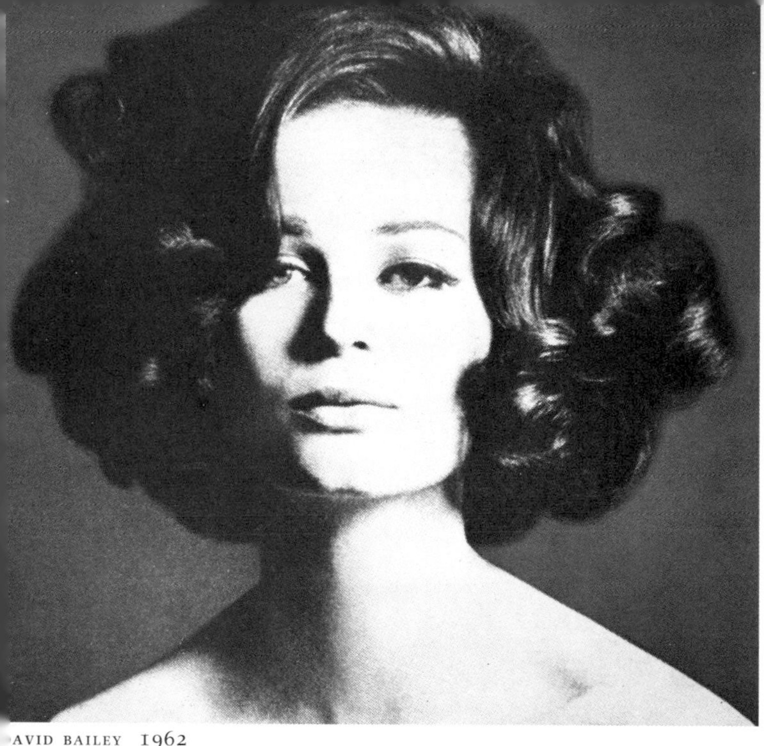

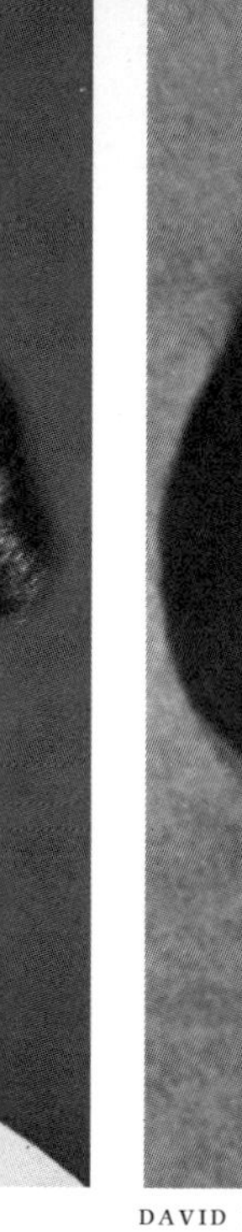

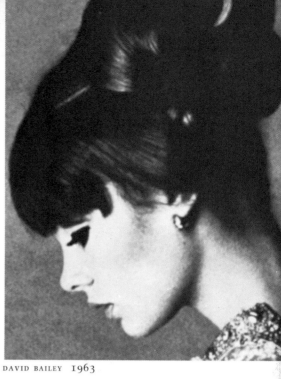

AVID BAILEY 1962

DAVID BAILEY 1963

EOMBRUNO-BODI 1964

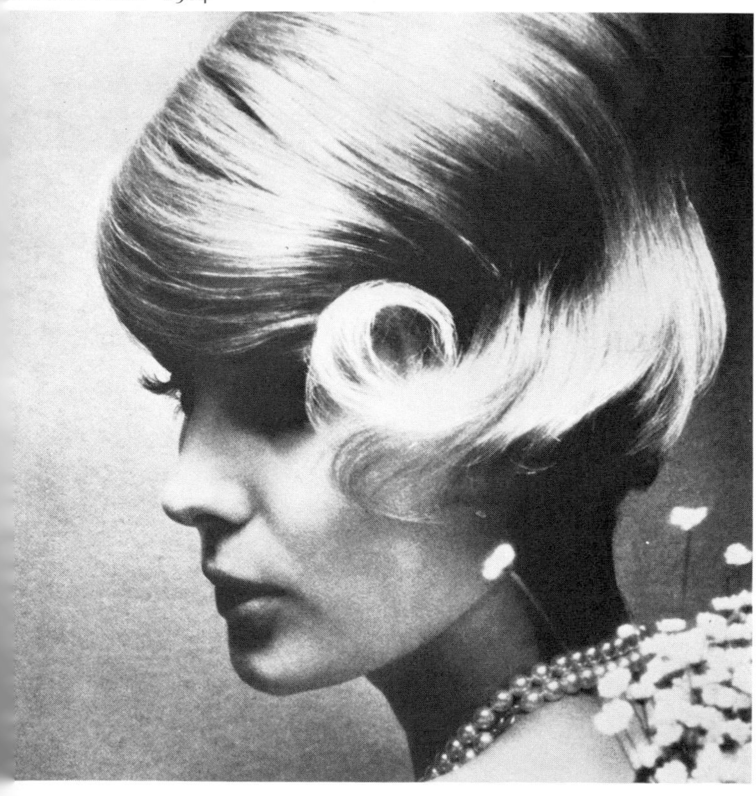

DAVID BAILEY 1964

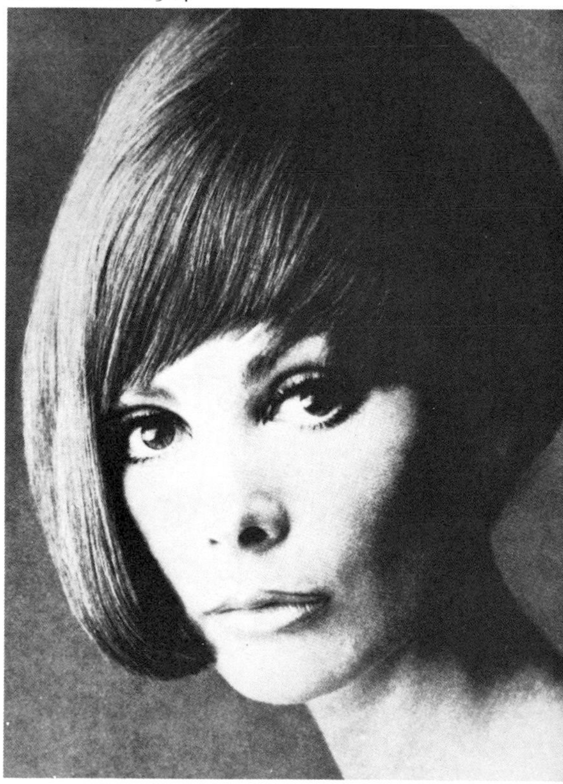

posite: The Vidal Sassoon cut. DONOVAN 1962

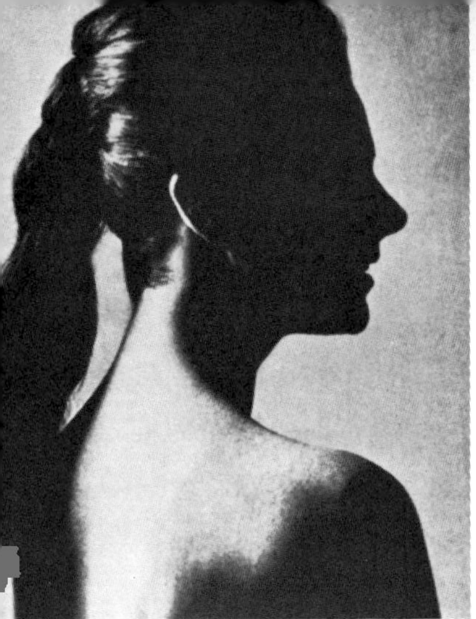

LEOMBRUNO-BODI 1964

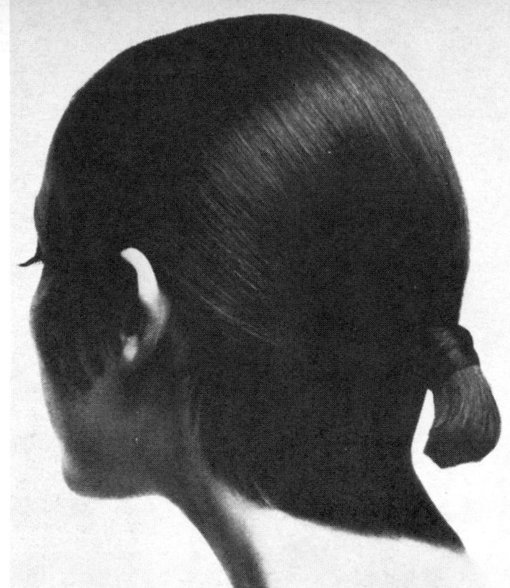

STEPHEN BOBROFF 1968

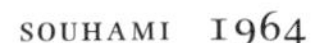

SOUHAMI 1964

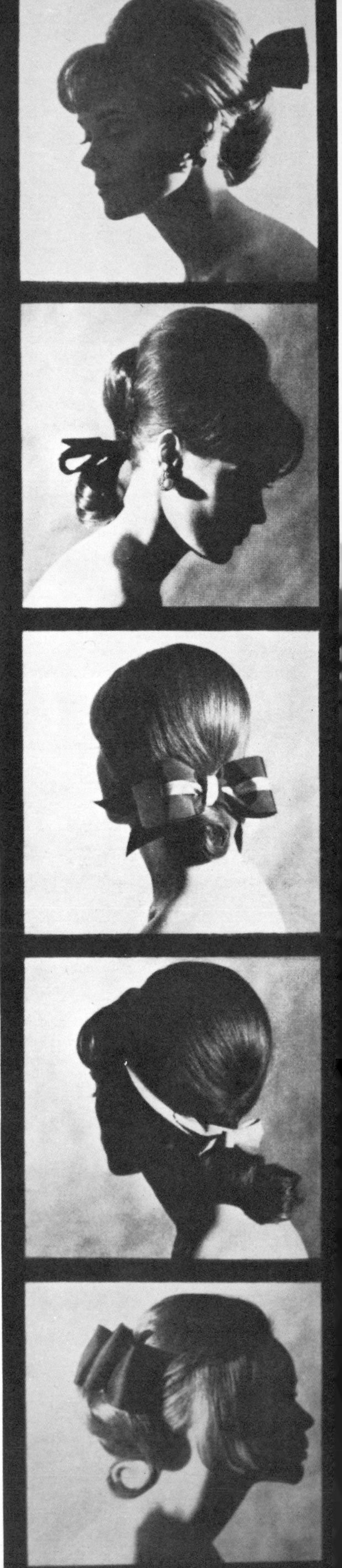

PETER RAND 1964

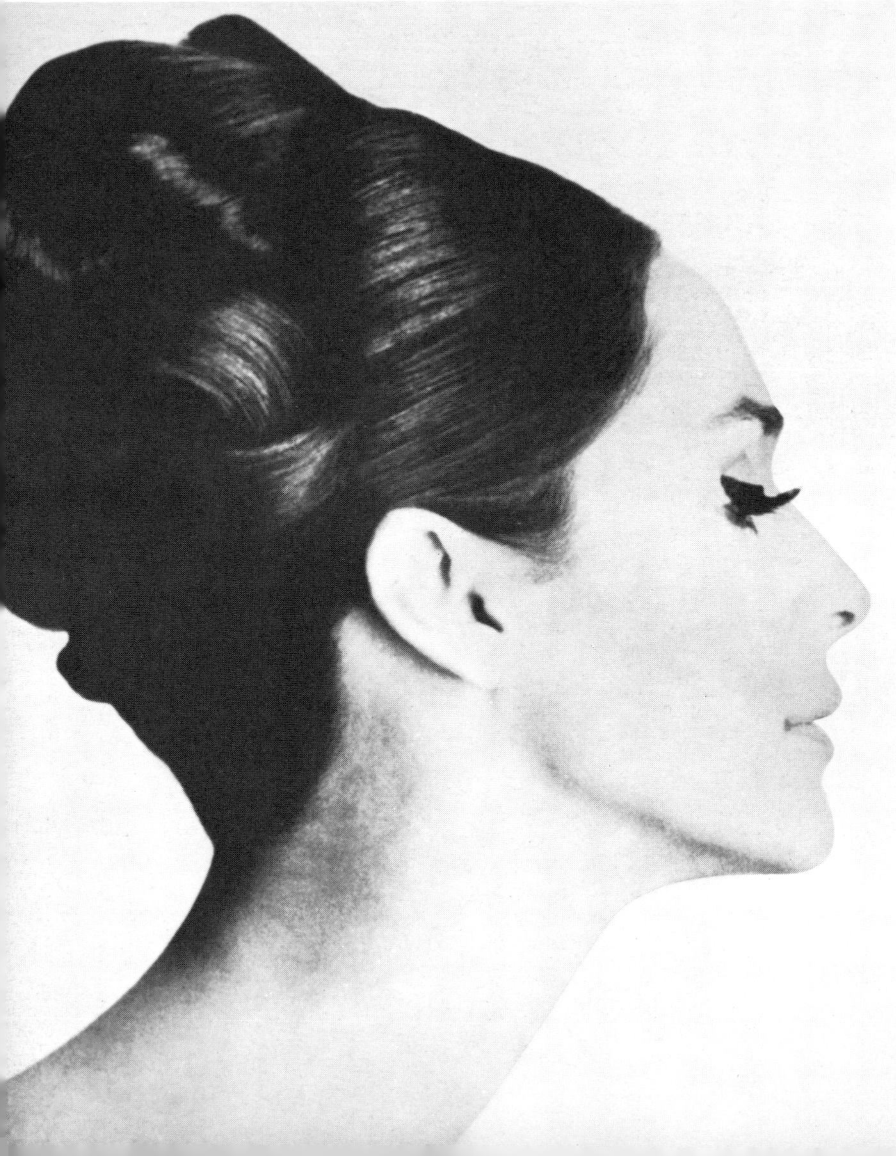

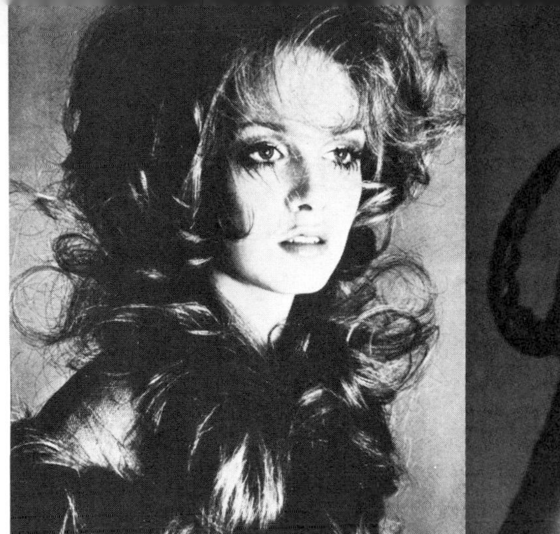

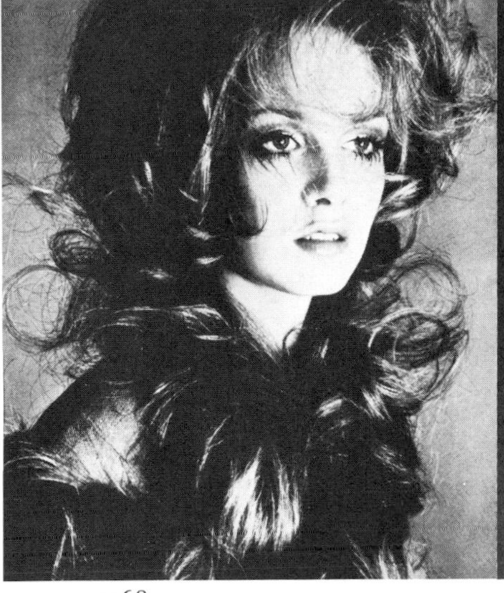

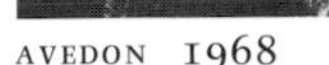

AVEDON 1968

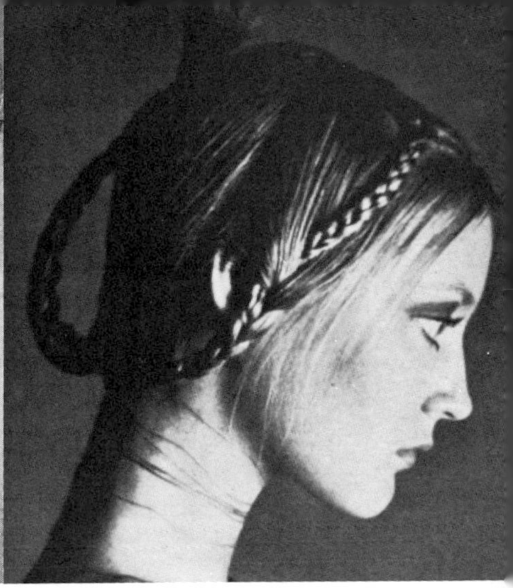

AVEDON 1969

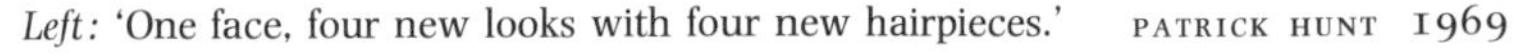

Left: 'One face, four new looks with four new hairpieces.' PATRICK HUNT 1969

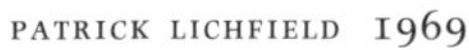

PATRICK LICHFIELD 1969

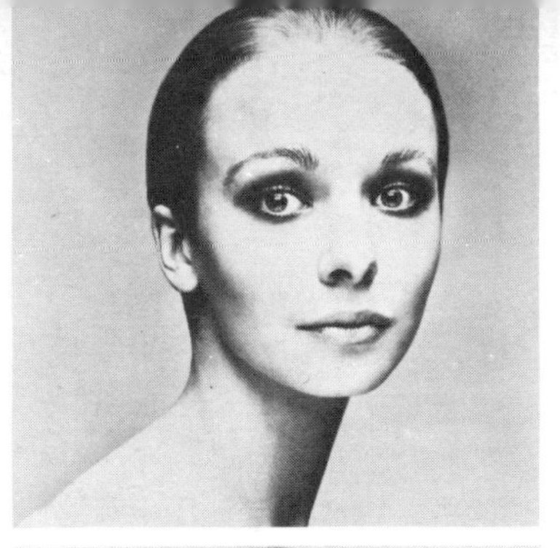

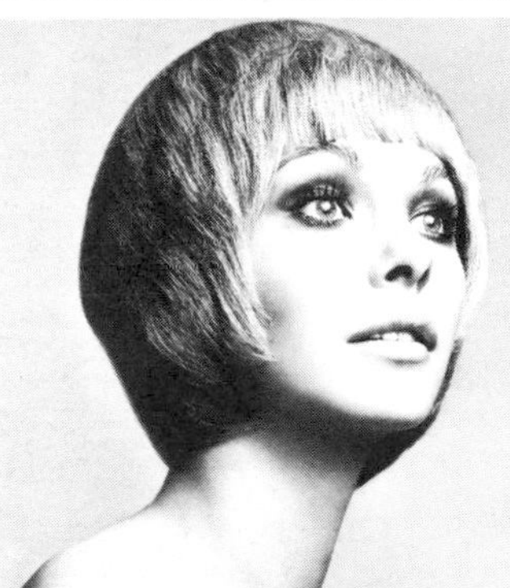

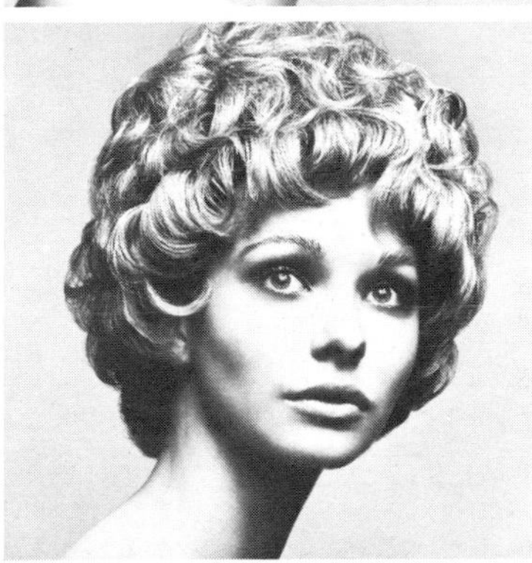

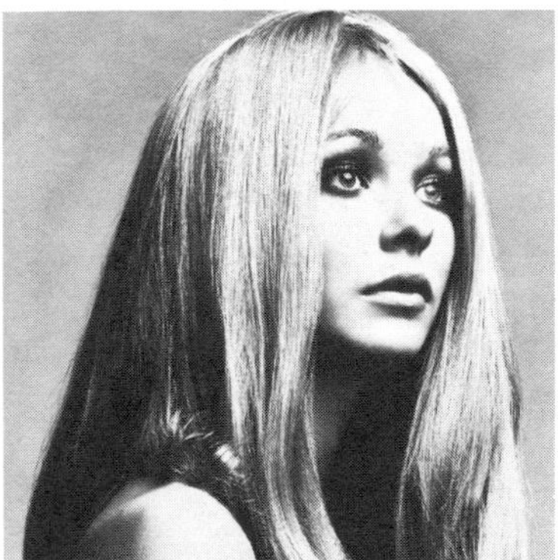

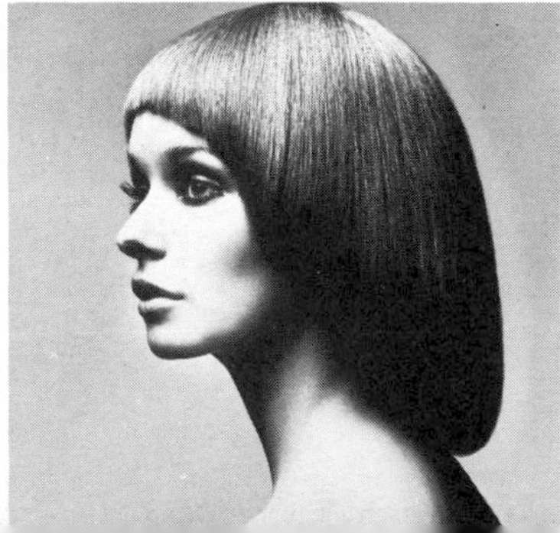

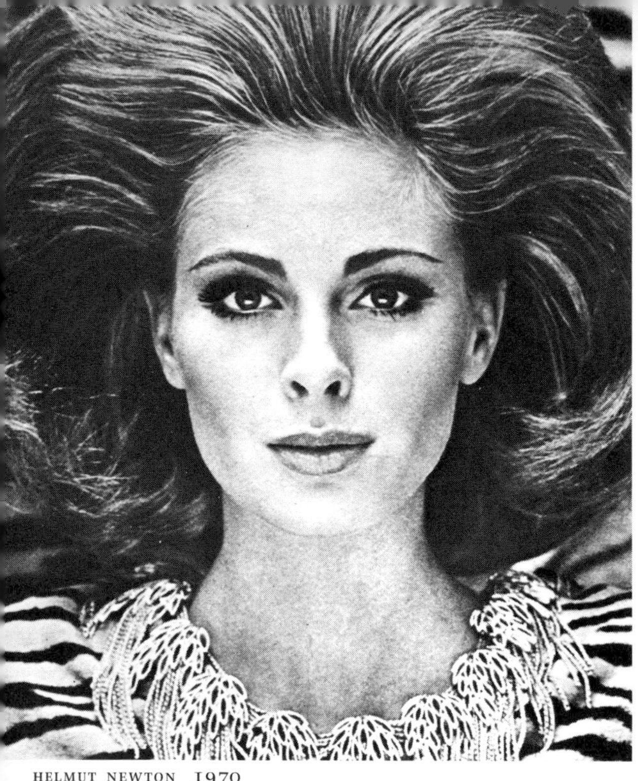

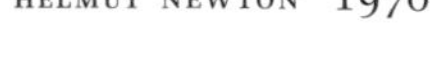

HELMUT NEWTON 1970

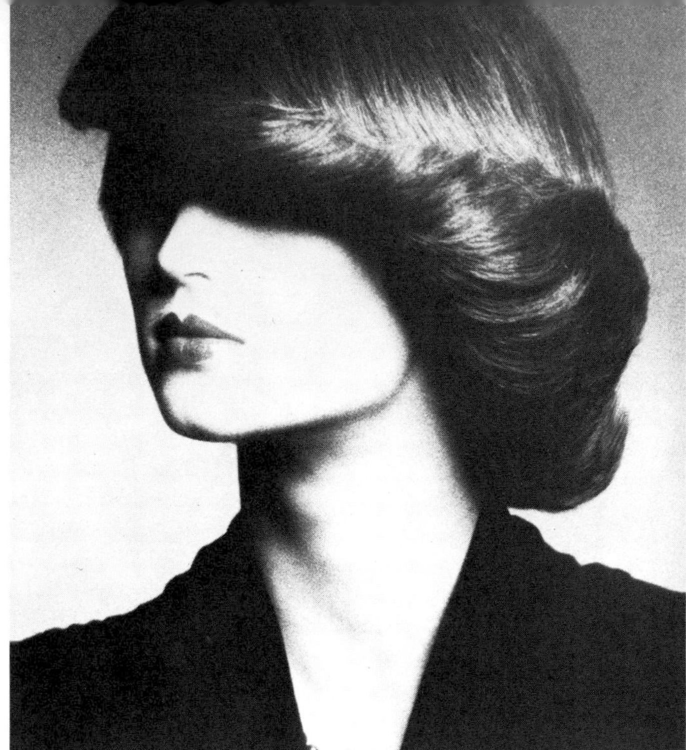

SARAH MOON 1973

Opposite: JOHN SWANNELL 1976

STUART MACLEOD 1975

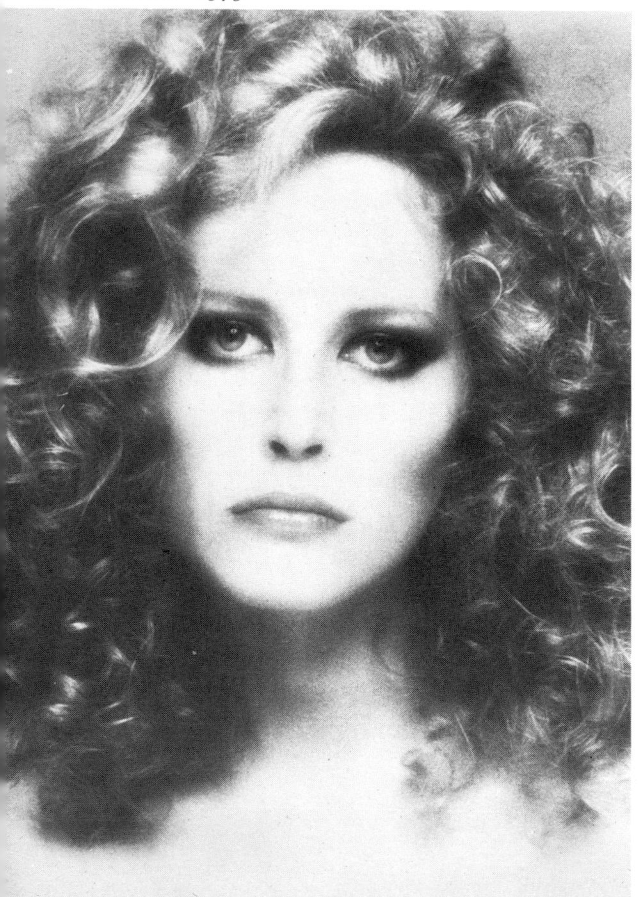

DAVID BAILEY 1976

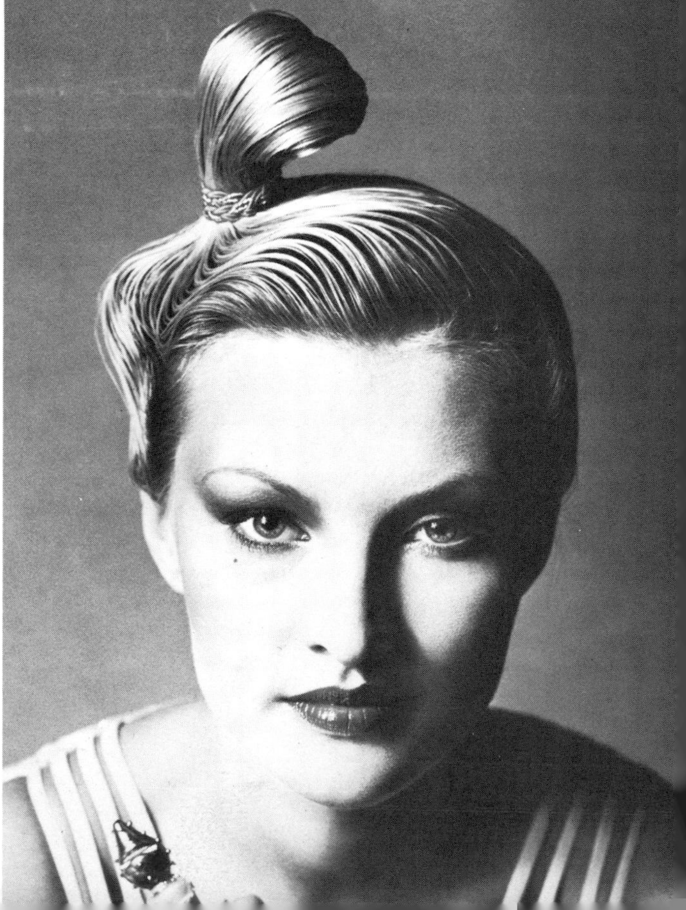

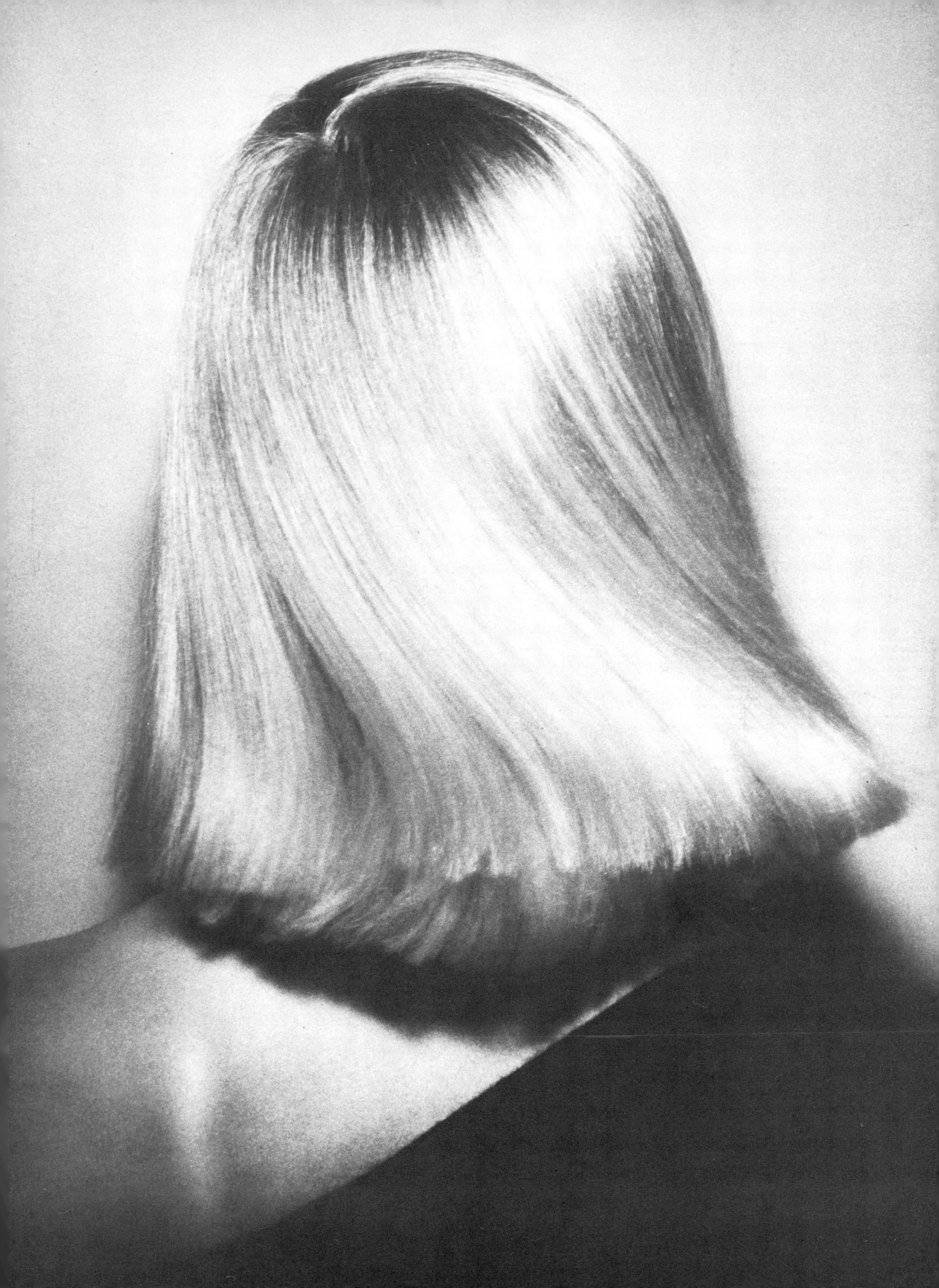

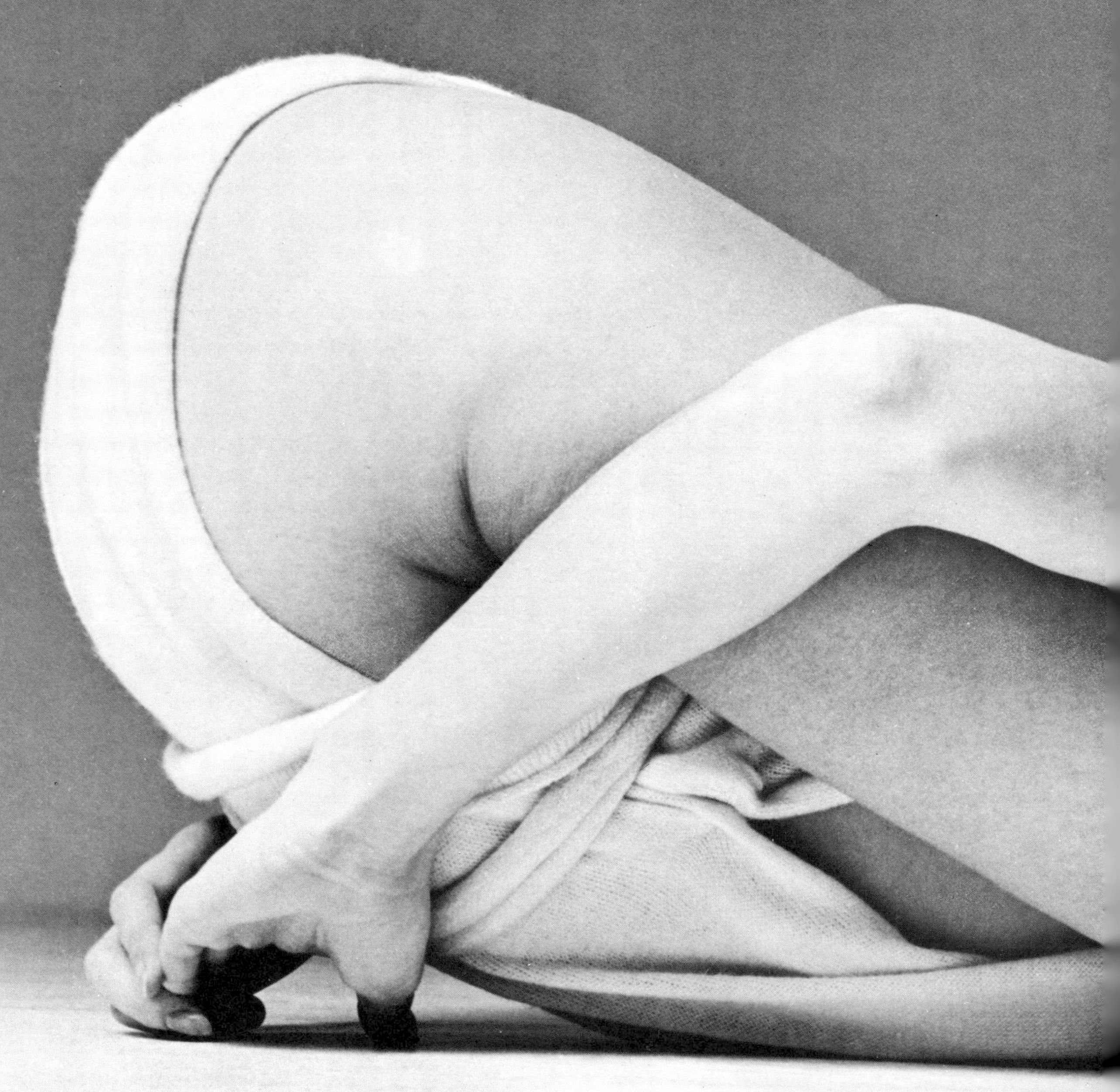

AVEDON

PART III THE SCIENCES

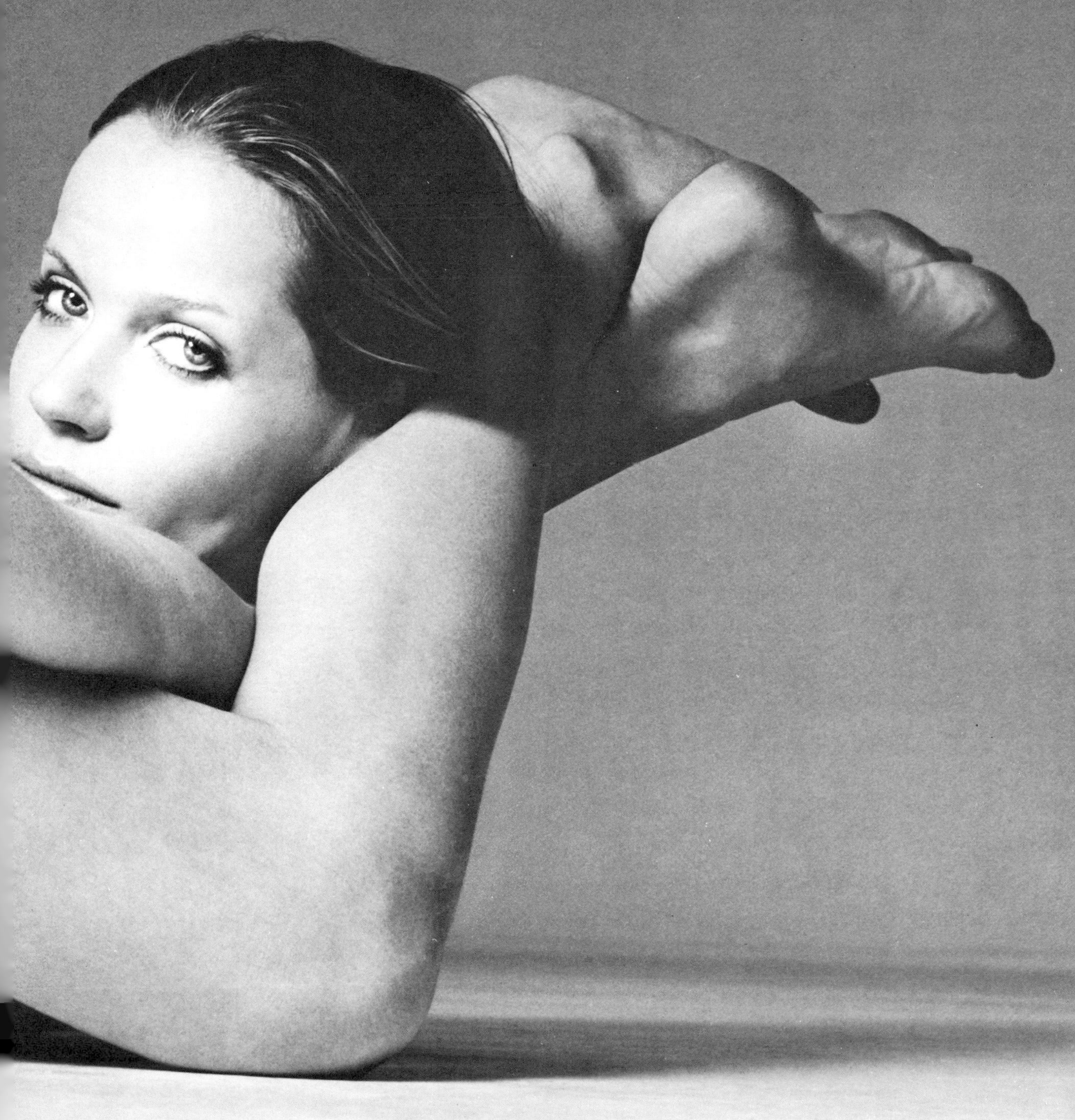

1

NATURAL AIDS

Experiments have shown that the breaking down and building up of cells – the essential body metabolism – is helped by the consumption of plants and their juices. This vegetable matter has an influence on gland activity. Juice and human blood are closely associated in their metabolic function, and roots, barks, foliage, and herbs are restorative in building up health and resistance to disease. They are used in various ways – eaten raw or cooked, infused, distilled, and applied externally.

VEGETABLES

A knowledgeable use of vegetables is a preventive measure, and if some minor trouble should interfere with organic function, certain vegetables can often correct the problem and help restore the body's equilibrium.

Artichoke: Particularly beneficial for the liver; it can purify the blood and act as a diuretic (an increased flow of urine). It can provide protection against urea, cholesterol, arthritis, and certain intestinal viruses. It is bitter when not cooked or as a juice but it is certainly worthwhile taking. Press the juice from stem and leaves, or steep the root in wine. Either liquid will help keep away rheumatism if two or three teaspoons are taken before meals – perhaps in a glass of wine to improve the taste. A tea brewed from the fresh leaves is good for a liver attack.

Asparagus: Can improve a sluggish liver and help diabetes; kidney ailments and bladder stones often benefit. Its tonic properties are said to affect the brain, heightening both mental and emotional faculties, while it has a calming effect on heart ailments and palpitations.

Cabbage: When boiled, it is sometimes difficult for delicate stomachs to digest, so steam it or eat it raw. It can be put through a juicer, and, if lemon is added, makes an appealing and nutritious drink. Valuable for cirrhosis of the liver, especially when caused by alcoholism, and a preventive against arthritis and gout. Cabbage water brewed as a tea with sage is a soothing night cap, and gargle with it for a sore throat. Externally, a hot compress – cabbage leaves, finely chopped and sandwiched between muslin – can relieve various muscular aches and pains, neuralgia, sciatica, and rheumatism. It can be placed on any painful area to help alleviate liver attacks, intestinal pains and period pains. On the head it can reduce a migraine; on the chest and throat it helps colds and asthma. It is a first-aid item; for a burn or insect bite, a crushed cabbage leaf will reduce the pain and facilitate healing. It will help to heal any cuts or sores, lesions, pimples, abscesses, boils, skin eruptions, and superficial infections and swellings.

Celery: Helps to purify the blood, and said to be useful in cases of diabetes, gout, and rheumatism. During a rheumatic attack a small glass of pure celery juice can work wonders. It is a good tonic, produces perspiration and is a diuretic, therefore often included in slimming diets.

Cucumber: Has the ability to get rid of excess fluid and is highly valued for cleansing the body of its toxic matter, and for slimming. The juice, or merely the vegetable cut in fine slices, is soothing for burns and sunburn.

Dandelion: The most superlative diuretic; it purifies the blood by destroying excess acid; it increases the activity of the liver as well as that of the pancreas and spleen. It is beneficial for anaemia, diabetes, skin troubles, gout, and rheumatism. The leaves can be used in a salad; the root makes a good tisane when simmered for not less than half an hour in water; juice pressed from the roots is a tonic for the entire body. The white sap from the stalk can be used to dry out warts, and as an eye wash – one drop in each eye is recommended for minor infections.

Fennel: Soothes the stomach and is a mild laxative. Its principal asset is as an aid to the reproductive system. It helps to regularize menstrual periods, particularly normalizing an insufficient flow. It is said to increase the milk supply of nursing mothers, particularly if boiled with barley. Made as a tisane, it is a fine eye wash.

Garlic: Has become synonymous with good health, vitality and longevity. It contains powerful antibiotic elements, keeps germs at bay, is antiseptic, antibacterial, a laxative, and a diuretic. The smell of garlic puts many people off, but the more you eat, the less it seems to show and it is simple to counteract the odour by chewing fresh parsley or coffee beans. Garlic tonics are old folk lore – here are two: 1) mince a couple of cloves and steep in a glass of white wine for a few days; take a teaspoon on rising every morning. 2) steep chopped garlic in alcohol in the ratio of one part garlic to two of alcohol; allow to steep in warmth, preferably in sunlight, for two weeks; strain; begin by taking two drops in a glass of warm water before lunch or dinner, each successive day increase the dose by one drop until a maximum of twenty-five is added, then reverse the procedure, returning drop by drop to one. It is a tonic that can be taken several times a year, but allow an interval of six weeks between treatments.

Lettuce: Very calming, so much so that as a sedative it can have a hypnotic effect. It should be taken by those suffering from insomnia as a tea (simply boiled), or braised and eaten late in the evening. Better than any sleeping pill, say sufferers.

Onion: This close relative to garlic has much the same powers but to a lesser degree, and they are not lost in cooking. Raw onion is especially recommended for rheumatic patients. It is a good diuretic, acting not only against retention of fluids, but also helping to get rid of urea and sodium and is a particularly good tonic; helpful in combating colds and tonsillitis. A recipe for a tonic onion wine is: 5 oz. (150 g.) grated onion, 3½ oz. (100 g.) honey; mix together and add a quart (1 l.) of good white wine, cover and steep for two weeks; strain; take four teaspoons a day – it may taste strange, but it is very strengthening.

Radish: In small quantities stimulates digestion, but in large doses can produce violent contractions. Good for anaemia. The mucous tissues of the throat and lungs react to its sting, so it can be helpful in cases of respiratory infections. For bronchitis a teaspoon of a mixture of one part radish juice to two parts honey will help clear away phlegm and a sore throat, if taken before every meal and before sleeping. For a hangover: a plate of sliced radishes lightly sprinkled with salt and olive oil. As a poultice it can help aches – if you have rheumatism try it.

Watercress: Good for circulation and the liver; a glass of watercress juice first thing every morning is really bracing. It can help clear the lungs and relieves catarrh and congestion of the bronchi.

HERBS

Our ancestors profited from the secrets of herbal medicine, and now we are simply rediscovering the healing teas, infusions, gargles and poultices that were used to treat the minor illnesses in the family. Certain herbs have certain curative effects, and there are many of them. However, it is not necessary, nor is there usually the time, to become an expert on the subject before you start. Do it gradually, build up your botanical knowledge slowly and surely.

Begin by limiting your selection to familiar herbs, to the garden and field varieties that flourish locally. Garden herbs are aromatic and can be used in cooking as well as for medicine. Field and floral herbs are almost always purely for medicinal purposes.

Herb gathering is an art; not only do you have to know what part of the plant to gather, but the time of day and the time of year for the best results. The best hours are usually in the early morning or late afternoon, as the foliage should be dry but not scorched by the sun. It is useless to gather wet plants, for instead of drying out they are apt to mildew. Roots should be pulled in the spring or autumn when they are most juicy. Stalks are particularly full of goodness in the autumn when the rest of the plant has dried out or become inactive. Leaves are generally picked before the flowers appear, exceptions being the aromatic garden herbs, as their active essences do not diminish during flowering. Flowers are better gathered immediately they appear and certainly before pollination.

When drying herbs be absolutely sure they are put in a dry and airy place: the top of a cupboard, a shelf, a table in the attic. Clean them carefully first; usually leaves and flowers are dirt free, but roots need washing and patting dry. Put the herbs on paper, separate the varieties and turn them from time to time.

If not used in cooking or applied externally in natural form, herbs give off their active elements in water or in alcohol. For healing purposes, water is usually used, alcohol compounds being for external use only. There are two techniques, known as infusion and decoction.

Infusion – made as tea. Basic recipe: 1 oz. (30 g.) of the essential ingredient to a pint (6 dl.) of boiling water. Leaves and flowers should not be boiled, so pour the boiling water over them. The herb should be steeped for a minimum of half an hour and a maximum of 3 hours. For a simple tea, leave the pot or cup covered with a cosy for 10 to 15 minutes depending on the strength you prefer. Use only china, glass, or ceramic pots, stainless steel or unchipped enamel pans – never aluminium or copper. The container must be kept covered during steeping; afterwards strain the liquid into a jar or bottle. A herb can also be infused with milk: cold milk absorbs the essences of most herbs without heat. The general recipe is one tablespoon of the herb to every cup of milk; steep for several hours.

Decoction – simply boiling and usually necessary with seeds, wood, bark or root of a herb. Put 1 oz. (30 g.) into a saucepan with a quart (1 l.) of cold water. Bring to the boil slowly, then simmer until the water has been reduced by about half – this usually takes about half an hour. Keep the lid on during boiling, and use only stainless steel, earthenware or glass containers. Remove from heat, stir well and allow to cool before straining.

GARDEN HERBS

Basil: Soothing, helps calm the nerves. An infusion of basil taken hot at night encourages perspiration and stops a cold in its early stages. It will help relieve menstrual pains and fend off intestinal infections. The leaves can be effective when applied to snake bites and insect stings.

Bay Leaf: Antiseptic qualities, hence its wide use in marination and pickling of food; also stimulates the digestion.

Marjoram (or oregano): An excellent tranquillizer. Good as a tonic and particularly recommended for loss of appetite. Helps cure a headache and hepatitis. People with rheumatism should apply marjoram compresses to the painful areas. For a cold, boil marjoram in water and inhale the vapours. For toothache, drop oil of marjoram on the tooth.

Mint: A very strong antiseptic – even the smell of mint keeps away flies and mosquitoes. Beneficial for the entire digestive system, liver, gall bladder and intestines. Mint can stimulate the heart and the nervous system – it can revive the mind and counteract the enervation of hot weather. Its antiseptic properties make it a good respiratory medicine. At the start of a cold, inhale the vapours from a boiling infusion.

For asthma sufferers and other diseases where shortness of breath is involved, put a few drops of essence of mint in a cup of warm water, mix thoroughly then bottle and tightly cork. When breath becomes strained, a few drops sprinkled on a handkerchief and held to the mouth and nose, will give relief. Mint is a marvellous remedy for headaches – just placing freshly gathered leaves on the forehead can help. Mint tea can help to cure a headache, and if accompanied by stomach aches, as during menstruation, add half a teaspoon of ground ginger and a pinch of bicarbonate of soda before pouring on the water. Also for the head – a warm compress of mint infusion placed on the brow. A drop of essence of mint on the sensitive spot can soothe toothache.

Parsley: One of the easiest herbs to grow and should be used liberally. Apart from being rich in vitamin C, it has stimulating properties and is valuable in all liver ailments, particularly jaundice. It makes a pleasant tea, and is good steeped in warm milk. An infusion helps eye ailments. It is known to relieve gout and rheumatism and this recipe for parsley jelly will help those aches and also purify the blood: wash a large bunch of parsley, press it down firmly in a stainless steel or earthenware pot, cover with water. Bring to the boil then simmer with lid on for two hours. Strain. To each pint (6 dl.) of the liquid add a pound (½ k.) of sugar and the rind of a lemon. Bring to the boil and simmer until it sets.

Rosemary: Can alleviate nervous conditions, quicken the senses, clear the vision and help a weak memory. It is helpful in cases of malfunction of the liver and gall bladder; an infusion is a good mouth wash for gums, bad breath, and a sore throat. A hot tea morning and night is recommended for rheumatism and arthritis and a handful of rosemary boiled for 15 minutes in a quart (1 l.) of water, makes a good poultice for rheumatism. Rosemary wine is a marvellous tonic for the entire system. Steep 1¾ oz. (50 g.) in any Bordeaux for a few days – have a glass with every meal.

Sage: Strong antiseptic properties. Wounds heal rapidly when washed with sage tea and an infusion can be used as a gargle or a vaginal douche. Effective for fevers as it reduces night sweating and will help prevent flu developing. It has a regulating effect on the hormones, so it is considered important for pregnant women and during the menopause. A mild tea is useful for girls during puberty. Above all sage will enrich the blood and tone up the system. An after-dinner drink can be made by steeping 1¾ oz. (50 g.) of sage in a pint (6 dl.) of wine; leave for a week; take a small glass after meals – it is great for the digestion. Sage is well known for its anti-flatulent properties and can counteract any ill effects foods might have, particularly rich and fatty ones. A cup of sage tea is as effective as any pill, and if you are inclined to feel a little sick, add a quarter of a teaspoon of ground ginger; drink boiling hot.

Sage wine is particularly good for those suffering from anaemia and other blood disorders. Make it this way: take half a peck of freshly picked sage leaves, 3 lbs (1·5 k.) seedless raisins, finely chopped, 3 lbs (1·5 k.)

brown sugar; put these ingredients into a large earthenware pot and cover with 8 pints (4 l.) warm water; stir until sugar is dissolved then add $\frac{1}{4}$ oz. (7 g.) yeast. Let it stand for a week, stirring each day. Strain and, when fermentation is completed, bottle.

Thyme: Very strong antibacterial qualities and is a protection against catching colds and flu. Its tonic properties are considerable and it is recommended to sufferers from catarrh or a sore throat. Here's a recipe for a cough medicine: boil 1 tablespoon whole linseed in a quart (1 l.) of water, while boiling pour this over 1 oz. (30 g.) thyme and a finely sliced lemon; sweeten with honey; stir well and strain when cold. The dose is a tablespoonful five or six times a day. Externally it is a dependable disinfectant; cuts and gashes don't fester if washed with an infusion of thyme. It helps rheumatism and arthritis, particularly as an oil essence in a warm bath. Chopped thyme makes a good poultice for rheumatism; warm a mash of it and apply.

FIELD HERBS

At first it is not easy to recognize field herbs. Check in an illustrated guide. The most common for medicinal purposes are:

Borage: One of its more peculiar properties is that it banishes melancholy and comforts a heart saddened with grief; in today's terms, this means depression. Make a borage tea from both flowers and leaves and use for sudden fevers due to measles, scarlet fever, bronchitis or flu. It is rich in calcium and potassium and influences the entire glandular system. The juice of fresh borage is a good purifier, and is claimed to thoroughly revive the kidneys. Seeds and leaves are said to increase mother's milk.

Celandine: Limit this to external use, because it can be poisonous. If you break the stem, an orange juice trickles out, and if you put this on a wart – three or four applications – it will dry out, discolour and finally drop off. It is equally effective against corns and callouses. The sap, diluted with water, can be used as an eye wash against conjunctivitis.

Camomile: An infusion taken in doses of one or two tablespoons three times a day is excellent for most nervous conditions and if added to hot water and drunk before retiring, will induce sleep. It strengthens digestion and is recommended to sufferers of spasmodic coughs due to indigestion. As a lotion it can soothe toothache or neuralgia – make an infusion of equal parts of camomile flowers and poppy heads (altogether about 1 oz. [30 g.]) with a pint (6 dl.) of boiling water. A poultice of camomile is said to prevent gangrene and remove it when present. If you sponge a weak infusion all over the body, it prevents any type of insect from biting you.

Comfrey: A powerful remedy for coughs, sinusitis, lung trouble, asthma, ulceration of the kidneys, stomach or bowels. Boil 1 oz. (30 g.) of crushed root in a pint (6 dl.) of water for 10 minutes, add an equal quantity of milk, simmer for a quarter of an hour. A wineglassful should be taken every 3 hours. An infusion of the leaves is also good, sometimes flavoured with lemon juice to improve the taste. Poultices of muslin or cloth wrung out in a strong infusion relieve the pain of bruises, sprains, and fractures. Poultices of fresh leaves are excellent for ruptures, flesh wounds, burns, and moist ulcers. A poultice can relieve pain in the joints.

Nettle: Contains iron, sulphur, potassium and sodium and is helpful for kidney trouble. A poultice of the green leaves can relieve pain; the boiled leaves applied externally will stop bleeding almost at once. Nettle tea is good for rheumatism and directly affects the circulatory system, helping to arrest haemorrhages, nosebleed and reducing a heavy menstruation. An infusion of the leaves can be used as a gargle for a sore throat, and as a wash for such skin conditions as eczema, acne, and herpes.

Shepherd's Purse: Rather like a cress. The whole plant can be picked and dried, though it can also be put directly through a juicer – in this form it is most beneficial for all disorders of the blood. It can help to check haemorrhages, spitting of blood and nosebleed; it eases excessive menstrual flow of girls during puberty or women at the menopause. Poultices of Shepherd's Purse affect both varicose veins and haemorrhoids.

Yarrow: If the tea is taken freely at the beginning of a cold – preferably mixed with elderberry blossoms and peppermint – it will clear it very quickly. An infusion is a very good douche for leucorrhoea. The juice of the yarrow if applied to a cut will stop bleeding and aid healing.

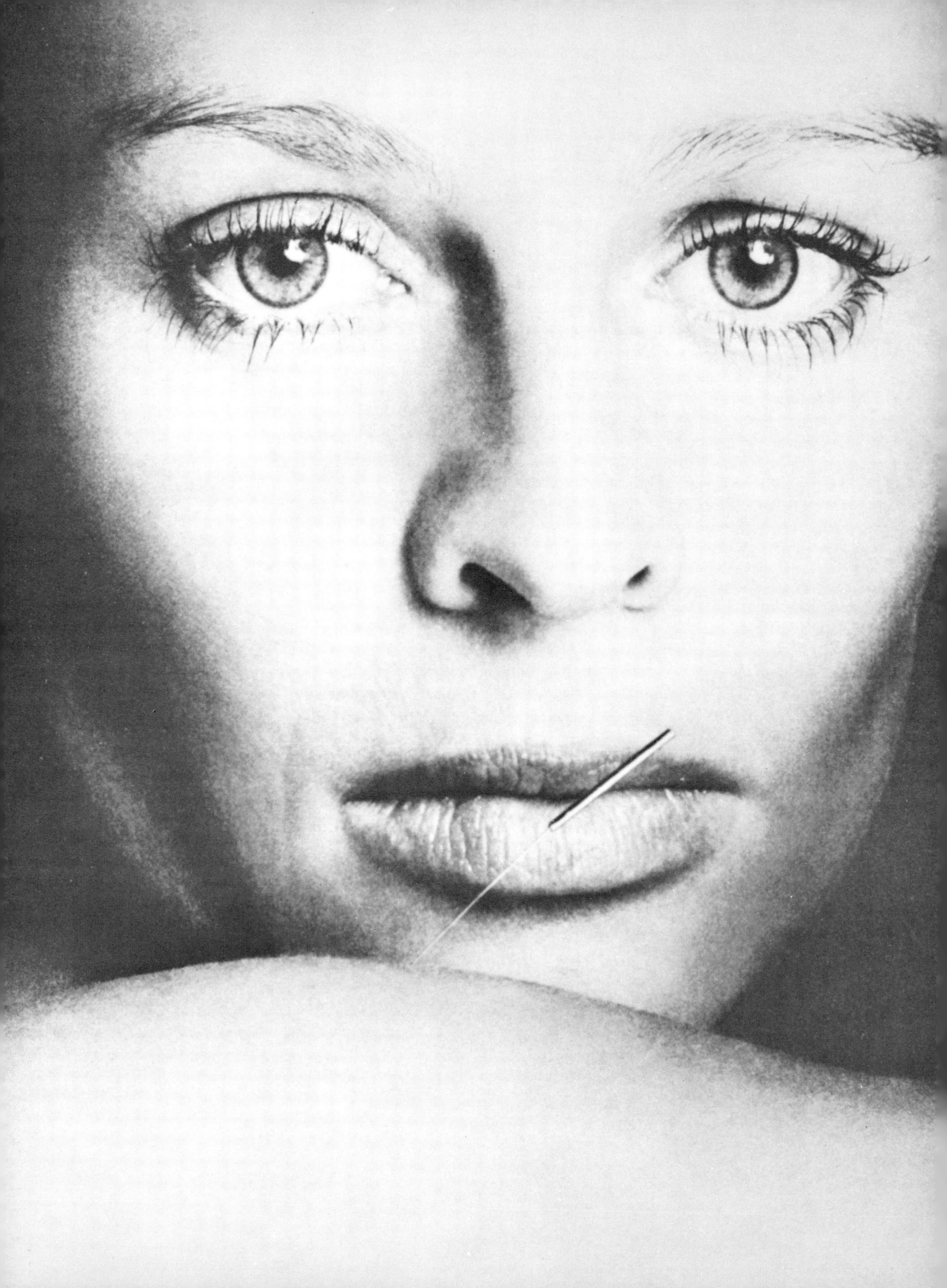

2

ALTERNATIVE MEDICINE

Fundamentally there are two distinctions between orthodox and alternative medicine. Orthodox treatment relies mainly on combating disease with the help of drugs or surgery; unorthodox treatment concentrates on encouraging the body to fight for itself, saying that it is a person's life force that determines the outcome. Orthodox medicine usually isolates a disease or a disorder and treats solely that; alternative practitioners consider the body as a whole, and treat the cause rather than the result.

The life force is a combination of the biological, mental and spiritual will to survive. The mechanism by which it works is little understood and the events that force it into action are varied and often unpredictable. Although the ideas and techniques of the alternative group vary they all rely mainly on this life force, and try to accelerate its action. We have built-in recuperative powers which can be seen at work on such a simple thing as a cut, which quickly heals into a scar, then fades.

Apart from the life force, the life of the person is taken into account. Alternative medicine deals with people, not symptoms. All systems stress the importance of detailed history, not judging by outward signs alone. Rapport between patient and doctor is of prime importance – if there is trust and confidence in a cure, it often works. One of the most effective forces is the power of suggestion. People who become fringe practitioners do so because they are convinced of their beliefs and this is contagious.

AVEDON

Diagnoses of the various disciplines are often quite different and specialized. A herbalist, for example, cannot work from the same type of diagnosis as an orthodox man because his conception of disease is totally different. He does not attempt to find out which germs have attacked the body, but which organs are failing in their function so they no longer can resist. Chiropractors and osteopaths make diagnoses from touch and X-rays, acupuncturists from pulse points.

ACUPUNCTURE

Acupuncture has been the standard form of medical treatment in China and other Eastern countries for 5000 years. To the Chinese the health of the body depends on the action and interaction of the invisible forces of life; their disharmony is revealed by disease, their disappearance by death.

Acupuncture aims to correct imbalance and is based on the belief that the body contains channels through which energy flows. They are called meridians and should not be confused with the physical nervous system though one affects the other. If the body is healthy the life force moves continuously through the meridians. If there is any bodily malfunction, the flow in the relevant meridian will decrease as though 'blocked', thus disturbing the body's equilibrium and causing illness, not necessarily at the place of the disturbed organ. The acupuncturist's skill lies in his ability to free the meridians for an even passage of energy.

This he does by lightly inserting needles of pure gold, silver or copper in the flesh at specific points along the lines of the meridians. The needles penetrate just below the skin and with a good therapist do not hurt at all.

The needle sets up a current of impulses along the line of the meridian which is picked up by the central nervous system, passed to the lower centres of the brain and passed out again to the stricken area. There are nerves in every part of the body controlling body processes and when stimulated some will increase or decrease the flow of digestive juices, the rate of the heart, contraction of blood vessels, secretion of hormones etc. There is little likelihood of the wrong organ being stimulated, as acupuncture is a self-regulating system and it is rare for the stimulation of an acupuncture point to produce a reaction if it is not needed.

The Chinese claim to have proved the presence of meridians by electronic aids and by a specialized form of photography. Choosing the meridian is traditionally done by following carefully detailed charts and by feeling the pulse in a special way and in specific areas.

Diagnoses are done with three fingers and the body is divided into twelve segments, each of which is checked separately.

The needle is not inserted where the pain is. For general work there are 365 points along the twelve meridian lines and it is up to the doctor himself to find the exact point – which is only a bit larger than the point of the needle. This is the factor that establishes the calibre of practitioner. Mastering such a technique cannot be learned from books, it is a combination of a sixth sense and years of experience. Some people are more sensitive and receptive than others, and they sense a small nodule of power at the exact point that needs stimulation.

Unfortunately for Western practitioners, most patients only consider acupuncture as a last resort, having found no relief in orthodox methods. But the particular value of acupuncture is in its preventive capacity. In China patients pay their doctor to keep them well and not when they are sick. Regular check-ups make it easier for symptoms and conditions to be detected and corrected before they are allowed to develop seriously.

The pulse diagnoses enable the acupuncturist to track down illness months, at times even years, before any physical manifestation appears. For such preventive measures it is necessary to check pulses every six months. Treatment at an early stage is said to maintain general health at a higher level, giving a positive feeling of well-being and increased physical and mental energy.

A patient with a disease of several years standing needs about seven treatments to be cured or given maximum relief. Acupuncturists report that some patients notice a response after the first treatment, others feel a difference minutes after the needle has been inserted.

A new development of acupuncture is the way it can be used instead of anaesthetics. Needles are inserted to numb certain areas of the body so that operations can be carried out without pain and without pain-killing drugs. It means less shock for the patients. The same method is successfully used in childbirth.

AROMATHERAPY

Oils and essences were the backbone of Egyptian medicine but aromatherapy as we know it now has only been developed in the last fifty years.

The system consists of massaging an aromatic blend, occasionally specially formulated, into the main nerve points of the body where it infuses cellular matter, acting as a stimulant to restore the body's rhythm. To know your rhythm, and maintain it, is a basic rule in aromatherapy and essential in combating the infiltration of illness. Growing old, say aromatherapists, is but a slowing down of body rhythm.

It is a safe, inoffensive and easy method to accept. It restores the defences of the body and normalizes the dominant functions. It tries to bring to the blood the sweet-smelling elements which aromatherapists believe are necessary to rectify defects.

The regeneration of tissue is seen in the fresher, livelier look of skin after treatment. Acne and eczema can be greatly helped but the capacity to rebuild cells and tissues is demonstrated most clearly when wounds are treated: scars disappear and burns leave no trace. Some orthodox surgeons have worked in cooperation with aromatherapists not only to alleviate scars, but to prepare the skin before an operation to prevent the formation of a raised scar in cases of grafting and plastic surgery. In the same way the skin can be preserved during X-ray treatments. One of the more remarkable results of restoring normal rhythm is the way it stimulates bone reconstruction.

Of particular interest is the effect of fragrance on the psychic and mental state. Scents can cause a state of relaxation, relieving tension and making it easier to dispel traumas. They can make powers of perception clearer and more acute.

Absorption takes place through the skin, so that the volatile elements work their way into the blood and come into contact with the central nervous channels. The temperature at which aromatics are applied is significant. In most cases they should have the same temperature as the skin; then, after the initial massage, a warm damp compress is applied to aid penetration. Application and massage concentrate in the spinal area.

Essential oils comprise organic molecules with free electrons – free to activate beneficially with other molecules. Essential oils are the vital elements of plants. They are extracted from the roots, stalks, leaves, flowers or fruit. The amount of essence varies, and – like wine – vintage essences exist. According to the part of the plant from which they come, the oils have a different composition and fragrance. The age of the plant affects their power. The production of the essential oil is active in young plants, increases up to the time of flowering, but then seems to stop.

The aromatherapist is interested primarily in restoring the natural rhythm of the body so it can help itself at the most efficient level; he prepares the aromatic formula from his knowledge of the physical and mental condition. He may examine reflex zones, use crystallography and blood spectography; personality and emotional patterns are as important as the physical ones.

The mixture is designed to compensate for deficiencies and reduce excesses, i.e. it is a stabilizing force. It will contain essences of various densities and variable times of evaporation. Oils evaporate in the direction of the skin and penetrate it in the order of their fluidity. Heavy resin-bearing scents and dense oils influence the quality of the tissues and the assimilation of food. Essential oils of average tonality influence function, while the very fluid oils seem directly to influence the mind.

The aromatic formula relates absolutely to the individual and might have little beneficial effect on another person. Formulation of individual mixtures is complicated; combined physical and mental conditions have to be taken into consideration. Treatment involves a series of sessions, the number and frequency depending on the diagnosis.

Some of the common essences in the aromatherapist's dispensary are: rose – this has many healing virtues and particular influence on the female sexual organs; it does not stimulate but cleanses and regulates; it also helps cardiac rhythms and blood circulation. Lemon Grass (Indian verbena) – has a preventive quality, a very important ingredient in the care of the skin, claimed to assist in arresting tumours. Palmrosa (Italian geranium) – essence acts on the intestinal flora. Benzoin – helps dispel anxiety. Sandalwood – for renal and cardiac deficiencies.

CHIROPRACTIC

This is an entirely manipulative art based on a particular approach to the spinal column and pelvis in relation to the nervous system and its influence on organic function. The chiropractor believes disease appears in the body because of interference in the nervous system at its main connective centre: the spine. Pressure, strain or tension upon the spinal cord caused by segments of the vertebral column being out of place, however slightly, affect nerve transmission and expression. Minor derangements through an accident or faulty posture can cause nerve inflammation and hinder nerve passage through the small openings of the joints. This results in an unhealthy state of the parts of the body controlled by the nerves in question. The aim of the chiropractor is to find the exact spot of joint and nerve trouble – usually with the help of X-rays – and by skilful manipulative adjustments to properly realign the joint or the spine. The nerves are then once more able to function freely; normal transmission is restored and the body's own resources restore healthy function.

To most people chiropractic is little known and only heard of in cases of 'slipped disc'. It is the link between bone position and nerve channels that is its vital element. Activities of the tissues, organs and limbs are coordinated and regulated by nerve response. Mechanical pressure or irritation of a nerve causes inflammation and, say chiropractors, causes waste and disease of tissues served by that nerve.

It takes only a minor spinal displacement – or subluxation as it is called – to irritate a nerve. Pressure can be caused not only by bone but by muscular contractions and toxins which aggravate sensory nerves.

Chiropractic was founded by Daniel David Palmer in North America at the end of the last century. It was an accidental discovery. He had heard his janitor explaining how he had lost his hearing many years previously after bending over and feeling something 'go' in his back. On examination, Palmer found a vertebra out of place. He adjusted it gradually by manipulation and the janitor recovered his hearing. This remarkable recovery was dismissed as a scientific impossibility, but Palmer decided to pursue the principle behind it. He experimented and developed the technique he named Chiropractic.

Neither drugs nor surgery are used. X-rays are closely studied to find out the extent of the deviations of bone structure. A physical examination of great precision is given to locate lesions. To help endorse findings, chiropractors often use a machine which detects small differences of temperature along the spinal column – on the assumption that it is the inflammation set up by the lesions that registers temperatures.

Practitioners are the first to acknowledge that the success of their treatment often depends on rapport with the patient, and they achieve the best results when their hands take over, and the 'feel' of the patient unconsciously directs manipulation.

There is no fundamental difference between chiropractic and osteopathy. Chiropractors follow Palmer's rule that it is the obstruction of nerve forces that causes illness, while osteopaths assert it is a blocking in the artery that is the contributory factor. Nerves and blood are interlinked and both can be freed to heal through spinal manipulation. The chiropractor uses thrusts or direct techniques that demand precision, high speed and minimum force.

Chiropractors believe that disease is essentially functional – it becomes organic only if the life force is not put back into healing action in time. Apart from headaches, back complaints, disc syndromes and postural defects, chiropractic also helps acne, arthritic complaints, bursitis, mysitis, neuralgia, hypertension, constipation and conditions of the urinary tract. The idea of having spinal manipulation for such diverse ailments may seem odd, but if it is a free flow of nerve power from the spine which enables organs to function it becomes comprehensible and logical.

HERBALISM

Herbalism is believed to have originated about 5,000 years ago in the Far East. It was the mainstay of Roman medicine until the Middle Ages when it lost its original nature-cure character by an infiltration of astrology and magic, though the monks continued to cultivate gardens for the benefit of the sick. The use of herbs continued, too, as the basis of country cures and recipes were handed down from generation to generation. An invaluable guide – still on sale today – was Culpeper's *Complete Herbal*, a translation from the Latin of the herbalists' pharmacopoeia.

Herbalists have never claimed that herbs cure in the same sense as antibiotic treatments. All that the herb or its distilled essence can do is assist the body, stimulate its reactions and strengthen the life force so it may heal itself.

There are about 400 herbs classified into groups which singly or jointly bring about body fortification. A herbalist diagnoses symptoms and uses botanicals directly to influence the function of a particular ailing organ or of organs in need of attention. There are herbs to help every area of the body and they need not necessarily be distilled into medicine to be healing. They can be eaten raw as in the case of vegetables and cooking herbs; they can be applied externally as poultices or emollients to help inflammations and eruptions.

Herbs embrace all botanical matters that can be used for therapeutic purposes – plants, vegetables, fruits and flowers. Herbalists often treat patients whom orthodox doctors have dismissed and many of their cases centre around arthritic and rheumatic conditions, heart ailments, skin complaints, headaches and digestive troubles (see 'Natural Aids', page 281).

HOMOEOPATHY

Homoeopathy is a combination of natural healing and medical science. It embraces the knowledge of orthodoxy but rejects its method of drug prescription. There are three basic elements: the belief that like cures like, the high potency of a microdose and the treatment of the patient rather than the disease. It considers disease as the outward manifestation of the body's struggle to overcome antagonistic forces. Consequently rather than attempting to reduce the disease, it encourages it. The theory is that if you put into the body more of the disease it is exhibiting, then you are encouraging the body's healing mechanism and the natural defences are fortified and supported. What something can cause, it can cure, say homoeopaths, in much the same way that vaccines immunize by stimulating natural resistance to a particular disease.

Great emphasis is placed on diagnosis and history. The physician tries to build up a multi-dimensional picture, based on personality and emotions as well as the medical history of the patient and his or her family.

Remedies are prepared from pure animal, vegetable or mineral sources. They are given in highly diluted doses, easily absorbed by the sick body. What is often deadly in large quantities can be valuable in small. Iodine, for example, added in minute amounts to a diet lacking the essential minimum, is most beneficial – though clearly marked poison.

The system is to put one drop of the actual substance in 99 drops of spirit or water. This is mechanically and violently shaken to produce a distribution of properties. Then one drop is taken from this, further diluted and shaken. The process is repeated many times until the actual amount in solution is infinitesimal. It is claimed that the more diluted the material becomes in the ultimate dose, the greater its effect on the vital force.

Homoeopaths use herbs and botanical medicines. They also use drugs like morphine, cocaine and arsenic – again in highly diluted form so they are no longer poisonous, but beneficially effective. Other curative poisons are: snake venom for blood poisoning, spider poison for angina pectoris, belladonna for scarlet fever.

Homoeopathy was established just over 150 years ago by Samuel Hahnemann, from Saxony. He had trained as an orthodox doctor and had done considerable research in pharmacology. The cruelty and ineffectiveness of medicine at that time forced him to look for another way to help the sick. He believed the patient's life force was usually sufficient to cope with illness, if the doctor could give it some help. He also reasoned that as the patient's life force mattered most, any treatment had to consider the nature of the patient as well as the disease.

He came to the conclusion that illness was a process of purification, a form of cure in itself. His theory of 'like cures like' was revealed to him while testing the effect of quinine on a healthy person – himself. Quinine was used to cure the ague, and to Hahnemann's surprise he discovered that it produced in a healthy body the same kind of feverish symptoms.

He reasoned that it was only by their power to make sick that drugs cured sickness, and that a medicine could only cure such conditions as it produced when tested on a healthy body. If the ague were the body's way of fighting malaria, not malaria's way of fighting the body, a drug which produced the same kind of feverish symptoms could serve as an ally – as did quinine.

It was a whole new approach to disease and he set out to demonstrate the principle, subjecting all drugs he used to intensive 'provings' on healthy people before they were tried out on the sick. His remedies were all single compound substances and most of them have remained in the homoeopathic *materia medica* that is used today. Hahnemann also found that by decreasing the amount used in a dose its effect was not decreased – in fact quite the opposite, even when diluted almost to vanishing point.

Compared with allopathic treatments, homoeopathy does not give a speedy cure. It often seems slow, but the microdoses put the patient on a gradual road to recovery. It is an alternative and complementary method to the orthodox one. Usually homoeopaths are trained first in the traditional way, including surgery; they are not against orthodox treatments but object to the belief in a different drug for every disease.

NATUROPATHY

This is the branch of alternative medicine that is most understood. Awareness of the dangers of body pollution has turned an increasing number of people to naturopathy as an antidote. It is an age-old philosophy which teaches the principles of healthy living and is now part of what is called natural therapeutics. It encompasses many of the marginal theories of medicine, for anything that encourages the natural life force to heal the body comes under the regime of the naturopath. Thus many practitioners are also osteopaths or chiropractors while some hold qualifications in herbal medicine and homoeopathy. The entry of unnatural elements is considered the cause of disease; these could be toxins that upset body chemistry, structural faults or pyschological factors due to stress.

Some of the earliest naturopathic principles are to be found in Hatha Yoga which teaches simple diet, breathing, exercise, mental, emotional and spiritual tranquillity. The main basis for the modern revival was made by Dr Henry Lindhar. He believed that disease is a healing effort of nature and that the suppression of acute illness by drugs, serums or surgery could be the cause of chronic disease in later life.

Naturopathy has two aims: it treats disease and builds up health. It is a practical system of health restoration without the possibility of dangerous side effects – but it is also a way of living which ensures the optimum level of physical, mental and spiritual well-being.

Naturopaths diagnose by methods similar to orthodox ones but include a thorough spinal investigation and a more intensive appraisal of psychological aspects. They classify causes into three groups: chemical – due to faulty eating, drinking, elimination and breathing; structural – misplacements in the spinal column, muscular lesions, incorrect posture, stiff joints; psychological – hampered reactions because of emotion, fear, tension and frustration.

The way to restore the balance of the body through self-healing consists mainly of dietetics, fasting, hydrotherapy and structural adjustment. Structural adjustments can take the form of postural re-education, remedial exercise, osteopathic, chiropractic or neuro-muscular techniques. Rest and tranquillity are very important, so is the therapeutic use of water as in Sitz baths, sprays, massage.

A fundamental naturopathic argument is that for the body to be nourished only with the ingredients it needs, is its best defence mechanism. The first necessity, therefore, is to eat foods which are natural and whole, grown without fertilizers, unrefined and uncontaminated. Pre-cooked foods should be avoided, and all foods should be cooked for as little time as possible. It is not necessary to be on a vegetarian diet, though sometimes flesh-free diets are indicated.

Restoration of health depends to a large extent on a build-up of energy. Far from eating more, this may necessitate eating less, even fasting, to give the body a rest and the opportunity to devote all its energies to the elimination of toxins.

OSTEOPATHY

Osteopaths believe that disease arises from interference with the circulatory system stemming primarily from blockage in the spinal area. The method was founded in the U.S.A. by Dr S. R. Still around 1870. Osteopaths state that wherever blood is circulating normally disease cannot develop – because blood is capable of manufacturing all matter necessary for disease immunity. If blood becomes static it toxifies and illness follows. Osteopathy is the study and practice of certain principles applied to functional and organic disease – those not generally recognized by orthodox practitioners. The basis is that any deviation from normal in structure of bones, joints or soft tissues is capable of affecting the natural organic functions of the body.

These abnormalities are referred to as lesions and are centred on the spinal column. Their detection and removal is said to counteract both physical disability and organic ill health. It may not necessarily be an out-of-line bone that causes trouble; tension and contraction in muscles, overstretching or contracting of ligaments, tightened bands of connective tissue – all can obstruct normal blood flow. Of equal importance is the smooth functioning of the lymphatic system, which Dr Still coupled with blood as comprising the fluids of life.

Osteopathy demonstrates that many illnesses have a relationship to disorders of the spine and can be reversed by manipulating joints back into correct alignment. All Still's original researches emphasize that illness is due to the condition of the whole body and not an isolated outbreak in one part of it. He looked at the symptoms, but did not treat them directly. He traced them back to structural disturbances – the malposition of bones, strains and dislocations which he adjusted by manipulation and allowed the life force to do the rest.

The same method applies today. The theory is that a body cannot function properly unless it is structurally sound, and if the structure is sound then the vital force will take over to help restore health, whatever the disorder. Osteopathy involves the normalizing and adjustment of spinal lesions, the massage of soft tissue, muscles and ligaments. Modern osteopaths work with X-rays to examine the position of the joints, paying special attention to spinal lesions. Past medical history is studied. A method of diagnosing the condition of the blood in certain areas was established by Still and is an important part of the osteopathic assessment: areas of the body are touched to judge the speed, heat and quality of blood palpitating beneath them. It is similar to the pulse diagnosis of the acupuncturist.

Once the cause is removed the conditions set up are said to disappear. Osteopaths know of deficiencies which often cause the loss of muscular tone – bad diet, lack of essential vitamins and minerals – and the consequent falling out of alignment of bones. If such deficiencies are not compensated the body will revert to misalignment. Lesions can be caused by accidents, falls, twists, blows, bad posture, bad diet, prolonged tension.

If an illness has reached the organic stage it may be too late for manipulation to work satisfactorily. Certain arthritic conditions, slipped discs, asthmatic-bronchitic ailments, muscular atrophy, the Parkinson syndrome, pneumonia and some skin diseases can be helped – apart from every form of dislocation.

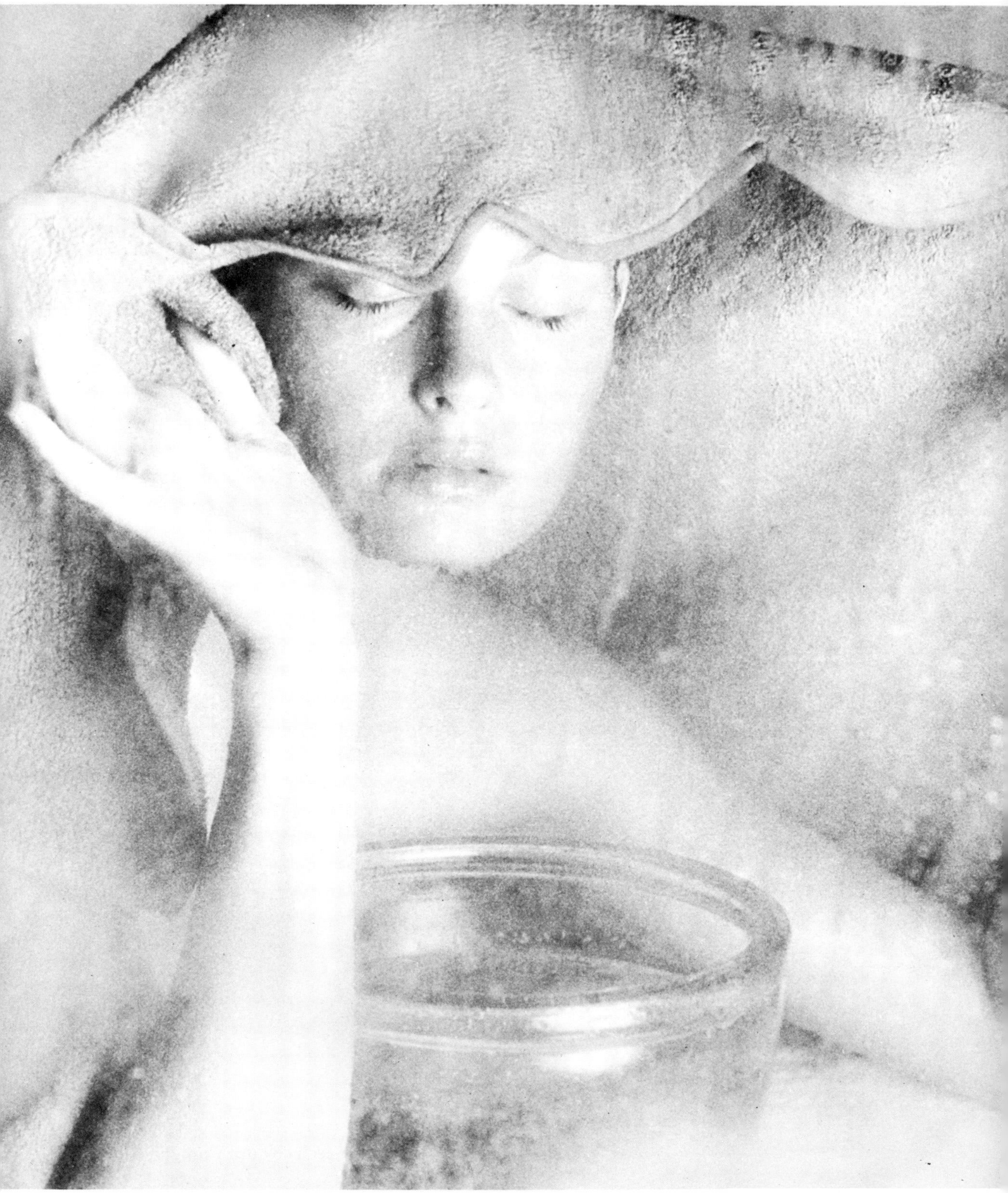

PENATI

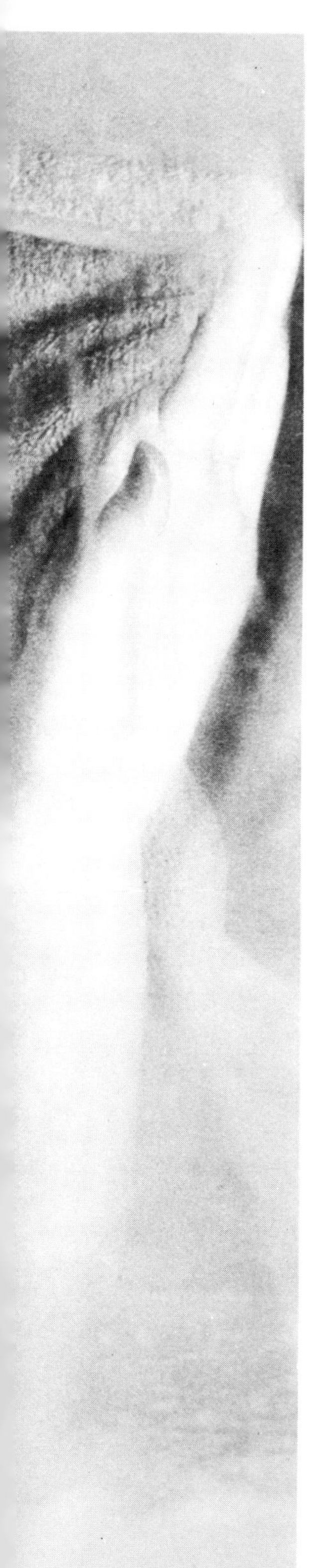

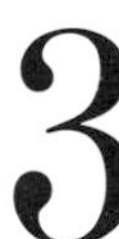

COMMON AILMENTS

Good health depends on many things – establishing regular physical and emotional patterns, coming to terms with hereditary inclinations, being conscious of the 'feel' of your body and being able to detect anything out of order. Most of us are midway between being sick and truly healthy. We are subject to many ailments which have become so common that they are often accepted as inevitable. Most of these common disorders – colds, headaches, backaches, asthma, constipation, high blood pressure, rheumatism – invariably have no one known cause, nor any definite cure. Treatment often falls back on rest, relaxation, warmth and positive thinking.

Listed here are some common complaints, their possible causes, symptoms and treatment.

ABDOMINAL PAIN: The stomach is in the upper left part of the abdominal cavity; the liver is above and to the right, the pancreas, spleen, bladder and intestines are below the stomach, and lower still, tucked away behind the pelvis, are the ovaries, womb and Fallopian tubes; the kidneys are towards the back of the stomach and protected by the last two ribs. Unless you know your body well, it is difficult to locate the pain exactly, though many aches are often caused by indigestion, wind and bowel upsets. If ordinary remedics fail, and if the pain continues for more than twenty-four hours, see a doctor.

ALCOHOLISM: A few years ago only one alcoholic in nine was a woman, now the ratio is one in four in Western countries. They are younger, the majority being under forty. Women are becoming problem drinkers because of boredom, frustration, the social acceptance of women drinking like men, the availability of alcohol. A drinker can be classified as medically alcoholic if she drinks the equivalent of two pints (1 l.) of whisky a day, has amnesia, and loses weight. A warning sign is the feeling that you must have a drink, not just at the end of the day, but early in the morning. Usually alcoholics can drink beyond the limit of others without appearing drunk. Heredity may play a part in problem drinking according to some experts. Others say that a biochemical factor is the influence, while others emphasize that stress and strain drive a person to drink. Whatever the cause, alcoholism is a real illness; it is a progressive disease which, unless arrested by total abstinence, inevitably leads to the deterioration of body and mind.

It takes time and patience to deal with alcoholism and an enormous amount of self discipline and control. One drink is like dynamite, and to abstain from that one drink is not easy. Group therapy seems to work better than any other treatment, and there are Alcoholics Anonymous branches all over the world. Here the drinker finds an atmosphere where there is no criticism, no hostility, only sympathy and understanding. Long-term plans are not even thought of; one day at a time without drinking is the aim.

Drugs can be used which, if followed by drinking within three or four days, make the patient feel extremely ill, with symptoms resembling heart-attack warnings. There is also aversion therapy, where injected emetic drugs make the alcoholic feel sick and vomit at the sight, taste or smell of alcohol. Neither treatment is pleasant, nor always successful.

Abstinence is the only cure. After a drinking bout an alcoholic can feel dreadfully ill for about a week, and it needs maximum courage and encouragement not to take the first few drinks that seem to cure the extended hangover. Unfortunately the compulsion to continue is usually too strong to resist.

ALLERGIES: Allergens or antigens are the medical names for the substances that cause allergic reactions, and they fall into four main groups: inhalants – pollens, grasses, plants, perfumes; ingestants – food and drink; contactants – dust, fabrics, cosmetics; injectants – insect stings and bites, injected medicines. Their effect is inconsistent: you can get a severe reaction to something you have eaten or inhaled for years without any problem. Sometimes the combination of allergens causes the reaction, and it is believed that several of the so-called allergy illnesses – asthma, migraine and eczema – could have emotional associations. In

Opposite and overleaf: Barry Lategan, 1975

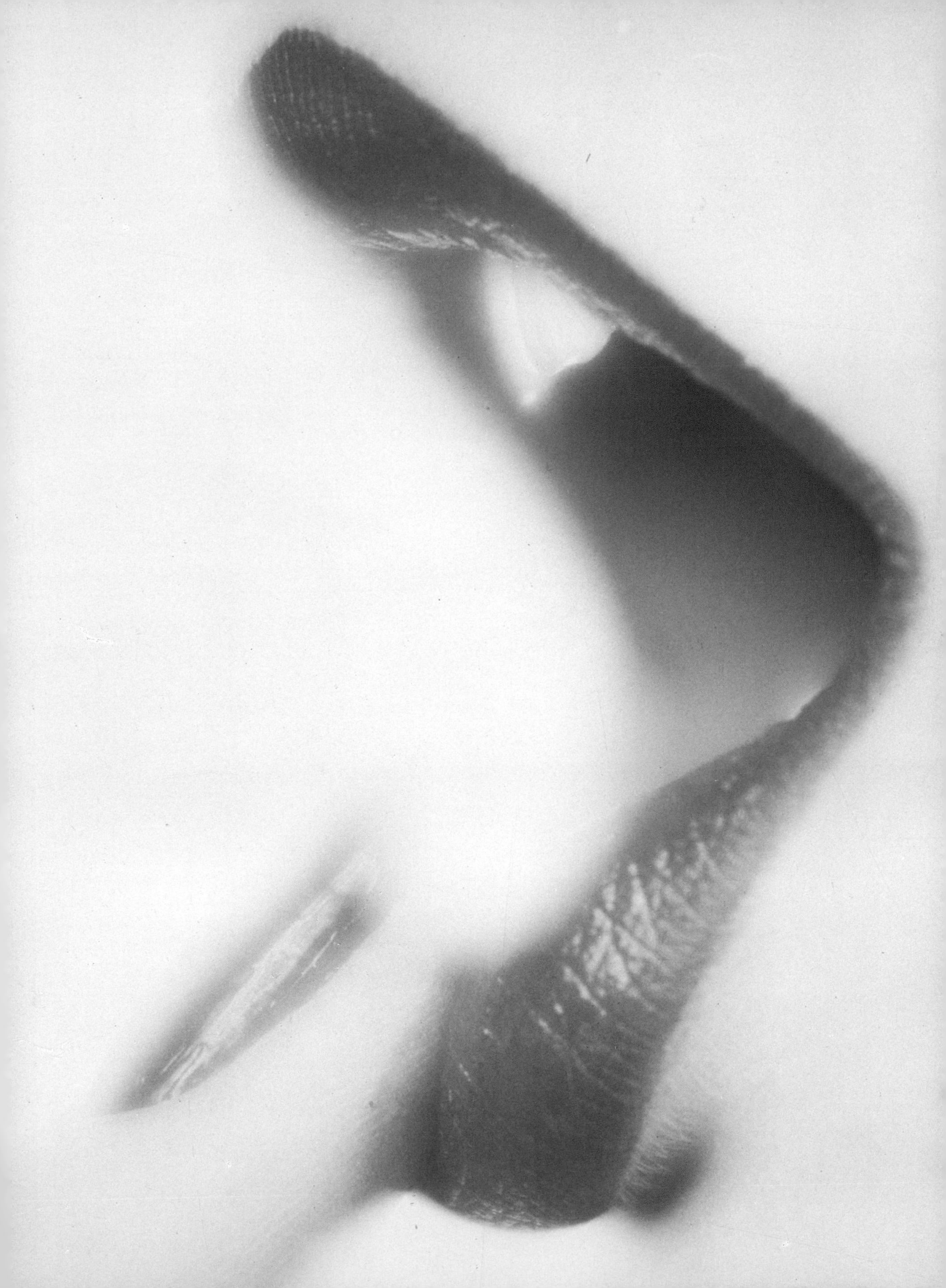

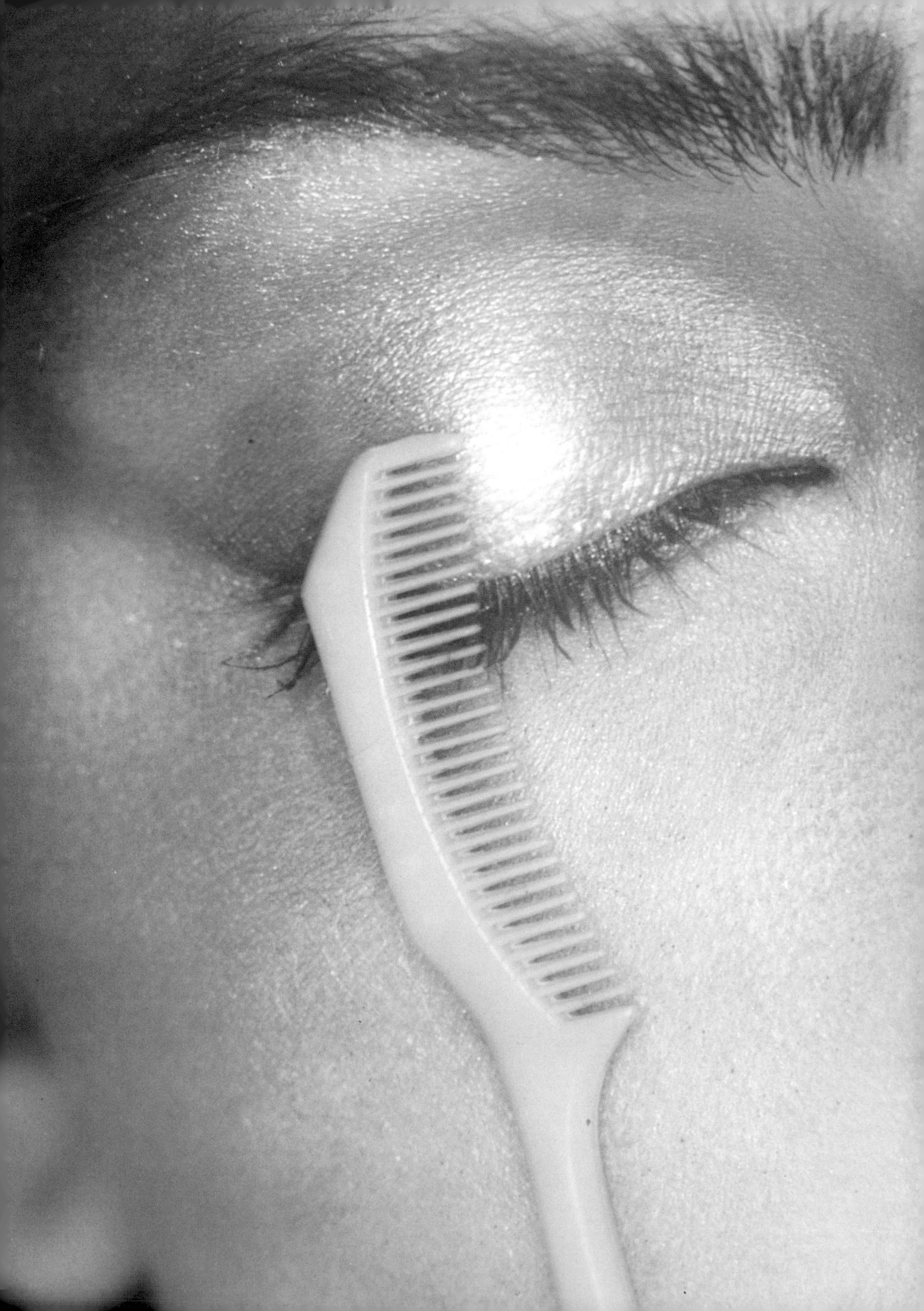

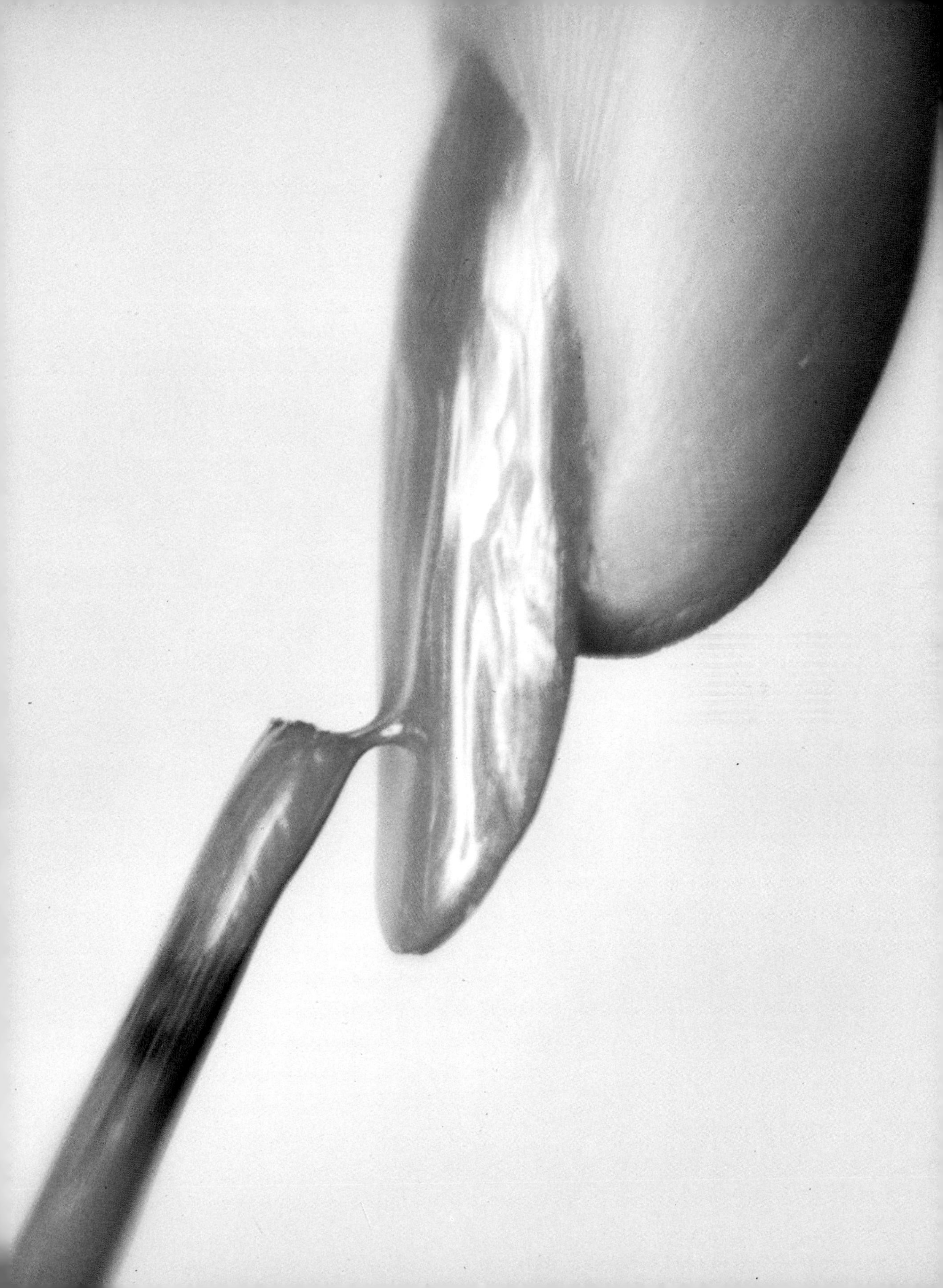

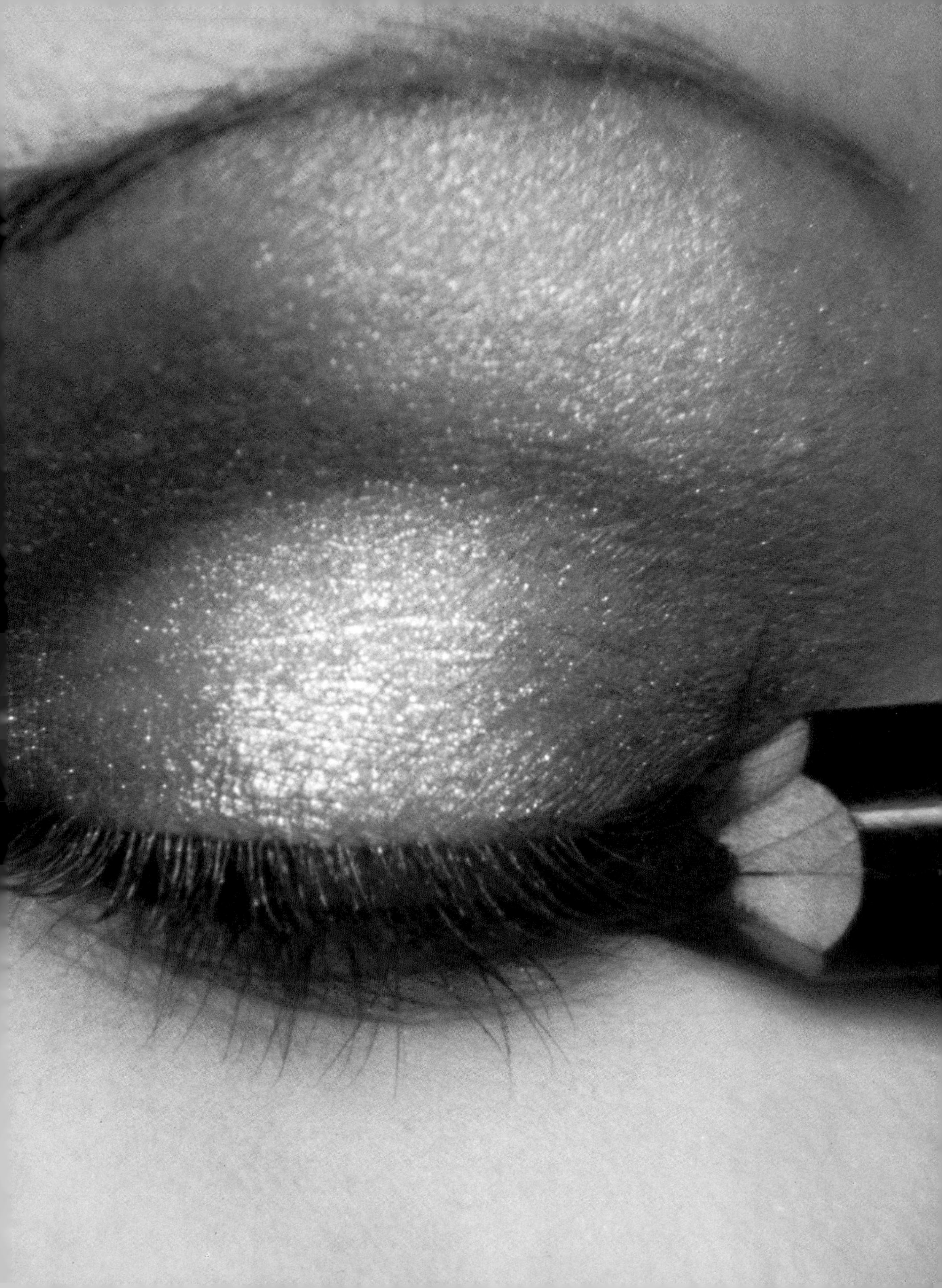

serious conditions, exhaustive tests are often necessary to trace the source.

The most common reaction is hay fever caused by pollen. Small amounts of pollen carried by the wind enter the nose and cause sensitization. Chemical substances in the body react with the pollen to produce the allergic reaction: blood vessels dilate causing red eyes, mucous glands secrete causing a running nose and muscles of the bronchial tubes contract causing wheezing.

During this allergic reaction, histamine is released into the tissues: this is a defence substance against the pollen but also responsible for the distressing outward symptoms. Many hay fever sufferers are put on medication known as antihistamine which stops the symptoms but there is a risk of a degree of sedation.

About one person in six reacts badly to stings from bees and wasps. If you are stung, apply ice to reduce the absorption of poison, removing the sting as carefully as possible. If swelling continues or is severe, check with a doctor or chemist.

Moulds are a common allergy producer. If damp, musty places make you sneeze, it is probably due to mould. Also be wary of aged cheese, wines and beers.

ANAEMIA: This covers a wide range of blood disorders, and is not always indicated by a pale skin. If you get tired easily it may be due to anaemia, so go to your doctor who will probably take blood tests and check the colour of the interior of your eyelids and gums. The most common version is a low haemoglobin count due to lack of iron. It can be caused also by an excessive loss of blood because of a heavy period, after childbirth or an accident. A diet of iron-rich foods is essential; and all the B vitamins should be supplemented, particularly B-12.

ASTHMA: It can begin in childhood and the sufferer may grow out of it, or it can appear in middle age. Its cause is not always known and it may be induced by an emotional upset or by an allergy to pollen, dust or animal fur. It affects the respiratory system: the bronchial tubes narrow due to muscle contraction and the linings of the tubes swell. Attacks cause wheezing and gasping for breath. Medication can reduce the swelling so that breathing becomes easier; in mild cases antihistamines are used, in severe cases drugs of the cortisone family.

BACKACHE: Almost everybody has backache at some time or another. In the majority of cases it is caused by lack of exercise resulting in

Opposite: Barry Lategan, 1975

muscular weakness, stress and strain. The wrong kind of exercise or spurts of excessive exercise often result in a bad back. Overweight, pregnancy, emotional tension and even sexual frustration are other causes. Real diseases are comparatively rare, though biological causes can be malfunctioning kidneys, arthritis, neurological damage or intestinal ailments; inflammation in the uterus and the ligament connecting it with the spine can also cause pain.

A 'slipped disc' is a misnomer as it is not so much a case of slipping as leaking. The rubbery disc covering herniates and some of the jelly-like substance escapes and presses on a sensitive nerve ending. It is the inflammation of the nerve that causes the severe pain. Many so-called slipped discs are often muscular problems. Disc trouble can also develop in the neck resulting in acute pain, stiffness and a frozen shoulder. Neck pain is frequently caused by anxiety and tension.

The causes of backaches are often complex and many people suffer from depression even if the pain is not of psychosomatic origin. It is a vicious circle: backache makes one depressed, one moves and sits in a slumped position, walks slower, aggravating backache and depression.

For all conditions, rest is essential. For low back pain and sciatica, rest in bed is advisable, always on a firm bed or a bedboard, while for the back pain, often called lumbago, heat is a help – preferably from an infra-red lamp or short-wave diathermy at a clinic. In severe cases, traction is helpful and this means hospitalization: the patient is anchored at the hips on a sloping bed so that the spine is stretched and the discs given a chance to readjust themselves. Or a surgical corset can give support to the lower back, a medical collar to the neck. The risk is that if these are worn too long or too often, muscles become even weaker through lack of use.

Treatment by an osteopath or chiropractor can be rewarding as spinal manipulation is the basis of their science. Massage and readjustment of vertebrae and lesions have been known to bring immediate relief.

Surgery for bad backs is very rarely performed and only when all other treatments have failed. One should never have back surgery without very careful consultation, probably with several physicians. Not all operations are entirely successful.

Prevention is the best solution. This includes keeping weight down, sleeping on a hard mattress, exercising smoothly and regularly. Be particularly conscious of posture and never bend forwards so the spine is used as a crane. When picking up something bend the knees to save the back. When sitting, sit well back in the chair so that the small of the back is supported.

To ease back muscles and aches, try these exercises:

1. Stand in a relaxed position, feet slightly apart; tense the buttocks, drawing them inwards and holding tightly for as long as possible; release slowly; tense again.

2. Lie face down with torso on a flat, firm support – a table or desk top; with hipline on the rim of the support, raise legs with knees straight to horizontal position; hold for a few seconds; drop feet to floor. Repeat many times. Turn over, repeat exercise, lying on back.

3. Sexual activity is good exercise and relaxing.

BLOOD PRESSURE: The concern is with high blood pressure, known as hypertension. Low blood pressure with no other abnormal clinical findings is less serious. Hypertension does not hurt and in the early stages produces no symptoms. Most hypertensive people feel fine, relaxed, energetic and generally cheerful. This means that high blood pressure can go undetected for decades, yet if left untreated can damage blood vessels all over the body and be a major cause of heart attacks.

High blood pressure is widespread and only a small number of people are aware they suffer from it. The method of taking blood pressure could be taught in about ten minutes and after practice you can become competent at reading the pressures. Two pressures are recorded, the upper (systolic) and the lower (diastolic) – the latter being the more important as this denotes the pressure in the circulation and strain on the heart muscle. Around 80 is normal, anything over 100 is abnormal. Blood pressure tends to increase with age and there may be occasional rises to abnormal levels which if transient are not significant.

Women tend to suffer more from hypertension than men but they tolerate it better. This means that women with high blood pressure probably can live longer without severe medical complications. There are times when it is important to check blood pressure regularly. First, when you go on the Pill. Second, during pregnancy: if it rises too drastically it can harm both mother and child. Third, at the onset of menopause: women tend to become hypertensive then and researchers believe that the physical and emotional stresses may be the reason, also the reduction of the oestrogen level.

Among the suspected causes are genetic factors, food habits, constant emotional strain. Although tension and anxiety may increase blood pressure temporarily most doctors feel the disease is not primarily psychosomatic. A few patients suffer from some specific disease – such as malfunction of the kidneys – which may be cured by surgery.

In treating hypertension, the aim is gradually to lower the blood pressure to near normal without producing distressing side effects. It is not always possible to do this as sometimes the circulation becomes geared to operating at a higher level and cannot function efficiently at a lower one. Moderate hypertension is treated easily. Keeping weight down is important; smoking is usually forbidden since this puts strain on the heart and alcohol allowed in moderation as this releases nervous tension. A low sodium diet is often prescribed and salt cut to an absolute minimum. Potassium supplements are sometimes necessary. If hypertension is very mild, diet alone may control it, with the possible addition of a diuretic to stimulate the kidneys to eliminate excess fluid.

There are drugs that depress the activities of the sympathetic nervous system but they may have uncomfortable side effects such as temporary fatigue, dizziness, weakness, depression or diarrhoea. These can often be eliminated, as at first it is difficult to judge the correct balance of drugs and dosage to control the disease while minimizing the side effects.

BLOOD SUGAR DISORDERS: There are two irregular conditions to do with blood sugar; one when it is too high (diabetes) and the other when it is too low (hypoglycaemia). They are often interrelated. Anyone who has consistently low blood sugar and no obvious biological problem should watch out for symptoms of diabetes. The diabetic is warned of the effects of hypoglycaemia – an overdose of insulin or an inadequate supply of food after an insulin injection may incite an acute attack of hypoglycaemia that can lead to mental disorientation, coma and even death.

Blood sugar disorders originate in the pancreas where either an over supply of insulin (meaning low blood sugar level) or an under supply of it (diabetes) can prevent the body from using glucose properly. Either condition has side effects – in the kidneys, arteries and, most significantly, the brain. This accounts for the mood swings, anxiety, depression and emotional outbursts that invariably go along with blood sugar disorders.

Tests easily reveal these conditions, which often can be treated by diet alone if detected early. The cause of blood sugar dysfunction is not clear. Heredity may be a factor and in the case of diabetes an overweight person seems more likely to become a victim. Diets too rich in carbohydrates and fats are said to bring on both conditions; also those too rich in sugar. Hypoglycaemia often comes from constantly mistreating the pancreas by skipping meals, excessive smoking, drinking instead of eating and by eating high-carbohydrate snacks in place of nutritious protein meals. Sometimes a weight-reduction regime does not provide adequate nutrition and an irresistible craving for something sweet precipitates a blood disorder. Hypoglycaemia can be cured by diet unless over production of insulin results from a tumour in the pancreas (which would demand surgery) or a liver disease. A diabetic needs to find the correct balance of insulin to be injected, and can then lead a normal and healthy life.

BRONCHITIS: Usually found only in cold, damp climates, very prevalent in industrial areas. It is an inflammation of the mucous membrane of the bronchial tubes and all too often called a chest cold: yet many people die from it every year. In the beginning there is a fever, dry cough and raw feeling behind the breastbone. As the cough progresses, mucus is produced, and if it becomes chronic, shortness of breath occurs. It is not hard to treat, but should not be neglected as there is always the possibility that it will develop into bronchial pneumonia. Also if the cough persists and is more or less permanent, it could be the symptom of a more serious condition such as TB or cancer.

Treatment consists of staying in bed and keeping warm; any vaporization system is recommended. Breathing in the fumes from Friar's Balsam (benzoin) freed in boiling water gives relief. Coughing and spitting up the mucus has to be encouraged, as this is the body's way of getting rid of the infection. Some cough mixtures and homoeopathic remedies help. The old-fashioned remedy of honey and lemon juice not only relieves the bronchial tubes but provides useful vitamins and minerals. Vitamin A is also of value.

COLDS AND 'FLU: A cold involves the upper respiratory tract and may be caused by any one of twenty viruses. A sore throat, running nose and a cough are the usual symptoms, while some viruses produce fever and weakness to become influenza. Vaccines have been developed for some strains of 'flu, particularly the epidemic kind that sweep through whole continents from time to time.

Colds are common and contagious. Why some people catch them and others not is unclear but it is thought to be a combination of biological weakness and psychological receptiveness. You invite colds by behaviour patterns; for instance resistance may have been lowered by poor eating, lack of rest, adverse weather conditions. There is said to be a connection between colds and depression, and although most people say they are depressed because they have colds, it may be vice versa. But catching a 'chill' is only too real and can give way to a more severe cold or 'flu. If the body is not adequately clothed or kept warm, the fighting force is fully occupied, leaving little power to fend off the cold germ.

There is no known cure for colds. Countless commercial remedies relieve the symptoms but do not keep you from catching cold again.

The best way to treat a cold is to let it run its course, making yourself as comfortable as possible. Stay in bed and keep warm; if there is a fever starve it and try not to take fever-suppressing drugs. Encourage perspiration by drinking warm drinks – citrus juices sweetened with honey are the best. Take large doses of vitamin C, 500–1,000 mg every hour. Vitamin C does not suppress a fever but it helps the body to win its own battle over the virus. Even large doses are non-toxic and harmless.

CONSTIPATION: Although it is ideal for the bowels to move smoothly and regularly each day, this is by no means essential to good health. A day or two can be missed without worry and without taking drastic measures. Artificial means of emptying the bowel disturb body chemistry and most doctors feel that a change of diet is better than medicine. A small dose of health salts is considered harmless, but a strong weekly dose is quite wrong; so is the use of mineral oil; either can result in colic, diarrhoea and dehydration. Medical opinion has come around to the old belief that constipation is largely due to a lack of 'roughage', so a diet of high fibre content is advisable – salads, leaves, stalks and skins of vegetables, fruit, wholewheat flours and breads.

CRAMP: Almost everyone gets this at some time – usually at night. It is frequently in the calf muscle and the pain can be extremely severe though often only lasting a few minutes. It is due to the shortening of the muscle fibres at a much higher rate than is usual. It can be caused by loss of salt through sweating, a calcium deficiency or sluggish kidneys. It often occurs during pregnancy. The pain can be relieved by forcibly stretching and massaging the affected muscles. It can sometimes be prevented by taking quinine sulphate tablets or building up calcium levels.

CYSTITIS: This is an inflammation of the bladder from which four out of five women suffer at least once in their lives. Symptoms include low backache, pain when passing water and an increased need to do so, occasionally some blood loss. It is caused primarily by an infection which lives naturally and harmlessly in the bowel but produces cystitis when it gets into the vagina and travels upwards to the bladder. Doctors usually prescribe antibiotics which may clear up the symptoms but attacks may re-occur. Keeping warm and resting in bed will aid a mild attack.

DRUG ADDICTION: A drug can be classified as any substance that has the capacity to produce measurable changes in mental and biochemical processes. There are many – botanical and chemical: some are valuable as medical therapeutics, others merely stimulate the brain and nervous system. The precise reaction within the body remains obscure, but whether beneficial or purely exhilarating most drugs can become addictive. This is a serious matter, for withdrawal symptoms are almost always fearful and can be severe enough to induce fits and finally kill. Even seemingly useful drugs such as barbiturates are able to produce different electrical brain patterns in different people. Many anti-depressant drugs interfere with hormonal metabolism; there is a group of prescriptive drugs that reduce depression, but change the amino-acid metabolism to a point where they may induce fatal results if eaten with cheese.

Addiction means you reach a point when you cannot do without a certain drug – you crave it, you do anything to get it. The mind directs the body to get what it wants and if this means giving up food for a drink, or walking across town to get a drug in the middle of the night, then you are addicted.

It is not advisable to self prescribe any drug. Once in the stomach anything we ingest must pass through the liver which attempts to render it harmless before it can pass into the blood stream. Because it has this capacity, many drug addicts prefer to use veins to get a quicker reaction.

Listed below are some of the more important drugs, their effect, use and addictive possibilities:

Amphetamines: Speed, meth, crystal, crank, dexies, ups, black beauties, 'pep' pills, Christmas trees. Chemical compounds that stimulate the nervous system. In medicine they are used mostly for depression and as an appetite suppressant. Their addictive power is moderate but an overdose can be fatal. They can produce high blood pressure and psychosis.

Barbiturates: Goofers, goof balls, downers, red devils, yellow jackets, yellow birds. Chemical compounds used as a depressant for the central nervous system, therefore given as a treatment for insomnia and as a sedative. Moderate to severe addictive possibilities, and an overdose can result in death. Especially dangerous in conjunction with alcohol.

Cocaine: Coke or snow. Increasing in popularity, for at first it gives quite pleasant perceptive side effects. When natural, it comes from the leaves of the coca bush found in Peru and Bolivia but can be synthetically produced. Stimulates the nervous system and can be used as a local anaesthetic. Addiction danger, plus a tendency to violence.

Hashish: Hash. The resin from the flower of the hemp plant and a more concentrated form of marijuana's active ingredient. Powers of perception are affected.

Heroin: H, horse, junk, skag. A derivative of the opium poppy. Acts as a depressant to the central nervous system and as a respiratory sedative. Opiates of the same botanical gender, such as morphine, are used as pain killers. Great danger of addiction.

LSD: Acid. Its compound has the complicated name of lysergic acid diethylamide. It produces intense hallucinations, changes perception of environment to a degree where faulty judgement of habitual surroundings can cause death. No known medical use. Dangers are psychosis and bad trips, suspected genetic damage.

Marijuana: Pot, weed, broccoli, grass, hemp tea, boo, mary jane. Comes from the female leaves of the hemp plant and alters perception of reality. Considered reasonably mild with possible dangers of psychological habituation, but rare psychosis.

Tranquillizers: Influence the emotional brain by calming it but do not affect the cortex where thinking, judgement and preservation instincts reside. Used medically to relieve emotional upsets and help insomnia by removing anxiety. Addiction to tranquillizers is rare, but the danger is combining them with alcohol; this can prove fatal, particularly in the case of excess of either.

DYSMENORRHOEA: The medical term for painful periods (see page 104).

FLUID RETENTION: This can cause bloating of the tissues, which is not only responsible for a degree of overweight but is the main reason for the formation of cellulite. It can be due to excessive salt in the diet, an underactive kidney or to a congenital defect. It can be helped biologically. First, keep salt to a minimum. Second, drink at least four glasses of water a day: this helps the elimination of salt and other minerals that require water in order to leave the body; a diuretic mineral water is of additional value. Anyone who drinks a fair amount of liquid other than water – even tea – is subject to fluid retention. It is more obvious in heavy drinkers.

HAEMORRHOIDS: Known as piles they can be agonizing, and are varicose veins of the anus – and like varicose veins are often hereditary. As soon as it becomes painful to evacuate or you notice blood, get medical advice: they sometimes occur as a secondary symptom of another disorder – such as a growth or liver disease – and should never be self-analysed and thought of as 'just piles'. The earlier they are treated, the better. In the initial stages, it may only be necessary to use ointments, suppositories or injections. If they continue to develop, surgery usually has to be used. This is not as painful as some people believe, though the first few bowel actions after the operation may be difficult. The veins that are clotting and bleeding are tied off or cut away. There is an alternative, a technique called cryosurgery – here piles are removed by freezing and this does not necessitate hospitalization. Another method which some doctors claim is as effective as surgery is this: the anus is dilated and the patient shown how to repeat the stretching process at regular intervals over a period of six weeks together with the use of a special laxative.

HEADACHE: Probably the most common type of pain in the body with causes ranging from a hangover to eye strain, from tension or too much sun to a brain tumour. Headaches can be divided into three types: vascular – includes migraine and cluster headaches; organical – from infections, tumours, eye and ear problems, nose and focal disorders; psychogenic – caused by tension, anxiety and depression. The clinical explanation is this: blood vessels in the head increase in size, and as these arteries are usually accompanied by nerves, when enlarged they press on the nerves and cause pain. Migraine starts this way and the warning signs of worse to come are visual disturbances and a general feeling of perception weakness. The blood vessels not only increase in size, but thicken and possibly release a fluid. At this stage, the pain is steady and agonizing and in extreme cases can continue for days.

What starts this activity is unclear. Heredity plays a part particularly in the case of migraine. Emotional strain and stress are possibly contributory causes; also food and allergies. For example, a chemical called tyramine that is found in some foods and drinks has been known to start headaches. It occurs naturally in cheese, chocolate, chicken livers, brown vinegar, yoghurt and most fermented food. Drinks with tyramine are beer, red wine, whisky, gin and vodka which may explain the typical hangover headache. A fast way to reduce such a headache is to take teaspoons of honey, slowly, one after the other – and as many as you like.

Headaches can be caused by low blood sugar, which is nothing more serious than bad eating habits. Many a headache has been cured by a good meal – protein, green vegetables, olive oil and garlic are recommended. Tension headaches are milder forms of the psychogenic variety and usually caused by fatigue and temporary stress. The more severe psychogenic ones usually require thorough tests and life-history research.

Cluster headaches are a form of migraine, but instead of being long and sustained, they manifest themselves in short violent attacks. They are considered the same as migraine when being treated. The migraine-prone person is usually highly intelligent, ambitious, creative and with a strong drive for perfection. Often the headache arrives after completion of an arduous task – musicians, writers, actors, may find themselves stricken once their creative work has been accomplished.

A change of weather is said to induce headaches – before a thunderstorm or a particularly strong wind the barometer drops sharply and weather-sensitive people develop severe headaches. This is because the atmosphere is positively charged. When the storm is over the air molecules become negatively charged and bring relief to the sufferer.

Most people rely on aspirins and their like to relieve headaches. Migraines respond unpredictably to treatment. Most relief drugs are based on ergot but they can have side effects. The heavier, habit-forming painkillers such as morphine should be avoided. A redirection of blood often helps; moving hands to make them warmer can lessen dilation of cranial blood vessels. Try lying on your side with the weight of your head resting on a thumb placed at the centre base of the skull (between the two muscle tendons); just a few seconds of pressure on each side can relax and relieve the headache. Acupuncture and spinal manipulation are considered helpful.

HEPATITIS: From time to time this disease can reach epidemic proportions. It is extremely contagious and also carried by persons who have no sign of it. Initially the virus is picked up in food, such as shell fish, that has become contaminated. There are two types of hepatitis – infectious and serum. Though caused by different viruses, they are both called viral hepatitis. One significant difference is the period of incubation. Infectious hepatitis (once known as epidemic jaundice) takes between 15–40 days to appear and serum hepatitis between 60–100 days.

Infectious hepatitis is easily transmitted by the faecal-oral route. Therefore it can spread quite rapidly within a family, school or an office. Isolated cases can appear. Children frequently get the disease but so mildly that it is not diagnosed as such – but it is equally contagious.

Serum hepatitis can be carried in adults as well and herein lies its epidemic danger. Healthy carriers can be detected by certain tests, but few healthy people take them. In northern Europe and north America carriers compose about 1% of apparently healthy people, but the number is much higher in tropical, Eastern and some Mediterranean countries.

One of the early symptoms of hepatitis is depression. Often there is sweating for no apparent reason – of the palms, the face. Usually there is inflammation of the liver, and it is frequently possible to feel it, somewhat enlarged and tender. Loss of appetite and nausea are often signs. Not all patients go yellow. It is essential to have a blood test.

There is no effective treatment for hepatitis. It can cause a day or so of discomfort or necessitate months in hospital. Rest and relaxation in bed is essential. Alcohol is forbidden, not only during, but for a long time after, an attack. This is because the liver cannot break down alcohol with its usual efficiency. Rich and fatty foods should be avoided.

HERPES: There is one strain of herpes that is closely linked with chicken pox and shingles, but the other one is the common annoyance that frequently crops up in connection with colds – this is the Herpes Simplex. It begins as a small area of irritation around the mouth or just inside the nose and generally makes its appearance towards the end of an ordinary cold, sore throat or chest infection. It can become very painful and raised, then forms a blister. This can take from forty-eight to seventy-two hours. Frequently the blisters burst and a watery fluid is emitted. The affected area usually crusts over and heals within two weeks. Sometimes the sores become re-infected and need treatment with an antibiotic ointment. Once a person is subject to a herpes infection it is frequently re-activated when another cold virus enters the system.

HYPERIDROSIS: Excessive sweating which cannot be controlled by anti-perspirants. It can be helped by surgery.

In the case of the underarm area, two to three days are generally required in hospital. The area of trouble can be as large as 3 inches (75 mm.) by 2 inches (50 mm.); the skin is excised and stitched. There is a scar, but in such an area it is of little significance. The operation for treating the hands and feet is more complicated and could mean up to 10 days in hospital. It involves removing the part of the sympathetic nerve chain that supplies the affected area. For the hands, the procedure is either through an incision on the side of the chest underneath the arm, or above the collar bone. For the feet, an incision is made in the abdomen at the level of the navel.

INSOMNIA: The word really means total inability to sleep, but this is virtually non-existent as a medical condition. People who say they can't sleep at all, usually do to some degree, but believe they lay awake night after night without closing their eyes. There are two main causes – anxiety, depression and psychological disorders of all sorts, and pain or discomfort.

Doctors usually prescribe a sleeping pill, barbiturate or tranquillizer, which often only adds to the problem. Barbiturates may interfere with REM sleep (see page 329). They make you drowsy and usually help to get you to sleep but because they interfere with natural body rhythms, the sleep is very light, so you wake up easily and often in a state of anxiety. The next step is usually to take another pill, then another. Barbiturates are dangerous because not only are they addictive, but one can wake up suddenly and not be entirely rational or conscious. A small overdose, especially in combination with alcohol, can be fatal.

Loss of sleep undermines physical and mental health. Not everyone needs eight hours of sleep at night but if a person is constantly exhausted during the day – because of insufficient sleep – it has to be made up somehow. The insomniac is fully aware of this, and trying to force sleep is a prescription for sleeplessness. It is a vicious cycle. Lying in bed at night, rigid and tense, waiting for relaxation and drowsiness, can be psychologically painful and physically exhausting.

Most people should be able to put themselves to sleep by a form of self-hypnosis or auto-suggestion. Here is one method. Lie looking upwards at the ceiling, hard enough to put a slight strain on your eyeballs. Untense hands by clenching and stretching alternatively a few times. Next focus eyes inward as well as upward, as though looking down your nose. Close eyes slowly, counting backwards from ten to one in rhythm with breathing. On the last count, take a deep breath and let it out slowly. Relax the entire body and imagine yourself asleep in the most pleasant way. Open your eyes and think of relaxation only.

MONONUCLEOSIS: Also called glandular fever or the kissing disease. It is actually a non-malignant leukaemia, where the white blood cells increase over the red. It is self limiting although it can continue in a mild form for months, and sometimes recurs.

The cause is not known, though it is suspected to be a virus. It is often incorrectly diagnosed at first, as the symptoms are like those of scarlet fever, german measles or undulant fever. There is always a definite fever, high temperature, fatigue, aches and pains, sore throat and headache. A chemical analysis of the blood can accurately detect it. It is infectious.

There is not much to be done except to allow the illness to take its own course. Stay in bed while the fever continues, eat nourishing food and take vitamin B-complex supplements. Antibiotics are useless against viruses though the side effects can be relieved.

MOTION SICKNESS: Some stomachs react adversely to movement, giving a series of shocks to the nervous system resulting in nausea, giddiness and vomiting. Anti-travel pills are not always recommended. As a precaution don't begin a trip on an empty stomach – a bowl of warm soup into which has been stirred a quarter of a teaspoon of cayenne pepper is beneficial. Keep the bowels open.

RHEUMATISM: Arthritis and gout are all different manifestations of the same disease – inflammation of the connective tissue in the joints. While not fatal it can cause a great number of disabilities. As it progresses the involved joints are moved less and less because of the pain. In consequence, the surrounding muscles begin to atrophy, resulting in crippling.

There are several causes: heredity, an accident which can leave a joint vulnerable, an improper diet. Medicine is largely unable to cure rheumatism. Drugs can relieve the pain but not the condition. It is always worse when the weather is cold and damp. Warmth is one of the best remedies and a thermal cure can often considerably help a chronic condition. Spinal manipulation can give relief. Exercise, rest, relaxation, proper food, vitamin and mineral therapy, plus vitamin B-12 supplements will help reduce the pain and discomfort. Fruit and vegetable juices are good, particularly raw carrot juice. Celery, cabbage and parsley are also recommended. It has been found that many arthritics have oil deficiencies, so should add a good vegetable oil to their diet.

ULCERS: Affect 10% of the population mostly between the ages of forty-five and fifty-five, though symptoms may begin quite young. Women are more subject to them after the menopause. Ulcers occur because the lining in the stomach or duodenum in certain spots is unable to withstand the digestive action of acid and pepsin. A duodenal ulcer tends to afflict those who produce an excess of acid, while a gastric (stomach) ulcer is developed by those who produce less acid than normal. The main symptoms are upper abdominal pain and hunger feelings. Vomiting sometimes occurs and may be tinged with blood. The diagnosis is confirmed by barium meal X-ray or by passing a flexible telescope through the mouth into the stomach to look at the ulcer directly.

Stress and pressure are said to incite a duodenal ulcer, also smoking, alcohol and spasmodic eating; people of Blood Group O appear to develop it more frequently than those of other blood groups.

Treatment involves removal of stressful situations, often a change in diet, alkalis to relieve the pain and sometimes a liquorice derivative which is claimed to increase the rate of healing. Surgery is a last resort.

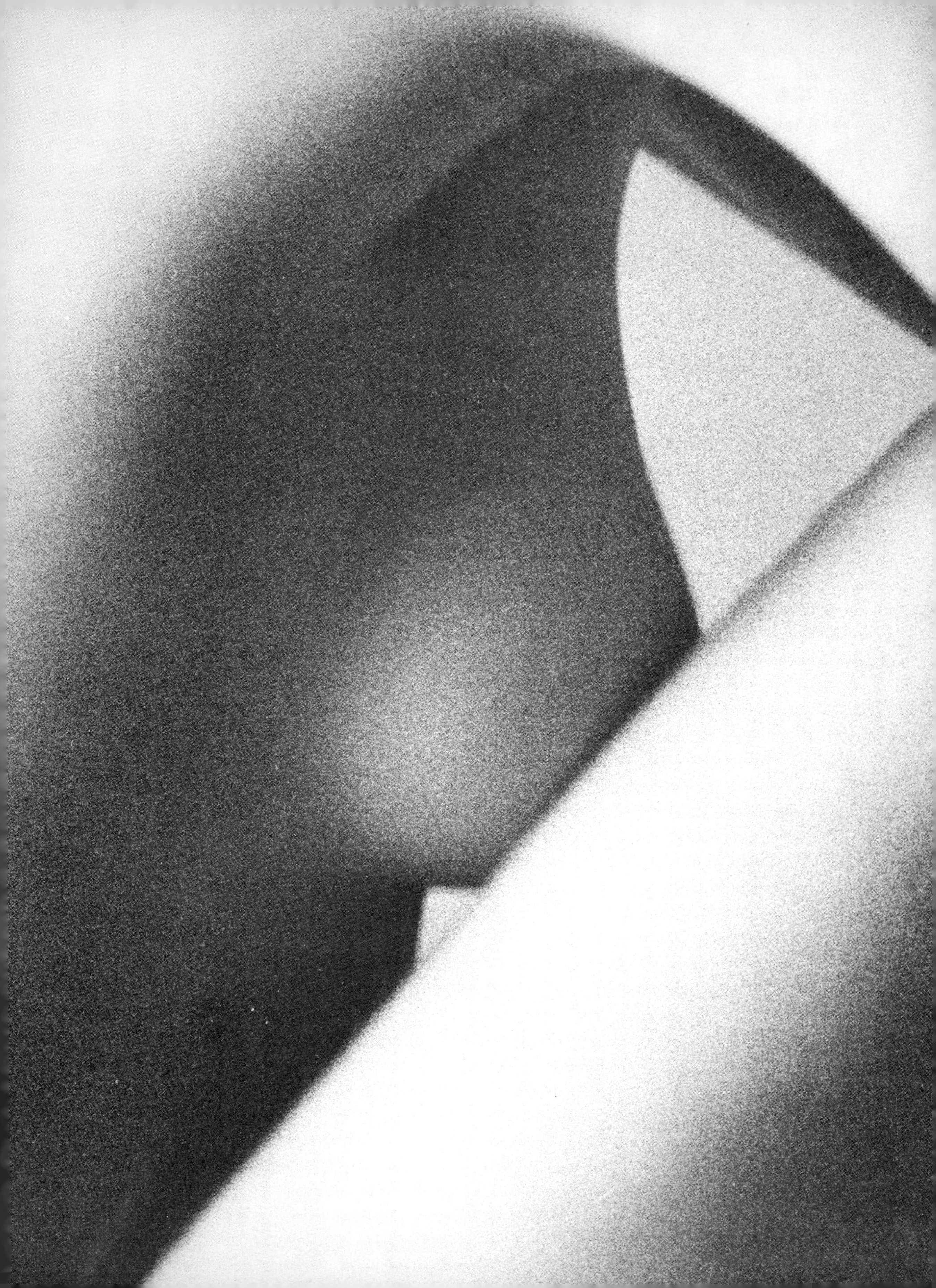

4

PLASTIC SURGERY

As a science and an art, plastic surgery has developed incredibly over the last twenty years or so. It can give young people more confidence, and for many adults it can provide a new lease of life. It is a natural follow-up after considerable weight loss. Although many improvements last a lifetime (nose structures, ear and chin corrections for example) even those that last a matter of years can be rewarding.

The modern plastic surgeon is one of the most interesting of medical specialists. In addition to being highly competent, he must have a certain amount of artistic ability if he is to perform his work with any degree of distinction. There is every reason to have confidence in him as the qualified plastic surgeon has had to go through a rigorous training.

Plastic surgery is basically either cutting away or adding – the former normally costs more than the latter. Surgeons, as might well be expected, are highly individual, sometimes using different methods or techniques. Bones, skin and fat can be reduced by simply taking part of them away. In lifting techniques (which also pull out wrinkles and lines) the skin is drawn into natural folds where it will be least conspicuous.

Inserted substances can build out an area. Human bones and cartilage are still widely used in corrective surgery, but in several cosmetic procedures, silicone prostheses (artificial implants) are popular and most effective, particularly the sponges which are constantly being improved, and for example too-small breasts can have implants of fluid silastic encased in a plastic bag (see details later). No more liquid injections are given as in earlier years when they were also used to fill out face and hand wrinkles as well as expand bosoms. Whereas the bulk silicone and the encased fluid can be safely secured and isolated, the liquid silicone was simply injected and did not always stay where it was put.

One of the most frequent questions asked is: how long will it last? It depends – on the person, the age, the metabolism, future care and stress. Some things once done are there for ever: those that have to do with bone structure or areas entirely uninfluenced by muscles or fatty deposits such as noses, chins, ears.

There is a new theory that a prevention-lift in the late thirties or early forties will keep a face in better, younger shape relatively longer: on the basis that the face can be re-arranged before muscles lose too much of their elasticity. However, not many people are so far-sighted. Nor can you have surgery and forget to care for the skin and body from that time on. One of the leading body-surgeons never ceases to emphasize that a sensible diet, exercise and skin care must be continued after surgery.

At an interview the surgeon will examine, advise and explain, and it is terribly important that you ask him about everything: what he will do in the operation, how long it will take, what about anaesthetic, how long is the hospital stay, when do the stitches come out, how soon can you use make-up, will any marks finally disappear – and the cost. It is impossible to give an estimate on fees for operations as they fluctuate not only from country to country, but also from doctor to doctor.

Here are the main corrective possibilities, which give a general idea:

EYES

Operating time: 1½ hours
Hospital time: 1 to 3 nights
Recuperation: 7 to 10 days
After-care: moderate
Benefit duration: 5 to 10 years

Eyes are a fair barometer of health, age and how a person feels. They are also possibly the most important focus of beauty and personality. This together with the fact that an eye job is one of the simplest, cheapest and most successful in the plastic surgeon's repertoire, accounts for the fact that this operation is one of the most popular.

Often facial ageing or disfigurement is nothing more than problems centred around the eyes. As one surgeon says: 'I'd have anyone who is considering a face-lift come first for the eyes. Having these done alone can make an enormous difference and it is frequently unnecessary to consider a total lift for many years.'

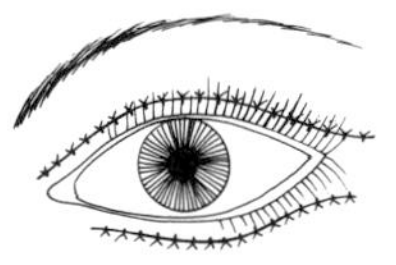

Under-eye bulges or crêpy, puffy skin on the upper eyelids can be removed. It is not only women in their middle years who are candidates, but quite young women too. This is because the so-called bags under the eyes may be an inherited family feature and nothing to do with age, late nights or a dissipated life. No amount of sleep or healthy living will rectify them. In this case, it is little hernias (ruptures) that are causing the swellings – pads of fat which escape the control of muscle surrounding the eye. These fatty ruptures can also appear above the eye, creating puffiness, but are not likely to be as noticeable as the underlid bags. In later years, it's another matter. Skin loosens whether there are hernias or not, while the upper eyelid can become as much of a problem as the lower; to such an extent that vision may be affected.

For either above or below the eye, the operation is relatively brief – about an hour and a half under local or general anaesthetic depending on the doctor. The surgeon makes a fine incision just below the lower lashes and/or in the hollow where the eyeball curves inward to meet the arch of the bone. In the case of the younger patient with smooth skin, he removes the fat and sews up. With an older patient whose skin is sagging and lined, he removes a section of the skin – so the puffiness, looseness and wrinkles are eliminated at the same time.

The healing of the tissues around the eye area is so accommodating that scars almost never occur, and if they do are no more than lines so fine as to escape the naked eye. Healing depends on the individual, but in general the patient can be out and about in three to four days (with dark glasses). Stitches can be taken out after five days. Bruising and discoloration usually remain for three to four weeks. Eyes are inclined to swell as they heal, though this is purely temporary and can be helped with ice application. Discoloration progressively becomes paler and make-up can usually be used after ten days to camouflage.

FACE

Operating time: 3 to 4 hours
Hospital time: 3 to 5 nights
Recuperation: 2 to 3 weeks
After-care: moderate
Benefit duration: 5 to 10 years

The face ages progressively. As a rule, at thirty, personality lines usually appear; around thirty-five or forty, muscle lines show up near the eyes, and from then on skin lines, wrinkles, neck marks, folds and pouches appear due to the general progressive degeneration of tissues.

The aim of the face-lift is to achieve exactly what its name implies: to pull up anything that is sagging and at the same time pull out the lines that invariably are concentrated around the eyes, mouth and on the forehead. In an older skin, the loss of supporting fat pads contributes to the increase in wrinkles, even over the cheeks, and also accounts for much of the folding. In a complete lift, the skin of the throat is smoothed if necessary, and the tightening of a double chin may also be included.

Originally a face-lift consisted of simply making an incision in the skin diagonally above the temple in the hairline. The skin was pulled, the

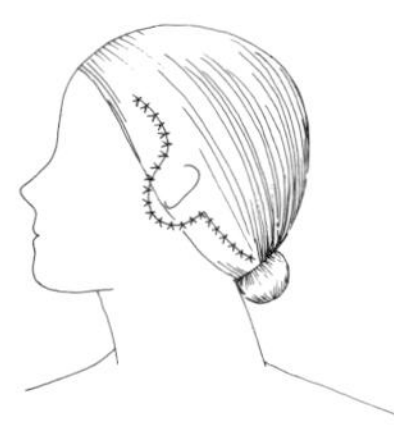

excess cut off, and all sewn together again. However, the pull of the facial muscles on the stretched skin soon caused the face to relapse. This is why the so-called mini-lift is a waste of time and money.

To do a good face-lift, it is essential to work also on the underlying muscular bed. Involved in this is considerable undercutting of the skin, and facial muscles are re-attached to minimize their pull. The secret is to decide which muscle action to eliminate or reduce. Unfortunately, although this greatly extends the life of the lift, it can cause a loss of expression. So it is possible to end up looking very much younger, but also with a rather blank face.

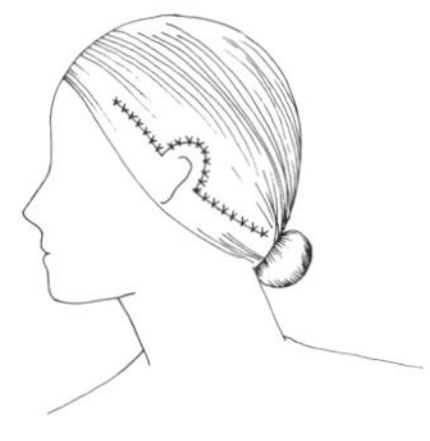

An incision is usually made in the natural fold in front of the ear, running under the lobe, up behind the ear and then diagonally into the scalp, though some surgeons prefer to make all incisions inside the hairline or behind the ear. In these ways a really good lift can be made. Some surgeons don't even shave the hair, but simply divide it. The only scar that shows, even in the early stages of healing, is the one in front of the hair, but this should fade completely within a couple of months. The others are hidden by hair right from the start. A local anaesthetic is often used even though the operation is a long one, three to four hours, but this is the joint decision of the doctor and patient. Some surgeons also prefer to divide the face, and work on a section at a time.

The stitches are removed after five to seven days, then there's another five days for full healing. There may be some swelling at first, but you are usually quite presentable after a week or two to go out with make-up. Sometimes puffiness and bruising can be prolonged; this depends on skin chemistry.

NECK

Operating time: 1½ to 2 hours
Hospital time: 2 to 3 nights
Recuperation: 2 to 3 weeks
After-care: moderate
Benefit duration: 5 to 10 years

This is really a partial face-lift and involves smoothing out the neck and getting rid of a double chin. The skin is taken upwards and the incision is made behind the ears in the shape of a long inverted hairpin. It is not often that this operation is considered alone, as most faces in need of such treatment usually require other improvements. However, there are women who don't mind facial lines, but have a complex about a double chin. Also many young women are affected this way.

NOSE

Depending on skin texture and on thickness, the nose can be straightened, shortened, softened, narrowed and built-up. The operation is performed

Operating time: 1 hour
Hospital time: 3 nights
Recuperation: 2 weeks to 1 month
After-care: moderate
Benefit duration: for ever

from the inside, so there is absolutely no scarring. For reduction, the surgeon chisels away to remove excess bone, cartilage and superfluous tissue. Cartilage and silicone implants are used for enlarging. Afterwards there's a little discomfort as a plaster cast is put on the nose and you have to breathe through the mouth, but it is no worse than having a heavy cold. The cast is removed after 7 to 10 days. There will be sensitivity, pinkness and swelling, as well as bruising around the eyes. This discoloration lasts for a few weeks, but it is usually possible for a patient to go back to everyday life after 2 weeks. It may take a month for all swelling and sensitivity to disappear.

This is one cosmetic operation that may be desirable for the adolescent. If a young person clearly has a nose of such shape or proportion that it is bound to have deep psychological effects, it is well worth while getting it corrected as early as possible.

BOSOM (*Lifting or enlarging*)

Operating time: $1\frac{1}{2}$ hours each breast
Hospital time: 3 to 4 nights
Recuperation: 3 weeks
After-care: moderate
Benefit duration: up to 10 years

Breasts that droop are rarely corrected by simply taking a tuck in tired muscles. After excess skin is removed, the breasts would probably be small. So they are enlarged and filled out where necessary to achieve an even, rounded bosom. The same technique is used as that for providing a reasonable bosom for the flat-chested. In this instance, the stretching property of skin is for once an advantage, as the skin expands smoothly to cover any additional matter that is put in. The usual method is to insert prostheses (implants) made of gel or saline-filled sacs that sometimes have mesh backs; these come in many sizes and feel, and look, completely natural. They are firmly stitched to the chest wall. Incisions are usually made in a half-moon curve under each bosom; sometimes sacs are inserted through incisions in the armpits. In the case of flat-chested patients, some surgeons prefer to secure an empty sac, then inject saline afterwards. This method is particularly advantageous when the operation is for breasts of unequal size. Small breasts should not be tampered with until after childbirth.

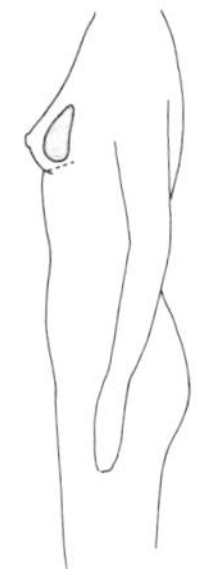

BOSOM (*Reduction*)

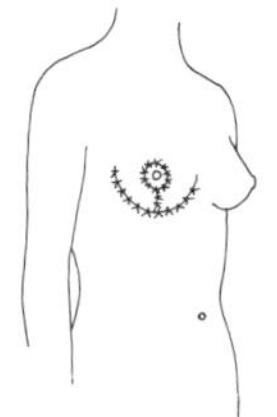

Besides being the cause of much embarrassment, the large bosom can be a health hazard, not to mention the strain on the spine. Many doctors consider it more susceptible to malignancies.

Reduction is a complicated and delicate operation and can take up to two hours for each breast. It is done under a general anaesthetic and the

Operating time: $1\frac{1}{2}$ to 2 hours each breast
Hospital time: 4 to 5 nights
Recuperation: 3 to 5 weeks
After-care: considerable
Benefit duration: up to 10 years or longer

surgeon's task is to remove excess fat and skin, and to replace the nipple if necessary – and it usually is. There are several methods of incision, but generally it involves a vertical cut from the nipple down, another that curves under the breast's fold, and a third around the nipple. Scars come close to disappearing in a few months but rarely go completely. The operation sometimes involves the risk of hampering the nipple's normal function, such as lactation, but surgeons are terribly careful to control this whenever possible. Depending on each case, the doctor will always give implicit instructions for post-operative care. After three to five weeks the bosom should be in shape and the scars reasonably faint. However, the nipples take some adjusting and will settle into their final, natural position about ten to twelve months after the operation.

CHIN *(Receding, prominent or double)*

Operating time: 1 to 2 hours
Hospital time: 2 to 3 nights
Recuperation: 2 weeks for minor surgery, up to 12 weeks for major surgery
After-care: moderate
Benefit duration: for ever

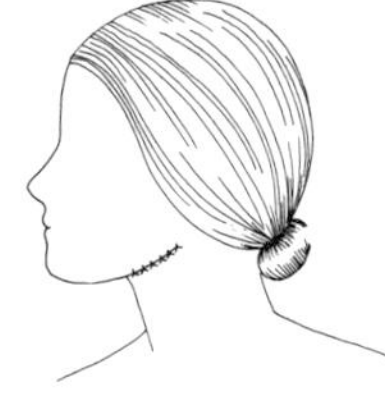

A receding chin can be built up by adding bone and cartilage or inserting a shaped silicone implant. An incision is made inside the mouth in front of the teeth. Often a nose irregularity and a receding chin go together, but an operation to bring the chin forward may balance the profile to such a degree that a nose correction is unnecessary.

A double chin is usually corrected as part of a face-lift or a neck operation, but if the trouble is just a pad of fat under the chin, flabbiness or loose 'turkey' skin, there is a simple operation that is done under local anaesthetic and takes about an hour. A Z-shaped incision is made directly under the chin, excess tissue removed, excess skin is cut away. Stitches come out after a few days.

EARS

Operating time: 3 to 4 hours each ear
Hospital time: 2 nights
Recuperation: 2 weeks
After-care: moderate
Benefit duration: for ever

Fly-away or 'bat' ears can be easily repositioned to the head, leaving behind each ear an almost invisible fine-line scar. A tiny incision is made behind each ear, the excess cartilage is removed and the skin correspondingly tightened. All is then stitched up. The ear is bandaged flat against the head. Healing takes about two weeks and the bandages must remain in place during this time. Children can suffer undue teasing over this defect, and because this operation is one that can be successfully performed at an early age – from the age of four on – the sooner it is done the better. For adults, the technique and result of the operation are exactly the same.

BUTTOCKS AND THIGHS

Operating time: 2 to 3 hours
Hospital time: 7 to 10 nights
Recuperation: 3 to 4 weeks
After-care: considerable
Benefit duration: 5 to 10 years

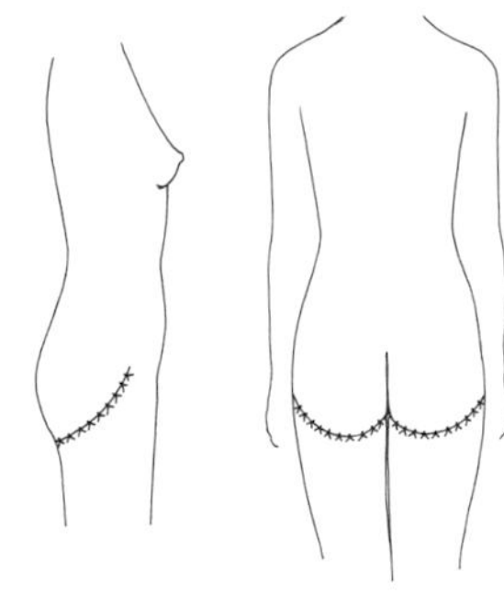

Buttocks and thighs can be operated on together under general anaesthesia, to remedy what is known as the 'riding breeches' problem. It is a long and complex operation, for the young and middle-aged only, and not all surgeons will do it. It is recommended to try to lose some weight first, though usually this is the area where fat refuses to budge and is in the form of cellulite. The first step is to calculate the quantity of tissue to be cut away; this is done standing, for maximum accuracy and better aesthetic assessment. Two lines are drawn on the buttocks – one above and one below the original gluteal folds – to indicate the section to be taken away. The upper line establishes the new level of the fold and is the first line of incision. The lower one is the second incision and the adipose tissue is removed from under this crescent-shaped flap. The skin line is pulled upward and backward towards the inner side of the upper thighs, excess cut off, then sutured to the upper skin line. This means that the flabbiness of the inner thigh is corrected along with the outside figure line. The final stitching line is tucked neatly within the buttock fold, but extends to the outer thighs curving around a little in front to almost reach the hip-bone. After the operation, it is usually possible to walk without too much discomfort within two days but to sit down normally takes about two to three weeks. The scars do pale, but very slowly.

STOMACH

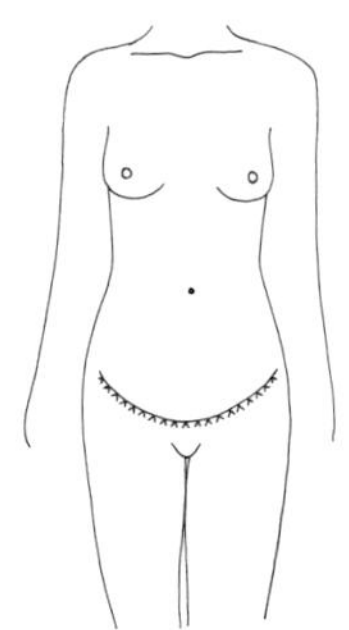

Operating time: 2 to 3 hours
Hospital time: 5 nights for stretch marks, 8 nights for more extensive surgery
Recuperation: 3 to 4 weeks
After-care: moderate
Benefit duration: 5 to 10 years

Fat can be removed from the stomach, though not every surgeon will perform the surgery. It is a most delicate procedure and can also include the reconstruction of an ugly, malformed navel. To a much lesser degree, the concern of many women lies in stretch marks that come from pregnancy or drastic loss of weight. These can be smoothed out by basically the same procedure – at considerably less time and cost. Stomach reduction works on the same principle as a face-lift, except that it goes in the reverse direction. It is a matter of taking away excess fat and skin and controlling the muscles. The incision is low on the belly and is carried in an upward curve over the hips. The scar coincides with the pubic hairline so it is virtually invisible. In time the scar on the hips will pale but it rarely completely disappears. Sometimes the navel has to be repositioned.

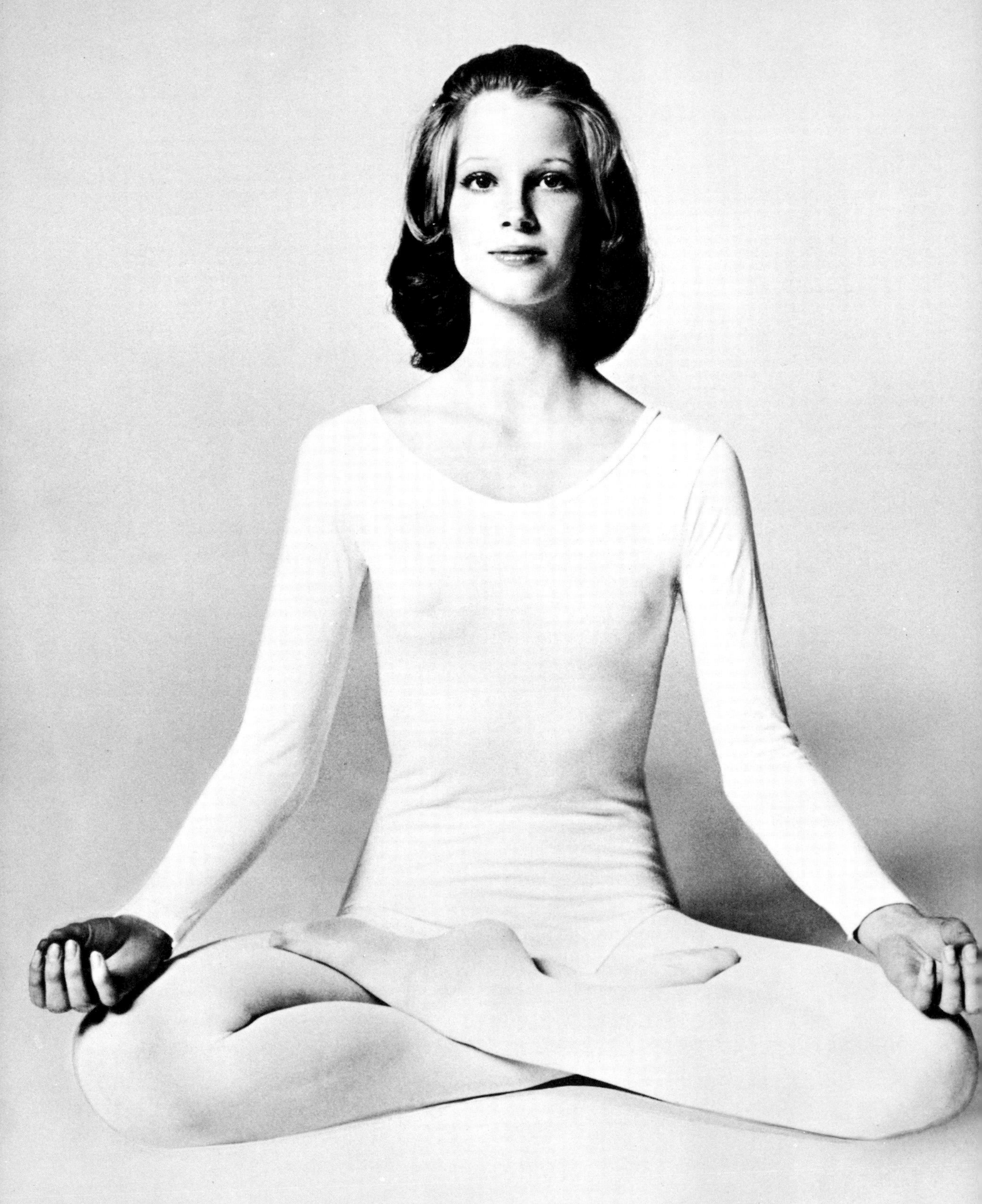

5

NERVES AND TENSION

Tension is not an illness; it is a symptom, a reaction to stress. It can, however, trigger off a real illness, finding its outlet in physical, nervous and mental disturbances.

How does it start? Tension is primarily the result of unresolved inner conflict. It indicates a clash between impulses that demand action and a counterforce that stops it. Whether this involves a physical or mental process is of little importance as nerve reactions are basically the same.

Whenever stress signals go out to the brain, the nervous system prepares the body to react on a fight-or-flight basis. Adrenalin is poured into the bloodstream, the muscles flex, blood pressure rises and the body is equipped for attacking or retreating. Then comes the counter signal of civilized training and reason: stop, it's wrong, a bad decision, too emotional, too aggressive, risky, selfish. The result is no action and no outlet for accumulated energy; tension follows.

Many people can be unaware that they are in a state of neuromuscular tension though congested nerve channels can cause headaches, backaches, fatigue, insomnia, dizziness and general inertia. Do you find your hands are clenched, palms sweating, your feet tapping? Such nervous reactions in themselves can create further anxiety by altering the chemistry of the blood. It is a vicious circle.

Stress levels are individual. Each of us has a limit as to how much stress we can stand before the brain is alerted and changes take place in

FRANCES MCLAUGHLIN-GILL

the hormone system. Our stress quotient is the barometer of our reaction to environment. Stress always has to have a stimulus. Some people find ordinary everyday life so full of stimuli that their over-reaction to living is a permanent trial and even seemingly harmless stimuli can cause stress and become 'the last straw'. Morbid depression and mental illness lie at the end of this path; both are essentially an alienation from society and environment. Indecisive or negative reaction can cause stress. This is where inner conflict is at its zenith and can become paralysing. When there is no positive action, physical or mental, tension remains and builds up. Indecision is fed by anxiety, guilt and fear. Negativeness is expressed in self doubt about emotions, ability and judgements. To help yourself means slowly to accept everything for what it is, your limitations and those of others too. With positive actions you can ease the stress gradually and alleviate the tension; sometimes medical help is necessary through psychotherapy and drug relief.

Anxiety is extremely common, particularly in women. It is different from fear, which is a normal emotional reaction to a definite real danger. Anxiety is a neurotic response, for it anticipates a catastrophe that is invariably imagined. Most women who suffer from anxiety are never quite sure exactly what it is they are so anxious about, although they will list generalities such as money, the future, security, losing a job, husband, the home, growing old. All nebulous, but such is the power of the imagination that it can direct the brain into action as though real ordeals were imminent, and a stress and tension pattern follows.

The hypothalamus reacts immediately to anxiety and drugs that depress this can help but do so only by suppressing the symptoms, not eliminating the cause. Diet is thought to play a role in anxiety: anyone deficient in any of the vitamin B complex shows signs of nervousness. Even missing a meal can put some people in a stressful state.

To help control anxiety, try rationing yourself. List the most important things to worry about and concentrate on those. Live from day to day; don't look back, don't peer into the future. Balance your anxiety with physical and mental recreations that leave little time and thought for fretting. Women with time on their hands worry more, and the more you worry the less inclined you are to go out and take action. Try to make one positive decision a day, starting with little things such as choosing a new lipstick. It is surprising how quickly confidence can build up to enable you to face a major decision without the nagging anxiety that you have made the wrong move.

Unbalanced emotions can cause considerable stress. You have to know when to let go and when to restrain. Bottling up some things is a sure way to build up tension. The problem is often fear – fear of showing emotions beyond the bounds of what you consider to be proper; or more correctly, beyond the bounds of what you think others consider proper. Fear of letting go sexually runs under the surface of most psyches. Fear of aggression follows closely and is related. Both often simply represent the wish to admit to an inner need for some form of self-expression.

People are afraid to cry, to unleash their feelings of loneliness and loss in case they get carried away in a flood of emotion. A good weep has its limits, and whether you are crying for someone, something or just out of self pity, it can ease stress and tension. By the same token, if anger has no outlet, you can look and feel washed out from inner exhaustion.

Jealousy is one of the most stressful and destructive emotions; it can maim the spirit and almost paralyse the will. You can be jealous of a person, a thing, a situation. At its most intense it cannot be sustained without nerves going to pieces. The cure for jealousy is to see it exactly for what it is: a dissatisfaction with oneself, a complex of inadequacy and insecurity. Your energy is better directed into doing something constructive and positive. Another emotion, frustration, stems from envy. It thrives on unhappy compromise and can turn into habitual resentment. Again action is the answer.

Guilt is closely akin to anxiety as it is a clash between an inner urge and a fear of its consequences. It is particularly insidious because it is unconscious with quick automatic response. On an emotional level it appears as anxiety, confusion or depression. On a physical level it is manifested in aches, pains, fatigue, digestive and circulatory disorders.

Its roots lie in right-and-wrong guidance during childhood. It is like a computer in the super-ego ruling actions with all that has been fed into it, and handing out punishments. It judges the conscious rational self, the ego, and the deeper intuitive raw self, the id. There is no choice but to come to terms with guilt, putting it in perspective. Whatever the specific situation – an action, a misdeed, a break-up of a marriage, ending of an affair or friendship – to live healthily means to learn to accept reality and to make peace between an inbred sense of morality and immediate needs for survival. It is not selfish, it is practical.

Depression is a morbid sadness accompanied by a sense of futility. All these stress factors can lead to depression, but it doesn't mean necessarily you are going to get depressed if you suffer from any of them.

Psychiatrists say it is unconsciously motivated by a loss of some kind – a person, a thing, a possession, a job, security, confidence, looks, money.

The loss can be spontaneous or anticipated, but the depression is an inner reaction to the events that led up to it. It is quite different from grief, which is a realistic and appropriate reaction to a loss. Once in a state of depression every move seems to take you down further. It needs the most determined will and constructive methods to get out of it.

Women are more prone to depression than men. Many feel frustrated, bored and trapped in house-bound monotony. Boredom is the surface state; underneath is conflict supported by thoughts of repression, rebellion and dreams. A woman may feel she is lacking something important if she is satisfied with the traditional female role – and this depresses her. Or she may expect more out of her life – but what is not altogether clear. She feels inadequate, ineffectual and frustrated. Women are more prone to depression after childbirth, in the mid-thirties and at the menopause when hormone disturbances are significant. Failure in sexual relations is often a cause for depression, so is criticism or rejection.

The signs of depression are only too apparent. Sleep is often affected – sometimes there is difficulty in getting to sleep and early waking; sometimes sleep is an escape and you simply can't get enough of it. Psychosomatic illnesses are often a cover-up for depression. Intellectual lucidity diminishes, concentration is low, conversation dull and listless, reflected in passive facial expressions and a general air of boredom and indifference.

A depression can be stemmed if you recognize the symptoms and tackle them early enough. It means making a tremendous effort to meet people, to go out, to get involved. Psychic fatigue is part of depression. Loss of interest and apathy makes you too exhausted to do anything. It is necessary to force yourself to do something stimulating: specific exercise or sport is good; energy creates energy.

All causes of stress are connected with nervous response. Excessive control of stress builds up tension, and if you live under conditions of great strain, you have to find a way of relaxing. The best way to discharge neuro-muscular tension is through pleasure. The more absorbing and more physical the better.

RELAXATION

Just learning to relax and let go is the basic way to combat tension. Try some or all of these methods, but always one a day:

Breathing: Nature's way of releasing tension is to bring oxygen to all parts of the body. More important than breathing in is learning to breathe out so that the lungs are completely emptied of stale air. Breathe out longer and harder than you breathe in. Standing or sitting cross-legged on the floor, inhale to the count of four, breathe out to the count of eight. Breathe in through the nose and out through the mouth, which should be partially opened with jaw relaxed.

Lying at a slant: This is a Yoga position of relaxation, where the head is down and the feet raised twelve inches above the floor, so the body goes in a smooth backward slope. Use a firm board – a plank covered with a towel is perfect – propped or secured at the correct angle. Relax for fifteen minutes every day, eyes closed, hands by your sides. At this angle the spine straightens out and muscles, ordinarily tensed while standing, sitting or walking, are relaxed. A good time to relax like this is after a day's work, before a bath or an evening out.

Head rolling: With arms behind your back, breathe in deeply, then slowly rotate head from left to right making a complete circle. Be conscious of muscles in neck and shoulders. Do very slowly, twice in each direction.

Dangling: With legs wide apart, allow the body to fall over from the waist, so the head becomes a weight at the end of the spine. Hang and sway from side to side for about half a minute. Slowly lift up, using stomach muscles to raise the back, one vertebra at a time.

Slapping: Throw your arms alternately across your body, over the shoulder to give yourself a good slap on the back in the area of the shoulder blades. 10 slaps with each hand.

MEDITATION

This is the next step after relaxation because it releases from tension the mind as well as the body. While the body is at rest, the mind empties itself and you emerge from meditation physically revived and more mentally alert. It can also serve as a self analysis session, for when you meditate, you are forced to observe your thoughts. The process can be difficult. At the beginning it is a great strain to sit still for fifteen or twenty minutes and to clear the mind of all trivia. After practice it can be achieved. During meditation there is a drop in the rate of breathing and heart activity, brain patterns change to a more relaxed form. Experienced meditators say that you can begin to see problems objectively and dependence on forms of relief such as drugs, alcohol or cigarettes, is considerably lessened. The two most prevalent forms of meditation are Raja Yoga and Transcendental, both of which use a 'mantra' (a sound to be spoken aloud or in the head) to clear the mind. It is advisable to go for initial instruction as this gives you a better understanding of the philosophy behind meditation plus practical help on technique.

The rules are simple:

Choose a comfortable position. It is not necessary to sit cross-legged, but once accustomed to it, it helps achieve regular relaxed breathing.

Breathe slowly and rhythmically, taking twice as long to breathe out as to breathe in.

Now determine which 'mantra' you will use. The traditional ones are like our vowel sounds of ah-eh-ih-oh-uh. Repeat them all and decide which one suits you best. It is said that ah relieves anxiety, eh tension, ih aggression, oh pain and uh sexual excitement.

Introduce the chosen sound into your mind, saying it aloud at first if it helps you to concentrate. Repeat it over and over again in your head, pushing out every other thought – not with force, but with detached observation of the mind's wanderings. At first the mind runs wild and other thoughts refuse to go; both practice and patience are needed. If you find it difficult to meditate with eyes closed, focus on some object, a picture or a sculpture. This sometimes increases concentration.

Make yourself sit and learn the technique for a minimum of fifteen minutes a day. Make it a regular habit. In time you will begin to look forward to it, and find it absolutely necessary.

SLEEP

Sleep is imperative for mental and physical health. Deprived of it, we can become tense and nervous. It has always been a physiological necessity but only recently has the significance of various aspects of sleep come to light. The repose of sleep and lowered metabolism may rest and revive the body, but dreams restore the mind and discharge tension.

When we fall asleep, the eyelids close and the pupils become small. Breathing is diminished, blood pressure falls, the heart slows down, the temperature drops and the digestive juices and saliva decrease. Consciousness is lost, but only temporarily; a noise, a light, a jab can cause wakefulness. There are several stages from drowsiness to oblivious sleep where all muscles are relaxed and it is difficult to be woken. The brain still receives every sound and touch, but though it responds, it does not express messages in actions – unless you are prone to sleepwalking. Sleep is not a tranquil posture; a normal person may change position from twenty to sixty times a night.

There are two kinds of sleep – slow-wave sleep, which is dreamless and usually starts the sleeping sequence, and dreaming sleep, known as REM sleep, as it is characterized by Rapid Eye Movements. The two types alternate during the night.

REM sleep is the deepest and most refreshing, for it is both a physiological and psychological process. Dreams are said to restore the central nervous system but how is still not quite clear. They may help in the working out of emotional problems, and are necessary for psychic survival. Research has shown that if one is deprived of slow-wave sleep, it does little physical damage, but if REM sleep is interrupted it can be more serious, resulting in increased tension and nervous reactions. The natural recuperative reaction is to dream more during the next sleeping period – making up for lost dreams and lost tension relief. Dream activity therefore is good for mental health which is why you often wake up depressed after taking alcohol, barbiturates or tranquillizers – because all these decrease the amount of REM sleep.

Eight hours sleep a night is considered average and necessary to restore normal body functions and alertness. It is possible to get sufficient sleep in short spurts, provided all the benefits from the full slow-wave and REM sleep cycle are obtained. Some people claim they need more sleep than others and studies have been done on the personality types: short sleepers are usually active and outgoing, flexible, sociable and relatively high on social conformity. Long sleepers tend to be more introverted and creative but are successful at sustained work.

It doesn't matter when you sleep provided it is daily, regular and within a twenty-four hour cycle. It is the rhythm that is important, and each body has its own inner clock known as circadian rhythm – a cycle in which a 90 to 120 minute period of sleep – or wakefulness – alternates with a 5 to 10 minute dream period. It goes on unceasingly twenty-four hours a day like breathing. It is combined with an almost clocklike regularity in the rise and fall of the body's temperature. The highest points are when you feel most alive and alert, the lowest when you are day-dreaming or sleep-dreaming. It is much easier to get to sleep during one of the low points in temperature, and many sleeping difficulties could be circumvented if we kept track of them. Try this, and relaxation exercises, and check other remedies detailed under 'Insomnia' (page 311).

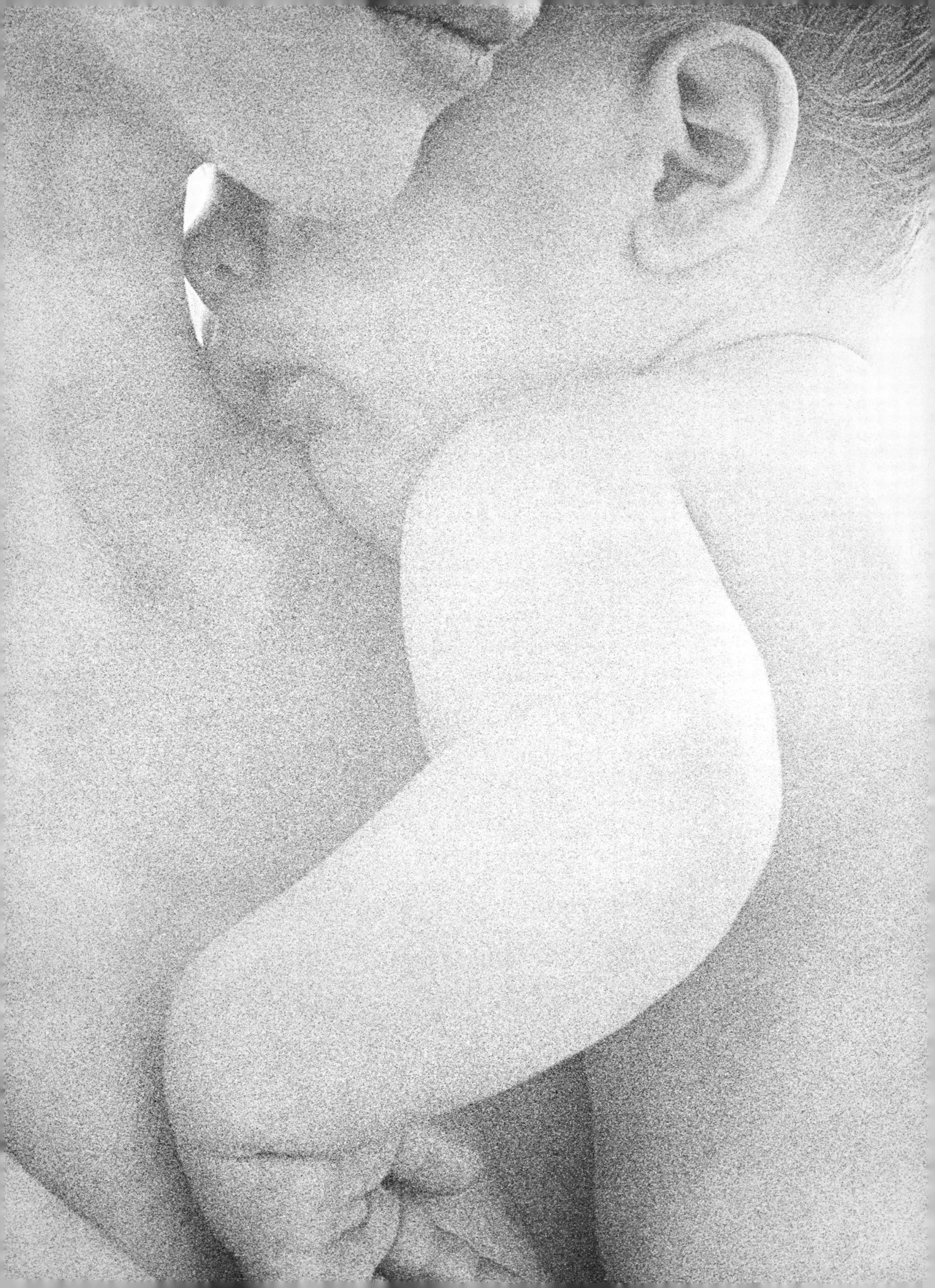

6

AGEING

Fifty years ago a woman of forty was finished. Now the boundaries are extended, but although the surrender to ageing no longer has a deadline, the ageing crisis starts earlier and lasts longer due to the emphasis on extreme youth. There is a survival instinct that pushes women through each decade with determination to keep things at a status quo; this plus a supply of survival equipment enables women to look younger, longer. What we call ageing is not the same for everyone; one woman's forty is another's sixty. Doctors cannot determine with any assurance whether a person is thirty, forty or fifty; they may misjudge by as many as fifteen years. Biological age is what matters and this can be self-determined and adjusted.

There is no mysterious fountain of youth but there is a great deal that can be done to make you look and feel younger at any age. Rejuvenation therapies are going on in many different fields – cosmetics, nutrition, psychology, surgery, endocrinology and chemistry, but the most remarkable have been in the hormone and chemical fields. The aim is not so much to prolong life as to make it more vital and rewarding though added years are often a bonus. Various elixirs of youth have claimed unbelievable things, now the approach is more realistic.

Visible ageing varies and there is no way of estimating when it will start. As we get older, the cells' capacity to reproduce, grow and renew themselves decreases – clearly seen in the way our bodies cannot heal a wound as quickly as they used to. This happens at different rates throughout the body but it is a progressive reduction which means a decline in the regulation and intensity of the vital processes. There comes a point when cells not merely fail to reproduce but actively destroy themselves. No two people age at the same rate and different cells have different life

LATEGAN

spans. A cell forming part of the tissue that lines the alimentary canal lives only thirty-six hours, while nerve cells may live until you die. Blood cells show early changes, cartilage cells change little in form during life and may even survive death by several hours.

There are many theories as to why cells become disorganized but the precise reason is by no means established. It is possibly a combination of several factors:

We age because we wear out and cells produced later in life are inferior to those produced earlier.

We are programmed to age. This is determined by heredity; we have an inbuilt mechanism scheduling cells to divide a certain number of times, after that the body reaches its limit of renewal.

A mistake in biochemistry causes dysfunction. This is connected with the theory that metabolism is maintained and directed by catalysts such as minerals, vitamins, enzymes, micro-elements and amino acids. If we succeeded in substituting the catalysts, then the cells would begin to reactivate normally and youthfully.

The accumulation of harmful hinderants blocks the tissues to such an extent that the cells are unable to perform efficiently.

The connective tissue deteriorates – the colloid theory. Many of the symptoms typical to ageing such as wrinkling and flabbiness of the skin, hardening of the arteries are related to the properties of the colloid molecules in the connective tissue.

The body loses its ability to differentiate between its own proteins and foreign ones and begins to reject its own new ones.

Whatever the reason, cell growth slows down because of the decreasing ability of the organism to renovate itself. If the laws governing activations were known, nature could be forced into regeneration. Only the control and regulation of human chemistry can lead to the final conquest of age.

PREVENTION: SELF-CARE

Growing older and staying younger is not entirely dependent on chemical control. There is a whole range of aesthetic and skin aids ranging from plastic surgery and dermabrasion to the reviving effects of fragrances but all these depend on the skill of others. Heredity, habits and environment all play a part in the way we age. The best way to look young and feel good for decades is to start early building health and care habits to last a lifetime. But it is never too late to improve – start with diet, exercise and attitude:

Diet

Keep your weight down; you will not only look younger but will have a good chance of by-passing such ageing maladies as diabetes, high blood pressure and hardening of the arteries. If blood pressure and cholesterol levels are too high you may be biologically ten years older. Not all people who are overweight die young, just as not all people who smoke get lung cancer, but statistics show that excessive weight anticipates an earlier death.

You need less food as you get older, usually no more than 1,800 Calories a day. You need the right food – vegetables, fruit, lean meat, milk, cheese, fish, little or no animal fat. You need to weigh yourself daily, even if you've never been in the habit of doing so before, as the secret is never to put on more than a few pounds above your norm. These can be taken off without too much effort or sacrifice. Starvation and crash diets are not a good idea, as these tax temper and nerves, shrivel the body and collapse the face, because the skin is no longer capable of re-adjusting its elasticity and coverage.

Be sure you are getting an adequate supply of vitamins and minerals. Supplement your diet with brewers' yeast, kelp, rose hips, yoghourt and honey. Use garlic and onions a lot; include ginseng tea in your beverages; make apricots, fresh or dried, one of your most important fruits. Vitamin E is thought to be particularly good as a regenerator, and one of its best natural sources is wheatgerm. Vitamin C is recommended to help regulate hormones and keep the collagens of connective tissue healthy.

If you have a sweet tooth, substitute these honey balls for commercial confectionery.

1 cup sesame seeds
1–2 tablespoons solid honey

Grind sesame seeds, pour into honey and knead until a firm dough; make into balls, sprinkle with coconut if you like.

Pollen tablets as a diet supplement are considered by many to help build up stamina and body resistance. They are made from pollen, which is the male sex cells of flowers and contains a concentration of essential food elements. Pollen, together with unstrained honey, is an integral part of the diet of the longest-living peoples such as the Hunzas and the Caucasians.

Exercise

Life-long exercise is ideal not only in the interests of a young figure, but for keeping circulation at its peak and thus maintaining the overall health of the body. Anyone who wants a thirty-year-old figure at sixty had better start early. Don't take up exercise suddenly, it can do more harm than good. If you've never exercised much, start gradually and with the more gentle regimes. The Mensendiek routines aren't strenuous, nor are those done in the bath or in water. Massage and electrical stimulation are relaxing. Active sports are the most enjoyable way to exercise and usually the most consistent. And walk – with a spring and with good posture; don't get into the habit of dragging yourself along – it looks and is ageing.

Attitude

Boredom and lethargy will age a person almost as quickly as poor diet or lack of exercise. Keep optimistic and interested. Never retire from living, even if you have to retire from a job, but progress from one stage to another. Remaining sexually active is an important youth preserver. It is a myth that sexual desire and ability decline in the course of ageing.

Research reveals that those who live longest do not appear to be endowed with much competitive spirit and have a pragmatic fatalism about life. This does not mean sitting back and letting things happen, but an absence of exhausting aggressive characteristics. The body needs a certain amount of stress but the amount must be controlled.

Puritans claim a relationship between a short life and a merry one. They couldn't be more wrong. Happiness and gaiety are interwoven with health and vitality.

Appearance

Looking younger doesn't mean clinging to an image of earlier days. It means accepting your age without giving in to it. Uniformity is essential: body, attitude, camouflage. It is pointless to have a young face on an old body, or bright hair over wrinkles, or to act like a young girl when you look more like her mother.

Your personality shows when you are older. What you have been thinking for years is revealed in facial expressions, gestures and sounds. Your faults can become exaggerated and permanent.

The attention a mature woman gives to her appearance must be specialized and consistent. Looks are not luck but a daily responsibility.

You need not spend a great deal of time each day, but it must be every day. The good-looking vital woman with the young figure, the smooth skin, the shining hair is a study in discipline.

THE MENOPAUSE

Women are the only animals who outlive their capacity to reproduce. Throughout adolescence and maturity, female hormones affect a woman's sexuality, appearance and temperament. There are two hormones involved – oestrogen and progesterone – and for the duration of a woman's productive life they appear in a cyclical pattern. Oestrogen is more plentiful in the first half of the cycle and progesterone during the second. Primarily they cause the lining of the womb to thicken each month in preparation for a possible pregnancy and lead to menstruation if conception does not occur.

When most women reach their middle or late forties, the supply of oestrogen in the body is greatly reduced and finally stops altogether. This is known as the menopause and has far-reaching effects. No more than 20% of normal women are fortunate enough to undergo a menopause free of symptoms.

Strictly speaking, the menopause is the date of the last menstrual period, and the climacteric is the transition phase of ovarian function which can extend for some two years before or some two years after. The average age is 48, with a normal range from 45 to 52. No two women have the same experience. The more rapidly the ovaries fail, the greater the likelihood of severe symptoms. A few women menstruate as usual and then suddenly never have another period. Often periods gradually become scanty and irregular, sometimes disappearing only to return before ending completely. Signs and symptoms can begin before any alteration in the menstrual pattern; sometimes they come at the same time as cessation or may not occur until years afterwards. One symptom usually appears first, to be joined by others:

Hot flushes and sweating – probably the most distressing of the early symptoms; a feeling of heat rises from the chest to the head and the face becomes red; it may be accompanied by excessive perspiration; in many women, stress or excitement tends to bring on these symptoms.

Emotional changes – include feelings of nervousness, irritability, depression, weepiness, difficulty in concentrating, loss of memory and confidence, apprehension.

Sexual implications – loss of vaginal tissue and less plentiful secretions can cause dryness to a degree of atrophy so severe that intercourse is often impossible; in addition there is often a decrease in sexual responsiveness.

Bone alterations – changes often take place in the skeleton; bones may lose some of their protein, slowly becoming more brittle with a tendency towards osteoporosis (weakened bones). This is why women often break their hips or wrists even in minor accidents. The spine often becomes weak and curved, a condition known as dowager's hump. Bone aches and associated muscle pain are common.

Body and skin changes – skin as a whole becomes thinner, less firm and loses its elasticity; breasts shrink and lose their contour as muscle and skin tone diminishes; hair becomes brittle and thinner.

Until recently women have had to put up with the menopause with little help except aspirins, tranquillizers and reassurance that it was 'normal'. It is now becoming accepted in medical circles that hormonal supplements are of enormous value in counteracting all the effects of the menopause.

HORMONE REPLACEMENT THERAPY (HRT)

In recent years, oestrogen has had considerable publicity as a factor in controlling the adverse effects of ageing, particularly the menopause. It has been a controversial issue, but now doctors are more convinced that this is a correct and indicated treatment.

Replacement oestrogen does not make a woman fertile again but it does continue its protective and constructive jobs. It keeps bones strong and prevents osteoporosis, it helps to keep tissues healthy and preserves muscle tone, it keeps the vagina in shape and lubricated, it cures the hot flushes and the sweating, and by raising the level of tryptophan (an amino acid) in the blood, emotions are once more better balanced, most notably depressions are lifted. It is also believed to help prevent heart disease to which women are as prone as men after feminine hormones begin to decrease. In fact, replacement of oestrogen reverses the effects of the menopause.

For some women, the glandular imbalance may appear to make little or no difference for some years because oestrogen continues to be produced by other glands. But it is estimated that up to 50 per cent of women do need HRT and another 25 per cent would look better and feel happier with it. Specialists, however, stress that it should only be used under medical control, and that each patient must be individually assessed for treatment and dosage. A simple test establishes oestrogen level. There is sometimes a little weight gain at first, and the breasts can become larger and more active. Usually both return to normal in time.

The correct administration is extremely important. Oestrogen should be prescribed on a cyclic basis of three weeks out of every four and preferably with the addition of progestagen. The doctors who pioneered HRT advocate the combined therapy. It works this way: replacement oestrogen not only restores normality to many body functions, but builds up the lining of the womb. Although impregnation is impossible, it is not a sound idea to thicken the walls of the womb for a long period. Abnormal thickening can lead to a condition called hyperplasia, which has been known to precede or coexist with early cancer. The answer is to stop oestrogen for one week in four, thus allowing the level to drop and usually permitting any build-up to shed – more or less in the old menstrual pattern. To be sure of this the second female hormone of progestagen should be used for five days at the end of each cycle. However, many women are reluctant to accept obligatory withdrawal and subsequent bleeding. It is a rather short-sighted attitude. An additional point for the case of progestagen is that regulated bleeding prevents a possible break-through of blood and any subsequent examinations and tests to find out why it happened.

There is no evidence that HRT increases the risk of cancer in the breast or uterus or elsewhere. At first this was a fear, together with apprehension about it being a contributory factor in thrombosis. These doubts have no clinical support. These hormones have been submitted to many tests and questions – and survived. Some are manufactured from extracts in the urine of pregnant mares, others are chemical compounds.

CELLULAR THERAPY

This treatment is reactivation for the whole body. Organs are stimulated into renewed action and thus motivate metabolism back to its earlier more vigorous state of activity, avoiding the necessity of medical supplements or substitutions.

It began with Professor Paul Niehans in the early 1930s, and despite constant and current scepticism on the part of orthodox medicine, it still ranks high among rejuvenation methods. Niehans died (in his eighties) in 1971 but his exclusive La Prairie Clinic in Vevey, Switzerland continues treatment. There are other centres scattered over Europe, and in Germany alone there are 500 doctors registered as cell therapists, though not necessarily devoting their entire time to it.

Early in his career, Niehans was regarded as an outstanding expert in endocrinology. By chance he stumbled on a way for the body to accept organ replacements. A patient arrived in a parathyroid condition with no time left to be helped by surgery. On impulse Niehans chopped up the parathyroid gland of an ox, put it in a saline solution and injected it. The patient tolerated the intrusion, recovered and lived on for a quarter of a century.

From this example of human tolerance and acceptance of an animal organ (hitherto denounced as impossible and unsafe), Niehans reasoned that the body might be able to accept, or at least in some way exploit, animal cells. He decided to use embryonic cells where regeneration power and possibilities were strongest. He worked on the old medical principle of like heals like, and injected the identical cell to that in the human body in need of revitalization. For example, if the patient has a liver condition, fresh liver cells are used to stimulate the patient's own liver; heart cells combat heart disease; placenta cells alleviate angina and after-birth exhaustion. The fresh embryonic cells come from the foetus of a lamb, and Niehans preferred to use them as fresh as possible, literally minutes after extraction. Whether they are assimilated or whether they act as a catalyst is not understood, but they do help to begin a reactivation process, and it has been photographically shown that injected cells do migrate to the corresponding organ in the body. The recharging only works so long as organs have not deteriorated beyond a certain point.

The case for cellular therapy is still based on empirical evidence. Positive subjective reports or analysis of individual case histories showing before and after findings, are not sufficient for orthodox acceptance. Patients are first examined and a thorough diagnosis is made of what organs are ailing, confirmed by special analytical tests. The appropriate extracts are prepared and injected into the patient's buttocks. Treatment lasts 3–5 days usually. A diet is given, some restrictions imposed, such as no alcohol for several months, no sun, no saunas. Patients often claim to feel better at once but this improvement is usually temporary and frequently in the mind. The real benefits are not experienced for about three months, when visible and physical improvements appear.

Not all cellular therapists inject fresh cellular matter; some use dried cells in solution, others extracts of cells comprising the essential ribonucleic acids which contain the blueprints for renewal. Treatment can be used as a preventive measure, to ward off the effects of oncoming age rather than help counteract them. Treatment is not a once-in-a-lifetime project. A repeat is recommended every five years or so depending on how early you received the first treatment and how old you are. Niehans never claimed that his therapy could help keep anyone alive and younger indefinitely, but stressed that a better, more youthful life was possible throughout the natural span.

Organically the system can be improved; digestive disturbances respond well, so do conditions involving the heart and the arteries. Liver and kidney ailments are frequently treated. It is possible to treat any part of the body where malfunction or slow metabolism is the problem. The best results are seen in glandular disturbances, degenerative and stress disorders. The most frequent demands are for help with impotence and frigidity, menopausal and menstruation difficulties. In the case of the menopause, improvement is claimed in all the usual resulting disorders.

Despite the resistance of medical authorities to these ideas and claims, many women continue to seek out cellular therapists. One thing is a fact: the records of cellular therapy since Niehans began in 1931 have shown that it is certainly safe. Whether effective or not is a personal judgement.

PROCAINE THERAPY

Another approach to age retardation is a drug called Gerovital (also known as GH-3) which has the reputation of diminishing almost all the inflictions of ageing. The discoverer of Gerovital is Professor Ana Aslan of Romania, who over the years has treated more than 100,000 patients in her clinic in Bucharest. Gerovital is a white soluble crystalline substance known as procaine hydrochloride, commonly familiar as novocain and used as a local anaesthetic in dentistry and minor surgery.

Like other revitalizing agents, it was not the result of planned research at all. Professor Aslan was treating elderly patients suffering from rheumatism with procaine injections to alleviate pain and discomfort. She found and observed over a period of seven years that it also made them more active in mind and body, in addition cleared up many skin troubles. From these incidental findings developed Gerovital, which also contains other ingredients including benzoic acid and potassium salts which alter the action of procaine, expanding and prolonging its effect.

Professor Aslan was put at the head of a special geriatric clinic and large-scale experiments were initiated. She did not know exactly how and why it worked, but it did, and she was able to produce substantial clinical evidence to back her claim. The first change is normally in mental functions and physical changes occur shortly afterwards. One of the earliest visible signs is improvement in the skin – it softens, wrinkles smooth out, colour brightens and pigmentation improves. Hair has been known to grow more thickly again. Its effect on psycho-mental functions is particularly significant because the depression so often associated with ageing causes many other diseases. Once this is alleviated the related disorders are often removed. Professor Aslan and other protagonists of Gerovital say it is successful in stimulating cell renewal, in stimulating the circulatory system, in strengthening bones and joints, heightening the endocrine glands, and has a mobilizing effect on cholesterol.

Initially it was met with doubts by the medical hierarchy though the interest and support of the public were overwhelming. The Romanian government gives its complete approval to the treatment and dispenses the drug in 150 centres throughout the country. Patients at the Bucharest Clinic need a series of 12 injections over a period from 10 days to 2 weeks. Effects wear off, so it is advisable to repeat them before a year has passed. In some countries the drug is considered acceptable as an anti-depressant measure but discounted as an anti-ageing method.

The Germans recognized the potential of Gerovital and developed the drug in tablet form, quickly named 'The Youth Pill'. It is known as KH-3 and is a combination of procaine and haematoporphine which acts as a catalyst. It is readily available in European pharmacies, and the prescription is one capsule a day for five months. Its effectiveness has still to be substantially proved. It is not advisable for women under 30 or pregnant women; no side effects are known, but it is a cautionary measure. Generally speaking KH-3 is said to have the same effect as a super-vitamin, but it is also believed to have a direct catalytic effect on the chemistry of the cell itself. No one really knows.

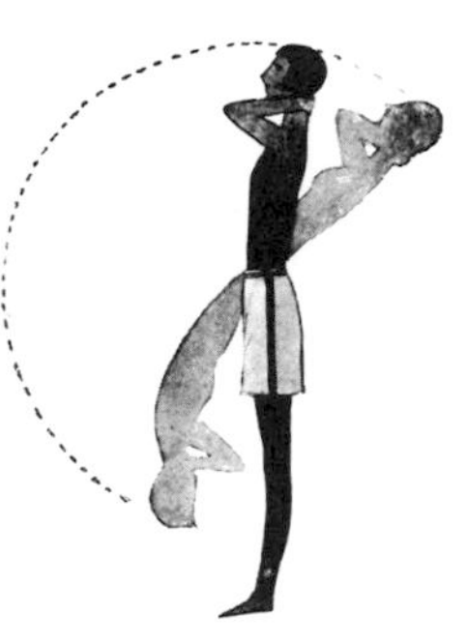

THE BODY

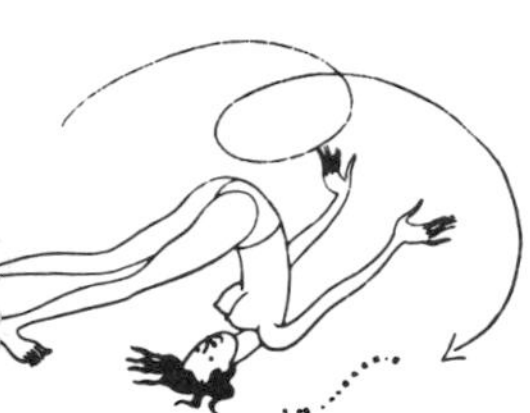

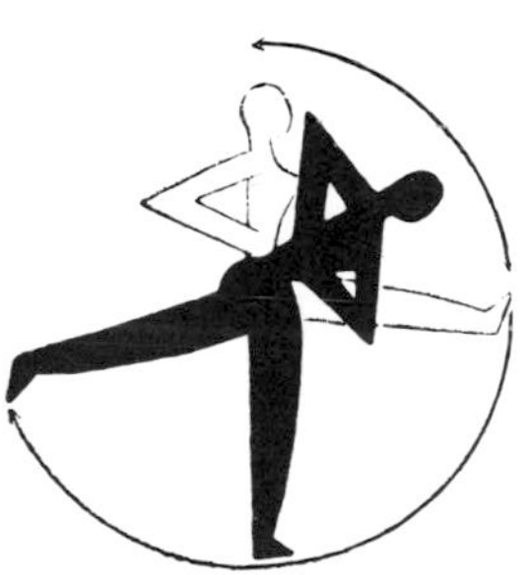

In the 1920s women sailed, swam, skied and played tennis – poker face Helen Wills and temperamental Suzanne Lenglen were the idols. It was chic to be thin – and for thinning legs, ankles and for tired feet 'Sculpto Crystals' were 'unsurpassed'. 'A new aid for those who are troubled by excess of avoirdupois is the Rub Away, an excellent massage roller composed of hollow cylinders of rubber.' 'Excessive underarm perspiration' was the 'menace to every woman's daintiness' and you could send for a sample of ODO-RO-NO for only 3d. With the 1930s came the great open-air cult. Sunbathing was the craze and stripped, oiled sun worshippers lay on roofs and beaches, toasting each side. Kensington's 'perfect spa' for the culture of health and beauty had 'every kind of bath ever invented – Vichy, Brine, Wax, Pine Needle, Foam, Aeration and Sulphur'. To the question, 'Please Vogue my brow is wet with honest sweat. And not only my brow. What can I do to keep fresh?' the reply was, 'We, personally, swear by Perstik and Perstop.' The 1940s was the age of health care and the 'diary of a bright young thing': feed the glands, the body reduces itself . . . and don't rely on the War to 'slim away' stoutness. Vogue *said: 'The new beauty has stiffened her spine and improved her figure.' The psychologists moved into the beauty field and recommended the overweight to think less about 'how delicious' and more about 'how many inches'. With the 1960s came the health food kick, growing your own vegetables and eating pure foods without preservatives or additives. More and more of the body was bared and by 1966: 'Bikinis have never been more minimal, nor the chance of a smooth tan from head to foot more possible.' Comfort was sacrificed to the youth cult and the ideal was to look like a thin coltish child in the early teens. What now, what next? People look less self-conscious, more natural, more relaxed. 'Today people are more than just aware of being overweight, they are doing something about it. To be obese is an offence – against society and yourself.'*

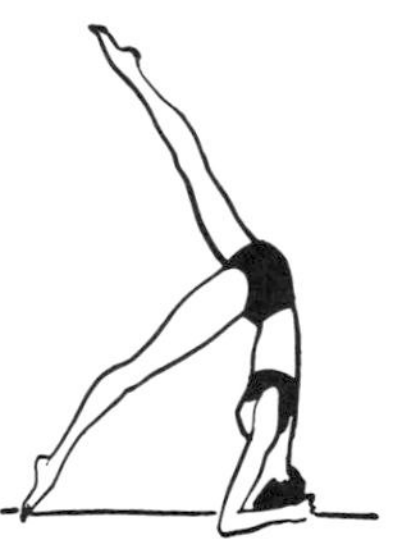

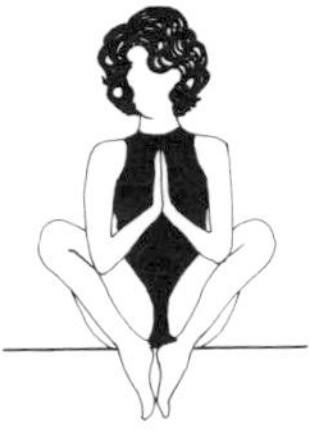

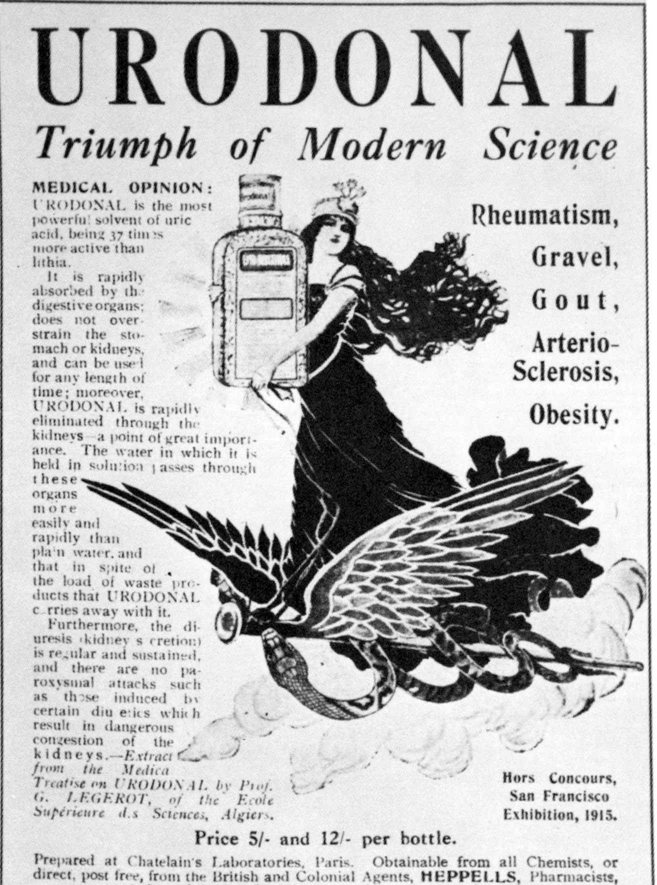

URODONAL
Triumph of Modern Science
MEDICAL OPINION: URODONAL is the most powerful solvent of uric acid, being 37 times more active than lithia.
It is rapidly absorbed by the digestive organs; does not overstrain the stomach or kidneys, and can be used for any length of time; moreover, URODONAL is rapidly eliminated through the kidneys—a point of great importance. The water in which it is held in solution passes through these organs more easily and rapidly than plain water, and that in spite of the load of waste products that URODONAL carries away with it.
Furthermore, the diuresis (kidney secretion) is regular and sustained, and there are no paroxysmal attacks such as those induced by certain diuretics which result in dangerous congestion of the kidneys.—Extract from the Medical Treatise on URODONAL by Prof. G. LEGEROT, of the Ecole Supérieure des Sciences, Algiers.
Rheumatism,
Gravel,
Gout,
Arterio-Sclerosis,
Obesity.
Hors Concours, San Francisco Exhibition, 1915.
Price 5/- and 12/- per bottle.
Prepared at Chatelain's Laboratories, Paris. Obtainable from all Chemists, or direct, post free, from the British and Colonial Agents, HEPPELLS, Pharmacists, 164 Piccadilly, London W. Write for explanatory booklet.

1917

'To achieve beauty without make-up
by means of electricity
and gentle massage is the secret
of a beauty specialist.'

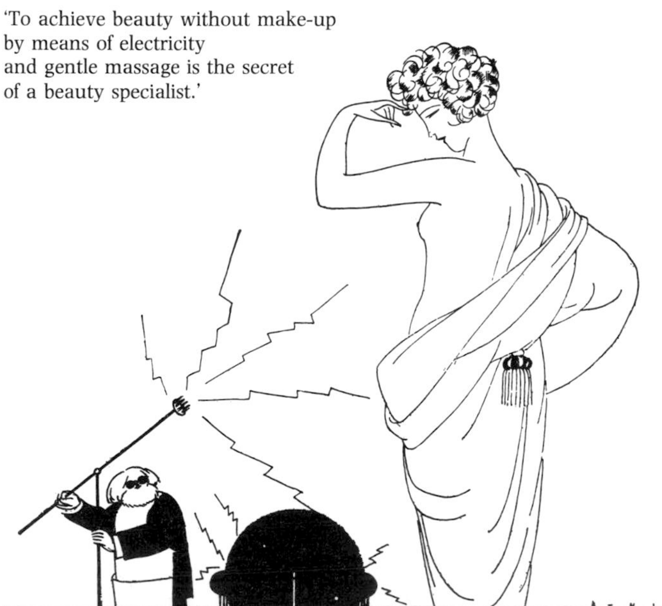

BENITO 1922

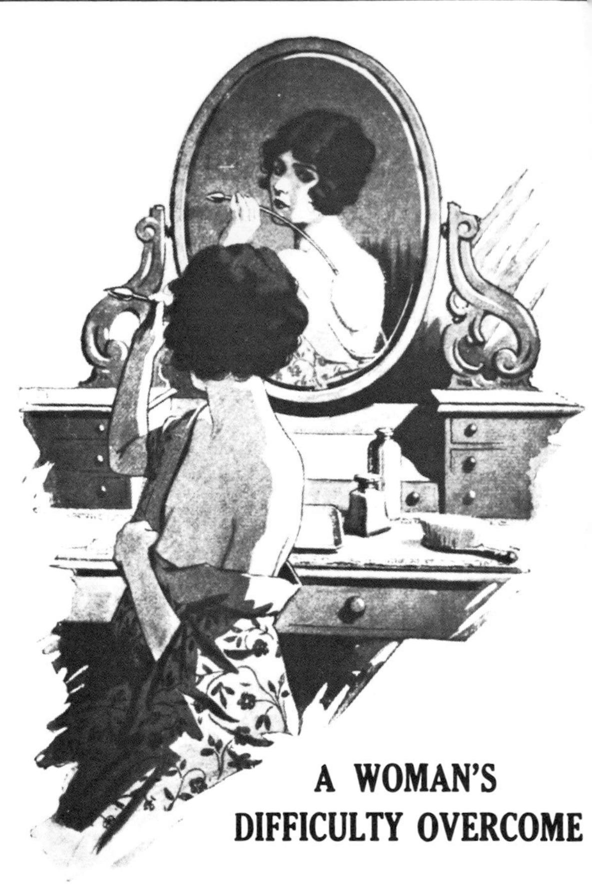

A WOMAN'S
DIFFICULTY OVERCOME

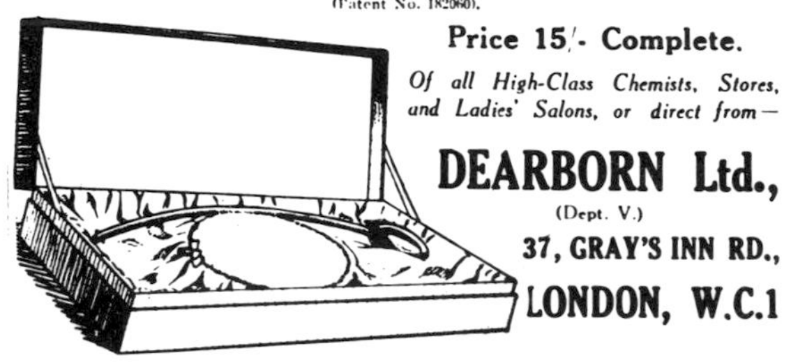

1922

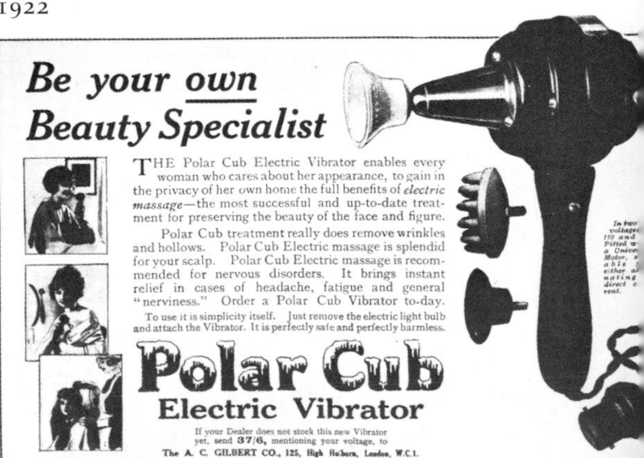

Be your own
Beauty Specialist
THE Polar Cub Electric Vibrator enables every woman who cares about her appearance, to gain in the privacy of her own home the full benefits of electric massage—the most successful and up-to-date treatment for preserving the beauty of the face and figure.
Polar Cub treatment really does remove wrinkles and hollows. Polar Cub Electric massage is splendid for your scalp. Polar Cub Electric massage is recommended for nervous disorders. It brings instant relief in cases of headache, fatigue and general "nerviness." Order a Polar Cub Vibrator to-day.
To use it is simplicity itself. Just remove the electric light bulb and attach the Vibrator. It is perfectly safe and perfectly harmless.
Polar Cub
Electric Vibrator
If your Dealer does not stock this new Vibrator yet, send 37/6, mentioning your voltage, to
The A. C. GILBERT CO., 125, High Holborn, London, W.C.1.

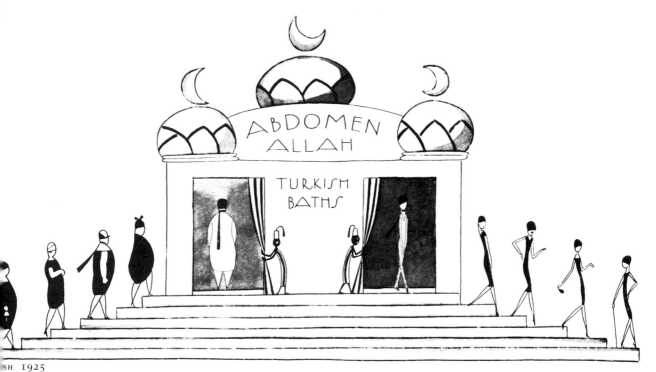

SH 1925

ntering the left hand portal of Abdomen Allah's fashionable aquarium, e see the portly female clientele on their way to take the waters, the eam bath, the hot room, the massage and other tortures prescribed by e terrible Turkish regime. Notice that the ladies resemble five of the ost upholstered ottomans in the Ottoman Empire. But wait . . .

Incredible as it may seem, the quintette of slim *Vogue* silhouettes, making their exit at the right, are the same monumental matrons who, at the left, occupied more than their full share of cubic space. The Turkish Bath has done it. Now they can face their modistes unashamed and slip into small size frocks without ignominy, shame, or rubber girdles.'

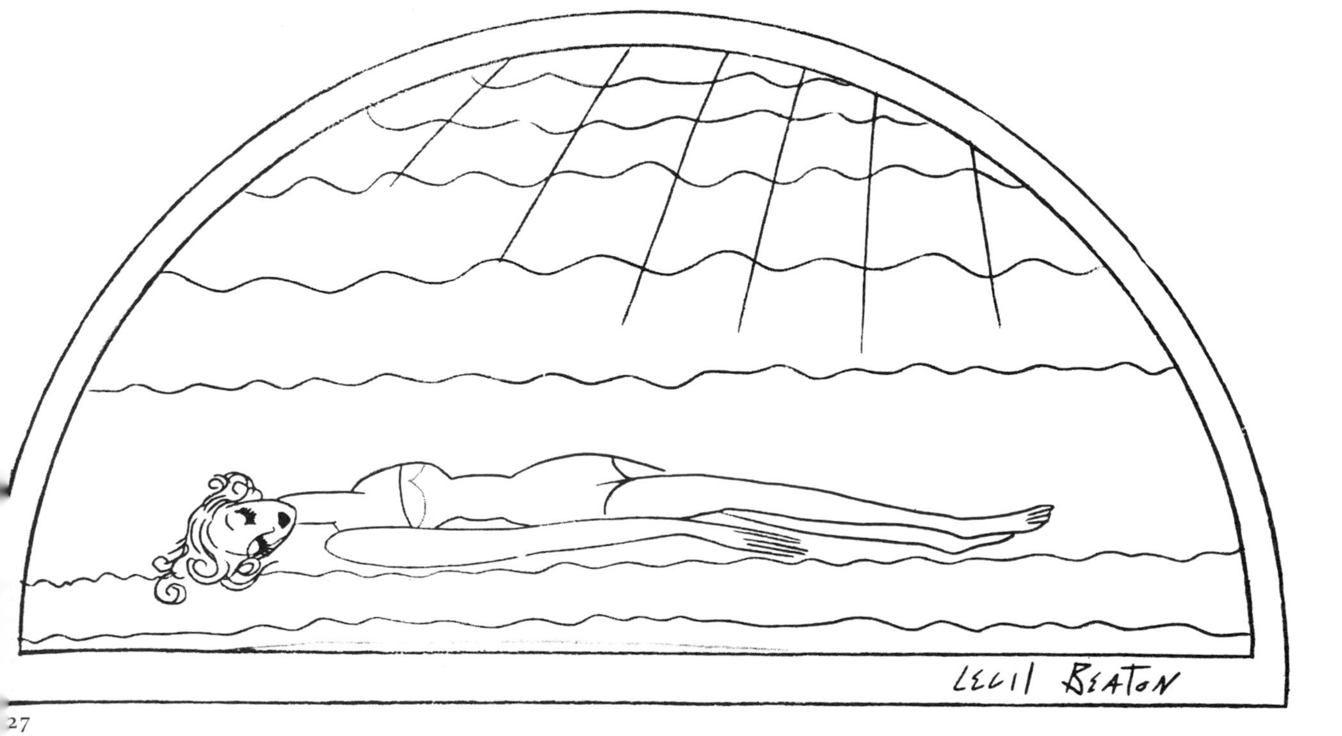

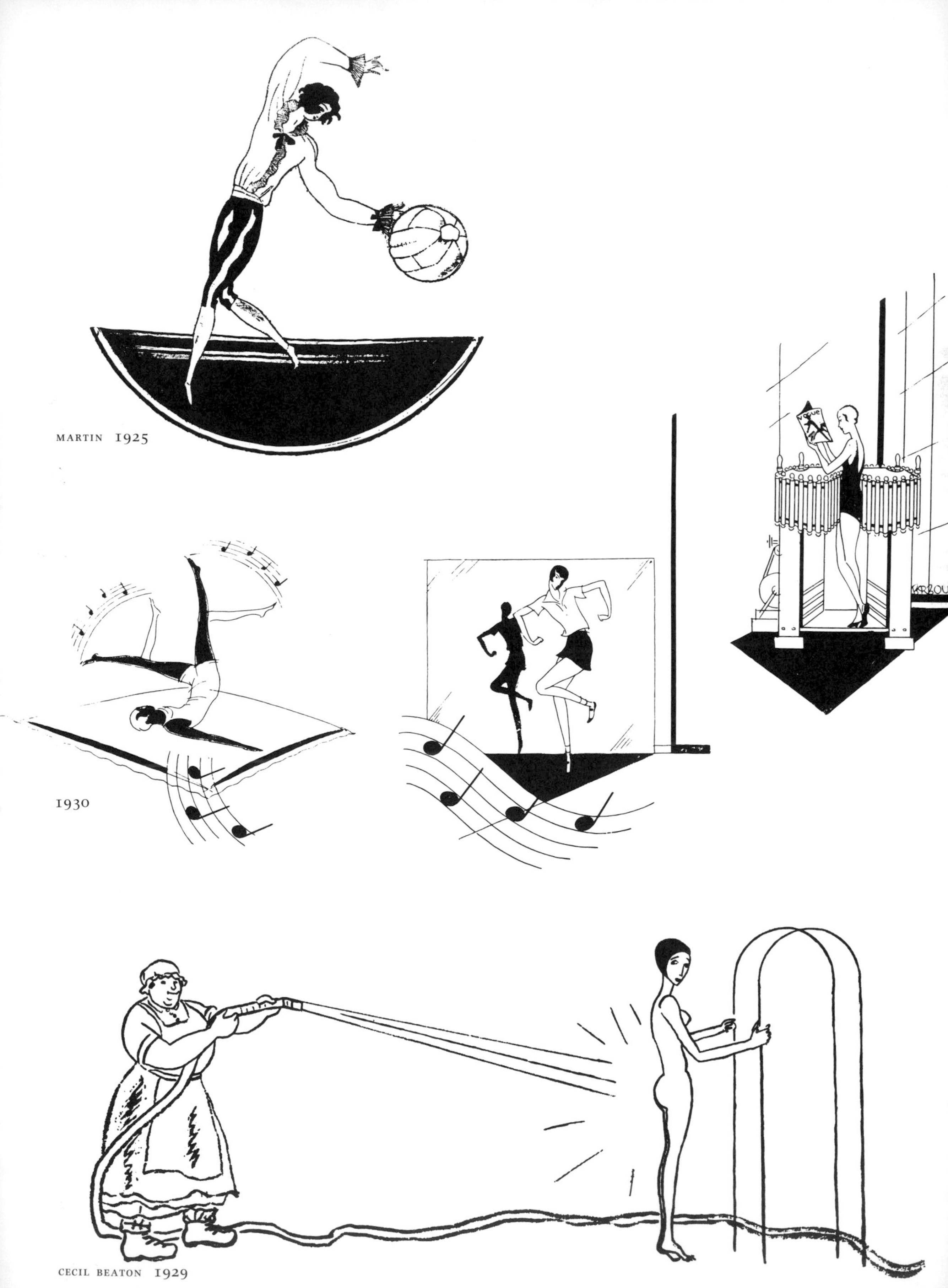

MARTIN 1925

1930

CECIL BEATON 1929

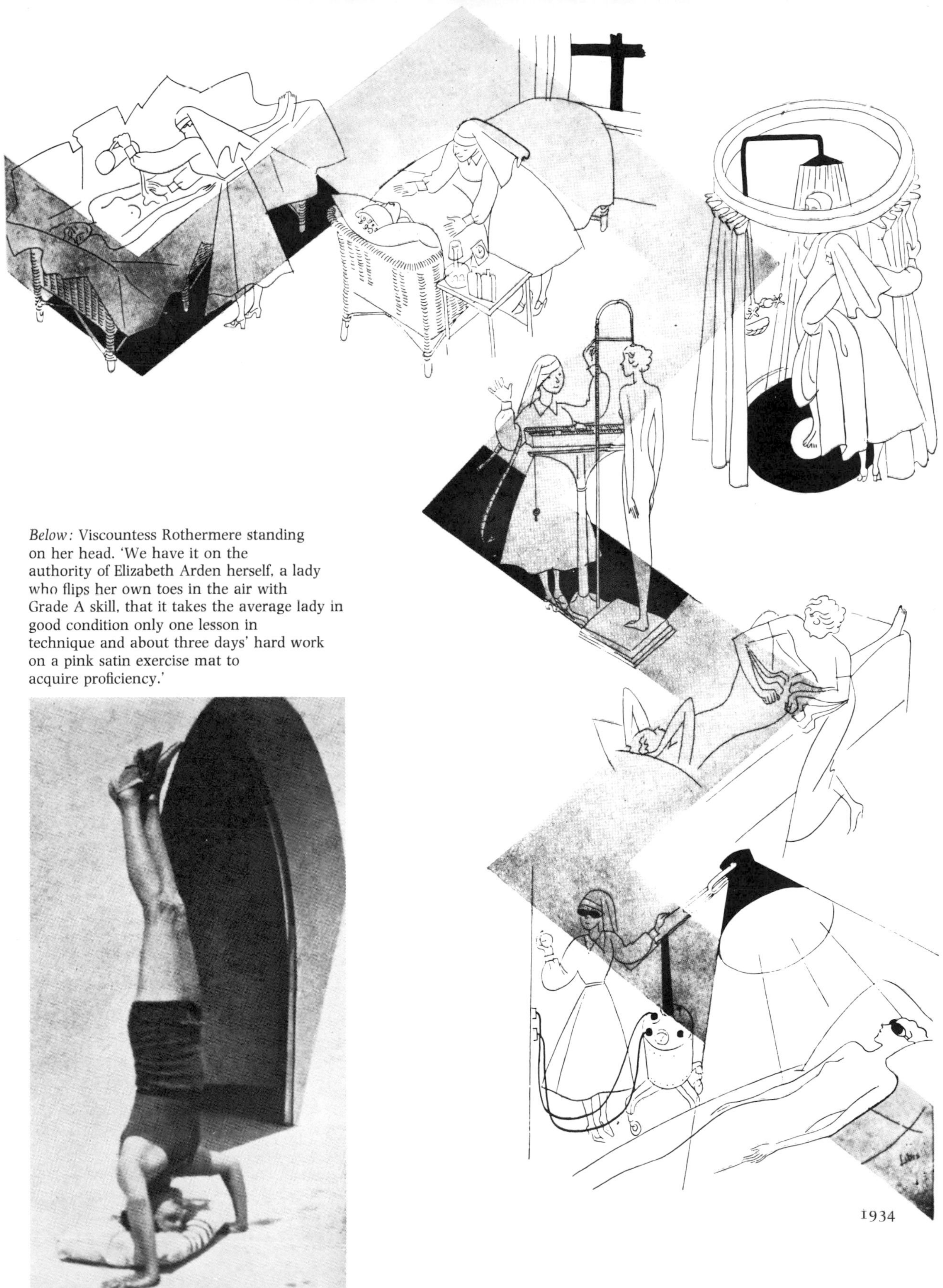

Below: Viscountess Rothermere standing on her head. 'We have it on the authority of Elizabeth Arden herself, a lady who flips her own toes in the air with Grade A skill, that it takes the average lady in good condition only one lesson in technique and about three days' hard work on a pink satin exercise mat to acquire proficiency.'

1934

1932

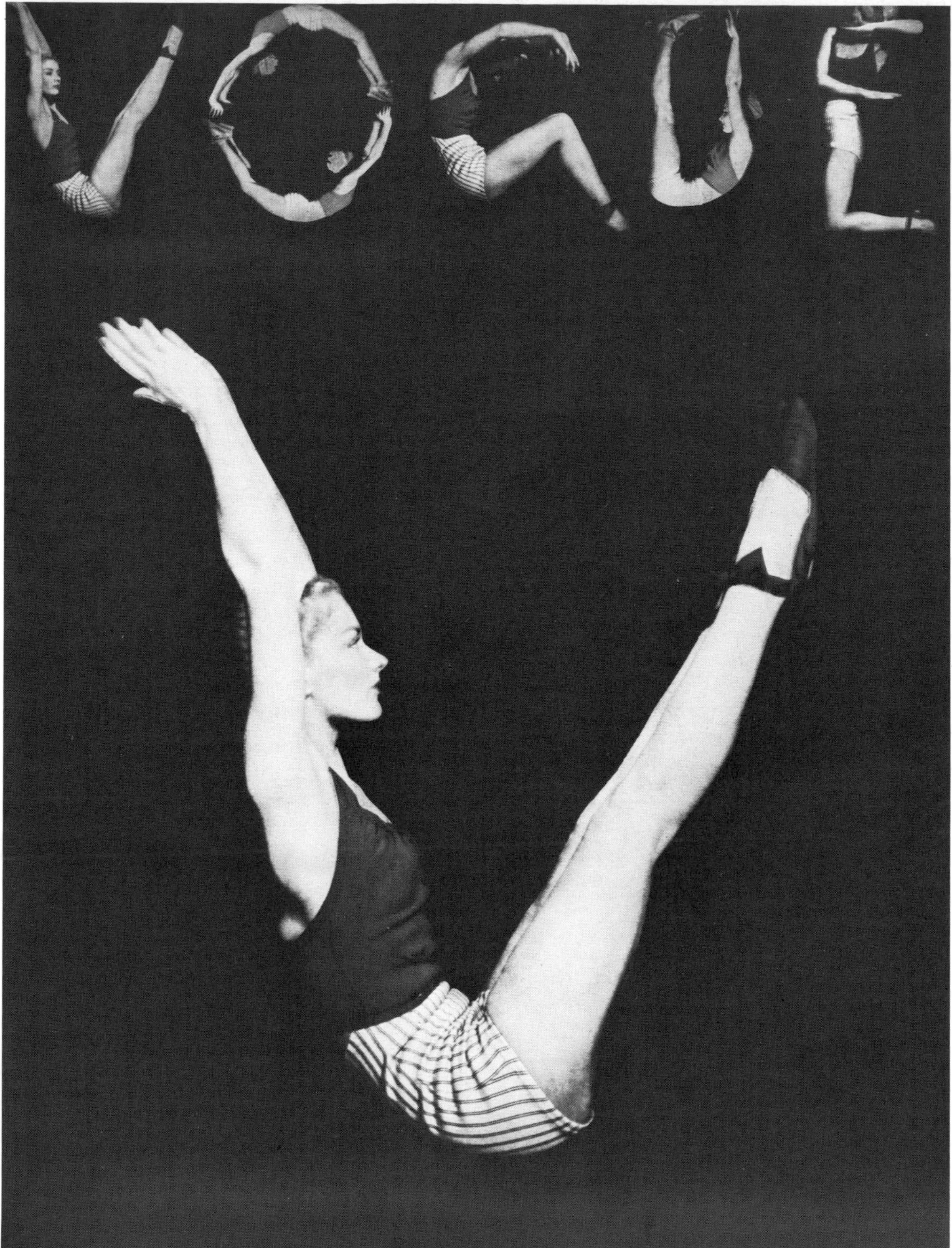

HORST 1940

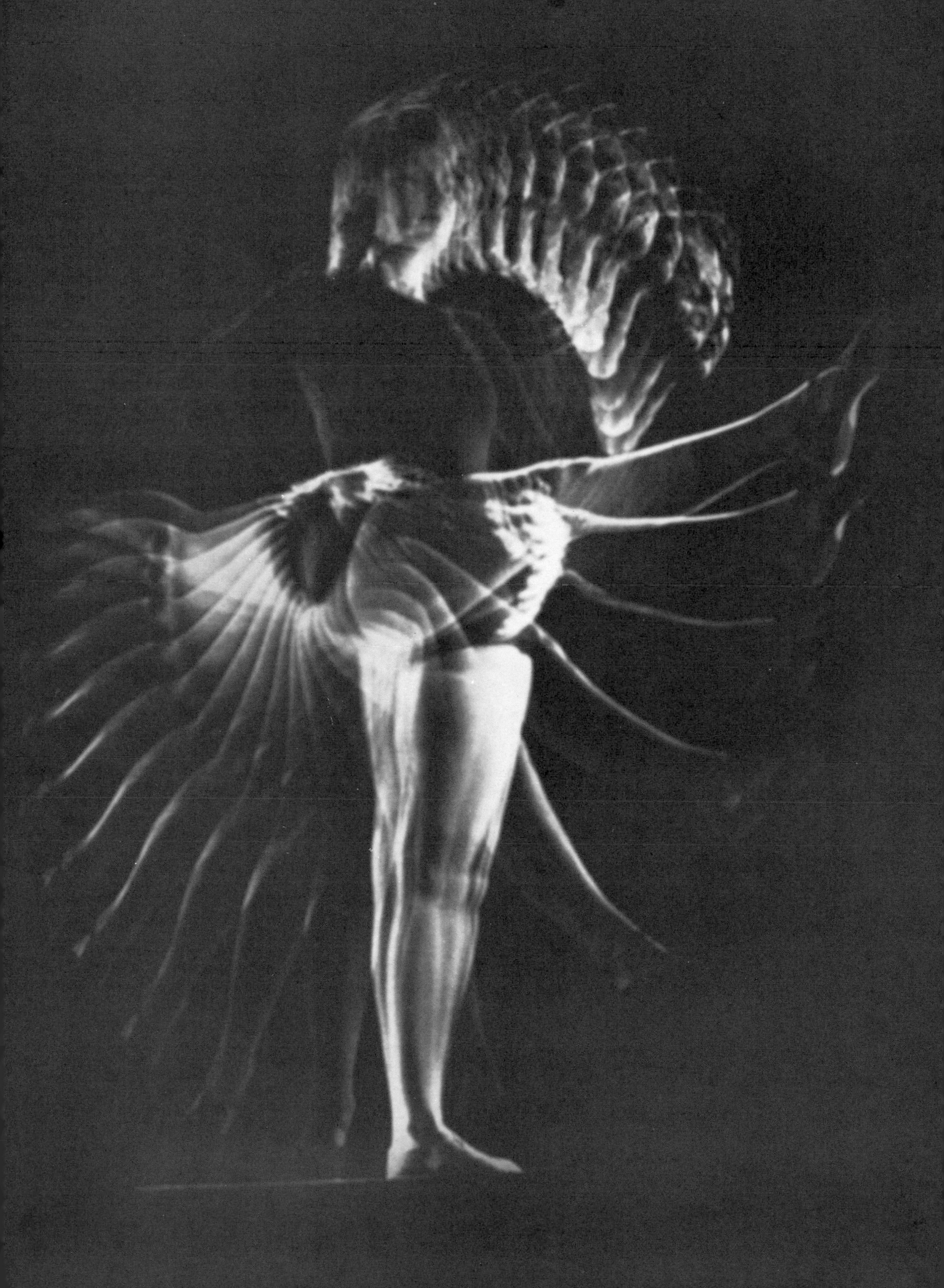

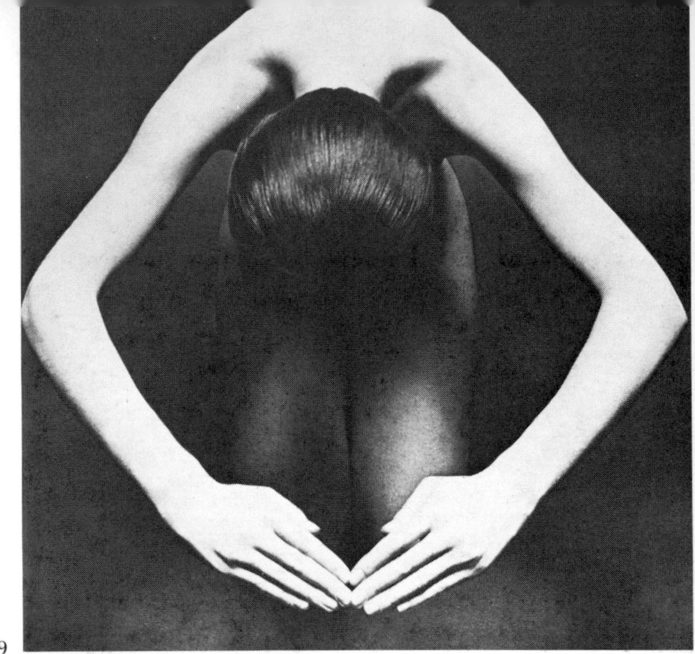

GUY BOURDIN 1969

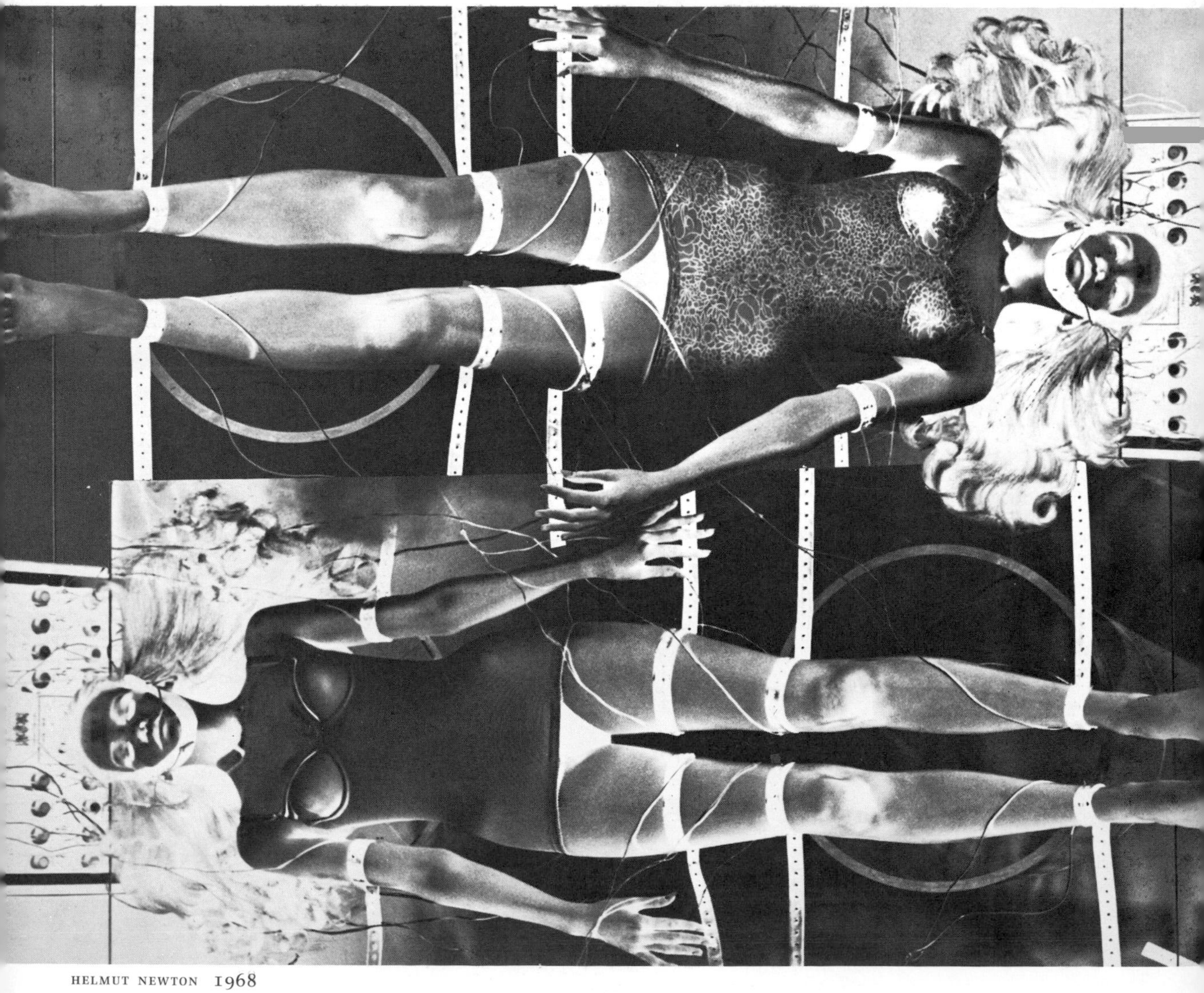

HELMUT NEWTON 1968

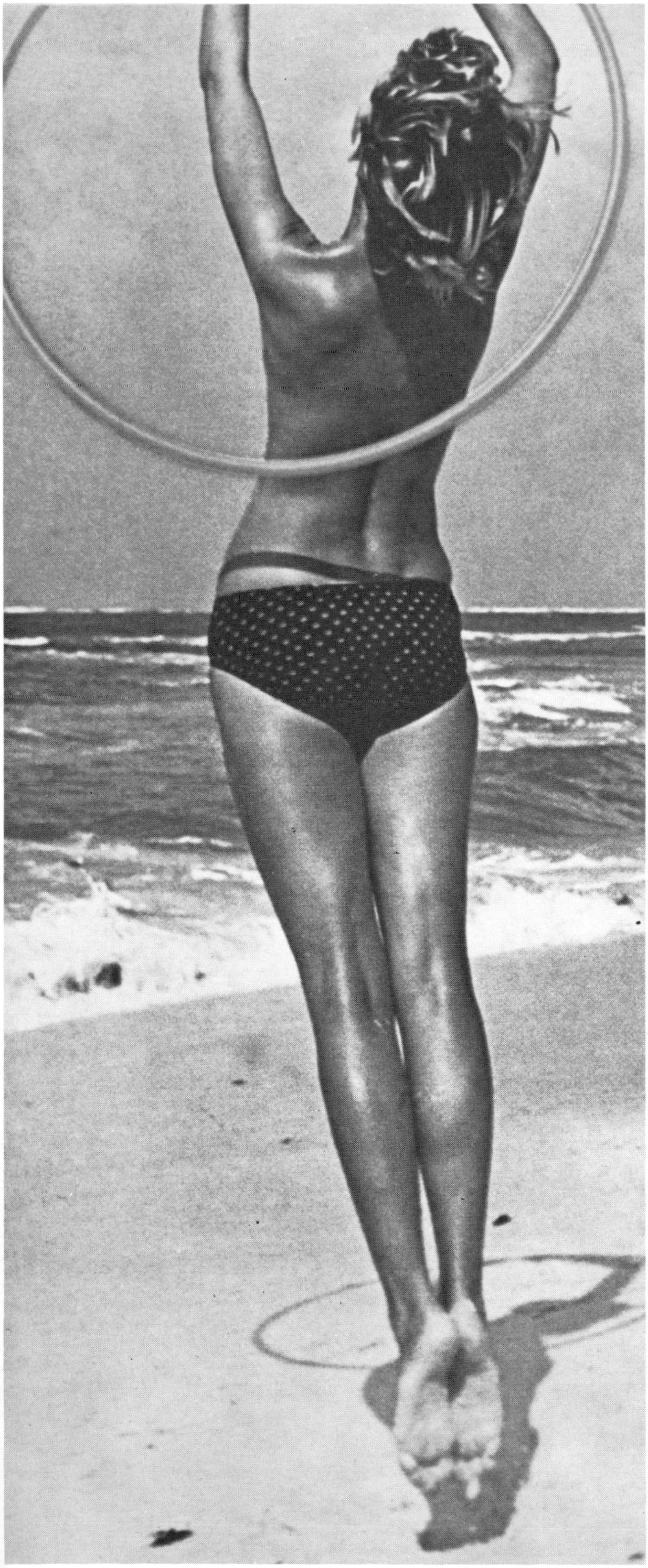

MIKE REINHARDT 1972

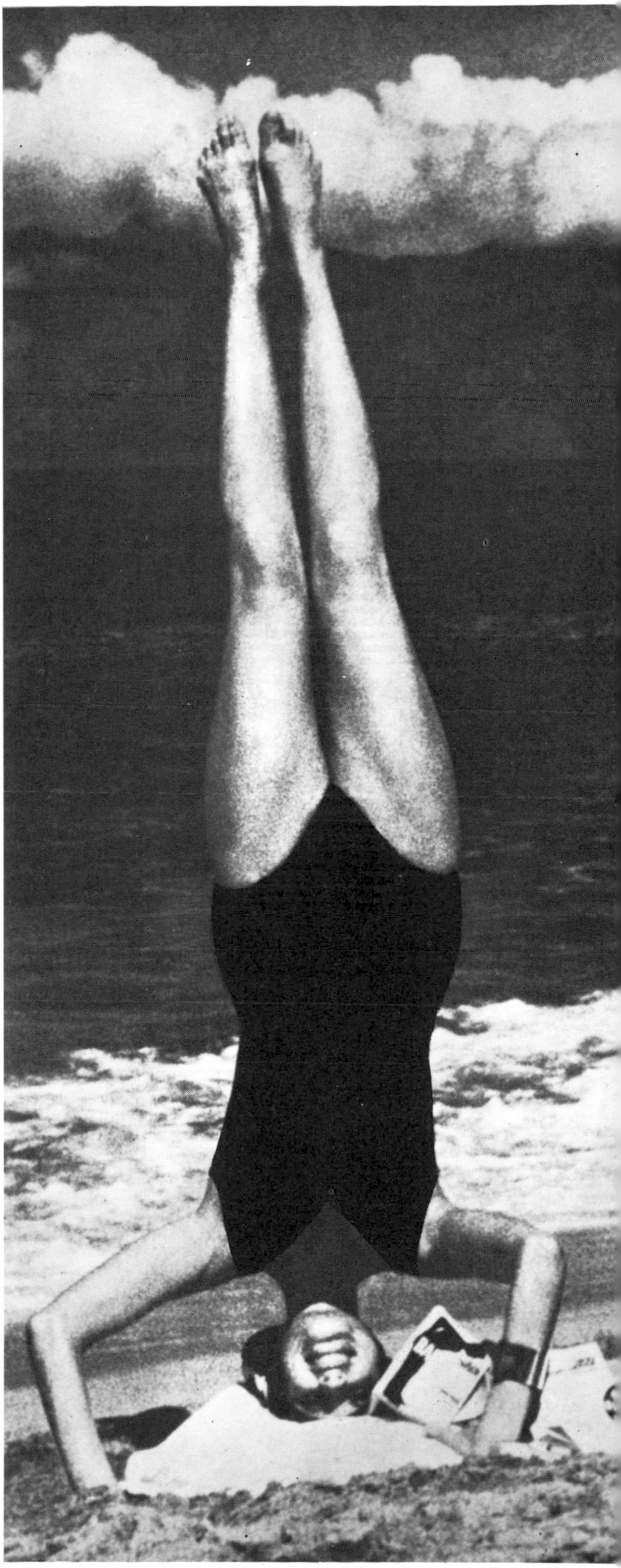

HELMUT NEWTON 1972

INDEX

The Scottish Islands

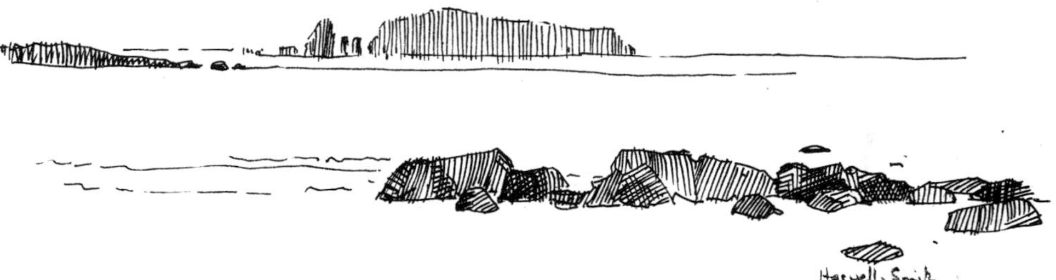

The Scottish

The bestselling guide to

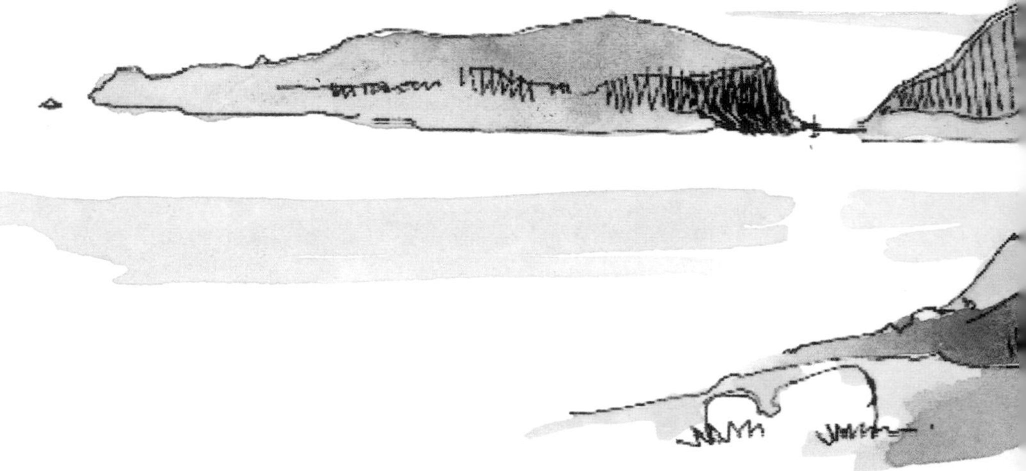

Islands

HAMISH HASWELL-SMITH

...every Scottish Island

FULLY REVISED EDITION

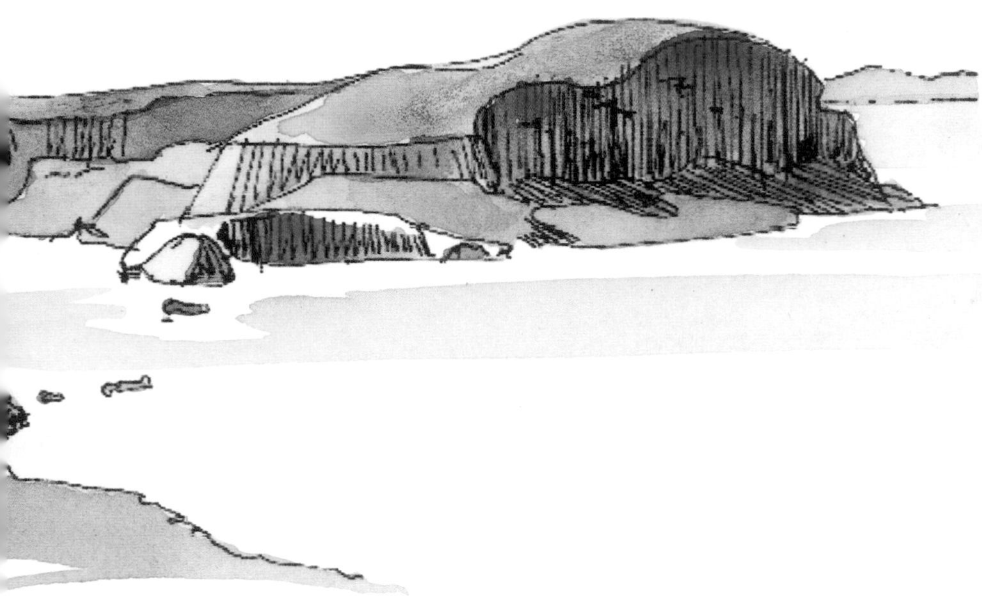

CANON GATE
Edinburgh · London · New York · Melbourne

First published in Great Britain
in 1996 by Canongate Books Ltd
14 High Street, Edinburgh EH1 1TE
Fully revised second edition 2004
Fully revised and updated 2008
1

ISBN 978 1 84767 277 3

British Library Cataloguing-in-Publication Data
A catalogue record for this book is available on
request from the British Library

Art Direction by James Hutcheson
Design and Layout by Barrie Tullett
Set in Photina MT and Gill Sans

To Jean

Author's Note

My original intention was merely to compile, for my personal satisfaction, a list of the Scottish islands equivalent to 'Munro's Tables of the 3000ft Mountains of Scotland' (published by the Scottish Mountaineering Trust). This factually interesting little book satisfies the aspirations of 'Munro-baggers' and I considered that, as someone who enjoyed landing on islands, to grade islands by size instead of mountains by height, would be an interesting exercise and serve me well.

It was during the long labour of calculation that I realised that, like most island-collectors, the pleasure of landing on 'new' territory becomes secondary to the desire to explore and appreciate the island for itself alone. The research became more and more absorbing as the years rolled by. My original simple statistical database of island names and areas grew into an amorphous mass of information from many sources. In the end I had to call a halt and try to return to the logical structure with which I began the quest.

I am only too aware that the information contained here will always be incomplete. Sometimes it has been abbreviated for reasons of space; more often the scarce facts have had to be wrested with difficulty from diverse sources. I have endeavoured to check them assiduously and where possible referred back to original records but, even so, I know there will be errors and omissions. If you are an island resident or owner, I apologise if I have omitted something of particular interest, and if you are a specialist (and in Scotland we are particularly fortunate in having experts in every conceivable field) your comments and corrections would be appreciated for the next edition.

It is quite astonishing how many of our islands were still populated a few decades ago and whose inhabitants are no longer easily traced. All their unrecorded wisdom will vanish with them and so, with every passing year, more and more of our common heritage is being forgotten or lost by neglect.

Edinburgh 1996

Since writing the above note in the first edition of this book, I have come to realise that it has been assumed that all the material needed to list our islands was already available. This was not the case. Because there was no exact and universally applied definition of an island there were two problems:

1) NO ONE KNEW HOW MANY SCOTTISH ISLANDS THERE WERE,

and there was

2) NO ACCURATE RECORD OF THE AREAS OF OUR ISLANDS.

This meant that, unlike Munro, who at least had contour maps showing all the separate regions which were above 3000ft and no need to calculate them, I had to start from scratch. And I had to solve these problems in sequence, i.e. until I had a definition I couldn't work out how many islands there were, and until I had established the individual islands I couldn't work out what their areas were. Needless to say, if there are any errors they are entirely mine.

Edinburgh 2008

Contents

Acknowledgements

This book would not have been possible without *Jandara* – a 41' Moody sloop – who, like every woman, has few faults and many virtues. She possesses four of us – a farmer, a baker, a quantity-surveyor, and me. Three of our wives are called Jean and one is called Ann so, by convoluted reasoning in kitchen Gaelic, her name derives from 'Jean-Ann-andara' – the second wife.

Our partnership has survived for more than twenty years and its success is probably due to our diverse personalities. The farmer, Craig Hutcheson, has a boyish sense of humour, a healthy appetite, and a considerable practical aptitude when he cares to apply it. He plays the 'daft laddie' to perfection but is nobody's fool. The baker, Ian Terris, is a business man and world traveller who wakens everyone at five in the morning and doesn't know the meaning of sotto voce. But he is a competent seaman, a genuine friend, and always steady and reliable in a crisis. Peter Crabb, the quantity-surveyor, is a meticulous handyman who has a steady and considered approach to every problem and a love of the great outdoors. Being 6'5" tall, he is also our spare mast. Peter shares my star-sign – if one accepts such nonsense – and coughs discreetly at our occasional minor divergences of opinion. My only comment on my own personality is to thank my partners for their indulgence.

I am fortunate that my partners share my enthusiasm for exploring islands and that my other sailing friends also accept the challenge wholeheartedly. Among the latter I must particularly mention Harry Holmes, an energetic Yorkshireman and erstwhile Commodore of the Royal Forth Yacht Club, and his wife Brenda, a marvellous cook among her many other attributes; George Steedman, a fellow architect, and steadfast crew on some memorable voyages; and my cousin, Dr Ronald Howie, who has recently taught me a thing or two.

We try to explore every island 'in depth' but conditions are sometimes difficult. A heavy swell and seaweed on the rocks can be a considerable hazard but a conquest doesn't 'count' unless one has truly landed, even if detailed exploration in such cases has to await the next favourable opportunity.

I would like to thank the many kind people who have been so generous with their help. In particular, I wish to record my appreciation for the invaluable information given to me by:

Kenneth John Smith of Earshader, Mrs Anna Mackinnon of Ardroil, Angus McLean of Brenish, Norman Buchanan and his son of Valtos, Uig, and D Murdie of Bernera, all of the Isle of Lewis; Donald Macdonald of Lingerbay, Isle of Harris; Donald MacKillop of Berneray, Sound of Harris; D J Campbell of Lochmaddy, Isle of North Uist; Dorota Rychlik of Vaila (No.11.10); Margaret Wilkes, Head of the Map Library of the National Library of Scotland, and members of staff; Dr David H Caldwell, National Museums of Scotland; the Census Division of the General Register Office of Scotland; Anne Taylor of Scottish Natural Heritage; Mary Miers of South Uist; Nancy Scott of Westray; E Mairi MacArthur (author of *Columba's Island*); Stephen P Newall DL LLD of Shuna (No.3.12); Alan C Millar of Tighnabruaich; Richard Fresson of the

CCC; Angus Duncan; R A Ingham Clark; Major B E Sykes; Dr John Holden; A S Halford-MacLeod of Mulag (No.8.14); Torquil Johnson-Ferguson of Lunga (No.2.11).

My sincere thanks also to:
Betty Kirkpatrick, Albert Morris, Norman G Masson, and Barbara MacLeod for their encouragement and friendly advice; Kenneth Mackenzie for his information on Scottish birdlife; the late Bobby Tulloch of Yell for his vast knowledge of Shetland, which he divulged so generously, and the late Norman MacCaig for his ready support and permission to include some lines from his poems.

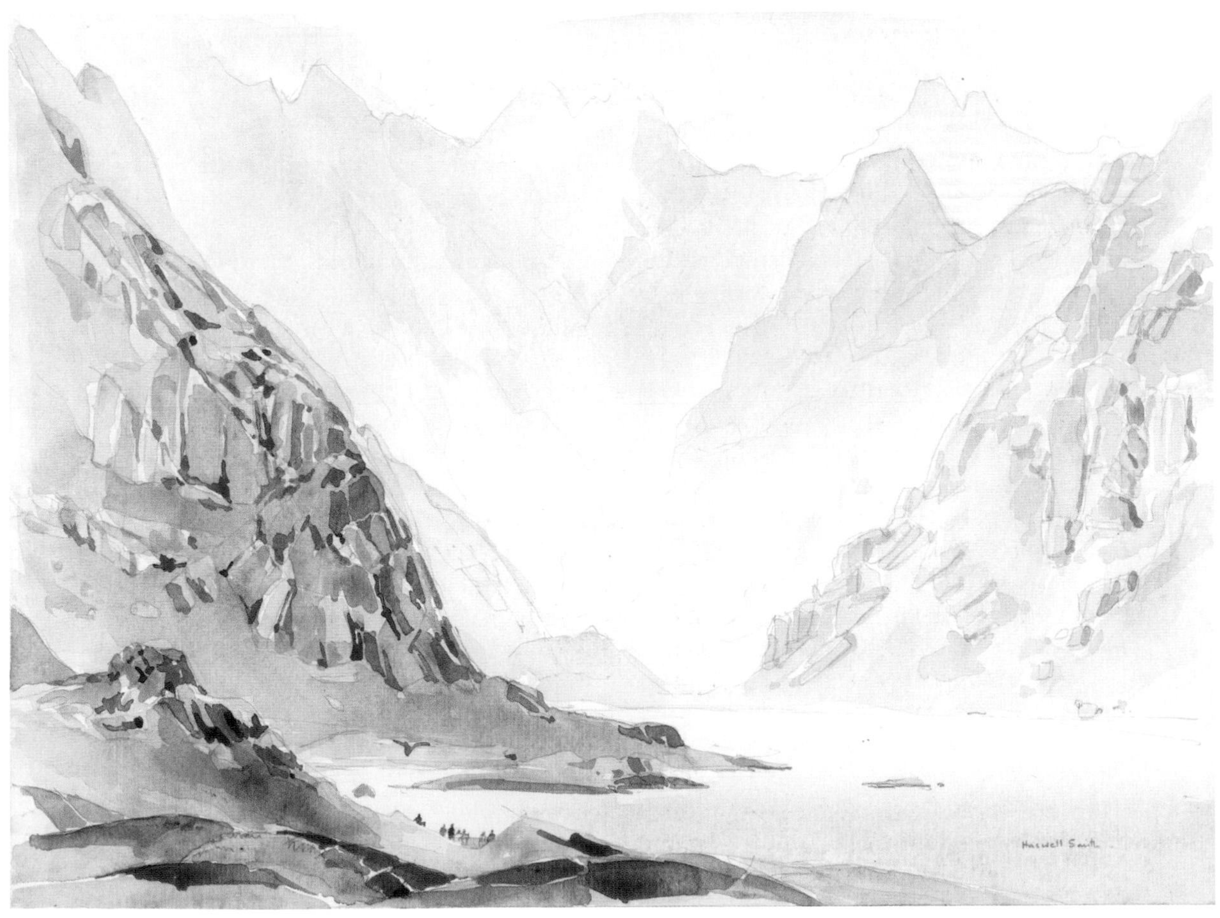

AWESOME LOCH CORUISK, SKYE

Preface

There are few parts of the world which possess such magic and mystery as the seas around Scotland. Some six thousand miles of contorted coastline (69% of the total United Kingdom coastline) create a wonderland of islands and mountains and rocks and stacks and secret inlets and remote, uninhabited places. This is an area of breathtaking beauty with a character formed not only by the proximity of mountains and sea but also by the complexity of the geography and the geology, of the climate and the social history. It is a serene yet chaotic landscape in which every isle has a distinct personality. Each is an individual entity with differences so remarkable that the mere crossing of a short stretch of water can be like visiting another continent.

What is the fascination of an island?

Why do we experience such a thrill at being surrounded by water, cut off from the rest of mankind, imprisoned on a miniature world? Is it because an island is of human scale, easy to comprehend, safe and defensible when the world beyond is big and terrifying? Who hasn't dreamed of being marooned on the proverbial desert island? For generations islands have been a theme of literature and poetry and, more recently, of radio and film. Utopia, Atlantis, *Robinson Crusoe, Treasure Island, Desert Island Discs* – to name a few. It is a long list.

I have found Scottish islands so intriguing that the lack of a ready source of information on them has been a great frustration. The sheer excitement of landing on – and exploring – another island can be tempered by having little fore-knowledge of what to look for and where to go. Is there an archaeological ruin worth seeing? – a cave worth visiting? – uncommon birdlife? It is the '– you mean to say you were in Venice and you didn't even see St Marks?!' syndrome. This is particularly true as the available time ashore is usually severely limited.

Reach for a book on Scottish islands – there are any number of excellent ones – and time after time the same subjects turn up: Mull, Arran, Lewis, Islay, mainland Orkney or Shetland (because they are large), Staffa (because of Fingal's Cave), Iona (for its history and mystery) . . . and so on: possibly thirty or forty islands in all.

But what about the rest?

What about Hellisay or Killegray? Fuday or Fuiay? Uyea or Wiay? Hascosay or Mingulay?

Scotland has 162 islands of forty hectares and over (i.e. approximately one hundred acres), a figure I arrived at after many months of measurement and classification of each and every separate land mass. My very restrictive rules of classification will be explained later but they don't include 'bridged' islands like Skye, or Seil, or Scalpay (Harris); they count the whole of the Uists and Benbecula as only one island; they exclude the hundreds of islands which are less than forty hectares (even islets like the Bass Rock and Staffa); and, yet, they still produce a list of *162 islands* to be described in greater detail and, hopefully, visited?

'Islandeering' isn't easy anywhere but Scottish islands present a particularly difficult, but exciting, challenge – arguably more difficult than the collection of mountains. Most of the large islands are well-served with transport and accommodation but it's a different matter for the smaller, or more remote, islands. Is there a place to land? Will the weather or tides permit a landing? Once having landed, how long dare one stay ashore? And what is the opportunity for exploration and getting to know the island's individual characteristics?

However, this is no reason not to take each island one at a time and still build up a handsome score. A few general statistics may highlight how easy it is to start. Of my 162 listed islands: sixty are still populated and many others have at least one part-time resident; forty-six have scheduled ferry services (and at least ten more provide informal services on request or by agreement); twenty-five have airstrips or airfields, and twenty-two have scheduled air services; most of the populated islands provide bed-and-breakfast, hostel accommodation, or campsites and twenty-three also provide hotel accommodation.

When this book was first published in 1996 I challenged anyone to land on every one of my list of 162 islands (what my islandeering friends have chosen to call, in the Munro tradition, 'Haswells'). Islandeering isn't always easy as some islands demand a combination of ideal tidal and weather conditions, confidence, perseverance, agility and a head for heights.

The problem with writing about remote and uninhabited places is that doing so can destroy just what we find so attractive. I remember meeting a couple on an island visit who were from the south coast of England. 'We sail and explore these waters every year,' they said, 'but we don't tell anyone about it. These are secret places, far away from people. Why attract the crowds?'

I understand this viewpoint, yet I am taking a calculated risk that newcomers will visit these secret places, not just to chalk up another conquest, but because they have poetry in their souls and a true love of islands; that they will appreciate that it takes only one castaway beer can or cigarette packet to destroy the next visitor's pleasure; and that they will understand that it is common courtesy to respect the privacy of the island's inhabitants, avoid causing damage, and when possible ask permission to land and explore.

Before I could start collating information about islands I was faced with a difficult problem of definition.

What, exactly, is an island? The dictionary says it is 'a mass of land, but not a continent, surrounded with water'. That defines maximum size, but do remember that size changes with every ebb and flow of the tide. The 1861 Census defined an island as 'any piece of solid land surrounded by water which affords sufficient vegetation to support one or two sheep, or is inhabited by man'. That is not a very scientific definition for minimum size – if one is needed – but it again confirms that an island must be surrounded by water. But does this mean permanently surrounded by water? What if there is a linking sandbank when the tide is out? The definition also seems to allow a bridge or tunnel connection whilst definitely precluding a causeway because that would interrupt the surrounding ring of water.

In the end I had to arrive at my own definition: *An island is a piece of land or group of pieces of land which is entirely surrounded by seawater at Lowest Astronomical Tide and to which there is no permanent means of dry access.*

This satisfies my belief that the quality of insularity requires isolation.

In other words, if you can walk across to a piece of land without wading through seawater, even if it is only at the time of the lowest of tides, then that piece of land is not an island. And, similarly, land accessible by bridge, causeway or tunnel is not an island.

Likewise, if a number of 'islands' are accessible to each other at low water, or by bridge, tunnel or causeway, they should be considered one, single island.

By this definition the Uists, Benbecula, Berneray, Eriskay and their many adjoining satellites ('drying' or 'tidal' islands) count as one large island. And Skye, with a bridge to the mainland, no longer counts as an island. Although some, I know, will disagree with this definition because it may seem unduly restrictive, loosening the parameters leads to so many unresolvable situations that the exercise becomes pointless. Take a close look at the coast of Benbecula to see what I mean.

One requirement in my definition, however, is quite arbitrary: 'seawater'. I have restricted myself to ocean islands. There are plenty of Scottish islands which meet the above definition in every other respect but happen to be surrounded by fresh loch or river water. Maybe, someone someday will want to list them. My only excuse for not doing so is that there is already more than a lifetime's interest in the seaward islands.

Format and Overview

The Scottish islands have been divided into twelve geographical areas or sections.

Every island of forty or more hectares in area (i.e. approximately 100 acres or more) has been separately classified and tabulated.

On each island map:

> The sea area is overlaid with a grid of 5-cable squares (i.e. half a nautical mile or nearly one kilometre) to allow instant comparison of scale and distance.
>
> Darker blue colour indicates approximate sea areas of less than 2m depth or areas of potential risk.
>
> Grey-blue colour indicates tidal areas of rock, sand, or foreshore which cover at high water.
>
> The scale shows kilometres and statute miles (– not nautical miles).

Every piece of land which is less than the minimum area for classification but which could still justifiably be called an island or an islet is at least mentioned together with any information of interest. If there is a lot of interesting information

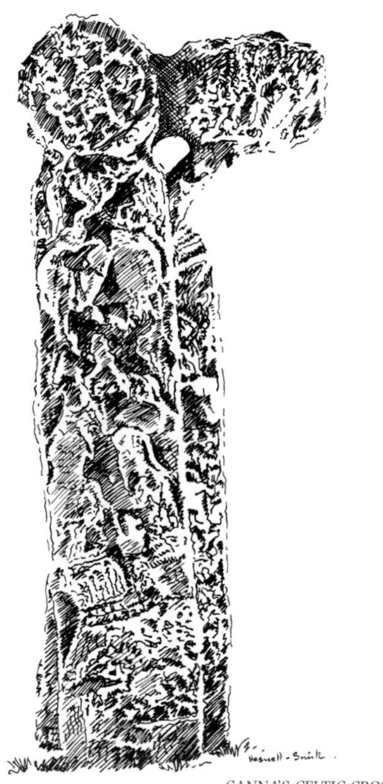

CANNA'S CELTIC CROSS (4.4)

then this is either given in the introduction to the section or put in a separate appendix. Occasionally, some of the 'drying' or 'tidal' islands have also merited this treatment.

Information for each of the 162 classified islands has been presented in the following manner:

NAME
There were four main language groups from which Scottish place-names have evolved:

> *Brythonic (or P-Celtic).* This was probably an older Celtic language than Gaelic. It was spoken by the ancient Britons of the Clyde valley and the Picts may also have spoken it, or a language closely allied to it. It is represented today by the Welsh, Cornish and Breton languages.
>
> *Gaelic (or Q-Celtic).* This is the Celtic language still spoken today in Scotland and Ireland, although in many different forms. It originated in Ireland, came over with the Scottish settlers and Christian missionaries, and by the 9th century was spoken in much of Scotland.
>
> *Norse.* Many Viking invaders settled in the Western Isles bringing their language with them and these islands eventually came within the dominion of Norway in or about the 9th century. Even after the Lord of the Isles took control, the Norse language lingered on for a considerable time. The Orkney and Shetland Islands had been part of Norway from a much earlier date and only became part of Scotland when they were annexed by the Scottish Crown in 1471. The vast majority of Scottish island names end in '-ay', which means 'island' (-øy in Norse) and tends to illustrate the strong historical influence of this language.
>
> *English.* Although English (or a Scottish form of it) is the language of most of Scotland today, having been widely established since the 12th century, there are areas of the Western Isles where Gaelic is still the native tongue and the language of choice. The English language was late in reaching the islands and it has had very little influence on most Scottish island names.

Many of the Western Isles have a local Gaelic name as well as the normal Norse-derived or Anglicised-Gaelic name. The Gaelic names are usually, but not always, closely related to the common-usage name given on the Ordnance Survey maps. I have for simplicity given only the 'Ordnance Survey' name (with occasional necessary corrections such as Rum instead of Rhum) but the Gaelic or Norse name is sometimes referred to in the notes on derivation.

The following abbreviations have been (loosely) applied:

B	Brythonic	E	English
EI	Early Irish	G	Gaelic
OE	Old English	S	Scottish
Sc	Scandinavian		
ON	Old Norse, Norse, Norn.		

PRONUNCIATION

In a few cases pronunciation is given in square brackets after a name. There are wide variations so this is no more than a very rough guide to normal-usage.

The following simple key has been used:

Pronunciation of Vowels

ë=th**e**, moth**er**	o=l**o**t
a=s**a**t	u=h**u**t
a:=f**a**ther	oa=b**oa**t
ay=d**ay**	oo=sch**oo**l
e=f**e**d	aw=cr**aw**l
ee=w**ee**k	ow=f**ow**l
i=fit	a-oo=as **ow** but longer
Y=**i**sle or b**y**	oy=b**oy**

oe=approximately French **oe**ufs or German G**oe**the

Pronunciation of Consonants

Most consonants similar to the English but for Gaelic pronunciation there are the following approximations:

s=**s**ee	b=nearly **p**
g=**g**et but nearly **k**et	d=nearly **t**
ch=German Ba**ch** or i**ch**	l=variable
gh=as **ch** but voiced	

When an island's name ends in '-ay' the ending is often pronounced either as [-ay] or as [-ë]. For example, Berneray is either Berneray [-ay] or Bernera [-ë], and usually the latter. This may have originated because the Old Norse '-øy' was a sound which was neither [-ay] nor [-ë].

An exception is Islay which is always [Y-lë], and never [Y-lay].

MAP REFERENCES

References are given for the Landranger series of maps at a scale of 1:50,000 (2cm to 1km) and the Explorer series at a scale of 1:25,000 (4cm to 1km), both published by the Ordnance Survey and readily available. References are also given for the applicable Admiralty Charts.

AREA

Shakespeare defined England as 'this scepter'd isle . . . this precious stone set in a silver sea, which serves it . . . as a moat defensive'. This is inspiring stuff, but untrue because the moat is interrupted when it reaches Scotland. England is not an island and nor is Scotland. Britain is an island.

Scotland is for our purposes here, the mainland. It has an overall area of roughly 4,800,000 hectares (30,000 square miles).

How big is an island? As the tide goes in and out, an island varies in size, which leads to many wild suppositions and few hard facts. So, once again, a definition is required but the requirement here is different from the definition of an island given in the Preface. The part of the island that matters is the part that is more-or-less always dry land. Quoting an overall area which included vast tracts of sand, mud and rocks only accessible at low tide would not be realistic. So I have come up with an arbitrary restriction:

An island's area is the total surface area lying above sea-level at Mean High Water Springs.

I have used averaged planimeter readings to estimate the area of each and every island within its MHWS perimeter as there is no consistent record elsewhere. With digitalised map data it will soon be possible to program a computer to provide this information. In the meantime I have been as accurate as possible but I certainly do not plead infallibility!

The tables include every Scottish island (or linked group of islands) which totals forty hectares or more in size. Not only is this a nice round figure, as forty hectares is roughly equivalent to one hundred old-fashioned acres, but if this limit is lowered the number of islands requiring inclusion grows rapidly out-of-control. The disadvantage in being so definitive is that it leads to the omission of some very small islands which are of notable interest: Staffa for instance. Such islets have therefore been included as appendices or within the foreword to the relevant Section.

Where applicable the areas of small tidal islands have been included in the total area for the main island even where this is not specifically mentioned.

HEIGHT
I have included a separate table of heights for interest. The Admiralty and the Ordnance Survey use different sea-level data to suit their differing requirements and even these can change as surveying techniques improve. For example my old edition of the Admiralty Pilot quotes Holy Island as 312.4m in height, the latest Admiralty metric chart shows 311m height whilst the latest edition of the Ordnance Survey gives 314m as the correct height. I have used the most up-to-date Ordnance Survey heights for consistency. There is, in any case, a large margin of error as all the heights are in round-figure metres without decimal fractions.

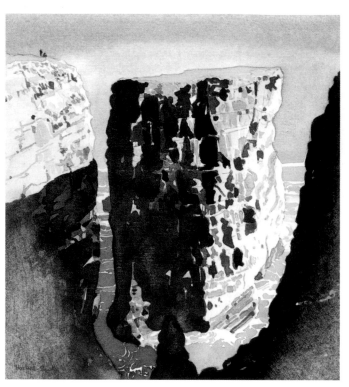

THE GREAT STACK OF HANDA (6.9)

OWNERSHIP
Some islands have been under one ownership for generations but many change hands with astonishing frequency.

Islands are often bought on impulse. They come on the market. The sun is shining, the seas are calm. This brings out three main categories of buyer: those who buy, visit a few times, intend to return, but never do; those who are hooked and change their entire lifestyle to suit the island; and those who get bored and quickly trade on to the next impulsive dreamer.

As there is a fairly quick turnover of some Scottish islands it is impossible to keep up to date on ownership. Furthermore, some islands are bought relatively incognito under a company name or that of a bank, or even as an unspecified small part of a large estate. However, ownership is obviously of interest for a variety of reasons and I have tried to establish it where I can. As the information has come from a variety of sources its accuracy cannot be guaranteed.

POPULATION
Historic figures – pre-1830 – have been gleaned from a number of sources such as travellers' accounts and old gazetteers. These are therefore uncertain and unreliable. More recent figures are taken from the ten-yearly National Census.

Some of the small 'uninhabited' islands are still occupied occasionally during the summer by herdsmen or fishermen or, in a very few cases, by an owner.

GEOLOGY
Although matters of individual interest have been covered in the text a general history of island formation gives a better overall picture. Most of the life-forms of today only appeared on the islands after the last ice-age, a mere 10,000 years ago. Prior to this, island development was almost entirely a geological phenomenon.

The First Three Thousand Million Years. . .
About 2500 million years ago, in an area of the earth which is now the far South Atlantic, there was a large slab of proto-continent. The Earth was no longer molten but its crust was still hot and in a state of violent geological upheaval. Great tectonic plates ground against each other and parts of them, often composed of common rocks rich in quartz and feldspar and mica, were forced deep down beneath the crust and subjected to enormous pressures and intense heat. The rocks folded and melted and twisted, separated into layers and were intruded by other igneous rocks. After a long time the activity slowly

subsided and the metamorphosis was complete. The reconstituted rock started to cool down, taking æons to do so, and forming a coarsely crystalline structure. We call this rock – gneiss (pronounced, nice [nYs]. It comes from an old German word meaning 'sparkling').

Through most of the subsequent 2500 million years the gneiss stayed deep beneath the crust, almost undisturbed, until it surfaced in comparatively recent times in the middle of the Outer Hebrides (**North Uist**, **Benbecula** and part of **South Uist**). This partially explains why the rocks there, although ancient, look so freshly scrubbed and clean: they have been kept under wraps until now. They have no fossils because they were formed before there was any recognisable life on earth.

There was a further similar period of upheaval in an adjacent part of the proto-continent about 2000 million years ago. This created gneiss of a different composition which forms the rest of the Outer Hebrides and patches of the Inner Hebrides. It is generally referred to as Lewisian gneiss.

The chunk of proto-continent was on the move, sliding slowly over the Earth's mantle in a northerly direction. By some 800 million years ago it had reached the latitude of South Africa. It had an upland region (which was eventually to become part of Greenland) eroded by rivers which spread alluvial deposits over a plain and into a shallow sea. These deposits built up increasing layers of red and grey sandstones, conglomerates, and shales. They are to be found today in the Torridon district of Wester Ross after which they have been named. Micro-fossils show that plankton and minute primitive life-forms were present in the shallow sea. Islands such as **Handa**, the **Summer Isles**, **Scalpay**, **Soay**, and parts of **Skye**, **Rum** and **Raasay** have all been sculpted from this dull red Torridonian sandstone.

The shallow sea grew and became the Cambrian Sea and the land which contained Scotland and its islands sank beneath it and lay there for 150 million years. During this time the north-western seashore suffered further deformation and metamorphosis due to the vast weight of some five kilometres thickness of sand and mud which was deposited over it. Siltstone became schist, mudstone became slate, limestone became marble and quartz sandstones became quartzites. The crushing and overlapping of strata formed a zone which runs from the north coast of Sutherland to the Sleat peninsula on **Skye** and forced outcropping on **Jura**, **Islay** and in the **Shetland Isles**. There were small outcrops on **Arran**, **Gigha**, **Skye** and **Mull** and, possibly, **Colonsay**. Much of Jura still has 5 kilometres thickness of quartzite which was laid down at this time in the form of clean river sand. Large extrusions of granite also occurred, particularly in Shetland and the Ross of Mull.

During at least one stage, while still far south of the Equator, the land and sea were covered with ice which deposited a bed of glacial boulders. Part of this bed can be clearly seen today at Port Askaig on **Islay**.

The remorseless northern movement of the plate of proto-continent continued until, about 490 million years ago, it came up against another rigid plate. The collision squeezed up a colossal mountain range which equalled the present-day Andes in size. This was the Caledonian Mountain Chain. It extended across the continental slab from the area which was to become Scandinavia, through Scotland and Greenland, into Newfoundland and southwards down the east coast of North America. Only remnants of this chain still exist, as erosion, continental drift and old age have steadily worn it down so that it no longer has the height and grandeur of the more recently formed mountain ranges – the Himalayas, the Andes and the Alps.

As the sliding plate approached the equator the violent upheavals caused by the collision waned, although volcanic activity was widespread. A huge lake stretched over the area of the future Orkneys and Caithness, sometimes extending as far north as Shetland. Layers of sand and limey mud were deposited in this lake forming sandstone strata. Fossils in the sandstone show that the lake was well stocked with fish. This Old Red Sandstone, as it is known, is particularly thick on **Hoy**, forming sea cliffs 350m high. The Old Red Sandstone of the Old Man of Hoy sits on top of a layer of volcanic ash and basalt.

A split in the plate similar to the San Andreas Fault in California started to form at this time, part of which eventually became the Great Glen.

About 350 million years ago the plate crossed the equator. Desert sand was compressed into sandstone on **Arran**. There was volcanic activity along an incipient rift zone forming between Great Britain, Norway and Denmark, which was eventually to become the North Sea. The North

Atlantic started to open up, causing a number of rifts, one of which started to split the British Isles away from Greenland and North America. As the gap between Greenland and Europe opened up at the rate of about 2cm per year there was intense igneous activity down the west coast of Scotland. Vast quantities of basalt lava poured out of fissures and volcanoes and piled up at intervals along the centre line between the two plates. This is still going on today but the centre of activity has now moved over to Iceland.

Basaltic lava poured out and rapidly cooled on **Canna**, **Eigg**, **Muck**, **Skye**, **Raasay** and **Mull**. On Mull the lava layer is 1.8 kilometres thick! As the magma reached the surface it cooled fairly quickly forming the well-known columns to be seen at their best on **Staffa** or the **Shiant Isles**. Other activity became concentrated around intrusive centres on **Skye**, **Rum**, **Mull**, **Arran**, the **St Kilda** group and **Rockall**. These centres often have nearly circular outlines of 10–15km diameter. Most of them are of gabbro and peridotite, but some are of granite. Coarse crystalline gabbro is formed from magma which has cooled slowly deep in the earth's crust. Other intrusions into cracks were later eroded to form dykes, stone 'walls' which can look almost man-made and maintain a constant thickness over long distances. There are dykes crossing Mull which continue all the way to the north-east coast of England.

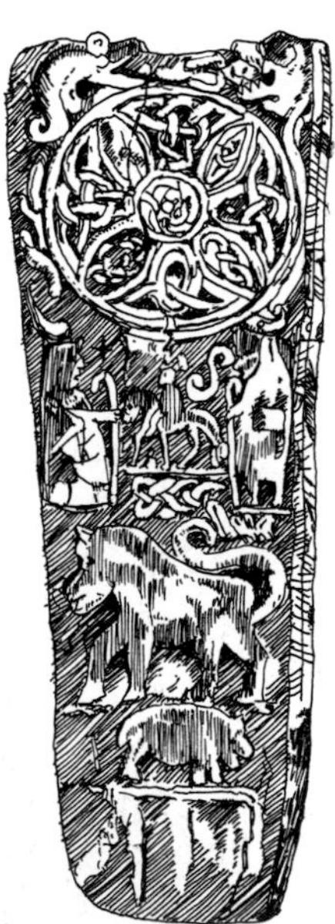

THE BRESSAY STONE (11.8)

All this violent volcanic activity died down about fifty-five million years ago as the fault centres moved elsewhere. It was at this time that another plate collision started the formation of the Alps in Europe, which tended to uplift Scotland.

For most of geological time the earth has been ice-free, even at the poles. There have been three major exceptions. There was the Ice Age in Precambrian times, which incidentally formed the boulder bed on Islay. Then there was an Ice Age during the Carboniferous period, but as Britain was near the equator she was unaffected. It is the most recent Ice Age which has had a profound influence. Ice sheets formed over the whole country, and glaciers carved out many features in the landscape. For example, Loch Coruisk on Skye was gouged out to a depth of 30m below present sea-level.

The last glaciation finished about 15,000 years ago, a mere blink of the eye in geological time. The immense weight of ice had squeezed the land downwards. When it melted the land rebounded raising beaches and sea-caves far above sea level. Particularly on **Jura**, but throughout the Inner Hebrides, the effect of this change of level is very obvious. It is as though a giant has pulled the plug and partly drained the sea. The same effect is not to be seen in the Outer Hebrides, nor Orkney as very little ice covered these areas.

HISTORY. . . or the Last Ten Thousand Years

After the great glaciers of the last Ice Age had receded about 15,000 years ago and while Britain was still linked to the European land-mass, the forests moved north with the improving climate. Man followed and about 8000BC small Mesolithic kinship groups of hunters, fishers and food-gatherers settled in the area south of Oban. They spread from there to **Arran**, **Jura**, **Oronsay**, **Rum**, **Skye** and **Lewis**. Evidence of their settlements are to be found in shell heaps, and the remains of their tools – antler mattocks, harpoons and fish-hooks, stone hammers and flints. Although the number of settlers at this time must have been very small they left a remarkable range and variety of artefacts. These show possible cultural links with earlier relics from the Basque and Baltic regions.

About 4000BC immigrants arrived in Scotland in larger numbers. These were Neolithic farmers and fishermen. They were skilled seamen who brought their seed-grain, planted crops and kept domestic livestock. They spread up the west coast using the sea and lochs as their highway to the Great Glen, on through the Glen to the north-east and across the sea to **Orkney**. Later they reached **Shetland**. They were an intelligent and hard-working people and their way of life was so successful that they found time to build communal and religious structures. These became progressively more sophisticated. There were chambered cairns and communal tombs of a variety of types and complexity culminating in the splendour of Maes Howe in Orkney. The spectacular village remains at Skara Brae with canopied beds and stone cupboards show how advanced even their domestic structures were. It should be remembered that the best-preserved and largest number of Neolithic remains in the whole of Europe are to be found on the Scottish islands and many of these structures predated the Egyptian pyramids.

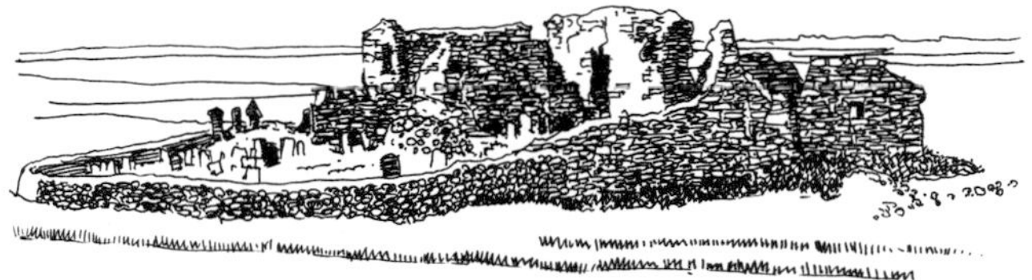

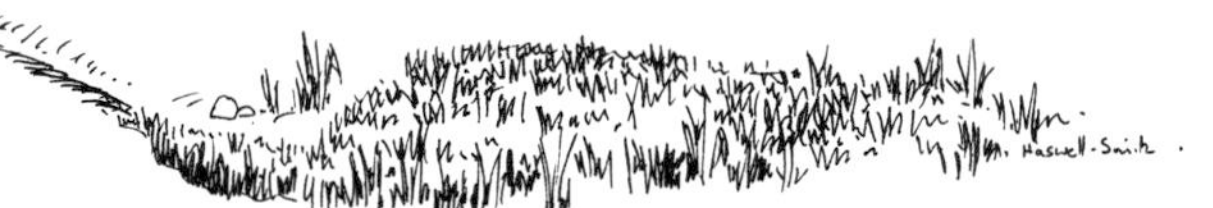

TEAMPULL NA TRIANAID, NORTH UIST (7.15)

Soon after Maes Howe was completed work began on the henges of Brodgar and Stenness. Hundreds of standing stones and stone circles were erected at this time to various mathematical models and apparently using a standard unit of measurement. Their purpose is still a matter of conjecture, probably religious, possibly astronomical, possibly both, but the engineering and geometric skills are clear to see. Callanish on **Lewis** is, of course, a supreme example.

By 2500BC new groups of people had arrived. They are called the Beaker people because of their distinctive pottery but their area of origin is uncertain. For some time they maintained a separate culture but eventually we find them adapting the tombs and structures of the earlier settlers for their own requirements. They introduced basic metallurgy, stone-carving, textiles and new concepts of social structure and political power. One of their prime settlements was the Crinan Plain in Argyll which strangely enough is also where the very first incomers to Scotland are thought to have settled. In due course the Beaker people introduced techniques for working in bronze, probably learnt from Southern Europe, heralding the demise of the Stone Age.

Between 1500BC and 700BC the climate, which had been mild and pleasant for many centuries, deteriorated. Wet, cold weather made arable farming less productive, causing economic and social change. In due course the old religions were abandoned and cremation became favoured instead of burial of the dead. Peat moss accumulated around the deserted monuments. The people had attractive jewellery but bronze weaponry and the building of hill-forts indicate that these were troubled times. Jarlshof in **Shetland** has the best-preserved example of a Bronze Age settlement dating from about 1000BC. There was also the development of timber-reinforced structures. Forts were built with timber posts sandwiched between stone skins (sometimes leading to vitrification) and timber, stone and soil were employed to build crannogs – artificial islands – in the lochs.

The strange and beautiful buildings called brochs were built between c.200BC and 100AD. Fine examples are on Mousa and at Carloway on Lewis. There are hundreds of them and they are found nowhere else in the world. Little is known about their purpose – were they really fortresses or watch-towers as has been claimed? – and, anyway, who built them? The Picts?

This mysterious race produced a wealth of beautiful stone-carvings with many strange, repetitive symbols. For a few centuries they dominated Scotland north of the central belt, but were eventually engulfed by the Scots and the Norsemen and disappeared from the world stage. Where they came from, what they looked like and what language they spoke is all conjecture. They are still one of the mysteries of our past although recent research has begun to produce a few answers.

About this time there was a great influx of newcomers from the south of Britain. Between 600BC and 500AD Celts came over the Channel in large numbers and steadily drifted northwards, bringing their language and culture with them. They had a stratified matriarchal society and a great love of warfare. The Romans said that in spite of cold, wet weather the Celts always fought stark naked, wearing only golden ornaments

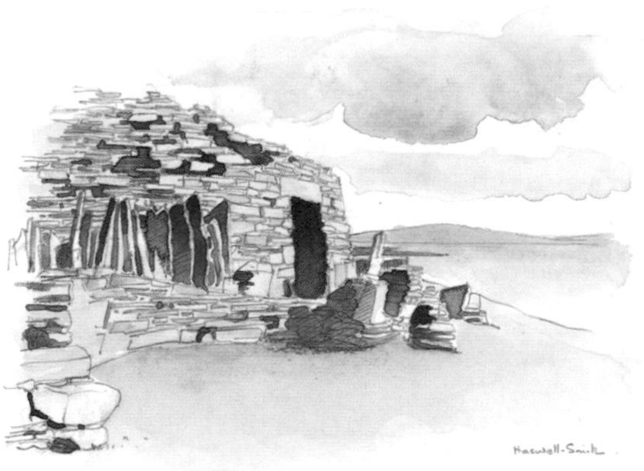

MIDHOWE BROCH, ROUSAY (10.20)

and a sword belt and sporting an elaborate hair arrangement. Because they were so quarrelsome among themselves they were often easily outwitted by a disciplined force. The Romans also said that even the women enjoyed a fight and were built like Amazons. Celtic priests, the druids, held great authority in society. They worshipped in oak groves and had no connection whatsoever with ancient Neolithic stone circles. Celts were skilled craftsmen who understood the technology of iron-working and were adept at carving stone. The Romans suppressed them in the south of Britain but they held their own elsewhere. Generally speaking, the Roman occupation of Britain had little or no influence on any of the Scottish islands or their inhabitants.

The pre-Celtic or Brythonic or, maybe, Pictish language which was prevalent at the time was displaced in northern Ireland – Dalriada – by the Celtic-speakers that settled there. These were Gauls, or Gaels, of Indo-Aryan origin fleeing from the Roman invasion of Central Europe. Modern Welsh is derived from the earlier tongue (known as P-Celtic) whilst modern Gaelic as spoken in the Western Isles is derived from the Irish version.

In the 4th century AD the Romans adopted Christianity and about the 5th century, after the legions had left Britain, a mission was set up by Ninian in the kingdom of Strathclyde. He had studied in Rome and he was followed by Patrick, another Romanised Briton from Ayrshire. Patrick could write Latin and spoke Brythonic (or Welsh). He went to Ireland where he learnt Gaelic and then spread the word in western Scotland. He was followed by Colum Cille O'Neill – the Dove of the Church and prince of the royal Irish house of O'Neill – better known as St Columba. Concurrently, Fergus Mòr, king of the Scots of Dalriada moved the seat of his kingdom from Antrim to Dunadd on the Crinan Plain of Argyll. In this way the Gaelic language, the Scottish name and the Christian religion were introduced to the islands of **Arran**, **Bute**, **Islay**, **Jura** and mainland Argyll. Incidentally, the name of the Scots kingdom of Dalriada came from Cairbre Ruadh (G. – red-haired Cairbar), nicknamed 'Red', who slew Oscar son of Ossian, and became king. Dal-ruaidh means the land of 'Red'.

In 563AD St Columba landed on Iona and founded the famous monastery which gained international recognition. Missionaries from Iona spread the Christian faith to many of the most remote islands, and scholars came from far across Europe to study at this famous seat of learning.

Around the year 800AD, the murderous Viking invasions began. The Danes mainly concentrated on England, but Norsemen could reach Shetland in thirty-six hours, or less, and spread south from there. The first Vikings were wealthy adventurers, expert seamen with good ships, weapons made of the finest Swedish iron, no respect for culture and an interest only in piracy. They plundered the monasteries including Iona and destroyed most of the historical records of the time. Where there was no treasure they could always carry the people off to slavery or hold them to ransom. The tender Scoto-Irish civilisation centred on Iona and recognised by Charlemagne as one of the most learned in Europe was virtually destroyed. Following the first waves of pure piracy a few of the marauders chose to stay and the Norse settlers who followed were better behaved. In due course this brought a modicum of peace to some areas.

In Orkney and Shetland the Pictish culture was all but wiped out before the islands gained a new economic significance as a springboard for Norse raiding parties travelling south. In 1098 another wealthy adventurer, King Magnus, sailed over from Norway on a campaign to plunder Lewis, the Uists, Skye, Mull, Iona, Tiree, Islay and the mainland of Argyll. He obtained an agreement from the King of the Scots confirming his ownership of all the islands. An island was defined as any piece of land which a boat could circumnavigate so he gained the Kintyre peninsula by having his men carry him across the Tarbert isthmus sitting in a boat.

He went on to pillage Ireland and came to a violent end in 1103.

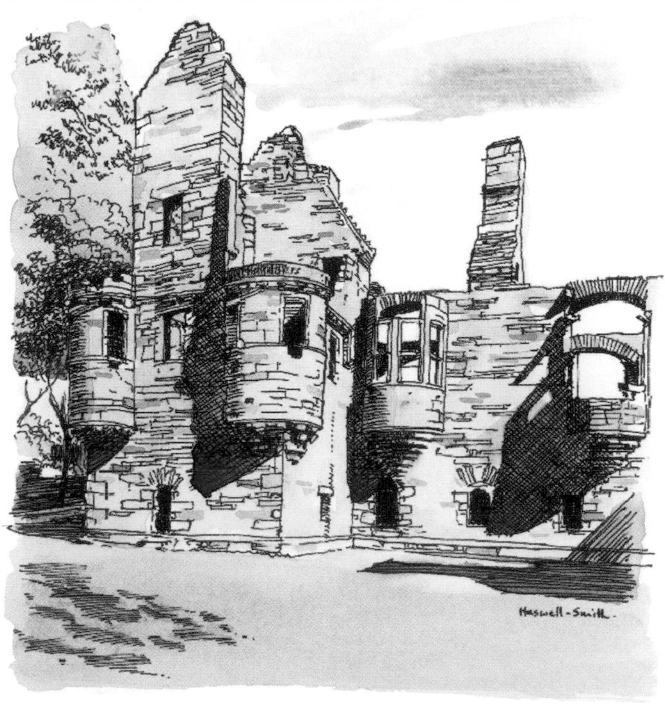

EARL PATRICK'S PALACE, ORKNEY MAINLAND (10.10)

the Isles to Ranald, and Lorn to Dughall. His grandson, Donald, gave his name to the Clan Donald which became the most powerful clan in Scottish history. The MacDonalds supported Bruce and the victory at Bannockburn confirmed their powerful position in Argyll and the Isles. In the end however they overplayed their hand and after repeated rebellions they had their inheritance forfeited in 1493. The Campbells then took over.

The Norwegians did not give up easily. They still held the **Northern Isles**, **Lewis**, **Skye**, and the Isle of Man. A son of the King of Man, Leod, inherited Lewis, Harris and Skye and made his home on Dunvegan rock. The King of Scots offered to purchase the Hebrides from King Haakon of Norway but he refused to sell. Furthermore, in 1248, Haakon shrewdly invited Ewen, Somerled's descendant, to Norway and formally accepted his status as King of the Isles. He thus gained Ewen's allegiance, but the Scots started raiding the Hebrides, which put Ewen in a difficult position as he also owed allegiance to the King of Scots for his lands in Argyll.

In 1117 on the island of Egilsay, a different Magnus, Earl Magnus of Orkney, grandson of Thorfinn the Mighty, was murdered by his cousin, Earl Haakon. Earl Magnus was something of a pacifist and pilgrims to his tomb later claimed they had experienced miracles, so he was canonised and Kirkwall's beautiful cathedral was dedicated to him.

Although Shetland was under direct Norwegian rule and Orkney was a Norse earldom, all the Western Isles were a Norse sub-kingdom controlled from the Isle of Man by a king who was subordinate to the Norwegian sovereign. A Scots prince of the kingdom of Argyll, Somerled (the name means 'summer-sailor' in Norse), married a daughter of King Olaf, King of Man. In 1130, Somerled, who had built a fleet of ships of improved design and shown himself to be much more than a 'summer-sailor', succeeded to the throne of Argyll. He first drove the Vikings out of Morvern and in due course outmanoeuvred and defeated them in a brilliant sea-battle in 1156. He then set about restoring the monastery at Iona and founded the House of Islay. He, and the next five generations of his family called themselves 'King of the Isles', but changed this to 'Lord of the Isles' in deference to the King of the Scots. Somerled had three sons. He gave the Lordship of Bute and Arran to his son Angus, Kintyre and

In 1263, King Haakon IV, an old man by then, decided to demonstrate his authority. He gathered a large fleet and sailed down the west coast of Scotland. Ewen refused to join him, but to be honourable he relinquished his Norwegian title of King of the Isles. There was an inconclusive Scottish-Norwegian skirmish between Largs and the Cumbraes when bad weather persuaded the Norwegians to withdraw. This was a disastrous decision and returning northwards their ships were battered by severe storms. Soon after they reached the haven of **Orkney** King Haakon died and, within two years, sovereignty of all the Western Isles and the Isle of Man had passed to the Scottish Crown.

Alexander III of Scotland offered his daughter's hand in marriage to the new Norwegian King as a diplomatic gesture of friendship which was accepted. But twenty years later Alexander died in an accident with the result that the sole direct heir to the Scottish throne was the King of Norway's baby daughter, Margaret – the Maid of Norway. Unfortunately, on her way to Scotland in 1290, she died at **Orkney**, just as King Haakon

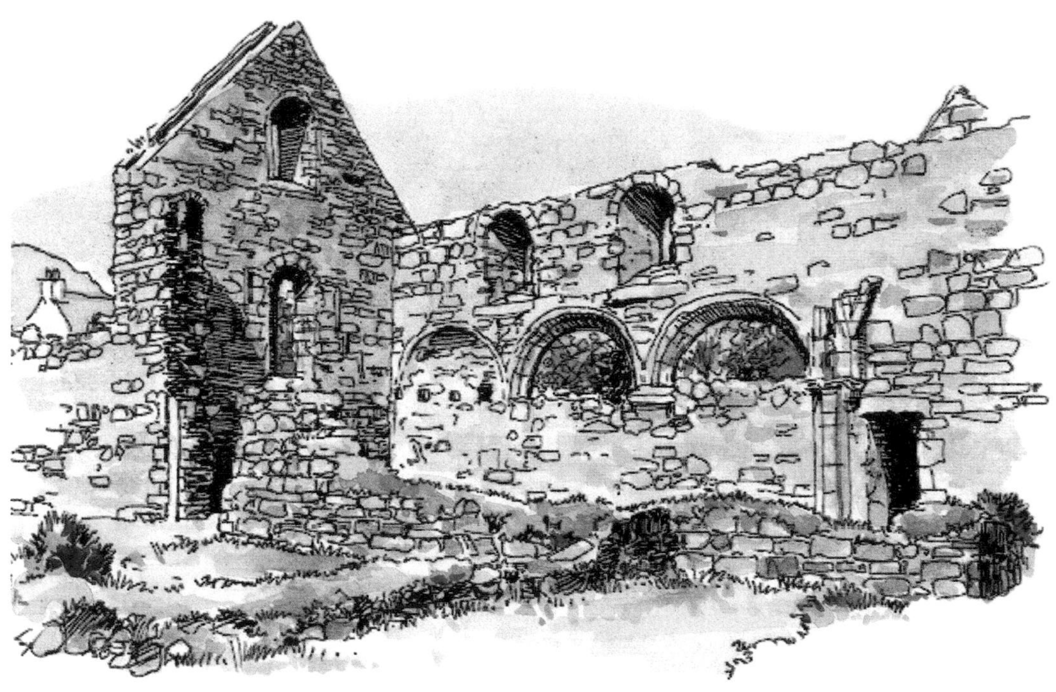

THE NUNNERY OF ST MARY, IONA (3.1)

had done, and this gave Edward I of England an excuse to claim the vacant Scottish throne. The consequence was Scotland's lengthy war to maintain its independence.

Shetland and **Orkney** remained Norwegian possessions for two more centuries until Margaret, daughter of King Christian of Denmark and Norway, was betrothed to James III, King of Scots, in 1468. The islands were pledged as security for an agreed dowry of 60,000 golden florins. Christian could not find the dowry money so the Scottish Crown foreclosed and took over the islands instead.

Although the Lord of the Isles lost his mini-kingdom during the Haakon intervention the MacDonald clan continued to exercise a powerful and peaceful influence on island affairs from **Islay** where they held councils of Hebridean chieftains once a year. Their territory encompassed the **Uists**, **Benbecula**, and Sleat on **Skye**. The complex history of the isles at this time saw the formation of vassal clans through marriages and treaties which eventually became interlaced with skirmishes and treachery. The Clan Iain held most of **Jura** and part of **Islay** and **Mull**; the McLeans of Duart held **Coll**, **Tiree** and most of **Mull**; Clan Neil held **Barra**, **South Uist** and **Gigha**; the McPhees held **Colonsay**; the MacLeods held **Lewis**, **Harris** and a large part of **Skye**; the MacKinnons also held parts of **Skye** and **Mull**. All these clans disliked and often disobeyed the Norman feudal system of lords and vassals which was being imposed by the Scottish kings; they preferred the Celtic (and Norse) system of lords and freemen. Eventually an exasperated Stewart King, James IV, broke the last remnants of Donald overlordship: but this only resulted in a lack of adequate leadership and a widespread breakdown of law and order. Clan fought clan, churches were burnt down, and the islanders suffered appalling cruelty and hardship.

James VI was ashamed of his lack of control of this troublesome territory when he succeeded to the English throne in 1603 and decided to prove his authority. So he invited the Hebridean chiefs to a friendly meeting on Mull, imprisoned them all on his flagship and brought them to Edinburgh. They were released a year later but only after having agreed to specific conditions of behaviour. Remarkably, this rough and ready method worked. Relative peace returned to the islands although there were still some minor feuds, in one of which the Campbells wrested control of **Islay** from the MacDonalds. Generally speaking, however, this was a time of reasonable prosperity.

Many of the clans joined forces in a common

cause in 1745 when Prince Charles Edward Stewart landed on **Eriskay** to lay claim to the British throne. By the following year, the collapse of his cause at Culloden effectively broke the power, and the wealth, of the clans for ever. Some distressed clan chiefs sold land which in ancient Celtic terms had belonged communally to the members of the clan as a whole, others looked to other means of raising money. By the early 19th century new absentee landlords, and some of the less scrupulous chieftains, were turning their land over to the new, profitable business of sheep-farming. The crofters, who had occupied their own land for centuries but held no written title, were mercilessly evicted. The Clearances had begun and huge areas, and many islands, were depopulated.

Crofters' rights of tenancy were only safeguarded by law in 1886 – too late – for by this time thousands of families had emigrated or been shipped off to Canada, Australia and the United States. Further depopulation was caused by potato blights, the decline of the fishing industry, two world wars and mainland attractions for the young.

WILDLIFE

The Scottish islands have a particularly interesting and diverse natural history mainly due to wide variations in climate and geology. Lime-rich alkaline soils occur on areas of calciferous rocks and acidic soils are found with granite and gneiss. The soil and the climate dictate the plantlife and the ground cover – moorland, meadow, woodland, peat bog, bare rock or sand – and the ground cover dictates the wildlife habitat.

These are the main considerations but there are other factors such as the influence of man or the geographical position of the island. Most islands have the same common plant forms as the nearest mainland regions but islands which lie in the warmth of the Gulf Stream and which are well sheltered, like **Gigha** or **Arran**, have varieties of primula normally only found in the south of Britain and other unusual plants such as the rare whitebeam of Arran.

Scottish islands have few endemic plant species but there are a number of interesting sub-species or specialities. The Hebridean orchid, a sub-species of the common spotted orchid *Dactylorhiza fuchsii*, is found in the **Outer Hebrides**, **Coll**, **Tiree** and **Shetland**, and there is a unique sub-species of the heath spotted orchid *Dactylorhiza maculata* found on **Rum**. One of the few endemic species is the gold and orange flowered hawkweed found only in **Shetland** in a number of varieties.

The outlying islands have the most difficult climatic conditions, yet **Hirta** has around 140 different botanical species and even **Rona** in the far north has nearly fifty species. This can be contrasted with Shetland which has over a hundred times the land area of Hirta yet supports only three times the number of native species. This is partly due to the presence of man, as grazing and burning of the scrub have been going on for over 5000 years. Peat digging has also had a serious effect on many Scottish islands as the top layer is rarely replaced and in the end the landscape is reduced to bog or bare rock. After the Ice Age most of the islands acquired woodland cover. Even storm-ridden St Kilda had sparse birch and alder scrub. Subsequent climatic changes upset the balance but man was the greatest culprit as trees were cut for buildings or fuel, land was cleared for planting and overgrazing, and erosion then took over.

Atlantic gales have been a mixed blessing to the west side of the 'Long Island', as the

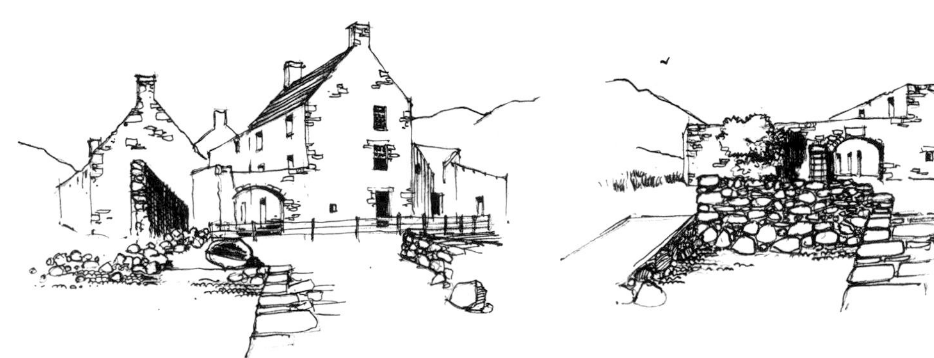

TIGH AN QUAY, 1938 (FROM A FRASER DARLING PHOTOGRAPH)

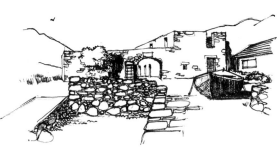

TIGH AN QUAY, TANERA MOR, 1994 (6.7)

almost continuous line of islands in the **Outer Hebrides** is known. They flatten and tear up any vegetation which dares to stand above the rest but they also scatter shell sand from the beaches – a valuable lime fertiliser. Interestingly, early records show much of the west coast of the Long Island as a sandy desert. It was by ploughing in seaweed to bind the sand and provide potash that man created the machair, welcome evidence that our species is not always destructive! In spring and summer the machair is a carpet of tiny wildflowers and particularly in the areas which have not been grazed by sheep this creates an unrivalled spectacle. Level as a billiard table and framed by pink thrift, white sand and deep turquoise sea the colours change with each passing week – daisies, buttercups, silverweed, birdsfoot trefoil, kidney vetch, white and red clover, wild pansies, corn marigold, spotted orchids, purple-tufted vetch and yellow pepperwort. And beyond the machair in the desolate peat bogs are butterfly orchids, bogbeam, pink ragged robin, mare's tail, marsh cinquefoil, kingcups and cotton grass. Contrast all this colour with the east coast which has little else but sedges, grass, heather and sphagnum moss in peat pockets on the bare rock.

Behind the sand dunes of **Orkney Mainland** there are great drifts of white clover, eyebright and birdsfoot trefoil. There are Arctic alpines in the Cuillin of **Skye** and in some of the nearby islands such as **Soay** and **Raasay** which are to be found nowhere else in Britain; while **Mull**, **Orkney** and **Shetland** and the **St Kilda** archipelago have examples of mountain sorrel, mountain everlasting catsfoot, white globe flower, purple saxifrage, meadow rue, roseroot and moss campion. **Rum** has a rare alpine saxifrage and both **Orkney** and **Shetland** support the unique purple-flowering Scottish primrose. In the peaty lochans of **Jura**, the **Uists**, and some of the smaller islands a distinctive and beautiful subspecies of the white waterlily *Nymphaea alba* can be seen. Unfortunately, such plants are at serious risk from thoughtless collectors and common thieves.

The remaining natural woodlands are mainly thickets of oak, hazel, birch, willow, pine, alder and rowan. Examples can be found on **Soay**, **Raasay**, **Ulva** and (south) **Rona** to name a few. Cultivated woodland in limited areas can also be found on **Canna**, **Gigha**, and **Lewis**, and **Arran** has large tracts of planted imported conifers.

In some ways animal life on the islands is as varied as the plantlife which supports it. Most of the island mammals were first introduced by man. The Soay sheep of the **St Kilda** group have been there for at least a thousand years. They were domesticated by Neolithic man but their place of origin is unknown. Their population fluctuations are the subject of scientific study at present. There is another Neolithic strain of short-tailed sheep, also of unknown origin, to be found on **North Ronaldsay**. This breed lives mainly on seaweed.

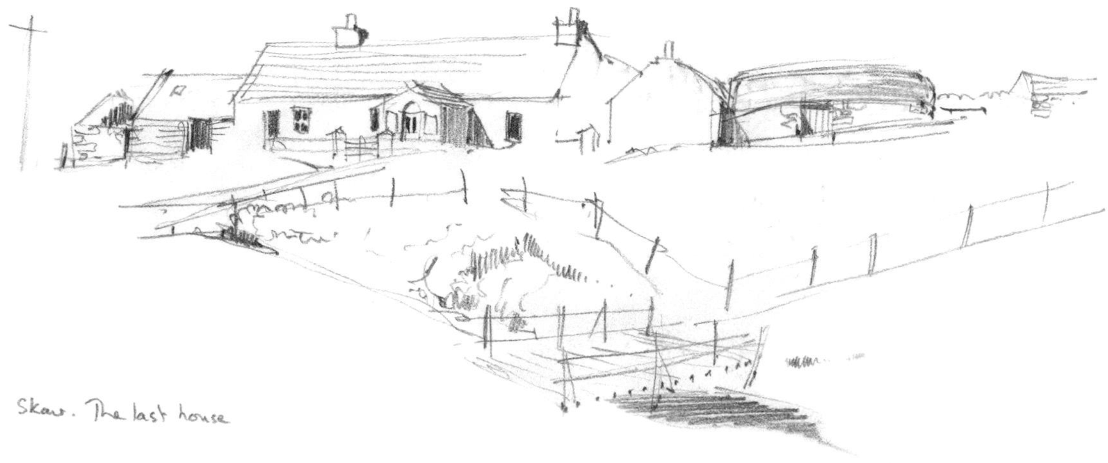

SKAW, THE LAST HOUSE IN BRITAIN

Many islands have feral goats which have been traced back to Middle Eastern stock but how they were introduced to the Scottish islands is entirely speculative. Red deer are fairly widespread and as they can swim a considerable distance they may have colonised some of the inshore islands by their own effort. The original population was almost exterminated by destruction of the forests and by hunting. But in the 19th century landlords encouraged their reintroduction for sporting purposes and the deer themselves have learned to adapt to the lack of forest cover. On **Rum** the deer are carefully protected and studied for ecological research. Rum's own breed of ponies is used to bring the deer carcasses in for examination. The breed is the result of the islanders crossing Highland mares with Arab sires. The **Shetland** pony is also the result of selective breeding in the distant past.

The common fox *Vulpes vulpes* has never been native to the Outer Hebrides although a few misguided people still defy common sense by introducing the occasional specimen. Foxes would have a devastating effect if they gained a foothold, particularly on communities of ground-nesting birds such as greenshank, dunlin and tern. These have already suffered from the deliberate introduction of mink, hedgehogs, ferrets, and domestic cats.

There are no frogs or adders in the **Northern Isles** but the adder is very common in parts of the Inner Hebrides such as **Jura.**

Rabbits were first introduced to some of the islands as a source of meat and Boswell mentions in particular the warren on **Coll** in 1773. Rabbits are not indigenous to the British Isles and were originally imported by the Normans who enjoyed their tasty meat. They posed no problem initially as they were kept successfully in defined warrens, culled and savagely guarded by the gentry. Then came the Industrial Revolution and the Clearances; the warrens were left to fall into disrepair and the rabbits were left in peace to do what rabbits do best. Strangely, there are no rabbits on Coll's near neighbour, **Tiree** and thankfully **St Kilda**, **North Rona** and **Berneray** in the Sound of Harris are bunny-free.

Among the other small mammals there are a number of unique sub-species such as the **St Kilda** mouse, the **Rum** mouse, and the **Bute** mouse. Short-tailed voles are a general Hebridean sub-species and there is also an **Orkney** vole but bank voles are only found on **Mull** and **Raasay**. Otters are common in most of the islands and especially on some of the **Northern Isles**.

Many grey or Atlantic seals frequent the west coast of the **Outer Hebrides** and the Scottish Islands generally are home to about half the world's population of this species. The common seal is less common and tends to prefer east-facing coasts. Numbers of porpoises and dolphins were in decline for many years but quite recently there seems to have been some recovery and it is rare to sail any distance in these waters without seeing them. The same goes for the basking shark and schools of killer or minke whales may also be seen.

Insect life is probably no more and no less varied on the islands than it is on the mainland but thanks to a lack of use of insecticides on many of the islands some of the less common species have had a better survival rate. This is particularly true of butterflies. Flodday by **Sandray**, south of Barra for example, boasts a unique sub-species of the dark green fritillary, **Rum** and **Eigg** have a number of species, and the **Northern Isles** also have a good assortment.

Without doubt, though, the most memorable island insect is the midge. There are thirty-four known species in the UK but only the females of five species bite and the worst belong to just one species, *Culicodes impunctatus.* It has been suggested that the forced depopulation of the islands in the 19th century may have been partly responsible for an increase in these tiny, voracious creatures which can make life so miserable in the mid-summer months. Discounting chemical

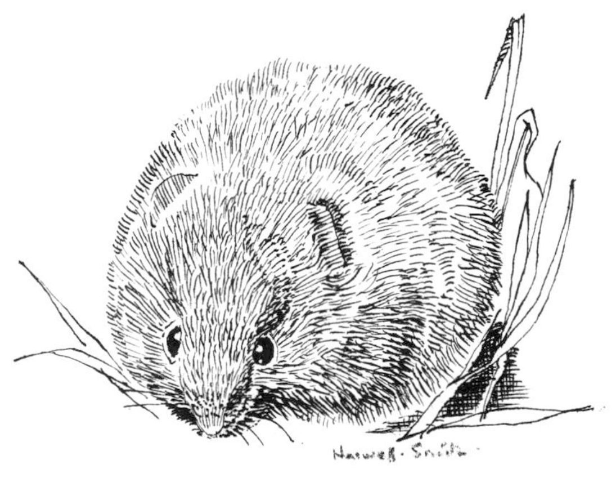

THE ORKNEY VOLE

insect repellents, which are only effective for a very short time, there are only two recognised antidotes – wind and whisky. The former blows them away and the latter makes them bearable. It is probable that, when the population was removed and the land reverted to rough grazing and sporting estates, midges would have found the change to their liking. Bracken, for example, protects them from the wind while cultivation destroys their breeding grounds. Compare well-managed and relatively midge-free **Canna** with the clouds of man-eating midges on wild and boggy **Rum** or **Jura.**

For the birdwatcher the islands are unsurpassed. For seabirds in particular, the remote or uninhabited islands are perfect sanctuaries. About 70% of the world's entire population of razorbills nest on the Scottish islands. In the **St Kilda** group, Stac Lee is home to some 100,000 pairs of gannets, which is probably the biggest gannetry in the world. And this particular island archipelago has a greater number and more species of seabirds than any other island group in Europe. Runners-up on a smaller scale are the **Treshnish** archipelago off Mull and the **Shiant** Islands north of Skye. Apart from also having magnificent seabird communities, the **Northern Isles** are the birdwatchers' finest hunting-ground for rare migrants blown there from far-off places.

Two of Britain's rarest birds, the corncrake and the chough, are now only to be found in the Western Isles: proof, if such were needed, that this is a last corner of paradise.

ACCESS

Where there is any regular form of public transport to an island this information is given but all details should be verified before use. There are a number of excellent annual guides which give more detail than there is room for here and VisitScotland (the Scottish Tourist Board) can also be of assistance (0131-332 2433). Although all the larger and more populated islands are served by public transport my main interest is with the smaller, and mainly uninhabited, islands. These are never easy to visit and means of access are not covered by the normal tourist guides.

Most hotels and guest-houses on the larger islands, or the adjacent mainland, are very willing to make arrangements with a local boat-owner. But even if weather conditions are suitable be prepared for some uncertainty.

Anchorages

It is, of course, much easier to arrange an island visit if you have your own boat. For this reason I have tried to provide a comprehensive list of all recognised (and some unrecognised) island anchorages with a brief note of their advantages or shortcomings. This is intended solely as an aid to pre-planning. It provides a simple means of selecting an anchorage to suit one's purpose – a quiet night with the family aboard, a visit to some particular site, a quick run ashore, a sketch, photography, a stop for lunch, a safe haven, etc. Difficulty of access, poor holding, or excessive exposure, will all influence one's choice.

In my attempt to be comprehensive I have compiled the list from a variety of sources – from the authority of Admiralty Pilots to the comments of local fishermen. ***Neither these notes, nor the illustrative maps in this publication, should be used for navigation – they are intended only for passage-planning.*** Where anchorages are indicated on the maps in this book by an anchor-symbol it is usually because they are well-recognised anchorages for that island. Most of the listed anchorage positions are described but not shown for reasons of scale. The navigation charts should always be consulted.

British Admiralty Charts and the sailing directions of the CCC, which include the Northern Isles (Clyde Cruising Club Publications Ltd, Suite 408, The Pentagon Centre, 36 Washington Street, Glasgow G3 8AZ (0141-221 2774)) are virtually essential. The CCC also supplies the FYCA sailing directions for the East Coast, Martin Lawrence's excellent West Coast Pilots which I highly recommend, and Imray Yachting Charts (Imray Laurie Norie & Wilson Ltd, St Ives, Cambridgeshire).

Where an anchorage is labelled 'temp' or 'temporary' it must be approached with caution and only used in daylight and under ideal conditions (slack tides, gentle winds, etc). Always maintain an anchor watch and normally use a tripping line.

An 'occasional' anchorage is slightly better and in ideal conditions could be used overnight. However it may only offer shelter from a limited wind direction and if conditions change should be vacated promptly.

The Geographical Sections

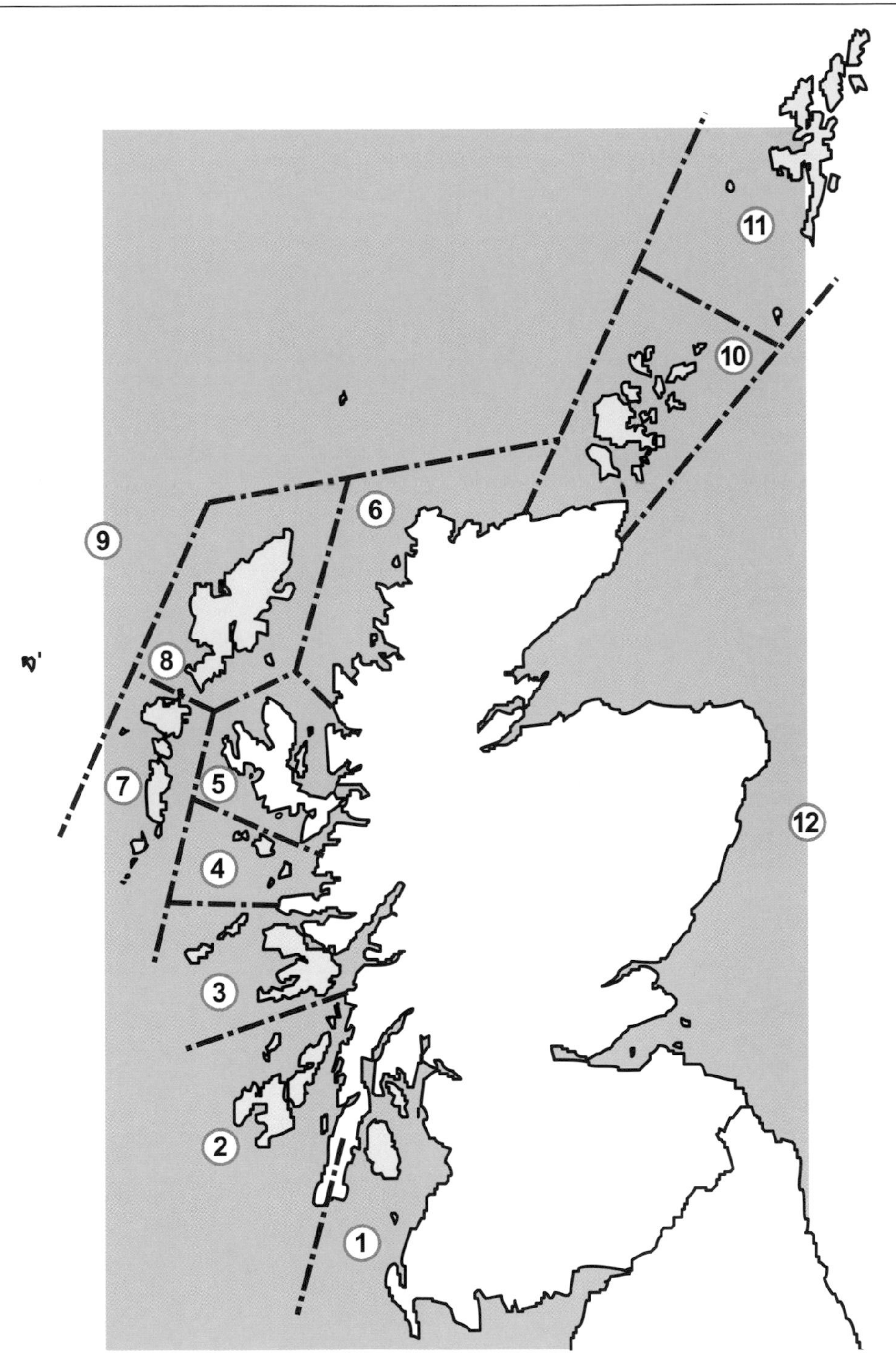

SECTION I

The Solway Firth to the Firth of Clyde

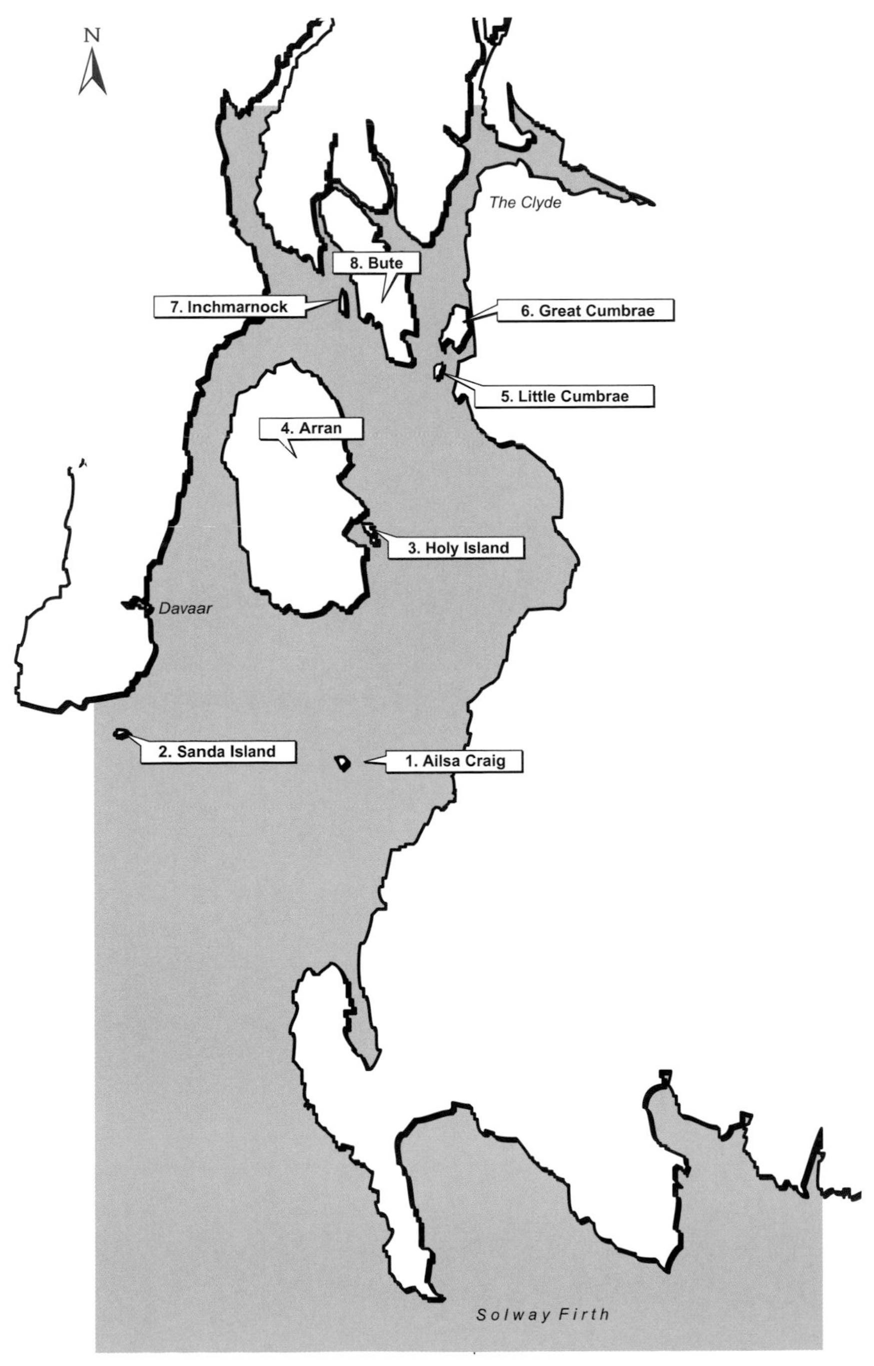

Section 1, Table 1: Arranged according to geographical position

No.	Name	Latitude	Longitude	Table 2* No.	Table 3** No.	Area in Acres	Area in Hectares
1.1	Ailsa Craig	55° 15N	05° 07W	111	19	245	99
1.2	Sanda	55° 17N	05° 35W	93	54	373	151
1.3	Holy Island	55° 32N	05° 04W	75	20	625	253
1.4	Arran	55° 35N	05° 15W	7	2	106750	43201
1.5	Little Cumbrae Island	55° 43N	04° 57W	64	53	773	313
1.6	Great Cumbrae	55° 46N	04° 55W	39	49	2886	1168
1.7	Inchmarnock	55° 47N	05° 09W	73	104	657	266
1.8	Bute	55° 49N	05° 06W	11	24	30188	12217

*Table 2: The islands arranged in order of magnitude
**Table 3: The islands arranged in order of height

Introduction

Here, within a short distance of Scotland's greatest conurbation, are eight fascinating and diverse islands. Turn left on the Clyde at Cloch Point and travel 'doon the watter' to Bute, guard of the western entrance, with Inchmarnock tucked behind it. The eastern sentinels are the Cumbraes, Great and Little. Ahead and beyond, the towering serrated ridge of Arran dominates the entire Firth, dwarfing even the high peak of Holy Island. Further out, lonely and conspicuous in the southern reaches of the Firth, stands Ailsa Craig – familiarly referred to as Paddy's Milestone and on the horizon, a speck at the foot of the Mull of Kintyre, is mysterious Sanda Island.

This area, with its long sea-lochs, offers a marvellous environment for inshore sailing. The longest of these lochs – longer than Loch Long – is Loch Fyne, stretching from the north of Arran to well beyond Inveraray. The fishing town of Tarbert is the main port on this loch and source of the world-famous Loch Fyne kippers. The larger 'islands' in the vicinity, Barmore and Eilean Aoidhe, are in fact peninsulas and the only islets possibly worthy of the name are **Eilean Buidhe** and **Eilean a' Bhuic** opposite Tarbert and **Eilean a' Chromhraig** just south of the entrance.

Halfway up the loch in Loch Gilp is **Duncuan Island** with, to the east of it, another drying island – Eilean Mór. However, alongside Eilean Mór is the strip of **Liath Eilean** with a pleasant anchorage in between.

In the upper reaches there is **Glas Eilean** off Port Ann with **Eilean Aoghainn** in the centre of the loch and overlooked by Minard Castle.

The islets of the Kilbrannan Sound are equally insignificant – two tiny islets on the coast of the Mull of Kintyre – **Thorn Isle** and **Island Ross**. **Davaar**, which guards the entrance to Campbeltown Loch and issues its own postage stamps, is not by definition a true island as it can be reached at low water over a shingle causeway (dangerous when the tide comes in). It is worth a visit because there are seven caves and the fifth conceals a famous mural of Christ crucified which was painted in secret by a local artist, Alexander MacKinnon in 1887.

On the Ayrshire coast by Ardrossan harbour five species of gull nest on low-lying **Horse Island** and, likewise, colonies of common, sandwich and arctic tern nest on **Lady Isle** off Troon. There are no other islets on this coast and the Solway Firth is also short of islands. The largest group is at Fleet Bay – **Murray's Isles**, **Ardwall Island** and **Barlocco Island**. At Kirkcudbright Bay **Little Ross** is off the Ross headland and **Hestan Island** is in the centre of shallow, tidal Auchencairn Bay. Little Ross supports a Stevenson lighthouse which has been automatic since 1961. Two lighthouse-keepers' houses are, or were, owned by Dr S R Wild of Edinburgh. The islet was the scene of a nasty murder in 1960: but that's another story.

1.1 Ailsa Craig

(G. aillse creag – fairy rock). Referred to locally as Paddy's Milestone but sometimes known as creag Ealasaid (G. – Elizabeth's rock). In the old Irish tale of 'Buioe Suibne' it is called carraig Alastair (G. – Alastair's rock).

OS Maps: 1:50000 Sheet 76 1:25000 Sheet 326 1:10000 (NX 09)
Admiralty Chart: 1:75000 No.2126

Area: 99ha (245 acres)
Height: 338m (1109 ft)

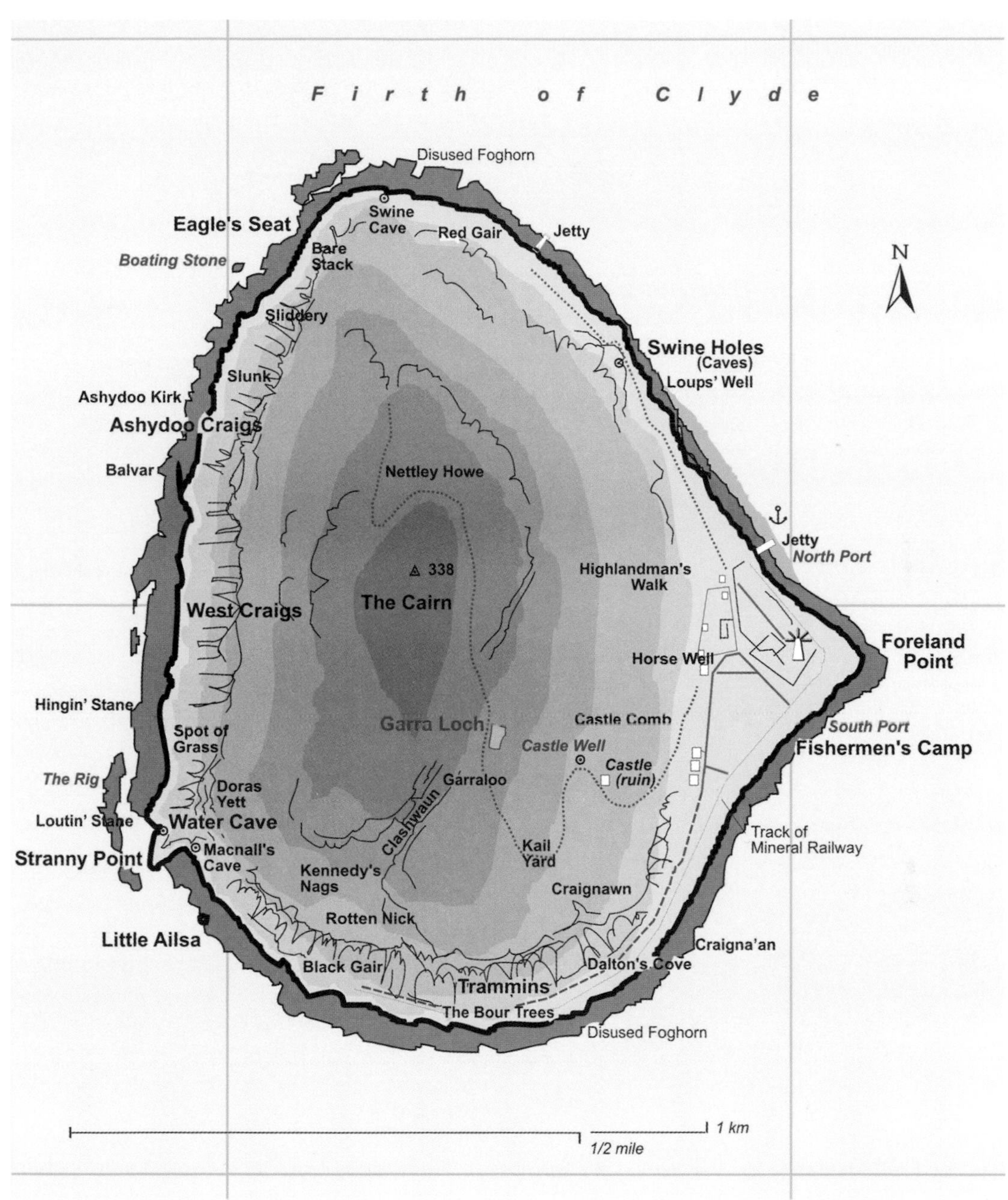

Owner: Cassilis Estates (Marquess of Ailsa). The lighthouse compound, helipad and pier are in separate ownership.

Population: From 19th century to mid-20th century a small population of quarrymen and families. 1881–29. 1891–27. 1931–11. 1961–10. 1971–3 (lighthouse keepers). 1981–2. 1991–0 (lighthouse automatic). 2001–0.

Geology: Mainly an acid igneous rock containing fine-grained crystals of quartz, mica and feldspar, known as microgranite. In the south-west corner there is a seam of reibickite, a fine-grained micro-granite, which was considered ideal for the manufacture of curling stones. These were cut on the island but polished on the mainland. The floor of the Chapel of the Thistle in St Giles Cathedral, Edinburgh, is made of this beautiful Ailsa Craig granite but the quarries are now disused. Much of the island is columnar basalt, sometimes forming columns 400 feet in height.

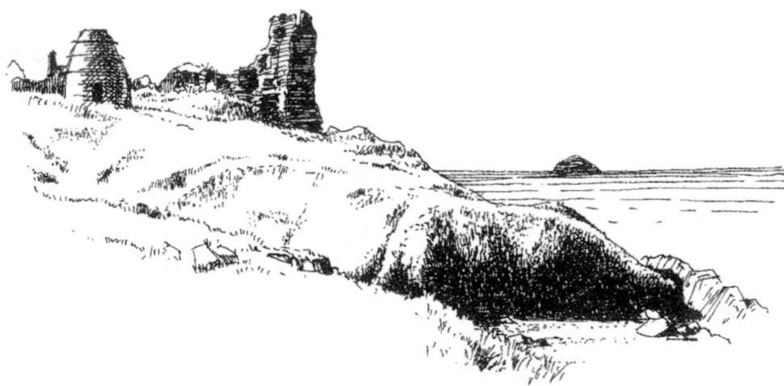

AILSA CRAIG FROM DUNURE CASTLE, SEAT OF THE KENNEDYS

History: An old square peel-tower on the island was almost certainly built by the Hamiltons but there is no record of why it was built nor how long it was occupied. It is however said that the monks of Crossraguel Abbey (near Maybole in Ayrshire) eventually used it as a retreat. The Catholics also once held it on behalf of Philip II of Spain.

The lighthouse was built in 1868 by the Stevensons.

Wildlife: In 2004 the island became an RSPB Reserve by invitation of the Marquess. It was already a Site of Special Scientific Interest and a European Special Protection Area.

At one time some Soay sheep from St Kilda (neolithic, dark-brown, small and hardy) were bred here. Rabbits were said to have been brought in by the quarrymen to supplement their diet. These have not been as big a problem, however, as the brown rats which arrived in 1889 when ships were ferrying materials and supplies to the newly built lighthouse. (The quarrymen later claimed that the rats and rabbits were interbreeding!)

Before the brown rats moved in there were at least 250,000 pairs of puffins on the island. An ornithologist, Robert Gray, reported in the 1860s that when he disturbed the puffins 'for a time their numbers seemed so great as to cause a bewildering darkness.'

By 1990 the rats had successfully driven many birds off the island and not a single puffin had been seen since 1984. So in 1991 a rat eradication programme was instituted by the Marquess of Ailsa, Glasgow University and Scottish Natural Heritage. Poison to kill the rats, three tons of Warfarin, was airlifted by helicopter from *HMS Gannet*, Prestwick, and distributed on the island in the Spring. 'Some of it was put in bait boxes and a lot went straight into the rat holes,' said Dr Zonfrillo, a leading ornithologist member of the working group. The rats died in their burrows so there were no rat carcasses strewn about. The treatment seems to have worked and it has also (temporarily?) reduced the rabbit population.

By 1996 black guillemots and shelduck had returned to nest and occasional puffins had been seen, but it was not until 2002 that it was certain that a few puffins had at last established nest-burrows on the island and started breeding again.

Ailsa Craig is noted for its immense gannet colony which has been there since at least 1526. Recently nearly 40,000 breeding pairs of gannets were reported which is about 5% of the gannet population of the world. They are mainly on the south-west side. Numerous guillemots, kittiwakes and gulls are also to be found and blackbirds, song-thrushes, wheatears and willow warblers have been seen. Pipits may be found on the steep slopes above the smooth rock walls.

The island's slow worms, which hide under the rocks, are considered the largest in Europe and there is a wide variety of plant life. In places the cliffs are white with the scented flowers of scurvy grass spotted here and there with red lychnis. The rose-coloured flowers of the tree mallow, *Lavatera arborea*, can be seen growing 2–3m high near the buildings but warmer weather is now unfortunately encouraging this plant to spread across the island and block the puffins' nesting holes (See Bass Rock, Section 12-Appendix).

* * *

AILSA CRAIG is the Lowlands' answer to the Hebridean and Orcadian stacks, those great chunks of rock rearing out of the sea. Its basalt and columnar trap rises abruptly from sea level and soars to a height of nearly 340m – over 1100 feet. When its ethereal shape materialises

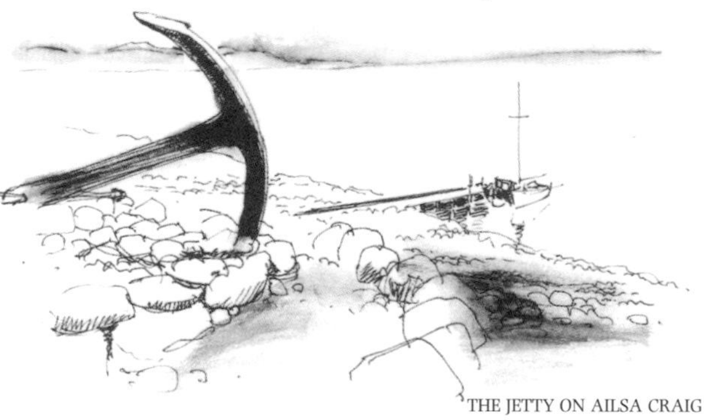

THE JETTY ON AILSA CRAIG

out of the mist one can understand it being named fairy rock by some ancient Celt. Except on the east side which has an accessible slope it is so precipitous that even the seabirds are unable to nest on some of the cliffs. Wordsworth and Keats were impressed by it, but Burns' only comment (in 'Duncan Gray') was that 'Meg was deaf as Ailsa Craig'!

Twenty-five thousand years ago when Scotland lay smothered under a thick sheet of ice a glacier flowing down the Clyde valley broke off pieces of Ailsa Craig granite and carried them south to the English Midlands where they still lie around today scattered between Wales and the Pennines. Much more recently the same fine-grained granite was again distributed widely, but this time in the form of curling stones. For many years there was no other source.

An old anchor bedded in the pebble beach by the broken jetty marks the path to the group of white buildings clustered round the lighthouse.

A rusty narrow-gauge railway line runs from the pier and past the quarrymen's cottages to the abandoned quarry on the south side. A forge and disused foghorns are also in evidence and there are heaps of waste granite pieces from which the spheroidal curling stones have been cut leaving fascinating shapes like miniature Henry Moore sculptures. I am told the heaps are dwindling as the offcuts are being sold as curios. The Andrew Kay company still has the sole quarrying rights on Ailsa Craig.

A well-defined zig-zag path climbs to the top, starting near the lighthouse and passing the old square **peel-tower** about 100m up the slope [NX023995]. The three stars of the Hamilton coat of arms are carved on a stone set in the walls.

Further up, the path passes over the shallow valley of Garraloo and beside the tiny **Garra Loch** with the cleft of Rotten Nick below before making its way to the top. Here the precipice plunges straight to the sea; **Bare Stack**, in the north-west, with two ferocious brown overhangs and **Ashydoo** cliff lying just south. Far below to the south-west is Spot of Grass, Doras Yett and the outcrop of Kennedy's Nags. And beyond the white lace of the surf lie the wide stretches of the Firth of Clyde with the long dark shape of Ulster on the south-western horizon.

It is possible to make an exciting and relatively easy two-mile circumnavigation of the island beneath these cliffs. The only minor obstruction is at **Water Cave** in the south-west cleft. The exposed corner of Stranny Point has to be negotiated to reach this mini Fingal's Cave when coming from the east around the shore, past **Little Ailsa**. Try and time it for low water.

Climbers may prefer to go directly up the slope from the landing place on the east shore. There is no difficulty in the ascent but in places the route leads over steeply inclined slabs. No rock-climbing routes on any of the dramatic cliffs have been recorded but this is just as well as the island is a bird-sanctuary.

* * *

Access: Crossing time approx. 1 hour. Boat trips from Girvan by arrangement, Mark McCrindle, 01465-713219 or ASW Charters *Rachel Clare*, 01465-715934.

Anchorage:
1. A timber jetty or pier of sorts in the north-east beside the lighthouse at Foreland Point has only 0.6m at its head. Temp anchorage possible close N of jetty but beware ruins of old jetty close NW of existing jetty. Bottom of granite boulders shelves steeply. Use tripping line and do not leave yacht unattended.

1.2 Sanda Island

(ON. sandtange – sand spit) island. There is a large sand spit near the harbour called Oitir Buidhe (G. – yellow sand spit). According to the Ordnance Gazetteer Sanda was called 'Avona Porticosa' by the Vikings and known as 'Aven' in Gaelic (?G. abhainn – river). But Dean Munro says the Danes called it 'Havin', i.e. anchorage – which makes much more sense.

OS Maps: 1:50000 Sheet 68 1:25000 Sheet 356
Admiralty Charts: 1:75000 Nos. 2126 or 2199

Area: 127ha (314 acres)
Height: 123m (403 ft)

Owner: Bought in 1989 by Meg and Dick Gannon (formerly of Lundy Island) for a reported £250,000. Former owners were Jack Bruce of the rock group Cream and James Gulliver (Argyll Group).

Population: 1841–11 (1 house). 1871–32. 1881–14. 1891–36 (7 houses). 1931–14. 1961–7. 1981–0. 1991–0. 2001–1.

Geology: Lower Old Red Sandstone in red and yellow varieties, and undifferentiated schists.

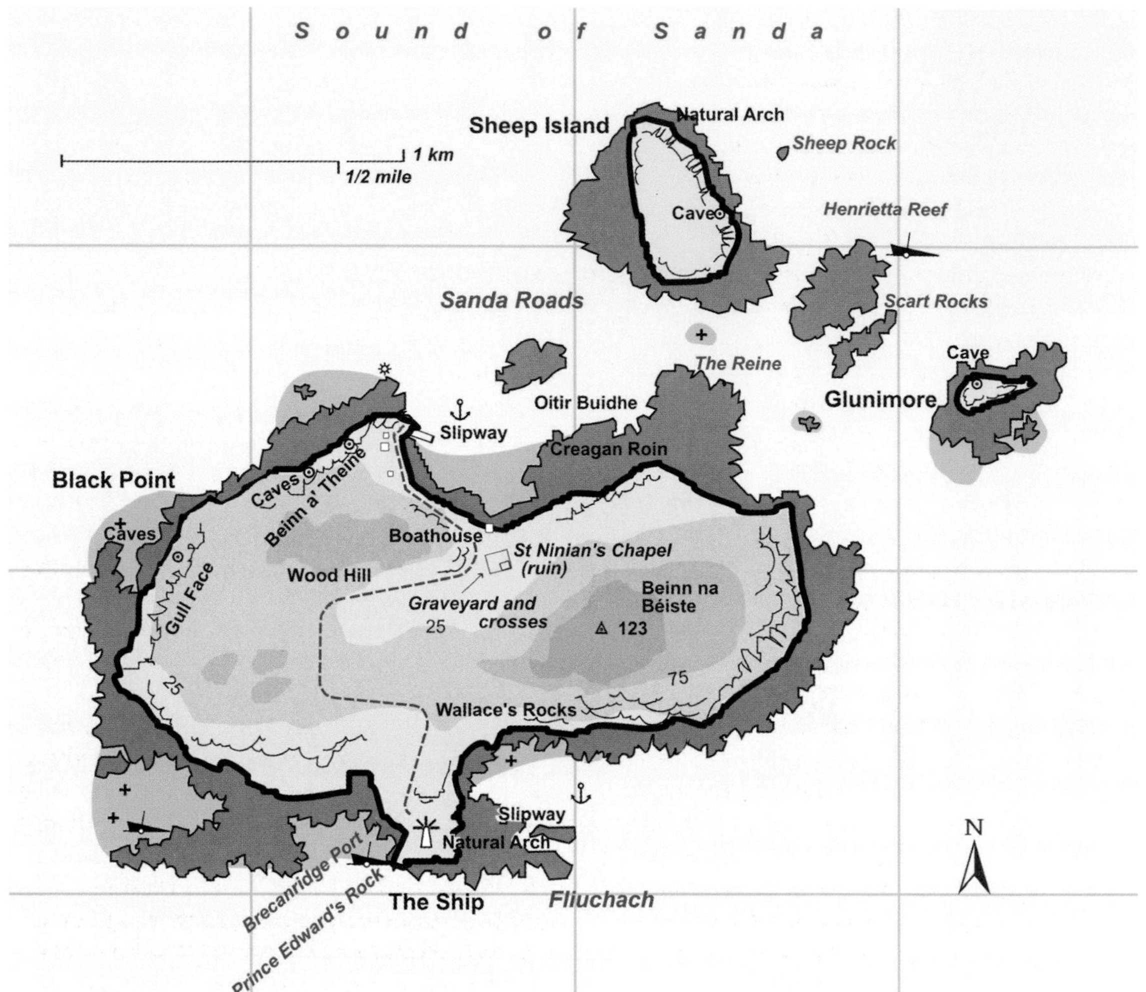

History: In 1306 Bruce may have landed here. Angus II, fifth King of the Isles, sheltered him at Dunaverty Castle which stood on the headland at Southend overlooking Sanda Island [NR688076]. When the English fleet drew closer he slipped away to Ireland.

The end of the lighthouse promontory on the south of the island is called Prince Edward's Rock after Edward Bruce, Robert the Bruce's impulsive brother, who was, very briefly, King of Ireland.

At this time Sanda was part of the lands of the Priory of Whithorn in Galloway and remained so until the late 16th century, when it became the property of the MacDonalds of Sanda with the Earl of Argyll holding the superiority.

In 1647, Dunaverty Castle again entered the history books when 300 MacDonalds of Kintyre, Catholic royalists and supporters of Montrose, made their last stand against the Covenanter general, Leslie. Among them were Archibald Mor, chief of the MacDonalds of Sanda and his son and heir Archibald Og. Sir Alexander MacDonald had left them to defend the castle when he withdrew to Ireland but they were besieged and short of drinking water. Leslie offered to spare them should they surrender. They did so whereupon he had every one of them massacred. The castle was razed to the ground, never rebuilt, and from then on it has been known as Bloody Castle.

The MacDonalds' estates were forfeited but in 1661 they were restored by Act of Parliament. Ronald MacDonald inherited Sanda but died in 1679 when his son, Archibald, became the 6th Laird of Sanda.

In 1946 the Campbeltown lifeboat *The Duke of Connaught* (brought out of retirement as the new boat was under repair) went to the assistance of the 7000-ton *Byron Darnton* stuck on a reef on the south of Sanda. The skipper of the wrecked ship apparently considered it safer to stay aboard and keep below decks, but the lifeboatmen knew that the ship was bound to break up before long with the almost inevitable death of everyone on board. Unfortunately the old lifeboat had no radio. Conditions were appalling and communication with the ship was impossible as no one was on deck so the lifeboat sailed back round the island to the north harbour, where one of the crew ran overland to the south side. There was a radio transmitter at the lighthouse by which he eventually persuaded the captain of the stricken ship to allow those aboard to be taken off. Once again the lifeboat set out into the violent storm, rounded the island, and in spite of a very unreliable engine risked going into the chaotic sea among the rocks. It took eighteen long hours of almost foolhardy bravery but all fifty-four passengers and crew (and even a dog) were saved. Just as the lifeboat pulled clear of the rocks the ship finally disintegrated. But all was not over for while struggling home the old engine at last sputtered out. It seemed a losing battle as they were blown out to sea but after an hour they coaxed her into life again and at last reached the safety of the harbour.

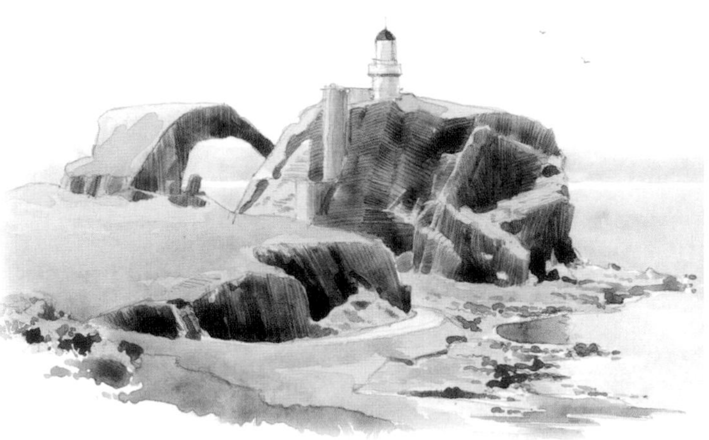

'THE SHIP' LIGHTHOUSE, SANDA

Wildlife: Two of Sanda's small neighbouring islands, Sheep Island and Glunimore Island, are important breeding grounds for puffins in the Clyde area but many seabirds also breed on Sanda Island's crags. The converted boatshed is a visitors' centre.

* * *

Although **SANDA ISLAND** is a useful stopping-off point for a yacht waiting for the tide to round the Mull of Kintyre it is also well worth visiting for its own sake. The farmhouse, which has been restored by the owner for his own occupation, is just beside the jetty and slipway. There is also an old schoolhouse and various farm buildings which were converted in 2003 for letting as holiday cottages as well as a small licensed restaurant, the Byron Darnton tavern. This is a Site of Scientific Interest (SSI) and also an RSPB Reserve since 2005 and the Nature Conservancy Council have the seabirds monitored and ringed both on Sanda and on its two little neighbours, **Sheep Island** and **Glunimore Island**. Glunimore is a tiny lump of rock but Sheep Island is large enough to provide some grazing for sheep. It has a cave on it and a natural stone arch at its north end.

The road which runs round the bay and across the island to the lighthouse had been macadamed in the past and there are still patches of tar lying in the ruts. The roofless ruin of little **St Ninian's Chapel**, about 10.3m by 6.3m, is on the south side of a knoll within the burial enclosure [NR727046]. Fordun noted this building in the second half of the 14th century. The side walls, of local rubble dressed with local sandstone, are still standing to roof level, but the gables have partly collapsed. There is an intact wooden lintel over the entrance doorway. One of the three window embrasures is still in reasonable condition and it has a stone basin or piscina set in the wall beside it. A matching basin has not been seen since 1873. There is a stone altar slab with a rectangular slot in it – possibly used for relics and an inscription on a grave slab set in the floor refers to 'Archibald – son to MacDonald of Sanda' and 'Cirstin Stewart'. Cirstin Stewart was the widow of Archibald Mor MacDonald who died in the Dunaverty Massacre.

By the north-west corner of the chapel a worn Early Christian slab is incised with a cross and near the centre of the burial ground there is a large much-eroded cruciform-shaped stone nearly 2m high and a few scattered headstones. Heraldic memorials to the MacDonald lairds show that Archibald, the sixth laird, was alive in 1731.

Just west of the chapel are the footings of a

small square structure. A 1630 record states – 'at the syde of that Chappell there is a litle well or compass of stones. . . And they say that the bones of certaine holie men that lived in that Illand is buried within that place.' The same record also refers to a 'spring of fresh water called St Ninian's Well' which had therapeutic powers but this has not been identified.

In the past there was an active fishing community living on Sanda. Apparently, by tradition, if there was a severe storm and the men were still at sea, the families would gather in the burial ground by a particular unmarked grave, say a prayer for the fishermen, and then solemnly pour a cup of fresh water on the grave. The origin of this ceremony is unknown.

Legend has it that St Ninian himself is buried on Sanda and that anyone who steps on his grave will die within a year. This dangerous spot once had an alder tree marking its whereabouts but that has long since disappeared.

The island had not been farmed since 1946 but in 1991 the new owner had neatly repaired the fences and sheep were grazing in the central valley. There are no trees but this was not always the case; the hill above the farmhouse is still called Wood Hill. The lighthouse, on a promontory on the south shore (called **The Ship** because it has that appearance from the sea), was built in 1850 by Alan Stevenson. The skerries here are littered with the wrecks of ships. There is a striking wide-span natural stone arch alongside the lighthouse and many cave-riddled crags and rock formations in the vicinity. On a sunny summer day there are few more enjoyable experiences than a walk across Sanda. The central valley traps the heat as it is sheltered from all the prevailing winds.

* * *

Access: Byron Darnton tavern (07810-356278). Kintyre Marine Charters sails from the Old Quay, Campbeltown, Kintyre (01586-554667) daily throughout the summer, weather permitting.

Anchorages:

1. Off Sanda Roads just NE of slipway/jetty, 4–5m, sand. Strong nearby tidal stream requires care. On W side of anchorage a reef extends about ¾c N from Beinn a Theine marked by a perch. Note sunken rocks in centre of the Roads. Some swell likely but well-protected from SW.
2. South Bay, small bight on S side of Sanda. Temporary anchorage and shelter from NW winds about 3c ENE of The Ship light-tower. Rocks dry up to 2.5c E of SW point of the lighthouse promontory.

1.3 Holy Island

Formerly eilean Molaise (G. – Mo Las' island) corrupted to Lamlash. Was also known as Holy Island and this became its official name in 1830 when the village on Arran adopted the name of Lamlash.

OS Maps: 1:50000 Sheet 69 1:25000 Sheet 361
Admiralty Charts: 1:20000 No.1864

Area: 253ha (625 acres)
Height: 314m (1030 ft)

Owner: At one time part of the estates of the Duke of Hamilton. Bought in 1991 by a group of Scottish Buddhists, the Samyé Ling Buddhist Centre, for about £400,000 from Mrs Catherine Morris. The price was agreed on the understanding that there would be no commercial exploitation and that the archaeological and spiritual amenities, and the distinctive flora and fauna would be protected.

Population: 1841–no separate record. 1881–15. 1891–16 (3 houses). 1931–19. 1961–7. 1971–10. (These figures include the lighthouse keepers.) 1981–0. 1991–0. Now populated by a small community of Buddhists.

Geology: Mainly igneous rock of a rhyolite type in the north and basalt in the south. The steep patches on the west slopes are of porphyry and claystone.

History: The island's one-time resident and patron saint, St Mo Las, was born in Ireland in AD 566.

In the 12th century Somerled established a monastery on the island and it was visited by King Haakon's Norsemen before and probably also after the Battle of Largs in 1263.

In 1548 the ship carrying the five-year-old child who was to become Mary Queen of Scots sheltered here on its way to France.

Wildlife: The island is a nature reserve. It was once covered with trees and the present owners, following their passionate interest in the environment, have already planted some 35,000 native species at the north end.

Wild Saanen goats, once common on Arran but

now extinct there, still roam free on the island. In Victorian times it was fashionable to drink their milk which was thought to bestow longevity.

There is also a flock of Soay sheep, a herd of Eriskay ponies and, of course, thousands of rabbits on the island. All roam free, forage for themselves in peaceful co-existence with humans and are left to their own devices. Feeding or disturbing them is forbidden. Peregrines breed on the rocky cliffs and many birds, including eider duck, nest on the shores.

The 18th century traveller, Thomas Pennant, said that the island was 'infested with vipers' but this is certainly not true today.

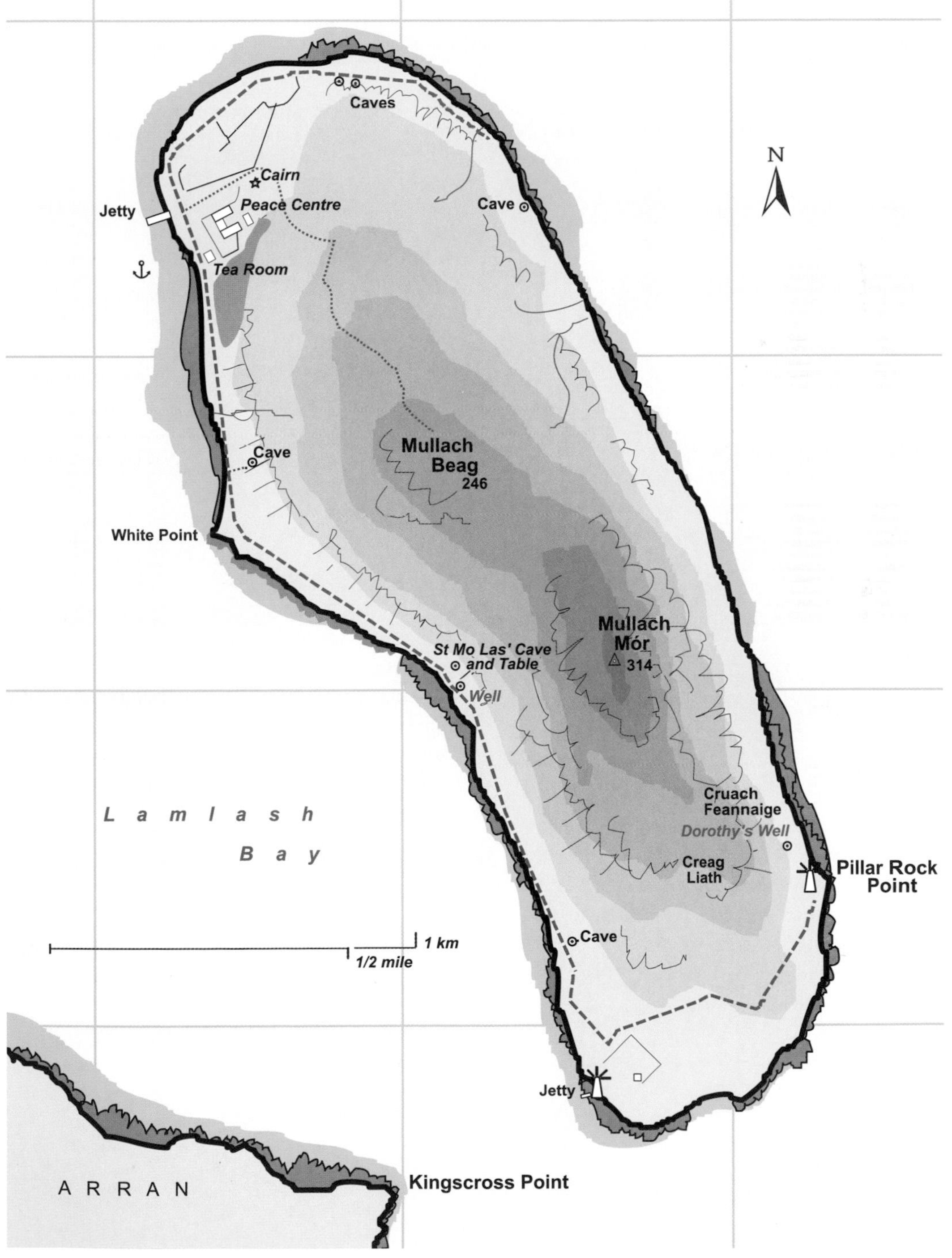

* * *

HOLY ISLAND shelters one of the finest of naval anchorages and the large mooring buoys used by the great warships of the Royal Navy in the First World War are still in place. This was the home in the 7th century of St Mo Las, or St Molias (or St Luserian in some accounts). The saint lived and meditated comfortably in **St Mo Las' Cave** [NS059297] well-furnished with every 'mod. con.', – a fireplace, a fresh water supply from a nearby spring, drainage carved out of the rock and, beside the front door, a large stone dining-table with stone seats which is known as the Judgement Stone because he sat there to settle local disputes. The saint was said to be a strict disciplinarian. The spring is called **St Mo Las' Well** and the cave contains runic and early Christian inscriptions. The former are thought to have been carved by King Haakon's defeated followers returning home after the Battle of Largs. The latter is a 'signature' thought to refer to Nicholas the 11th century Bishop of Man. It is marked with an episcopal cross. On my last visit there was an iron grille protecting the cave entrance and the (absent) owners' assistance would have been required to obtain access to the interior. In view of the damage that vandals have done to the King's Cave on Arran this is a sensible precaution.

St Mo Las is reputed to have lived to the ripe old age of 120 in spite of deliberately contracting thirty nasty diseases to expiate his sins. It is said that his bones were taken over to Arran, carried through the central valley and buried under a rough stone in a wall of the church at Shiskine, near Blackwaterfoot.

There are supposed to be a few traces of a 12th-century fortress built by Somerled, Lord of the Isles, and in the 13th century a monastery was established in a position south-east of the present Peace Centre. The small chapel was used for burials until 1790. The monastery is said to have been founded by Ranald, son of Somerled, but it was in a ruinous state by 1594.

Mullach Mór (G. - big top) is the descriptive name of the central peak and summit of the island at 314m, with Mullach Beag (G. - little top) to the north of it. This is the easiest route for a scramble up the mountain but avoid the precipitous east flank. Apart from the two lighthouses in the south of the island the Peace Centre, outbuildings and known archaeological remains are all in the north beside a mature woodland copse. The plan, however, is to build a Retreat Centre recessed into the southern hillside by Dorothy's Well and overlooking the sea. This will be a 'simple wall of rooms, Potala-like' and will accommodate a community of about 200 adherents looking for 'inner peace'. Meanwhile the renovated lighthouse-keepers' cottages serve as a Retreat.

This is part of the Samyé Ling Buddhist Order's twenty-year plan to create Europe's biggest non-denominational spiritual sanctuary on the island. Their Peace Centre, which incorporates the original farmhouse, was opened in 2003 with accommodation for 60 people, dining room, library, and multi-purpose Peace Hall. The old boathouse is now an Information Centre and tea room and the existing lighthouse-keepers' cottages have been renovated. Dry-stone dykes have been repaired, the one-time orchard has been replanted with traditional varieties, and there is an extensive vegetable garden as all meals served on the island are strictly vegetarian. Environmental considerations have been paramount: springs supply the fresh water, heating is by solar panels, sewage is treated in state-of-the-art reed beds and a large portion of the island has been reforested with native species.

A coastal circuit, half by path and dirt road, makes an interesting and not too demanding walk.

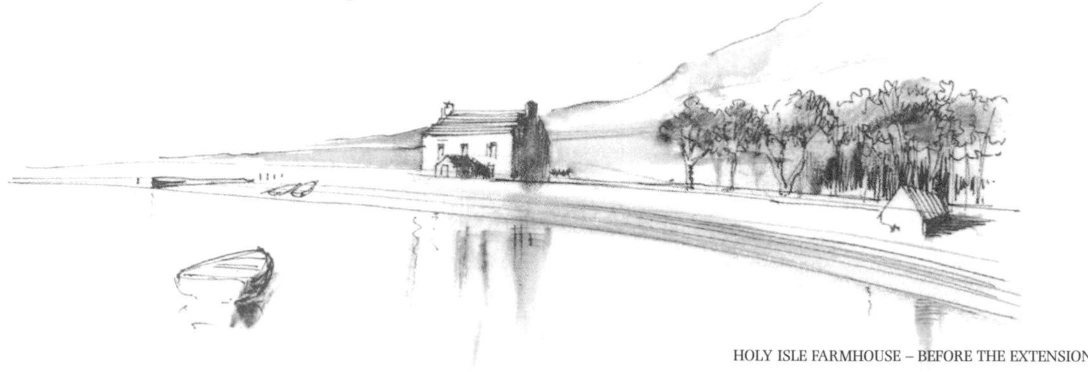

HOLY ISLE FARMHOUSE – BEFORE THE EXTENSION

I have been unable to discover the significance of the name of **Dorothy's Well** which is in the south-east [NS068292].

On the way back from such a walk, if the sun is setting over Goat Fell and Mullach Mór brooding in the evening light, rest for a while by the dry stone dyke and admire the view. Once upon a time, it is said, there was a farmer living in the original farmhouse whose wife bore him fifteen daughters. He was so disgusted at not having a son that he murdered her and buried her body under the stone-flagged kitchen floor.

Access: There is a regular private ferry service (01770-601100) to Holy Island from Lamlash pier (weather and tide permitting). Lamlash is 10 minutes' bus ride from Brodick. The crossing takes 10 minutes. Accommodation and meals available on Holy Island (01770- 601100) for persons of all Faiths but visitors are asked to respect and abide by the Five Golden Rules of Buddhism.

Anchorage:

1. Opposite the Peace Centre in 6m to 8m, well SW of the jetty and as near the shore as reasonable. Weed on pebbles. Check that anchor well bedded. Good shelter.

1.4 Arran

(B. aran – high place).

O S Maps: 1:50000 Sheet 69 1:25000 Sheet 361
Admiralty Charts: 1:75000 Nos.2126 and 2131 1:36000 No.2220 Pladda to Brodick and No.2221 Brodick to Cock of Arran 1:25000 No.1864 Brodick 1:20000 No.1864 Lamlash

Area: 43,201ha (106,750 acres) **Height:** 874m (2867 ft)

Owner: Multiple ownership but the principal owners are the heirs of the Duchess of Montrose, the Forestry Commission, the National Trust for Scotland (NTS), Stephen Gibbs (Dougarie) and J K & C Bone (Glenkiln). The Duchess of Montrose's inheritance came when the direct line of the Hamiltons ceased in 1895. Mary, Duchess of Montrose died in 1957 and in 1958 her daughter, Lady Jean Fforde gifted Goatfell and the neighbouring mountains to the NTS while Brodick Castle was accepted in lieu of estate duty by the Inland Revenue and transferred to the NTS.

Arran, oddly enough, appears to have three earldoms: Earl of Arran (No 1), is the Duke of Hamilton – title granted in 1389; Earl of Arran (No 2), title granted in 1467 and including 1000 acres and Lochranza Castle was sold by Lady Jean Fforde to an anonymous purchaser in 1994; Earl of Arran (No 3), title originated in Ireland, is held by the Gore family in Hertfordshire.

Population: 1755–3646. 1792–5804. 1821–6600. 1841–6241. 1881–4730. 1891–4824. 1931–4506. 1961–3700. 1971–3564. 1981–3845. 1991–4474. 2001–5058.

Geology: Arran is a geologist's paradise. It was described by the eminent geologist Sir Archibald Geikie as a complete synopsis of Scottish geology and it was here that James Hutton in the 18th century confirmed his theories of igneous geology. It is regularly visited by parties of students to study the rock formations. Goat Fell is an igneous intrusion into the surrounding Devonian sandstones and schists giving a ring of upturned strata around a granite core – the dramatic high peaks and corries are a direct result of this. The early settlers used local pitchstone for their artefacts and Cruttwell (18th century) claimed that topaz were to be found in the area.

In the north-east of Arran there is a region of carboniferous limestone whilst the south is composed of new red sandstone. Where there is hard granite the many basaltic dykes have eroded to form fissures but in the softer rock in the south of the island the dykes form conspicuous ridges. There are many erratics – boulders which have been moved a considerable distance from their source by Ice Age glaciers, particularly in the south. In the west below Dougarie Lodge there are interesting terraces of glacial material while in the north great rockfalls on the coast date back to the Mesozoic and Palaeozoic periods. The northern tip is a large sandstone outcrop called the Cock of Arran. A raised beach almost 8m above sea level virtually encircles the island.

History: Whoever the first inhabitants may have been several thousand years ago, Arran was probably invaded in 200BC by Britons speaking a Celtic language (Brythonic) related to present-day Welsh. (Dumbarton, meaning Fort of the Britons, was another similar enclave left by the Romans when they departed in 400AD.) Scots arrived from Ireland in the 6th century and included Arran in the Kingdom of Dalriada (roughly the extent of present-day Argyll, but for a time stretching further south). Norsemen then moved in about the 9th century and separated the island from Dalriada but Somerled, when founding the monastery at Saddell in Kintyre where he was eventually buried, took it from the Norse in 1156. After the Battle of Largs in 1263 Arran (still under the dominion of the Lord of the Isles) became part of the Scottish Kingdom but, as with Bute, it was considered the personal property of the Stewart kings – not Crown property. It was eventually awarded to the Hamiltons by Royal Charter in 1503 and at the end of the 18th century the Duke of Hamilton was still sole proprietor except for five small farms. After 1745 villages and crofts were deserted through massive emigration and large areas were later laid waste by the introduction of sheep farming. The Gaelic life and culture of the island was shattered. James Hogg wrote: 'Ah! Wae's me, I hear the Duke of Hamilton's crofters are a' gaun away, man and mither's son, frae the Isle o' Arran. Pity on us!'

Wildlife: Palm-lilies, a sub-tropical native tree of New Zealand, grow in the mild climate of the south and west. Most types of deciduous trees can be found with two unique species of whitebeam found nowhere else: *Sorbus arranensis*, and, with only two known specimens, *Sorbus pseudomeinichii*.

Some less common species of wildflowers flourish on Arran – alpine enchanter's nightshade in areas of deep shade and alpine lady's mantle which grows in Glen Sannox.

At present Arran has a population of about 2000 wild red deer. This is a recovery from the end of the 18th century when the herds had been hunted almost to extinction. There are no foxes, grey squirrels, stoats, weasels or moles and both adders and badgers are now fairly rare.

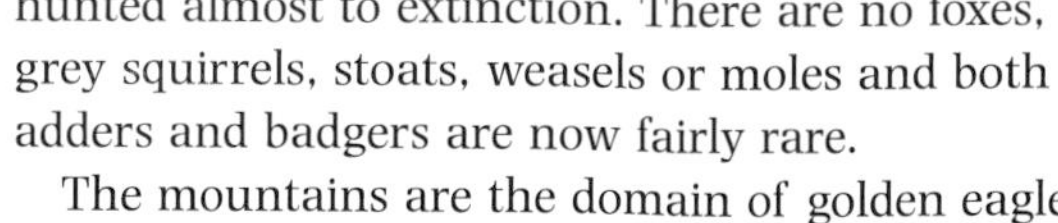

The mountains are the domain of golden eagles and all the characteristic moorland birds are to be found.

* * *

Sheltering behind the Mull of Kintyre and sitting snugly in the busy Firth of Clyde, **ARRAN** has the blessing of a mild climate and easy access to populous Glasgow. There is an average annual rainfall of 1250mm (50 ins) in the west, and double that figure up in the mountains. This has been a popular holiday resort since the early 18th century – and tourism is still the main industry, but agriculture and a whisky distillery play their part. This is also an island steeped in legends and ghosts, folklore and fairy tales.

A circuit of the island is about 92 Km (55 miles). The **Isle of Arran Heritage Museum** at Brodick is in an 18th-century croft farm, complete with smiddy, stables, bothy and coach house. It has a tea room and demonstrations of local crafts.

To the north of Brodick Bay (ON *breidr vik* – broad bay) and beneath the highest mountain, Goat Fell (G. *gaoth* – wind, ON *fjeld* – mountain) (874m) stands **Brodick Castle**. The walled garden was started in 1710 and the woodland garden, with one of Europe's finest collections of rhododendrons including some propagated from the plants at Achamore Gardens on Gigha (No.2.3), was started in 1923. Both castle and mountain belong to the National Trust for Scotland.

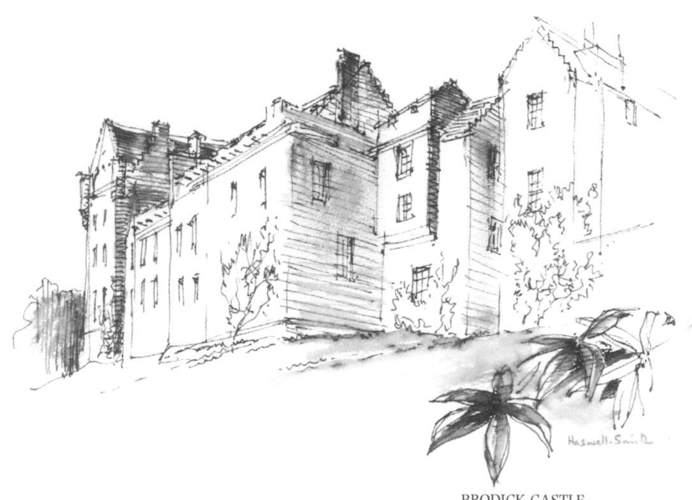

BRODICK CASTLE

Part of the Round Tower at Brodick Castle dates from the 13th century but the main building was constructed by the Hamiltons who started the work in 1558. In 1652 Cromwell's forces, normally renowned for destruction, built the Battery and an extra wing but the troops were later massacred by the islanders. In 1844 Gillespie Graham was the architect for the final work including the Great West Tower. He was commissioned by William, son of the tenth Duke of Hamilton, and his wife, Princess Mary of Baden, who was a great-niece of the Empress Josephine. The castle is worth visiting as a fine example of Scottish baronial

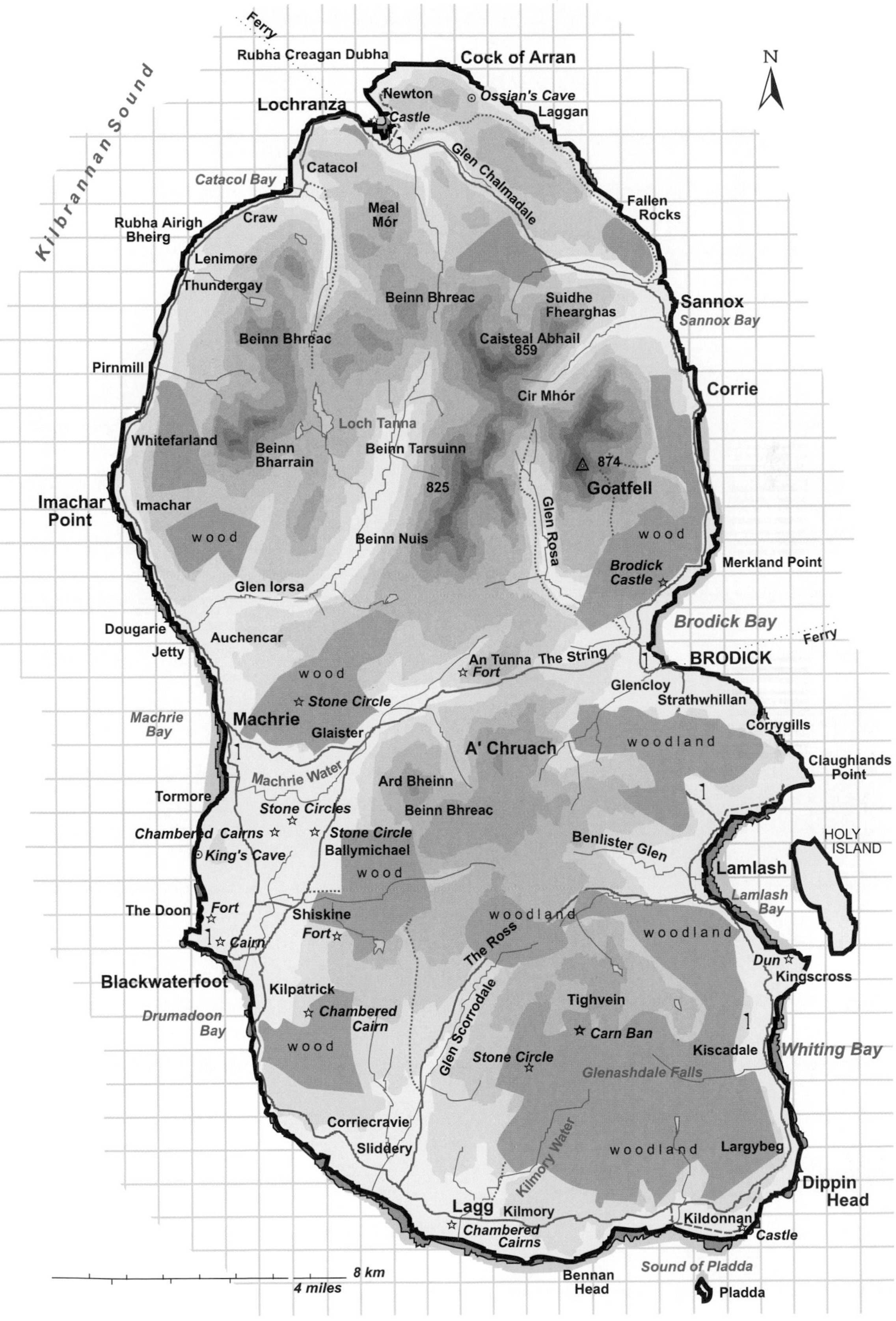
Ferry
Rubha Creagan Dubha
Cock of Arran
N
Kilbrannan Sound
Lochranza
Newton
Ossian's Cave
Castle
Laggan
Glen Chalmadale
Catacol
Catacol Bay
Meal Mór
Fallen Rocks
Rubha Airigh Bheirg
Craw
Lenimore
Thundergay
Beinn Bhreac
Suidhe Fhearghas
Sannox
Sannox Bay
Beinn Bhreac
Caisteal Abhail 859
Pirnmill
Cir Mhór
Corrie
Loch Tanna
Whitefarland
Beinn Bharrain
Beinn Tarsuinn
874
825
Goatfell
Imachar Point
Imachar
Glen Rosa
wood
wood
Beinn Nuis
Brodick Castle
Merkland Point
Glen Iorsa
Brodick Bay
Dougarie
Auchencar
Ferry
Jetty
An Tunna Fort
The String
BRODICK
wood
Glencloy
Stone Circle
Strathwhillan
Machrie Bay
Machrie
Glaister
Corrygills
A' Chruach
woodland
Claughlands Point
Machrie Water
Tormore
Ard Bheinn
Stone Circles
Beinn Bhreac
Chambered Cairns
Stone Circle
HOLY ISLAND
King's Cave
Ballymichael
Benlister Glen
Lamlash
wood
Lamlash Bay
The Doon
Fort
Shiskine
woodland
woodland
Cairn
Fort
The Ross
Dun
Kingscross
Blackwaterfoot
Kilpatrick
Tighvein
Drumadoon Bay
Chambered Cairn
Glen Scorrodale
Carn Ban
wood
Stone Circle
Kiscadale
Whiting Bay
Glenashdale Falls
Corriecravie
Sliddery
Kilmory Water
woodland
Largybeg
Dippin Head
Lagg
Kilmory
Kildonnan
Chambered Cairns
Castle
8 km
4 miles
Sound of Pladda
Bennan Head
Pladda

architecture with richly designed interiors, many art treasures, and a restored Victorian kitchen. The grounds are open throughout the year and the castle is open from Easter until late September.

There is a superb scenic hill-walk of 18km (11 miles) which starts near Brodick [NS004368] and goes up Glen Rosa, across the saddle at 460m (1500 ft) by Cir Mhór (G. – big comb) then down through the wild landscape of Glen Sannox and the remains of old barytes mines (abandoned 1938) to **Sannox Bay** [NS016454].

North of Brodick is the pretty village of **Corrie** (G. *coire* – a cauldron-shaped hollow) with two tiny harbours. The quarry in the hills behind provided stone for the construction of the Crinan Canal. The road continues through Sannox to Lochranza but, if the weather's good, there is a fine 15km (9 mile) walk along the shoreline passing Ossian's Cave and, the most northerly point, the **Cock of Arran**. The mountain side here once resembled an enormous crowing cock with its wings spread but its head has now eroded away. There is an alternative path at the mid-point, Laggan [NR979508], which goes over the hill ridge. Daniel MacMillan, founder of the publishing empire, spent his childhood here.

The little village of **Lochranza** spreads along the southern shore under the ramparts of ruined Lochranza Castle standing in the centre of the loch on a shingle spit. This is where Bruce is reputed to have landed in 1306 or 1307 on his return from Rathlin Island. His sister is also supposed to have sheltered here in a nunnery but no trace of one has been found. Fragments of Lochranza Castle are from an early fortification mentioned by Fordun in the 14th century but most of the existing ruin dates from the 16th century. In the early 15th century it belonged to John de Mentieth and it was then granted by James II to Alexander Lord Montgomery.

For the yachtsman the delightful anchorage of Loch Ranza has something of a reputation for anchor-dragging. I can recall one evening when the wind picked up to gale force and swung into the north-east and sudden violent squalls came down the glen. By midnight every one of the nine boats anchored in the loch was playing ring-a-ring-a-roses in the dark as they tried to find a sound bottom. We missed our normal visit to the excellent pub!

At **Catacol** (ON – *ravine of the wildcat*) south of Lochranza the terrace of cottages at the mouth of the glen is known as the Twelve Apostles [NR911497]. Loch Tanna, the largest loch

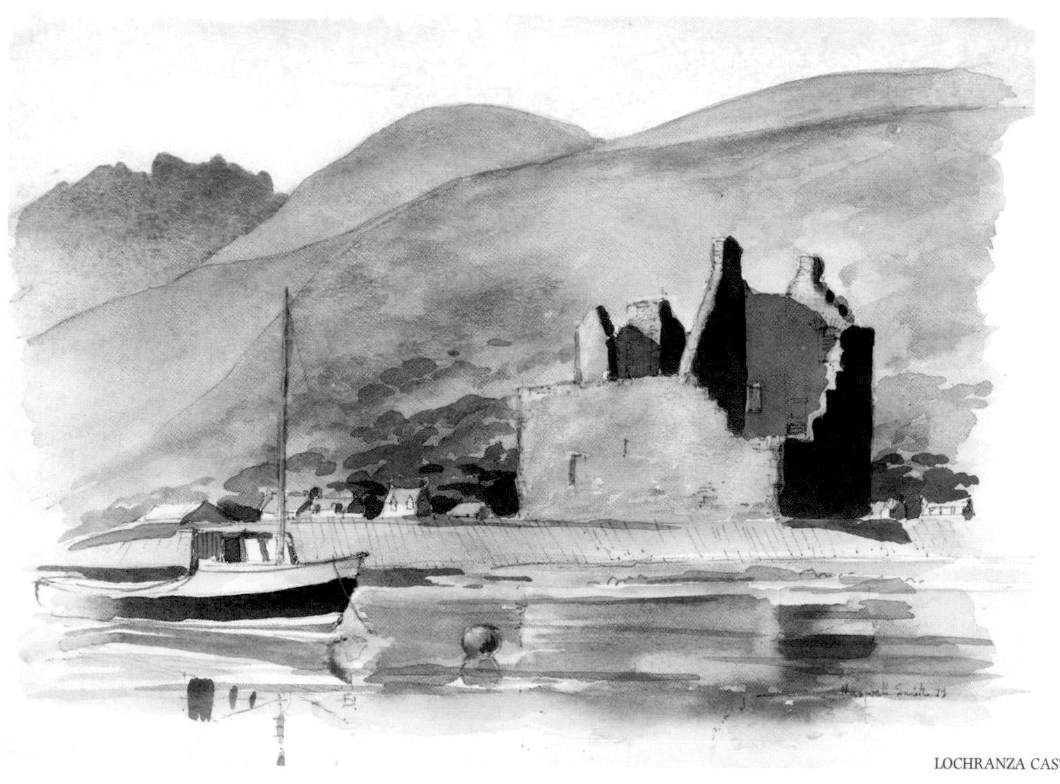

LOCHRANZA CASTLE

on Arran, is at the summit of Glen Catacol in the wild landscape beneath Beinn Bhreac (G. – speckled mountain) – 711m high (2332 ft). Further south by the fine beach at Pirnmill [NR873445] pine bobbins or 'pirns' were made for the Paisley mills – until there were no more pines.

The road runs on past the palm trees of Whitefarland and Imachar to **Dougarie Lodge** where Iorsa Water tumbles into the sea. The lodge [NR884371] was built by the Hamiltons and the first island telephone was installed here in 1891.

At Machrie Moor (G. *machair* – low, level land) where the central valley opens out there is a feast of archaeological remains. Some of the standing stones were unfortunately turned into millstones but many undamaged stones remain as well as chambered tombs and cairns (3500BC–1000BC) both here and in the southern coastal areas [eg. NR9032 and 9132]. Bronze Age burial chambers or cists have been found inside one of the many stone circles on Machrie Moor and there is a 15-stone circle round a burial cairn in the woods above the road at Auchagallon [NR908351]. Arran has no less than ten such henges or stone circles.

An interesting walk above the shore from **Tormore** leads to the **King's Cave**, a large, dry, sandstone cave, 30m deep and level with the raised beach [NR884309]. In the 18th century the Kirk Session met here and in the 19th century it was used as a school. The cave entrance (protected by a grille in 1995) can be seen when sailing in the Kilbrannan Sound. It was said to have been occupied by Fingal, Fionn MacCaul, the legendary Irish King, who, to prove his manhood, rebuffed a Viking raid by Manos, heir to the Swedish King. The cave was excavated in 1902 exposing early Christian or Viking wall-carvings of hunting scenes but vandals have now covered these with graffiti and caused a lot of damage. Incidentally, this cave is also supposed to have been lived in by Robert the Bruce when he was inspired by the well-kent spider but the cave on Rathlin Island off the north-east corner of Ireland has better credentials.

In 1817 Thomas Telford built the road (B880) which crosses the island to Brodick Bay. It was named '**The String**' by sailors because from the sea it looks like a piece of string laid across the bare moorland. South of Machrie Moor the village of **Shiskine** [NR913299] is reputed to be the burial place of St Mo Las of Holy Island (No.1.3).

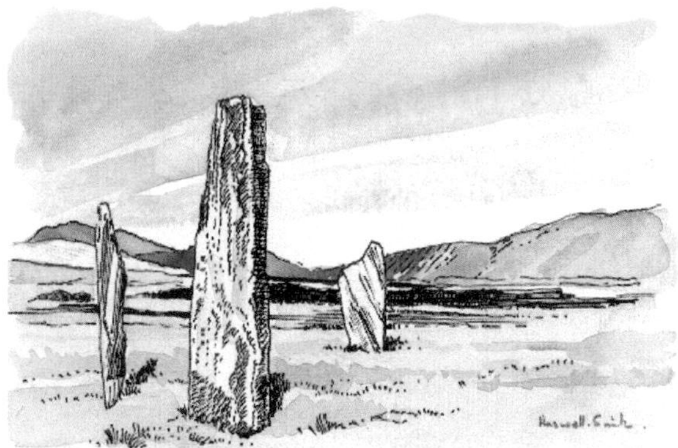
MONOLITHS AT MACHRIE MOOR

A large cairn [NR891288] at **Blackwaterfoot**, which was pillaged during the 19th century, contained relics including a dagger and this was thought to show a link with the culture of Stonehenge. The double ramparts of an iron-age fortress, Drumadoon (G. – fort on a ridge) are on a steep slope west of the village [NR886294].

In the south-east, a picturesque minor road called The Ross, follows Sliddery Water and the Green Glen to Lamlash.

Arran's oldest hotel, an 18th-century coaching inn, stands among the trees at **Lagg** (G. – a hollow) [NR956216]. It is haunted by a laird who sold his soul to the devil. Below the village and by the sea is the ruin of a prehistoric tomb which once held the remains of four adults and two children [NR955211].

Torrylin by **Kilmory** is the home of Arran cheese. The whole of this rocky south coast was once the haunt of smugglers from Ireland and wandering through the woods above the village are the ghosts of a young couple who were mistaken for smugglers and shot by coastguards. There is extensive forestry in the area with many interesting woodland walks. **Carn Ban**, a well-preserved Neolithic chambered cairn measuring 30m x 18m [NR991262] is by a burn in a high wooded valley – Allt an t-Sluice. It is 6½km (4 miles) up a forest track which starts just east of Kilmory and the site is 291m above sea level.

In the extreme south-east are the limited ruins of 14th-century **Kildonan Castle** [NS036209], which was granted by King Robert III to his bastard son, John, in 1406.

Kildonan, a place reputedly visited by St Donan after his training at Whithorn, overlooks the small tear-shaped island of **Pladda** (ON – flat isle). Owned by Arran Estate, it was up for sale in 1990 for £80,000, its first time ever on the market. Originally granted to the Hamiltons, the lighthouse was rebuilt by Stevenson in the 1820s and was manned until the 1980s. In spite of being only 11ha in area, Pladda is lucky to have its own fresh water supply.

Glenashdale Burn enters the sea by the youth hostel at **Whiting Bay**. There is an easy walk [NS046252] through the woods one mile up the glen to see the dramatic waterfalls which have a 30m drop over a lava sill. Nearby are the ruins of a fort, two chambered cairns and the 'Giants' Graves'.

The substantial remains of a Viking burial mound and fort [NS056283] are at **Kingscross Point**, south of Lamlash Bay. It was here that Robert the Bruce waited for a bonfire to be lit on the Ayrshire coast as the prearranged signal that his supporters were ready for his final attempt to claim the crown. There was a false alarm and he arrived too early, but his claim was successful nevertheless.

The High School at **Lamlash** [NS024307] stands on the ground where Donald 'Tattie' MacKelvie developed the world renowned seed potatoes, *Arran Chief, Arran Pilot* and *Arran Banner*.

For anglers the salmon and trout fishing in both the Machrie and Iorsa Waters has a high rating and, for general recreational activities, Arran provides swimming, boating, pony-trekking, and seven golf-courses.

For the mountaineer Arran is noted for its four 'Corbetts': Goatfell, 874m; Beinn Tarsuinn (G. – transverse hill), 825m; Cir Mhor [keer vor] (G. – big comb), 798m; and, Caisteal Abhail (G. – Castle ptarmigan), 859m.

It is, I am reliably told, possible to traverse all the main tops in the east and central groups in one day – 'as the going is so easy'. This amounts to a total height of about 2600m to be climbed. Many of the excellent climbs, ridge-walks and hill-walks of Arran are listed in the publications of the Scottish Mountaineering Club.

Incidentally, the name of the mountain called Suidhe Fhearghas (G. – seat of Fergus) [NR990455] recalls a day when the Fianna of Ireland were hunting red deer on Arran. They took time off to meet for a banquet on the mountain and to listen to their bard, Fergus of the True Lips.

Access: Car ferry: Ardrossan/Brodick takes one hour, 08000-66-5000. Train connections with Glasgow. Advance booking usually essential. Tourist Information Office near Brodick pier, 01770-302140. Car ferry: Lochranza/Claonaig Kintyre, summer only and subject to reasonable weather, 30 min. trip. There is a bus service on Arran, 0871-222-2233, and bicycles and cars can be hired. Local companies operate coach tours.

Anchorages:

Note: All anchorages except Lochranza and Lamlash Bay are exposed and only tenable in settled conditions.

1. North Sannox, between the southernmost measured-mile posts. Exposed temp. anchorage in 3m, sand, close inshore just N of the burn. Outstanding views.
2. Sannox Bay, sandy bay at entrance to the Sannox river. Temp anchorage off old stone pier in 6–12m. Beware Sannox rock near centre of bay. Very exposed NE to SE. Beautiful view.
3. Corrie. Exposed temp. anchorage in 4–8m off either of the old stone harbours N and S of Corrie Point.
4. Brodick bay. Visitors' moorings or good anchorage in light W'lies in 3–5m, sand, about 2c W of the pier. Anchor well off-shore to avoid moorings and ferry or, in NW winds, anywhere between Merkland Point and the Old Quay. Restricted temp. shelter within inner pier subject to HM's agreement. (*Access to Brodick Castle and grounds*).
5. Clauchlands Point. Anchor in Lamlash Bay 4c W of the Point. Exposed to E.
6. Lamlash. There are 25 visitors' moorings laid by Arran Yacht Club. Or anchor in 4–6m, E of stone pier but many moorings and bottom steep. Swell in E winds. Squalls in strong NW winds.
7. Cordon to Kingscross. Anchor anywhere from SE of the Cordon shoal to Kingscross avoiding moorings and fish cages. In S'ly gales best NW of old ferry pier.
8. Whiting Bay, between Largybeg and Kingscross Points, sheltered from W'lies only. Temp anchorage in 4–8m, well off-shore.
9. Pladda. Anchor on E side of island close in-shore just N of lighthouse jetty, in 5–8m, sand with thick weed. Sheltered N to W and partly from SW. Many dangers in channel between Pladda and Arran.
10. Blackwaterfoot (Drumadoon Bay), very exposed to S and W. Anchor in 4m near burn mouth but beware many rocks.
11. Machrie bay, mid-W side, temp. anchorage in 3–7m anywhere in bay but avoid Iorsa Patch at N end. Depths increase suddenly. At Machrie burn the shore shoals out for about 1c for 1M on either side. Exposed SW to NW.

12. Whitefarland bay, temp. anchorage in 6–12m, protected from S and E winds. Bay shoals for 2c off shore for about ½M N.

13. Catacol bay, temp anchorage at S of bay S of Catacol burn in 12m, some shelter from S.

14. Lochranza, small sea loch which dries about 2c from head. Ferry pier extends N from Coillemore point (the S entrance point). Exposed W through N to NNE. NE to NW winds cause considerable swell and there can be violent squalls. Enter closer to ferry pier. Visitors' moorings or anchor in centre of loch, off the ruined castle. Bottom soft mud with poor holding.

1.5 Little Cumbrae

Probably (B. cymri – Brythonic Gaelic people) i.e. the place of the Brythonic or Welsh-speaking Gaels. Formerly known as Little, Lesser or Wee Cumray.

OS Maps: 1:50000 Sheet 63 1:25000 Sheet 341
Admiralty Chart: 1:25000 1907 or 1:36000 2221

Area: 313ha (773 acres)
Height: 123m (403ft)

Owner: Property of the Earl of Eglington prior to 1913. Purchased in 1960 by Mr & Mrs Peter Kaye for £24,000 from the trustees of Ian Robertson

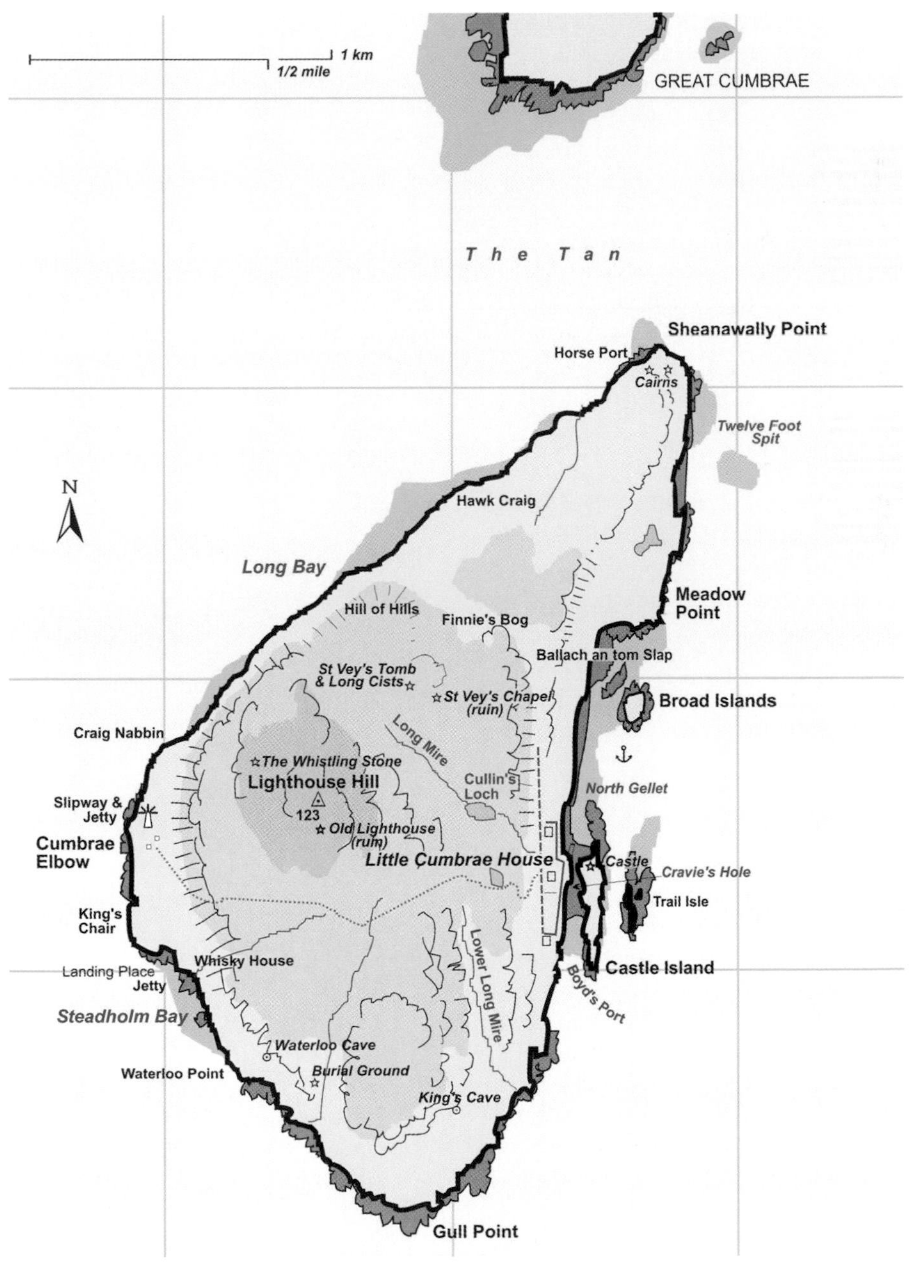

Parker of Cheshire. Bought by Stephen Worrallo in 2005. Sold in 2008 for £2.5m.

Population: 1841–8. 1881–23. 1891–17. 1931–21. 1961–8. 1981–6. 1991–6. 2001–0.

Geology: Mainly Carboniferous basalt and spilite.

History: Until 1515 the hereditary keepers of the island were the Hunters of Hunterston. During the 14th century Kings Robert II and Robert III used the island as a deer forest.

Cromwell's men landed and caused some damage to the castle in 1653.

Wildlife: In the 19th century over 5000 rabbits a year were 'harvested' and rabbits are still numerous. The island has been maintained as a nature reserve ('bugs, beasties, botany, etc.') and visited by occasional university study groups.

* * *

An attractive large house, **Cumbrae House**, overlooks the castle ruin and a bay which has some rocky outcrops on the north side known as **Broad Islands**.

Castle Island is linked by a drying strand to Little Cumbrae's east coast with **Trail Island** lying alongside like a moored ship. The original castle was possibly built by Bruce's son-in-law. A Royal Charter was signed there in 1375. The present square keep on Castle Island [NS152513] was erected in 1527, apparently to control deer poaching. It was wrecked by Cromwell's army but still stands as an imposing ruin. It is a twin to the keep on the mainland at Portencross. A short distance north of it [NS148518] are the remains of **St Veya's Chapel** and various antiquities which are worth inspection. St Veya (or St Beya) was a 7th-century nun.

The ancient lighthouse tower at the summit of the island [NS143515] is the type that had a fire of coals, or 'cresset', burning in an open grate. Presumably a fairly large fire had to be maintained. Imagine the effort of shipping coal to the island, carrying it up the hillside, hoisting it onto the open platform and keeping it burning during gale-lashed rainstorms! This particular light-tower was built in 1757 and is similar to the original design on the Isle of May (See No.12-1). The modern lighthouse (now automatic solar-powered) and landing place stands below it on the west shore. There is a path leading over 'Rest and Be Thankful' and skirting Tom's Loch before descending to Cumbrae House on the east side by the castle.

The island, which is easily accessible but infrequently visited, is rugged, with many rock outcrops and caves on the raised beach at the south end.

* * *

Access: Try Cumbrae Voyages, Largs Yacht Haven, 0845-257-0404 or a Largs or Millport boat owner.

Anchorages:
1. Give N end of island a wide berth because of shoals. Anchor on E coast in 2–4m between Castle Island and Broad Island or to the N of Broad Island. Avoid moorings and jetty. Uncomfortable in S and E winds.
2. There is a landing place for the lighthouse on the W shore.

1.6 Great Cumbrae

Probably (B. cymri – Brythonic Gaelic people) i.e. the place of the Brythonic or Welsh-speaking Gaels. Formerly known as Great or Greater Cumray.

O S Maps: 1:50000 Sheet 63 1:25000 Sheet 341
Admiralty Charts: 1:25000 No.1907 or 1:36000 No.2221

Area: 1,168ha (2886 acres)
Height: 127m (417ft)

Owner: Owned by the Marquess of Bute's family since the 12th century when King Malcolm reputedly awarded it to their ancestor, Walter Fitzalan, for defeating a mini-invasion of the Clyde. It was sold by the Marquess to his tenants in 1999.

Population: 1793–509. 1841–1413. 1881–1856. 1891–1784. 1931–2144. 1961–1638. 1981–1300. 1991–1393. 2001–1434. This is the most densely populated of the listed Scottish islands.

Geology: Most of the island is Old Red Sandstone but the area round Millport is Carboniferous limestone. There are many igneous dykes such as 'The Lion' near the south-east corner opposite Largs.

History: King Haakon is reputed to have set up his camp at Tomont End, the northern tip of Great Cumbrae, before the Battle of Largs in 1263.

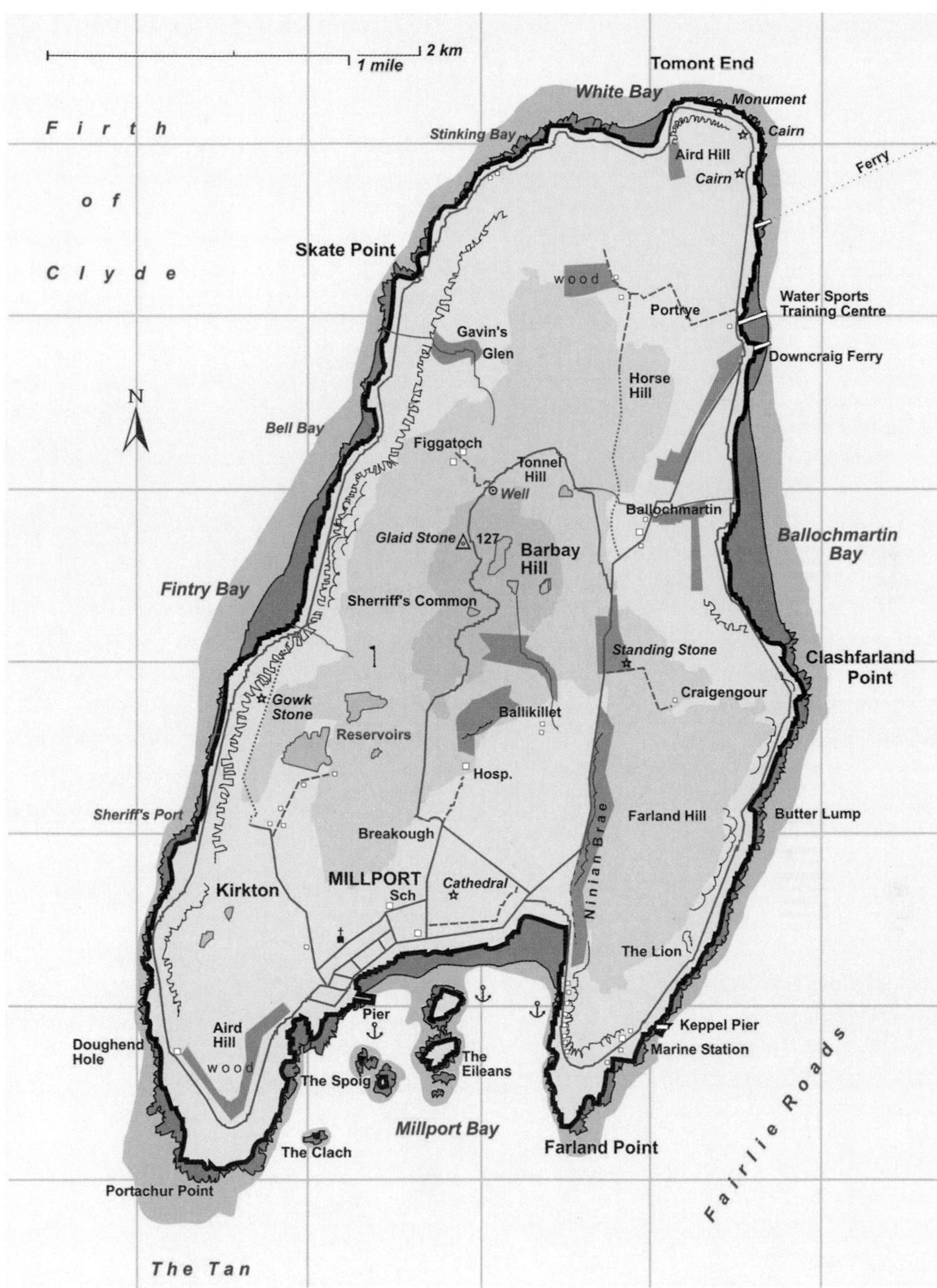

Millport was popular with trippers in the heyday of holidays on the Clyde but in 1906 the steamer companies boycotted the island because of excessive harbour dues. The island nearly died until Lloyd George stepped in and settled the dispute – just in time for the annual Glasgow Fair holiday.

Wildlife: The marine life round the island is very rich and has been studied since the 1840s. At that time David Robertson, the 'Cumbrae Naturalist', after many visits to the island, established a floating laboratory. In 1896 the headquarters of the Scottish Marine Biological Association were built to the east of the town at Kepple Pier but this was transferred to Dunstaffnage near Oban in 1970. The University Marine Biological Station controlled by Glasgow and London Universities then took over the buildings. They have diving facilities, research vessels, a decompression chamber and a well-stocked aquarium which is open to the public.

The roseate tern, *Sterna dougallii*, was first identified here as a separate species by Dr MacDougal in 1812.

* * *

At the start of the 19th century the Rev James Adam, a local minister, always prayed for the people of **GREAT CUMBRAE** and 'the adjacent islands of Great Britain and Ireland' – which gives some indication of this island's importance in the eyes of its inhabitants.

A ridge of green hills stippled with rose-red rocks runs down the centre with the highest point (127m) marked by the **Glaid Stone** [NS167570]. Alongside this ridge is a hill road with unrivalled views over the Clyde and, below it, a coastal road of about 20km (12 miles) which encircles the island. In summer it can almost rival Amsterdam with numerous holidaymakers on hired cycles in search of exercise and fun.

Millport spreading round the south-facing bay is a typical small seaside resort with fun-fair, cinema, museum and sandy beaches. It was developed as a resort by the Victorians before they turned their attention to Rothesay. The solid residences look out on the bay to one of the loveliest views of Arran. The rocky islets in the middle of the bay are known simply as **The Eileans** (G. – islands).

The 'city' boasts the smallest cathedral in Britain – the **Episcopal Cathedral of Argyll and the Isles**. It was started in the 1840s by the 6th Earl of Glasgow under the influence of the Oxford Movement and the stone was quarried from the site, forming terraced gardens. The architect was William Butterfield. The mini-cathedral has a 37m spire, a starkly simple nave and a highly ornate brightly-coloured tiled chancel. One feels it has a foot in both camps, Presbyterian and Catholic. The Earl ran out of funds but the project was completed and consecrated in 1886 by Bishop Chinnery-Haldane of Argyll and the Isles.

The village of **Kirkton** in the south-west, which is now almost a suburb of Millport, was the first centre of population on the island. There has been a chapel there since the 13th century or earlier.

Norsemen who died in the Battle of Largs in 1263 are thought to be buried at **Tomont End** which is the northern tip of the island.

Both freshwater and sea fishing can be arranged from Millport and the Scottish Sports Council's **National Water Sports Training Centre** near the ferry terminal in the north-east teaches sailing, sub-aqua and canoeing.

The golf course on Sheriff's Common, near the reservoirs, provides spectacular views as well as a stimulating game and for climbers the rock outcrops on the hill behind Millport and the basaltic dykes of Lion Rock and The Deil's Dyke near Keppel Pier can be fun. Millport also has facilities for bowling and horse riding.

* * *

Access: Car ferry: Largs (10-min crossing time)/ Cumbrae Slip, 08000-66-5000. Round island bus service to Millport timed to meet the ferry. Train connections: Glasgow/ Largs. Tourist information, 01475-689962.

Anchorages:

1. Millport Bay. Visitors' moorings in the anchorage near the pier or anchor clear of the moorings E of the northmost of The Eileans in a suitable depth. Millport pier leading lights bearing 333deg between the Eileans and The Spoig leads to the W anchorage. . Bottom shelves gradually. Tripping line advised.
2. Keppel pier with a T-head, on SE coast about 4c NE of Farland point, the SE extremity. Least depth of 4.9m alongside head of pier.
3. Ballochmartin or Balloch Bay N of Clashfarland Point on E coast has a T-headed pier at the N entrance point of bay. Anchor near Grey House in 8m.
4. National Water Sports Training Centre at N end of Balloch Bay. Suitable moorings may be available. If not anchor N of the slip but well off-shore.
5. Tomont End (Monument), White Bay. Good holding and well-sheltered from SW winds, 5–9m, sand. Bay dries out 1c.

1.7 Inchmarnock

(G. innis Marnoc – island of Marnoc)

OS Maps: 1:50000 Sheet 63 1:25000 Sheet 362
Admiralty Charts: 1:25000 No.2383 or 1:36000 No.2221

Area: 253ha (625 acres)
Height: 60m (197 ft).

Owner: Bought in 1999 from Sir Richard

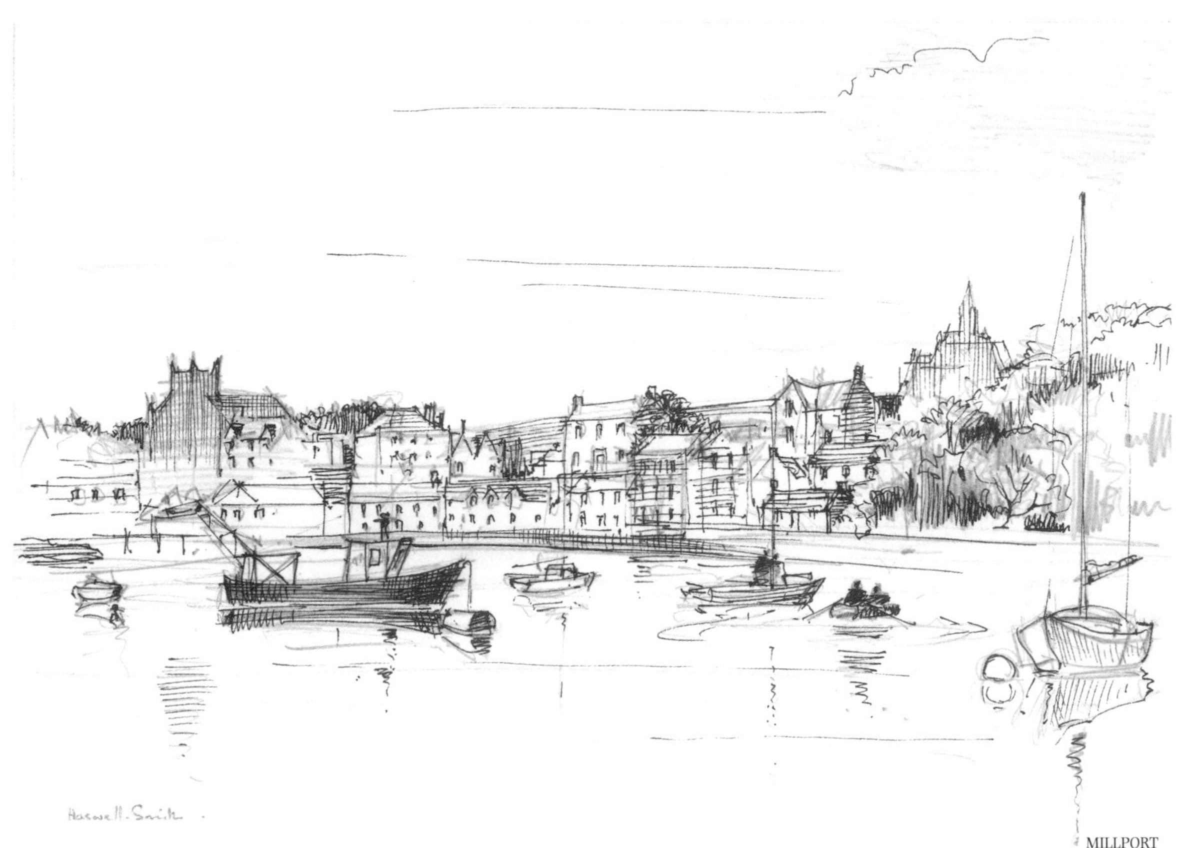

MILLPORT

Branson's brother by Sir Robert Haldane Smith, a Scottish merchant banker and BBC governor for, reportedly, £800,000.

Population: 1871–30. 1881–17. 1891–10 (3 houses). 1931–14. 1961–6. 1971–6. 1981–5. 1991–0. 2001–0.

Geology: Mainly Dalradian schistose grit similar to north Bute.

History: After the days of St Marnoc the Cistercians of Saddell in Kintyre owned the island.

It is a widely held belief that, in the 19th century, the people of Bute left their alcoholics here to cure them 'by deprivation and isolation' but this has not been verified.

Wildlife: Inchmarnock has the largest herring-gull colony on the Clyde and there is prolific birdlife. It is a popular wintering haven for greylag geese.

* * *

A derelict 'landing-craft' for ferrying material across to the island is beached beside the anchorage off Midpark Farm on **INCHMARNOCK**. The farm buildings are picturesque with hawthorn hedges on each side of the farm road and bluebells in the long grass verges. The view from the low ridge running down the centre of the island is panoramic, encompassing a great sweep of water stretching from the lower reaches of Loch Fyne to the high peaks of Arran. The hazy blue hills of the Mull of Kintyre are the backdrop. There is an overwhelming sense of peace and it is almost impossible to believe that the great city of Glasgow is only a few miles away as the crow flies.

Legend has it that there was a cheeky young Scots lad who pestered and interrupted St Columba with questions when he was preaching on the mainland. The monks were irritated and tried to silence him but St Columba chided them and prophesied that young Marnoc would become a great teacher. He had recognised a lively mind. The prophecy came true and Marnoc, later St Marnoc, settled on this island and built himself a chapel. People came from near and far to hear him preach.

A very few remains of the ancient **Chapel of**

St Marnoc, probably from a later building of the 12th or 13th century, can be seen just north of the **Midpark** farm buildings [NS024596]. Several stone fragments of Celtic crosses have been uncovered near it and also other sculpted stones including one commemorating the Viking, Gutlief. These are now in Bute Museum. The church existed until the 18th century but a farmer, Alexander McDonald, used the stone from it to build Midpark farmhouse in 1718. Only when the work was complete did he decide to play safe with eternity so he sent £10 to the Church Session and asked for atonement.

A century later the gravestones from the cemetery were used by another farmer to build a cowhouse. No Christian atonement was requested

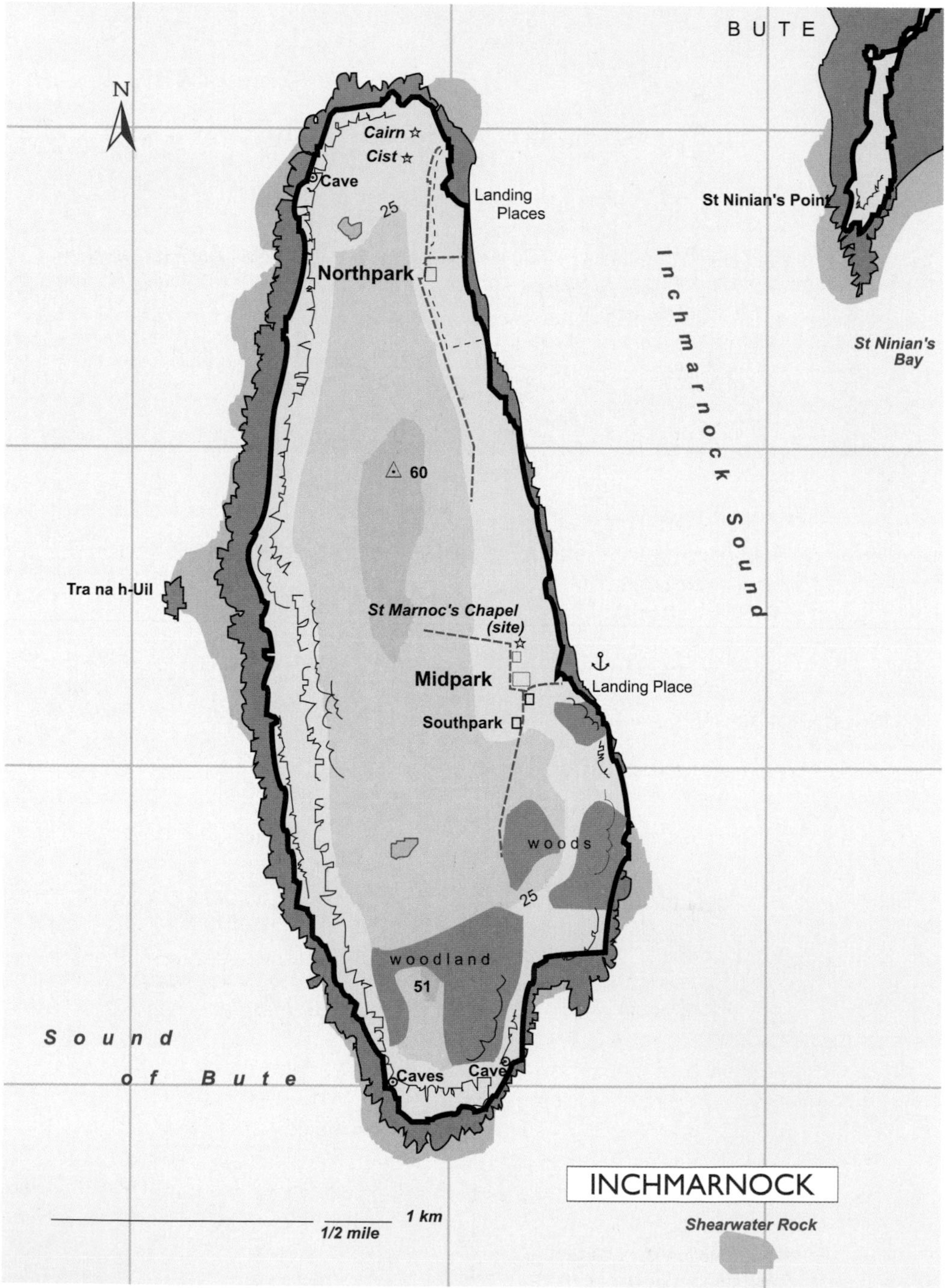

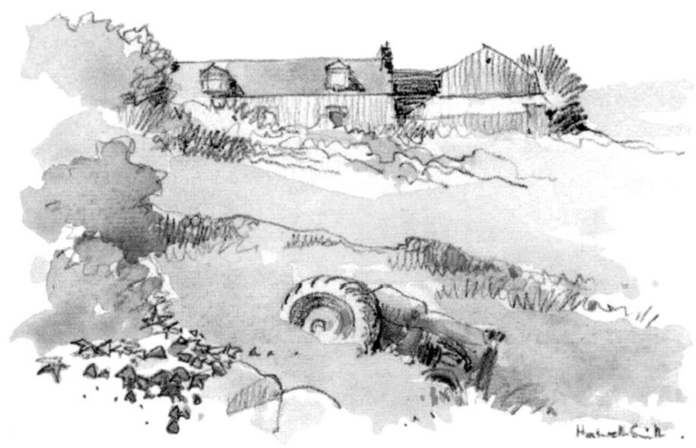
MIDPARK, INCHMARNOCK

in this case but it is recorded that his cattle all died. The farmer decided the devil was to blame so he made a burnt offering of one of the carcasses on the beach at dead of night.

The farmyard is reputed to have been laid out over the burial ground which was adjacent to the chapel, but **The Women's Burial Place** could still be distinguished in 1860 in a field adjoining the church.

In the extreme north of the island the skeleton of a young woman was found in one of three stone burial cists which were uncovered during archaeological excavation of a Bronze Age cairn [NS020612]. She was wearing a necklace consisting of 139 jet (lignite) beads, which can be seen in Bute Museum, and at her hand lay a flint knife. The tomb of the **Queen of the Inch**, as she is known, is close to Northpark, the owner's house. After the 3500-year-old skeleton had been radiocarbon-dated it was returned to its original tomb with a glass panel fitted to allow it to be seen. This was considered the best way to preserve the remains, rather than letting them moulder in a museum store. But walking past the tomb by torchlight at night requires a very steady nerve, said the previous owner. It is dark, it is quiet, it is lonely, and the shadows in the skull's eye-sockets follow every movement.

The island is divided into three farms – Northpark, Midpark and Southpark – although the latter buildings are now untenanted. The semi-derelict **Southpark** farm buildings adjoin Midpark.

Towards the end of the 19th century a tenant of Southpark was draining a 'moss' when he found in the peat a layer of preserved hazelnuts three feet thick. Investigation showed that although the island had been farmed for several thousand years, at one time it was covered with luxuriant oak and hazel forest.

The Inchmarnock islanders were evacuated during the Second World War to enable a commando training area to be created. A considerable amount of damage was done and a large area is still covered with craters. The land is generally fertile but largely uncultivated. Visitors to the island should try to obtain permission first or at least keep to the shoreline as the owner is understandably keen that the island should be disturbed as little as possible.

Inchmarnock issued its own first distinctive postage stamp in July 1999.

Access: Try Don Clark, MFV *Morag*, Tighnabruaich, ring 01700-811538 or ask in the local hotels (include time ashore to explore).

Anchorage:

1. Anchor near the middle of the E side of island off Midpark Farm in 5m sand. Sheltered from NW and W but subject to swell.

1.8 Bute

Probably (B. budh – corn, Sc. -aer – island), or, less likely, (ON bot – patch of land). For centuries, however, the island was called Rothes-ay (Roth's or Roderick's island) and the main town was called Baile Bhoid (G. – the town of corn). The Chronicle of the Scots, 1482–1530, says Bute is named after St Brandan but this is doubtful.

O S Maps: 1:50000 Sheet 63 1:25000 Sheet 362
Admiralty Charts: 1:75000 No.2131 1:25000 Nos.1906 and 2383

Area: 12,217ha (30,188 acres)
Height: 278m (912 ft)

Owner: Principal owner – Bute Estate (John Colum Crichton-Stuart, The 7th Marquess of Bute, who prefers to be known as Johnny Dumfries, or Johnny Bute. He was a world championship Grand Prix driver, who won the 24-hour race at Le Mans in 1988).
Sir Richard Attenborough owns 600ha at Rudhabodach.

Population: 1755–3220. 1792–4759. 1841–7147. 1881–10998. 1891–11735. 1931–12112. 1961–9793. 1971–8423. 1981–7306. 1991–7354. 2001–7228. There are about one million visitors each year.

Geology: Loch Fad, which cuts across the centre of the island, is a continuation of the

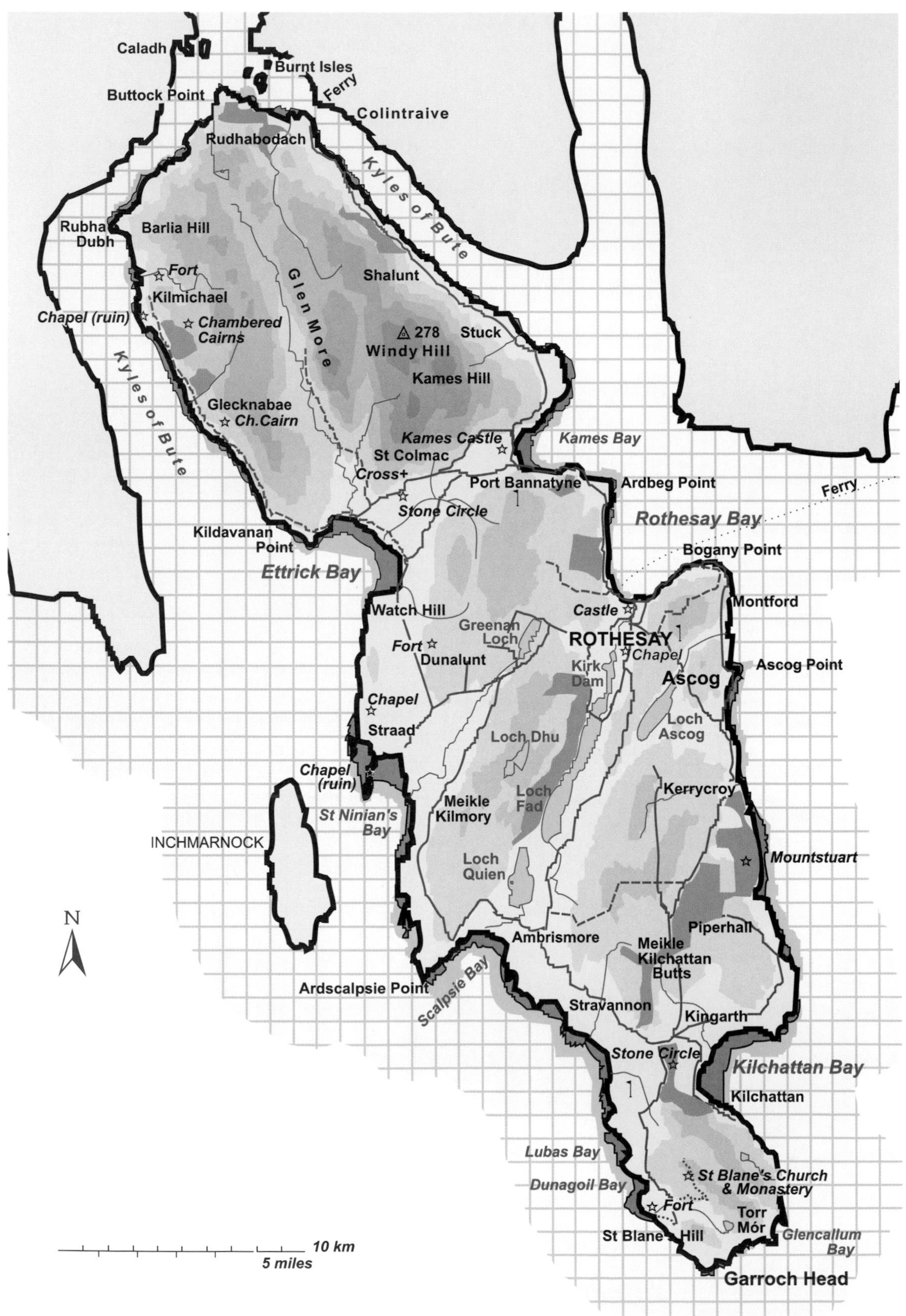
Caladh
Burnt Isles
Ferry
Buttock Point
Colintraive
Rudhabodach
Kyles of Bute
Rubha Dubh
Barlia Hill
Fort
Kilmichael
Chapel (ruin)
Chambered Cairns
Glen More
Shalunt
278
Windy Hill
Stuck
Kames Hill
Kyles of Bute
Glecknabae
Ch.Cairn
Kames Castle
Kames Bay
St Colmac
Cross+
Port Bannatyne
Ardbeg Point
Ferry
Stone Circle
Rothesay Bay
Kildavanan Point
Bogany Point
Ettrick Bay
Montford
Watch Hill
Castle
Greenan Loch
ROTHESAY
Fort
Dunalunt
Chapel
Ascog Point
Kirk Dam
Ascog
Chapel
Loch Ascog
Straad
Loch Dhu
Chapel (ruin)
Kerrycroy
Loch Fad
St Ninian's Bay
Meikle Kilmory
INCHMARNOCK
Loch Quien
Mountstuart
N
Piperhall
Ambrismore
Meikle Kilchattan Butts
Ardscalpsie Point
Scalpsie Bay
Stravannon
Kingarth
Stone Circle
Kilchattan Bay
Kilchattan
Lubas Bay
St Blane's Church & Monastery
Dunagoil Bay
Fort
Torr Mór
St Blane
Hill
Glencallum Bay
10 km
5 miles
Garroch Head

Highland Boundary Fault. To the south is Old Red Sandstone ('red pudding rock'), some basaltic lavas, and fertile undulating arable land; to the north is Dalradian schistose grit and hilly terrain.

A fine example of a raised beach can be seen from the road at Tormore Hill.

History: Bute has been continuously inhabited for at least 6000 years.

After the Roman period Bute and Arran may still have been Brythonic (Welsh-type language) kingdoms. Nearby Dumbarton means the 'Fort of the Britons'. Later, the Erse, or Gaelic language of the Scots spread into Bute.

How early Bute was personally acquired by the Stewart family is uncertain. Steward Walter married the daughter of Robert the Bruce and fathered Robert II, the first Stuart king, in 1316. The royal Stewarts were known as Sheriffs of Bute and Keepers of Rothesay Castle. Roberts II and III used the castle as a holiday home and Robert the High Steward owned the island in 1334. Rothesay became a Royal Burgh in 1403 with a further charter by James VI in 1584. Many of the Provosts of the Burgh have been members of the Bute family and much of the island's history centres on Rothesay Castle.

In the 19th century before the advent of tourism herring-fishing brought prosperity to the island and as far back as 1779 the first cotton mill was built in Rothesay. Robert Thom, an early mill-owner, realised that more water was needed for the cotton mills and built a canal to bring water from the west side of the island to Rothesay. The dry canal can still be seen below the road at Tormore Hill.

The island peaked in popularity in the Victorian and Edwardian era as a tourist centre providing holidays 'doon the watter' from Glasgow.

Wildlife: Bute has a unique long-tailed field-mouse which is a sub-species of the mainland variety. A trial reintroduction of the European beaver (extinct in Britain since the 13th century) took place on Bute in 1875 but the animals only survived until the 1890s.

Birdlife is not particularly noteworthy due to the amount of cultivation but there are some areas of pleasant mixed woodland habitat which encourage a variety of species.

With bog cotton in the marshes and heather on the upper slopes, all the common botanical species are in evidence but there is little in the way of distinctive plant life. However, Bute Natural History Society in the Bute Museum, Rothesay

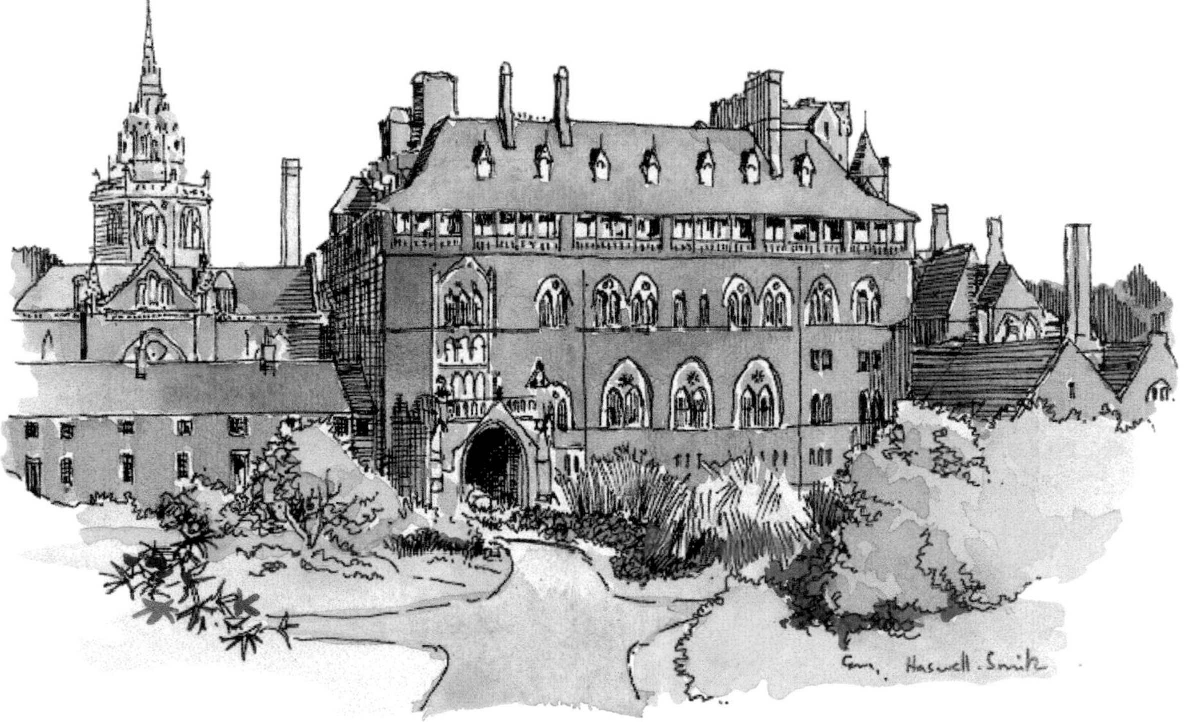

MOUNTSTUART – ERSTWHILE HOME OF THE MARQUESS OF BUTE

provides excellent information on nature trails, paths, plants and birdlife, and there is much of interest.

* * *

BUTE is first and foremost an island catering for the needs of visitors and there are many recreational facilities. Coarse fishing for pike and perch, sea angling, cycling, sailing and pony trekking are only a few of the many popular diversions.

The existence of **Rothesay Castle** was first recorded in 1230 when it was besieged and taken by the Norsemen. The breached east wall can still be seen in the massive, circular sandstone structure surrounded by a moat. The English took the castle on one occasion and it was taken in about 1334 by Sir Colin Campbell for Edward Balliol. It was also attacked by the Lord of the Isles in the 15th century. James IV and James V used it as a base for their campaigns to subdue the Hebrides and it was then that the great tower was built (1541). In 1498 the Bute family were appointed hereditary keepers of the castle and the present Marquess still holds that office. The rebel Master of Ruthven attacked the castle in 1527 but failed to take it so he destroyed the surrounding burgh. In 1544 the Earl of Lennox had more success when he took it for the English. Cromwell kept a garrison here but when it withdrew in 1659 much of the building was dismantled and during the Duke of Monmouth's rebellion in 1685 the rest of the castle was burned down by the Duke of Argyll.

The story goes that shortly after this the Duke of Argyll married off one of his daughters to a Bute. When the newly-wed bride reached the island the first thing she did was to complain bitterly to her husband that he did not have a castle fit for her to live in.

The 2nd Marquess of Bute began restoring the castle in 1816 and further work was done by the 3rd Marquess. The great hall was renovated by the 6th Marquess in 1970 and the government now maintains the property. The castle is open daily and well worth a visit.

The harbour at Rothesay was constructed in the 17th century and eventually rebuilt and extended during the heyday of holidays 'doon the watter' from Glasgow. The bay was a naval anchorage from 1940 to 1957. Nearby, the Victorian Winter Garden on the sea front, at one time the haunt of music hall performers and comedians, has recently been restored.

This is the only Scottish island which had a tram service. This was electrified in 1902 but buses eventually took over in 1936.

The ancient **Church of St Mary's**, which was once part of the Bishopric of Man, is on the road just south of Rothesay at the foot of Loch Fad [NS086637]. It contains two canopied tombs.

Most of the north of the island is wild, hilly and unpopulated. The road runs up the east side to **Rhubodach** with its ferry to Colintraive on the mainland. It passes Kames Bay where there is a tower house, **Kames Castle**, which had its origins in the 14th century [NS064675]. And sitting below Kames Hill, is **Wester Kames**, a 17th-century keep which has been restored [NS062680]. A scramble up Kames Hill (267m) is rewarded by a striking view across to Arran, and a short distance further to the north-west is **Windy Hill** (278m), Bute's highest point.

The bare northern tip of Bute which divides the Kyles is aptly named **Buttock Point** with, opposite it, the delightful little anchorage of Caladh Bay (G. *caladh* – haven) tucked behind **Eilean Dubh** (G. – black isle). On this islet [NS006757], which has been owned by the family of Ingham-Clark for over a century, is the family graveyard. The Stephenson family of locomotive fame owned Caladh before the Ingham-Clarks. Loch Riddon to the north has one tiny islet, **Eilean Dearg**. Its castle was blown up by the English fleet in 1685. There is a sheltered anchorage between it and the shore.

At the head of the East Kyle are three more attractive islets, the **Burnt Islands**, one of which has the remains of a vitrified fort on it.

At the north-west extremity and south of Rubha Dubh there is a fort [NR995713], the ruins of little **Kilmichael Chapel** which was destroyed by the Norsemen [NR993706], and the chambered burial cairn of Glenvoidean in the hills above [NR997706]. Further south there are two more chambered cairns.

All these can be seen on a pleasant but long walk (about 20km total, there and back) along the quiet and narrow coastal road from **Ettrick Bay**. There are beautiful views down the Kyles, and mature woods of birch and oak below the shapely ridge of Barlia Hill (105m).

Near Ettrick Bay there is a stone circle [NS044668] about 1km north-east of the shore

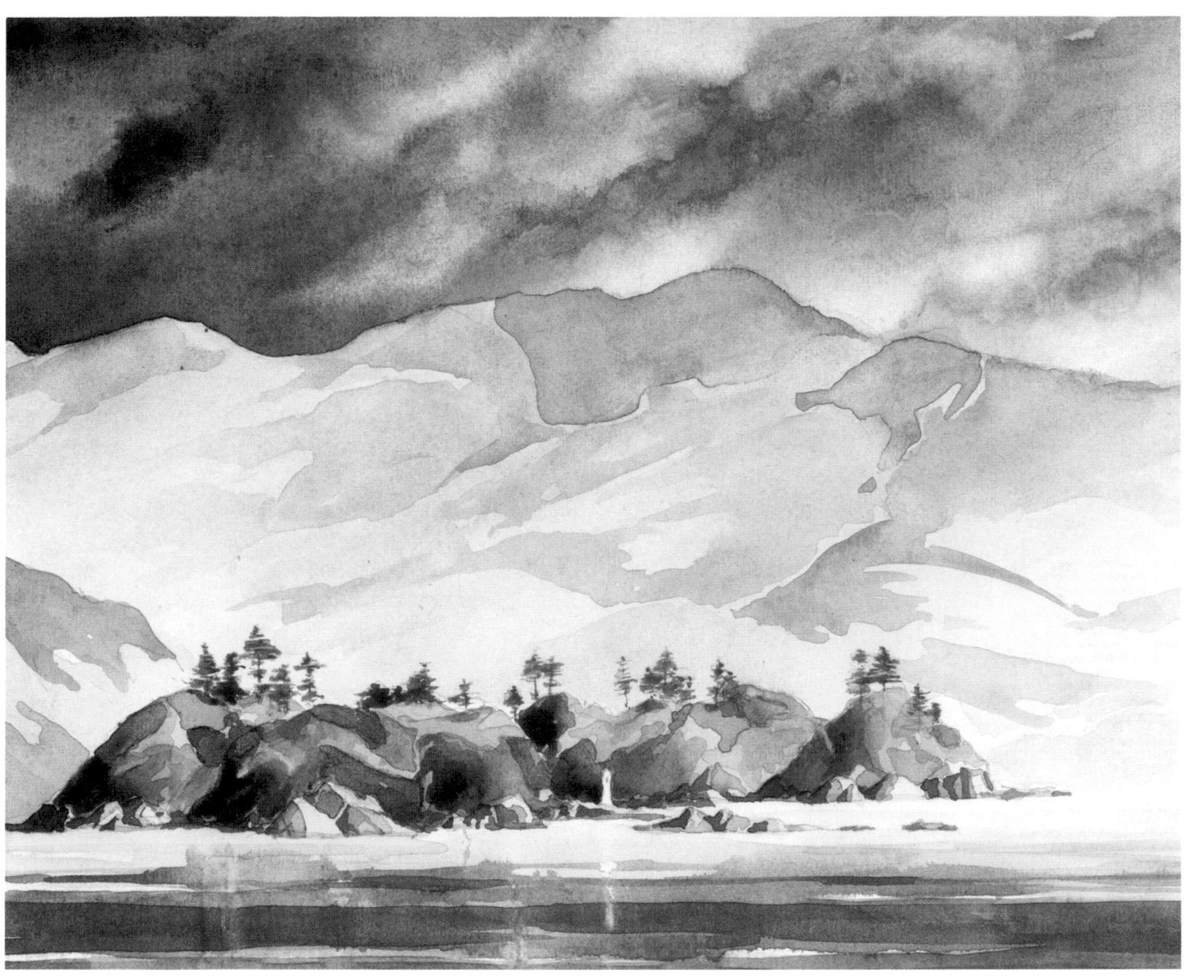

EILEAN DUBH AND CALADH BAY IN THE KYLES OF BUTE

and a Celtic cross near St Colmac [NS045672]. At the bridge over Glenmore burn concrete frames built for the army exercises on Inchmarnock (See No.1.7) represented practice landing craft for D-day.

A ruined chapel [NS035613] just north of St Ninian's Point was excavated in 1953. Standing stones can be seen in the north-west corner of St Ninian's Bay with another chapel 1km north of them [NS036626].

Tourism is the main industry but dairy farming and cheese-making are also of major economic importance. The agricultural part of the island is south of the 'rift valley' between Rothesay Bay and **Scalpsie Bay**. This valley is partly filled by **Loch Fad** (G. – long loch) with its wooded shores, and Loch Quien which has a crannog in it. Several duns and forts are near Scalpsie Bay and where the road winds round Tormore there are some of the finest viewpoints on the island.

A stone circle stands starkly on the narrow neck of land near Kingarth [NS092556] beyond the cemetery on the south side of the road. Across the golf links on the other side a row of standing stones looks like stunted exclamation marks [NS084553].

At the extreme south of the island, which culminates in Garroch Head, St Blane's Hill rises steeply 124m (403ft) above the shore. Here a path leads to **St Blane's Chapel**, a 12th-century Norman church [NS095534]. Its green garth is set in a wooded glade amid the well-preserved ruins of a 6th-century Celtic monastery established by St Catan but named after his nephew St Blane who died in 590. The circular stone building is known as the Devil's Cauldron. Remains of the monks' cells are still visible. On a promontory to the west and above a secluded cove with a beach of clean sharp sand is the vitrified Dunagoil fort dating from about 100BC [NS086531]. The whole of this area of tumbled landscape, bristling with antiquities and surrounded by the great expanse of the Firth of Clyde, is a rambler's delight.

On the east coast, approaching Rothesay and the rustic-English-style 19th century village of Kerrycroy from the south, the road passes **Mountstuart**, traditional home of the Bute family for over 250 years. This magnificent building is now open to the public. The church and cottages at **Ascog** [NS108633], a few miles further north, were designed by David Hamilton in 1845.

* * *

Access: Car ferry: Wemyss Bay/ Rothesay (30 mins), 08000-66-5000. Train connections: Glasgow Central/ Wemyss Bay. Also car ferry: Colintraive/ Rhubodach (5 mins), 08000-66-5000. Tourist information, 08707-200619 or 0845-2255-121.

Anchorages:

1. Rothesay bay. Visitors' moorings (pay) off sailing club or anchor anywhere in bay, clear of moorings, holding generally good. W side of bay is best. Considerable swell with NE winds.
2. Rothesay harbour. Pontoon berths (pay, 01700-500630).
3. Kames Bay, Port Bannatyne. E gales can cause heavy swell. Anchor in 5–7m between disused pier and yacht slip.
4. Eilean Mór, Burnt Islands. Good anchorage E of S extremity of En Mór in 4m, sand. Avoid rocky patch to N.
5. Balnakailly Bay. Anchor S of Eilean Mór and clear of Wood Farm Rock in 3m to 4m.
6. Wreck Bay. Anchor between Beere Rock (off Bear Craig) and Buttock Point in 3–4m.
7. Blackfarland bay, about 1½M SW of Buttock Point, good anchorage about midway between entrance points in 4–7m. Protected from S winds. The coast on both sides of entrance to bay is foul.
8. Ettrick Bay is seldom used as open SW and W Head dries out 2c and depths of less than 5.5m extend about 2c farther off-shore. Underwater obstructions reported.
9. St Ninian's Bay, well sheltered except SW. Head of bay dries out 3½c. There is a broad sandy beach. Avoid spit S of St Ninian's Point. Anchor in 6–8m.
10. Scalpsie Bay. Give Ardscalpsie Point a very wide berth. Anchor near centre of bay and well offshore. Sheltered for all points N.
11. Dunagoil Bay. Clear sandy bay. Exposed, but occasional anchorage in light E'lies. (*Useful for visit to Dunagoil fort and St Blane's*).
12. Glencallum Bay (Callum's Hole). NE entrance marked by white beacon. Avoid rocks slightly NE of centre of bay. Occasional anchorage at head or clear of SW shore in 2m to 6m. Exposed to S winds.
13. Kilchattan Bay. Moorings for hotel patrons or anchor NW of disused pier in 4m to 6m. Head of bay dries out about 4c. Exposed SE to NE.

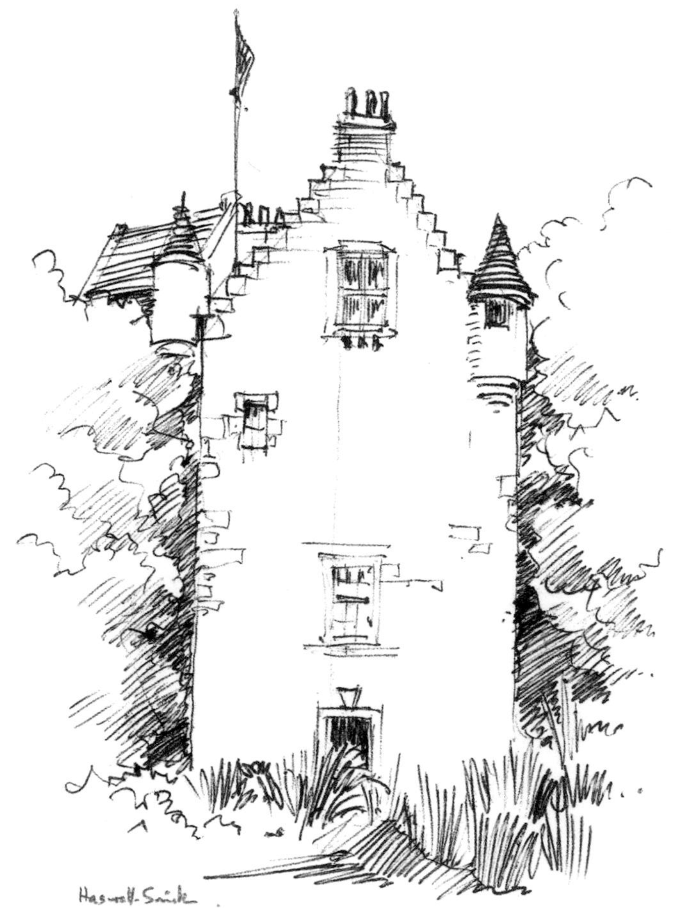

WESTER KAMES – A 17TH CENTURY KEEP

SECTION 2

The Mull of Kintyre to the Firth of Lorn

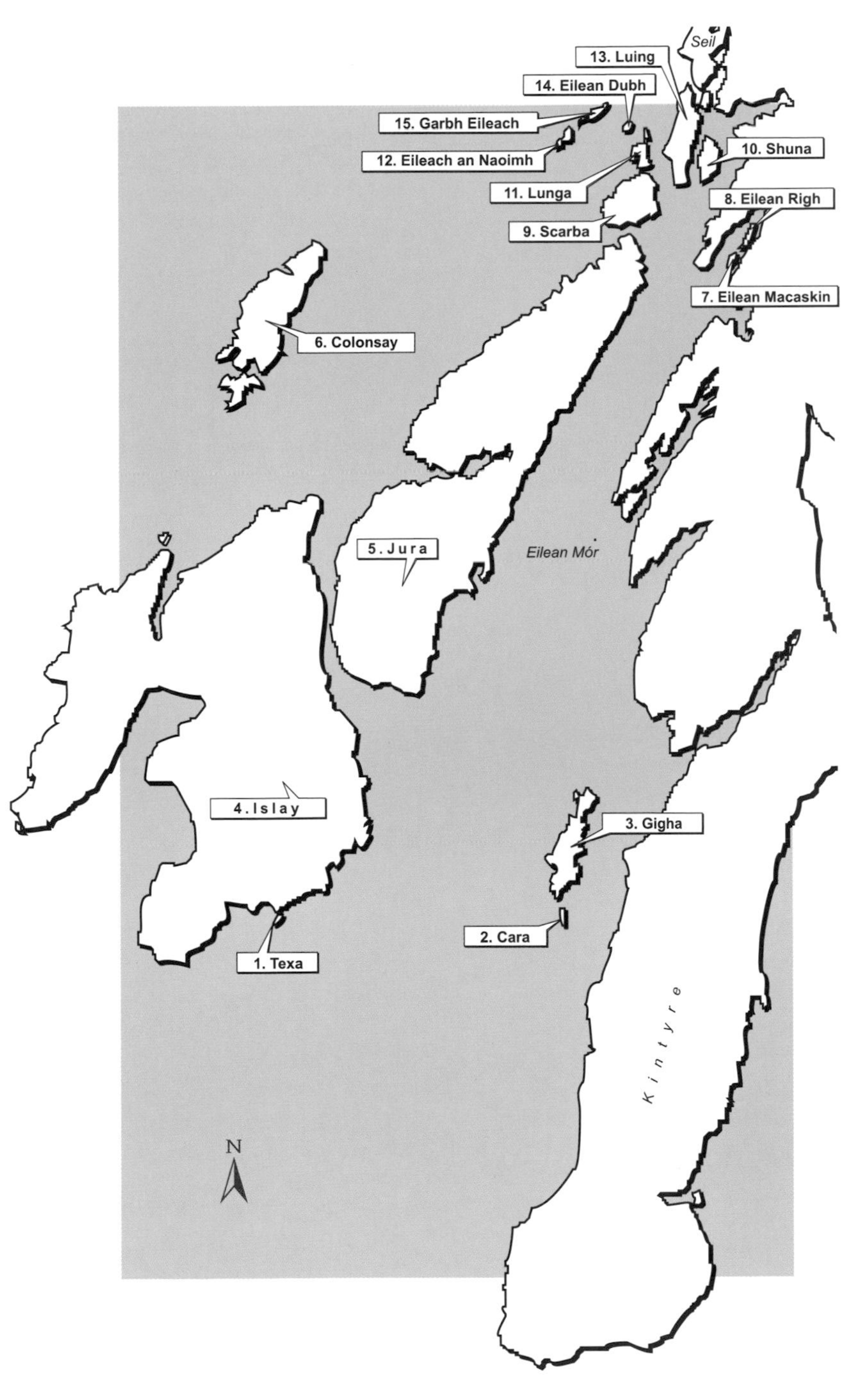

Section 2, Table 1: Arranged according to geographical position

No.	Name	Latitude	Longitude	Table 2* No.	Table 3** No.	Area in Acres	Area in Hectares	
2.1	Texa	55° 37N	06° 08W	151	121	119		48
2.2	Cara	55° 38N	05° 45W	134	109	163		66
2.3	Gigha	55° 41N	05° 45W	35	69	3447		1395
2.4	Islay	55° 45N	06° 16W	5	7	153093		61956
2.5	Jura	55° 58N	05° 50W	8	5	90666		36692
2.6	Colonsay	56° 04N	06° 12W	21	45	10067	4074	
	Oronsay	*56° 01N*	*06° 14W*			1342	543	4617
2.7	Eilean Macaskin	56° 08N	05° 33W	148	97	124		50
2.8	Eilean Righ	56° 09N	05° 33W	116	111	213		86
2.9	Scarba	56° 11N	05° 43W	34	10	3642		1474
2.10	Shuna	56° 13N	05° 36W	55	77	1114		451
2.11	Lunga	56° 13N	05° 42W	74	71	628		254
2.12	Eileach an Naoimh	56° 13N	05° 48W	142	82	138		56
2.13	Luing	56° 14N	05° 38W	32	75	3534		1430
	Torsa	*56° 16N*	*05° 37W*			279	113	1543
2.14	Eilean Dubh Mór	56° 14N	05° 43W	136	112	161		65
2.15	Garbh Eileach	56° 15N	05° 46W	97	60	351		142
2.A	*Seil*	*56° 18N*	*05° 37W*			*3283*		*1329*

*Table 2: The islands arranged in order of magnitude
**Table 3: The islands arranged in order of height

Introduction

The islands to the west and north of the Mull of Kintyre have a long history as they were possibly the very first Scottish islands to be colonised by man. (In fact they may have been settled before anyone dared to colonise the mainland.) In medieval times the area gained particular importance when the Lord of the Isles established the 'capital' of his island empire at Finlaggan on Islay.

The Sound of Jura is a natural highway up the west coast as it is protected from the worst fury of the Atlantic gales. After passing Gigha on the route north, the Kintyre peninsula is broken by a succession of sea-lochs which give some shelter even although they are aligned to the prevailing wind coming from the south-west. The first of these – West Loch Tarbert – has an islet at its head, **Eilean dà Ghallagain**, and likewise the second, Loch Caolisport, has **Eilean Fada**. The latter loch also has two islets nearer the entrance – **Liath Eilean** (G. – grey island) and **Eilean nam Muc** (G. – isle of the pigs).

It is the next loch north, Loch Sween, which has more of interest. Long and narrow, it runs past forbidding Castle Sween and into the wooded hills of Argyll. Here in the creeks among the trees beyond an inhabited islet called **Eilean Loain** (G. – pack-of-hounds isle), are some colourful patches of mossy rock known affectionately as the **Fairy Isles**.

Apart from **Taynish Island** halfway up Loch Sween, all the islets are gathered around the entrance to the loch and the large bridged and tidal island of **Danna**. They are known as the MacCormaig Isles and consist of **Carraig an Daimh** (G. – isle connected to the rock), **Liath Eilean**, **Eilean nan Leac** (G. – island of the grave), **Eilean Gamhna** (G. – island of the farrow cow), **Corr Eilean** (G. – tapering island) with a prehistoric cairn, and the most important island in the group, **Eilean Mór** (G. – big island) which has the distinction of being owned by the Scottish National Party.

Scots-born John Paul Jones sailed in these waters during the American War of Independence and visited Eilean Mór. In ancient times this holy island was the retreat of St Abban mac ui Charmaig, otherwise known as St Cormac, who founded a monastery at Keills and who died in 640. It is worth exploring. A tiny inlet on the north side still has part of a submerged rock in it, despite army 'exercises' to blow it up in 1996, but is a well-sheltered anchorage in all but northerlies.

The medieval chapel, dedicated to St Cormac, is close to the anchorage. It is relatively well preserved although it was once used as an ale-house and illicit still. The saint was buried nearby. To the south beyond the two standing crosses, one of which is a replica, there is a cave which was an anchorite's retreat. This deep, damp grotto has two 8th-century crosses incised on its rock walls. Outside are the ruins of a second chapel proving the veneration in which this little island was held.

North again past **Eilean nan Coinean**, another rabbit island, **Eilean Fraoch**, another heather island, and **Eilean Dubh**, another black island, brings one to **Carsaig Island** with a delightful anchorage behind it. On a visit there, while a young seal was showing off in front of its admiring elders, I was lucky to see a chough. This area is possibly the last Scottish home of the chough, an attractive member of the crow family – rather like a raven with a red beak. It is thought that there are only about one hundred breeding pairs left.

Eilean da Mhèinn sits in the centre of crowded Crinan Harbour surrounded by so many moorings that it is no longer possible to anchor to the south or east of it, but Crinan is such a pleasant spot that one can understand its popularity.

2.1 Texa

(EI tech – house, ON -øy – island). Thought to have been the island referred to as Oidecha insula by Abbot Adomnan. An alternative possibility is a monastic seminary – (G. oideachd – instruction).

OS Maps: 1:50000 Sheet 60 1:25000 Sheet 352
Admiralty Chart: 1:75000 No.2168

Area: 48ha (119 acres)
Height: 48m (157ft)

Owner: In 1614 'Ilantasson' (Island Texa) was chartered by the crown to Sir John Campbell of Cawdor (see No.2.4). The Ramsays of Kildalton had ownership from 1855 to 1915, Philip Morel from 1915 to 1951, followed by Ian Hunter and Elizabeth Williamson of Laphroaig. The island was sold in 1983, resold in 1995 to Mr & Mrs Bolmeijer of Chevy Chase, USA, and up for sale again in 1999 for £120,000.

Population: 1625–29. Late 18th century–8. Still populated in early 19th century but uninhabited since then.

Geology: Mainly interstratified quartzose-mica-schist, grit, and some hornblende.

History: Adomnan refers to the 'island of Oidech' as a stopping place for St Cainnech on his journey from Iona to Ireland in the 6th century and most scholars think that this refers to Texa. Cainnech, or Kenneth, was said to have left his pastoral staff on Iona. Columba found it, blessed it, and cast it into the sea and Kenneth later discovered it washed up on the shore of Texa.

It is assumed that Texa's present chapel, which may be on the site of an earlier one, was built in the late 14th century by Reginald, son of John of Islay. It was dedicated to St Mary the Virgin and generously endowed and the well, Tobar Moireig, was similarly dedicated.

The earliest sculptured stone portrait of a member of the house of Somerled was part of the shaft of a 14th-century cross which stood east of the chapel. It was removed in the early 1900s for safe keeping and can be seen in the National Museum of Scotland in Edinburgh. It is of Ragnald, eldest son of John the Good and progenitor of the MacDonalds of Clanranald. The inscription reads, 'This is the cross of Reginald, son of John, of Islay'. It was Ragnald's younger brother, Donald, who succeeded his father as Lord of the Isles. Ragnald inherited some of the Western Isles and also Castle Tioram beside Loch Moidart and it was there that he died. About the same time (1385) Fordun mentioned 'the monks' chapel' on 'Helan ttexa'. Early 16th-century records show that the church was generously endowed with the lands of Texa, Cragabus and 'two Kilbrides'.

In 1608, Andrew Knox, Bishop of the Isles, wrote from 'Ilintexa' to King James VI asking to be retired – '. . .seeing my ould aige dayle crepis on. . . .'

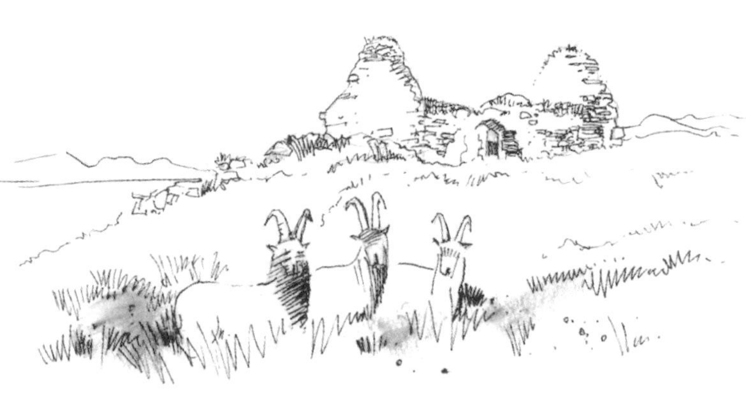

WILD GOATS BY THE RUINED CHAPEL

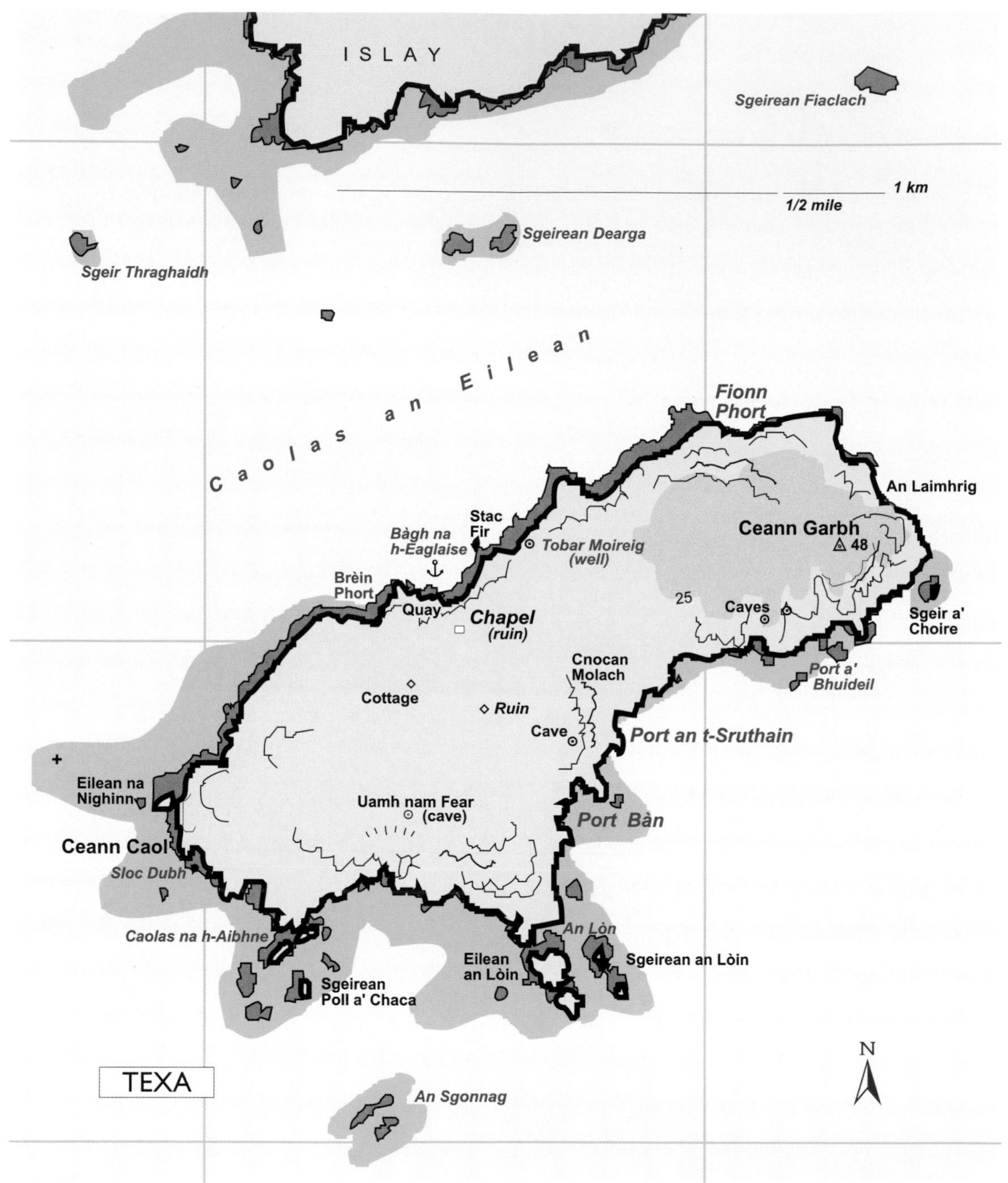

Strangely, a report dated 1614–15 lists only six active churches in the parishes of Islay and there is no mention of Texa. In 1625 Father Cornelius Ward, a Franciscan missionary, also fails to mention the church when he landed on Texa and found that most of the inhabitants were Catholic. He converted the six who were not.

A century and a half later the *Statistical Account 1791–99* records that the inhabitants were 'formerly wont to bury those who were of the popish religion' in the chapel, '. . .but the whole inhabitants now belong to the Established Church, so that there are none now buried. . .'. But, even so, there is a burial enclosure beside the chapel which appears to date from the 19th century.

Wildlife: In early summer the rough ground

is so covered with bluebells that it is like a mist collecting in the hollows. Groups of the eighty or so feral goats watch visitors warily and woodmice and otters are other resident mammals.

* * *

TEXA is a wee rocky hump of an island with many caves, good pasturage and a small white concrete beacon at the highest point, Ceann Garbh (48m) (G. – rough headland). It is part of the Islay parish of Kildalton. The traditional monastic islands sited round Islay are thought to have been – Texa to the south, **Nave** with **Eilean Beag** to the north and **Orsay** to the west. All three are tiny in size, Texa being the largest, but they all have religious relics.

On the slope overlooking **Caolas an Eilean** (G. – the island channel, or kyle) and some distance beyond the jetty there is a renovated cottage. On terraced ground about 100m north-east are the walls of an ancient chapel, built of rubble but with ashlar sandstone trimmings [NR391438]. There is evidence that this formed the centre of an area of continuous agricultural settlement. There is also a burial ground with the footings of at least five buildings and an enclosure to the south and another structure to the north. None of these buildings is thought to be of an early date but they have not been examined in detail. Detailed investigation is needed to establish whether or not a monastery or seminary ever existed but at least this tiny island could support a population for it is fortunate in having its own water supply, **Tobar Moireig** (G. – Mary's well).

The early Celtic church had no parochial organisation. Any small Christian community could build a chapel for the purpose of communal worship. There would be a lay custodian, but no resident priest, although occasionally one might attend from a neighbouring monastery. It is possible that this was no more than just a primitive 'clachan' church, although it seems unlikely that Texa would support a large enough lay community of farmers and fishermen to undertake such a building.

There are some minor landing places – An Laimhrig (G. – the landing place) in the east, and Port an t-Sruthain (G. – tidal port) and Port Ban (G. – fair port) in the south-east bay. Texa also has a number of caves including Uamh nam Fear (G. – the men's cave).

Across Caolas an Eilean at the entrance to Port Ellen on Islay is tiny **Eilean nan Caorach** (G. – sheep island). In the 12th century Somerled's fleet anchored in nearby Lagavulin Bay beside Dunyvaig Castle. Loch an t-Sàilein provides a better anchorage beyond Lagavulin Bay. It is sheltered by tidal **Eilean Imersay** and the rocks of **Iseanach Mór** while, standing well out to sea like a sentinel, is **Iomallach**. Further up the coast are the lovely Ardmore Islands. They are treeless **Eilean Craobhach** (G. – tree-covered island), **Eilean a' Chuirn** (G. – heap-of-stones island) with a light beacon on it, **Eilean Bhride** (G. – Bridget's isle), and the long reef of **Eilean Mhic Mhaolmhoire**.

* * *

Access: No regular access but Islay Sea Safari at Port Ellen (01496-840510) may be able to help

Anchorages:
Note: Approach with caution, preferably 1½c clear of E end of island, and then keep nearer to S side of the Kyle. Note submerged rock about 3c WNW of En na Nighinn off W extremity of island. All anchorages are exposed.
1. Fionn Phort on the N face of the NE extremity in 5m.
2.Bàgh na h-Eaglaise (G. – Church Bay). Off the quay and chapel ruins near the centre of the N coast in 5–6m, sand. This is the traditional anchorage.
3.Port an t-Sruthain, in centre of open bay on SE coast. There are a number of off-shore rocks and a large 7c reef extending S from the SW extremity. Best avoided.

2.2 Cara

Various possible derivations. (G. carr ON -øy – island of the projecting rock or rock ledge) or (G. cor ON -øy – island of the rounded hill) or (ON Kari-øy – Kari's island), Kari was a Norse hero. A (B. caer – fort) derivation is improbable.

OS Maps: 1:50000 Sheet 62 1:25000 Sheet 357
Admiralty Chart: 1:25000 No.2475

Area: 66ha (163 acres)
Height: 56m (184 ft)

Owner: For centuries Cara has been part of the Macdonald estate of Largie on the Kintyre peninsula. It is not part of the Gigha estate. The Macdonalds of Largie claim direct descent from the Lord of the Isles.

Population: Alexander Macdonald of Largie married Jane McNeill in 1798 on Cara according to the parish register and there were several families living on the island at that time. 1881–4. 1891–3. 1931–3. Last person to be born on the island was Mrs Charlotte McAlister who was living on Gigha in 1991. Last farmed by Angus McGuigan in 1932 and uninhabited since the 1940s but a Londoner was renovating Cara House in 1991, possibly with a view to living on the island.

Geology: Cara is a continuation of the geology of Gigha (No.2.3).

At the south end, below the Mull of Cara, there are two interconnecting caves each about 12m deep which shows signs of human – and goat – habitation. The strata has also created a number of rock shelters under overhangs, such as at Poll an Aba.

History: As King Haakon's huge fleet was anchored in Gigalum Sound for two or three weeks in 1263 it would be surprising if the Norsemen had not landed on Cara Island. But no definite evidence has been found.

In 1615 Sir James Macdonald escaped from a Crown prison and enlisted many islanders to help him free his lands from Campbell (Argyll) control. Hector MacNeill of Taynish and Gigha, Chief of the Southern Clan Neill, was thirled to Argyll and the rebels were keen to capture him. The rebels set up their base on Cara as this belonged to their ally, Macdonald of Largie, whilst their army of about 1000 men camped on the Kintyre coast opposite Gigha. MacNeill sent a raiding party to Cara but the Largie servants warned the rebels by beacon and they thwarted the attack. They were however generally undisciplined and Argyll's forces soon had them all in retreat. An uncorroborated story says that the MacNeill and Campbell lords then had a dinner in the Cara mansion-house and finished it by hanging eight captured rebels in front of the house. The corpses were later buried in the chapel.

These were strange times, for only three years later, in 1618, it was Argyll who was disgraced 'for open defection from the true religion' and 'suspicious dealings' with Sir James Macdonald. He was proclaimed a traitor whereas Sir James Macdonald was pardoned and given a pension.

Flora Macdonald was related to the Macdonalds of Largie and some time after the events of 1745 she stayed at Largie for a year before emigrating to Carolina. Her brother was also a guest at Largie but he was mortally wounded in a shooting accident on Cara.

Wildlife: Rabbits (particularly noted for their numbers by Dean Monro), otters, goats, nesting seabirds and peregrine falcons are Cara's specialities. In the days of falconry the Macdonalds would collect chicks from the cliff nests – ' but never more than one chick from a nest having two or more' according to an octogenarian whose grandfather used to collect them. Shags, guillemots and terns with a few razorbills, and herring, common and great black-backed gulls breed on the coasts. Elsewhere are nests of ringed plovers, rock and meadow pipits, mute swans and buzzards.

The herd of wild goats is quite large and a considerable number of goat skeletons are scattered about, but the goats themselves can be difficult to see when the bracken is high.

There are many wildflowers but no trees.

Poll an Aba 'is always good for a sea trout near the white shore' says a local man.

* * *

The peaty ground below the house on **CARA** in the month of June is a sea of wildflowers. The marshy nature of the soil here keeps the bracken at bay. Cara House itself is a dour two-storey stone building with a slated roof standing lonely and conspicuous, staring across the Sound towards Kintyre. It was built about 1733 as a residence for the tacksman. There is a well-preserved corn-drying kiln close by.

Behind the house is the ruined chapel which could easily be mistaken at first for a sheep pen [NR640443]. It is about 9m long by 5m broad. It originally had a lancet-shaped window with splayed ingoes near the east end of each side wall as well as the west gable, and the door on the north side was Gothic-arched. It is said that the chapel was used for burials and that a priest is buried in the north-east corner where there is a broken greenish stone slab which was originally part of the pulpit. There is no record of a burial ground. The chapel fell into disuse in the late 18th century and was used for a time as a kitchen for the house.

According to a record dated 14 June 1456 it was called 'the chapel of St Finla in the island of Kara beside the Monkshaven'. St Finlay (G. *Fionnlugh* – fair hero) was a contemporary of

St Columba and evidently the patron saint of the House of Islay. It appears that the chapel was built about this time by the Macdonalds although in the Latin 'Scotia Sacra' there is the entry – 'Insula Carray, where there is a shrine of the Most Holy Trinity. It is doubtful who first founded it.' Dean Monro said the chapel belonged to Icolmkill (Iona) with the island being used as a monks' retreat. This may be corroborated by there being a pleasant round pool on the south-east shore called Poll an Aba (G. – the pool of the abbot) and an anchorage called Monkshaven.

It was at Poll an Aba in later times that the Macdonalds rolled their fishing boats up the beach during the winter months as there was no shelter for them over on Kintyre. The men would stay in huts below the brow of the hill while carrying out maintenance work on the boats. The Brownie's Well close by provided fresh water and it has never run dry.

East of the main house there is another well which serves the house. A track leads from the chapel ruin to Port an Stòir (G. – stormy port) at the north extremity where there are some ruined

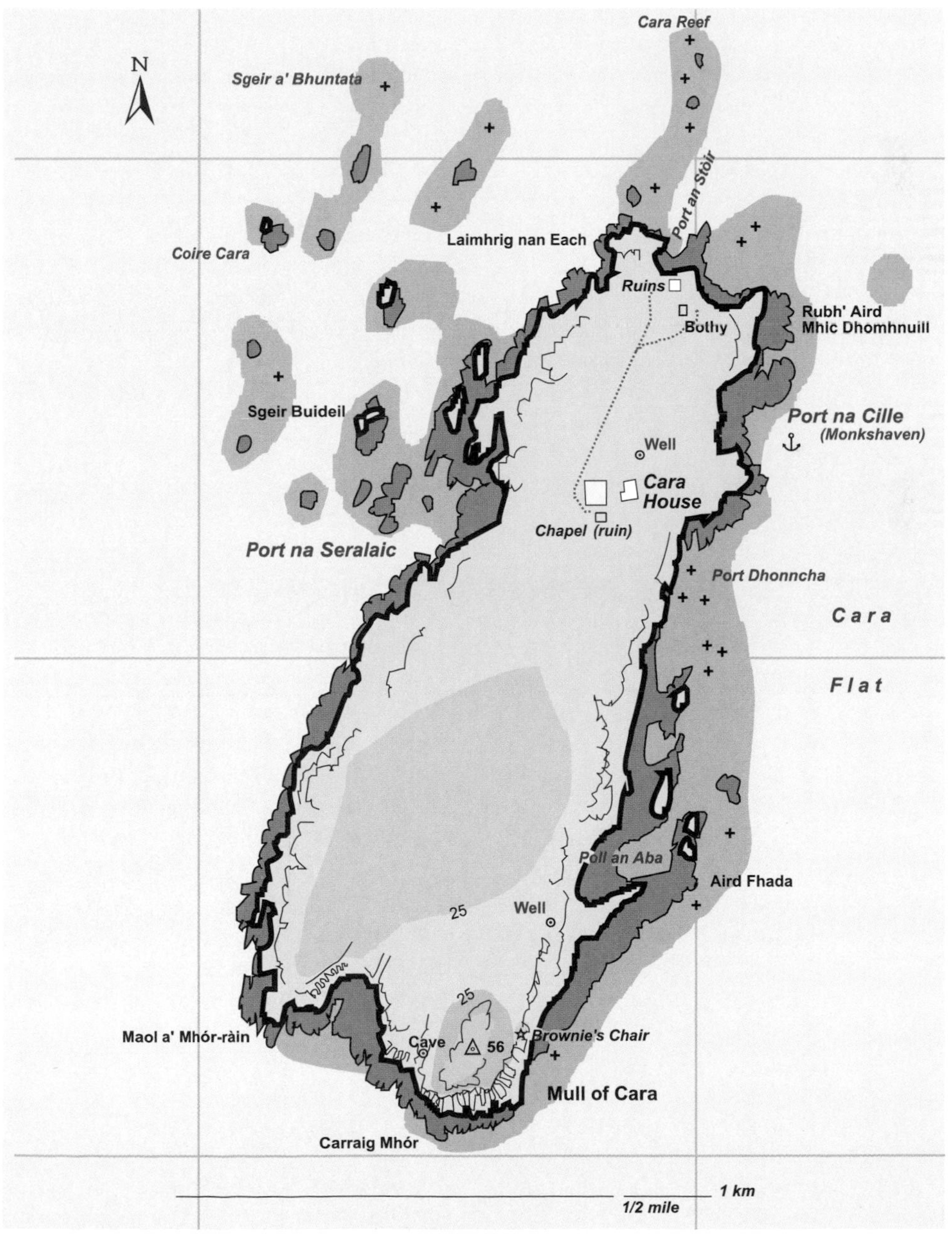

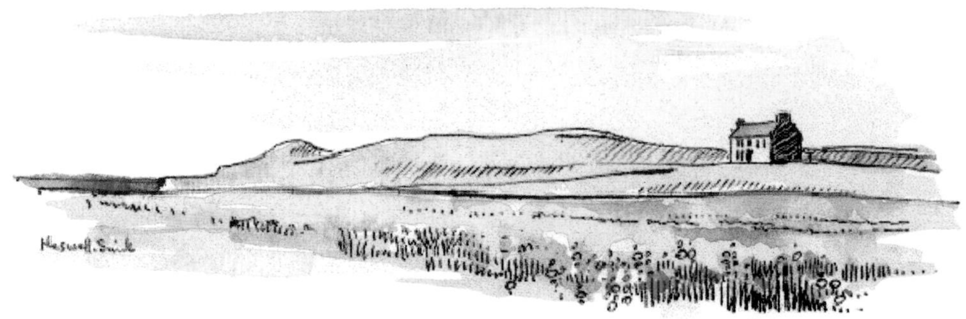

CARA HOUSE – LONELY AND CONSPICUOUS

enclosures. About two hundred years ago the track also extended southwards to a large building of unknown purpose according to an old map.

During the Second World War a newly-built P & O ship with a cargo of copra on board was hit by a German bomb which went straight down its funnel. The blazing hulk drifted for two days before coming to rest in the bay on the west side of Cara where she burned for a further six weeks.

At the south-west corner, Maol à Mhór-ràin, a cleft in the rock conceals part of a lifeboat and an embedded anchor, and the bay on the south side seems to attract all the flotsam and jetsam in the area. This was the area that was always searched first for the bodies of sailors drowned in the vicinity.

In the autumn of 1756 there was, according to the *Statistical Account of Scotland – 1791–99*, a great storm in this area. Lightning struck the southern headland called the Mull of Cara breaking off large pieces of rock, 'which has a lot of iron ore in it', and the shock was felt in all the islanders' houses. The sea rose so high on the west side that the waves swept right across the island. All the houses – which may have been of turf construction – were severely damaged and stacks of corn were ruined. The people 'were obliged to take shelter in the only slated house on the island, which fortunately suffered no damage.' Other reports claim that it was not lightning but a meteorite which struck just below the southern cliff on the Mull of Cara. This seems more probable. If the bulk of the meteorite hit the sea to the south-west, this could account for the freak wave. The broken cliff face can still be seen.

The Brownie's Chair is a huge stone 'armchair', with only one arm, set on a ledge above the sea on the east side of the highest point – the Mull of Cara [NR639434].

The Brownie of Cara is said to be the ghost of a Macdonald murdered by a Campbell. Tradition says that he inhabits an attic room in Cara House, and that the laird and minister have always raised their hats to him when they step ashore on Cara, and so should everyone else. The Macdonald's gallery in the church at Ardminish on Gigha built in 1780 was known as the Brownie's gallery. The *Observer* reported in 1909 that Morton Macdonald of Largie claimed that the Brownie was often seen, or heard, moving about in his room, – 'A neat little man, dressed in brown, with a pointed beard.'

The Brownie has a characteristically impish sense of humour. One story tells how the Laird of Largie sent two of his men over to fetch a cask of wine from the big cellar in Cara House. Whilst they were arranging a gangplank to roll the cask up from the cellar they were joking about the Brownie. They then found they were unable to move the barrel so, in the end, they offered a sincere apology for the remarks they had made. Suddenly the barrel ran up the plank by itself, bounced and rolled across the ground to the sea and came to a stop beside their boat.

There are many stories telling how the Brownie would wash the dishes and tidy up the kitchen to help the housewife and maids – yet couldn't resist an occasional practical joke.

It was essential that the main house had a good view of the mainland because Cara was the centre of smuggling activity for Gigha, Jura and Islay. In 1786 the *Prince of Wales* revenue cutter dug up eighteen casks of foreign spirits at Poll an Aba. No wonder that twinkling lights were often to be seen on dark nights in the window of the Brownie's room!

* * *

Access: Boat trips may be arranged with a local fisherman through the hotel or store at

Ardminish on Gigha (but not for anyone with Campbell blood in their veins!).

Anchorages: There are no permanent anchorages but Gigalum Sound is fairly close and sheltered from the E by Gigalum Island (see Gigha No.2.3).
1. Port na Cille or Monkshaven on E coast. Temp. anchorage. in 9m sand, with the house bearing approximately 240deg. Exposed NNE to SSW.
2. Port an Stòir at the N extremity. Used as a landing place but local knowledge essential.

2.3 Gigha

*[***gee***-ë:] (ON Gud-øy – God's island or the good island) This is the normally accepted derivation but possible alternatives are (ON gja-øy – island of creeks or geos) or (ON – Gydha's isle). Gydha was a woman's name.*

O S Maps: 1:50000 Sheet 62 1:25000 Sheet 357
Admiralty Charts: 1:75000 No. 2168 or 1:25000 No. 2475

Area: 1,395ha (3447 acres)
Height: 100m (328ft)

Owner: Bought from David W Landale by English property developer Malcolm Potier's company, Tanap Investments, for £5.4m in 1989. This purchase included all Gigha's main businesses and a fish farm. In 1992 it was attached for debts by Interallianz Bank of Zürich and then sold to Holt Leisure Group (owners of Kip and Craobh Marinas) for a reported £2.3m. As is always the case, however, these continual changes of ownership were most unsettling for the islanders so in 2001, when Mr Holt chose to put the island – but not the fish farm – back on the market, he accepted the islanders' bid of £4,000,250 (reported to be £1 million less than the best offer). Unlike the island of Eigg (No.4.2) where there was an anonymous donation of £1 million towards the cost, the islanders' bid broke new ground by being almost entirely paid by Scottish taxpayers (£500,000 from Highlands and Islands Enterprise) and the National Lottery (£3,500,000 from the Lottery-based Scottish Land Fund subject to £1 million being repaid within two years). One million pounds was repaid on time partly financed by the sale of Achamore House in 2003 for a reported £640,000 to Mr Don Dennis, an American. Present indications are that the island's rather idealistic form of collective ownership is succeeding well and as Willie McSporran, chairman of the community trust, enthusiastically said: 'There have been good lairds and bad lairds, but at last we have stability and security of tenure.'

Population: Including Cara: 1755–514. 1792–614. 1801–556. 1841–550. Gigha only: 1881–378. 1891–398. 1911–326. 1931–240. 1951–190. 1961–163. 1981–153. 1991–143. 2001–110. 2007–154.

Geology: Some of the best examples of glaciated rock in Scotland are on Creag Bhan (G. – white or sacred rock). The summit appears to have escaped being covered with ice during the Ice Age. The island has a long spinal ridge and hummocky hills of epidiorite with basalt intrusions. In the north and west the rock is clean and less riven – like the Cuillin – and there are many caves along the coast, some at sea level, some at old raised beaches. Sloc an Leim (G. – squirting pit) is a long subterranean passage through which the sea rushes violently during westerly gales and jets up to a great height. The south and east coast are of quartzite and grit and this stratum continues through Gigalum and Cara.

History: Occupancy stretches back five thousand years as proven by the archaeological remains. Gigha's key position on the sea route along the Kintyre peninsula had a profound influence on its history.

One of the earliest recorded visits was in the autumn of 1263 when King Haakon's fleet of more than one hundred ships anchored in Gigalum Sound on the way to the Battle of Largs

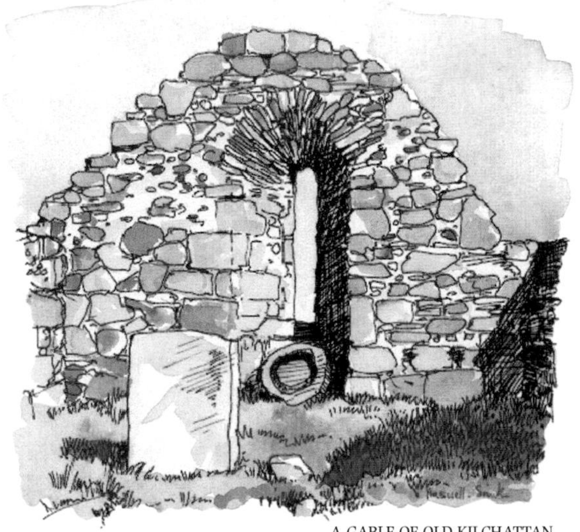
A GABLE OF OLD KILCHATTAN

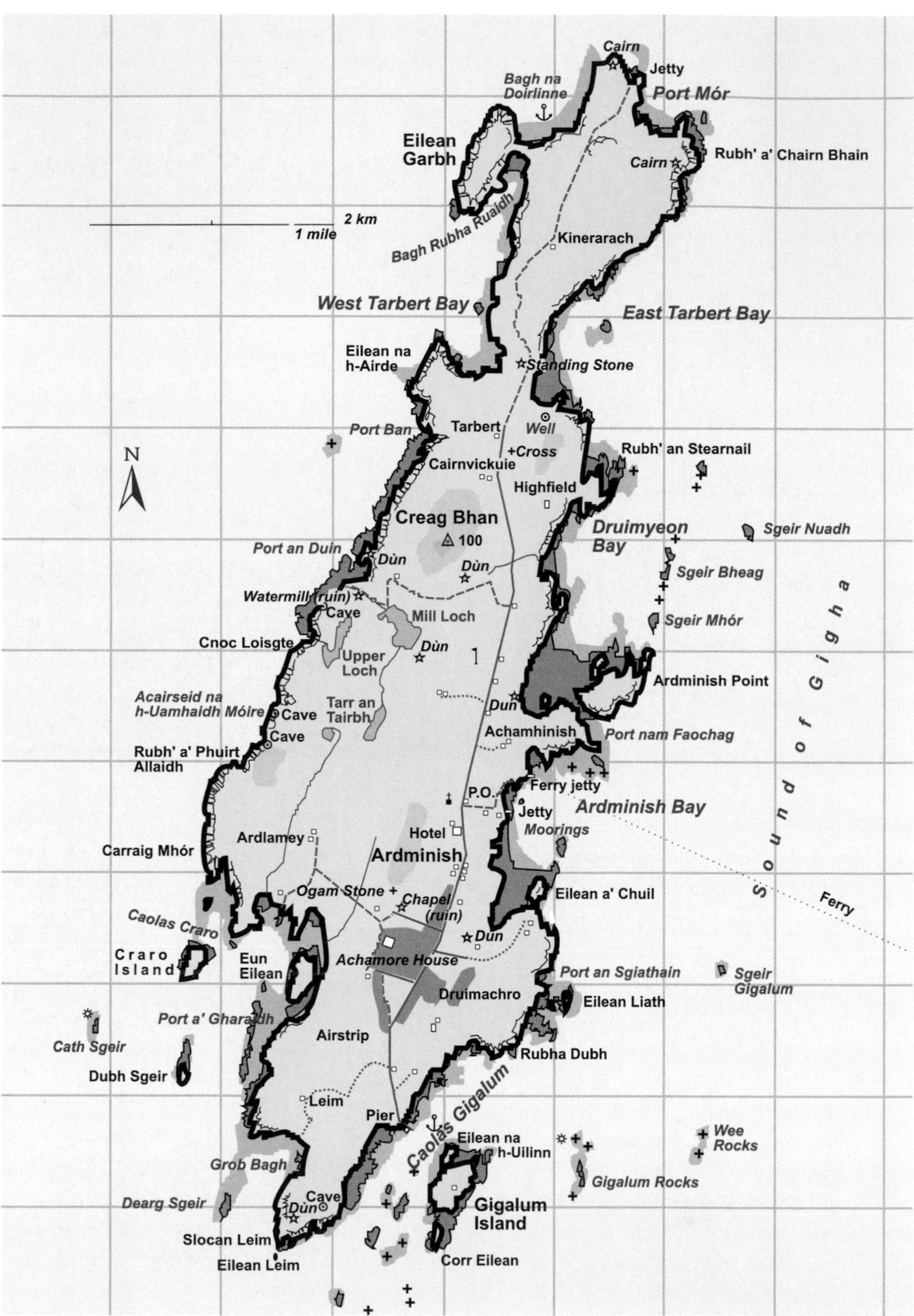

and were delayed there for some time by bad weather. On board the King's longship was Ewin, Lord of the Isles (called King John in the Haakon Saga). He had come on board at Oban to ask to be excused taking up arms against the Scots' King Alexander. Haakon eventually agreed and Ewin returned to the north. While on the island Haakon received the allegiance of Murdoch and Angus of Kintyre – the Lairds of Gigha, a peace mission from the Abbot of Saddell, and a request from the Irish for his assistance against the English. He sent a cutter to Ireland to investigate.

The King's return to Gigalum Sound after his defeat was not so triumphant. He still considered assisting the Irish but his men wanted to return home to Norway without further delay.

In 1309 the 'island of Gug' was made over by Bruce to the Earl of Mar. In 1335 Edward Balliol formally granted Gigha to John, Lord of the Isles and this grant was 'confirmed' by Edward III when he occupied Scotland in 1336. When the Kings of Scotland had regained their position in 1343 David II also confirmed the grant of the 'island of Githey' to John, Lord of the Isles and Chief of the Macdonalds. In 1449 Alexander, Earl of Ross and Lord of the Isles died having granted part of the island to Torquil MacNeill of Taynish and 'two merklands' to the Monks of Paisley. In 1493 the whole island came into the hands of the MacNeills of Taynish, but a pirate, Allan McLean (Allan-na-Sop), plundered Gigha in 1530 and slew Neil MacNeill of Taynish and many of the inhabitants. However, James V conferred the title on MacNeill's son, also called Neil, and elevated Gigha to a Barony. In 1542 the title deeds of the Thaindom of Gigha were 'lost' when eleven Gigha gentlemen were slain by unknown assailants. Dean Munro wrote in 1549 that 'the auld thane of Gigay should be Laird of the same, call it MacNeill of Gigay and now it is possessed by Clan Ranald' (i.e. the Macdonalds). Sure enough, by 1554 the deeds had reappeared in Macdonald hands. The following year Neil MacNeill was restored as Lord of Gigha by Mary, Queen of Scots, but he then sold the island to the Macdonalds of Islay. They in turn sold Gigha to Sir John Campbell of Calder but McNeill of Taynish repurchased most of it in 1590 for 3000 merks (£170 sterling).

William of Orange landed on Gigha in 1689 and had the support of MacNeill of Gigha. MacNeill also remained loyal during the 1745 uprising but this is not altogether surprising as the Duke of Argyll was his overlord.

About 1779 MacNeill of Taynish sold out to John MacNeil of Colonsay, probably a relation, who became the first resident owner. The remaining part of Gigha was owned by another member of the MacNeill family of Taynish.

In 1865 Captain William Scarlett of Thryberg in Yorkshire, the third Lord Abinger, bought Gigha for £49,000 and built a mansion at Achamore. This was the first time that the entire island had been under single ownership and it remained in the Scarlett family until 1919 when it was bought by Major John Allen. He sold it to R J A Hamer in 1937 and his son-in-law Somerset de Chair sold it to Sir James Horlick in 1944. David W Landale purchased it from the Horlick estate in 1973.

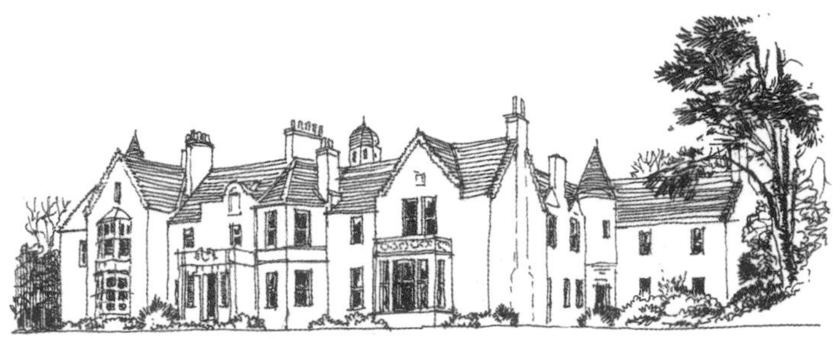

ACHAMORE HOUSE

Wildlife: Gigha has an abundance of wildflowers. In late spring the Achamore woods are a sea of bluebells and the rocks and ridges are crowded with dwarf whin scented like honey and competing with the honey-scented flowers of the Grass of Parnassus. Apart from the main woodland at Achamore, Gigha has more trees than many small Scottish islands, with scrub willow, prostrate juniper, sycamore, thorn, alder, birch and hazel.

When the Scarletts were the proprietors from 1870 to 1919 they regularly stocked the Mill and Upper Lochs with trout – but these are now very scarce. Deer, weasels, stoats, moles and foxes apparently never reached the island but there are many rabbits. There were hares but they became extinct in the 19th century, probably due to the great black-backed gulls.

Over 70 species of bird have been recorded on Gigha, including great northern and black-throated divers, mute and whooper swans, snipe, eider, fulmar, and shelduck by Eun Eilean in Craro Bay on the west coast. There is a gullery on Eilean Garbh in the north-west with eider and guillemot nesting on the western ledges. Hen harrier nest in the central moorland.

* * *

GIGHA is a fertile and hospitable island with good arable land on 25% of its surface area and a mild climate. In fact the rich soil produced such beautiful potatoes that the Irish used to buy them to place on top of their own potatoes on the way to market. This wonderful island supports a stable community and a relaxed way of life. Electricity is supplied by three second-hand wind turbines with the surplus sold to the Grid.

When William James Yorke Scarlett, owner in the 1890s, was away on the mainland and his servants were taking time off for a round of golf on the island's course, a fire unfortunately burned down most of the Mansion House. It was eventually rebuilt and renamed **Achamore House** [NR642479].

Sir James Horlick (of the well-known beverage) purchased Gigha in 1944 and is remembered by the islanders as a very fine and generous benefactor who did a lot to make the island viable and stop depopulation. He modernised the farms and built-up dairy production to 250,000 gallons of milk a year. He converted some deciduous woodland around Achamore House into one of the finest gardens on the west coast of Scotland planted with many rare species which he had collected for his garden near Ascot. Apart from the varied deciduous trees there are rhododendron (including the famous Horlick hybrids), azalea, laburnum, *Primula candelabra*, and various sub-tropical plants such as palm lilies (*Cordyline australis*), palm trees and flame-trees (*Embothrium longifolium*). Sir James used to drive through his gardens in a dragon-caparisoned motorised tricycle. He died at Achamore House in 1972.

The beautiful gardens of Achamore (the plants were gifted to the National Trust in 1962), are open to the public from April to September inclusive. May is probably the best month to see them.

In the scattered little village of **Ardminish** there is an attractive hotel (which won an architectural award) and about eighteen new houses have been built by the Island Trust – 'for people with special needs'. The well-known local character, Mr Seumas McSporran, who, with his wife, ran the island's only general store and post office, was also the postman, Registrar of Births, Marriages and Deaths, coastguard, fireman, policeman, and holder of numerous other official duties before enjoying a well-earned partial retirement.

The parish church, whose congregation includes all denominations, has several good stained-glass windows, one dedicated to Kenneth MacLeod who was born in 1872 on Eigg (No.4.2). He composed, among many other songs, the 'Road to the Isles'.

The red and yellow sandstone ruins of the 13th-century **Kilchattan** (St Catan's Chapel) are south of Ardminish [NR643481]. St Catan was an Irish missionary of the 6th century who settled in Bute but travelled widely. There are a number of interesting carved grave-slabs in the churchyard dating back to the 14th century. The original octagonal stone font has been moved into the Parish Church at Ardminish for safe-keeping. Opposite the lower end of the graveyard and south of the road is St Catan's Well.

The ogam stone above the church ruins is the only example of its kind in the west of Scotland. Ogam is an ancient Celtic writing which is still largely undeciphered. There are also some unusual standing stones and 'cup-marked' stones at different parts of the island.

The beaches at Ardminish and in the many attractive coastal bays and inlets are of fine white sand. The pier in the south-east corner at Caolas Gigalum was the only ferry pier until the ro-ro ferry access was constructed at Ardminish in the 1980s. Gigalum Island, which gives its name to the kyle, is tiny but has a modern house in the dead centre. The two largest lochs, **Mill Loch** and the **Upper Loch**, are very ancient artificial lochs and the small islands in the latter may be crannogs.

Gigha is rich in folklore. At the north end of the island is Raven's Rock where it is believed that Noah's raven (not a dove) landed after the Flood.

Just south of East Tarbert Bay is Tobar a' Bheathaig (G. – Beathag's well). If a sailor wants a fair wind he must throw the well-water in the required direction and leave some payment by the well. A Viking Burial is thought to have taken place in East Tarbert Bay.

The very narrow loch west of and above North Ardminish, Tarr an Tairbh (G. – the tail of the bull), hides a shy bull-like monster reputedly seen by the islanders.

There are a number of interesting caves around the coastline. **Uamh Mhor** (G. – big cave) [NR633495] is on the coast to the west of Tarr an Tairbh and difficult to approach from the land. It was probably occupied in prehistoric times and was also a favourite hide for smugglers. It has the same well-worn legend as other Hebridean islands; that a dog disappeared down it and reappeared, not as usual on the other side of the island, but on the mainland. This cave has never been fully explored. South of it is a large bay, full of rocks, skerries, and two islets, **Craro Island** in the centre which now belongs to Mr Don Dennis – the new owner of Achamore House, and tidal

Eun Eilean (G. – bird island). (Mr Dennis runs a small business producing flower essences which has provided some useful employment.)

In 1991 the Russian factory ship *Kartli* was hit by a freak wave off Islay. Her crew was rescued but the wreck drifted on to the rocks off the coast of Gigha. Although the islanders had to live with the smell of rotting fish for several months after the disaster, with their customary generosity they collected a substantial sum to assist the injured captain.

* * *

Access: Every day frequent ro-ro ferry from Tayinloan, Kintyre (20 mins), 0990-650000 or 08000-66-5000. Caravans not permitted. Cycles can be hired from the store near the ferry pier and also from the hotel. Tourist info. 08707-200600

Anchorages:

1. Gigalum Sound (Caolas Gigalum). Approach is easy provided all visible rocks are identified and given a reasonable berth but best avoid S approach in fresh S'lies. The shore is foul. Anchor off the pier, sand.
2. Ardminish Bay. The most popular anchorage. Extensive reefs on both sides of the bay. Kiln rock, 1c off thc jetty covers. Visitors' moorings available or anchor clear of the moorings, sand. Can be unpleasant in E'lies.
3. Drumyeon Bay. Has been much obstructed by a fish farm. Sand and weed.
4. East Tarbert Bay. Occasional anchorage avoiding rocks and shellfish floats in middle of the bay.
5. Port Mor. Pleasant occasional anchorage if breeze is southerly and weather settled.
6. Eilean Garbh. Good anchorage N or S of the sand spit as close as depth permits, sand. Exposed N or SW respectively. N side was favourite picnic stop for *RY Britannia*.
7. West Tarbert Bay. Approach is clear. Exposed W. Reasonable in E'lies but swell likely. Anchor in 4–8m, sand and shingle.
8. Craro Bay. Temp. anchorage in settled weather, best approached from due W. Anchor about 2½c E of the centre of Craro Island in 8m.

2.4 Islay

*[**Y-lĕ**] Possibly, (ON Yula-øy or Jle-øy – Yula's isle). Yula was a Norse princess who is reputed to be buried under a standing stone on the east side of Port Ellen.*

OS Maps: 1:50000 Sheet 60 1:25000 Sheets 352 and 353

Admiralty Charts: 1:75000 No.2168 Sound of Islay 1: 25000 No.2481 Port Ellen 1:15000 No.2474

Area: 61956ha (153,093 acres)
Height: 491m (1610 ft)

Owner: Multiple ownership. Robert Fleming & Trusts, the Duke of Argyll and Lord Margadale have the largest holdings but the RSPB reserves take up a substantial area including the Oa (purchased 2003).

Population: 1755–5344. Pennant estimated 7000–8000 in 1772. 1792–9500. 1841–15772. 1881–7559. 1891–7375. 1931–4970. 1961–3860. 1981–3792. 1991–3538. 2001–3457.

Geology: Complex. In 1798 it was recorded that 'Ila has mines of lead mixed with copper: . . . iron called Bog Ore, veins of emery, and some of quicksilver'. Lead and silver were being mined in the 19th century near Port Askaig, with copper and manganese also present.

The northern part of the Rinns is calcareous Torridonian sandstone with good loamy agricultural soil, whilst the southern part is Archaean gneiss with patches of hornblende; rough, rocky and treeless. The far north of the island is Cambrian quartzite with Dalradian limestone belts running through it. A strip of mica schist with limestone cuts right across the island from Port Askaig to the Mull of Oa. South-east of this is a continuation of the geology of Jura with a similar landscape, and in the extreme south-east coast between Port Ellen and Ardtalla there is mica schist and hornblende creating a beautifully shattered coastline backed by woodland and scrub.

History: The island was formerly the 'capital' of the Western Isles. Written records go back further in time for Islay than for any other Hebridean isle. The Irish settled here in the 3rd century and for some three hundred years the island was part of the Scots kingdom of Dalriada. The Norse were in charge from about 850 to 1150, then Somerled, King of Argyll, defeated them in a sea-battle off Islay, took over the southern Hebrides, made the island his home and his headquarters and founded the immensely powerful Clan Donald. His main Macdonald stronghold, Dunyvaig Castle, overlooks Lagavulin Bay where his war-galleys would lie at anchor.

Islay, as the seat of government of the Lord of

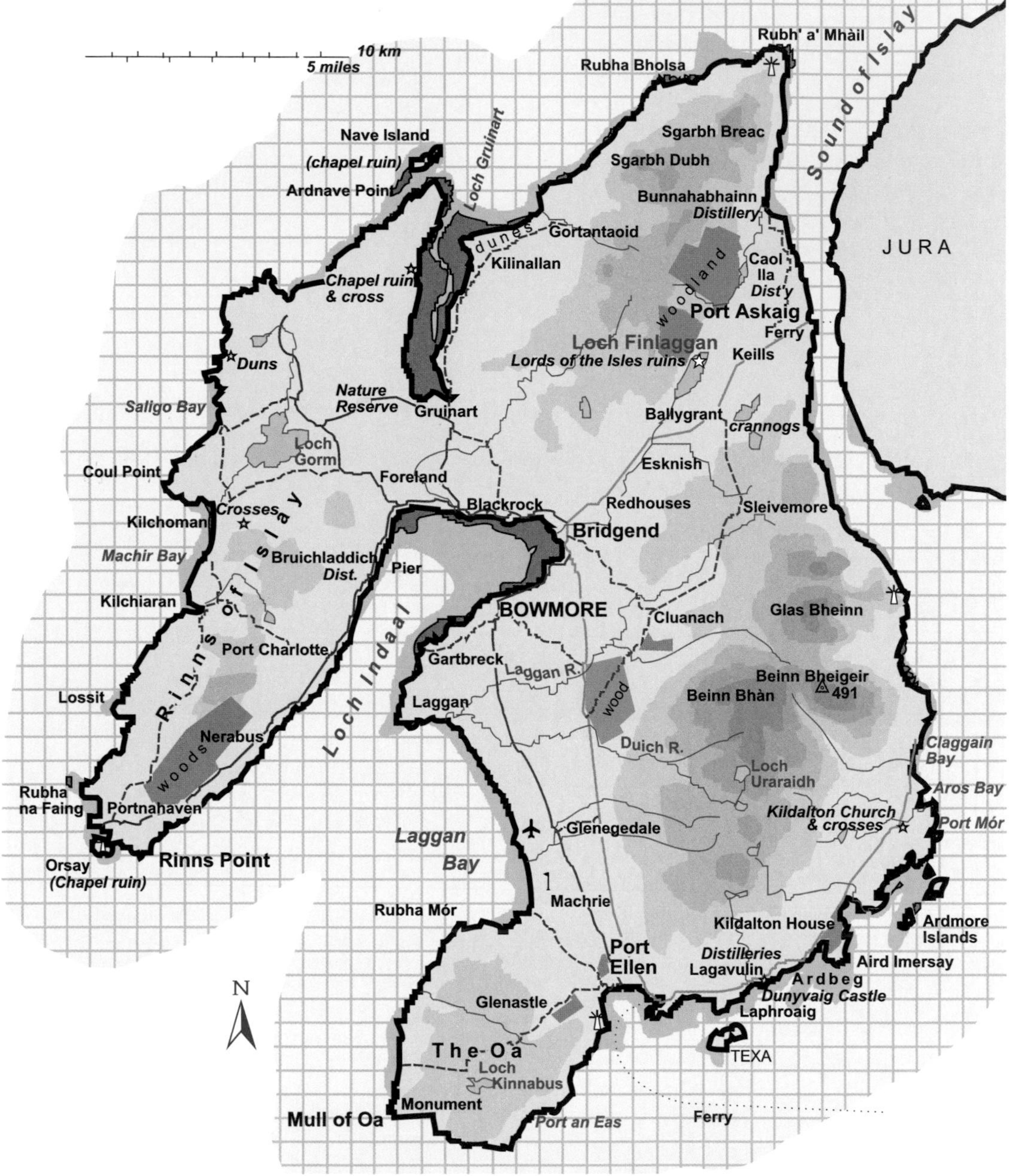

the Isles, thus became an autonomous principality powerful enough by the 14th century to have made its own treaties with England, France and Ireland, sometimes against the Scottish interest. New chiefs were proclaimed at the administrative headquarters at Loch Finlaggan near Port Askaig. This continued until 1493 when King James IV stripped John of the Isles of his titles and forced him to spend the rest of his days as a pensioner at the Stewart court.

In 1598 there was a vicious clan battle commemorated by a stone at the road junction south-west of the head of Loch Gruinart. James VI had granted land in Islay to the quarrelsome Sir Lachlan MacLean of Duart on Mull. The local Macdonalds understandably would not accept this so about four hundred MacLeans, with their chief, invaded the island. Nearly all of them, including Sir Lachlan, were slain. About thirty took sanctuary in the ancient church of Kilnave (G. – church of the saints) by Loch Gruinart but the Macdonalds set fire to the church and they were all burned to death.

In 1614 the Scots King granted Islay to Sir John Campbell of Cawdor but he had to fight for more than four years to gain possession from the Macdonalds. Sir John then gave Islay to his son as a wedding present, but his son was declared insane in 1639, and his grandson died young. All this strife and unrest devastated the island and impoverished the islanders. It was not until the early 18th century that the island was bought by a Daniel Campbell and his family who did a great deal to restore it to its former glory and make it a 'leader and model of the other isles'. This testimonial was actually given by a Macdonald and with widespread agreement.

By 1847 the owner's philanthropy had bankrupted him. His son, John Francis Campbell (1822–85), spent his life recording Gaelic traditions, poetry and folklore for posterity and there is a monument to him overlooking the house at Bridgend on the island that he never inherited.

Wildlife: Otters can often be seen on the shores of Loch Gruinart. There are red deer in the south-east and wild goats in the Oa.

Islay has the richest birdlife in the Hebrides with over 180 recorded species, and over 100 breeding on the island including the rare and elusive chough. Although it is particularly noted for its geese – about 20,000 barnacle geese and 6000 Greenland white-fronted geese have been recorded – there is much more of interest. Some sites noted by the RSPB are:

Loch Gruinart: Geese, waders, and black and red grouse. Occasionally golden eagle, peregrine, hen harrier and merlin can be seen hunting.

Ardnave Loch: Oct–May. Mute swan, wigeon, teal, mallard, pochard and tufted duck.

Bowmore: Many sea-fowl including scaup, eider, common scoter and Slavonian grebe can be seen from the pier. Glaucous and Iceland gulls frequent the rubbish tip. Dabbling duck and waders are in the shoreline shallows.

Head of Loch Indaal. Shoveller in the small saltmarsh lagoons. Marvellous spectacle of barnacle geese at dusk coming in to roost. Pintail in the river channel.

Bruichladdich Pier. Rocks at distillery for purple sandpiper in winter and many divers and sea-duck.

Frenchman's Rocks. Sooty shearwater, gannet, storm petrel, Leach's petrel sometimes, arctic and great skua, kittiwake galore.

Saligo Bay-Sanaigmore coast: Sea-birds, buzzard, golden eagle, merlin, kestrel, hen harrier, peregrine, red grouse, stonechat, chough, raven, twite. Also whinchat and wheatear.

The Oa: Snow bunting in winter. Many breeding sea-birds on the cliffs.

Loch Ballygrant: for wildfowl and common woodland species.

Claggain Bay: for great northern divers Oct–May.

Port Ellen for gulls and sea-fowl.

In 1993 Duich Moss – Eilean na Muice Duibhe – was made a National Nature Reserve by Scottish Natural Heritage.

* * *

ISLAY is probably better known for its whisky than for its birdlife. There are extensive peat deposits which are used as fuel and whose dark waters are used for the preparation of malt whisky. Working distilleries, famous for their distinctive flavours, are Ardbeg, Bunnahabhain, Bruichladdich, Bowmore, Lagavulin, Caol Ila, Laphroaig, and Port Ellen which only produces

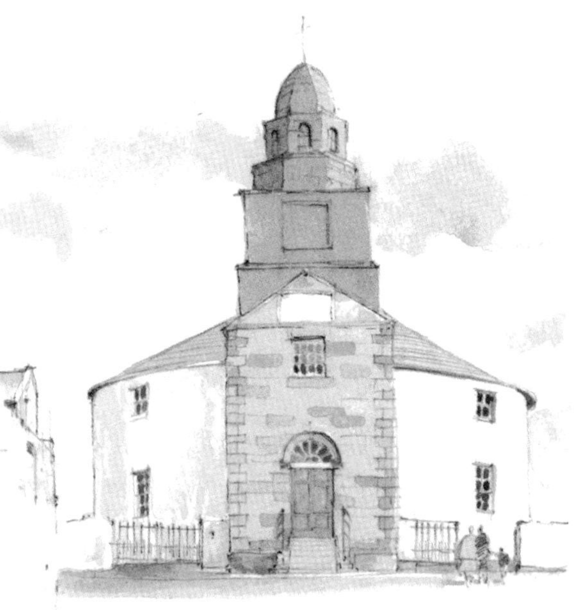

BOWMORE PARISH CHURCH

maltings for the others. And newly opened – Kilchoman (2005) and Port Charlotte (2007). About 180 years ago many of the illicit stills were legalised but no duty was payable on local whisky. As a result there was such widespread drunkenness that the parish ministers demanded government action. Today Islay produces about four million proof gallons of whisky each year, most of which is exported overseas. Even so, the duty collected by the Government from sales on the home market alone is the equivalent of a generous income for every man, woman and child on the island.

The climate is relatively mild but it is difficult to avoid the Atlantic winds which constantly funnel through Loch Indaal. The landscape is generally undulating except where the line of Jura mountains cross the Sound of Islay and peter out in the south-east corner. The island has quite an extensive farming industry and there is rich machair grassland on the west coast.

Historically Islay was once the most important of all the Scottish islands and it has much of archaeological interest. The elegant, 2.4m high Celtic cross at Kilchoman on the Rinns south of **Loch Gorm** was erected by John, first Lord of the Isles in the 14th century in memory of his second wife, Margaret. The wishing stone beneath it in a worn stone basin has to be turned by any mother who wishes to have a son. The legendary pipers, the MacCrimmons of Skye, are thought to have originated from near here.

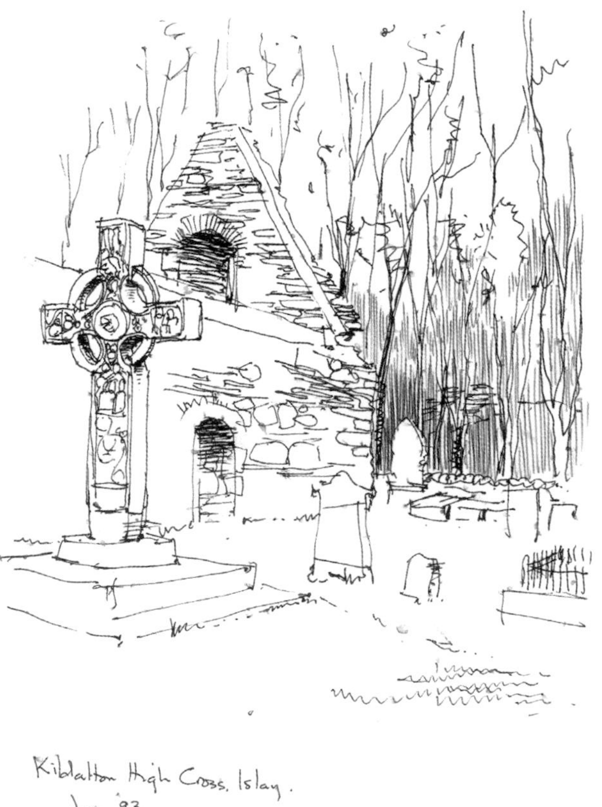

THE HIGH CROSS IN KILDALTON CHURCHYARD

On the west coast peat-bog of the Rinns (G. *rinn* – promontory. 'Rhinns' is the incorrect spelling) between Loch Gorm and **Saligo Bay** is an area where thousands of barnacle, greylag and Greenland white-fronted geese winter every year. The birds cause considerable damage to surrounding farms and peat-cutting is essential for the whisky industry so there was a rousing disagreement between islanders and conservationists in 1985. The area, **Duich Moss**, or Eilean na Muice Duibhe, was eventually made a National Nature Reserve in 1993 after agreement was reached with the distillers to use peat from an alternative site. This has safeguarded a rich variety of wildlife associated with peatland and is a boon to the budding tourist industry. United Distillers actively assisted Scottish Natural Heritage in measures such as damming drainage ditches to allow the water table to rise to its normal level.

At the head of Loch Gruinart, which separates the Rinns from the rest of Islay, a bloody battle between the MacLeans of Duart and the MacDonalds of Islay in 1598 was won, according to the MacDonalds, thanks to the magical intervention of the black elf, *Du-sith*.

The north-east part of the island has sporting estates well stocked with deer, pheasants and trout streams and very few roads. This is hill-walking country. **Sgarbh Breac** (364m) is a good climb reached by way of Beinn Thrasda's summit (260m) with a stunning view down the Sound of Islay and over to West Loch Tarbert on Jura.

Port Askaig is a tiny indentation which just avoids the fierce tides in the Sound of Islay. Its hotel dates from the 16th century. Ferries call here from Kennacraig on the mainland and Feolin on Jura. To the south is a wild and trackless mountain region with sport for the climber and hill-walker and wonderful views for the artist or photographer from the slopes of Beinn Bheigier (491m), Glas Bheinn (471m) and Beinn Bhàn (471m).

A main road cuts across the island from Port

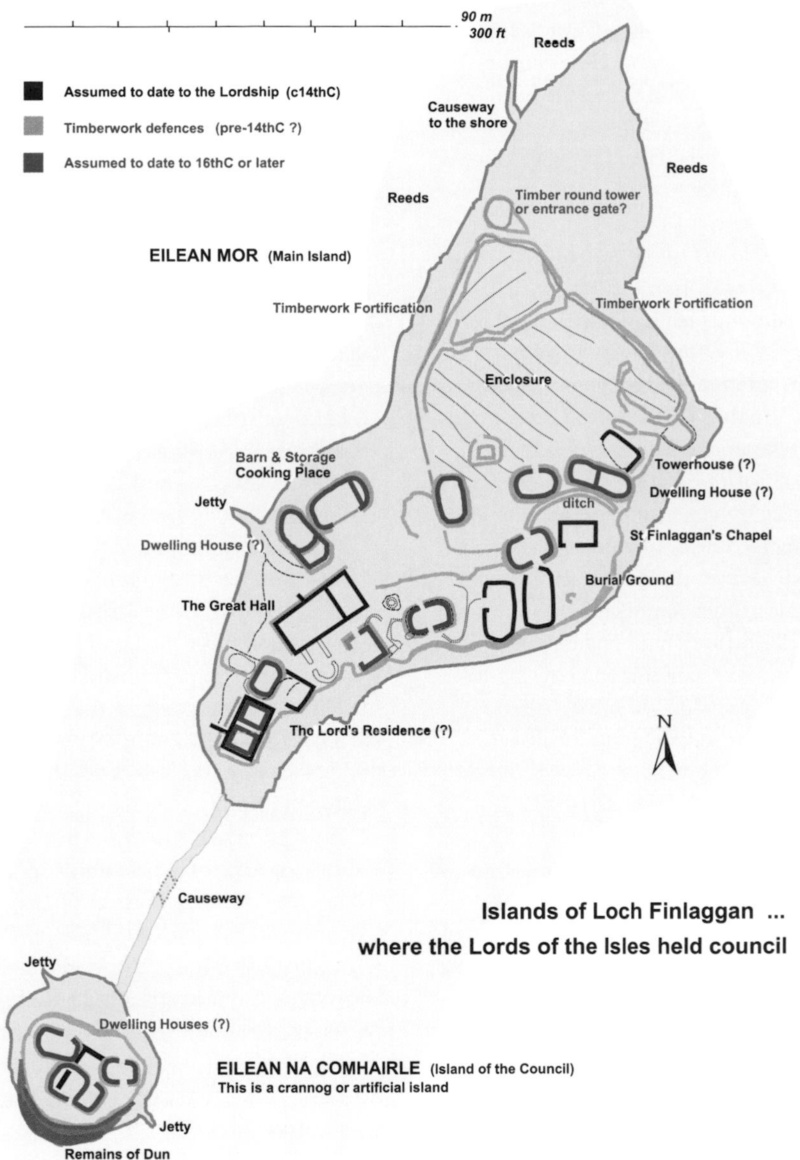

Askaig to Bridgend on Loch Indaal. Each of several lochs near Ballygrant has its own crannog. **Loch Finlaggan**, north of the village, was the Lord of the Isles' headquarters and is one of Scotland's most important archaeological sites, although little attention was paid to it before 1989. There are two islands (crannogs) in the loch, Eilean Mór (G. – big island) and Eilean na Comhairle [co**a**-oorloo] (G. – council island), both covered with ruins [NR389681]. In among the profuse wildflowers are the remains of at least 28 buildings of this ancient centre of Scottish Gaelic culture and administration including the Great Hall of the Lords, the chapel, scattered carved gravestones, buildings which held the 'parliament' of ecclesiastics and chiefs, living quarters, and many other crumbling ruins still to be identified. Excavation continues and the Finlaggan Trust now has a visitor centre on the site.

Bridgend is the home village of the former laird's mansion – Islay House, which is carefully screened from view by trees [NR334628]. The farm buildings have been beautifully renovated as craft workshops and together with the nearby Woollen Mill (1883) are worth visiting. The road on the north pebbled shore of **Loch Indaal** runs round to Bruichladdich with its distillery and on to the charming little fishing village of Port Charlotte, known as the **Queen of the Rinns**. This was built at the turn of the 18th century by a local minister, Rev Maclaurin. Every house is of identical plan and measures 9m x 7m. In the old Free Kirk is the Museum of Islay Life with a lot of interesting exhibits.

At **Nerabus**, two ancient burial grounds contain some of the finest medieval grave-slabs to be found in Scotland and 3km further on there are exotic wildfowl ponds at the Rodney Dawson Memorial collection of birds. The main road ends at **Portnahaven**, an old fishing village, which faces the islands of **Mhic Coinnich** and **Orsay** with its ancient chapel and Stevenson lighthouse. This is now the site of the world's first commercial wave-energy electricity generator, a remarkable example of Scottish innovation. About 9km north of Portnahaven on a very rural road **Kilchiaran** (G. – cell of St Ciaran) was founded by St Columba in honour of his Irish tutor who had died in 548. **Eilean Liath** forms a reef beside the bay.

Turning south from Bridgend brings one to **Bowmore**, the present-day 'capital' of Islay, with a population of about 900. It was founded by the laird, Daniel Campbell, in 1767. The rounded church of Kilarrow here [NR312596] was designed 'so the devil could find no corners to lurk in'.

Between Bowmore and Port Ellen a 10km shell-sand beach borders **Laggan Bay** with the airfield and a golf course on the machair at its southern end.

Port Ellen is the largest centre of population. The port construction was started in the 1820s by Walter Campbell, 4th of Islay, who named it Port Elinor after his wife. To the east of the town is the vestigial ruin of a chapel dedicated to St Lasar, an obscure 6th-century Irish nun, marked by two curious upright stones with holes cut through them. A pub near the harbour has several walls covered with excellent murals of island scenes and depicting local people. These were painted by an Irish artist, each character being placed in the composition in return for a dram – or two – or maybe three. I understand the poor chap died of drink – but he has left a fascinating memorial.

To the west of Port Ellen is **The Oa** – pronounced 'oh' – and on the Mull of Oa is an American Memorial [NR270415] commemorating US servicemen lost when the *Tuscania* was torpedoed in February 1918 and the *Otranto* was wrecked in a gale the following October. Many bodies were washed ashore beneath these cliffs. This is a storm-lashed area which overlooks the grey Atlantic but mountaineers appreciate the cliffs. A clean granite arête from sea-level to the cairn of Beinn Mhor provides an exciting 150m climb. Other good ridges are nearby to the east and also beyond the Memorial.

The southern road from Port Ellen to **Ardbeg** runs through one of the most archaeologically interesting parts of the island. It passes the Laphroaig distillery overlooking the island of Texa (No.2.1). Further east, by Lagavulin, are the ruins of 14th-century **Dunyvaig Castle** (G. – fort of the little ships) [NR406455], built either by Donald I or John of Islay, Lord of the Isles. This castle has a long and bloody history very similar to another Macdonald stronghold, Dunaverty Castle, on the Mull of Kintyre overlooking Sanda island (No.1.2). Further on, **Kildalton House** in a woodland setting is beside magic Loch a' Chnuic. This estate was owned by John Ramsay MP, who deported all his tenants to America in the 19th century. He was cursed by an old woman as she was dragged away and before long both he and his wife died and the estate fell into financial ruin.

Three kilometres further, the renowned **Kildalton High Cross** stands by a ruined chapel (G. *cille daltan* – the church of the disciple) [NR458508]. Carved in c.800 out of bluestone by a sculptor from Iona, it is considered by many to be the finest Celtic cross in the whole of Scotland. Beside it are some magnificent carved grave-slabs of the 15th century. The road dwindles to a track by Trudernish Point near a vitrified dun and standing stones.

Apart from the beautiful scenery, beaches, birdlife, and prehistoric and medieval remains, Islay also offers the visitor golf, riding, hill-walking, sea angling, freshwater fishing, diving, and any amount of subject matter for the artist. And although the island attracts many visitors in the summer months it never appears crowded.

* * *

Access: Car ferry: Kennacraig on West Loch Tarbert (Kintyre)/ Port Ellen or Port Askaig. Crossing 2¼ hours. Several services daily, 08000-66-5000. Regular air service from Glasgow, 0870-850-9850. There are regular island bus services, 01496-840273. Tourist Information,

Bowmore, 08707-200617 or 0845-2255-121.

Anchorages:
Note: The tidal range here is less than 2m and sometimes only 60cm – less than anywhere else in the British Isles. The movement at neaps is barely distinguishable.
1. Port Ellen. Hazards at entrance and west of harbour pier. 22-berth self-service pontoon in harbour in 3m dredged area; shelter good. Visitors' moorings NW of pier, but poor shelter in all S'lies. Kilnaughton bay W of harbour has better shelter from southerly swell or W winds and holding moderately good. Anchor N of Carraig Fhada lighthouse in 6–9m. This is a busy harbour so keep the approaches clear.
2. Lagavulin. Tricky approach and entrance. Two visitors' moorings at distillery or anchor in 3m in middle of pool, mud. Very restricted area and subject to swell.
3. Loch an t'Sailen. Approach to Lagavulin then follow a course 2c off the coast and leave the Ardbeg islet to port. Anchor NNE of Sgeir Dubh in 3m, rock and sand, good holding. Well sheltered.
4. Loch a' Chnuic (Kildalton Bay). Only suitable if no chance of winds from E to S, and in any case subject to heavy swell. Hazards on approach. Anchor near above-water rock in 3m, hard sand.
5. Ardmore Islands. A fascinating hideaway teeming with wildlife. Anchor SW of Eilean Craobhach or, with care, in the rocky but snug Plod Sgeirean behind a submerged reef.
6. Port Mór. Avoid N side and give S entrance point a wide berth. Head is shoal. Anchor in SW where depth suitable, sand. (*Best for visit to Kildalton Church and Cross.*)
7. Glas Uig. Between Port Mór and Aros Bay. Attractive but a number of dangers inside the anchorage and very restricted. Exposed to E and subject to swell. Anchor N of centre, 3m, sand and weed.
8. Aros Bay. A wide sandy bay with no off-lying dangers. Exposed N and E. Anchor in 3m in centre. (*Useful for visit to historic Kildalton Church and Cross but longer walk than No.6 above*).
9. Port Askaig. Strong tide and limited space. Alongside ferry pier sometimes possible.
10. Caol Ila distillery. Better holding than Port Askaig but avoid obstructing pier.
11. Bunnahabhain Bay. Temporary anchorage in 4m ½c N of pier.
12. Tràigh Baile Aonghais bay near Gortantaoid point. Exposed. Occasional anchorage in suitable weather.
13. Nave Island. Anchor SE of island opposite church ruin, sand, good holding but very little shelter. Occasional anchorage in suitable winds.
14. Portnahaven (Orsay). Well-sheltered channel. North entrance foul with rocks. Approach from S but beware strong tides across the entrance. Anchor NW of Portnahaven quay, sand.
15. Port Charlotte, Loch Indaal. Temporary anchorage.
16. Temp. anchorage off pier at Bruichladdich, Loch Indaal, in suitable weather. Pier has 3m depth at head.
17. Bowmore, Loch Indaal. The loch head dries out about 7½c and shores are shoal. Indifferent shelter. Anchor well offshore N of the N'most of the two beacons.

2.5 Jura

(ON jur-øy – udder island) – to a Viking sailor the Paps of Jura would be the obvious identification. All expert sources, however, give the derivation as (ON dyr-øy – deer island) and one 7th-century document refers to the island as 'Doiradeilinn'.

O S Maps: 1:50000 Sheet 61 1:25000 Sheet 355
Admiralty Charts: 1:75000 Nos.2168 and 2169 Sounds of Islay and Jura 1:25000 Nos.2481, 2396 and 2397 Gulf of Corryvreckan 1:25000 No.2343

Area: 36,692ha (90,666 acres)
Height: 785m (2575ft)

Owner: Multiple ownership. In 1938 a large part of the island was sold to five separate purchasers and most of these estates are still intact. The Fletchers (of Ardlussa) own the north; the central portion around Loch Tarbert is split between Viscount Astor and Lindsay C N Bury; Lord Vestey owns the area overlooking Craighouse Bay; A W A Riley-Smith owns the south of the island around Jura House and north to Craighouse, and Sir William J Lithgow's family own the western area centred on Feolin.

Population: 1755–1097. 1794–929. 1831–1312. 1841–no separate census figures. 1881–773. 1891–619. 1931–364. 1961–249. 1971–210. 1981–228. 1991–196. 2001–188.

Geology: This is the largest area of metamorphic quartzite in the Highlands producing poor soil and a lot of peat. A narrow strip of schist runs along the east coast and no other coast has so many arches, caves and raised beaches as the west side of Jura. The rocks are mainly white and red granite with fine blue slate and micaceous sandstone in the north. Iron ore is plentiful and the good silica sand deposits on the west coast were once used for glass-making. There are about fifty very large caves – some were used as mortuaries for the dead before the bodies were shipped to Iona or Oronsay for burial.

History: About 678AD, in Dalriadic times, there was a great battle fought on Jura between the native Picts and the Scots from Ireland.

During the time of the Lords of the Isles and Macdonald power, Jura's importance was due to its proximity to the headquarter territory of Islay. This lasted until the Clan Donald sold Jura to the Campbells of Argyll in 1607.

In 1647 during the Wars of the Covenant the Macleans of Jura were attacked by Campbell of Craignish and there was a fierce battle. 'MacLaine saved his lands with the loss of his reputation' according to Sir James Turner. General David Leslie arrived from Islay and Maclean promptly gave him his castle, his son, and 'fourteen prettie Irishmen who had been all along faithful to him' as hostages. Leslie had the fourteen hanged.

In 1767 fifty islanders sailed from Jura to settle in Canada and islanders continued to do so during the next seventy years. Walter Campbell of Jura inherited Islay in 1777 and sold his lands in Jura to concentrate his assets on Islay. About this time the island was divided into twenty-seven separate farms. In the 18th century and the early 19th century Jura was a centre for breeding Highland cattle. There was also a small number of hardy little sheep with a particularly fine wool, a lot of wild goats and some horses. In 1812 experiments were conducted on Beinn An Oir to determine the boiling point of water in relation to altitude.

After 1840 there was widespread introduction of sheep and the crofters were cleared from the land. The grassy glens deteriorated in consequence and much of the ground is now only of use for deer stalking.

Wildlife: By the end of the 18th century the deer population had declined seriously but numbers have slowly increased again with encouragement from the hunting fraternity and today there are about 5000. There are also some wild goats.

It is dangerous to wander about after mid-August when the stag shooting season has begun and at any time it is sensible to request permission. (Enquire at the Isle of Jura Hotel at Craighouse.) There are many adders so wear sensible footwear. During a 3km walk on a hot summer day, I passed seven different rocks with adders sunbathing on them.

North along the beach from the ferry landing at Feolin is the largest heronry on the island and a favourite haunt for otters. At least fifteen pairs of golden eagles are resident in the hills and hen harriers sweep over the lower ground. At the end of the 18th century it was reported that the 'many eagles... are very destructive to the lambs.' Loch Tarbert is a favourite haunt of mergansers and divers. Common seals frequent the skerries,

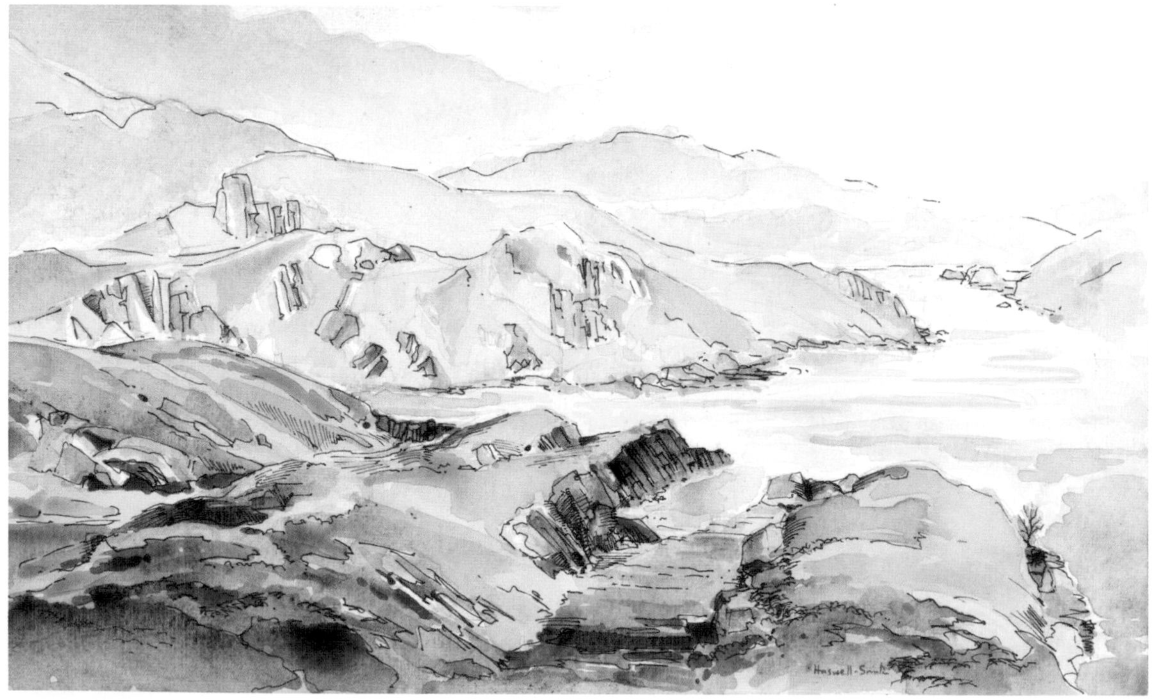

THE PASSAGE TO INNER LOCH TARBERT

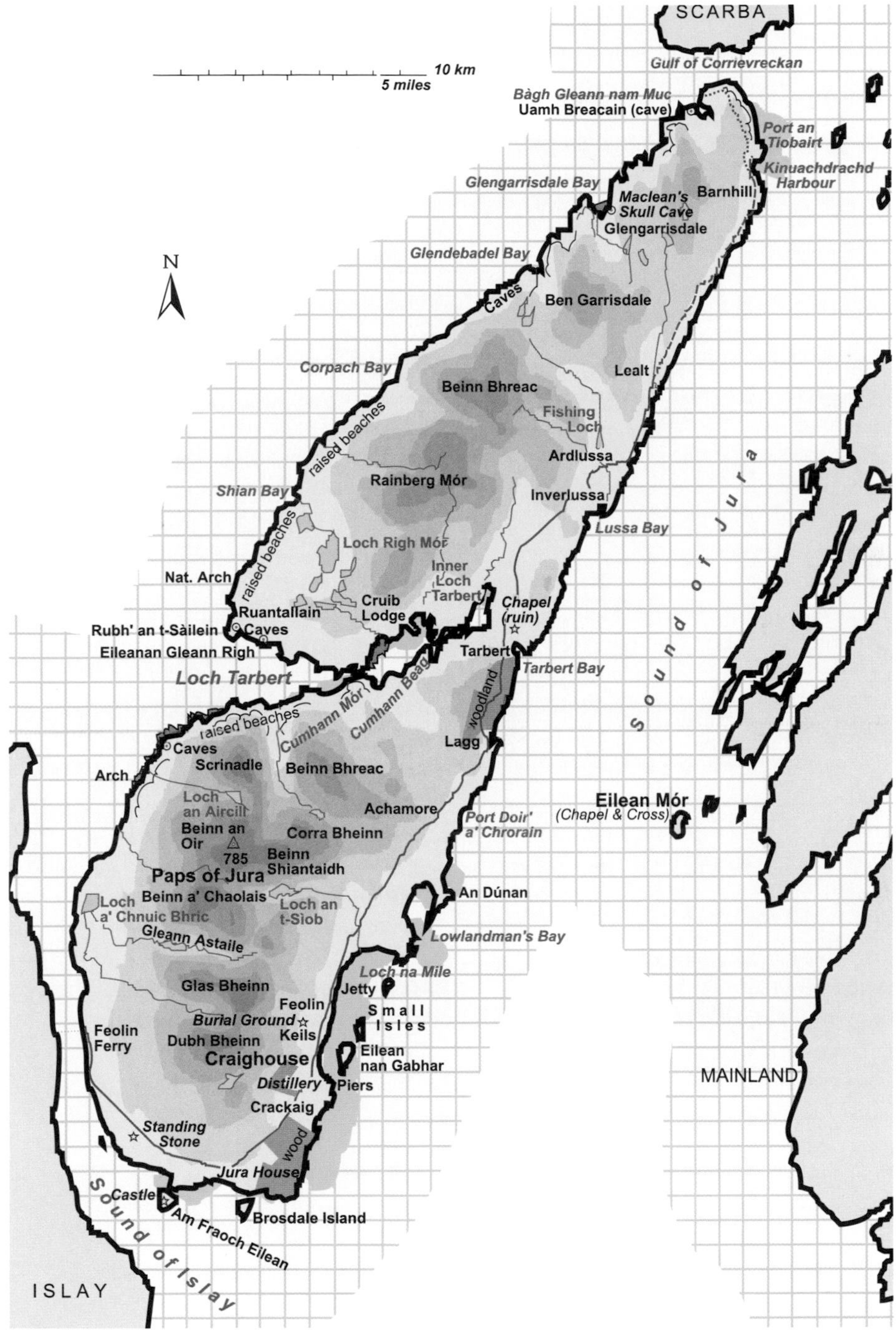

mainly on the south shoreline.

The wild terrain is almost too coarse to encourage a great botanical variety but there are unexpected finds to be made. Many of the marshy pools are covered with water-lilies and an interesting variety of alpine plants thrive on the higher slopes. Palm trees grow around Craighouse as a reminder of the mildness of the climate when sheltered from the wind.

JURA is the wildest island in the Inner Hebrides. It is a vast area of rock and blanket bog, most of it without roads or habitation of any kind and the haunt of deer and wild goats. Crossing this terrain of rough ankle-twisting rock and scree, or knee-high grass, heather, and bracken, is painfully slow. But this gives it added fascination. On Jura it is easy to believe that there is no such thing as the human race and that exploration of this remote environment is bound to yield some earth-shattering discovery. And scattered along the west coast of the ragged lonely landscape are spacious caves with dry floors and lofty vaulted roofs, great natural stone arches and pillars, and raised beaches which are almost artificial in their perfection.

Loch Tarbert nearly bisects the island. South of the first narrows, Cumhann Mór, there is a raised beach possibly ¾km in length and about 15m above sea-level with a lochan beside it. It is clean, with no weeds and the surface looks as though a gardener has just finished raking the smooth round pebbles. And yet it has been lying there for some 10,000 years!

Exploring Loch Tarbert by boat for the first time is an exciting experience. Negotiating the outer loch past the **Eileanan Gleann Righ** (G. – islands of the royal glen), through the narrow Cumhann Mór into the large middle loch with **Eilean Ard** to the north and finding, and passing through, the concealed entrance to the dog-leg passage leading to the inner sanctum. This entails slipping past rocks and tidal eddies, squeezing past little **Eilean an Easbuig**, and then, at last, the shallow inner loch opens up with its one deep patch in the centre.

Some of the many large caves include rudimentary altars which were built by the islanders when they stopped there while transporting their dead to Iona or Oronsay for burial, and there is one cave in **Bàgh Gleann Righ Mór** (G. – large bay of the valley of the king) in West Loch Tarbert which has a royal connection and an ancient history, but is the subject of conflicting scholarly argument [NR518824].

The **Paps of Jura** are almost as high as Goat Fell and almost as famous as the Cuillin – painted by McTaggart and many artists. There are, strangely, three paps: **Beinn an Oir** (a Corbett) at 785m (2575ft) (G. – the mountain of gold), **Beinn Shiantaidh** at 755m (2476ft) (G. – the holy mountain), and **Beinn a' Chaolais** at 734m (2408ft) (G. – the mountain of the kyle). North-west of Beinn an Oir is Sgriob na Caillich (G. – the witch's broom) – a large rock scar. A causeway was erected on Beinn an Oir by the Ordnance Survey in the mid-19th century.

For climbers who want to conquer all the Paps, there is a favourite steep scramble up Beinn Shiantaidh from the river outlet of Loch an t-Stob, down to the pass and lochans to the north-east and then a steep ascent of Corra Bheinn (575m) and a 5km round trip back to Shiantaidh: down the west ridge and across the 450m col and up to Beinn An Oir. Then descending the south spur, avoiding the steep ground overlooking Na Garbh-lochanan corrie to the col at 370m, and on up to Beinn a' Chaolais, the lowest of the Paps: after this a descent to Feolin on the west coast via Cnocbreac or to Keills near Craighouse via the shoulder above the head of Glen Astaile, under the east slope of Glas Beinn. Finish by passing the St Earnadail graveyard – if you are still able.

The west coast has always been underpopulated. It is now deserted but there used to be a small settlement at **Glengarrisdale** and another at **Ruantallain** at the entrance to West Loch Tarbert which was only abandoned about 1947. At Glengarrisdale Bay, in the far north-west, **Maclean's Skull Cave** contained a human skull and bones mounted on a cairn [NR647970] but about twenty years ago it was removed. This gruesome relic was alleged to be the remains of a Maclean who was slain when Jura was attacked by Campbell of Craignish in 1647 during the Wars of the Covenant.

Nowadays all the inhabitants of Jura live on the east coast, mostly in the vicinity of **Craighouse**. The distillery was built in 1963 and bottled its first malt in 1974. It replaced one built by the Campbells in the mid-19th century. Craighouse also has a post-office, shop, hotel, school and doctor. One of the two piers was built in 1814 by Thomas Telford. A string of islets known as the Small Isles form a breakwater to the bay. They are **Eilean nan Gabhar** (G. – island of the goats), **Eilean Diomhain** (G. – idle island), **Eilean nan Coinean** (G. – island of the rabbits), **Pladda** and **Eilean Bhride** (G – Bridget's isle).

At the south end of Jura, by the road running round from the ferry on the Sound of Islay, Jura House stands in a woodland estate with its beautiful walled gardens open to the public, just a short walk from the boathouse opposite Heather Island. Offshore is the small island of **Am Fraoch Eilean** (G. – the heather isle) on which are the ruins of Claig Castle [NR471627], a Norman-style square tower with 3m-thick walls built in 1154 by Somerled to defend the Sound of Islay

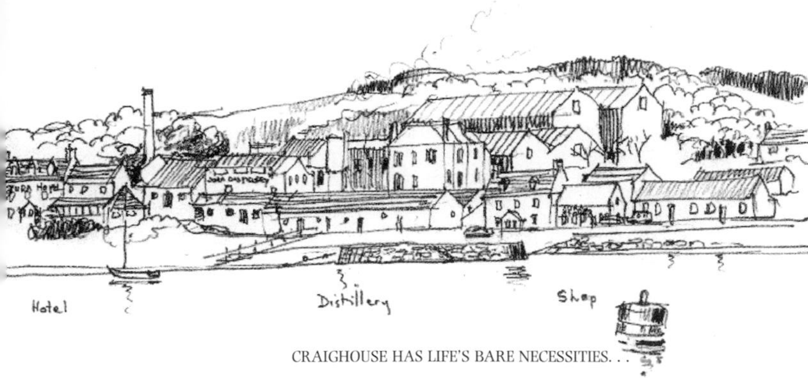

CRAIGHOUSE HAS LIFE'S BARE NECESSITIES. . .

and also used by his descendants as a prison. The Macdonald clan slogan is still 'Fraoch Eilean'. Jura House is a short walk from the boathouse opposite Heather Island and has beautiful walled gardens (open to the public). To the east of Am Fraoch Eilean by the Sound of Jura is **Brosdale Island** and to the west, in the Sound of Islay, are the sharp rocks of **Glas Eilean**.

In this area and up the east coast standing stones prove that early man also favoured the east of the island.

Jura's one and only public road continues north from Craighouse and passes the crofting hamlet of Keills with its **Chapel of St Earnadail** [NR524687] who was a little-known early Celtic missionary from Iona. Although he lived on Islay he insisted that he should be buried on Jura, and that a ball of mist would guide his mourners to a suitable burial place. A gravestone in the churchyard commemorates Gillouir MacCrain who died in 1645. Another MacCrain, Mary, died aged 128 in 1856 and is buried at Inverlussa. The tombstone inscription says that she was a 'Descendant of Gillouir MacCrain who kept One Hundred and Eighty Christmasses in his own house. And died in the reign of Charles I.' There is a wry sense of humour here! Until the 20th century Jura chose to recognise both the old and the new calendar (see Foula, No.11.6) so two Hogmanays and two Christmases could be celebrated each year.

The road continues up the east coast passing a wide stretch of beach at the head of **Loch na Mile**. Then it climbs and crosses a stretch of moorland before entering an area of attractive woodland at **Lagg**. Tarbert Bay, at the narrow low-lying neck of land adjoining West Loch Tarbert, has a small enclosed beach, standing stones and a ruined chapel and, a further 6km on, the road runs out at **Inverlussa**. Ardlussa estate, of about 6900ha, was once the only independent property on Jura. The present house was built by Lord Colonsay about 1840. A track continues up the coast from here to the north of the island passing Barnhill [NR705970] where George Orwell stayed when he wrote his famous novel *1984*.

From the most northern point of the vehicle track there is a fairly undemanding 3km hill-walk to a point above the clifftops overlooking the notorious **Corryvreckan** (G. *coire bhreacain* – the speckled cauldron). This is a marvellous vantage point to watch the swirl of the waters 100m or more below, although the finest view point is on Scarba (No.2.9) on the opposite side. The most dramatic sight is when a spring tide is in flood (i.e. running westwards at a speed of up to 10 knots) against a strong west wind. There have been many shipwrecks and disasters and Orwell recorded how he also nearly lost his life here in 1949 when trying to circumnavigate Jura.

It is often said that the tidal race was named after Breacan, a Norse Prince, who foundered with his entire fleet of fifty ships. But from Adomnan's *Life of St Columba* it would appear that this calamity occurred in the tidal race between Rathlin Island and Antrim. Nevertheless, Breacan is reputed to be buried in the 55m-deep cave [NM685005] on the south side of Bagh nam Muc (G. – bay of the swine), at the north-western tip of Jura and guarded by **Eilean Mór** and **Eilean Beag**. Martin Martin reported in 1695 that 'Breacan's stone', a tomb and an altar were in the cave.

* * *

Access: Car ferry Kennacraig/ Port Ellen or Port Askaig, Islay, 08000-66-5000. Scheduled air service: Glasgow/Islay, 0870-850-9850.
Bus service, Port Ellen/Port Askaig, Islay, 01496-840273. Car ferry, Port Askaig/Feolin, Jura, 01496-840681. (Petrol is not available on Jura). Ferry services by arrangement: Craobh Haven/ Craighouse, Farsain Cruises, 01852-500664 or Islay Sea Safari, Port Ellen, 01496-840510.

Anchorages:

1. Craighouse. Avoid Goat Rock, E of Eilean nan Gabhar, and enter bay centrally between beacon and perch.

Visitors' moorings, or anchor in 3m off old stone pier. Alternatively, in E'lies anchor as close as depth permits to the centre of the W side of Eilean nan Gabhar. Sand and kelp in both cases, holding poor.
2. Loch na Mile, N end. Sand and kelp, but cleaner than Craighouse. Subject to swell.
3. Drum an Dùnan bay. Small bay at S side of entrance to Lowlandman's Bay. Good anchorage in SW winds. Anchor in centre when the small islet off its point closes with the point, hard sand.
4. Lowlandman's Bay. Good shelter in W winds, but exposed to S and N winds which bring fierce squalls and a swell. Head dries out 1c and shoals a considerable distance. Best near E side, off stone jetty, thick kelp.
5. Lagg Bay is a shallow bight 3¾M NNE of Lowlandman's Bay. Temp. anchorage. Avoid central cable and anchor either side of it. Kelp and subject to swell.
6. Tarbert Bay, 1½M NNE of Lagg Bay is small inlet with central reef. Enter close to Liath Eilean on W side of inlet and anchor just N of it in 2–3m, sand. Everywhere else is dense kelp. Can be subject to swell.
7. Lussa bay, temp. anchorage with good shelter from N. Avoid reefs about ¾c from W shore. Anchor in centre, 2–4m, sand. Subject to swell.
8. Ardlussa bay, 1M NNE of Lussa bay, temp. anchorage midway between En Traigh and Ru an Fhaing, kelp.
9. Kinuachdrach harbour in NE of Jura. Temp. anchorage, close off N shore, in depths of 4–7m, cabbage kelp. Subject to swell.
10. Port an Tiobairt, at NE extremity, good occasional anchorage except for NE winds. Anchor centrally in 2–5m, sand and kelp. Subject to swell.
11. Bàgh Gleann nam Muc, in NW next Gulf of Corryvreckan, pleasant and safe, but with rocky shoals off both entrance points. Anchor at head of the larger bay off the small headland to port, firm sand. No swell except during NW wind at slack water.
12. Glentrosdale bay, the next bay SW of Bàgh Gleann nam Muc and 9½c NNE of Bàgh uamh nan Giall. Temp. anchorage, open NW.
13. Bàgh uamh nan Giall, about 8½c NE of E entrance point of Glengarrisdale Bay, is free from dangers, 4–6m.
14. Glendebadel bay and Glengarrisdale bay, 6¼M and 8¼M respec. NE of Shian Bay are small but easily accessible. Temp. anchorages when wind suitable.
15. Shian Bay, 3½M NNE of Loch Tarbert. Small, shallow, several rocks, exposed, and usually a heavy swell, but possible in fine weather.
16. Brein Phort, N of Ruantallain. Temp. anchorage in light E'lies in 6m inside the reef.
17. Rubh' an t-Sàilein, rocky headland at N entrance point of Loch Tarbert has small rocky cove on E side and bight close E again which are good landing points but poor anchorage.
18. Bàgh Gleann Righ Mór is an indentation E of Eileanan Gleann Righ, N side of outer Loch Tarbert. Easy access and good holding in 3–4m off W side of bay. Bay shoals. Heavy swell with W'lies but reasonable in N'lies.
19. Bàgh Gleann Righ Beag, a bight immediately ESE of Bàgh Gleann Righ Mór and NE of Aird Reamhar, gives occasional anchorage except in W'lies.
20. Cuan Mór Bay in outer West Loch Tarbert immediately NW of the Cumhann Mór (the narrows). Approach using leading lines. Anchor in centre avoiding reef on E side, mud, holding and shelter good.
21. Cairidh Mhor, S shore of Inner Loch. Most of bay dries. Good holding in mud and reasonable shelter in most conditions..
22. Cruib Lodge (bothy). Anchor well off-shore on N shore of the centre loch, S of lone cottage and drying rocks in the bay, mud.
23. Eilean an Easbuig pool (Halfway Anchorage). Fairly hazardous entry through the Cumhann Beag using several leading marks but good anchorage slightly N of centre of the pool in 4m.
24. Inner Loch Tarbert. Further passage to remote top pool. Anchoring in 'The Hole' is not advised as depth changes suddenly and bottom probably foul. (*1½ km track from boathouse to the east coast of Jura*).
25. Glenbatrick bay between Sgeir Agleann and Rubh' a' Bhaillein on S shore of Outer Loch Tarbert. Anchor in suitable depth, near Sgeir Agleann, sand. Sheltered SW. Mouth of river shoals 2c.
26. Whitefarland Bay. Opposite Caol Isla distillery in Sound of Islay. Clean, open bay out of main tidal stream. Anchor N of anchor-painted boulder in 3m. The boulder has a mooring ring.
27. Am Fraoch Eilean. Approach carefully as many foul and shallow areas. Occasional anchorage NNW of Am Fraoch Eilean and W of nearby boathouse and pier on Jura in 3–4m, sand and weed. (*2km walk to Jura House*).

2.6 Colonsay

(ON – Columba's island).

Oronsay

(ON – Oran's island). Normally this is the Gaelic name for a tidal island (which this is) but here the name derives from St Oran who founded the island monastery in 563AD.

O S Maps: 1:50000 Sheet 61 1:25000 Sheet 354

Admiralty Charts: 1:75000 No.2169 Scalasaig Harbour 1:12500 No.2474

Area: 4617ha (11,409 acres)
Height: 143m (469 ft)

Owner: Colonsay, with the exception of the church and the ferry pier, has been in the family of the one-time Minister of Defence, Lord Strathcona and Mount Royal, since 1905. Oronsay, except for the Priory, was also owned by the Strathconas but was sold to Adam Bergius, an American, for about £100,000 in the 1970s and another American, Ike Colburn, bought it in the 1980s. Mrs Francis Colburn of Massachusetts has now leased it to the RSPB but still visits it annually.

Population: Approximate figures for Colonsay and Oronsay combined: 1792–718 (134 families). 1841–987.

	1881	1891	1931	1961	1981	1991	2001
Colonsay	387	358	232	164	133	98	108
Oronsay	10	23	6	2	3	8	5
	397	381	238	166	136	106	113

Geology: Lower mudstone strata with Torridonian sandstone containing lime, which breaks down into good soil. There are some basalt dykes, white limestone at the north end of Bheinn Bhreac, and a particularly fine raised beach north of Kiloran Bay which is worth a visit.

History: The Macphees or MacDuffies, archivists to the Lords of the Isles, were the islands' owners from at least the 15th century but they were dispossessed by the MacDonalds soon after 1615. The Campbells of Argyll then ousted the MacDonalds. Malcolm MacNeil of Knapdale acquired the islands (i.e. both Colonsay and Oronsay) from the Campbells in 1700 for an agreed exchange of land. This was one of the few Hebridean islands which was fortunate enough to escape the 19th-century clearances as the laird at the time, John MacNeil, had a liberal approach. Even so, many families had already emigrated to America in the summer of 1791 and the *Statistical Account* lamented, 'Pity it is that such numbers should bid farewell to their native country, when there is so great a demand for useful citizens.' By 1905 mounting debt forced the MacNeil family to hand over the island to Lord Strathcona (Donald Smith, a Canadian Scot) in lieu of £44,000 which they owed him.

Wildlife: There are many seals, particularly among the skerries of the grassy Ardskenish peninsula on the west coast, and also on Eilean nan Ron (G. – seal island), which is a nature reserve. Rabbits were introduced 200 years ago to provide fresh meat and as there are no foxes, weasels or stoats they thrive enthusiastically. A few wild goats exist in the more remote areas and Hebridean sheep were introduced to Oronsay by the RSPB in 1999.

When Lord Strathcona bought Colonsay he was able to take advantage of the woodland planted in Kiloran valley by the MacNeils. He cultivated many rhododendrons, magnolia and azalea, and extended the tree cover with acacia, maple, poplar, sea-buckthorn, and eucalyptus. The woods include sycamore, beech, elm, ash, spruce, aspen, hazel, willow, larch, silver birch and pine. The sheltered valley is almost sub-tropical.

In late summer at Garvard by the Strand field gentians bloom and rock samphire hide in the clefts. Colonsay has, possibly, the greatest variety of flora in the Hebrides – some five hundred species.

Loch Fada and the lesser lochs in the centre of the island have a great variety of birds and also provide good fishing (permits from the hotel). Around the coast eider are so common that they are known locally as 'Colonsay duck'. Kittiwakes, guillemots and razorbills breed on the west coast and Oronsay is a wintering ground for barnacle geese. There is also – rare sight! – a small number of resident choughs.

* * *

COLONSAY and ORONSAY are separated by a wide expanse of shell sand called The Strand which can be walked across when the tide is out, following a defined route. Halfway across is the sanctuary cross: any Colonsay fugitive who reached it was immune from punishment provided he stayed on Oronsay for a year and a day.

These islands have been inhabited for 8,700 years. On the south side of **Kiloran Bay**, in Uamh Uir (G. – the cave of the grave-dust) the bones of domestic animals and Neolithic flint tools have been excavated. There are many pre-Christian and early Christian relics. A Viking warrior who had been given a ship burial in 855 with his weapons, horse and coins, was uncovered in the sand dunes here in 1882. Although it was a pagan burial two crosses

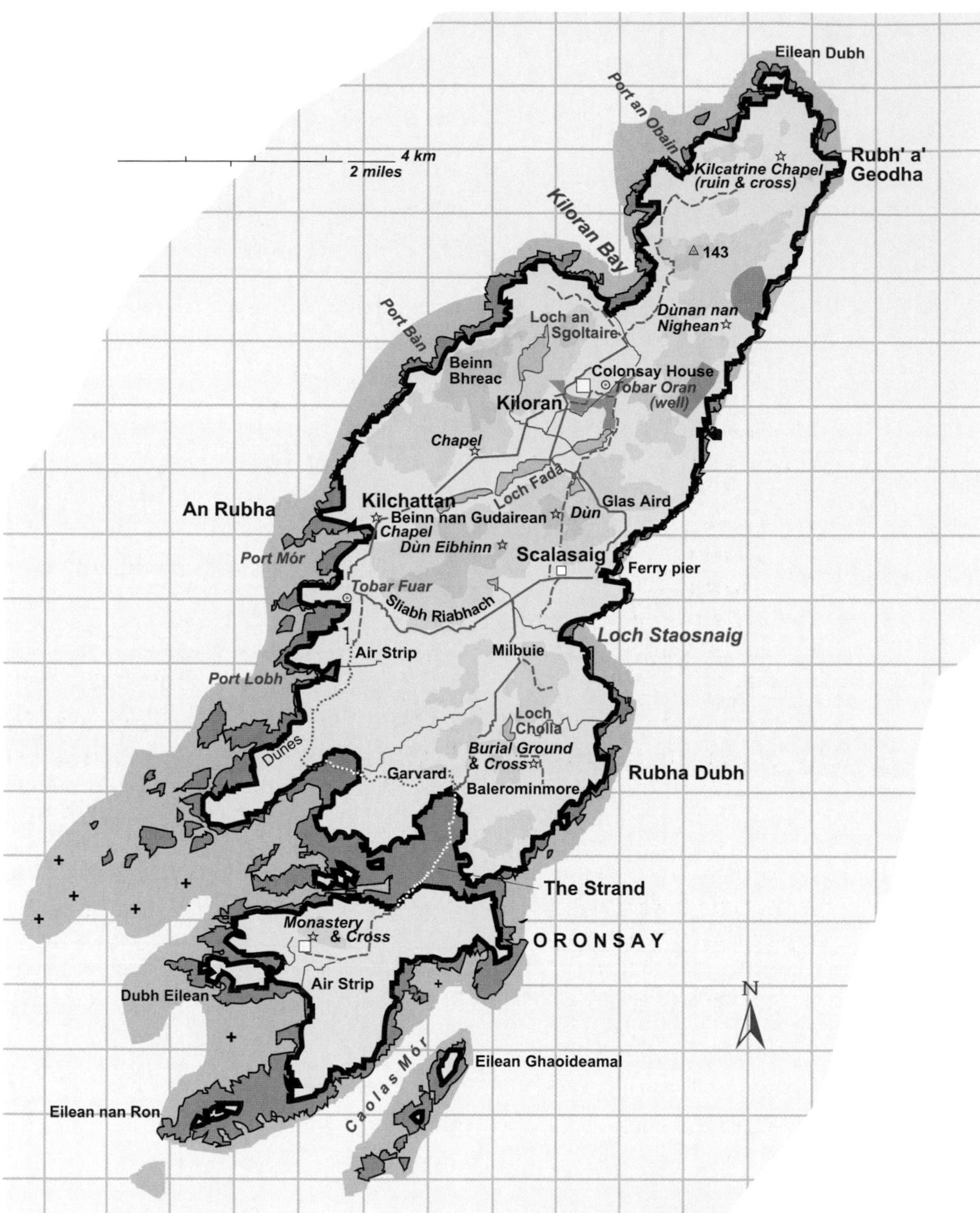

incised on stone slabs were included as an additional guarantee.

Both islands have deeply indented coasts with numerous rocks and reefs and the west coast backed by machair. Colonsay is generally of good soil although the higher ground is moorland and scrub. Raised beaches on the west coast and sea beach debris in the interior mark a time when the land was lower in the sea and these were four separate islands. The economy depends on crofting, farming, a little fishing and tourism. Visitors may wander freely throughout the island, although cars are restricted in some parts.

In the extreme north, in a low valley of sand-dunes running down to a fine beach, the remains of **Kilcatrine** (G. – Catherine's chapel) are marked by a standing stone and cross [NR421999]. This may have been the site of a 13th-century convent.

According to legend the MacNeils first came to the island with their cattle in an open boat. MacNeil's wife gave birth during the voyage and to keep her and the baby warm they slaughtered a cow so that mother and child could shelter inside the carcass.

Palm trees and bamboo now grow in the mild

and sheltered Kiloran valley where Malcolm MacNeil built Colonsay House in 1722. He is said to have salvaged stones from an old church or abbey which was nearby. The gardens were once considered equal to Inverewe, Crarae, and Achamore on Gigha (No.2.3), and are still beautiful, but Colonsay House is now partly converted to holiday flats and the work of eighteen gardeners is done by one man.

The inevitable Piper's Cave where a piper and his dog went to hunt for hell is on the coast at Port Bàn. Only the dog reappeared but from a cave four miles south with his hair burned off. (One wonders why this legend occurs on so many of the Scottish islands, see Barra, Gigha, etc.)

The ferry pier was built at **Scalasaig** (ON – shieling bay) in 1965. This is the main village and two other centres of population are Kilchattan and Kiloran. The island has a junior school, a minister of the church and a resident doctor, but no policeman. There is a hotel, some summer cottages, bed-and-breakfast accommodation and a brewery. The hotel at Scalasaig provides all the local tourist information. By the road between the hotel and the harbour is the Well of the South Wind where fishermen used to pray for a south wind and overlooking the village is an Iron Age fort, the most important of many on the island, called **Dun Eibhinn** [NR382944]. There is another one just to the north-east on Beinn nan Gudairean and this is also possibly the best viewpoint on the island [NR388950].

On the west coast opposite Scalasaig between **Tobar Fuar** (G. – cold well) and **Port Lobh** (G. – the port that smells of seaweed) is an 18-hole golf course. This stretch of Colonsay coastline has many skerries and off-shore islets – **Eilean nam Ban** (G. – women's isle), **Eilean Dubh**, **Eilean a' Chladaich** (G. – shore isle), **Eilean na Bilearach** (G. – sea-grass isle), **Eilean Leathan** (G. – broad island) and the inevitable **Glas Eilean** (G. – pale grey-green isle). This is in contrast to the east coast which boasts only one islet – **Eilean Olmsa**.

Across the sea from the old burial ground at **Balerominmore** [NR384914] in the south-east of Colonsay, which has a cross and carved slab, the Paps of Jura glow in the summer evening sun. Nearby at Garvard, overlooking the Strand, are the foundations of a cell or chapel, with a dun, and a standing stone.

* * *

ORONSAY has a very fine ruin, possibly second only to Iona in importance, of an Augustinian **Priory** built in c.1380 which is probably on the same site as St Oran's original monastery of 563 [NR350890]. This is a fascinating group of buildings in a reasonable state of preservation although, unfortunately, part of the stonework was removed by the MacNeils to build the adjacent farmhouse. Some human bones from the neighbouring graveyard are kept by the high altar in the chapel and beautifully sculpted medieval

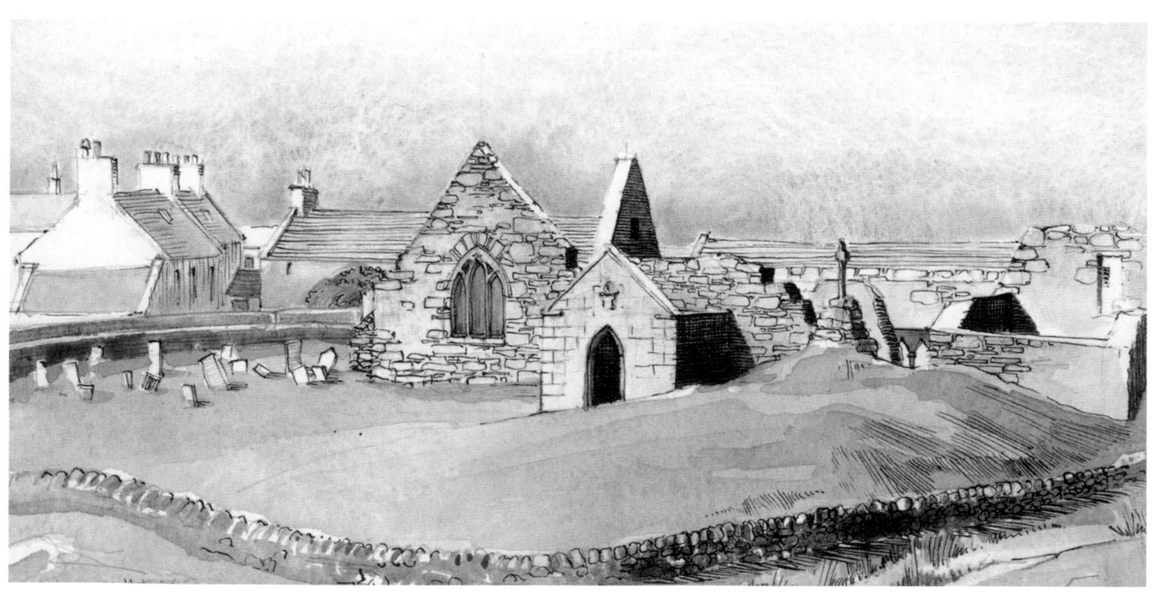

THE AUGUSTINIAN PRIORY ON ORONSAY

tombstones are protected in the Prior's House beside the delightfully-proportioned miniature cloisters. Outside there are two notable Celtic crosses, one of 3.7m height featuring a relief of the Crucifixion in commemoration of Prior Colin, who died in 1510. Oronsay is suffused with a feeling of tranquillity and it is easy to understand why St Oran chose it for a retreat (Columba is said to have rejected it because it was within sight of Ireland.)

Archaeological excavations on Oronsay have shown evidence of a Middle Stone Age settlement and there are a number of Mesolithic shell mounds. The grass airstrip by the monastery fights a losing battle with the rabbits.

A reef of islets, **Eilean Ghaoideamal** (G. – the blemished isle), **Eilean an Eoin** (G. – bird isle), and some skerries, lies parallel to the east coast of Oronsay creating a channel, Caolas Mór, which is the only partially sheltered anchorage in the area. A small sandy beach called Tràigh Uamha Seilbhe (G. – beach of the caves used as stock-pens) faces the kyle.

On **Eilean nan Ron** (G. – seal island) at the most southern tip, beyond the sheep and ponies grazing on the landing strip, is the ruin of an old kelp-gatherer's cottage. The huge expanse of skerries round this islet is a favourite breeding ground for the grey Atlantic seal. A thousand or more converge here in the autumn each year and the roar of battling bulls can be heard for miles.

* * *

Access: Vehicle ferry from Oban five times a week, 01631-566688; and from Kennacraig on Wednesdays only, 01880-730253. No caravans allowed. Boat excursions, Farsain Cruises, Craobh Haven, 01852-500664. There is an island post-bus and bicycles can be hired at the hotel.

Anchorages: There are no good anchorages.

1. Caolas Mór, Oronsay. Occasional anchorage in the bay opposite Eilean Ghaoideamal on a line between N extremity of En Ghaoideamal and boathouse on Oronsay. Beware reef Leac nan Geadh to the N which covers. (*1¼km easy walk to Priory*). Better shelter sometimes in the bight N of En Ghaoideamal behind the reef extending S from Eilean Treadhrach which is sometimes favoured. 4–6m in both cases, bottom sand, but swell from S and E.
2. Eilean Treadhrach. Occasional anchorage in N bay, sheltered from SW but negotiate with care, preferably at LW.
3. Loch Staosnaig. Anchor near head of bay towards S side, sand. Avoid line of submarine cable. Subject to swell but more room than Scalasaig.
4. Scalasaig harbour, tie alongside N side of pier at the wave screen, if there is room. Or anchor N of pier, but space very limited, sand. Open to E and subject to swell.
5. Balnahard Bay at NE tip of Colonsay. Occasional anchorage on S side in 6–10m sand and shingle.
6. Kiloran Bay. Occasional anchorage off sandy beach but can be subject to severe swell at times and dangerous in W'lies.
7. Port Mór, a bay central on W coast. Keep at least 5c clear of coast until line of the road passing the cemetery is completely open, then approach carefully on this line. The head shoals about 2c. Good shelter from E but subject to heavy S'ly swell.

2.7 Eilean Macaskin

(G. – Macaskin's Island)

OS Maps: 1:50000 Sheet 55 1:25000 Sheet 358
Admiralty Chart: 1:25000 No.2326

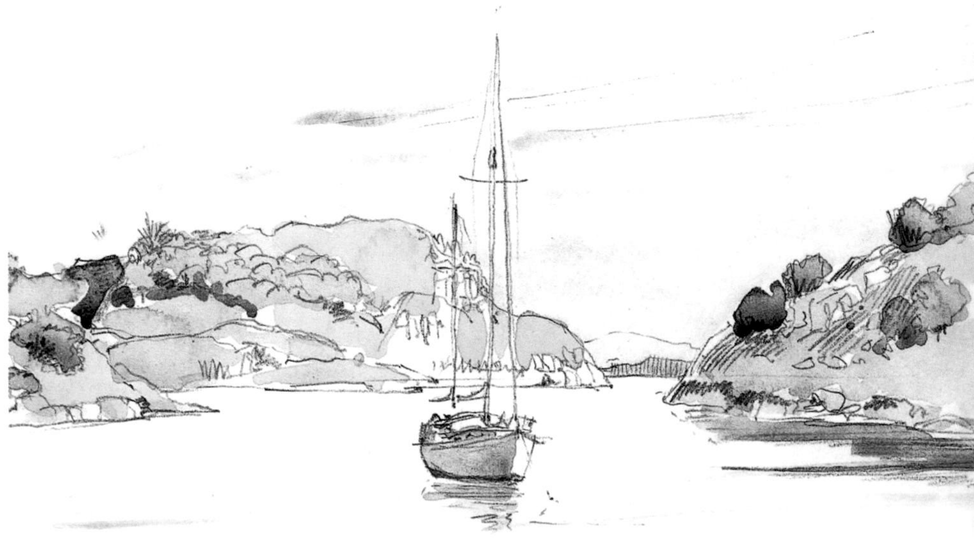

THE ANCHORAGE BY GOATS ISLAND

Area: 50ha (124 acres)
Height: 65m (213ft)

Owner: Was bought in 1934, together with Eilean Righ (see No.2.8) and Eilean nan Gabhar, by Sir Reginald Johnston for £1200. Now owned by Mr David P G Sillar of Winscombe, Somerset.

Population: 1841–no separate Census figures. 1881–6. 1891–0. No permanent habitation since.

Geology: Metamorphic epidiorite with some Dalradian quartzite at the south end.

Wildlife: Many wildflowers although not as prolific as on Eilean Righ (No.2.8).

EILEAN MACASKIN lies at the entrance to Loch Craignish and has a narrow rock-strewn but easily navigable channel up the east side. The island consists of a long ridge running parallel with the loch, 65m high at its highest point, steep on the west side but with a strip of relatively level ground on the east. It is comparatively well wooded and comfortably sheltered except for the southern end which can catch the blast of the prevailing wind rushing up the Sound of Jura. A reef of skerries extends further south towards an islet called **Eilean nan Coinean** (G. – isle of the rabbits).

Eilean nan Gabhar (G. – island of the goats)

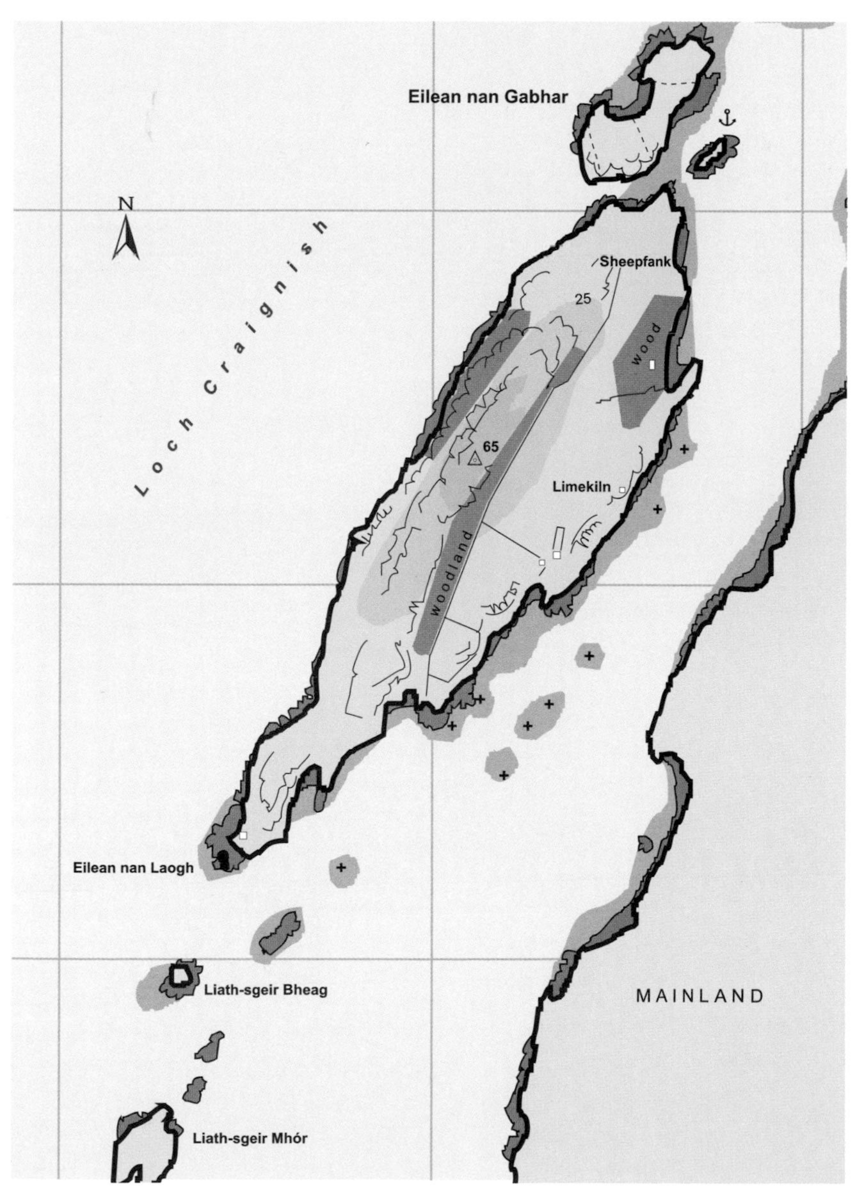

lies between Eilean Righ (No.2.8) and Eilean Macaskin giving shelter to a pleasant little anchorage. It is steep, with patches of scrub cover, and more suitable for goats than sheep although the latter seem to cope quite well. The landing place for Eilean Macaskin is on a rocky grey sand beach at the north extremity which fringes some swampy ground. Beyond, old wooden sheep pens stand in a bed of foxgloves. Well-built dry-stone dykes run along the ridges and the patches of woodland and scattered mature trees give the settled appearance of parkland.

To the south-west of Eilean Macaskin is the powerful tidal race of the Dorus Mór (G. – great door) which tumbles with force through the gateway between Craignish Point and the small island of **Garbh Rèisa** (G. – the rough one in the tidal race). At 43m height this could almost be considered a doorpost. Adjoining Garbh Rèisa is **Eilean na Cille** (G. – chapel island). West of Craignish Point is **Rèisa an t-Sruith** (G. – the tidal-race island in the current) and north of it is **Rèisa Mhic Phaidean** (G. – McFadyen's island in the tidal race). These little islands are all fairly insignificant rocks but they are worthy of respect when the tide is in full flood.

* * *

Access: Farsain Cruises, Craobh Haven, 01852-500664 or enquire at Ardfern.

Anchorages:

1. Eilean nan Gabhar (G. – goat island), N of En Macaskin. Anchor in limited space between the N end of the skerry and the reef which lies alongside the E side of Goat Island, 3–4m, firm mud and clay.
2. Temp. anchorage in small bay at NE corner but restricted swinging space and bottom falls away rapidly.

2.8 Eilean Righ

[elan ree] (G. – royal island) May have been named after the Danish sea-king Olaf who is reputed to have died in this region, or one of the early Scottish kings who were crowned in mid-Argyll.

OS Maps: 1:50000 Sheet 55 1:25000 Sheet 358
Admiralty Chart: 1:25000 2326

Area: 86ha (213 acres)
Height: 55m (180ft)
Owner: Bought in 1992 by Viscount Chewton (a Somerset farmer and brother of William Waldegrave, the former Government minister) for about £250,000. He carried out many improvements to the property but, on inheriting the Waldegrave earldom, put it up for resale in 1996. It was sold in 1998 for about £400,000 to Mr Siva Jothy.

Population: 1841–no separate Census figures. 1881–0. 1891–5 (2 houses). 1931–7. No Census records since but occasional occupation.

Geology: Mainly epidiorite and allied metamorphosed igneous rocks.

History: Once belonged to Sir Reginald Fleming Johnston, son of an Edinburgh solicitor and ex-tutor of Pu Yi, the last emperor of China. He was the author of *Twilight in the Forbidden City* and he was portrayed by Peter O'Toole in the film, *The Last Emperor.*

Wildlife: A fairly large area of mature woodland with oak, ash, rowan, alder and hawthorn spreads along the east shore, attracting many birds. There is a small herd of wild goats and rich pasture for sheep, scattered with buttercups, ragged-robin, yellow flag, ubiquitous bracken and very little heather. Wintering divers and wildfowl can be seen here from October to March.

There are wild mussel beds by the shoreline.

* * *

EILEAN RIGH is snugly situated in Loch Craignish between Eilean Macaskin (No.2.7) to the south-west and the tidal **Eilean Mhic-Chrion** (G. – MacNiven's Island) to the north across the loch.

Although it is a fairly small island it was evidently of some importance in ancient times for it has the remnants of two Iron Age duns and a name with royal connections. It is not known if the forts were contemporaneous or not but there is a further fort on the tiny Eilean na Nighinn which is part of **Eilean Dubh** on the north side of the loch. These would have controlled access to the head of the loch.

On Eilean Righ, the most northerly dun is 650m NNE of the house, set on the grassy summit of the ridge. It is oval-shaped and a number of minor artefacts were uncovered during excavation in 1982 [NM804022]. The second dun is south-west of the house at the summit of a flat-topped ridge. It is rectangular in plan with an oval structure in the south corner [NM800014].

The south side of the highest point, Dun Righ, has an interesting example of a large cup-mark on the lichen-covered rock [NM798010].

The former owner, Sir Reginald Johnston, with his female companion, modernised the island's two houses in 1934 with the addition of a Buddhist temple and lantern. The pleasant buildings, set round a courtyard with a central flagpole, have now been extensively and attractively renovated with a new helipad and hangar concealed to the south. The road from the rebuilt jetty has been widened where it climbs through a dense belt of mixed woodland, stippled with primroses amid a tangle of brambles.

It is said that when Sir Reginald died in 1938 (aged 65) valuable porcelain and china were

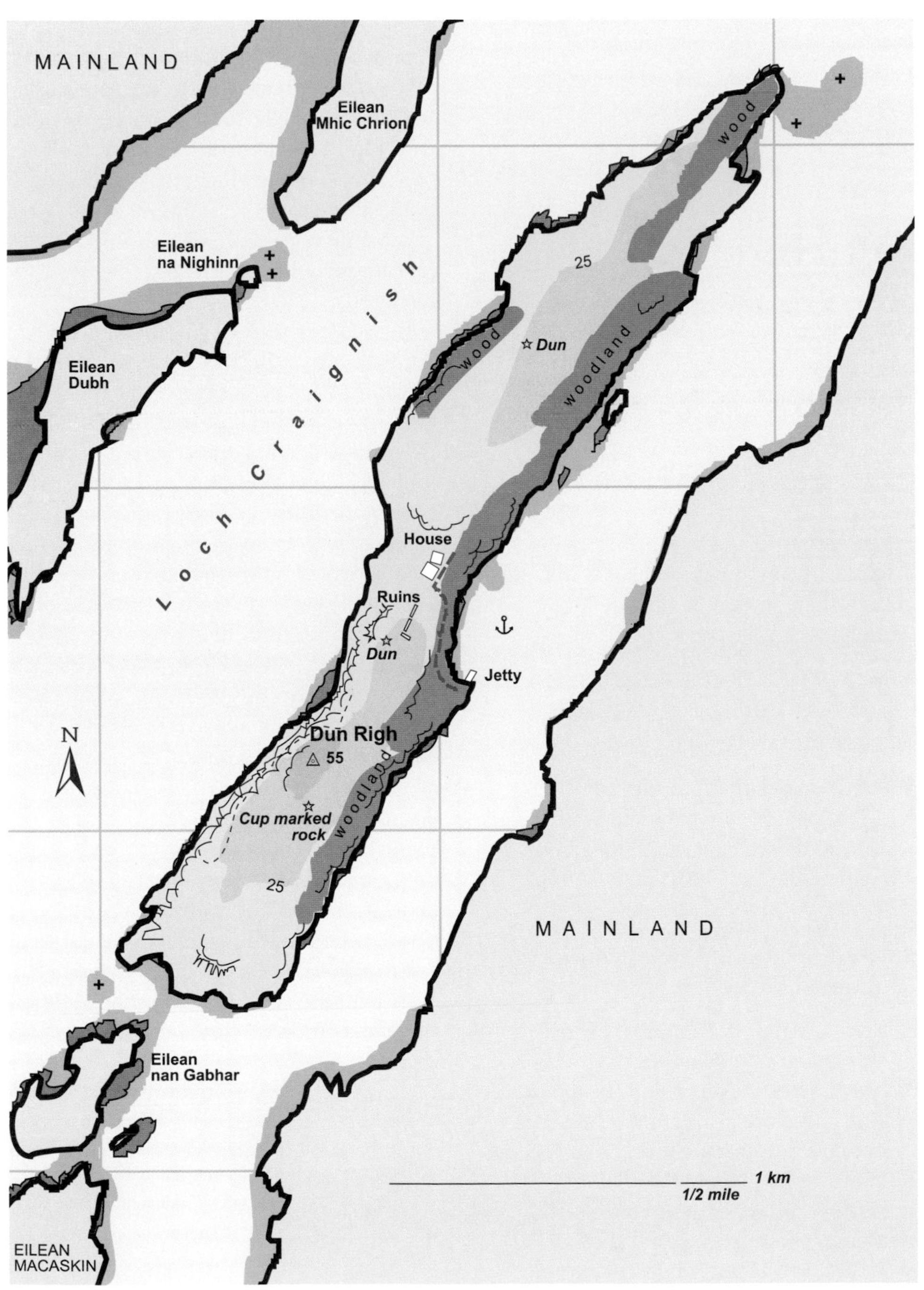

thrown into the loch, but I have been unable to establish whether the story is true or not. However, it has been recorded that his last lover, Elizabeth Sparshott, on hearing of his death destroyed many of his documents and artefacts.

* * *

Access: Farsain Cruises, Craobh Haven, 01852-500664, or enquire at Ardfern.

Anchorage:
1. Good anchorage centre of E coast of the island, below the farmhouse, 5m. Anchor at S end of the bay, NNE of the jetty, as N end is foul with weed. Shoal runs out for 50m in line with 2-storey gable of farmhouse.

2.9 Scarba

(ON skarpoe – sharp, stony, hilly terrain). Alternatively, but less likely, (G. sgarbh, or ON skarf – cormorant, ON -øy – island).

OS Maps: 1:50000 Sheet 55 1:25000 Sheet 355
Admiralty Charts: 1:25000 Nos.2326 or 2343

Area: 1474ha (3642 acres)
Height: 449m (1473ft)

Owner: Lord Richard Sandys, Worcestershire (the family of Lord Duncan Sandys, a former Minister of State). Previously owned by the late Mrs Yvonne Studd-Trench-Gascoigne of Leeds.

Population: 1794–50 (14 families). 1881–19. 1891–9. 1931–5. 1961–5. Only occasional habitation since the 1960s.

Geology: Schist and slate in the east and quartzite in the west. A conglomerate of quartzite, limestone, and shale lies between, known as 'Scarba Conglomerate'.

History: This was the site of an early Christian settlement. At the end of the 18th century the island was divided into two farms.

Wildlife: There are many red and fallow deer, some wild goats, and otters among the rockfalls below the coastline cliffs. Sheep and the famous breed of Luing cattle are grazed here. Although drainage channels have been cut and new fencing erected to improve the grazing the ground is still very rough with heather, bracken and tufts of boggy grass and sphagnum moss. Ragged-robin, cotton grass, and at least two different varieties of orchid give vivid splashes of colour among the tussocks.

Natural oak woodland and scrub are scattered over parts of the east coast below the 50m contour. Together with some patches of planted conifers at a higher level, these attract a variety of birdlife.

* * *

SCARBA is a single mountain top which rises straight out of the sea to a height of 449m. It is set between two notoriously dangerous tidal races, the Corryvreckan to the south and the Grey Dogs to the north. Its coasts are bleak and rugged with many great caves. The west flank is the most precipitous, the heather slopes tumbling steeply to the shore rocks with many unstable boulders covered by vegetation. Cut into this face is an exceptionally high raised beach – over 30m above sea level.

Above **Port nan Urrachann**, a bay on the west coast, the faint remains of Iron Age dwellings have been reported at the top of an ancient path which zig-zags up the steep slope.

The east side is gentler, with a small patch of land fit for cultivation, and some scattered woodland. **Kilmory Lodge**, the main house, is situated here and it is occasionally occupied by members of the owner's family. Below the Lodge and by the eastern shore, south-west of Port a' Chaibeil, is an ancient chapel ruin, **Cille Mhoire an Caibel** (G. – the Virgin Mary's Church of the family graveyard) [NM718057]. The walls are still 1½m high but the only recognisable feature is the doorway. This was almost certainly the 'chapel of the Blessed Virgin, where many miracles occur' – mentioned by John Fordun in 1380 or thereabouts. The burial ground was abandoned in the mid-19th century. There are reports of nearby remnants of rudimentary beehive cells but I have been unable to confirm this. If true, then – who knows? – Scarba may have rivalled Eileach an Naoimh (No.2.12) as a favourite retreat for the monks of Iona. Just south of the chapel is a cave [NM718055], which had associations with the early Christian community and beyond it and above the coastline trees is **Blàr nan Sìth**, which could be freely translated from the Gaelic as the Elysian Field!

Beside the road which leads from the pier to the Lodge there is an empty cist with a dislodged capstone. The islanders' village settlement was

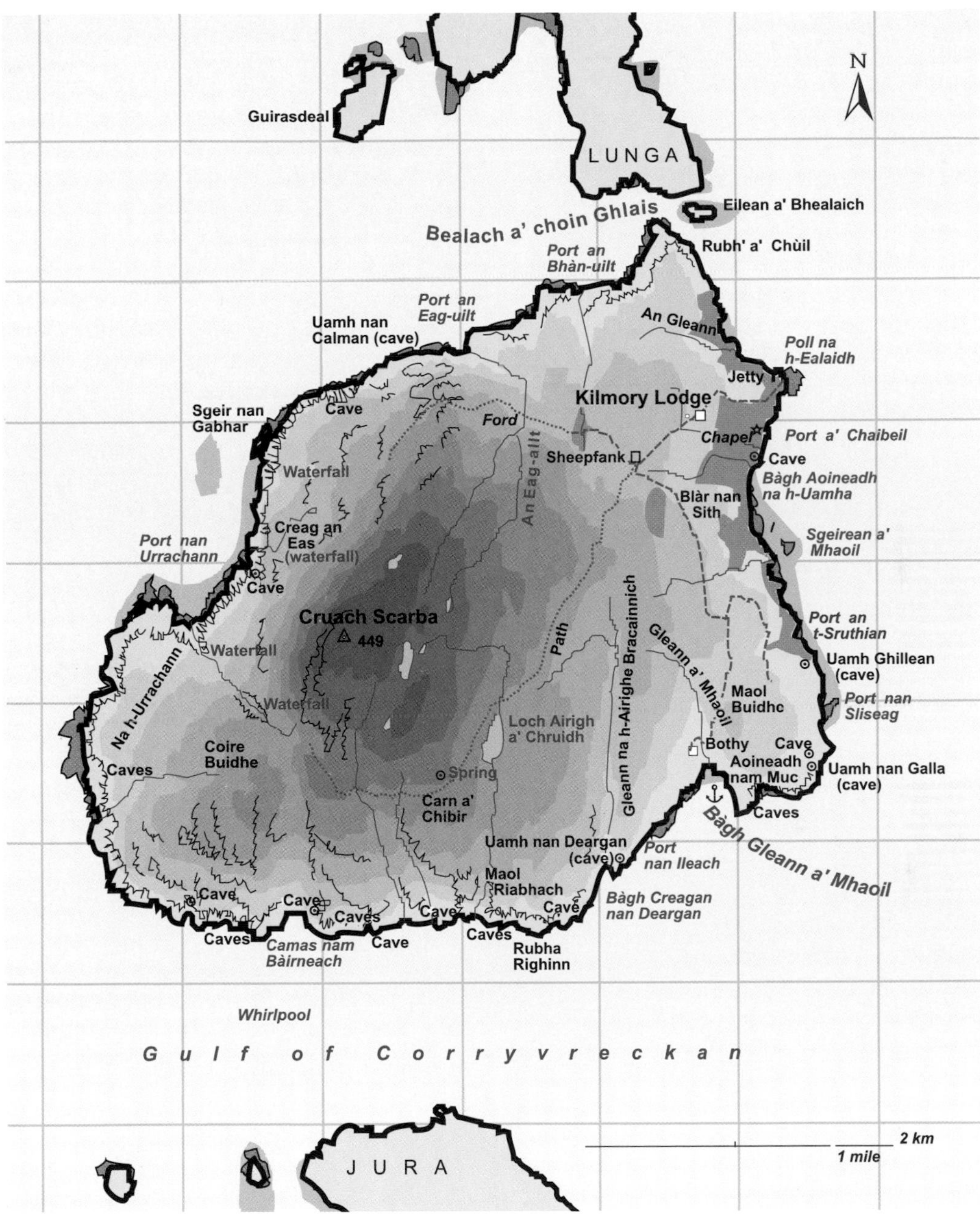

north of the Lodge.

Like so many of the Hebridean islands, Scarba had a reputation for healthy living and longevity – Martin Martin reported in the 17th century that an old woman had just died on Scarba aged 140, still having possession of all her faculties – but it also has its share of myths. The ghosts of evil sailors walk Scarba's cliffs as a penance. Others are chased by the Grey Dog which was drowned between Scarba and Lunga and which had belonged to Prince Breacan of Lochlann. To escape the dog's drooling fangs the phantoms must confess their crimes and these cries can be heard after dark on moonless nights.

There is a small cottage above the anchorage in **Bàgh Gleann a' Mhaoil** (G. – bay in the cleft of the mull), which was used for a time by an adventure school for children. The bay has a beach of large, multi-coloured pebbles. There is an interesting trudge up the ridge beside the bothy, then the next ridge and the next again. The going is rough: tufts of ankle-twisting grass, heather, and bracken with boggy patches between. Behind the ridges there is a small loch – **Loch Airigh a' Chruidh** (G. – loch in the horseshoe-shaped pasture) beside a vestigial path. Only a narrow earth barrier stops this loch emptying itself nearly 300m down the mountain-side. Following the path round the contours until it disappears brings you to the head of a steep gully which falls dramatically down to Camas nam Bàirneach (G. – limpet creek) and a deep-set cave. Beyond the creek is the main Corryvreckan whirlpool – a thrilling viewpoint! Deer spy on you from every rocky height.

The footpath, which encircles part of the mountain, starts from the sheep fank above Kilmory Lodge. The easiest climb to the peak, **Cruach Scarba** (G. *cruach* – stack or heap), and the low spine of rock at the top is from this path where it traverses the east side of the mountain. From the sheep fank it is also possible to reach the rough vehicle track which leads to Bàgh Gleann a' Mhaoil.

The tides run though the **Corryvreckan** (G. *coire bhreacain* – the speckled cauldron), west on the flood and east on the ebb, at speeds of up to ten knots. Beneath this channel is the rock-strewn record of some great primaeval cataclysm. There is a ridge running out from Camas nan Bàirneach on Scarba with a solitary rock stack on the end of it which rears up 44m and comes within 29m of the surface of the sea. When a westerly blows against the flood during a spring tide the noise of the violent overfalls can be heard many miles away. Local fishermen used to call the whirlpool which forms at these times over this submarine rock pinnacle, the Cailleach (G. – the old woman). According to legend a hag controls the maelstrom and decides which ships will sink and which survive. There are also enormous breakers and violent eddies elsewhere. Another submerged rock stack is in the centre of the Gulf and beside it a great narrow pit like a gateway to hell which descends 100m below the surrounding seabed to an overall depth of 219m.

The early writers' descriptions are interesting. Martin Martin declared: 'The sea begins to boil and ferment with the tide of flood, and resembles the boiling of a pot; and then increases gradually, until it appears in many whirlpools which form themselves in sort of pyramids and immediately after spout up as high as the mast of a little vessel and at the same time make a loud report.' And

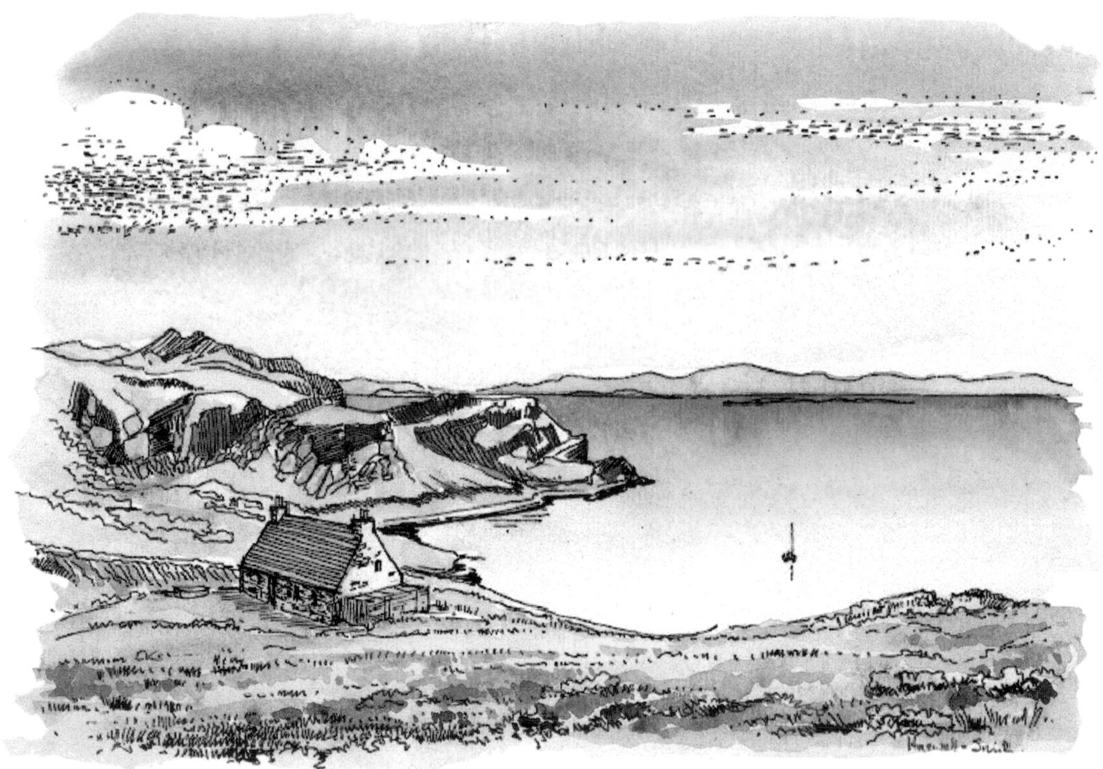

THE BOTHY IN GLEANN A' MHAOIL

John MacCulloch said: 'Impossible to be engaged in this place without anxiety... danger is always impending. The error of a few minutes might have been the price of as many lives... .'

There is a short period at slack water when it is safe to sail through the Corryvreckan but the timing has to be accurate. Even then, the turgid eddies, sudden movements and whorls sucking at the surface as the water spills over the irregular rock formations deep below create a palpable sense of menace.

* * *

Access: Farsain Cruises, Craobh, 01852-500664. Gemini Cruises, Crinan, 01546-830208.

Anchorages:

1. Bàgh Gleann a' Mhaoil, at the SE corner of Scarba. Occasional anchorage out of the tidal currents in 9m, sand with some weed. Exposed to S and SE and can be subject to swell. Avoid approach when tide is running strongly or conditions adverse.
2. Port a' Chaibeil. Temp. anchorage due W of Kilmory Lodge in 8–10m.
3. Poll na h-Ealaidh and jetty. A very restricted little landing-place on N side of promontory by Kilmory Lodge.
4. An Gleann. Temp. anchorage in quiet conditions off centre of inlet. *(Interesting walk to see the 'Grey Dogs'.)*
5. Port nan Urrachann, on W side. Approach from N using chart to avoid rocks and shallows, and anchor in 10–12m, sand. Exposed SW-N-NE, out of the tide but can be subject to swell.

2.10 Shuna

Possibly (G. sidhean – fairy, ON -øy – island), but probably of Norse origin.

OS Maps: 1:50000 Sheet 55 1:25000 Sheet 359
Admiralty Charts: 1:25000 Nos.2326 or 2343

Area: 451ha (1114 acres)
Height: 90m (295ft)

Owner: Edward Gully, the 5th Viscount Selby was co-owner with his uncle but, aged 33, he was killed in a car accident in January 2001. He has a son and Shuna is still owned by the Gully and Selby families.

Population: 1841–69 (10 houses). 1881–14. 1891–11. 1931–12. 1961–3. 1971–3. 1981–7. 1991–1. 2001–1.

Geology: Shuna was one of the small group of islands cut off from the mainland by the Firth of Lorn glacier in the last Ice Age. Unlike neighbouring Luing, there is no workable slate on Shuna – the rock is mainly phyllite and mica-schist – but on the west side a band of attractive blue crystalline limestone used to be worked.

History: A small rectangular enclosure just north of Shuna farmhouse holds a tombstone commemorating John McLean of Shuna and his wife Mary Campbell. This was probably the John McLean who died in 1787 and whose son, Alexander, was the last of the McLeans to own the island. The McLeans' original life-rent was granted by Lord Neil Campbell in 1679.

When the owner, James Yates, died in 1829 he bequeathed Shuna to the City of Glasgow with the stipulation that the income should be 'devoted to benevolent purposes'. The Corporation preferred the capital value and sold the island.

Wildlife: The very thick growth of alder, birch, hazel and scrub oak hides red, roe and fallow deer and attracts a variety of birds and woodland plants.

* * *

SHUNA lies between Luing and Craobh Haven. Shuna House, a castellated mansion stands at the north-west corner of the island with a view towards Loch Melfort. It is now in ruins but one of the owner's family occupies an adjacent estate house.

The island is grazed by sheep and there are fish farms at the north end with a resident manager. Some of the estate cottages have been renovated and are let for holiday use.

In the north bay there is an old stone quay on the west side at **Rubh' an Aoil** (G. – lime-plaster headland), no doubt named when limestone was being quarried on the island. The east side has a concealed reef and is called **Rubha Salach** (G. – foul headland). At the head of the bay, which floods at high water, the wreck of an old wooden ferry *The Maid of Luing*, with a turntable and a livestock hold, lies on the rocks. It is a difficult walk round the shoreline which requires scrambling over hard vertical slabs of grey aerated rock like petrified Dunlopillo. Striking inland is no easier as sheep tracks mysteriously disappear and the tangled growth of alder, birch and undergrowth in the mossy humps and ravines is almost impenetrable.

Round the corner, on the west coast, is **Port na Cro** (G. – the sheep-pen port) which is too small and shallow for anything but a dinghy.

Roofless Shuna House is more distinguished and substantial when seen from a distance. Its scale is misleading. An estate road runs diagonally across the island connecting it with **Shuna Cottage** (which is actually a solid two-storeyed house rather than a cottage) in the south-west. Roughly in the centre of the island it passes **Druim na Dubh Ghlaic** (G. – the ridge by the black hollow), which is the highest point at 90m. A burn runs down the 'black hollow' to Port an t-Salainn (G. – the salt port) on the east side. South of this is further dense woodland in the Coille Mhór (G. – the big wood) and Poll na Gile (G. – clear pool), a little cove on the east coast.

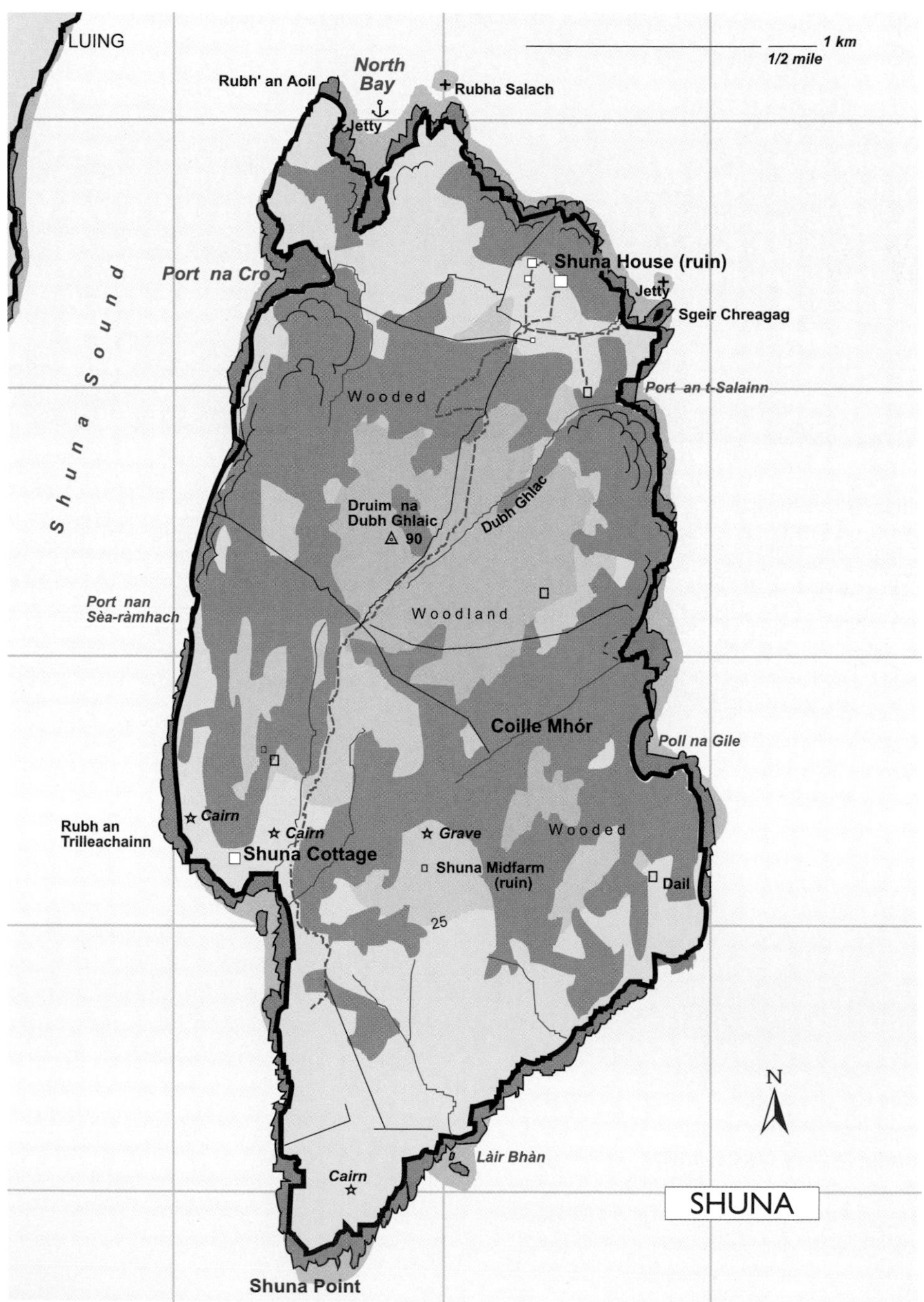

The southern extremity, called Shuna Point, is marked by a prehistoric cairn, and there are two more cairns at **Rubh an Trilleachainn** (G. – oystercatcher point) behind Shuna Cottage [NM759075]. One of these is a chambered cairn which has been extensively robbed in the past.

A remarkable hoard of three bronze swords, possibly dating from the 8th century BC, was discovered on Shuna sticking point-down in the peat. They may have been placed in this way as a votive offering.

There are several islets near Shuna – **Eilean Gamhna** (G. – farrow cow island) and **Eilean Creagach** (G. – craggy island) to the north west; **Eilean Buidhe** (G. – yellow island) and Eilean an Dùin (G. – island of the fort) to the west now form part of the Craobh Haven marina breakwater. Together with **Eilean Arsa** (G. – ancient island), they used to be known as the Craobh islands. The old fort on Eilean an Dùin was, regrettably, virtually demolished when the breakwater was built. Craobh, incidentally, means a tree in Gaelic but it can also refer to bubbles in a glass of whisky – a much more poetic interpretation.

* * *

Access: No regular access. Boat trips by arrangement, Farsain Cruises, Craobh Haven, 01852-500664.

Anchorage:

1. Bay at N of Shuna with remnants of a stone quay on its west side. Anchor no further in than abreast the quay, 3m, mud and sand. There is a drying reef on SW side and a large part of the bay is shoal. Note submerged rock about ¾c N of the E point of the bay.

2.11 Lunga

(N langr-øy – isle of the longships) or (G. long – ship, N -øy – island)

OS Maps: 1:50000 Sheet 55 1:25000 Sheet 359
Admiralty Charts: 1:25000 2326 or 2386

Area: 254ha (628 acres)
Height: 98m (321ft)

Owner: Torquil Johnson-Ferguson. Previously owned by the Cadzow family of Luing until about 1964.

Population: 1794–29 (6 families). 1881–17. 1891–15 (3 families in 1 house). 1931–5. 1961–0. 1971–0. 1981–3. 1991–2. 2001–2.

Geology: Schist and mica-schist run northwards towards the small 'slate' island of Belnahua, but the west, and part of the 'drying islands' to the north, are of 'Scarba conglomerate' (see No.2.9).

Wildlife: Grazed by domestic sheep and Luing cattle. Golden eagles have been reported over Bidein na h-Iolaire but buzzards are more common.

* * *

LUNGA is an untidy island, all humps and bumps, rocks and bogs, and a misshapen coastline which disintegrates into smaller tidal islands in the north – **Rubha Fiola** (G. – tidal island headland), **Fiola Meadhonach** (G. – middle tidal island) – these are sometimes called North and South Fullah, **Eilean Iosal** (G. – humble island) and **Fiola an Droma** (G. – drum-shaped tidal island). It is fortunate to have a reasonable anchorage sheltered from the prevailing wind just north of the skerry in Poll nan Corran (G. – the sickle-shaped pool) where there is a pebble beach. Birds of prey circle slowly above the dominant hill, Bidein na h-Iolaire (G. – pinnacle of the eagle) and seem to be acting a part – keen to prove that this really is eagle territory.

Walking on the island is not easy but the Luing cattle which graze there have trampled a number of muddy trails through the scrub. There are rock formations which could be mistaken for standing stones from a distance and many wildflowers in the crevices.

Tobar a Challuim-Chille (G. – the well of St Columba's church), a fresh-water spring bubbling into a mossy rectangular trough of ancient flagstones, is beyond the central ridge in the north-west [NM705091]. This has never run dry and in times of drought was used by the slate quarry workers from Belnahua. There are three houses on the main island, all in very poor condition and only one of which may still be habitable.

One of the tidal islands, Rubha Fiola, is run as an adventure centre by the owner and his family. It has a timber chalet for accommodation built beside the remains of an old blackhouse. Young people aged 9 to 16 are given training in survival techniques such as abseiling, cave-dwelling,

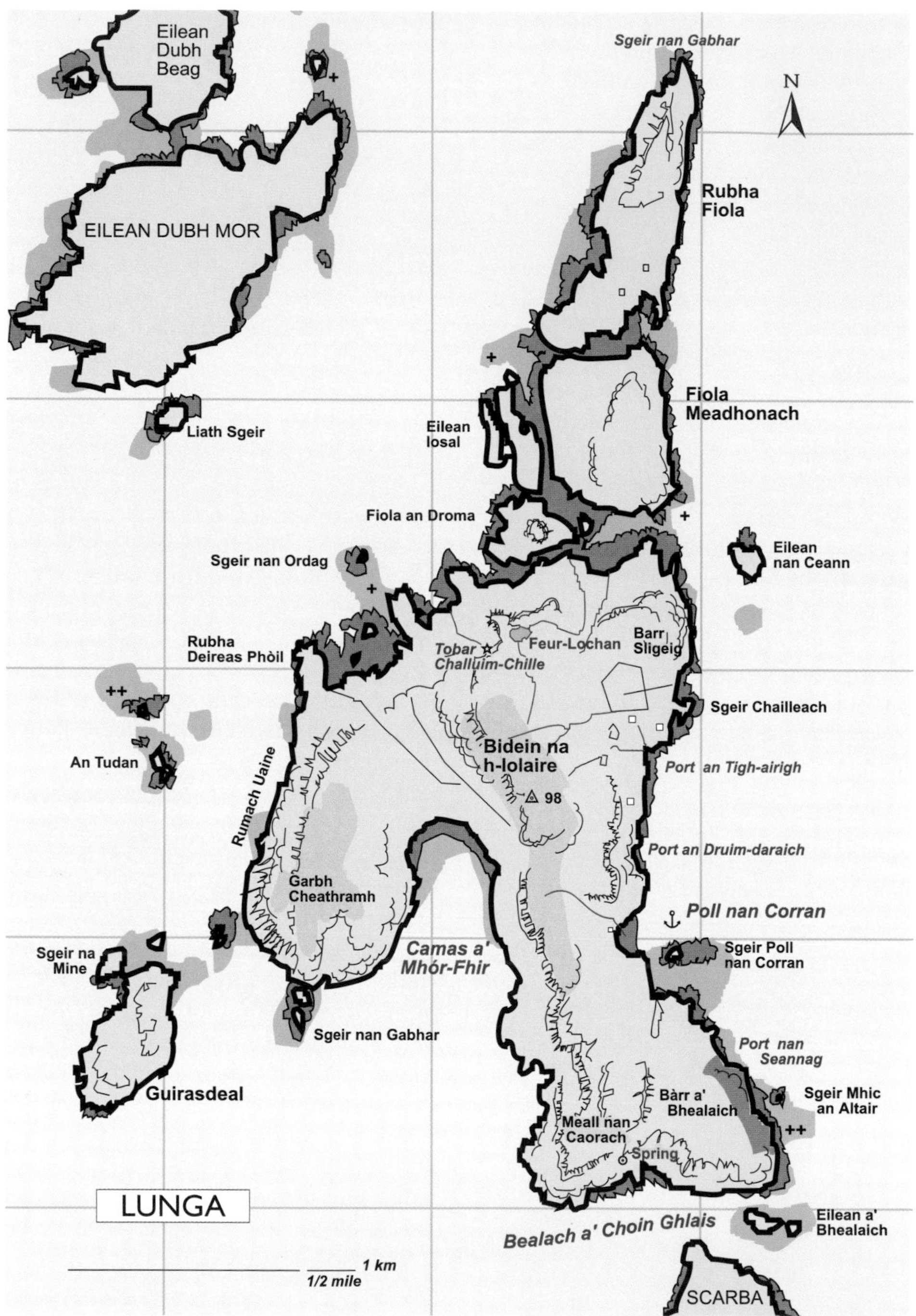

canoeing, fishing, climbing and beach-combing, and the experience of living on an uninhabited island unaccompanied by adults (see No.2.14). This must be every adventurous youngster's dream come true!

The graves of some of the past inhabitants of Lunga are to be found in the burial ground of Kilchattan on Luing (No.2.13).

The channel between Lunga and Scarba is the famous **Bealach a' Choin Ghlais** (G. – the pass of the Grey Dogs). This can be almost as dangerous as the Corryvreckan as a sly tide pounds through at over 8 knots. The channel is narrow and divided by **Eilean a' Bhealaich.** When the tide is at full flood the water south of the island is at two distinct levels with a spectacular downhill torrent. There is another dangerous overfall at the narrowest point, after which the race rushes westwards for another two miles passing the rocky islet of **Guirasdeal** (32m high).

Ormsa islet, also owned by the Johnson-Fergusons, lies directly north of Lunga and beyond it is the slate island of **Belnahua**. Belnahua, which belongs to the Carling family, has a very extensive drying reef to the north-west. In 1936 a Latvian vessel, *Helena Faulbaums*, struck this reef and sank with the loss of 16 lives. The visible part of the island is tiny and yet it supported a major slate industry. Now all that remains is the shattered quarry cutting deep into the heart of the island and the grey, deserted slate-workers' cottages. Beside Belnahua is the islet of **Fladda** (owned by the Platt family). Its lighthouse is a well-known sea-mark in the Sound of Luing.

* * *

Access: No regular access. By arrangement: Farsain Cruises, Craobh Haven, 01852-500664. Sea Fari Adventures, Oban, 01852 300003.

Anchorages:

1. Poll nan Corran (Puill a' Charrain). A bay on the E side. Approach from NE and anchor N of the Sgeir, off centre of pebble beach, 8–9m, mud. Partially exposed to E, otherwise reasonably sheltered.
2. Camas a' Mhór-Fhir. S-facing bay on W side of Lunga, outside Grey Dogs. Anchor near head of bay according to depth, 4–10m. Exposed S to W.

2.12 Eileach an Naoimh

*[**el**-uchěn **noe**:v] (G. – rocky place of the saint). According to Watson the correct name is na h-Eileacha Naomha (G. – the Holy Rocks).*

OS Maps: 1:50000 Sheet 55 1:25000 Sheet 359
Admiralty Charts: 1:75000 2169 1:25000 2386

Area: 56ha (138 acres)
Height: 80m (262ft)

Owner: Lord Richard Sandys, Worcestershire (the family of Lord Duncan Sandys, a former Minister of State). All the monuments are in the care of Historic Scotland.

Population: Uninhabited for many centuries.

Geology: The strata, mainly of limestone and Dalradian calcareous slate but with some sandstone, are severely tilted up to the north-west, where they are exposed as steep cliffs falling directly to a continuous rock-platform at sea-level. The south-east slopes are sheltered and fertile.

History: This is generally agreed to be **Hinba** [**een**-ba] the island mentioned by Adomnan: 'Inba' in early Gaelic means 'Isle of the Sea' and 'Hinba' is the plural. However Watson, in *Celtic Place Names of Scotland*, disagrees and considers that Jura has a much better claim to the title.

A monastery was founded here by St Brendan of Clonfert in 542AD, twenty-one years before St Columba founded Iona. Although continuing to enjoy some significance as a religious shrine, the island appears to have remained unpopulated ever since the monastery was destroyed by Norsemen, probably in the early 10th century.

Wildlife: The soil bedded on limestone gives an ideal growing medium and the verdant hillsides all face south. Provided no sheep have been grazing on the island, the grassy slopes and rocky crevices are covered with scarlet pimpernel, primrose, blue pansy, spotted orchids, spring cinque-foil, yellow iris, meadow-sweet, honeysuckle and many other species.

* * *

If the wind is light, and the portents good, one can risk an overnight stop although as a West Highland friend once claimed: '... only a very brave man would spend the night on **EILEACH AN NAOIMH**, it is so peopled by ghosts.' In spite of such ominous warnings *Jandara* spent a peaceful night there at anchor, although I must admit we did not venture ashore after dark!

The original Celtic monks searched for communion with God in the lonely deserts of the ocean, emulating the devotion of St John the Baptist. It was in the spirit of this search for solitude that St Brendan established his monastery here. Later it is supposed to have become the favourite retreat of his nephew, St Columba, who loved it as much as Iona and who came here for peace and contemplation. His mother, Eithne, Princess of Leinster, is also supposed to be buried here. A small upright slate slab roughly incised with a cross marks the spot near the top of a hillock south of the monastery ruins [NM639096].

The landing place is inside a lagoon formed by a line of skerries, **Sgeiran Dubha**. **Port Chaluim Chille** (G. – the port for Columba's church) is a tiny creek with a shingle beach, and a fresh-water spring in a stone basin overgrown with watercress. This is at the foot of a gully which leads up to a shallow amphitheatre below the slope of **Dun Bhreanain**, the spinal ridge. The hollow shelters the low, broken walls of the **Monastery** and **Church** [NM640097]. These are thought to date from the 9th century as St Brendan's earlier structures would almost certainly have been of wood. It has been suggested that the stone ruins might not have been the monastery at all, but a monk's farmhouse and byre although it is probably older than the church with its chancel and mortared walls.

Just north of these ruins is a small cell structure and beyond it the **Chapel**. Its walls are nearly 1m thick and it measures about 6.7m by 3.7m with only one indecipherable carved slab inside. There is open space by the chapel with a low vallum or rampart at the foot of the hillside.

Among other artefacts in the area are the remains of a stone oven or kiln with a fireplace and flue in which the monks baked their bread, or maybe dried corn. This is north of the chapel and to the east is a structure that may have been a winnowing barn.

A natural rock 'pulpit' stands by the landing place near the shore and on the slope above it (about 90m east of the chapel) there are two partly reconstructed 'semi-d' beehive cells [NM641097]. These are the finest Scottish examples of the ancient structures and only some cells on a cliff ledge of Skellig Michael Rock off Southern Ireland are better preserved. One of the cells of the **Clochain** – as this double cell is called – could have been an oratory with an underground cell beside it, like a Pictish souterrain, which may have been a wine cellar.

West of the landing place are two enclosures, the further being a herb garden. The burial ground beside it has a number of upended slabs, one of which bears a cross. It was reported in 1824, when the ruins were first publicised, that there were many carved tombs, ornamented stones and crosses but through the years these have been stolen.

The north end of the island sports a splendid natural sandstone arch, **An Chlàrsach** (G. – the harp), gouged out at the time when the raised beaches were being formed. This can be reached fairly easily by an interesting but rough walk

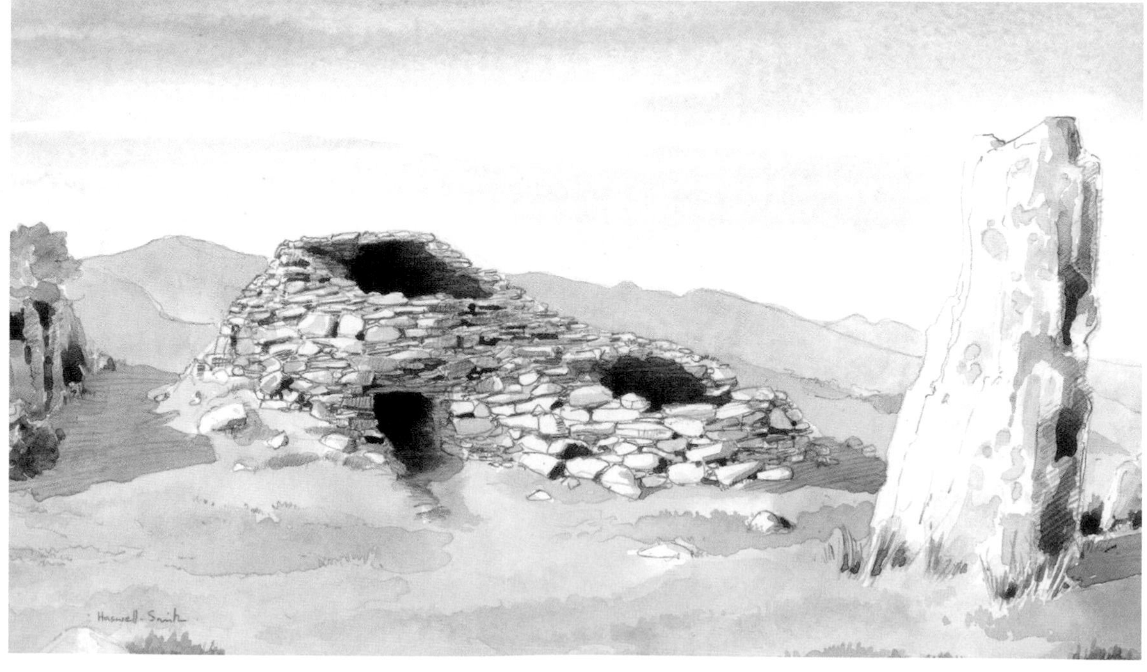

. . . SEMI-DETACHED BEEHIVE CELLS

(approximately following the 25m contour). Beyond the skerry of **Sgeir Leth a' Chuain** is the islet of **A' Chuli** (G. – the retreat), on which there was once a chapel. St Brendan is reputed to have been buried here. A bracing walk back to the landing place on the springy turf along the top of the ridge is rewarding. On one side – larks singing above the lush grass; on the other – the sea frothing at the foot of the cliffs.

Access: No regular access. Boat trips by arrangement with Farsain Cruises, Craobh Haven, 01852-500664.

Anchorage:

1. Occasional anchorage on SE side between island and line of skerries and islets. Approach from E through SW side of main gap in the skerries, or from SW keeping parallel to, and fairly close to, the line of skerries. Anchor off the old landing place, or E of drying/submerged rocks in NE pool. Not recommended for overnight stay except in settled conditions.

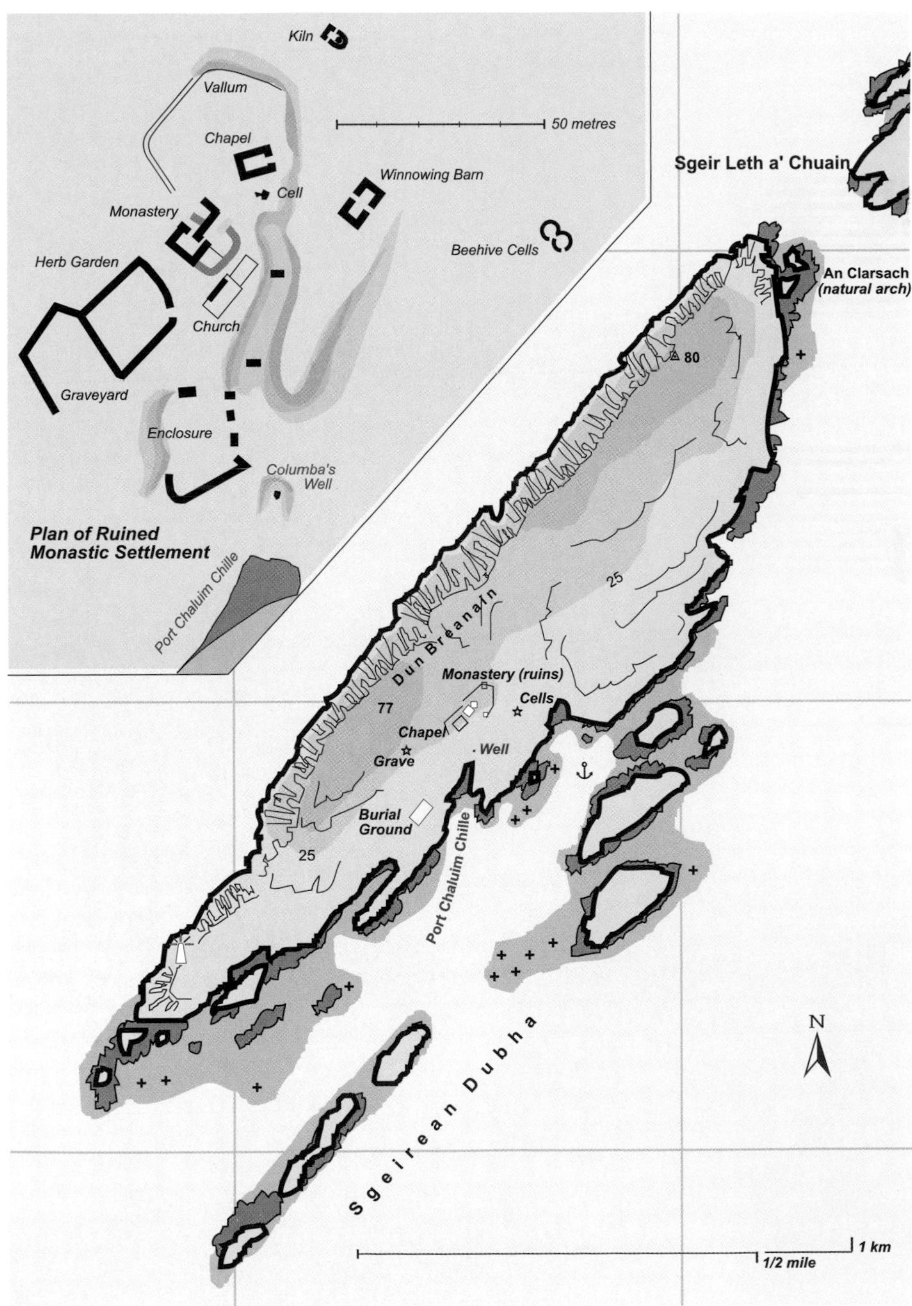

2.13 Luing

[ling] (G. long – ship) or (ON lyng – heather).

O S Maps: 1:50000 Sheet 55 1:25000 Sheet 359
Admiralty Charts: 1:75000 No.2169 1:25000 No.2326

Area: 1543ha (3813 acres)
Height: 94m (308ft)

Owner: Multiple ownership but most of the agricultural land has been owned by the Cadzow family of Duncrahill, East Lothian, since 1947.

Population: 1841–no separate Census figures. 1881–527. 1891–632. 1931–312. 1961–192. 1981–157. 1991–182. 2001–220. These figures include the tidal island of Torsa having one house.

Geology: Predominantly graphitic schists and

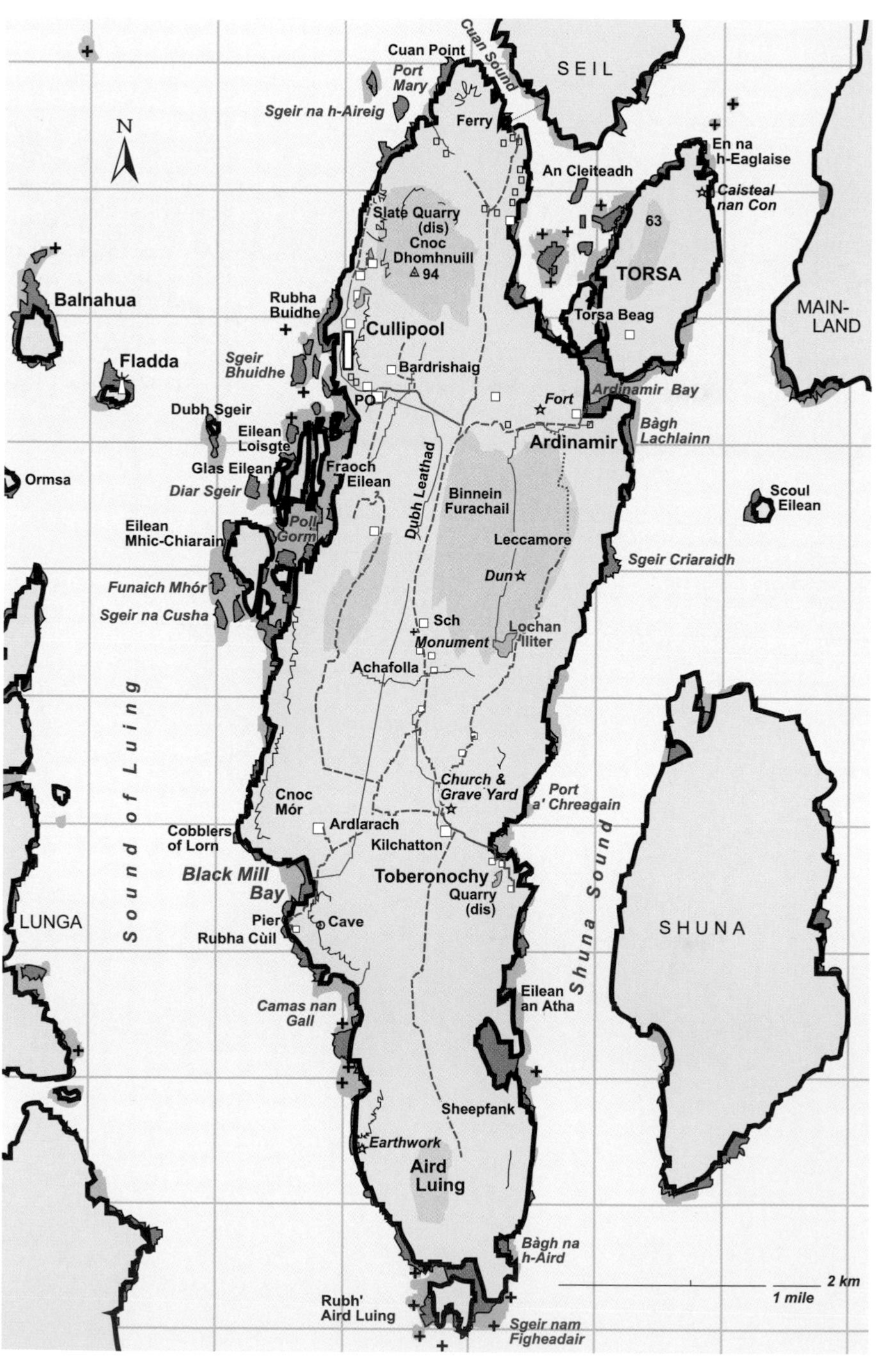

slate. The north end has large partially quarried slate deposits but the north part of the central ridge is of hornblende-schist.

Wildlife: There are no rabbits but there are stoats. The birdlife is similar to the adjacent mainland and pipistrelle bats can be seen at Ardinamir on summer evenings. Wild boar were once common on the Scottish mainland but Luing is one of the few islands on which remains have actually been found.

* * *

LUING is an easy island to reach from the mainland as there is a fast and regular vehicle ferry service across the 200m wide Cuan Sound which separates it from the island of Seil (Seil in turn is linked to the mainland by the famous Clachan Bridge.) The spring tides rush through the Cuan Sound at nine miles per hour creating a 'step' in the water as the flood builds up a difference of level.

Slate was the principal industry on Luing and was still being quarried here beside the main village of Cullipool until 1965. One hundred and fifty skilled men were employed and 700,000 slates were produced each year. Iona Cathedral is roofed with Luing slates. Now livestock farming is the principal activity, in particular the famous and unique herd of prize beef cattle bred by the island's owners since 1947.

Luing's other claim to fame is as a lobster-fishing centre. The lobster pond between **Eilean Loisgte** and **Fraoch Eilean** (G. – heather island) is one of the largest in Scotland.

Cullipool (G. – boat pool) is a pretty village of whitewashed cottages. These were the original slateworkers' houses but a number are now holiday homes or have been purchased by retired couples. In the evening the old slate workings to the north have a sculptural quality with subtle colours in the strata and to the west, across the many tiny islets in the Sound of Luing with Lunga and the Isles of the Sea beyond, there are the most magnificent Atlantic sunsets.

The secure little anchorage of **Ardinamir** (G. – headland by the bed of the river) is very popular but the entrance has to be negotiated

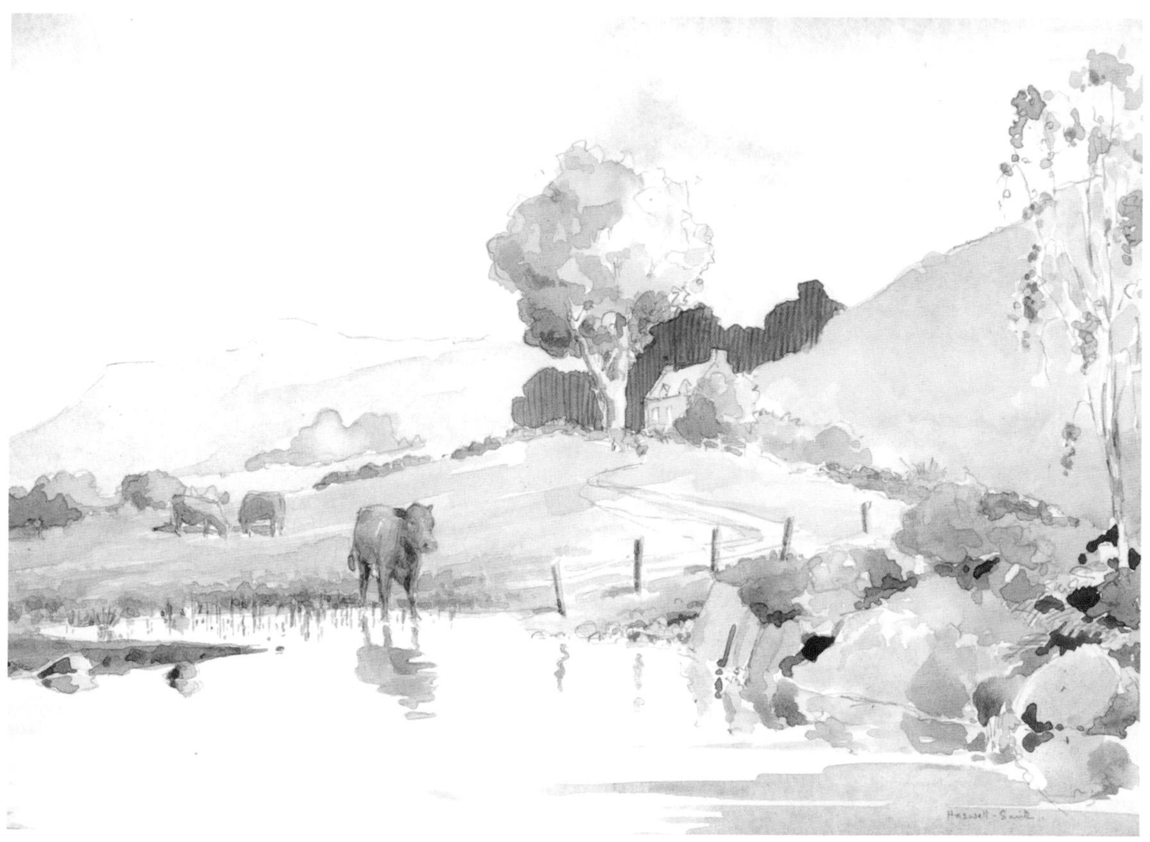

IRENE'S HOME AT ARDINAMIR

with great care. Until 1991 its popularity owed much to Irene McLachlin who lived alone in her croft beside it – with her cat, McElvie. She kept the leading mark freshly painted and should a yachtsman hit a rock she would offer friendly advice in a voice which could be heard on the mainland. As an honorary member of the Clyde Cruising Club she had a register of every visiting yacht since the 1940s and prided herself on never forgetting a name. Irene spent many happy hours sitting at the open window admiring the West Coast Drizzle. McElvie, a very big cat with pink eyes, always occupied the single armchair.

On the hill above Ardinamir, just north of Irene's house, is a large Iron Age fort, **Dun Ballycastle** [NM752121], and further south on the next hill is another one, **Dun Leccamore**, which has the remains of a stairway and several rooms [NM751108].

Above the attractive village of **Toberonochy** beside the bay and overlooking Shuna (No.2.10) stands the bleak well-tended ruin of Kilchatton chapel which was abandoned after 1685 [NM745091]. It is surrounded by slate gravestones including the grave of Covenanter Alex Campbell who 'digged my grave before I died'. On his tombstone he advises against '... women that wear Babylonish garments... men that have whiskers... Quakers, Tabernacle folk, Haldians, Independents, Anabaptists...' and so on.

At the centre of the island, near the ruined water mill, is the Fairy Knoll where visitors (who can spare one) are expected to place a hair on top to please the sprites.

The island's highest point, **Binnein Furachail** (G. – the outlook pinnacle) is 87m (285ft). It lies on the central axis midway between Ardinamir and Poll Gorm (G. – the azure pool).

Luing has a number of satellite islands linked to each other or Luing itself when the tide is out. **Eilean Mhic Chiarain** and **Glas Eilean** in the west, **Rubh' Aird Luing** in the south, and, in the north-east, **Torsa** (ON – Thor's island) and **Torsa Beag** which are permanently joined by a narrow strip of land. The sole habitation on Torsa is a farmhouse on the south side by Ardinamir which was occupied until the 1960s and is now once again inhabited. On the north side the ruined 16th-century fortress of **Caisteal nan Con** (G. – castle of the dogs) [NM766136] was the site of a hunting lodge for the Lords of the Isles and may also have given the Cuan Sound its name, although (G. *cumhainn* – narrows) is more probable.

* * *

Access: By passenger and ro-ro ferry from Seil, across the Cuan Sound. Frequent, daily service, 01631-562125. Five minutes crossing time.

Anchorages:

1. Kilchatton Bay (Toberonochy) on E side about 2M N of Rubh' Aird Luing, good anchorage in 5.5m to 11m; sheltered except from SSW winds. Bay shoals rapidly all round and head dries out about ¾c. Avoid disturbing scientific research buoys.
2. Ardinamir bay, between NE side of Luing and SW bend of Torsa. Popular small shallow cove. Very narrow entrance channel between a rock drying 0.3m and an extensive rock ledge and shoal off Torsa shore with similar rock drying 1.5m opposite on Luing shore. Holding uncertain due to weed.
3. Cuan Sound. More secure than Ardinamir in S winds. Anchor off boat house slipway on Luing, SW of the Cleit Rock, 5m, sand and rock, but avoid drying reef just N of boathouse and foul ground near the islet.
4. Port Mary, a small creek on the W side, about 2¾c SW of Cuan point. Fairly shallow and exposed but useful temp. anchorage between the shore and the closer of two off-lying islets.
5. Cullipool. An interesting anchorage provided sailing directions are followed carefully. Least depth in narrow N channel is 3.3m. There are leading marks for the W approach.
6. Glas Ford and Back o' the Pond, S of Cullipool. Needs careful negotiation at the right state of the tide. Secure anchorage but follow directions carefully.
7. Black Mill bay on W side, about 2M NNW of Rubh' Aird Luing. The head of the bay shoals ½c. Pier on S side of bay. Exposed to W.
8. Bàgh na h-Aird (Ard Bay) at SE corner. Temp. anchorage 1c off-shore but very exposed.

2.14 Eilean Dubh Mór

(G. – big black island) and **Eilean Dubh Beag** *[bek] (G. – little black island).*

OS Maps: 1:50000 Sheet 55 1:25000 Sheet 359
Admiralty Charts: 1:75000 2169 1:25000 2386

Area: 65ha (161 acres)
Height: 53m (174ft)

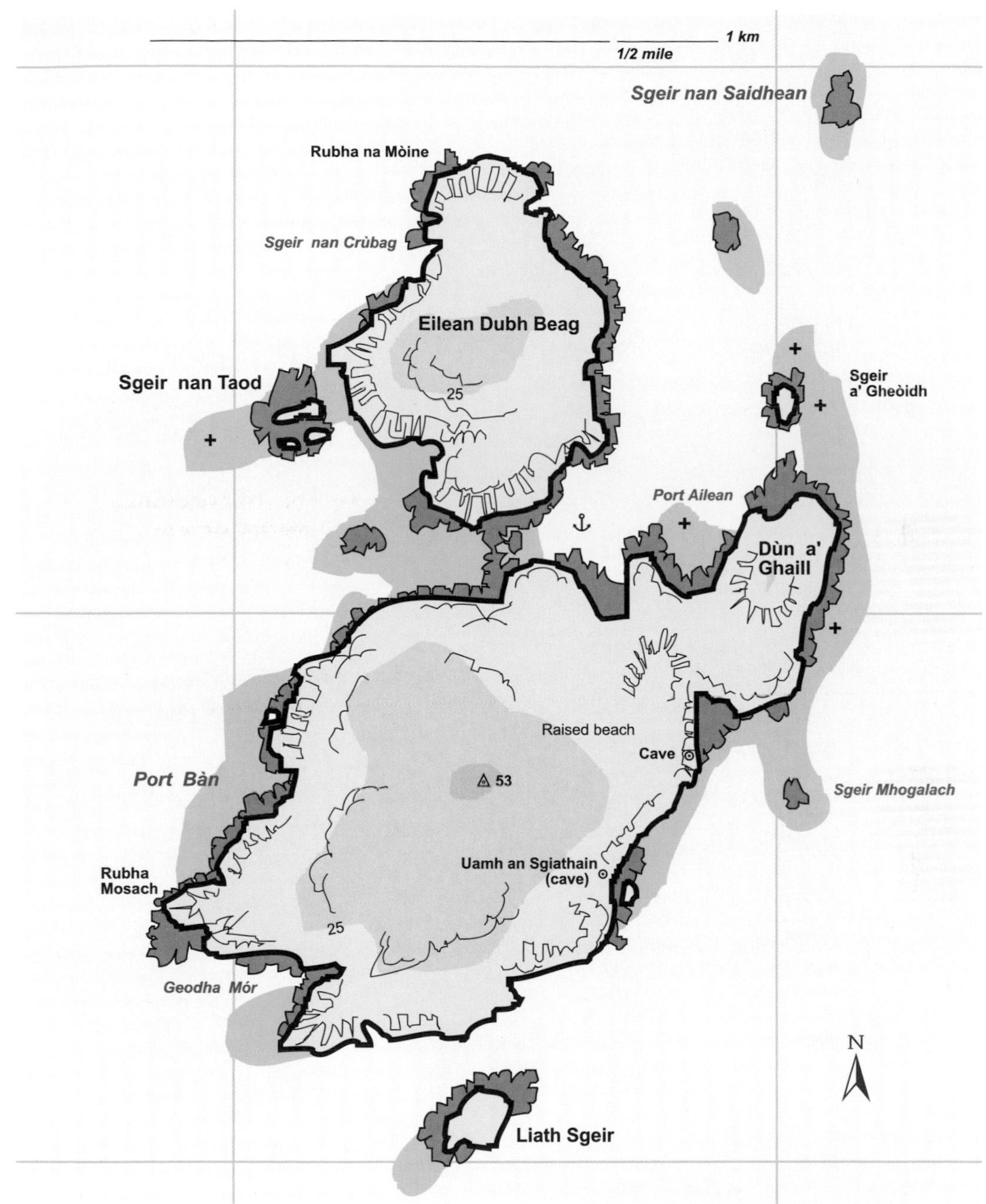

Population: No Census records and uninhabited.

Geology: Graphite schist with some quartzite interspersed with 'Scarba conglomerate'.

Wildlife: Droppings and bones would indicate that deer occasionally swim over from Lunga. There are many nesting herring gulls with black-backed gulls waiting to pirate their nests and fledglings.

Among the numerous wildflowers are large patches of the low-growing Burnet rose *(Rosa pimpinellifolia)*.

* * *

There are a few rocks in the sea to the north-east of the anchorage between **EILEAN DUBH MOR** and Eilean Dubh Beag which must be avoided so boats normally approach from due north or round the top of Eilean Dubh Beag. The amount of swinging room is misleading. I have been told that the Highland Yacht Club sometimes uses this location for musters and that on one occasion forty boats anchored here!

Eilean Dubh Mór is composed of a single mound-shaped hill, 53m high connected by a saddle to a promontory on the north-east side which also has a small hill on it. The terrain is heather, rocks, peaty bog-land and bracken. There is a very small raised beach in the central saddle, just a patch of pebbles which is bare of heather. On the south-west side of the saddle is a cove with cliffs round it and a cave. Further south another cave has a raised platform within it and a large quantity of dry bracken on the platform shows that it sometimes serves as a bed. This was unexpected on an uninhabited island until I learned the reason for it. The shoreline is rocky with small cliffs and indentations summed up by the name of the headland on the west side, Rubha Mosach (G. – the mean and nasty headland).

Eilean Dubh Beag (15ha) is almost a miniature replica of its big brother (or sister?) but it lacks the extra appendage. It is just a simple hump, 40m high, surrounded by lichen and seaweed covered rocks. The narrow channel between the two islands could almost be a man-made canal and is said only to dry out at the very lowest of tides.

Eilean Dubh Mór is sometimes used by the adventure centre on neighbouring Lunga (No.2.11). Youngsters are given the chance to test their survival techniques on an uninhabited island free of any direct adult supervision. They sleep and shelter in the caves with bracken for bedding. Whatever the rigours there are, no doubt, compensations and it is surprising how often in these beautiful surroundings one will awaken to a clear still morning with air like sparkling wine. What promise of excitement and adventure!

There is, by the way, a pole set on the top of the hill. Its purpose, in case you wonder, is that the castaways can tie something to it should they be in need of assistance...

* * *

Access: No regular access. Boat trips by arrangement with Farsain Cruises, Craobh Haven, 01852-500664.

Anchorage:

1. E end of the channel between the islands. Approach from N keeping ½c off En Dubh Beag. Anchor as near the channel as convenient, off E side of Dubh Beag, or N of the promontory between the two foul bays on Dubh Mór, 4–10m, good holding when the weed can be avoided. Exposed N to E and occasional swell.

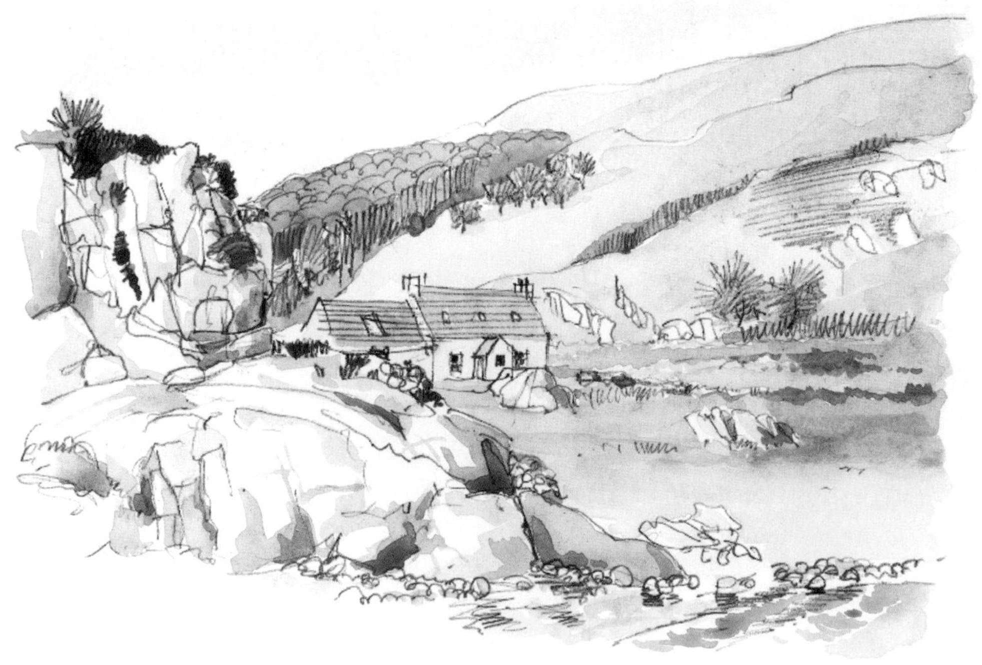

VIEW FROM THE LANDING PLACE, GARBH EILEACH

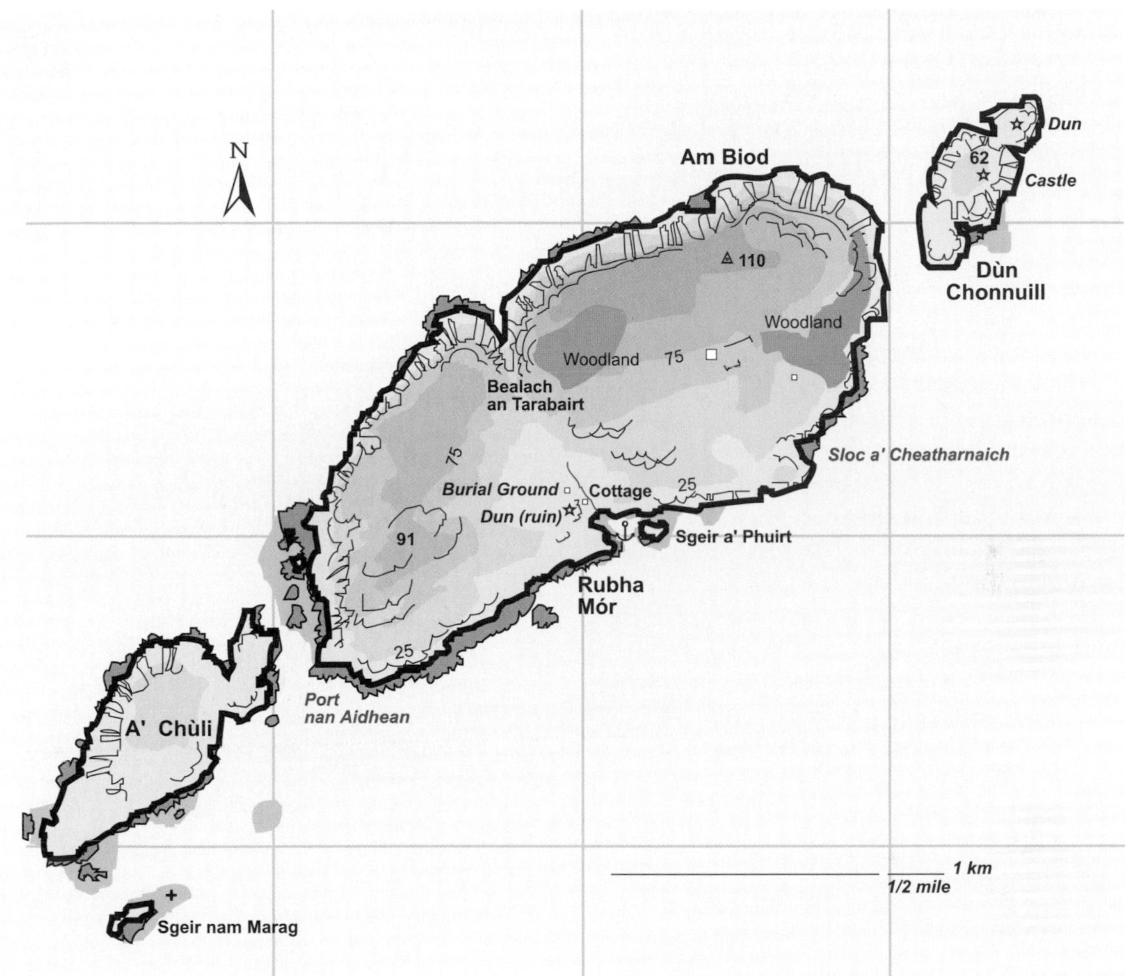

2.15 Garbh Eileach

[ga:rv ***el****uch] (G. – rough rocky mound).*

OS Maps: 1:50000 Sheet 55 1:25000 Sheet 359
Admiralty Charts: 1:75000 2169 1:25000 2386

Area: 142ha (351 acres)
Height: 110m (361ft)

Owner: Lord Richard Sandys, Worcestershire (the family of Lord Duncan Sandys, a former Minister of State).

Population: No Census records. Uninhabited.

Geology: This archipelago includes two members of the Dalriadan sequence, a white or pale limestone and a group which is largely quartzite and could be called the Boulder Beds. The strata are in a succession of sharp folds with white limestone at the core.

History: Signs of the past which prove that Garbh Eileach had its small place in history alongside its better-known neighbour are the remains of an ancient fort near the landing place and the historic indication of a small burial ground, Cladh Dhuban (G. – Duban's graveyard).

Wildlife: A small herd of red deer is resident and the scattered patches of birch woodland attract a variety of birds.

* * *

The largest of the Isles of the Sea, **GARBH EILEACH** has not the same historical interest as Eileach an Naoimh (No.2.12) but is still worth exploring. Just north-east of it, separated by a navigable channel, there is the small island of **Dùn Chonnuill** (G. – Conal's castle). Conal Cearnach was a minor 1st-century Ulster king. The present ruined castle was probably built by MacLean of Duart when he was given the island by Robert III about 1400. Sir Charles, son of the late, renowned, Sir Fitzroy Maclean, is 'Hereditary Keeper'.

The Isles of the Sea form a small archipelago of violently tilted rock-strata. As with the others, Garbh Eileach's north-western side is steep cliff whilst its south-eastern side has a grassy slope. The island is split almost centrally by a deep cleft, **Bealach an Tarabairt** (G. – the pass at the isthmus), where there is a small burn of clear water which has filtered through the limestone.

On the south side by the landing place, a stone bothy is still maintained in reasonable condition for occasional use as living quarters. Sheep (and, formerly, cattle ferried over from Luing) graze on the lush green grass, but apart from such times as the cottage is occupied the island is only inhabited by memories.

There are magnificent and extensive views from the summit of the ridge. The highest point is difficult to locate, but is at the most northern extremity with almost vertical cliffs tumbling down to the sea below. For rock-climbers the limestone ledges are like the Dolomites in miniature.

Access: By arrangement: Farsain Cruises, Craobh Haven, 01852-500664. Sea Fari Adventures, Oban, 01852-300003.

Anchorage:
1. Temporary anchorage in small bay in middle of SE side. There is a drying rock approx ¼c directly S of the islet, Sgeir a' Phuirt, on E side of the bay. Anchor E of concrete slip, thick weed over sand. There are mooring points on the islet, N of the islet and on the slipway.

2–Appendix Seil

Probably, (G. – sealg [sha:lg] – the hunting island) but maybe derived from the Indo-European root sal- meaning stream, flowing water, current (eg R. Shiel, Loch Moidart).

O S Maps: 1:50000 Sheet 55 (and 49) 1:25000 Sheet 359 (and 343)
Admiralty Charts: 1:75000 No.2169 1:25000 No.2386

Area: 1329ha (3285 acres)
Height: 146m (479ft)

Owner: Multiple ownership.

Population:1881–661. 1891–548 (122 houses). 1931–367. 1961–303. 1971–326. 1981–424. 1991–506. 2001–560.

Geology: Large deposits of slate at the southern end of Seil were quarried extensively until 1965. Most of the island is a slatey schist with a patch of hornblende-schist in the south and basaltic tuff bordering the Sound of Insh.

Wildlife: The joints of the mossy old masonry of the Clachan Bridge support a rare and tiny fairy foxglove, *Erinus alpinus*, a native of the mountains of central Europe.

* * *

SEIL is proud of its insularity but it has been very much a part of the mainland ever since 'the Bridge over the Atlantic' was built. The **Clachan Bridge**, as it is correctly called, was designed by Robert Mylne and built in 1792/93 at a cost of £450. It spans the narrow, shallow and tidal Clachan Sound which can only be navigated at high water by shallow-draught craft. Whales fail to appreciate this fact. In 1835 a whale of 78 feet in length was stranded in the sound and two years later a school of 192 pilot whales was also trapped.

At the north end of the Clachan Sound there are some islets which form the popular anchorage of Puilladobhrain (G. – pool of the otter). Unfortunately, the 'yachters' have frightened away the otters. At the end of a line of drying islets, **Eilean nam Beathach** (G. – isle of the brutes or beasts), **Eilean nam Freumha** (G. – isle of the roots) and **Eilean Buidhe** (G. – yellow or pleasant island) – which give good shelter from the west, is **Eilean Dùin** (G. – fort island) which has a central rock outcrop like a small fort.

A well-trodden footpath leads over the hill from Puilladobhrain to the famous pub, Tigh na Truish (G. – the house of the trousers), by the Clachan Bridge. When Highland dress was banned by law after the Jacobite Rebellion, shore-going islanders swapped their kilts here for a pair of breeks (or so it is said, but it may merely mark the site of a tailor's house).

Seil is noted for its slate which has been quarried for nearly three centuries. The fourth Earl of Breadalbane, who was the landowner, built picturesque villages for the workers. The main quarry on the south side went deeper and deeper into the ground as the men chiselled out the slate. Gunpowder was then used for blasting and by 1880 the pit was 75m deep (nearly 250 feet below sea-level) with only narrow walls of slate keeping out the sea. In November 1881 the

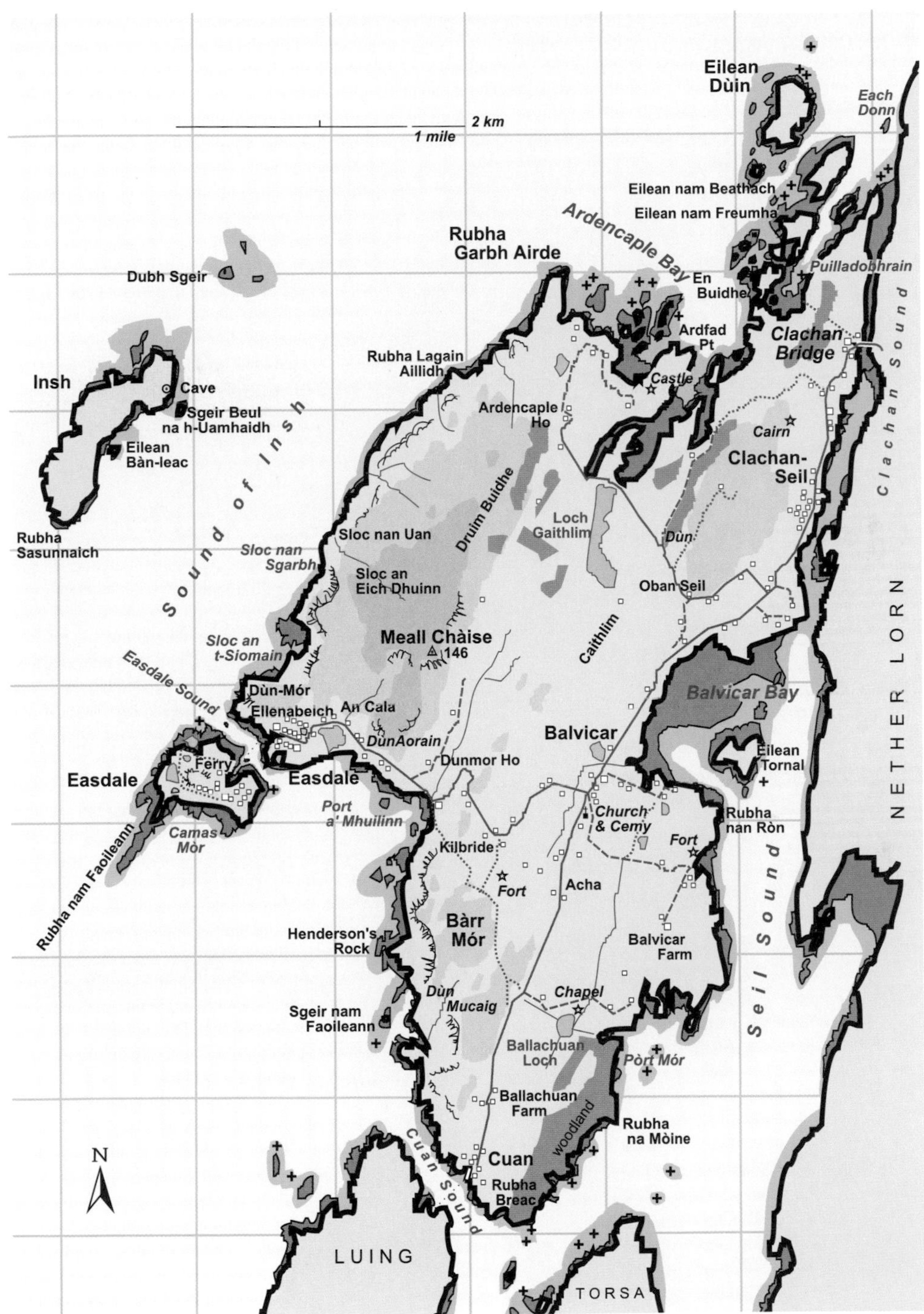

inevitable happened. There was a violent storm and the sea broke through. Luckily it was night and the pit was unmanned but 240 families lost their only means of support and severe poverty ensued. The place where the sea breached the wall can still be clearly seen.

The walls of Easdale harbour are of beautiful masonry work but with its disintegrating pier it is now a rather desolate place. In the 19th century this was a major port of call for ships collecting slate for transport through the Crinan Canal. 526 ships, including 245 steamers, used the harbour in 1825 alone.

The delightful village of trim white slate-workers' cottages was featured in the film *Ring of Bright Water* and now supports a thriving artists' colony. It is generally called Easdale although its correct name is **Ellenabeich** (G. – island of the birches) as it was an island separated from Seil by a narrow channel which was eventually filled in with quarry waste. On the slope above the east end of the village is **An Cala** (G. – haven or refuge) – a five-acre garden started in 1930 by Lord Elibank and his wife, the actress Faith Celli. Sweeping terraces provide dramatic views, and shelter belts of trees with an undercover of escallonia protect the garden from the prevailing sou'-westerlies. A burn tumbles over rocks and a high wall draped with clematis gives further shelter. The present owners, the Downies, open the garden to the public from April to September.

Seil's particular saint was St Brendan of Clonfert in Galway. He died in 577. The Kilbrandon Parish Church, with an interesting graveyard of ancient carved slabs, is south of **Balvicar** on Seil Sound. **Eilean Tornal** (sold for £100,000 in 2005) is the islet in Balvicar Bay.

The broken-off outlier, **Easdale** (G. *eas* – waterfall, ON *dal* – valley) was owned by Chris Nicolson of Coventry. He bought it in 1979 for £16,500 from Clive Feigenbaum, a former chairman of Stanley Gibbons, who introduced Easdale's own postage stamps. The population of this crowded piece of slate with its whitewashed slate-workers' cottages was 78 in 1931, only 16 in the 1961 Census, but had risen again to 58 by 2001 making it the most densely populated island. There is a regular ferry service across the harbour and an interesting folk museum which is worth visiting.

Rocky **Insh** (G. *innis* – island), also known as Sheep Island, lies west of Seil and separated from it by the Sound of Insh. It is reputed to be owned by a Londoner who occasionally occupies the cave.

* * *

Access: Follow the B844 over the Clachan Bridge. Tourist Information, 01631-563122. Ferry to Easdale island, 01631-562125.

Anchorages:

1. Balvicar Bay. Perfect shelter but restricted by moorings where it does not dry out. Approach by mid-channel S of Eilean Tornal.
2. Easdale Sound. Anchor off the slate wharf which is N of the ruined pier. Navigation in the Sound requires care and close adherence to the sailing instructions. Reasonable shelter in moderate winds.
3. Ardencaple Bay. Occasional anchorage off Ardfad Point in settled weather. No difficulties if approached carefully from due N. Exposed N. Mud and weed.
4. Puilladobhrain. Very popular anchorage and often crowded. Careful identification of all hazards and beacons is required on approach.

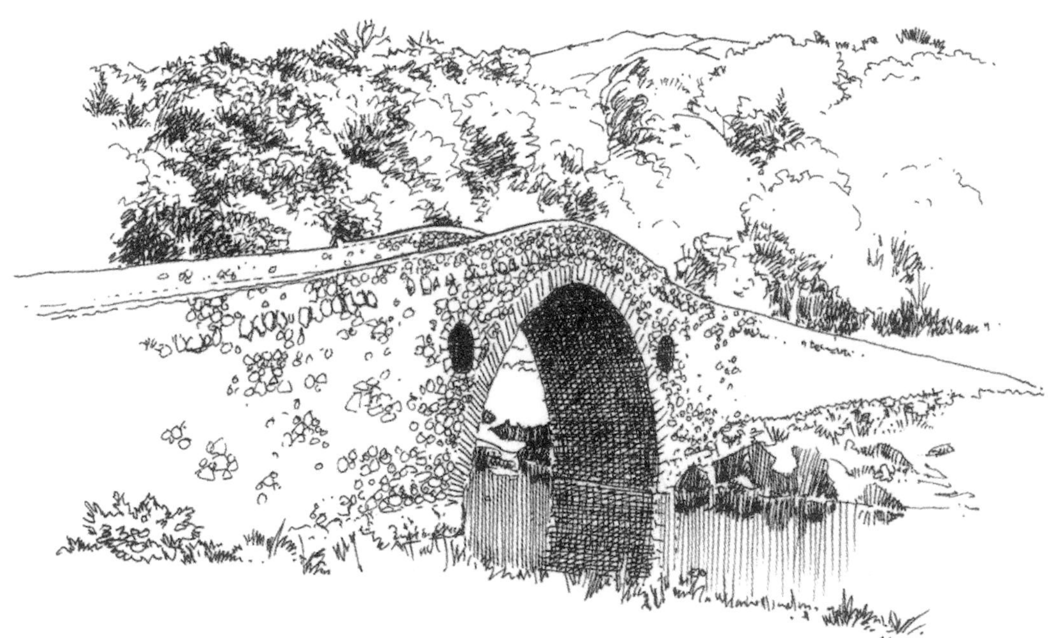

CLACHAN BRIDGE – THE 'BRIDGE OVER THE ATLANTIC'

SECTION 3

Mull and the Surrounding Islands

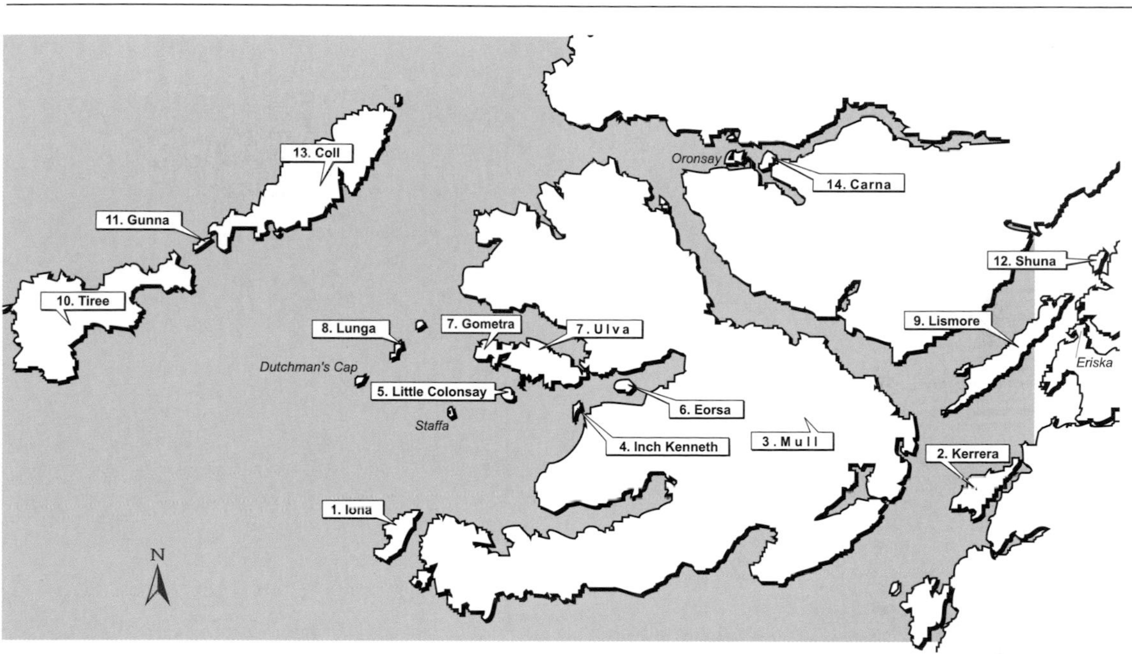

SECTION 3, Table 1: Arranged according to geographic position

No.	Name	Latitude	Longitude	Table 2* No.	Table 3** No.	Area in Acres	Area in Hectares	
3.1	Iona	56° 20N	06° 25W	44	70	2167		877
3.2	Kerrera	56° 24N	05° 33W	38	37	3000		1214
3.3	Mull	56° 27N	06° 00W	3	1	216299	87535	
	Erraid	*56° 18N*	*06° 22W*			462	187	
	Calve Island	*56° 37N*	*06° 02W*			178	72	87794
3.4	Inch Kenneth	56° 27N	06° 09W	143	120	136		55
3.5	Little Colonsay	56° 27N	06° 15W	115	102	217		88
3.6	Eorsa	56° 28N	06° 05W	106	72	301		122
3.7	Ulva	56° 29N	06° 13W	29	21	4917	1990	
	Gometra	*56° 29N*	*06° 17W*			1050	425	2415
3.8	Lunga	56° 29N	06° 26W	120	65	200		81
3.9	Lismore	56° 30N	05° 30W	30	50	5809		2351
3.10	Tiree	56° 30N	06° 52W	14	46	19358		7834
3.11	Gunna	56° 34N	06° 43W	131	137	170		69
3.12	Shuna	56° 35N	05° 23W	92	90	383		155
3.13	Coll	56° 37N	06° 34W	15	64	18990		7685
3.14	Carna	56° 40N	05° 53W	82	41	526		213
3.A	*Staffa*	*56° 26N*	*06° 21W*			*82*		*33*

*Table 2: The islands arranged in order of magnitude
**Table 3: The islands arranged in order of height

Introduction

With Mull in the geographical centre, most of the classified islands in this section are easily accessible and well known. Mull itself has such good communication with the mainland that it would be easy to forget that it is an island while its next-door neighbour Iona attracts tourists and pilgrims from all over the world.

There are a few tiny islets in the mainland firths which have not been mentioned elsewhere. **Eilean an Ruisg** (G. – bare island) in Loch Feochan, and **Eileanan Mór** and **Beag** at the entrance to lovely Loch Etive beside the castle, chapel and marina at Dunstafnage. On the loch itself are the **Abbot's Isles**, which are little more than scattered rocks with hardly a grassy foothold. **Eilean Choinneich** and **Eilean Munde** in Loch Leven are not much bigger but the latter islet, at the foot of Glencoe, is the traditional burial ground of the Macdonalds of Glencoe and close to it lies Eilean a' Chòmhraidh (G.- the meeting-place island).

Eriska (G. *ùruisg* – water-nymph island) is a flat tidal island at the entrance to Loch Creran with a bridge over the drying channel linking it to the mainland road network. It has a hotel and pleasant wooded grounds.

Staffa with its world-famous Fingal's Cave is well below the size limit of forty hectares which I have set for classification but it is much too remarkable to be ignored and is therefore included as an appendix to the section. The name of the legendary Irish hero, Fionn McCool, was given to the cave by Sir Joseph Banks because, so it was reported twelve years later, the local name for the cave was *An Uamh Bhinn* (G. – the melodious cave) and his interpreter mistook this for the Gaelic genitive form of Fingal – *Finn*. A plausible story, but not entirely convincing.

The traditional Gaelic term for a Norseman who had settled in the Hebrides was, and still is, *Fionnghall*, meaning a fair-haired stranger. (This is in contrast to *Dubhghall*, a dark stranger, for a Teuton or a Dane). Most Gaelic place names tend to be practical rather than poetic, so is it possible that the cave was simply known locally as the Norseman's cave?

3.1 Iona

In very early times called I [ee], IO, HII, HIA or IOUA – possibly from the Norse Hiöe [ee-ë] meaning island of the den of the brown bear. Later named ICOLMKILL (G. I Chaluim cille – island of Calum's monastery). Columba is a Latinised version of calaman (G. – dove), but the saint's given name was Calum. IOUA became corrupted to IONA in the 18th century through a typographical error.

O S Maps: 1:50000 Sheet 48 1:25000 Sheet 373
Admiralty Charts: 1:25000 No.2617

Area: 877ha (2167 acres)
Height: 100m (328 ft)

Owner: The sacred buildings and sites were presented to the Church of Scotland's Iona Cathedral Trust in 1899 by the 8th Duke of Argyll. The island as a whole was purchased from the Duke of Argyll by Sir Hugh Fraser in 1979 and given to the National Trust for Scotland.

Population: 1841–496. 1881–243. 1891–247. 1931–141. 1961–130. 1981–122. 1991–130. 2001–125.

Geology: Although Iona lies close to Mull it has a different geological composition. Much of it is Lewisian gneiss but on the east side there are clayey Torridonian beds, minor igneous dykes and glacial erratics from the Ross of Mull; raised beach deposits of late-glacial and post-glacial periods make up the western machair. On the south-east coast [NM268217] is the quarry for the original 'Iona marble' – actually a Lewisian gneiss with a large limestone content. The communion table in the abbey is made of it. The 'Iona marble' which is now sold on the island, and elsewhere, comes from Connemara in Ireland.

History: Iona was inhabited at least as far back as the Iron Age and it may have been a religious centre long before St Columba. It has been called Innis nan Druinich (G. – the Isle of Druidic Hermits) but any association is speculative.

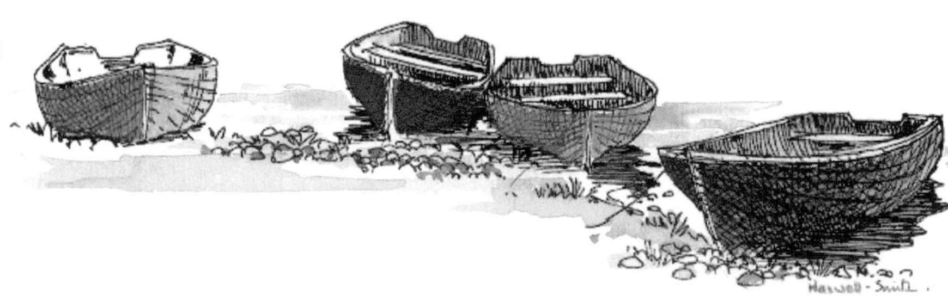

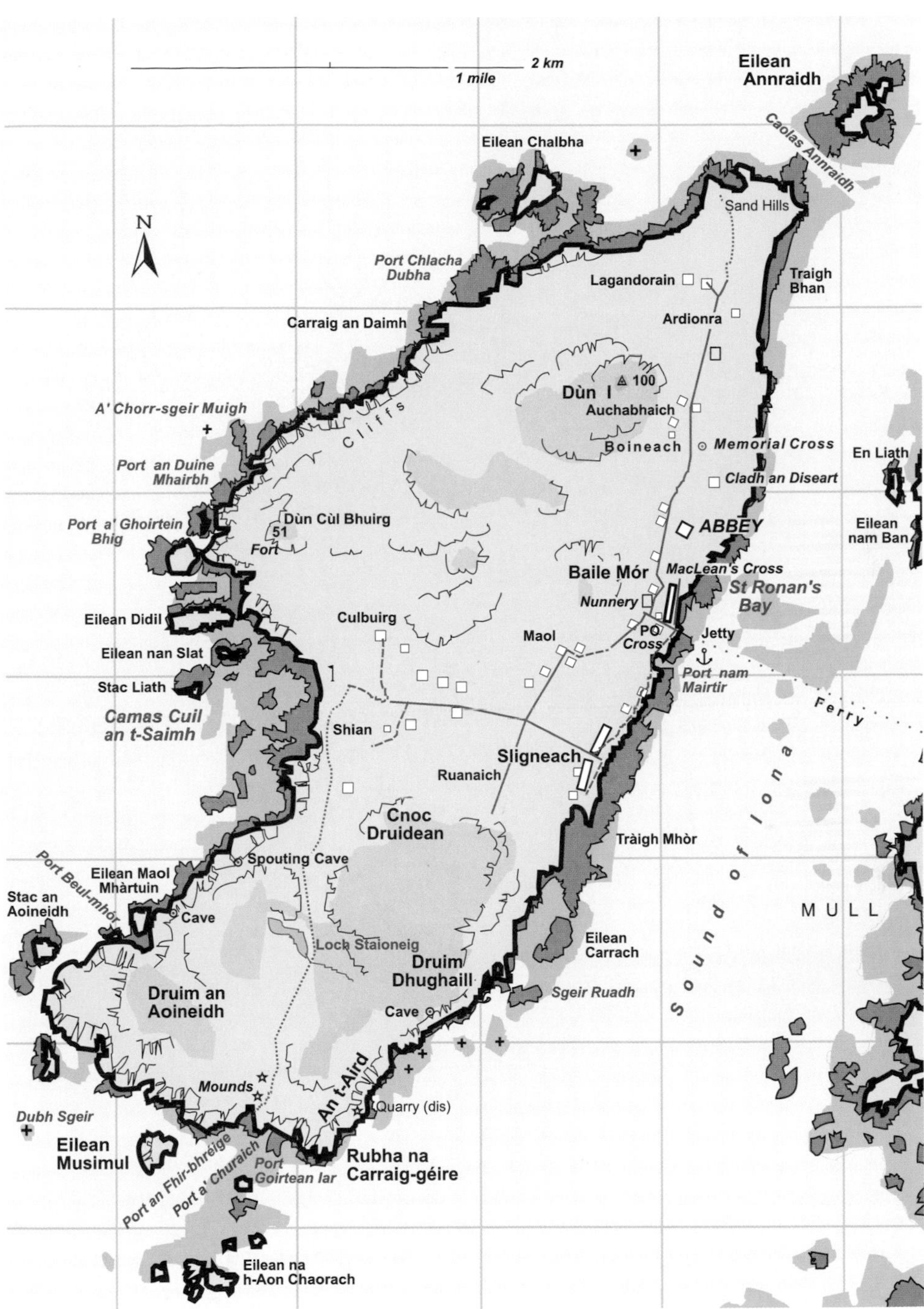

However, the Druid symbol of Bel – a circle – was later incorporated with the Christian Cross to become the well-known Celtic Cross.

Columba, an Irish prince accompanied by twelve companions, arrived in the year 563, when he was forty-two years old. He probably made his approach up the west coast of Islay in a large currach with a lug-sail. During the next thirty-four years he founded a monastery and turned Iona into a place of pilgrimage and Christian learning which was renowned throughout Europe. He died on the island in 597, having achieved his goal of conversion of the Picts to Christianity at a time when St Augustine had only started conversion of the English.

St Columba was not the earliest Irish missionary

to reach Scotland and may not even have been the greatest but he was a strong man with the confidence of a royal upbringing. When the king of Dalriada died Columba consecrated one of his relatives, Aiden, on the throne. With such powerful connections his fame grew and after his death it became established for posterity by the publication of no less than three biographies.

In 795 the first Norse raid on Iona took place with widespread destruction and pillaging. There was no defence. The monastery, which was built of mud, wood, wattle and thatch with an earthwork vallum and ditch to keep livestock out of the sanctuary area, was razed to the ground. It was rebuilt but the Norse struck again in 798 and 802, each time burning and levelling the buildings. Once more it was rebuilt. In 806 the Vikings again returned, destroyed the monastery, and murdered sixty-eight monks at Martyrs' Bay (200m south of the ferry jetty). In 849 after a further Norse raid in 825, the few remaining treasures were divided between Dunkeld in Scotland and Kells in Ireland including, it is thought, at least part of the beautifully illustrated *Book of Kells*, now in Dublin, and the Breccbennoch, a reliquary, now in Edinburgh. St Columba's remains were also moved after which they apparently disappeared, although it is possible that they were later returned to Iona and reburied in St Columba's Shrine next to the cathedral. Kells proved to be no safer than Iona and was ravaged seven times by the Vikings. Another murderous raid on Iona occurred in 986, when the abbot and fifteen monks were killed at the White Strand in the north of the island. It is little wonder that so few relics of this ancient seat of European culture have survived.

Queen Margaret is said to have rebuilt the monastery in stone and St Oran's Chapel in 1074 but whether this is true or not in 1203 Reginald or Ragnald of Islay, son of Somerled, founded a new monastery and abbey for the Benedictines on the site of the earlier monastery and also an Augustinian convent or nunnery whose fine pink granite ruins still remain. His sister became the first Abbess of Icolmkill. The greater part of the present cathedral was built in the 1500s on the foundations of Reginald's Benedictine abbey.

From the 14th century the Mackinnons of Mull were the hereditary Abbots of Iona. In 1499 the Benedictine church on Iona, which was the seat of the Bishopric of the Isles, was given cathedral status until the dissolution after 1570. The island was seized by the MacLeans of Duart in 1574 but it was taken over by the Earl of Argyll in 1688. It has been said that during the Reformation 360 stone crosses were smashed and thrown into the sea but this could be a myth. In 1609 the Hebridean chiefs swore loyalty to the Stuart kings in the church on Iona (documented as the Statutes of Icolmkill) and agreed to measures which curbed their powers but which were designed to improve island life. Unfortunately, later statutes were repressive and led to severe restrictions on Gaelic culture. In 1617 the church on Iona was annexed to the Protestant Bishopric of the Isles.

The roofless old abbey church was restored by the Church of Scotland in 1902–10. The general restoration and maintenance of all the monastic buildings was in the hands of the Iona Community, a body founded by a Govan minister, the Rev George Macleod (later, Lord Macleod of Fiunary). It is now the responsibility of the Iona Cathedral Trust.

Wildlife: Corncrake can often be heard on Iona these days, although rarely seen. Fulmar, shag and kittiwake breed here and also rock dove and jackdaw. Linnet, twite and yellowhammer can be seen and both the common and Arctic terns.

* * *

'That man is little to be envied,' said Dr Johnson, 'whose patriotism would not gain force upon the plain of Marathon, or whose piety would not grow warmer among the ruins of IONA!' He was referring to the island cradle of Scottish Christianity and learning, a place of pilgrimage with religious associations stretching far back into antiquity. Sir Walter Scott may have found it 'desolate and miserable' but it inspired Wordsworth in 1835 to compose three sonnets.

The island is austere and windswept yet remarkably fertile. The coastline has a magic and mysticism which, to me, rivals or even surpasses that of the acknowledged religious sites. The shell-sands are clean and white, the rocks have subtle colours tinged with rose and the sea ranges from deep violet to translucent emerald green. There is a sparkle and clarity in the air which is unique to this island and which has proved a challenge and delight to many artists.

The lone and distinctive hill in the north standing above the cathedral has the pre-

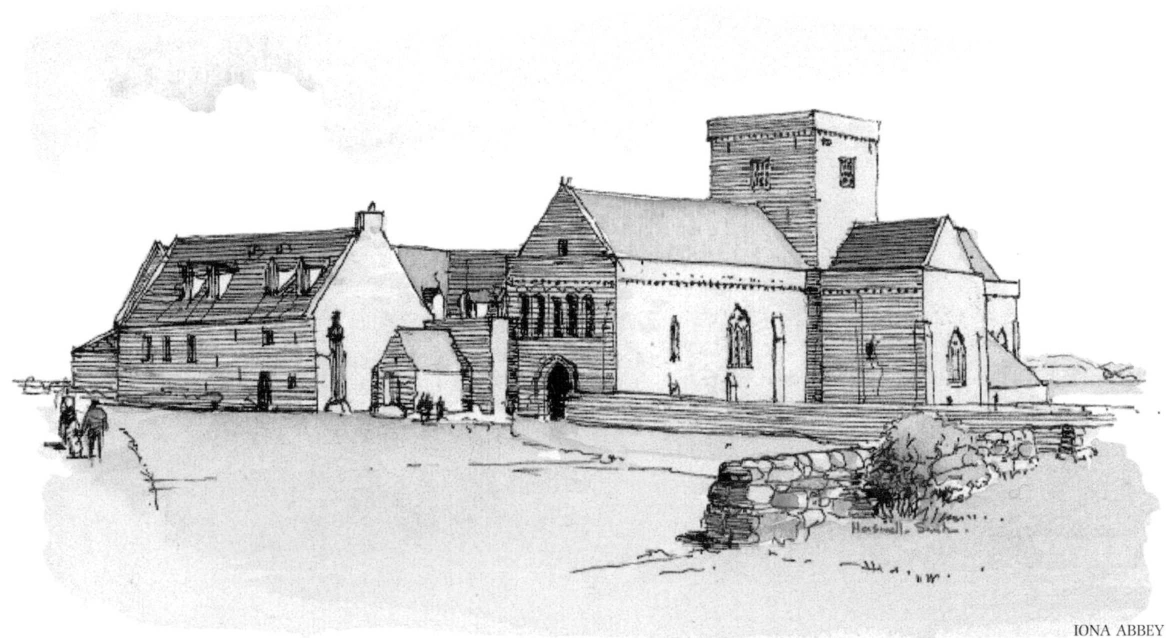
IONA ABBEY

Columban name of Dùn I [**doon**-ee]. In this case the 'dùn' probably refers to the mound-like shape rather than to a fort. It is an easy ten-minute climb to the top of this mountain in miniature which has its own 'north face' and rock chimney. From the top, at 100m (328ft), there is a marvellous view of coastline and islands stretching from Islay to Skye.

To the north is machair and the notorious but beautiful White Strand of the Monks with **Eilean Chalba** and **Eilean Annraidh** and, beyond, the islands of Staffa and the Treshnish Group.

The east coast, facing peacefully across the narrow Sound to the pink granite rocks of Mull, has a violent past. **Martyr's Bay**, near the ferry jetty, is where sixty-eight monks were massacred. The cathedral, solid and square, sits below the hill like a great supporting boulder. Further down the sound beyond Sligneach the white sands of Tràigh Mhór (G. – big beach) reach out to **Eilean Mór** and **Eilean Carrach**.

The south coast has cliffs and bays and green serpentine pebbles on the beaches. **Port a' Churaich** (G. – port of the coracle), or St Columba's Bay, was the saint's traditional landing place when he arrived from Ireland and it lies beside Port an Fhir-bhréige (G. – port of the manlike prehistoric mound). Entrance to the port leads past **Soa** (ON – sheep island) and between **Eilean Musimul** and **Eilean na h-Aon Chaorach**.

On the west, facing the Atlantic, there are fine farms and crofts on the machair while, out to sea, **Stac Mhic Mhurchaidh** stands proudly beside little **Réidh Eilean** (G. – levelled island). This is where tourists rarely go although there is a golf course overlooking Camas Cùil an t-Saimh (G. – ? the bay of twin recesses). South of this is Spouting Cave, beside an overhanging cliff. The bays here have semi-precious stones among the shingle.

The village, **Baile Mór** (G. – big town), facing the Sound of Mull sees half a million tourists a year tripping through it and like many tourist traps it is nothing to 'write home about'. However all the sacred sites are within easy walking distance of the ferry jetty.

Close to the jetty the first site to be reached, and the most beautiful, is the **Nunnery of St Mary** [NM284241]. It is of lovely mellow pink granite and the ruins, which are quite well preserved, include the church and choir, the Lady Chapel, cloister court, chapter house and refectory. Beside it the Romanesque **Church of St Ronan** (12th/13th century) serves as a museum.

Carrying on towards the cathedral you pass the 3m high MacLean's Cross dating from the 15th century [NM285242]. **Reilig Odhrain** (G. – graveyard of Oran) is on the right-hand side. A ridge in this simple cemetery was probably the burial place of many Scottish kings up to the time of Duncan and Macbeth in the 11th century and some West Highland chieftains in the Middle Ages were also buried here. The cemetery is said to hold the graves of many other kings but this is now thought unlikely.

The little Norman-style **St Oran's Chapel** [NM285244], which was probably built as a family mortuary by the Lords of the Isles in the 12th century, has been restored.

Crossing the meadow in front of the cathedral and beneath Dùn I is the **Street of the Dead** – a 13th-century pavement of red granite along which kings were borne for burial.

The 10th-century **St Martin's Cross**, 4.3m high, is opposite the west facade and to the left of it is a concrete replica of the 9th-century **St John's Cross**. Near the well is the broken shaft of **St Mathew's Cross**. St Columba's remains may be within **St Columba's Shrine** at the north-west corner of the nave or they may be in **Tor Abb**, the mound just west of the cathedral.

The **Abbey** or **Cathedral** [NM286245] is built of a rosy granite quarried from Tormore on Mull. It has a heavy square tower 21m high centred over arches on a cruciform plan. Much of the building dates from the late 15th century, when Reginald's abbey of 1203 was rebuilt but there have been many additions and alterations since then. In the north the Sacristy doorway of golden sandstone from Carsaig on Mull dates from 1500. The **Cloister**, entered through Norman arches in the north transept, contains two medieval pillars. Several of the monastic buildings have been restored such as the **Chapter House** (1955) with Norman doorway, the **Refectory** and the **Undercroft** (1949), the **Reredorter** (1944) and the **Caretaker's House** (1950) which has a gable of the old Abbot's House. **Michael Chapel** (rebuilt 1960) and the **Infirmary** are built on the original Celtic foundations.

The **Abbey Museum**, behind the Abbey, shelters many of the notable grave-stones. It is also the specially constructed site of the original **St John's Cross**. The **Iona Heritage Centre** (the former Telford Manse) has local and natural history displays in the summer.

Ferry access is not cheap and is occasionally disrupted by the weather causing inevitable stress on the population. This uncertainty has led to talk of the possible construction of a causeway or low-level bridge.

Access: Frequent passenger ferry from Fionnphort on Mull (5 min.), 01680-812343. Summer only or by request. No cars. Vehicle ferry Oban/Craignure on Mull, 08000-66-5000. Bus service Craignure / Fionnphort, 01546-604360. There is a taxi on Iona and bicycles can be hired.

Anchorages:
1. Martyrs' Bay, S of pier. Temporary anchorage in suitable weather, 3m, sand. Avoid cables and moorings and note that there can be strong tidal currents.
2. Port na Fraing (Traigh Bhan) N of abbey. Possibly better temporary anchorage, at least ½c offshore. Avoid power cable. Good holding when clear of weed.
3. Bull Hole, between Eilean nam Ban and Ross of Mull N of Fionnphort. Good, sheltered, but restricted anchorage in depths of 3–4m. Approach from S. Anchor near Limpet Rock if there is room or off ruined pier in entrance channel. 1M distance to Martyrs' Bay.

3.2 Kerrera

(ON Kjarbar-øy – Kjarbar's island) or (ON ciarr-øy – brushwood island).

O S Maps: 1:50000 Sheet 49 1:25000 Sheet 359
Admiralty Charts: 1:25000 No.2387 1:10000 No.1790

Area: 1214ha (3000 acres)
Height: 189m (620 ft)

Owner: Principal landowner, Mrs C H E MacDougall of MacDougall. 270 acres at north end were put up for sale by Lord Lovat in 1994.

Population: 1841–187. 1861–105. 1881–103. 1891–92. 1931–79. 1961–42. 1971–27. 1981–38. 1991–39. 2001–42.

Geology: The island is of secondary basalt, graphitic schists and red sandstone.

History: Kerrera has belonged to the MacDougalls since Somerled founded the clan in the 12th century. Alexander II and his fleet of ships anchored in Horse Shoe bay in 1249 to enforce suzerainty on Ewen of Lorn who was paying homage to King Haakon of Norway. Alexander died on the island before achieving his object. A few years later, in 1263, King Haakon's fleet also mustered in the bay on its way to the Battle of Largs. The remnants of his shattered fleet again gathered here after the battle before returning home to Norway by way of Orkney (where King Haakon died).

In 1647 during the Covenanting Wars

General Leslie's army destroyed Gylen Castle, the MacDougall stronghold at the south end of the island. The Protestant minister, John Neave, persuaded the troops to slaughter every MacDougall defender – there were no survivors.

Wildlife: Wild thyme, wild roses, meadow-sweet and honeysuckle festoon the hill tracks.

Mute swan, eider duck, black guillemot and white-winged gulls inhabit Oban Bay all the year round. Buzzards are fairly common and rare red kites have been seen circling over the island.

KERRERA is compact, rural, generally unremarkable, and forms a natural breakwater for the important harbour of Oban. Although it is so close to this bustling tourist centre it is a world apart, with lovely views, and many quiet and gentle walks. An easy climb up Càrn Breugach (G. – the false rocky hill) through shrub woodland is rewarding for its magnificent view of the Lorn coast. The island's main function for many years was as a stepping-stone for transporting cattle from Mull to the mainland.

The ferry channel leads between **Maiden Island** and the north end of Kerrera. Here there is a prominent memorial commemorating David Hutcheson, who was one of the founders of the ubiquitous Caledonian MacBrayne ferry service. Maiden Island, by the way, is one of many such islands around Scotland which were so-named

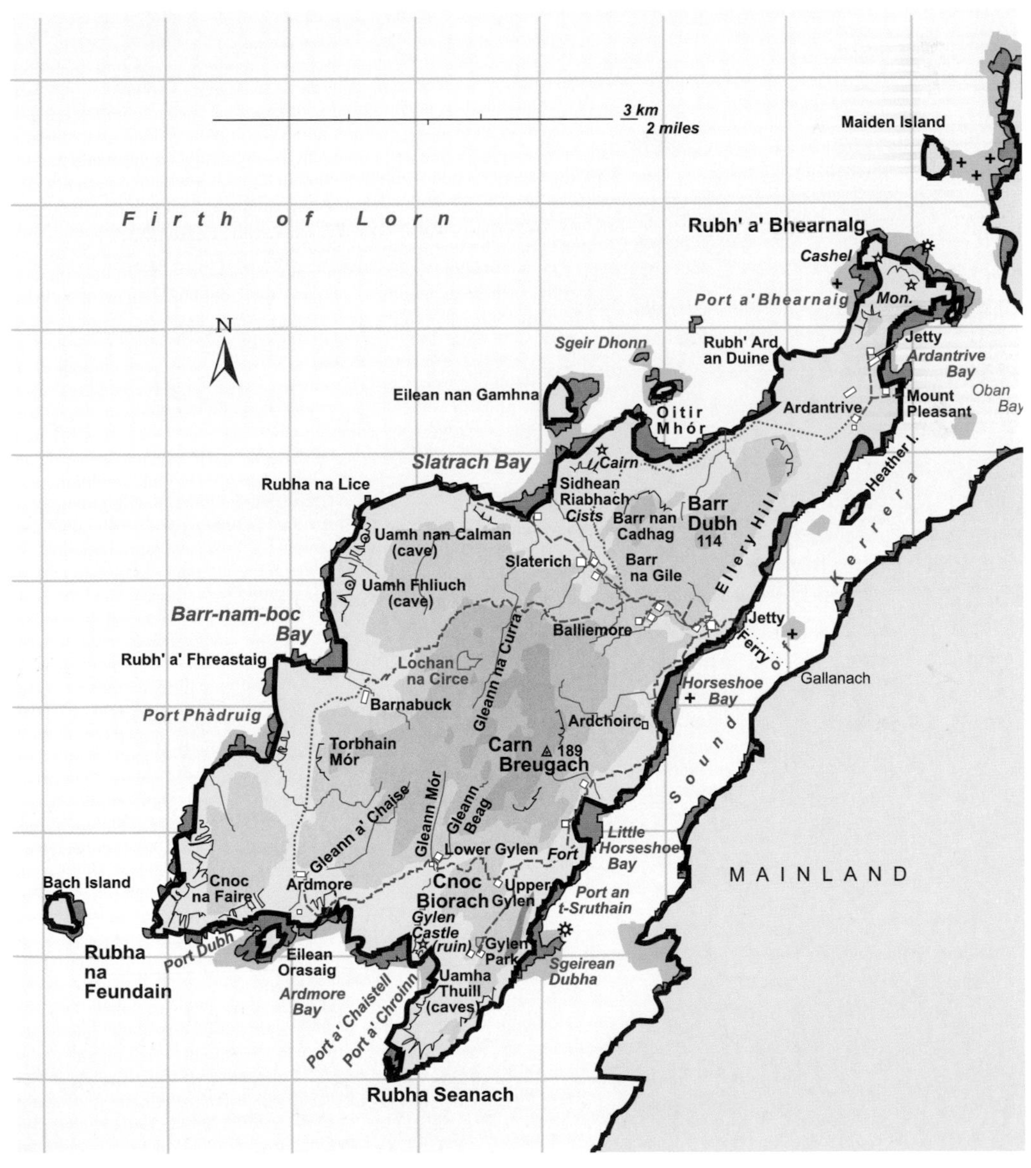

because they were used by chieftains as refuges for their womenfolk in time of war.

In **Ardantrive Bay** there are moorings, a boatyard, jetty and old slipway. The hillock south of the bay is called Mount Pleasant and **Heather Island** lies close by in the Sound of Kerrera. Across the island, on the north-west coast, is Oitir Mhór (G. – big shoal) – a large bay facing Lismore with several small islets on its west side. The largest of these is **Eilean nan Gamhna** (G. – island of the stirks). (A stirk is a year-old calf.)

The two-pupil school closed in 1997. Both it and the church were built in 1872 and the post-office was established in 1879. There is a lobster packing factory beside **Horse Shoe Bay** where lobsters from the storage pond at Cullipool on Luing (No.2.13) are packed for market. The ferry jetty is just north of the bay.

When Alexander II's fleet anchored in Horse Shoe Bay in July 1249 Alexander slept aboard ship. In the morning he mentioned that he had dreamed that St Columba had come aboard and told him to return home immediately. Alexander's nobles felt he should heed the warning but Alexander scoffed at the idea and went ashore. As soon as he landed he stumbled and before he could be carried back on board he died. The land behind the bay is still called Dalrigh (G. – the field of the King).

A road or track, which at times is little more than a footpath, runs from Horse Shoe Bay in a loop encompassing most of the southern half of the island. Càrn Breugach, the highest point, sits above **Little Horse Shoe Bay** and there is a pleasant walk past the hill to the wild rocky site on the south coast with the fairytale turreted ruins of **Gylen Castle** (G. *caisteal nan geimhlean* – castle of the springs) [NM805265]. It was built in 1587 by Duncan MacDougall of Dunollie, the 16th Chief, on the site of an earlier fortification. The natural springs beneath the castle provided ample fresh water for the inhabitants. The building was besieged and burned in 1647 by General Leslie during the Covenanting Wars. The castle, which can look formidable on a gloomy day poised above the steep and rocky coastline, has an interesting passage underneath it. Carved heads can still be seen on the walls and an inscription which may have read – 'Trust in God and sin no more'.

Gylen Castle was the repository for the MacDougalls' famous Brooch of Lorn. This is an 11cm (4½in) disc of Celtic silver with filigree ornament and a central dome concealing a cavity for sacred relics and supporting a large rock-crystal circled by eight jewelled obelisks. It is said to have belonged to Bruce.

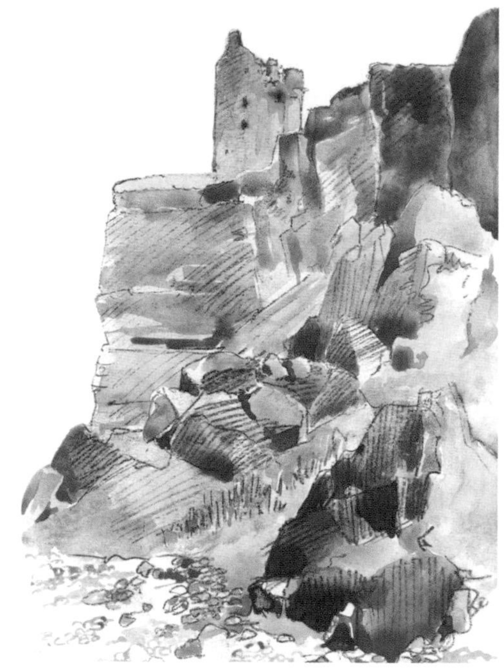

GYLEN CASTLE – SCENE OF A MASSACRE

When all the castle's defenders had been massacred, the Brooch was looted by one of Leslie's officers, Campbell of Inverawe. The castle was then burned down and for two centuries the MacDougalls believed their famous Brooch had been destroyed in the fire; that is, until 1825, when General Sir Duncan Campbell of Lochnell, who had inherited it, chose to present it to his neighbour, MacDougall of Dunollie, at a public ceremony.

The peninsula lying west of Gylen Castle which runs down to Rubha Seanach (G. – the venerable headland) has a number of caves in it and to the west is Ardmore Bay and the tiny tidal **Eilean Orasaig**. Lying off the western extremity and well into the Firth of Lorn is **Bach Island** (G. – windward island).

Another road and track leads directly across the centre of the island past Slatrach Bay on the west coast. Further south is Barr-nam-boc Bay (G. – billy-goat bay) and on the steep headland between these bays are two interesting caves – Uamh Fhliuch (G. – wet cave) and Uamh nan Calman (G. – the doves' cave) [NM802294].

Access: Frequent daily passenger ferry from Gallanach 3km S of Oban. Crossing 5 minutes, 01631-563665.

Anchorages:
1. Little Horse Shoe Bay about 4¾c NNE of Sgeirean Dubha light-beacon, 2.7–5.5m, good holding. Avoid shoal area marked by buoy and drying reef off S point. *(Best anchorage for walk to Gylen Castle).*
2. Horse Shoe Bay, 4c NE of Little Horse Shoe Bay, sheltered with good holding. Anchor between central covering rock spit and cable beacon on S point.
3. Heather Island. Possible anchorage off the bight on Kerrera and N of Heather Island. Use trip line.
4. Ardantrive bay, opposite Oban Bay. Visitors' moorings and pontoon berths (pay, 01631-565333). Well-sheltered with good holding but many moorings. Beware drying reef at S point with wreck which covers.
5. Oitir Mhór bay, on N coast, affords reasonable shelter in moderate weather. Straightforward approach from NW. SW side of bay dries 1c. Charlotte Bay to N is more exposed.
6. There are no other suitable anchorages on the W coast and the S coast is very exposed. Temp. anchorage in suitable weather S of Gylen Castle in centre of cove, 4–6m, sand and shingle. *(Useful for a short visit to Gylen Castle).*

3.3 Mull

(?G. meall – a lump or a rounded hill) This might refer to the rounded shape of Ben More. Alternatively, (?G. maol – bald). But the name is very ancient. 2000 years ago Ptolemy referred to Malaeos.

O S Maps: 1:50000 Sheets 47, 48 and 49 1:25000 Sheets 373, 374 and 375
Admiralty Charts: 1:75000 Nos.2169 and 2171 1:25000 Nos.2386, 2387, 2390, 2392, 2617, 2652 and 2771 1:10000 No.2474 Tobermory Harbour

Area: 87,794ha (216,939 acres)
Height: 966m (3168 ft)

Owner: Multiple ownership but with sizeable areas controlled by the Scottish Office (mainly the Forestry Commission). In the early decades of the 18th century the Kilninian and Kilmore parishes were controlled by the house of Argyll, and the Duke of Argyll still has considerable land-holdings in these parishes.

Population: 1755–5287. 1794–8016. Overpopulation by 1821–10,600 inhabitants led to some voluntary emigration before the Clearances. 1841–8316. 1881–5229. 1891–4691. 1931–2903. 1961–2154. 1981–2197. 1991–2708. 2001–2704.

Geology: Most of Mull is Tertiary basalt (trap) on top of Moine schist. In the mountain areas the basalt – volcanic lava flows of fifty million years ago – is weathered into terraces. These giant stepped formations are clearly seen round Loch Scridain and Loch na Keal. Ben More is the highest example of Tertiary basalt in Britain stepping down to a final 370m drop into the sea – the cliff at Wilderness on the Ardmeanach peninsula. Basalt cliffs at Ardtun have Tertiary leaf-beds petrified by liquid mud from the ancient volcano. Recognizable varieties are oak, hazel, plane, Ginkgo or maiden-hair tree, and various conifers – mainly Mediterranean varieties. The collapsed vent cores of volcanic eruptions centred on Beinn Chàisgidle and Loch Bà formed circular granite dykes 100m thick and some five miles in diameter. Columnar basalt is to be found near Tavool on Ardmeanach and also at Bunessan and Carsaig in the south. A sill of sapphires can be seen near the famous Carsaig arches. In this area the basalt sits on a chalk layer beneath which is an expanse of lias washed by lime-laden water.

North Mull is a basalt plateau with a volcanic plug at 'S Airde Beinn. On the headland overlooking the Treshnish Isles there is a fertile pre-glacial raised beach and raised beaches are also to be found on the east coast of Mull.

Between the masses of basalt there is a thin spread of Cretaceous and other sediments. This, and the friable rock, has given Mull well-drained and fertile soil.

Glen More, which has many glacial features and a terminal moraine, defines the southern part of Mull. Loch Spelve and Loch Buie in the south-east are at the end of the Great Glen fault.

The butt of the Ross of Mull is pink granite, with the largest mass of the mountain gabbro extruded in screes, or small outcrops and crags. The gabbro on Mull does not form the spectacular shapes it has on Rum and Skye and some of it contains olivine which gives it a sombre colour. Ben Buie has extrusions of breccias and ryolytes (volcanic granite). The south crags of Creach Ceinn are granophyres (almost granite but interwoven with quartz and felspar).

History: As with so many of the islands, Mull is rich in prehistoric remains – standing stones, circles, cairns and many large crannogs of both stone and timber construction in the fresh-water lochs. The island was known to the classical Greeks and Ptolemy referred to it in the 2nd century AD as Maleus. In the same century the Irish Celts appeared on the scene. One can infer from the visible remains of forts and duns (about thirty-five of them) that there were many battles and skirmishes. For a time Loch Spelve, Glen More and Loch Scridain is said to have formed the boundary between the kingdom of the Picts and Dalriada, kingdom of the Scots. Christianity was introduced after St Columba's arrival on Iona in 563.

The Norwegians exercised tenuous control from about the 8th century but, even so, King Magnus plundered the island in 1100. The Lord of the Isles gained suzerainty in 1266. In the following century the Macdougalls, the senior clan descended from Somerled, supported Balliol instead of Bruce and this misjudgement led King Robert to transfer control to the Macdonalds, the junior branch which had given him support at Bannockburn. Thus the Macdonalds became Lords of the Isles and the most influential clan, and it was not until 1543, after an abortive revolt, that the Campbells gained ascendancy. The Mackinnons of Mull and the MacLeans of Duart, although party to the uprising and allied to the Macdonalds, managed by various subterfuges to maintain status with the Campbells.

James VI (James I of England) was determined to destroy Gaelic culture which he thoroughly detested. In 1608 he sent Lord Ochiltree and the Bishop of the Isles to Aros Castle on Mull. All the Hebridean chiefs were summoned to meet there for a conference. An inaugural service was conducted by the Bishop on board a ship in Salen Bay whereupon the chiefs were all imprisoned in the ship and then sent to Edinburgh.

In Charles I's reign the Protestant Earl of Argyll chose to lead the Army of the Covenant. There were religious stresses throughout Mull as, for instance, the Maclaines of Lochbuie were Catholic while the MacLeans of Duart were Protestant. MacLean however refused to join Argyll only to find that Argyll bought up all his debts compelling him to sign away his castles of Duart and Aros. To enforce this, Argyll invaded Mull with 2000 men in 1674 and occupied the castles amid reports of needless barbarity. The Campbells rampaged through Mull and destroyed most of the priceless Gaelic library held by the Beatons of Pennycross.

Thomas Pennant observed in 1772 that although a Campbell lived in Aros Castle and government troops occupied Duart Castle, the MacLeans still retained about half the island. About this time the talented 5th Duke of Argyll, a very different man from some of his predecessors, was looking to the improvement of his estates. He instituted a system of nineteen-year leases for his tenants with fair rents related to means and as Governor of the British Fisheries Society he established the enchanting little port of Tobermory.

Wildlife: There is not much heather on the island due to the good soil but flag and meadowsweet and luxuriant fuchsia abound. The remaining patches of natural woodland are mainly oak, ash, birch and hazel. Carsaig is one of only two places in the western Highlands where watercress grows in the chalky streams, as it does in southern England.

Heavyweight stags can be seen in the mountain corries but red deer stalking in September and October restricts safe access to the hills. At least one family of otters feed on the brown trout in Loch Poit na h'I on the Ross of Mull.

Mull and Ulva are the last refuges of the beautiful red and black Scotch burnet moth which is now extinct elsewhere.

Ptarmigan nest on Ben Buie's slopes at under 700m – a lower altitude than they require in the Central Highlands and the white-tailed sea eagle can be regularly seen here. There is year-round interest for ornithologists with a wide variety of bird habitats and many interesting species. Sites worth visiting are:

Loch Frisa. Sea eagle viewing site.

Glen More, 16km from Craignure. Upland species: hen harrier, short-eared owl, golden eagle, kestrel, raven, buzzard. Also breeding curlew, cuckoo, whinchat. stonechat, and wheatear. Snow bunting in winter.

Mishnish Lochs near Tobermory: Little grebe, heron, goosander and red-throated diver. Hen harrier, buzzard, short-eared owl and golden eagle hunt in the vicinity. Whooper swan and goldeneye in the winter.

Loch Don has resident heron, mute swan, eider, red-breasted merganser, redshank, buzzard

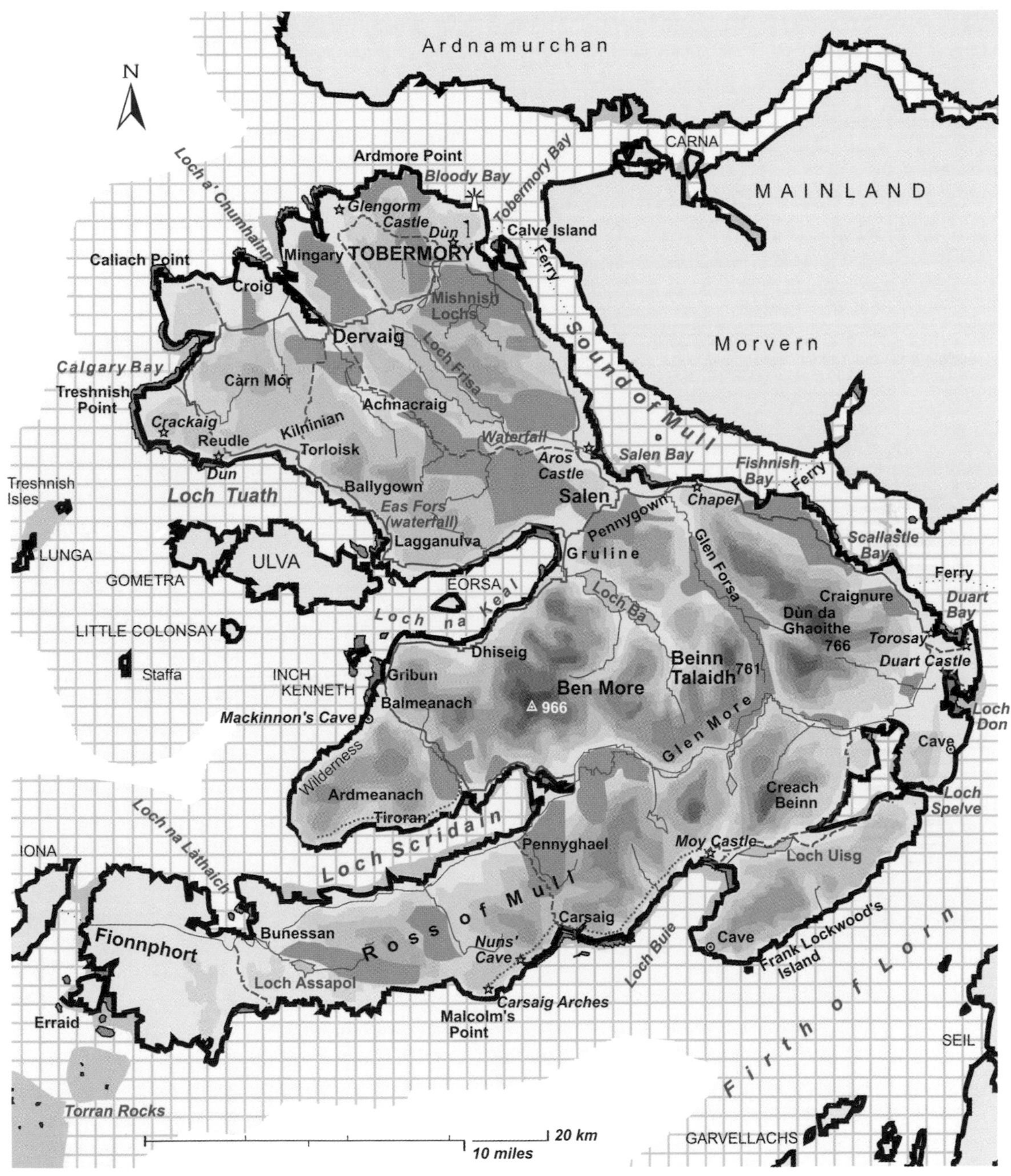

and hen harrier. Common and Arctic tern in summer. Red-throated diver, little grebe, cormorant, greenshank, wigeon, teal, mallard, goldeneye and shelduck in winter. Passage waders such as grey plover, knot, sanderling, bar and black-tailed godwits and whimbrel. Pectoral sandpiper, ruff, spotted redshank and green sandpiper have been seen.

Loch Na Keal: Excellent viewing of divers and the velvet scoter is sometimes seen. Also the Slavonian grebe.

Fionnphort and 1½km S at Fidden: Many migrant waders and passerines with Greenland white-fronted geese in winter. 1½km east at Loch Poit na h'I there are little grebe and, in winter, white-fronted geese, tufted duck and pochard.

Loch Scridain: In winter, red-throated, black-throated and great northern divers.

The main body of **MULL** is mountainous, rising to 966m at Ben More – the highest peak and

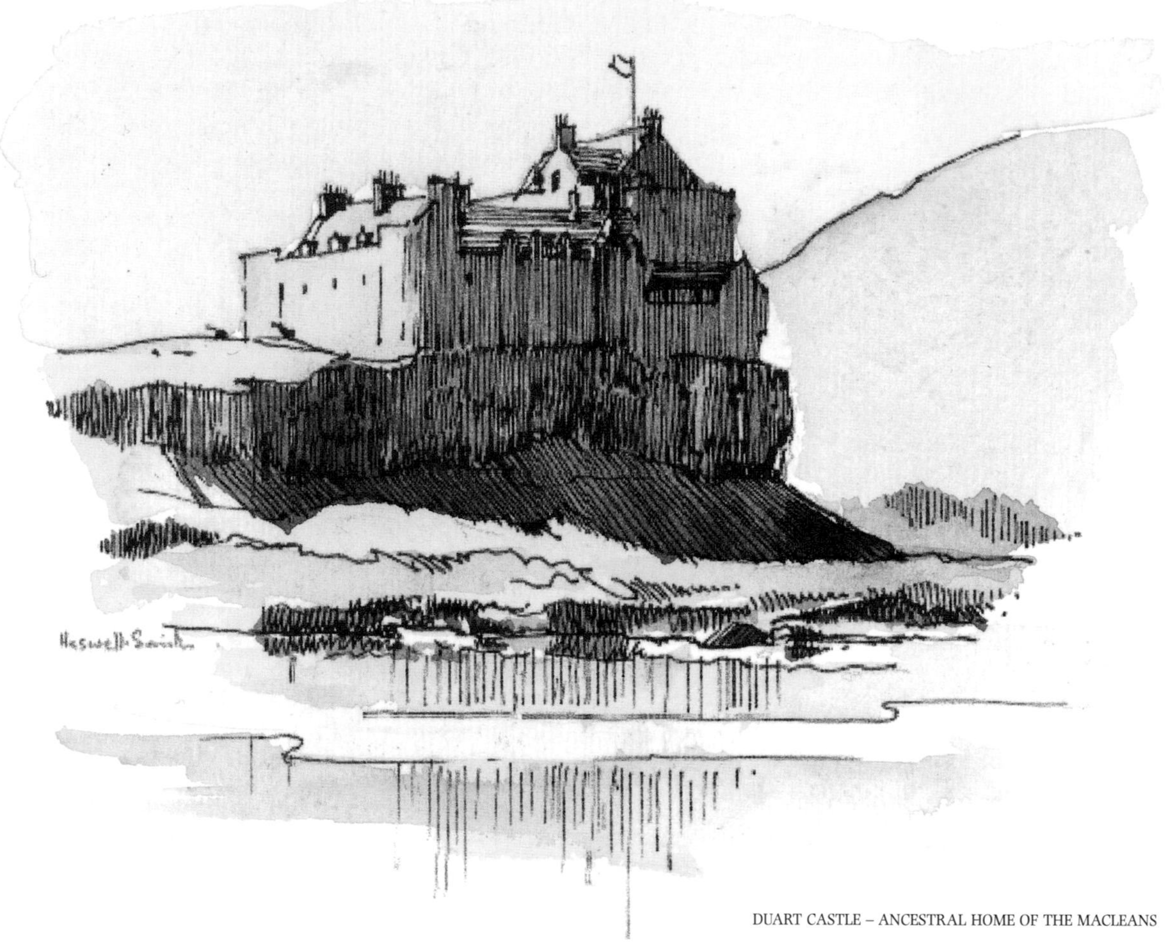

DUART CASTLE – ANCESTRAL HOME OF THE MACLEANS

the only Munro in all the Scottish islands. (Skye has twenty-two Munros but no longer qualifies for island classification since it is linked to the mainland by a bridge). Ben More from the west and Beinn Talaidh from the north are very shapely mountains. The non-mountainous areas had good agricultural potential but much of this was lost when large-scale sheep farming was introduced in the 19th century. The island is so heavily indented with sea lochs that there is about 500km of coastline but, due to good drainage, inland lochs are comparatively few – even though Mull suffers the wettest weather in the Hebrides. (May is the driest month.)

The vehicle ferry from Oban has its terminal at **Craignure** pier (built in 1964). On the way over it passes close by **Duart Castle** (G. *dubh aird* – black promontory), a much-photographed and perfect example of an island warlord's homestead [NM749353]. This has been the MacLeans' ancestral home since about 1250 although it was burned by the Duke of Argyll in 1691, and confiscated after Culloden. The 26th Chief, Sir Fitzroy MacLean, bought it in 1911 and with Sir John Burnett as his architect, carefully restored it. It is presently occupied by the 27th Chief and is open to the public.

Eilean Rubha an Ridire (G. – island at the promontory of the knight) is across on the Morvern shore, where the **Glas Eileanan** (G. – grey-green islands) guard the entrance to the Sound of Mull. During a gale on the 19 October 1690 the Royal Naval frigate *Dartmouth* dragged her anchor in Duart Bay and was wrecked on this islet. The wreck, which is now protected, was discovered by divers in 1973. There have been many such accidents. Until quite recently the mast of the wrecked 'puffer' *Ballista* could be seen, but it has now disintegrated.

It was on **Lady's Rock** opposite Duart Castle, which is submerged at each high tide, that Lachlan Cattanach, the 11th MacLean chieftain, had his wife, Elizabeth, tied up and marooned because he considered that their marriage was a failure. The next morning, seeing that she had been washed away with the tide, he sadly reported her death to her brother, the Earl of Argyll. Argyll was sympathetic and invited Lachlan to visit him at Inveraray but when Lachlan duly arrived, and was shown into the dining hall, he was horrified to see his wife (who had been rescued by a passing fisherman) sitting at the top table next to her brother. Nothing was said, the meal proceeded pleasantly, and at the end Lachlan was allowed to leave unharmed. Through the years that followed the subtle torture continued but Lachlan married twice more and by his third wife, a son and heir was born. It was not until thirty more years had passed (in 1527) that he was found murdered in his bed in Edinburgh.

A relatively modern Scottish Baronial castle, **Torosay**, is also in the vicinity and open to the public [NM728353]. David Bryce was the architect in 1856 and the building has beautiful terraced gardens designed by Sir Robert Lorimer in 1899 with a walk bordered by nineteen life-sized Venetian statues. It can be reached from Craignure by the Mull & West Highland Railway, a 10.25 gauge miniature line.

North of Craignure, beyond **Scallastle Bay**, is the terminal for the small Lochaline-Fishnish vehicle ferry which crosses the Sound of Mull and connects Mull with Morvern. Approaching the foot of Glen Forsa at **Pennygown** there is the ruin of a medieval chapel with the shaft of a Celtic cross in it [NM604432]. This area was once the haunt of benevolent fairies who would complete small tasks for people. Then someone left a twig with instructions to turn it into a ship's mast and the fairies have been on strike ever since.

Nearby is the island's airstrip which was built in 1966 in only fifty-four days by the 38th Engineer Regiment as a military exercise. The road leads on to the small village of **Salen** which lies in the 'waist' of Mull, the narrow strip between Salen Bay and Loch na Keal. On the north side of Salen Bay are the ruins of 13th-century **Aros Castle** built on the site of the first Norman-style castle to be completed by Somerled and last occupied in 1608 [NM563450]. One of the **Eileanan Glasa** (G. – grey-green islands) in the centre of the Sound of Mull opposite Salen, called **Dearg Sgeir** (G. – red rock), was hit by the cargo ship *Rondo* in 1935. The collision wrecked the ship and demolished the original lighthouse.

Tobermory (G. *tobar Mhoire* – Mary's well) is one of the loveliest and best-known small towns in Scotland. It was planned and built by The British Fisheries Society in 1788 and had burgh status from 1875 to 1975. The fine stone houses on the main street are brightly painted and form a cheerful backdrop to the beautiful harbour. Further up the hillside and among the trees is more recent housing. The town is well served with facilities. There are hotels, boarding-houses, a youth hostel, shops, bank, post-office, library, schools, museum and a tourist information office. The 1862 courthouse now serves as a police station and council offices. There is an attractive wooded public park and a nine-hole golf course. The eponymous St Mary's Well is at the top of the hill just west of the town beside a ruined medieval chapel. This was the original village in which Dr Johnson and Boswell stayed in 1773 in a 'tolerable inn'. As Boswell reported, 'Tobermorie is an excellent harbour. An island lies before it, and it is surrounded by a hilly theatre. The island is too low, otherwise this would be quite a secure port; but, the island not being sufficient protection, some storms blow very hard here. Not long ago, fifteen vessels were blown from their moorings'. Boswell's comments are correct but **Calve Island** (owned by the Cotton family who stay there during the summer), separated from Mull by a shallow tidal channel, is a fairly effective barrier nevertheless.

The famous wreck of a galleon or provision ship of the Spanish Armada, possibly *Almirante di Florencia*, is in the

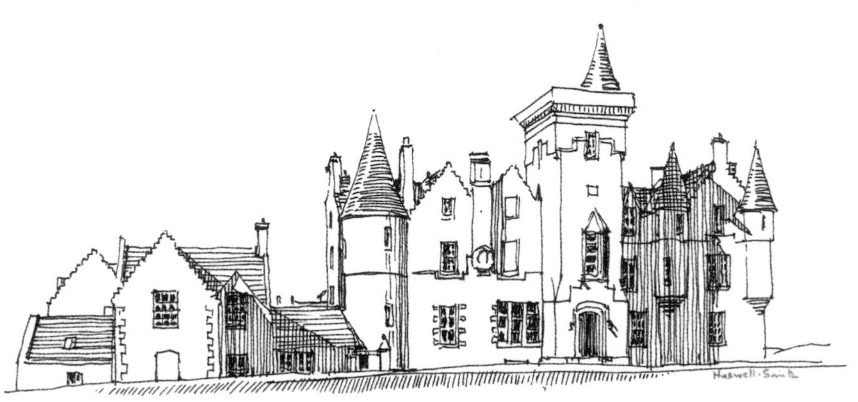

GLENGORM CASTLE

bay. Fleeing from the battle in 1588 she anchored here and took on provisions but when Donald MacLean went on board to ask for payment he was locked in the magazine and the Spaniards prepared to set sail. MacLean managed to escape but started a fire which blew up the ship. It was alleged that the ship carried thirty million ducats, and there have been many attempts to recover the treasure. These have probably been unsuccessful although there were rumours that part of the treasure was recovered and buried at Aros Castle. The wreck has now sunk deep in the mud and clay below the harbour.

Bloody Bay, between the lighthouse at Rubha nan Gall and Ardmore Point, was the setting for a sea battle between John, the last Lord of the Isles, and his son Angus. Ardmore Forest Walk, just north of the bay, is a popular cliff path with splendid views.

Dùn Urgadul, a vitrified fort, lies west of Tobermory [NM494553]. The minor road leading past it wanders through forests to **Glengorm Castle** [NM439572] in the north-west of the island looking across the sea to Ardnamurchan point. There was such an attractive haze in the air when the new owner arrived in the 19th century that he named it Glengorm (G. – the blue glen). He had not realised that the haze was caused by the smoke of burning crofts which were being 'cleared'. South-west of Tobermory the main road runs to Dervaig past the Mishnish lochs, well-stocked with trout, and on through open moorland.

Dervaig (G. *doire beag* – little grove) is a beautiful village built by the MacLeans of Coll in 1799. Kilmore Parish Church has an Irish style pencil-shaped steeple [NM431518]. Next door, the Mull Little Theatre, seating thirty-eight, was founded in this village. In the summer there are often boat excursions from here to Staffa and the Treshnish Isles. The minor road running south to Salen passes groups of standing stones and **Eas Corrach** (G. – steep waterfall) at the end of Glen Aros. Dervaig is at the head of Loch a' Chumhainn (G. – loch of the narrows), which has a narrow passage connecting it to the sea. The anchorage of **Port Croig**, where cattle from the outer isles were landed on their way to market, is in a rocky inlet.

A basalt dyke on its north side gives **Calgary Bay** its name (G. *caladh garaidh* – the haven by the dyke). In 1883 Col J F MacLeod of the Royal North-West Mounted Police, after an enjoyable holiday at Calgary House, gave the Canadian city the same name. (The bay is also incidentally noted for a 12lb lobster caught here in the 1920s.) On the moor to the south stands the lonely ruin of Reudle schoolhouse and beyond the hills on the peninsula to the west – overlooking the Treshnish Isles (No.3.8) – is the extensive deserted village of Crackaig. Two hundred people were cleared from here in the 19th century and a villager hanged himself from the ash tree in the walled garden beside the burn. Still Cave, where the local whisky was made, is further down the burn. Ruined **Dùn Aisgain** which dates from 1BC stands on a headland to the east [NM377453] while **Dun Bàn** is nearer the road [NM387453].

The road wends its way along the side of Loch Tuath (G. – north loch), the wide sea loch between Ulva and Mull through patches of natural woodland. In **Kilninian** burial ground [NM397457] there is a very fine medieval slab showing a kilted chieftain, and Torloisk (G. – burned hill) was the home of Alan of the Straws, a famous pirate. Many ancient artefacts are along the way and at Ballygown there is a broch, Dùn nan Gall, [NM433431] and an ancient fort [NM441431]. One kilometre further on is Mull's most spectacular waterfall, **Eas Fors** (G. *eas* – waterfall, ON *fors* – waterfall). At the head of Loch Tuath a group of tiny islets cluster in the narrow Sound of Ulva – **Eilean a' Bhuic** (G. – buck island), Eilean Garbh (G. – rough island), and Eilean a' Chaolais (G. – kyle island) are the largest. The road passes the

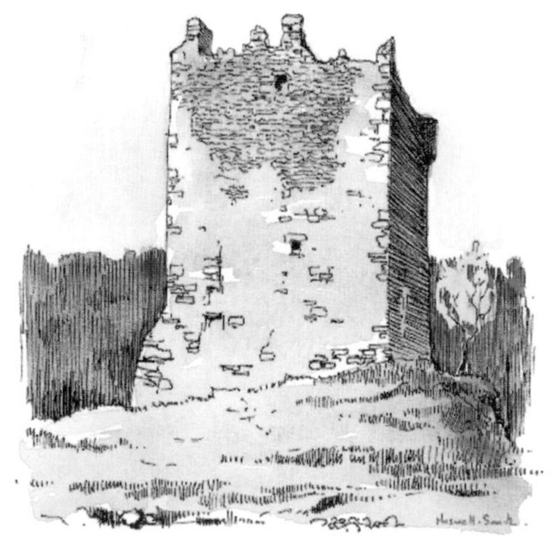

THE STURDY TOWER OF MOY CASTLE

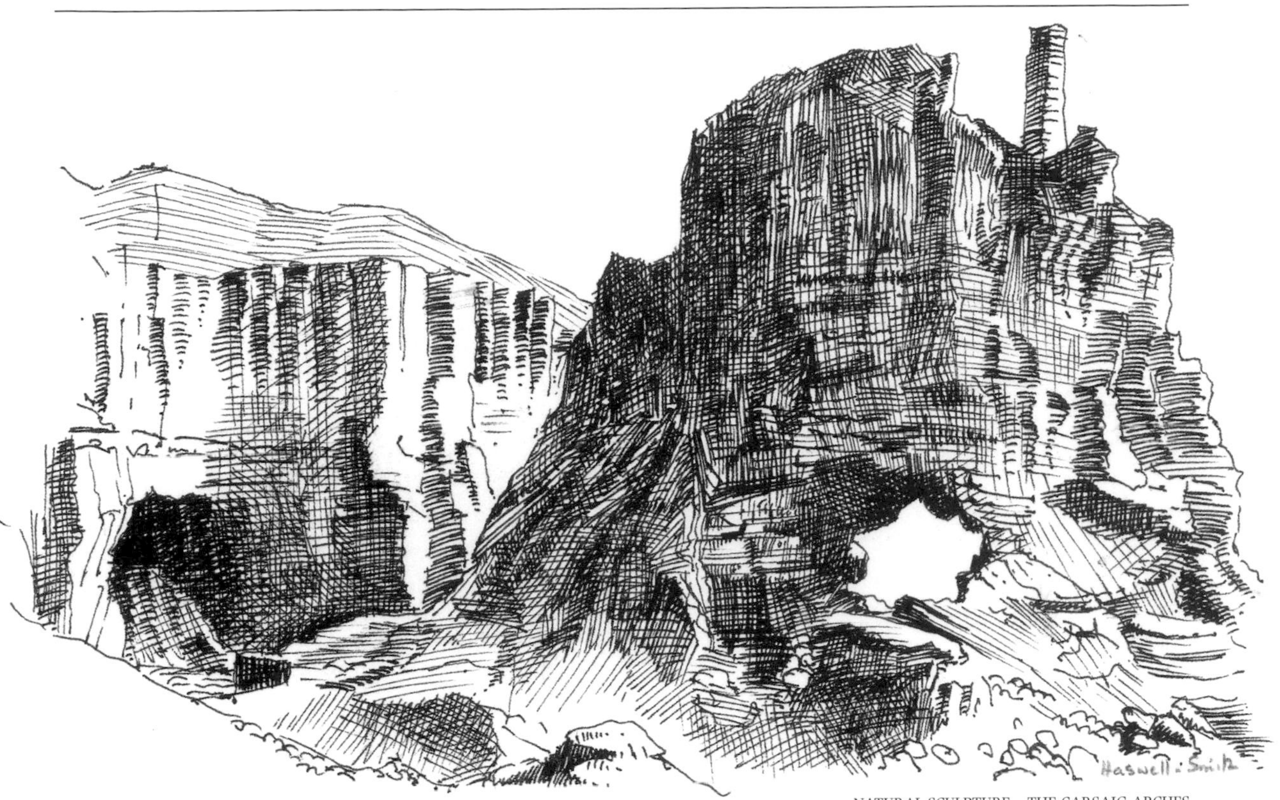

NATURAL SCULPTURE – THE CARSAIG ARCHES

turn-off to Ulva Ferry and carries on round the sides of Loch na Keal (G. – loch of the cliff) to Gruline, where a mausoleum is maintained by the National Trust of Australia for Major General Lachlan Macquarrie (1761–1824) of Ulva, the first Governor of New South Wales and 'father of Australia'. **Ben More** dominates the southern side of Loch na Keal and the easiest point to scramble up it is by Abhainn na h-Uamha (G. – river of the caves), 1½km NE of Dhiseig [NM507368]. Beyond its slopes the road skirts the cliffs overlooking Inch Kenneth (No.3.4) and turns southwards through the giant rockfalls at Gribun. One of these huge boulders, lying beside a stone wall, fell and crushed the entire cottage in which a young couple were enjoying their wedding night.

Opposite **Eilean Dubh Cruinn** (G. – round black island) the road swings across country to Loch Scridain (G. – loch of the screes) cutting off the wild and trackless Ardmeanach peninsula. A 2km path from the turn-off to Balmeanach farm leads to the renowned **Mackinnon's Cave**, which was visited by Dr Johnson [NM440323]. Some 30m high and probably the largest cave in the Hebrides, it can only be entered at low tide. As usual there is the well-worn legend of a piper and his dog entering the cave. The variation on this occasion is that a witch living in the cave killed the piper and the entire party which he was guiding through the cave to the other side of the peninsula. Only the piper's dog, scorched and hairless, appeared on the southern shore.

The most remote part of **Ardmeanach**, which Americans would call the Badlands but is known locally as the Wilderness, can be reached on foot from Balmeanach (a long and very strenuous walk) or partly by rough vehicle track from Tiroran above Loch Scridain followed by a 3km scramble with arrival timed for low water. The southern part belongs to the National Trust for Scotland and includes **MacCulloch's Tree**, a dramatic fifty-million-year-old fossil which is 12m high and a metre in diameter [NM402208]. Another lies toppled in a cave to the north. They can be located by two waterfalls on the cliff but ask for directions at Burg Farm. This area has a marvellous selection of wildlife and was given to the Trust in 1932 by A Campbell Blair of Dolgellau.

East of Tioran, at the head of the loch, the road meets the main Craignure-Fionnphort road which is the route to Iona.

Mull has many attractions for the sportsman

whether in hunting, fishing, shooting, pony trekking, riding, camping, exploring caves, wildlife expeditions or hill-walking. For the mountaineer, apart from the 'Munro' – Ben More (966m), and numerous sea-cliffs, there are also two 'Corbetts': Beinn Talaidh (G. – hill of Valhalla or allurement) (761m) and Dùn da Ghaoithe [doo:n da: goo-i] (G. – castle of the winds) (766m).

South of Craignure and Duart Castle a road runs down to the old ferry terminal at Grass Point by shallow **Loch Don**. This was the ancient pilgrims' way to Iona and also the drove road when island cattle were shipped from here to the mainland. On the coast between it and Loch Spelve is Port Donain, a small cove with a cave [NM741293] and chambered cairns above it.

Loch Spelve has two arms, a few skerries, and one islet, **Eilean Amalaig**. A minor road runs along the north side through mixed woodland and rhododendrons beneath the basalt heights of Creach Beinn and on past little Loch Uisg to Lochbuie. This valley is exceptionally fertile and used to be called the Garden of Mull. The sturdy tower of **Moy Castle** – near Mull's only example of a stone circle [NM618251] – overlooks the loch. The castle (now closed to the public) was built above a natural spring in the 14th century by the MacLaines of Lochbuie. It has a bottle-necked dungeon filled with water and a stone in the centre on which the prisoner sat in darkness.

The brother-in-law of the 21st MacLean of Duart was Solicitor General in 1894–5 and the tiny island east of the mouth of Loch Buie is named after him – **Frank Lockwood's Island**. Lord Lovat's bay at the entrance to Loch Buie has Lord Lovat's cave close north of it. On the east side of the loch is a medieval chapel reconstructed as a mausoleum for the MacLaines in 1864 [NM626236] and on the west side an 8km coastal path leads to Carsaig.

The main road runs beside the Lussa River in Glen More through a barren, glaciated landscape until one sees conifer forests on the way down to the head of Loch Scridain. At **Pennyghael** a cairn commemorates the Beatons, hereditary doctors to the Lords of the Isles. A minor road south meets the coast at the fertile farmland of **Carsaig**. This was a setting for the film *I Know Where I'm Going* which also featured the Corryvreckan whirlpool off Jura (No.2.5). Yachts find shelter behind the islet Gamhnach Mhór (G. – big cow) in Carsaig Bay. A long coastal walk to the west of Carsaig leads first to the **Nun's Cave** (G. – Uamh nan Cailleach) [NM524205], which has early Christian carvings and where nuns from Iona are reputed to have hidden during the Reformation. This is where sandstone was quarried in 1500 for dressing Iona Abbey and the masons' bankers with chips of stone beside them are still lying around. A further two hours walk beyond, at Malcolm's Point, are the spectacular rock formations of the Carsaig Arches [NM494185], one in the form of a very high pyramidal mass with arches in the middle and a solitary basaltic column on top. The arches are eroded sea-caves adjoining 220m-high cliffs lined with huge basalt columns.

The Ross of Mull is primeval moorland with scattered clumps of trees and a coast with many fine beaches and bays. **Bunessan** (G. – foot of the waterfall) on Loch na Làthaich provides a busy anchorage for fishing boats behind the shelter of **Eilean Bàn** (G. – pale island). The road finishes at **Fionnphort** [fina:foart] (G. – fair or holy port), the ferry terminal for Iona. Close by to the north, **Bull Hole** has a derelict stone jetty [NM301241] which was in use until the late 19th century, when the beautiful pink granite was quarried here for the construction of the Holburn Viaduct, Blackfriars Bridge and the Albert Memorial in London. The stone was also used for several lighthouses.

At the southern corner of the Sound of Iona, the tidal island of **Erraid** is accessible across the sands for two hours at low water. It featured in Robert Louis Stevenson's book, *Kidnapped*, which he is said to have written when staying on the island. This was the lighthouse shore station for **Dubh Artach** and **Skerryvore** until 1967 and the iron observatory at the summit of Crioc Mor {NM296203] was once used for signalling to the lighthouses. Erraid is surrounded by rocks and islets, including **Eilean Ghòmain**, **Eilean nam Muc**, **Eilean Chalmain**, **Eilean na Seamair** and, of course, the inevitable **Eilean Dubh** (two of them!).

South of Erraid lie the infamous **Torran Rocks** (G. *torrunn* – loud murmuring or thunder), which are scattered over a wide area like dragons' teeth. They lurk menacingly just beneath the surface, occasionally showing themselves in a froth of white spittle.

Access: Frequent vehicle ferries: Oban /Craignure: Lochaline /Fishnish: Kilchoan (Ardnamurchan) / Tobermory. All ferry information, 08000-66-

5000. Oban Tourist Information, 01631-563122. Tobermory Tourist Information, The Pier, 08452-255121. Island bus services, 01546-604360.

Anchorages:

1. Dòirlinn, Tobermory. Good anchorage in basin about 2c NW of the Narrows between Mull and Calve Island. Use anchor light.
2. Aros Bay, Tobermory. Far S corner of Tobermory harbour, by waterfall. Anchor between boathouse and fish farm in suitable depth.
3. Tobermory Bay. Busy, very popular anchorage, convenient for access to the town. Pontoons for approx 40 boats and 15-ton visitors' moorings (charged per night), or free anchorage in the area provided near the landing stage. Bottom can be foul in deeper water (20m) beyond the moorings. Exposed NE; swell after N'ly gales; otherwise protected.
4. Ardmore bay. Temp. anchorage W of Ardmore point, affords shelter from S winds.
5. Loch Mingary. Temporary anchorage in quiet conditions. Tricky but worthwhile.
6. Loch a' Chumhainn (Loch Cuan), between Rubha an Aird and Quinish point. Head dries out 9½c and both sides rocky and foul. Good shelter but a trap in onshore winds. Approach with care.
7. Calgary Bay. Temp. anchorage only suitable in N and E winds and when no onshore swell. Less attractive than Lochs Cuan and Mingary. Head dries out 2c. Keep 5c off coast to the N when approaching the bay and when rounding Rubha nan Oirean.
8. Port Rainich (56 31N 06 12W), behind Eilean Rainich reef, half-way down N side of Loch Tuath, about 7c beyond Traigh na Cille, the sandy bay at Kilninian and almost SSE of Torloisk House. Limited room but useful in N'lies.
9. Sound of Ulva (56 28.5N 06 08W), S of the ferry, WNW of Sgeir Beul a' Chaolais, can be squally. Alternatively, in settled weather, E of this anchorage in the bay on the Mull shore beyond the drying reef.
10. Scarisdale, Loch na Keal. Useful anchorage but submerged rocks to negotiate. Subject to squalls.
11. Dhiseig. Shore of Loch na Keal, SE of Eorsa. Temp. anchorage 5c ENE of the Dhiseig burn *(direct access to Ben More)*.
12. By Inch Kenneth. Approach with care. Temporary anchorage 4c SSW of Samalan Island in suitable depth. Exposed, subject to fierce squalls, holding poor.
13. Kilfinichen Bay, N side of Loch Scridain. Off burn at Tiroran House on W side of bay in 8–10m. Keep 2c clear of shore on approach.
14. Loch Beg at head of Loch Scridain is shallow but there is anchorage in 3.5m just within the entrance. Subject to swell and squalls.
15. Sgeir Alltach, S side of Loch Scridain. Good but restricted anchorage 1¾c SE of Sgeir Alltach, between Sgeir Chailleach and Sgeir na Rad. Careful attention to sailing directions required.
16. Bun an Leoib, on S shore of Loch Scridain entrance, E of Rubha Dubh. Anchor behind Sgeir Leathen and Sgeir Mor but not in N and NW winds as there is a heavy swell. Many drying rocks and reefs.
17. Loch na Làthaich (Bunessan). Well sheltered inlet on N side of Ross of Mull but busy and space restricted. Safest anchorage in this part of Mull. Visitors' moorings (pay at boatyard).
18. Bull Hole, between Eilean nam Ban and Ross of Mull. Good but restricted anchorage. Approach from S. Anchor off ruined pier in entrance channel avoiding water pipeline and ferry passage to night mooring. Alternatively, anchor between En Liath and En nam Ban.
19. Fionnphort. Occasional anchorage in suitable conditions midway between ferry jetty and entrance to Bull Hole, sand. Avoid obstructing ferry.
20. Tinker's Hole. Popular restricted anchorage between Eilean Dubh and W side of Erraid in Sound of Iona. Well sheltered. Alternative is pool 2c N of Tinker's Hole or temp. anchorage in 'David Balfour's Bay' to the E.
21. Ardalanish (56 16N 06 17W). Small inlet on W side of Rubh' Ardalanish, S coast of Ross of Mull. Restricted but attractive in settled weather. S side is steep-to. Sometimes subject to swell.
22. Carsaig Bay. Occasional anchorage close N of Gamhnach Mhór, a reef of islets opposite the pier or at a suitable depth off the beach in the bay.
23. Loch Buie, exposed and not safe except in fine weather.
24. Loch Spelve, E coast of Mull. Croggan pier, depths of 2.7m at head. Best anchorage is in bight on W side of head of N arm of the loch S of the Lussa River. Gusty in W'lies particularly in S arm of the loch.
25. Loch Don, narrow and shallow, with many rocks and extensive shoals but there is a sheltered pool within. The sailing instructions must be followed very carefully. Anchorage off pier is exposed.
26. Duart Bay. Temporary anchorage NW of castle, 5–6m, or well offshore opposite jetty on N shore in 4–6m (*Visit to Castle or Torosay House*).
27. Craignure bay, exposed N to NE. Anchor NW of ferry pier, or in S corner of bay in 4–5m. Avoid shoal water, moorings and ferry approach.
28. Scallastle Bay (56 29N 05 44W). Good anchorage in offshore winds but approach requires care.
29. Fishnish bay. Occasional anchorage near head of bay on 6m line. Head dries off 3c.

30. Salen (56 31N 05 57W). Approach with caution. Anchor SW of W'most ruined pier in 4m.
31. Aros Bay. Good anchorage if directions followed.

3.4 Inch Kenneth

Kenneth's island, named after Cainnech, follower of St Columba.

OS Maps: 1:50000 Sheet 47 1:25000 Sheet 375
Admiralty Charts: 1:25000 No.2652 or No.2771

Area: 55ha (136 acres)
Height: 49m (161 ft)

Owner: Owned for a time by Sir Harold Boulton, composer of 'The Skye Boat Song'. Bought by Lord Redesdale (David Mitford) in 1938 for £900 and remained the property of various members of the Mitford family until 1966. Present owner is Dr Andrew D Barlow of Kensington, London.

Population: 1841– no separate Census record. 1881–8. 1891–2. 1931–10. 1961–13. 1971–2. 1991–0. 2001–0.

Geology: Different from Mull as the rocks are sedimentary. Triassic conglomerates and limestone outcrops have been eroded and broken down into good soil.

History: Named after Kenneth, contemporary of St Columba, who is said to have saved the great man from drowning solely through the power of prayer. Kenneth became abbot of Achabo, in Ireland, and died in 600. The Prioress of Iona owned the island in 1569. It was considered second only to Iona in ecclesiastical importance.

Inch Kenneth achieved some fame, or notoriety, during the Second World War from its connection with the oddly dysfunctional Mitford family (related to the Churchills). It was purchased by David Mitford (Lord Redesdale) in 1938 when he, his wife Sydney and daughter Unity went to see it 'and loved it'. They had five other daughters and one son, Tom. Nancy, the author, and her sisters, Pamela, Jessica, and Deborah (Duchess of Devonshire) were bitingly witty but less concerned with politics. But their parents, Lord and Lady Redesdale, and siblings, Diana and Unity, and Tom for a time, were serious followers of the Fascist movement and great admirers of Hitler. Diana married Sir Oswald Mosley (the British Fascist leader and one-time Labour MP) in Germany in 1936. She was arrested and imprisoned in Holloway during the war.

Unity Valkyrie Mitford was a large and rather sulky girl, twice expelled from school – an exhibitionist with a coarse sense of humour. She idolised Hitler, followed him around and met him at last in 1935. Hitler was flattered by her attention and she spent many happy hours with him drawing up lists of Britons who would either cooperate or be shot. Hitler's entourage did not like her and called her 'Mitfahrt' (fellow traveller). When Britain eventually declared war on Germany Unity was so devastated that she shot herself in the head with a small silver pistol which Hitler had given her at the Nazi Nuremberg Rally. The bullet lodged in her brain and partially paralysed her. She returned to Britain, incontinent and brain-damaged. Inch Kenneth was listed as a wartime 'protected zone' requiring a special pass. David, who had repudiated Fascism at

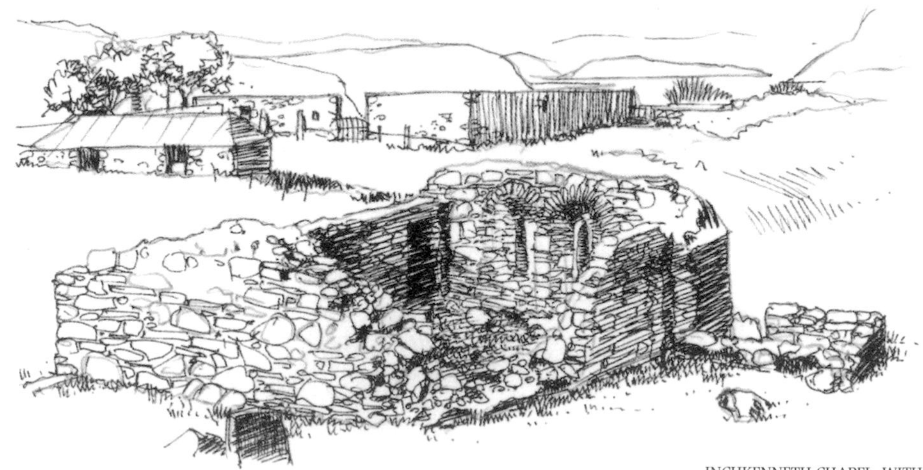

INCHKENNETH CHAPEL, WITH EORSA IN VIEW

the outbreak of war, was given clearance and spent six months each year living there. Unity, on the other hand, was originally denied a pass due to her political activities. Later, however, in 1944 she spent some time on Inch Kenneth improvising religious services in the ruined chapel and planning her own funeral. She died in Oban Cottage Hospital in 1948 of meningitis.

In 1945 David Mitford was in failing health so he made over the deeds of Inch Kenneth to Tom, his only son. Soon after this, Tom, who was serving in the Far East, was killed and David was astonished to find that under Scots Law, as he had died intestate, it was Tom's sisters who inherited the island. (Under English law his next of kin, i.e. parents, would have regained the title.) By this

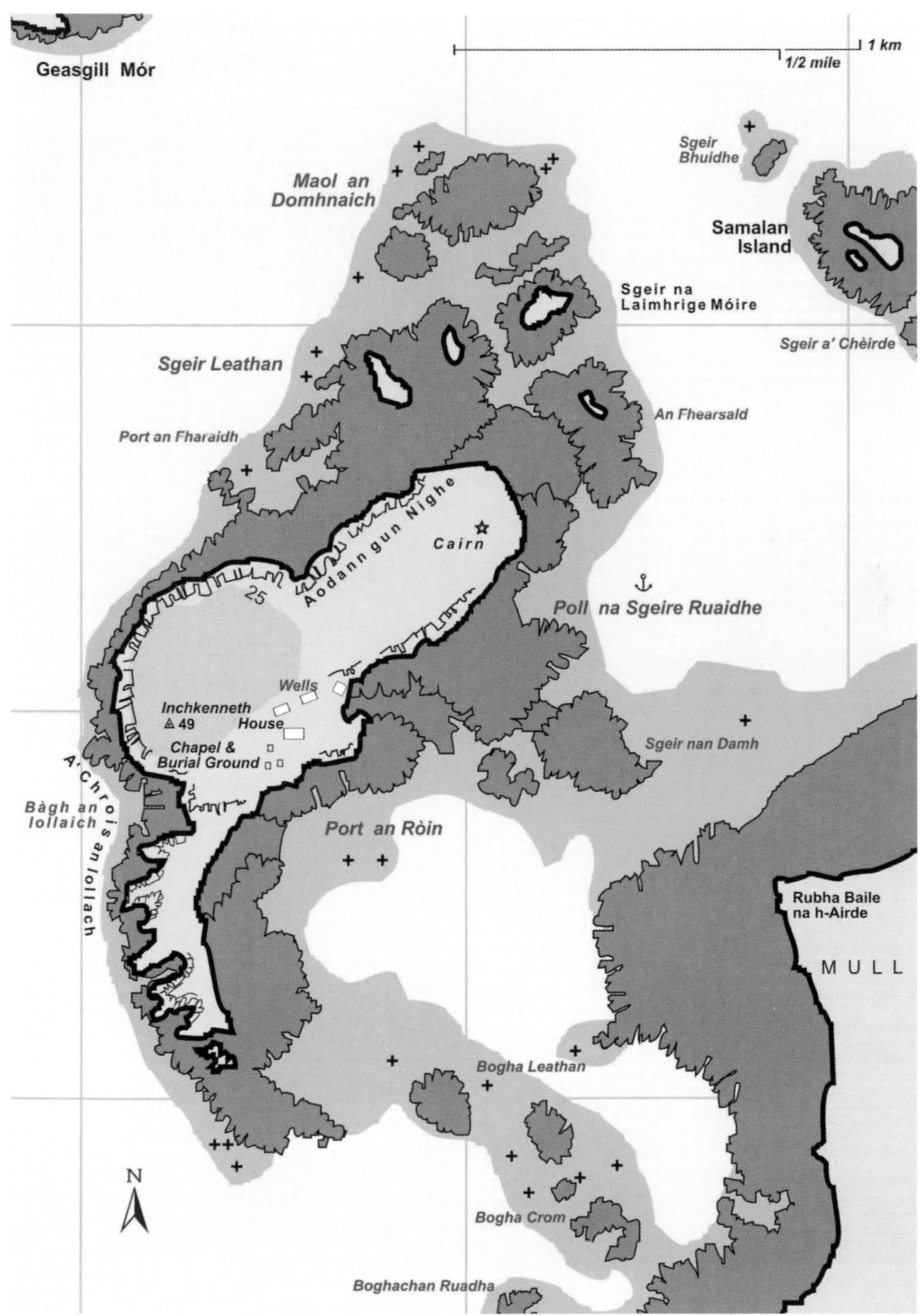

time, however, David had become a semi-recluse in Northumberland and had separated from Sydney and it was she who now spent more and more time on the island. 'The house is absolutely hideous,' she said, 'but comfortable inside. . . and the sea and rocks are so lovely.' She had a cook, housemaid, boatman, and three farm hands. She used no napkins (to economise) but ordered all her groceries from Harrods in London, sent them all her dirty washing to be laundered and dirty bank notes to be exchanged for crisp new ones.

Jessica, spitefully, tried to give her share of Inch Kenneth to the Communist Party – to 'compensate' for her family's Fascist leanings – but the Communist Party were not interested. Eventually, however she bought out her sister's shares so that their mother could live out her days on the island.

Sydney died in 1963 and Jessica sold Inch Kenneth in 1966.

Wildlife: The Statistical Account of 1845 reports that this was one of the main centres for kelp burning as the alkaline content of the ash was very high. The best seaweed was not the tangle, although this added bulk, but 'button wrack' which was prolific in the area.

In 1569 Dean Munro reported that rabbits were present in great numbers on Inch Kenneth so they have a long history here.

The island is popular with barnacle geese in winter. Shag, eider, red-breasted merganser, oystercatcher, curlew, redshank, razorbill and black guillemot are resident here all year round.

* * *

Like Tiree, **INCH KENNETH** is exceptionally fertile, and it once provided grain for the monks of Iona. There is a fine 19th-century three-storey mansion house and an attractive single-storey farmhouse.

Boswell and Johnson were entertained by Sir Alan Maclean, 22nd Chief of Duart, in the low-roofed stone building which is still standing but no longer occupied. Boswell considered Inch Kenneth 'a pretty little island'.

There is no trace now of the original monastery but there is an ancient ruined chapel of the First Pointed period, 12m x 6m (40' x 20'), with deeply splayed lancet windows [NM437354]. There are also the remains of a Celtic cross and many sculptured tombstones including that of Sir Alan Maclean who was Dr Johnson's host. It is the most elaborately carved slab in the Mull area and shows the Chief in armour with his dog at his feet. Many of the tombs are of Highland chiefs who were buried here when conditions were too wild to allow a crossing to Iona.

All the buildings are grouped centrally on the east side of the island.

Much of the island's economy is now provided by fish farming. Landing can be a problem unless the weather conditions are suitable as there is no ideal anchorage. The normal approach is close by the **Geasgill Islands**, avoiding **Maol an Domhnaich** (G. – Sunday rock, – but see No.7.5 Muldoanich derivation), and then between **Samalan Island** and **Sgeir na Laimhrige Móire** (G. – the rock of Mary's landing place). Inch Kenneth is encircled by wide areas of drying rocks, islets, reefs and skerries except for the west side where there is a 25m-high cliff above tumbled boulders. Just north of this is a low escarpment called **Aodann gun Nighe** (G. – the dirty face).

* * *

Access: No regular access. The owner's manager on Mull has private transport but try Turus Mara, Dervaig, Mull, 0800-085-8786.

Anchorages:

1. Red Skerry Pool (Poll na Sgeire Ruaidhe). E and N sides of the island are foul so approach with caution from N on given bearings. Anchor in bay on E side of island in 6–8m, holding poor. Subject to fierce squalls and landing can be tricky.
2. SE of Port an Ròin. Hazardous approach round the end of reef which extends SE of S extremity of island. Preferably only for shoal-draught vessels at mid-tide in quiet conditions.

3.5 Little Colonsay

(ON koln-øy – Columba's island) or (ON – Kolbein's island).

OS Maps: 1:50000 Sheet 47 1:25000 Sheet 374
Admiralty Chart: 1:25000 No.2652

Area: 88ha (217 acres)
Height: 61m (200 ft)
Owner: Lord Blakenham.

Population: 1841–16 (two households). 1881–0. 1891–2 (1 house). 1931–2. 1961–0.

1971–0. 1981–0. 1991–0. 2001–0.

Geology: Columnar basalt formations.

History: Between 1846 and 1851 Little Colonsay was cleared of its inhabitants by the owner F W Clark who also owned Ulva and Gometra (No.3.7). In the early 20th century the island was farmed by John McColum (known as 'Johnny Colonsay'). He had occupied the Victorian house on it for most of his life but he and his family were forced to abandon it because of a plague of rats.

Wildlife: Countless primroses, wild violets and celandine – no doubt due to the absence of sheep. A few seabirds nest on the cliffs and outcrops. We saw no wild goats but they were reported in the 1930s.

The anchorage on the north side of **LITTLE COLONSAY** is approached from the east through the channel between Sgaigein and **Garbh Eilean**, a tidal island south of Ulva. **Sgaigein** is a large

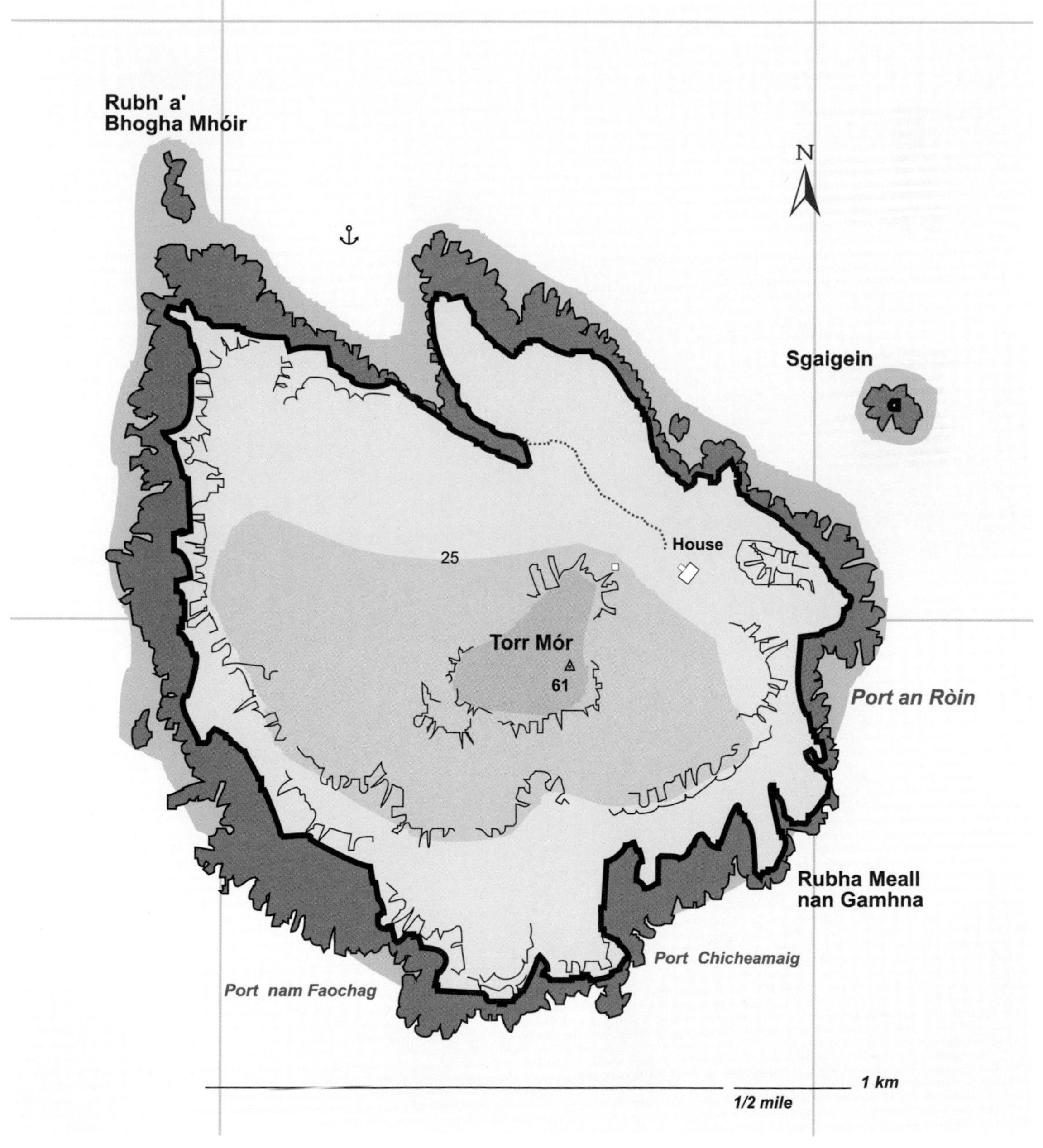

rock which only just shows at high water (0.6m high) and is about 1¾c north of the island. The householder keeps a lobster fishing boat on a private mooring. A path leads from the landing place through rocks covered with orange lichen. The lone house is surprisingly large and spacious with dormer windows and a slated roof. It is tucked into a hollow and protected from the prevailing sou'-westerlies by Torr Mór (G. – big hill), 61m high. It has recently been restored and an extensive water catchment system installed with storage tanks in a corrie on the hillside. Windbreaks of rowan tree saplings have also been planted but unfortunately many have not survived the gales.

This is a nice little island in a stunning setting with Ulva and Gometra close to the north, Inch Kenneth and the mountains of Mull to the east, **Erisgeir** islet and Iona to the south, and Staffa and the Treshnish Isles to the west. On a calm sunny day it is easy to be enthralled until you remember that the south-west is entirely exposed to the Atlantic with no sheltering land-mass between Little Colonsay and the shores of America.

The columnar basaltic rock formations of nearby Staffa are also to be found here, although in a considerably less dramatic form. The best examples are probably on the east side near **Rubha Meall nan Gamhna** (G. – humpy headland of the stirks). There are several small inlets called 'ports' in Gaelic, because it is possible to beach a small boat there. Two of them, **Port nam Faochag** (G. – port in the centre of the brow) directly south of Torr Mór, and **Port an Ròin** (G. – port of the seal) just north of Rubha Meall nam Gamhna may afford restricted anchorage in light northerlies but this has not been tested.

* * *

Access: Try Turus Mara, Dervaig, Mull, 0800-085-8786, or Ardnamurchan Charters, 01972-500208.

3.6 Eorsa

Derivation obscure. In the 18th century called Orsay. MacLean suggests (ON – Orri's island). Less likely, (ON Jorulf-øy – Jorulf's island) or a corruption of (G. àrsaidh – ancient).

OS Maps: 1:50000 Sheet 47 1:25000 Sheet 374 or 375
Admiralty Chart: 1:25000 No.2652

Area: 122ha (302 acres)
Height: 98m (321 ft)

Population: No Census returns and uninhabited.

Geology: Tertiary basalt bedrock.

History: Eorsa, together with Inch Kenneth, once belonged to the Priory of Iona.

Wildlife: The shores of Eorsa are sometimes the haunt of Great Northern, red-throated and black-throated divers. Very occasionally, velvet scoters may be seen and some Slavonian grebe can appear in early spring.

EORSA is a compact island in the centre of Loch na Keal (G. *loch na caol* – loch of the kyle or narrows). The west half of the island has a

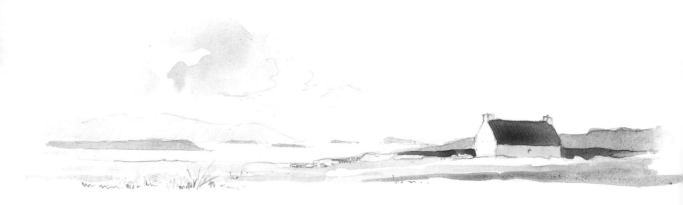

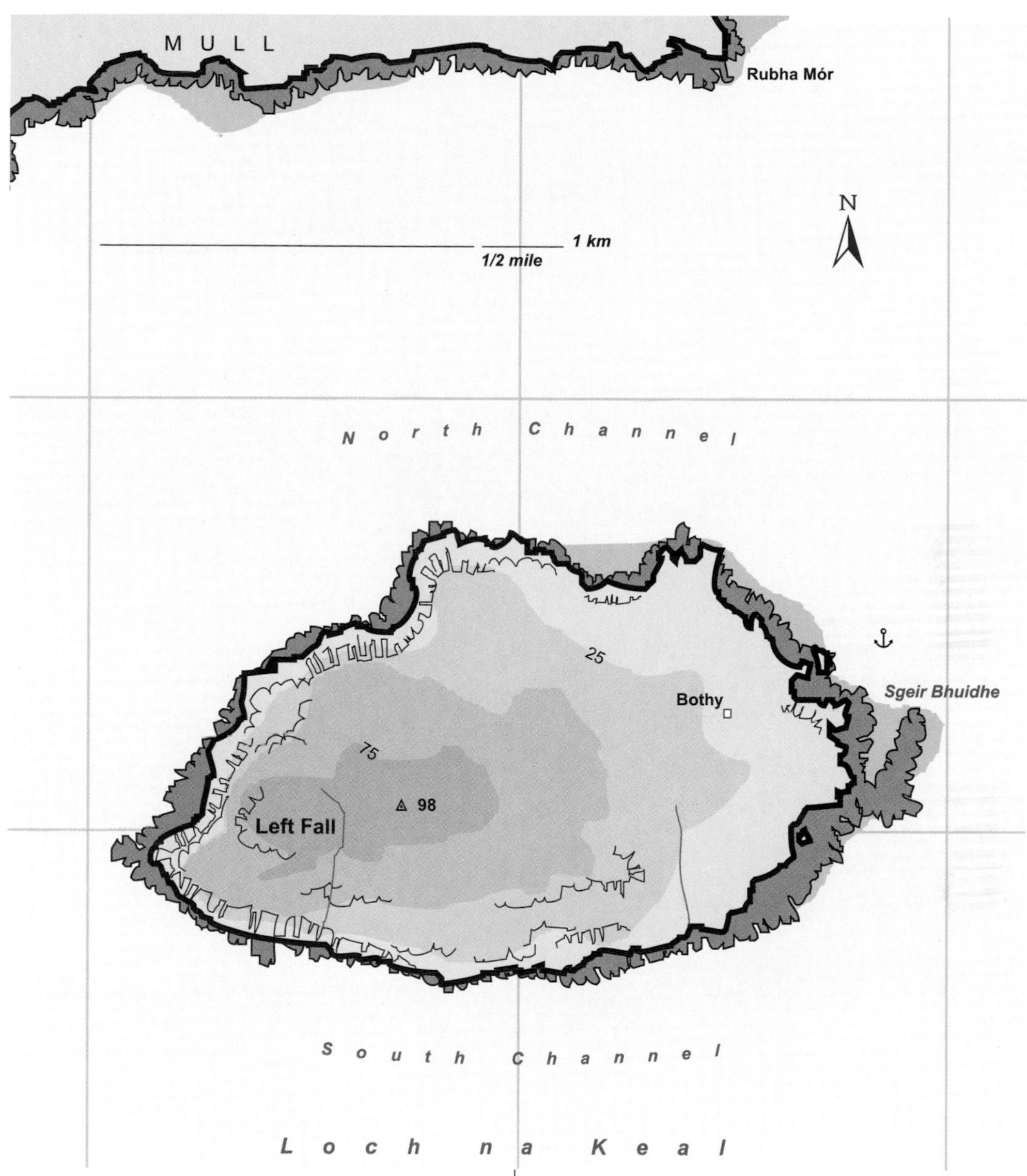

shoreline of high cliffs which were once frequented by wild goats but these moderate towards the east where a ruined bothy has a dramatic view of Ben More and the cliffs of Mull along the southern shore of the loch. There is the site of what may have been a hermit's monastic cell but there are no other features of note.

The island could provide reasonable grazing for sheep.

Eorsa served as a natural barrier across Loch na Keal during the First World War when the loch was used as a deep-water naval anchorage. During this period there were a number of visits by the Grand Fleet and it also provided a rendezvous for Atlantic convoys.

* * *

Access: Try Turus Mara, Dervaig, Mull, 0800-085-8786.

Anchorage:

1. Anchor ENE of the island on the 5m line. Loch na Keal is subject to squalls and W'lies cause a swell. Beware extensive reef S of anchorage.

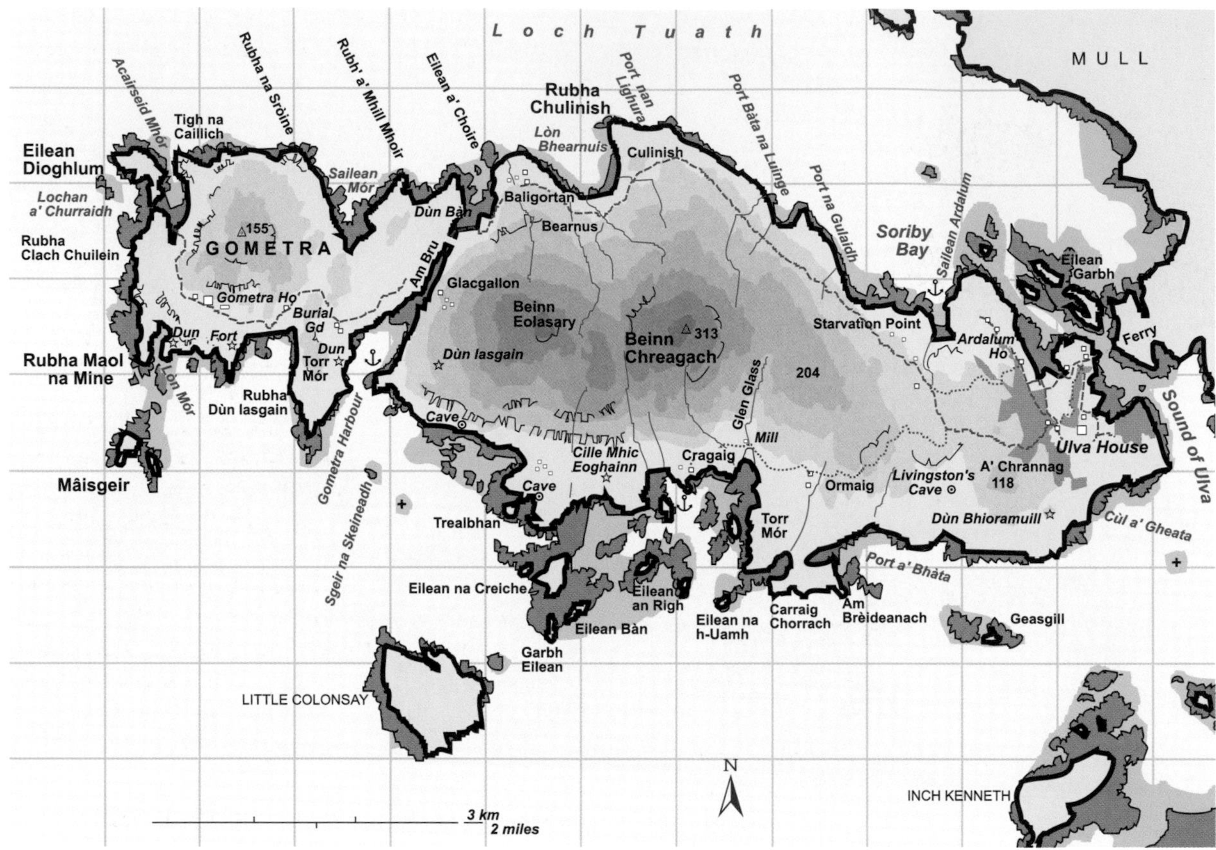

3.7 Ulva

(ON ulv-øy – wolf island) or (ON – Ulfr's island).

Gometra

Derivation obscure.

O S Maps: 1:50000 Sheet 47 1:25000 Sheet 374
Admiralty Chart: 1:25000 No.2652

Area: 2,415ha (5,968 acres)
Height: 313m (1,027 ft)

Owner: Owned by the Clark family from 1835 until sold to Edith Lady Congleton in 1945. Her daughter, the Hon Mrs Jean Howard, now owns Ulva and her son, Jamie Howard, manages the estate. They also owned Gometra but sold it in 1983. Gometra had previously belonged to Mrs Boo Henderson of Sussex who bought it from her great-aunt Lady Mary Evelyn Compton Vyner in 1947. Gometra was again put on the market in August 1991 for offers in the region of £650,000 and bought by Mr Roc Sandford, a close relation of Mrs Boo Henderson.

Population: 1841 – 570 for Ulva and 78 (15 households) for Gometra but in 1848 the potato famines followed by clearances reduced the population to 150.

	1881	1891	1931	1951	1961	1981	1991	2001
Ulva	53	46	25	19	33	13	30	16
G'etra	30	31	37	10	15	4	0	5
	83	77	62	29	48	17	30	21

Geology: Basalt domes reminiscent of the Pyramids and sea-cliffs of columnar basalt but generally a dark fine-grained igneous rock. The columnar formations on the south coast are particularly striking. There is no peat of any consequence.

History: Ulva belonged to the MacQuarries from the 10th century or earlier whereas Gometra belonged to the monastery of Iona before it came into the possession of the Duke of Argyll.

In 1543 Donald Dubh, aged sixty, recognised Chief of the Clan Donald and heir to the Lordship of the Isles, escaped from captivity in Edinburgh Castle after a total of fifty-five years' incarceration. This had been with the connivance of the First Earl of Argyll who was quick to exploit the situation after King James IV had decided to abolish the title of Lord of the Isles. It was the start of the Campbell takeover. The islanders rose to Donald's support – the Mackinnons of Mull, the MacLeans of Duart, the MacLeods from Lewis and Skye, the Macdonalds of Clanranald and the MacQuarries of Ulva. They held a Council at Finlaggan in Islay in 1545 in the traditional manner but Donald Dubh, weak from a lifetime in prison, died of a fever. He was duly buried with the honours of a Lord of the Isles and then the islesmen sadly returned home. 'It is no joy without Clan Donald, It is no strength to be without them...' said a Gaelic bard.

At one time the MacQuarries had a bright young piper called MacArthur who had been trained by the legendary MacCrimmons of Dunvegan in Skye. He founded his own piping college on Ulva which became renowned in its own right.

Lachlan McQuarrie had to sell Ulva to pay off his debts, just four years after he had entertained Dr Johnston and Boswell. It has been recorded that at this time every family on Ulva owned at least one boat and there was a surplus crop of potatoes for export, so the islanders themselves must at least have enjoyed, for a time, a reasonable standard of living. But with the increasing market value of kelp the islanders started neglecting their crofts and no longer used the seaweed for fertiliser.

In 1845 Ulva was again put up for sale and Gometra, which belonged to the MacDonalds of Staffa, was put up for sale simultaneously. Both islands were thus able to be purchased jointly by the notorious Mr Francis William Clark. It was also at this time that the kelp industry had foundered, followed by a severe potato blight on the impoverished land. Ulva was now seriously overpopulated with 604 starving crofters. In fairness, Clark tried various relief schemes before clearing the land and he did pay a proportion of the costs of emigration. But the heartless methods used by some of his employees, with or without his approval, are still remembered with disgust. In just four years – 1846 to 1851 – the new owner deported three-quarters of the total population. His factor and men turned some of the families out of their cottages without warning by setting fire to the thatch. They were not even given time to collect their few possessions and their livestock was forfeit.

Wildlife: A first impression of Ulva is of bracken galore and lots of rabbits but the island is in fact a feast of flora and fauna. There are plenty of mountain hares, red deer, seals, and an occasional otter, stoat and hedgehog. There are no foxes or adders. The island has a great variety of habitats for plant life and more than 500 recorded species.

Gometra has goats, a deer farm, and a small hardwood plantation on the east side.

Birdlife on both islands is varied, including buzzards, ravens, woodcock, snipe, occasional grouse and pheasant, common and Arctic tern, gannet, eider, oystercatcher, curlew, redshank and red-breasted merganser.

Ulva and Mull are the last refuges of the beautiful red and black Scotch burnet moth, which is now extinct elsewhere, and Ulva also is home to the exceptionally rare blue dragonfly, *Orthetrum coesilesceus*.

* * *

Dr Johnson and Boswell visited **ULVA** in October 1773. In Boswell's own words:

'. . .a servant was sent forward to the ferry, to secure the boat for us: but the boat was gone to the Ulva side, and the wind was so high that the people could not hear him call; and the night so dark that they could not see a signal. We should have been in a very bad situation, had there not fortunately been lying in the little sound of Ulva an Irish vessel. . . (which) ferried us over.

'M'Quarrie's house was mean; but we were agreeably surprised with the appearance of the master whom we found to be intelligent, polite and much a man of the world. Though his clan is not numerous, he is a very ancient Chief . . . He told us his family had possessed Ulva for nine hundred years; but I was distressed to hear that it was soon to be sold for payment of his debts.

'M'Quarrie insisted that the Mercheta Mulierum . . . did really mean the privilege which a lord of a manor had to have the first night of all his vassal's wives. Dr Johnson said the belief . . . was also held in England . . . by which the eldest child does not inherit, from a doubt of his being the son of the tenant. M'Quarrie told us that still on the marriage of each of his tenants, a sheep is due to him. I suppose Ulva is the only place where this custom remains.

'Being informed that there was nothing worthy of observation in Ulva, we took boat and proceeded to Inch Kenneth . . .'

There is actually a great deal 'worthy of observation' on these islands although possibly not to Boswell's taste. The MacQuarrie's 'mean' house was later rebuilt by the new owner to an Adam design and it was visited and praised by Sir Walter Scott. The present Ulva House stands in pleasant woodland on the site of the Adam masterpiece which unfortunately was destroyed by fire. Virtually all the present dwellings on Ulva are grouped at the east end of the island in the neighbourhood of the ferry and there is also a small chapel designed by Thomas Telford and built in 1827–28.

A rough farm road leads up through the trees by **A' Chrannag** (G. – the pulpit), a hill lying west of Ulva House. On the south side of the hill is a 'sea-cave' – now well-above sea-level – called **Livingston's Cave** which was occupied by prehistoric man more than 7000 years ago. The name of the cave is a reminder that the father and grandfather of the famous explorer lived in the cave while building their croft house nearby. This road leads along the north side overlooking Loch Tuath (G. – north loch) all the way to the causeway crossing **Am Bru** (G. – the gut), a narrow tidal channel, between Ulva and Gometra. **Beinn Chreagach** (G. – rocky mountain), the summit of Ulva and almost in the middle of the central ridge, is 313m (1027ft) high. Gometra's highest point which is in line with this ridge is 155m (508ft) high.

After the farm road has left the wooded area by Ulva House there is a track to the left which leads down to and along the south coast of Ulva. This passes a beautiful little ruined water mill with its lade connected to the burn tumbling down Glen Glass and the many sad ruins of the 'cleared' village of Cragaig. Some of the cottage doors still have their lintels in place. Beyond this point are standing stones beside the charming anchorage of Cragaig Bay, sheltered by tidal **Eilean Reilean** amid a peppering of skerries. A maze of sea-passages twist between the islets, **Eilean an Righ** (G. – royal island) and **Eilean na h-Uamha** (G. – cave island), and the many off-shore rocks. The track deteriorates further

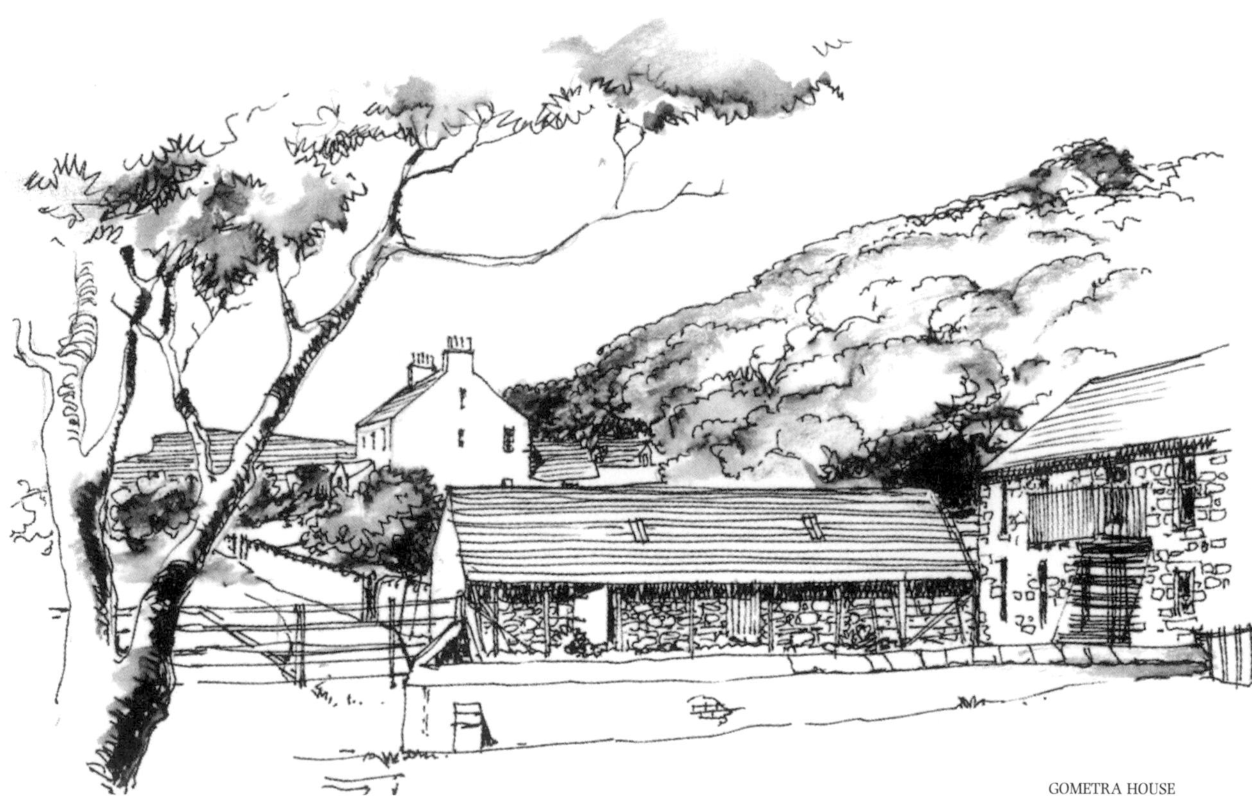

GOMETRA HOUSE

at this point but on the headland to the west are the remnants of **Cille Mhic Eoghainn**. A string of tidal islands, **Eilean na Creiche**, **Garbh Eilean**, and **Eilean Bàn**, form a natural breakwater for Cragaig Bay. In the west a dun on Ulva continues the chain of three duns stretching across Gometra.

General Lachlan MacQuarie (1761–1824), the 'father of Australia' was born on Ulva. He instituted liberal penal reforms in Australia while serving as governor of New South Wales. This made him so unpopular with the settlers that he was recalled. His mausoleum is at Gruline on Mull, by Loch na Keal.

Ulva was also the birthplace of some of the ancestors of the missionary and explorer, David Livingstone.

Thomas Campbell (1777–1844), in his famous poem 'Lord Ullin's Daughter', told the sad story of an eloping Chief of Ulva and his bride, who drowned when fleeing from her parents. They are reputed to be buried on the Mull shore in a grave between Oskamull Farm and Ulva Ferry. The channel at Ulva Ferry is very narrow and is even narrower where the islets **Eilean a' Chaolais** (G. – isle of the kyle) and **Eilean Garbh** restrict the passage, but it is navigable with care.

There is now a small tea room on Ulva – the Boathouse – which sells delicious fresh oysters from the home farm, and visitors are encouraged by an interpretive display to enjoy the island's many attractions with its beautiful walks and nature trails, 01688-500241.

* * *

GOMETRA was at one time, like Inch Kenneth, known as the granary of Iona. The land sheltering the tiny bay, Lòn Mór, in the south-west corner is still called Rhubha Maol na Mine (G. – flour-meal headland). The large low-lying skerry, **Mâisgeir** (ON – seagull skerry), is almost a continuation of this headland. There are the remains of at least three duns and signs of old settlements. A Roman coin was found here in 1958. Gometra House, with its six bedrooms, had been unoccupied since 1983 but it was renovated and reoccupied in 1993. It has extensive outbuildings and a walled garden. The old schoolhouse still stands near the shore and the most easterly of the cottages near Gometra House is called Teacher's Cottage. It has occasionally been occupied by a resident caretaker and his wife and family. The four dilapidated cottages beside Gometra harbour were formerly occupied by MacBrayne's Staffa boatmen, who used to row passengers out to the steamers which were unable to come alongside. Behind these cottages is an old graveyard.

Hugh Ruttledge, the Himalayan explorer, once had his home on Gometra.

A popular but shallow, confined, anchorage, Acairseid Mhór (G. – big anchorage) at the north-west corner has the never-failing attraction of a secret hideaway – a narrow passage past the rocks of tidal **Eilean Dioghlum** leads into an enclosed pool.

* * *

Access: Ulva Ferry – on request during normal hours except Saturdays, 01688-500226 or signal at pier. Crossing time about five minutes.

Anchorages:

1. Sound of Ulva (56 28.5N 06 08W), S of the ferry, WNW of Sgeir Beul a' Chaolais, can be squally in S'lies, 3m, sand and mud. Alternatively, in settled weather, E of this anchorage in the bay on the Mull shore beyond the drying reef.
2. Cragaig Bay. Pleasant sheltered (except for strong S'lies) anchorage NE of Little Colonsay among rocks and islets on S coast of Ulva.
3. Gometra Harbour. Sheltered anchorage between Ulva and Gometra entered from S. Well protected except S'ly gales. Anchor off E shore, mud and weed.
4. Acairseid Mhór, N coast of Gometra. A snug but very restricted anchorage behind Eilean Dioghalum. Anchor in 4m off E shore, sand and weed.
5. Soriby Bay (56 29N 06 11W), at SE of Loch Tuath. Good shelter except N'lies. Several hazards so follow sailing directions. Anchor at S end of W side of bay, or at inlet in SE corner.

3.8 Lunga

(ON langr-øy – longship island) or (G. long – ship, ON -øy – island). This is the largest of the Treshnish Isles, although Bac Mór, popularly known as the Dutchman's Cap, is much more prominent from a distance.

OS Maps: 1:50000 Sheet 46 or 48 1:25000 Sheet 374
1:10000 Sheet NM 24 SE
Admiralty Charts: 1:75000 No.2171 1:25000 No.2652

Area: 81ha (200 acres)
Height: 103m (338 ft)

Owner: The explorer and naturalist Col. Niall Rankin bought the Treshnish Isles in 1938. Put up for sale by Rankin family in 1994 for offers over £400,000. Sold in 2000.

Population: 1800 – about 20. Year-round occupation ended in 1824 when Donald Campbell and his family left the island but regular summer occupation continued until 1857. Uninhabited since then.

Geology: All the Treshnish group are of volcanic origin with the distinctive hat shape of Bac Mór being an ancient volcano with a lava platform brim. On Lunga the volcanic flows have eroded to form a lava plateau.

History: When the Lord of the Isles acquired the Treshnish Isles in 1354 they were on the frontier between the Nordreys and Sudreys – the Northern and Southern Isles. There is more Treshnish history on Lunga's northern neighbours than on Lunga itself. Cairn na Burgh More has the remains of a castle on the site of an earlier Norse building. The castle is thought to have belonged to the Lord of Lorn, Chief of the Clan MacDougall. Beside the fort are the remains of a small chapel and the Well of the Half Gallon. It is claimed that during a clan feud Maclean of Lochbuie was imprisoned in the castle on Cairn na Burgh More with only the ugliest woman in Mull for company but Lochbuie rose to the occasion and gave her a son who eventually won back his heritage. At

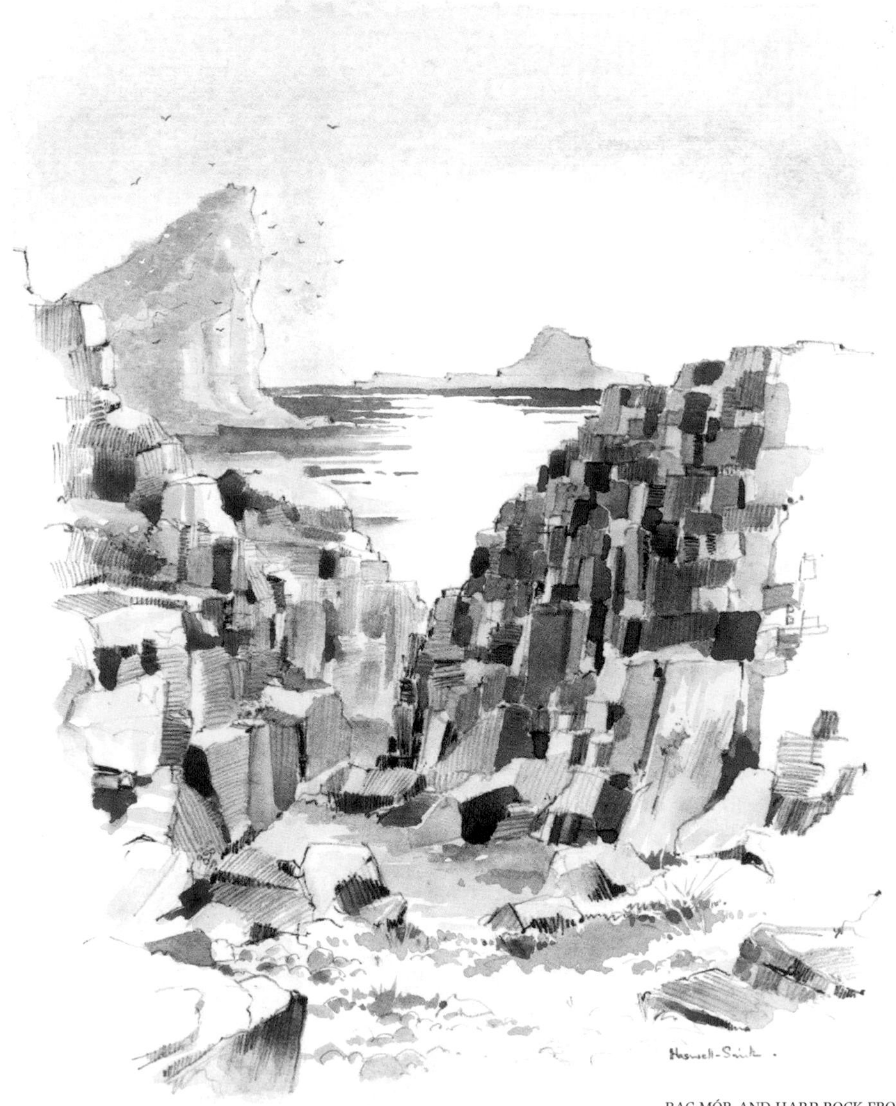

BAC MÓR AND HARP ROCK FROM CORRAN LUNGA

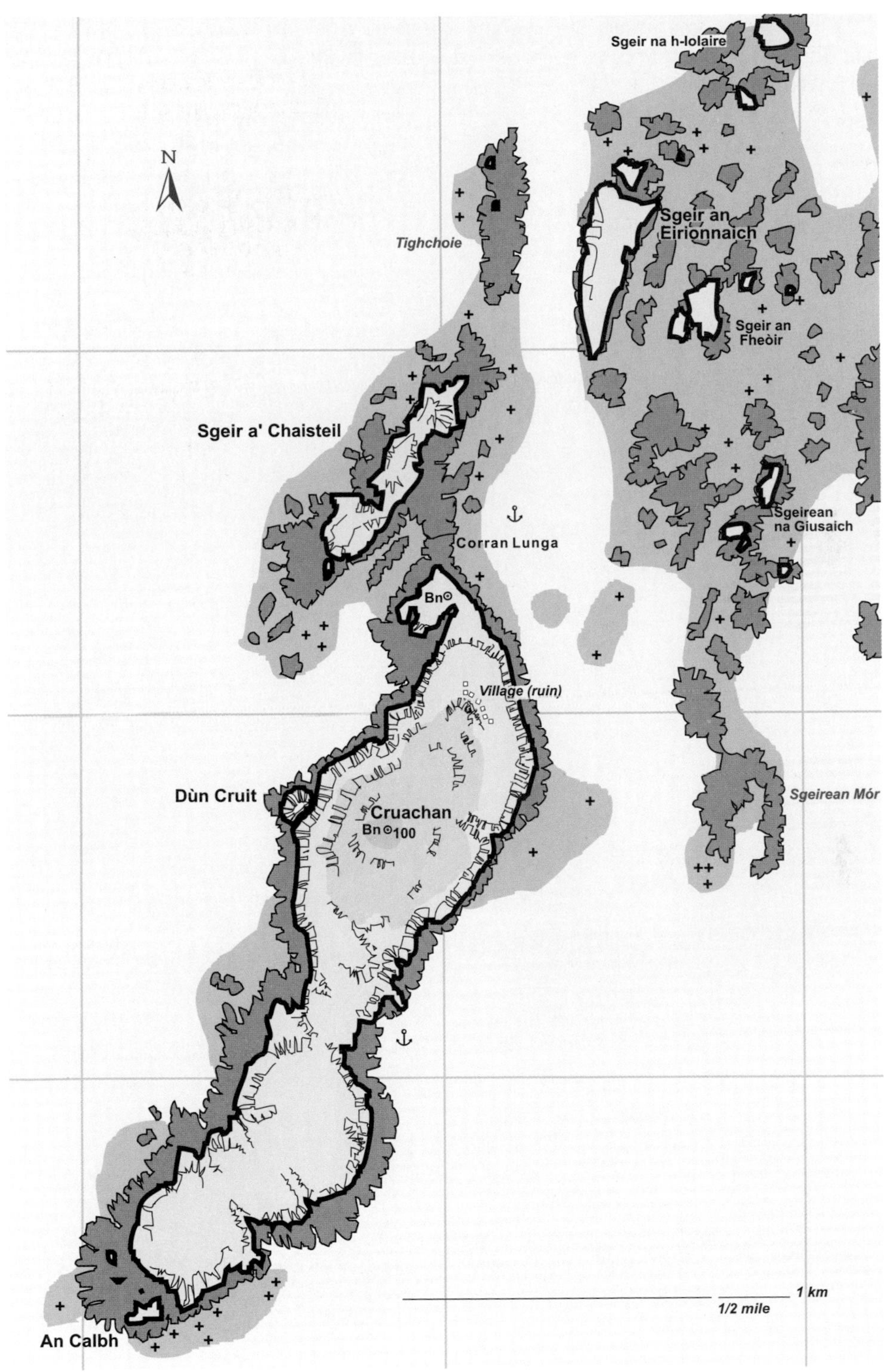

the Reformation of 1560 it is said that the monks of Iona buried their priceless library on Cairn na Burgh More for safety but it has never been recovered.

In 1680 after a prolonged attack by Argyll against the Macleans of Mull they retreated to the Treshnish Isles and held out for a long time but eventually had to surrender when Argyll obtained the King's support for his cause.

The ruins of a smaller castle or fort used during

the 1715 Jacobite rising are on the smaller island of Cairn na Burgh Beg. But on Lunga itself, below Cruachan's north slope, there are only the well-preserved walls of a small village of black houses last occupied in 1857.

Wildlife: Primroses, violets, birdsfoot trefoil, buttercups, daisies, bluebells, orchids, sea campion, sea pinks, wild rose, honeysuckle, brambles, scotch thistles, cotton grass, yellow flags, tormentil, silverweed, dandelion, and the scarce oyster-plant are all to be found on this delightful island. It is a designated Site of Special Scientific Interest.

This is a popular and important breeding ground for grey seals but only three land mammals have been recorded – mice, rabbits and domestic sheep. The mice may be descendants of the house mice that lived in the village in the mid-18th century according to Fraser Darling, who stayed for three months on Lunga in 1937. The mice ate his notes.

A thousand or more barnacle geese fly in each winter and there are hundreds of thrushes, blackbirds and starlings in the summer. Guillemot, razorbill and puffin breed on Lunga in large numbers, also fulmar, shag, kittiwake and other gulls. From May to September one can see Manx shearwater, storm petrel, gannet and Arctic skua and occasionally, pomarine, great skua, and great and sooty shearwater.

LUNGA has been described as 'a green jewel in a peacock sea', which sounds an extravagant description until one lands and realises the truth of it, for Lunga has a fresh and distinctive beauty all its own.

This is the largest island in the Treshnish group with a rounded hill called **Cruachan** (G. – conical hill) of 103m (338ft) and a magnificent view from its summit. To the south-west is the most conspicuous landmark of the Treshnish Isles, **Bac Mór** (G. – the big bank), or the Dutchman's Cap, which is an eroded volcanic cone encircled by a grassy rim of lava. It is only possible to land in the quietest of sea and weather and there is no safe anchorage either here or on nearby **Bac Beag**. This did not concern our ancestors for amid the wildflowers round the Dutchman's Cap can be found the remains of summer shielings.

Looking across the many rocks and skerries on Lunga's north-east side the smaller islands of **Fladda** (ON – flat island), **Cairn na Burgh Beag** and **Cairn na Burgh More** (G. *carn* – rock pile, ON *borv* – fort, – rock of the big fort) can be seen. Landing on both 'Carnburgs' is difficult and strong tidal streams don't help. It is easy to see how defensible they were. The larger Carnburg has its fortifications on the flat grassy top with a massive wall infilling a natural rock buttress on the perimeter. A further wall and stone gateway protects the castle and chapel.

On Lunga itself, **Dun Cruit** – Harp Rock – is a distinctive feature on the west side. It is a piece of sharply angled cliff, almost a stack, with a narrow chasm beside it into which the sea surges 30m (100') below. The shape is reminiscent of Boreray in the St Kilda group although the comparative scale is tiny and during the nesting season the rock disappears beneath a seething biomass of birds. The grassy summit and the edge of the surrounding cliffs are pitted with puffin burrows and the friendly, fearless, little birds will walk up to visitors, study them seriously, and pose for portraits.

In the past when sea-birds' eggs were an important item of diet, fishermen used to carry a mast up to Dun Cruit. They would lay this over the chasm and crawl across to collect the eggs and young birds (puffin mainly). There is only one record of a man falling to his death.

North of Lunga at the end of a drying spit of tumbled boulders – Corran Lunga – is **Sgeir a' Chaisteil** (G. – castle rock), a castle-shaped rock. This is a popular area for nesting gulls and oyster catchers. The boulder beach is also the most direct landing place for a dinghy from a yacht in the anchorage. Overlooking Corran Lunga there is a plateau beneath Cruachan with the ruined village on it and what appears to have been a walled vegetable patch. A fresh-water spring in fairly close proximity is quite difficult to find as it is under the shelter of a secluded overhanging rock on the hillside south of the village.

A rudimentary path runs round the entire island from Corran Lunga in the north to **An Calbh** (G. – the headland) at the southern extremity. On the south-eastern side it skirts the edge of a vertigo-inducing drop to the sea and rocks below. Almost central there is a cave, or 'gloup' [NM276415] which leads from a hollow to the western seashore, with rough steps leading into it. There are ferns in this mysterious, silent cavern which is shaped like a circular pit with a narrow dark passage through to the sea. The ravine nearby is called the Dorlinn

(G. – drying gravel beach). On the east side in the same area is a landing place for a dinghy.

Mountaineers may enjoy the challenge of a climb on Harp Rock. There is a possible line of ascent up a crack on the north side of the rock which is about 4m wide near the top, some 30m above the water. Remember, however, that this must never be attempted when the seabirds are breeding.

Access: Frequent summer trips: Gordon Grant Marine, Fionnphort, Mull, 01681-700338: Turus Mara, Dervaig, Mull, 0800-085-8786: or Ardnamurchan Charters, 01972-500208.

Anchorages:

1. E of Corran Lunga. The approach is from N or S but both directions require great caution. Anchor SE of Sgeir a' Chaisteil off the boulder beach in about 4m, sand. Subject to swell.
2. Below cleft on E side and off small boulder beach. Occasional anchorage in light W'lies, 10–15m.

3.9 Lismore

(G. lios-mór – big garden). As well as 'garden' the Gaelic word lios can also mean a residence, palace, fortified place or enclosure.

O S Maps: 1:50000 Sheet 49 1:25000 Sheet 376
Admiralty Charts: 1:25000 No.2378

Area: 2351ha (5809 acres)
Height: 127m (417 ft)

Population: 1798–900. 1841–1399. 1881–621. 1891–561. 1931–280. 1961–155. 1981–129. 1991–140. 2001–146.

Owner: The Duke of Argyll is the main landowner.

Geology: Mainly Dalradian limestone. Until the Second World War this was quarried at An Sàilein, a cove on the west coast. Lismore soil is exceptionally fertile.

History: There are a number of duns, forts and cairns which testify to the long period of settlement on Lismore.

St Moluag was an Irish contemporary of St Columba. For many centuries after he founded his monastery here in 561–564 the island was an ecclesiastical centre. About the year 1200 John the Englishman, Bishop of Dunkeld and Argyll, appealed to the Pope to disjoin the Argyll see because he was unable to learn to speak Gaelic. The Pope complied and Lismore was chosen as the seat of a separate diocese of Argyll and continued so until 1507 when the centre moved to Saddell in Kintyre. The bishops were called *Episcopi Lismorenses*. A manuscript collection of Gaelic and English poems which are of value as a guide to the works of Ossian, the *Book of the Dean of Lismore*, was compiled here in the 15th century.

Wildlife: There are many fine trees and shelter belts, mainly sycamore, ash, lime and chestnut, but little natural woodland although in 1596 the whole island was very thickly forested with oak. Thanks to the rich soil, wildflowers grow to larger

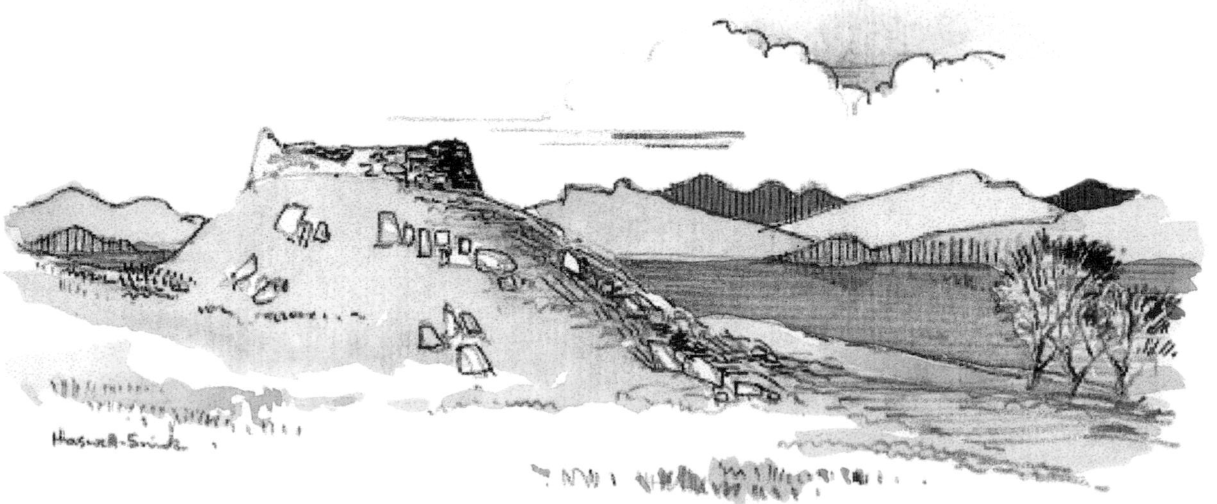

TIREFORE BROCH GUARDS THE LYNN OF LORN

than normal proportions; field gentians, rock rose (*Helianthemum*), mimulus, tutsan, ivy-leaved toadflax, wild orchids, yellow monkey-flower, cranesbill, brooklimes, water mints and speedwells are all to be found.

There are gulleries on the islets, Eilean nan Gamhna, and linked Eilean na Cloiche and Eilean Dubh in the Lynn of Lorn.

* * *

For delightful walking country **LISMORE** is supreme – a long narrow island with an undulating landscape of fertile soil in shallow longitudinal valleys. The highest hill is **Barr**

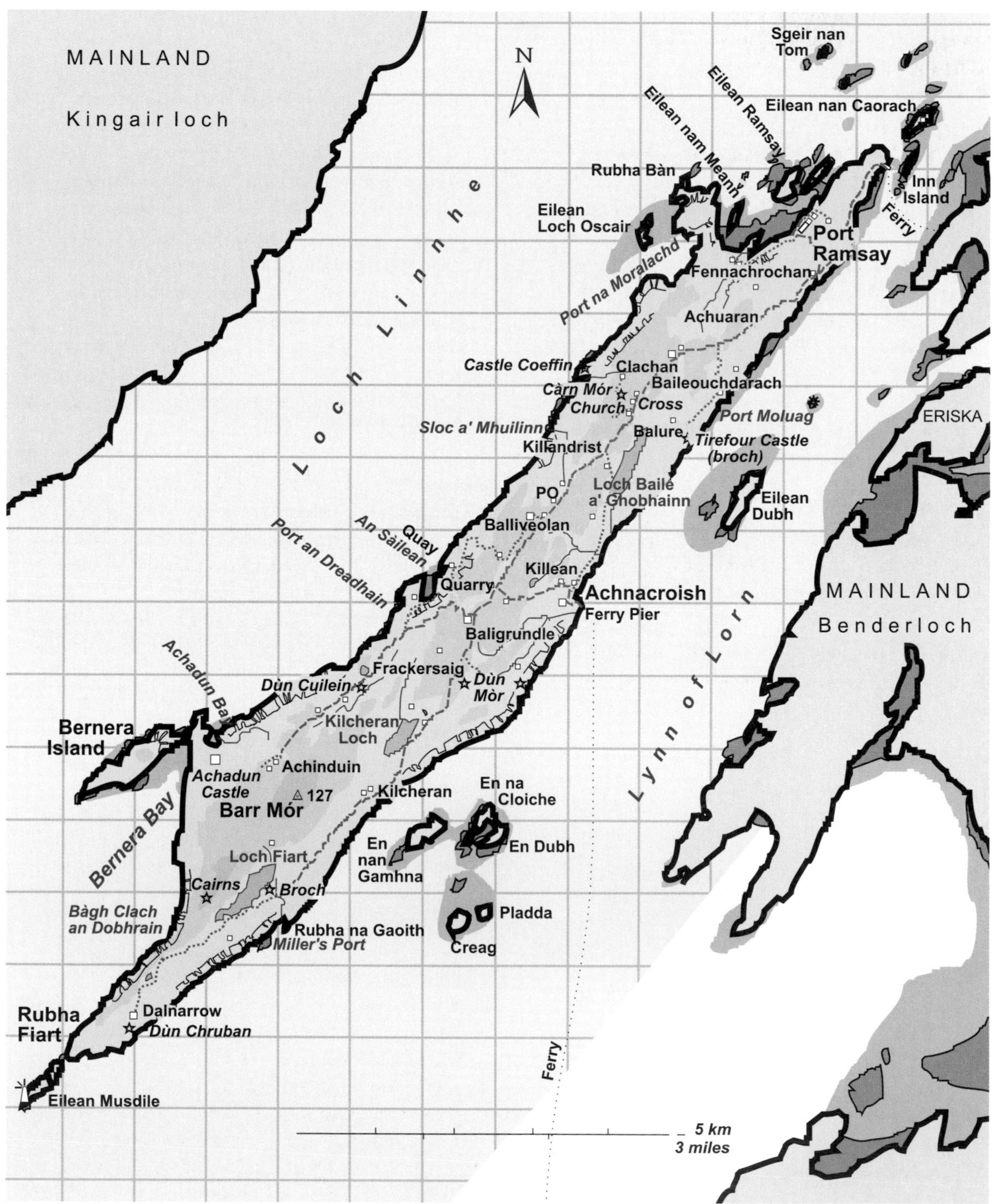

Mór (G. – big tip), a modest 127m, but right in the centre of the southern area with a stunning panoramic view from its summit – north to the mountains of Ardgour, Lochaber with Ben Nevis to the north-east, Port Appin and Lochs Creran and Etive to the east, Oban, Kerrera and the Firth of Lorn to the south, Duart Castle and Mull to the south-west and the mountains of Morvern to the west. The walk along the ridge, over the summit of Barr Mór and down by the reed-fringed lochan to the south must be one of the finest walks in Scotland with views which are unequalled anywhere.

The lighthouse on **Eilean Musdile** at the southern extremity was built by Alan Stevenson.

Lime was quarried on the west coast and lime kilns and quarrymen's cottages can still be seen on **Eilean nan Caorach** (G. – sheep island) among the skerries at the extreme north end opposite Port Appin and alongside **Inn Island** (G. ?*innis* – island). The boats carrying the lime operated out of Port Ramsay in the north. This sheltered anchorage between **Eilean Ramsay** and **Eilean nam Meann** (G. – kid island) is now used as an overnight stop by the occasional workboat from the giant quarry at Glensanda on the Morvern coast opposite Lismore. To the north is **Eilean Gainimh** (G. – island of fine sand) and **Eilean Glas** (G. – grey island). Port Ramsay is overlooked by a neat row of lime-burners' cottages most of which are now holiday homes.

The main road runs down the spine of the island with connections to the crofts and farms. In the 18th century the main crops were oats and barley but nowadays cattle and sheep are more popular. Most of the dwellings are in the north. The ruin of a tall galleried broch called Tirefour Castle, about 4km from the north-east end of Lismore, lies on the summit of a 50m-high grassy knoll close to the east coast [NM867429].

Almost opposite Tirefour, on the north-west coast, **Coeffin Castle**, a ruined 13th-century structure, was probably built by the MacDougalls of Lorn on the site of a Viking fortress [NM853437]. The MacDougalls were defeated by Robert the Bruce. There is an ancient tidal fish trap on the shore below the castle and above it are the remains of the largest cairn in Argyll [NM859435].

The ferry pier is at **Achnacroish**, near the centre of the east coast where there is a general store and a junior school. Lismore has no mains water supply. All the water comes from wells and springs and these can run dry at times.

The disused lime quarry at An Sàilein (G. – the creek), across the island from Achnacroish, is sadly deserted today with its ivy-covered kilns and roofless cottages. Carthorses from far afield used to be landed at the old quay as the Lismore men were noted for their ability to break them in.

Much of the shoreline is low sea cliffs with a few pleasant shingle beaches. The cliffs in the south-east opposite Eilean na Cloiche are only some 25m high yet they can present a severe challenge for mountaineers. **Eilean na Cloiche** (G. – island of the stone) is a boldly shaped rock rising almost straight out of the sea for about 21m with **Eilean nan Gamhna** alongside and a dumbbell-shaped islet formed by linked **Pladda** and **Creag**. **Eilean Dubh**, further north in the centre of the Lynn of Lorn is worth a visit but not for climbing as it is very loose rubble.

The man who built the great folly on the hill above Oban, John Stuart McCaig, was born on Lismore. He was a banker, essayist and art critic.

Bernera on the west coast can be reached at low water and was once known as Bernera of the Noble Yew, an ancient tree under which St Columba was said to have preached. This giant yew was felled in 1850 to make a staircase in Lochnell Castle on the mainland and traces of the small chapel and well have almost disappeared [NM795392]. **Achadun Castle**, the so-called Bishop's Castle, overlooks Bernera [NM804393].

The bishop lived at some distance from the small cathedral which was founded at the start of the 13th century on the ancient monastic site known as **Kilmoluaig** (G. – St Moluag's cell or church). It is on the main road near Clachan [NM860434]. Unfortunately there are few remains of the cathedral which was burned during the Reformation but in 1749 the walls of the cathedral choir were reduced in height and roofed to create the present tiny parish church – one of the earliest parish churches still in use. There are some fine medieval tombstones in the graveyard which is also reputed to be the burial site of St Moluag (523-592). **Eilean Loch Oscair** is in the bay to the north.

The story goes that two competitive saints, Moluag and Columba, had a boat race across the Lynn of Lorn after agreeing that the first to touch Lismore would be entitled to found his monastery on the island. Moluag realised at the last minute that he would not reach the land first so he cut off his finger and threw it ashore. It landed on the beach just north of the broch at Tirefour. This gained him the title and he duly founded his monastery in 564AD. His pastoral staff, a thorn stick nearly one metre long, is still held by the Livingstones of Bachuil, hereditary keepers for the parish.

Access: Two ferries serve the island: Port Appin is passenger only, crossing time 10 minutes, 01631-562125: Oban, Mon–Sat, car ferry, crossing time 50 minutes, 08000-66-5000.

Anchorages:

1. Port Ramsay, close E of Eilean nam Meann at N end of Lismore, a well-sheltered anchorage, bottom sand and shells. Use the north approach.
2. Port na Moralachd, at NW corner, reasonable shelter except for winds SW-W which can cause a swell. Anchor close in at S side of the bay. Only approach is from SW
3. An Sàilein, middle of W coast. Shallow inlet. Moderate draught in neaps or small craft able to take the ground. Obstructed by fish farm.
4. Achadun Bay, occasional anchorage NE of Bernera in E'ly winds.
5. Bernera Bay, by the SE side of Bernera Island, occasional anchorage in N'ly winds. Keep near the E shore to avoid rocks 1c from SE side of Bernera.
6. Achnacroish is the Oban ferry terminal; a stone causeway and pier extend from the shore; least depth of 3m alongside the pier.

3.10 Tiree

[tY-ree or tseeree] (G. tir iodh – land of corn). Watson disputes this derivation and suggests the name may be pre-Celtic.

O S Maps: 1:50000 Sheet 46 1:25000 Sheet 372
Admiralty Charts: 1:100000 No.1778 Sound of Gunna 1:25000 No.2475

Area: 7834ha (19358 acres)
Height: 141m (462 ft)

Owner: The Duke of Argyll owns most of the island.

Population: 1755–2200. 1794–2555. 1830–4450. 1841–4391 (805 houses). 1881–2730. 1891–2449 (537 houses).1931–1448. 1961–993. 1981–757. 1991–768. 2001–770.

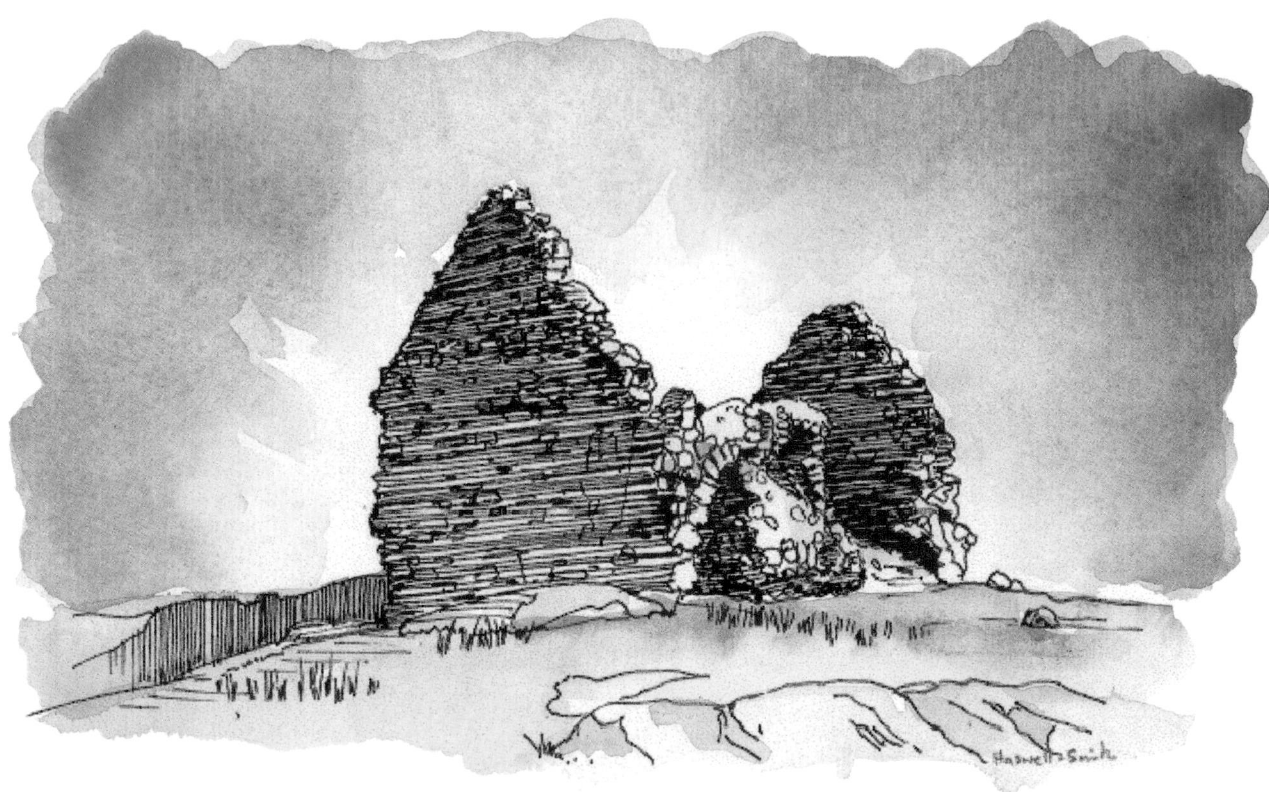

THE MEDIEVAL CHAPEL AT KIRKAPOL BESIDE THE LONG BEACH, TRÁIGH MHÓR

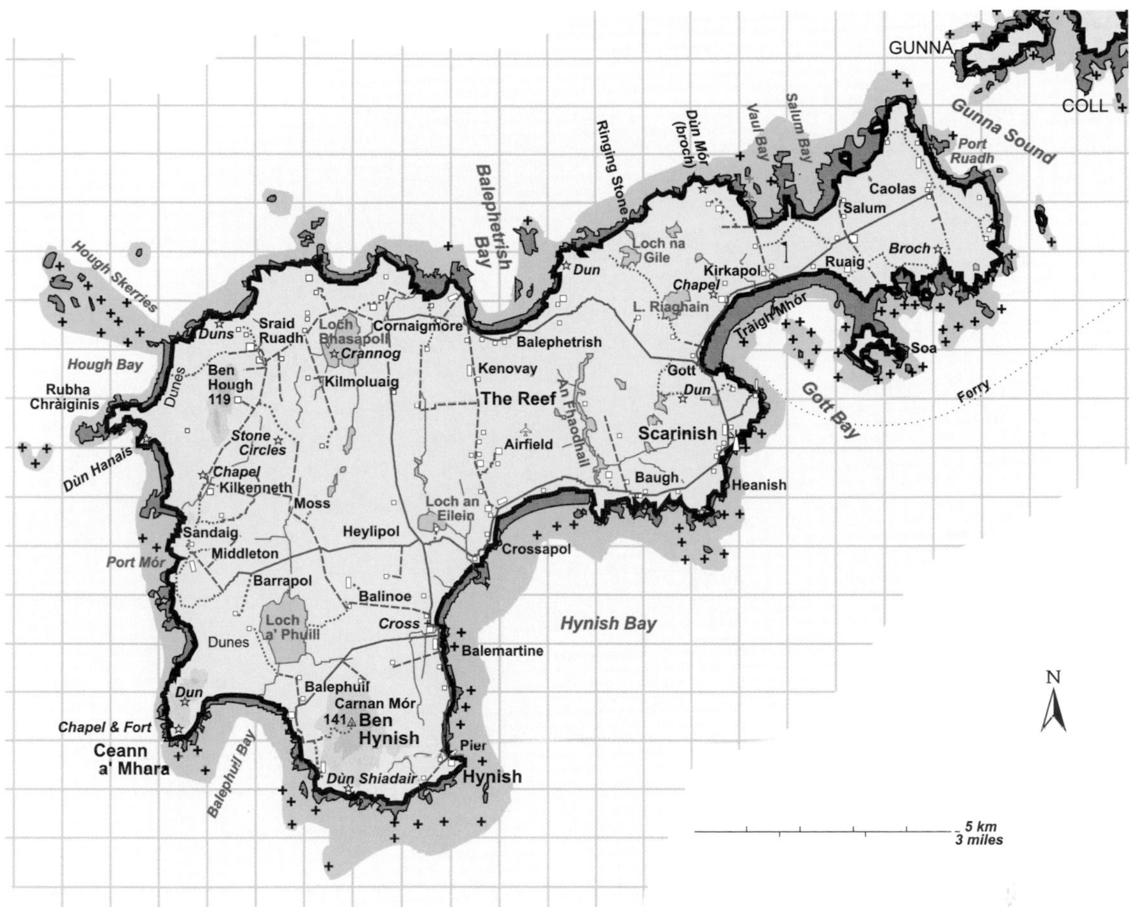

Geology: A flat fertile island with a bedrock of Archaean gneiss (a schist known as paragneiss). A limestone outcrop known as Tiree marble – pink flecked with green – was quarried at Balephetrish from 1791 to 1794 and briefly again in 1910. (Stones now sold as Tiree marble come from Connemara in Ireland.) East of the quarry is Clach a' Choire (G. – ringing stone) – a glacial erratic which originated on Rum.

History: Pottery and tools of 800BC have been uncovered at Dùn Mór Vaul where there is a broch. St Columba sailed into Gott Bay on his way to visit the monastery founded by his cousin, Baitheine, at Sorobaidh. Apparently, on arrival, he struck a rock which nearly sank his boat, so he cursed it. Most sailors still follow this tradition.

St Comgall, a Pict and an associate of St Columba, also founded a monastery on Tiree.

In 672 the Vikings burned down the monastery, but some decided that they liked the island and settled. This however did not stop King Magnus of Norway – twenty-five years old and a born arsonist – plundering the island at the end of the 11th century and setting it alight. According to one of his skalds, Bjorn Cripplehand, 'The glad wolf reddened tooth and claw with many a mortal wound in Tiree...' Control passed to the Kingdom of Man and then to Somerled, King of the Isles, and his heirs in 1164. After the Battle of Largs in 1263 Alexander III granted ownership to the MacDougalls but they were indecisive owners and there were continual disputes. By 1390 Lachlan MacLean was Bailie of Tiree and Coll, which led to his descendants claiming ownership. Eventually however, in the latter part of the 17th century, the Duke of Argyll took control.

It was at this time that much of the arable farming began to be replaced by cattle grazing, although barley was still grown for whisky. Tiree was exporting up to three thousand gallons of whisky a year at the end of the 18th century.

The population which had been 4450 in 1830

had dropped to 2700 fifty years later due to evictions and potato famines. In 1885 the Duke of Argyll prevailed on the Government to send fifty policemen and 250 marines on the *Ajax* and *Assistance* to evict the crofters. The crofters resisted and although the marines arrested and held five crofters for a token period they were generally sympathetic towards the islanders. The matter was settled in 1886 with the passing of the Crofters' Act which split the land into 270 crofts.

Wildlife: Tiree has hares, but no rabbits, foxes, stoats or weasels.

The machair has a dense cover of meadow flowers, particularly where there is restricted access for sheep. There is very little actual grass, the cover is mainly daisy, dandelion, red and white clover, buttercup, blue speedwell, hop and birdsfoot trefoil, eyebright, harebell, yellow and blue pansy, silverweed, wild thyme, and the common spotted orchid sub-species, *D. fuchsii hebridensis*.

A mat of sea thrift rings the coastline with marram grass tying down the dunes.

Tiree has great interest for birdwatchers all the year round and in spring and summer wildfowl, waders and seabirds breed there: skylark on the machair: sedge warbler, corncrake and reed bunting in denser vegetation. Exceptional sites are:

Loch a' Phuill: mute and whooper swans in autumn and winter. Oct – April Greenland white-fronted geese. Greylag geese all year. Wigeon, teal, mallard, pintail, shoveller, pochard, tufted duck, goldeneye, red-breasted merganser in winter.

Loch Bhasapol: Pochard, tufted duck and much more.

The Reef: The centre of the island. Greenland white-fronted geese.

Balephetrish Bay: ringed plover, sanderling, dunlin, purple sandpiper and turnstone. Great northern diver, eider and long-tailed duck in winter.

Salum and Vaul Bays: good for feeding waders.

Ceann a' Mhara: Breeders: fulmar, shag, kittiwake, guillemot and razorbill. Starlings nest in the caves.

* * *

TIREE is sometimes referred to as *Tir-fo-Thuinn* – the land beneath the waves. There are only two high points, **Ben Hynish** in the south (141m) with its 'golf-ball' radar station and **Ben Hough** in the north-west (119m). Over two-thirds of the island has been covered with wind-blown shell sand which has created a fertile, plough-deep and well-drained machair. It was this rich soil which earned Tiree the title of the land of corn. Tiree is virtually unique among Scottish isles in having no peat-bog. The rainfall is low and from May to September the climate is the sunniest in Britain, but the wind that brought the rich soil blows constantly and there is no natural shelter from it. This is the windiest place in the United Kingdom with an average annual wind speed of 17mph. No wonder that every October it is the venue for the world-renowned International Windsurfing Championships.

This is still a thriving crofting community (unlike its sister island Coll) maintaining a stable and viable population, although the smallness of the land-holdings make many of the crofts barely economic. Cattle and sheep are grazed, the arable farming being mainly for winter feed. The black houses (G. – *tigh dubh*) with dry-stone walls up to nine feet thick, rounded corners, a fire hearth in the middle of the floor and thatched roofs within the outer walls for wind protection are still here but most have been 'modernised' and are now white houses (G. – *tigh geal*), so called because the original walls have been cemented and whitewashed. Thatched roofs have been replaced with felt or corrugated iron and the houses now have fireplaces with chimneys.

In Gott Bay a fine sweep of sand (G. *Tràigh Mhór* – long beach) leads round from the tidal island of **Soa** (ON – sheep island) to the ferry terminal at **Scarinish** (ON – seagull headland). Here there is a post office, shops, hotel, and an old stone harbour (built 1771), now only frequented by the lobster boats, while on the beach lies the wreck of the *Mary Stewart*, one of the last sailing ships to trade in this area. West of Scarinish, in the flat centre of the island – called **The Reef** – is an airfield built by the RAF in 1941 for Squadrons 218 and 518 flying Warwicks and Halifax bombers. It is now used for commercial flights. The weather station here, which contributes to the shipping forecasts, was started by the Head Teacher of Consignor School who began keeping records in 1926.

At the southern tip, **Hynish** has granite houses and a small pier built for the workers on the **Skerryvore** lighthouse which is ten miles out to sea to the south-west. It was built by an uncle of R L Stevenson in 1838–43. It is 42m (138ft) high and sits on a rock only three metres above Mean High Water Springs. The 4000 tons of granite used in its construction came from the Bull Hole quarry on Mull. It was damaged by fire and has been unmanned since the 1960s. The granite tower at Hynish was used to send signals to the lighthouse, and is now a museum.

Tiree's largest loch, **Loch a' Phuill**, is near the west coast amid extensive areas of dunes which are grazed by sheep and cattle. The knuckle in the south-west corner, **Ceann a' Mhara** [kenë-va:rë] (G. – head of the sea) is littered with ancient relics while at the north-west corner numerous off-shore rocks and skerries surround the shell-sand bays.

Loch Bhasapoll is also in the north-west, with its two crannogs, marshy fringes, and wintering geese. A village called Baile nan Craganach (G. – place of the clumsy people) is said to have once stood on the loch's north shore, so called because the villagers all had six fingers on each hand. Further east, in the centre of the north coast, **Balephetrish Bay** (G. *baile pheadairich* – the place of the storm petrel) was the original source of Tiree marble.

Dun and broch remains (more than twenty of them), stone circles, standing stones, cairns and crannogs are scattered right across the island. **Dùn Mór Vaul** by Vaul Bay in the north-east is of particular interest [NM042492]. It was started as a timber structure in the 6th century BC and was later turned into a stone broch about the 1st century BC. Galleries are still visible in the 4m thick walls. The brochs of Tiree are the furthest south of all the island brochs.

The Ringing Stone, west of Vaul [NM027487], is covered with cup-marks and clangs eerily when struck. It should be treated with care as it is prophesied that if the stone is broken Tiree will sink forever beneath the waves.

Access: Vehicle ferry: Oban/ Coll/ Tiree, every day; continues to Barra, Thurs. only, 08000-66-5000. Air service from Glasgow, 0870-850-9850. There is a limited bus service for most of the island. Cars and bicycles can be hired locally.

Anchorages:

1. Scarinish. Both creek and drying harbour can occasionally be used if no swell is coming in. Near HW, or at neaps, temp. berth at old pier possible, or anchored in middle of creek.
2. Gott bay concrete pier has a depth of 3.4m (11') alongside. Landing slip on inner side. Foul ground extends 6c SE from pier.
3. Gott bay. Exposed but affords moderately good anchorage in settled weather or light W'lies in 4–5m, sand, N-NE of pier on SW side of bay. Several dangers both sides and in the fairway.
4. Clach Chuirr (Port Ruadh) off Gunna Sound affords some shelter from S and W. Anchor on either side of the power cable in 3m, sand.
5. Hynish pier. Some limited shelter from S in very settled conditions. Pier and dock dry out.

3.11 Gunna

(ON Gunni-øy – the island of Gunni the Dane) or, improbably, (?G Eilean nan Gamhna – island of the yearling cattle).

OS Maps: 1:50000 Sheet 46 1:25000 Sheet 372
Admiralty Charts: 1:75000 No.2171 Sd of Gunna 1:25000 No.2475

Area: 69ha (168 acres)
Height: 35m (115 ft)

Owner: Marcus de Ferranti. The owner has built a summer residence overlooking the anchorage.

Population: No Census records.

Geology: Paragneiss schist with a light sandy soil. Metasediments in the west, undifferentiated gneiss in the east.

Wildlife: The arctic tern, little tern, and possibly also sandwich tern plus three common species of large gull nest here but all these ground-nesting birds periodically suffer serious losses when brown rats, *Rattus norvegicus*, invade the island. Barnacle geese use the island for winter bed-and-breakfasting while large numbers of white-fronted and greylag geese occasionally appear. Shelduck are prolific in the spring.

This is a grey seal nursery and two dolphins have been resident for some years.

* * *

Lying in the sound between Tiree and Coll, **GUNNA** was probably once inhabited by an anchorite. It is now only grazed by cattle and wild geese. It is separated from Coll by a shallow rock-strewn passage. Gunna is a narrow little

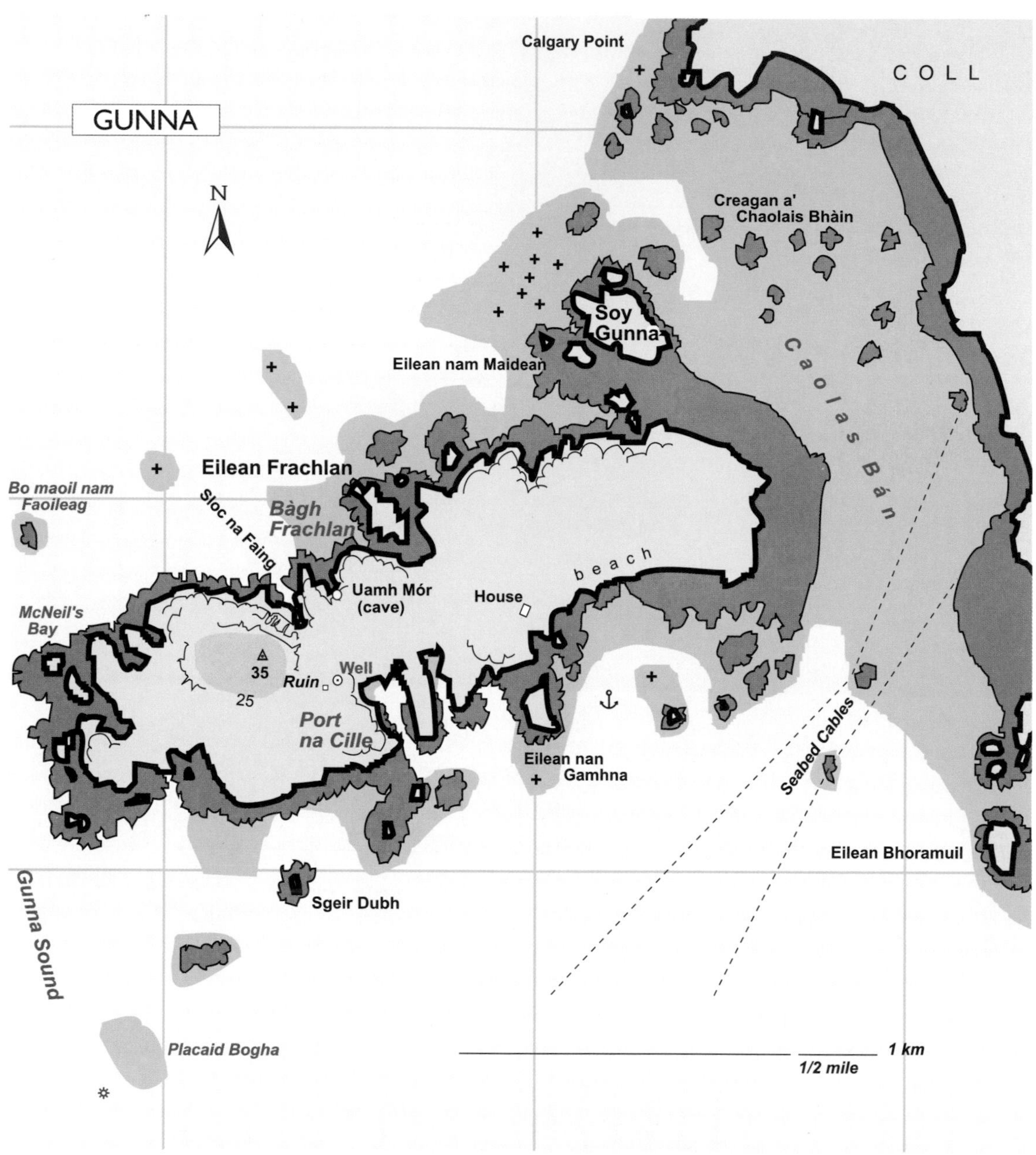

wind-blown island, no more than 500m wide for most of its length, and with few prominent features. There is a spring at Port na Cille (G. – port of the chapel), with the ruin of a small cell or shieling beside it. There are also other signs of early habitation. A cave in the centre of the north coast may have served as a hermit's shelter [NM099514].

Gunna Sound, between Coll and Tiree is a relatively shallow stretch of water. The area near Gunna is peppered with rocks and there are more rocky patches off the Tiree shore. Islets near Tiree include **Creachasdal**, **Librig**, **Eilean Liath** and **Eilean Ghreasamuill**, while **Eilean Bhoramuil** lies off the southern extremity of Coll.

Access: No regular means of access. Try Skipinnish Sea Tours, Tiree, 01879-220009 or Coll Hotel, Coll, 01879-230334.

Anchorage: Occasional anchorage E of Eilean na Gamhna, 4–5m, sand, good holding. Exposed to S'lies.

3.12 Shuna

Uncertain derivation, probably Norse but possibly (G. sidhean – fairy hill, ON -øy – island).

O.S.Maps: 1:50000 Sheet 49 1:25000 Sheet 376 or 383
Admiralty Chart: 1:25000 No.2379

Area: 155ha (383 acres)
Height: 71m (233 ft)

Owner: Stephen P Newall DL LLD,'Deputy Lord Lieutenant of Dunbartonshire, and his wife, Gay S Newall, daughter of the late Col. Tom Craig, who bought it in the 1950s.

Population: 1881–8. 1891–6. 1931–4. 1961–1. 1971–0. 1981–0. 1991–0. 2001–0.

Geology: Mostly Dalradian limestone giving a good soil.

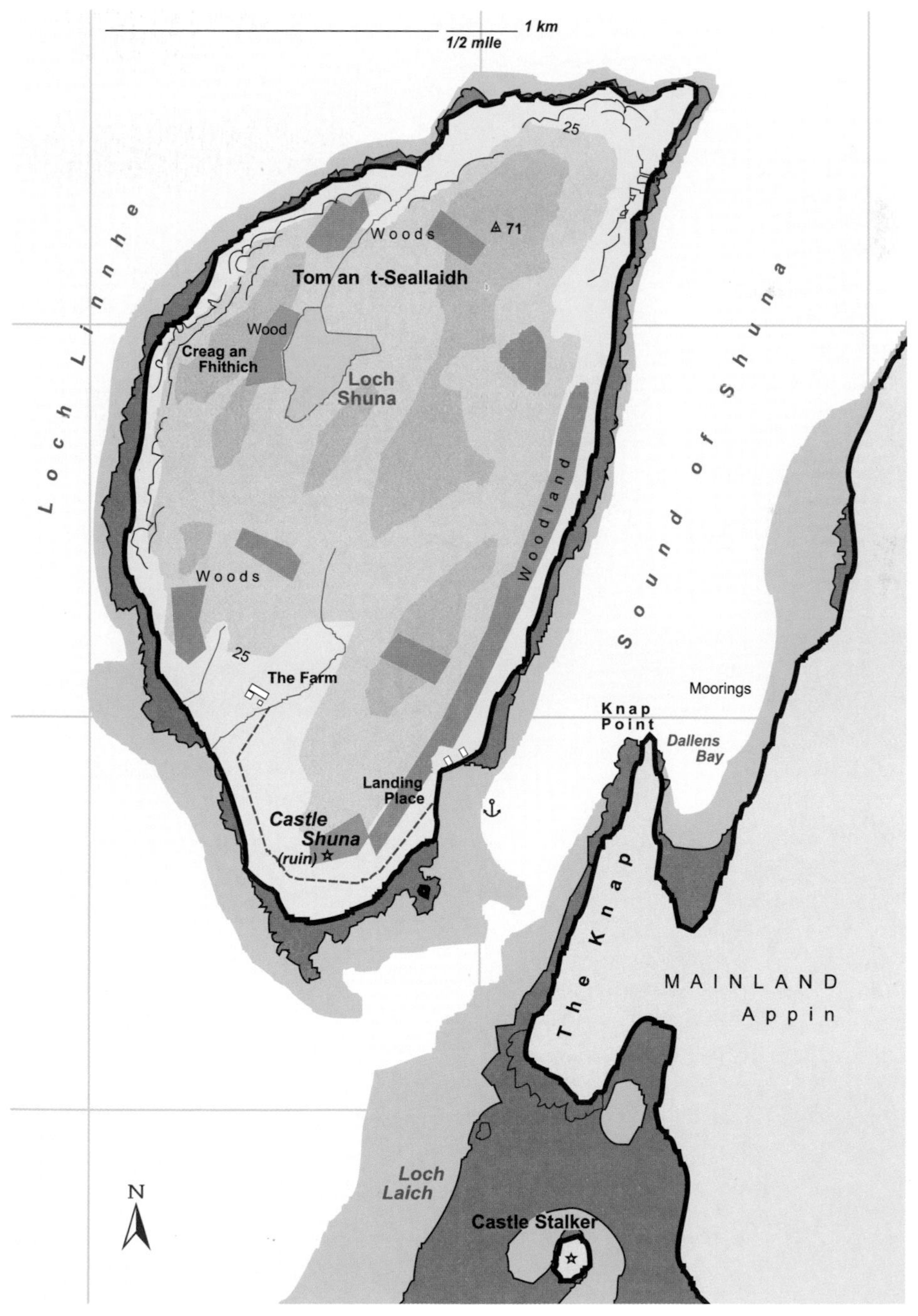

History: A document of 1577–1595 says that the island belonged to John Stewart, Laird of Appin. A further description in 1630 says that Shuna, property of the Laird of Appin is 'the most profitable and fertilest in all these Countries'.

SHUNA is sometimes rather needlessly called Shuna Island but this is probably to distinguish it from the other Shuna (No.2.10) which lies alongside Luing. It is a compact island separated from the mainland by the narrow Sound of Shuna and rising to a table-topped hill near the north-east end. In a hollow near the hill is a lochan with a stream running past some clumps of conifers. The view from here is dramatic, looking up Loch Linnhe to where the great flank of Ben Nevis can be seen beyond tiny **Eilean Balnagowan**.

Shuna (with 360 breeding ewes) is farmed by the owner, and the pleasant white farmhouse faces southwards towards Lismore (No.3.9) and Appin. At the southernmost extremity are the substantial ruins of **Castle Shuna**, a small square building about 10m high [NM915483]. This is actually a domestic tower house rather than a castle. It was probably built near the end of the 16th century by John Stewart, who died in 1595, or his son, Duncan Stewart. The building was abandoned at the end of the 18th century.

Across the sound is another island fortress, **Castle Stalker** in Loch Laich. It was built about 1500, also by the Stewarts of Appin, and James IV used it as a hunting lodge. It was a ruin for many years but has now been restored.

In 1958 near Tom an t-Seallaidh (G. – the knoll of the vision) a rock-shelter on Shuna was excavated and deposits of limpet shells, stone-scrapers, deer horn and flints were found.

Unfortunately, on our first visit many years ago, both the anchorage in the Sound of Shuna and the beautiful setting were spoilt by the unpleasant odour from a mink farm on The Knap, a piece of ground projecting into the Sound. I am happy to report that nowadays this is no longer a problem and that the abandoned and derelict farm is an interesting relic to be seen on a short walk through the attractive landscape in the area of the Knapp.

Access: No regular access but enquire at Linnhe Marine (Paul Zvegintzov), 07721-503981.

Anchorages:
1. In Shuna Sound, SW of Knap Point (N of the narrows).
2. Linnhe Marine. Visitors moorings (pay) in sheltered Dallens Bay (Shuna Cove), E of Knap Point.

3.13 Coll

(G. coll – a hazel). Adomnan calls it 'insula Coloso' from which Watson infers a pre-Celtic origin.

O S Maps: 1:50000 Sheet 46 1:25000 Sheet 372
Admiralty Charts: 1:100000 No.1796 1:75000 No.2171 Sound of Gunna 1:25000 No.2475 Loch Eatharna (Arinagour) 1:10000 No.2474

Area: 7685ha (18989 acres)
Height: 104m (341 ft)

Owner: The Stewart family, owners of Coll since 1856, sold about two-thirds of the island estate to Coll Properties Ltd in 1964 (the Dutch businessman, Jan de Vries), but Kenneth and Janet Stewart continued farming the rest until 1991 when they sold the remainder of the estate to Major N V MacLean Bristol of 'Project Venture' and Neil Smith of Ferndale Ltd. The de Vries estate was sold in two parts to the Royal Society for the Protection of Birds. Colin Kennedy owns the south end of the island.

Population: 1740– about 400. 1755–502. 1794–902. By 1841 it had reached 1442 (271 houses), which was greater than the island could support according to the laird, Maclean, and half the population emigrated to Australia or Canada. 1881–643. 1891–522 (111 houses). 1931–322. 1961–147. 1981–131. 1991–172. 2001–164.

Geology: Until comparatively recent times in geological terms, Coll and Tiree were one single island. Coll consists of low hummocks of a weathered rock called paragneiss, a schist metamorphosed from sedimentary rock, sticking through the grass and heather like currants in a bun, particularly in the eastern half. The south-western area around Gorton and Breachacha is of ancient sediments containing quartz and marble. High dunes and machair stretch along the west coast with raised beaches at Arnabost and Arinagour. Lead was mined in the south of the island in early times.

History: Coll and Tiree have a very similar early

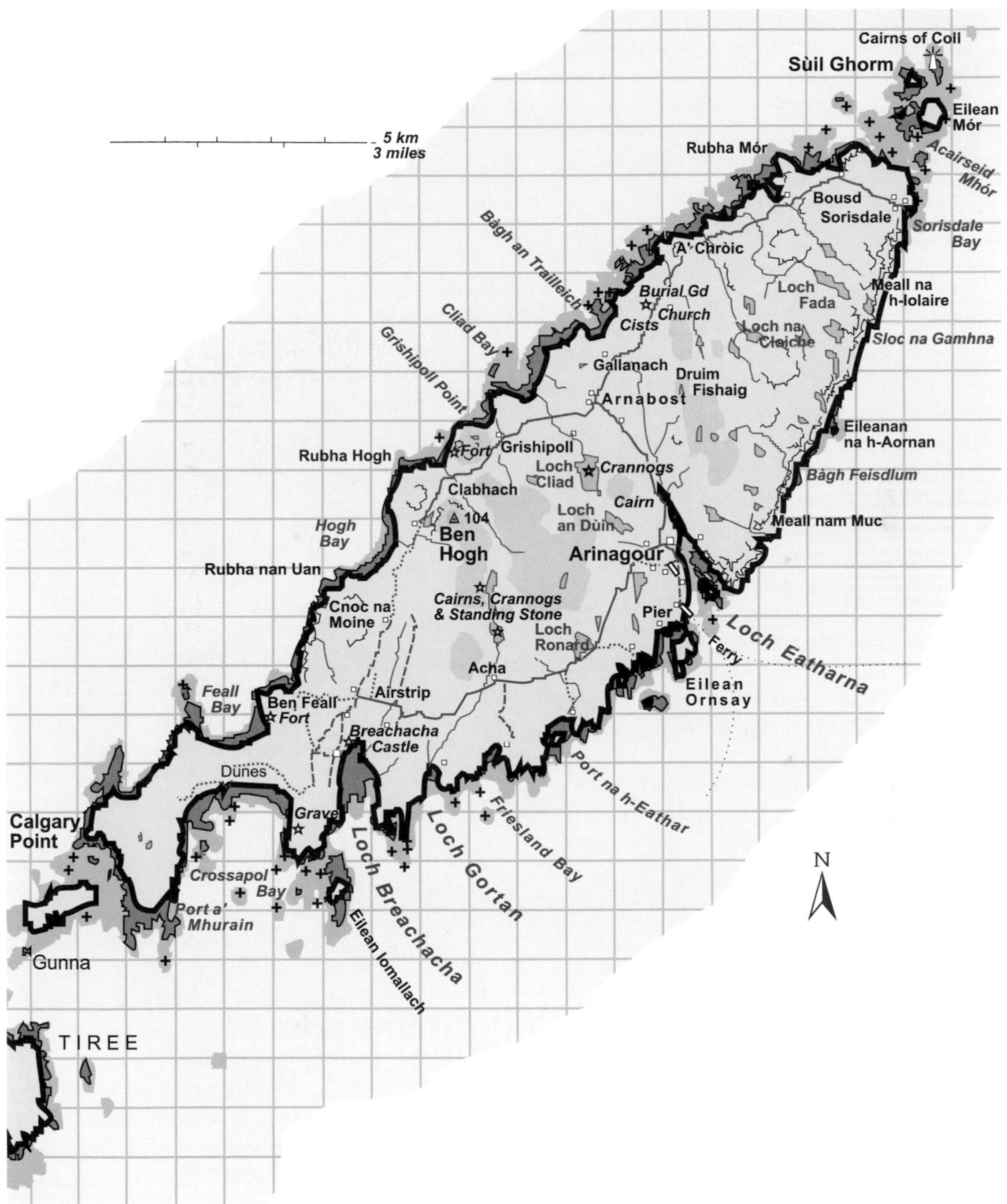

history. Angus Og of Islay, King of the Isles, was granted Coll by Bruce when MacDougall forfeited it around 1314. He was probably then responsible for building Breachacha Castle using the latest defensive techniques known to the Macdonalds.

The Maclean chieftains of Coll were an interesting and enlightened family. The 4th Chieftain, who died in 1560, was a bard who composed verse in both Gaelic and Latin. The 11th Chieftain, Lachlan Maclean, a renowned soldier, was drowned in an accident in 1687. His grandson, Hector, 13th of Coll, had a personal in-house harper at his new residence at Breachacha. He kept most of his clansmen from becoming embroiled in the 1745 rebellion and received a royal charter to his property so that he was not a vassal to the Campbells. He had two successive Campbell wives yet when the Duke of Argyll tried to lease two of his farms on Coll Maclean vowed that he would never let a Campbell move in. Neither of his Campbell wives gave him an heir, so his brother Hugh took over when he died in 1754.

Hugh maintained Neil Rankin, the last hereditary piper to the Macleans, in his household and constructed a mausoleum for his brother's remains. He subsidised a spinning school and the development of linen manufacture on the island. His son Donald, 'young Coll', embarrassed Boswell in 1773 by having to share his bed for the night when they met as guests on Inch Kenneth.

'He was a lively young man,' Boswell reported. 'We found he had been a good deal in England, studying farming, and was resolved to improve the value of his father's lands, without oppressing his tenants, or losing the ancient Highland fashions.' The young man tragically drowned the following year. His brother Alexander, who succeeded as 15th Chieftain in 1790, had many of the same ideals as his brother. He was Lieutenant Colonel of the Breadalbane Fencibles, a regiment which gave employment to many of his clansmen.

By 1841 the population had grown rapidly to over 1400 which was more than the island could support. The laird impoverished himself trying to feed the islanders during the potato famine and paying the fares of those who wished to go to Australia and Canada, and finally had to sell the island to John Lorne Stewart in 1856. The new owner, despite the crofters' protests, raised the rents so in 1861 the 'great exodus' took place. Virtually all the tenants, overnight, left their crofts and moved from the arable south-east to the rock-bound north-west of the island. This area was under Campbell ownership and the promised rents were reasonable but the families had to improvise shelter while they built their new homes. Unfortunately overcrowding led to many families leaving the island in the ensuing years.

Towards the end of the 19th century the Stewarts decided that they now had to repopulate the land and offered crofts at attractive rents to Ayrshire dairy farmers. This resulted in the production of the famous Coll cheese – a favourite delicacy at the House of Lords up to the time that the market for dairy produce collapsed near the start of the First World War.

Wildlife: In 1939 botanists were surprised to discover the Irish Lady's Tresses orchid growing on Coll. It grows in a few Irish localities but is actually a native of North America. Since then a few have also been found on Colonsay. The sub species, *hebridensis*, of the common spotted orchid also grows here and there is one sub-species unique to Coll called The Great Yellow Bumble Bee.

It is estimated that, due to modern intensive farming, less than 500 pairs of corncrakes now survive in Britain, mostly in the Outer Hebrides. The birds, which are more often heard than seen, like rough uncultivated conditions. There are about 120 pairs on Tiree and the RSPB has created a corncrake reserve for the twenty or so pairs on Coll.

Boswell gives an interesting account of the natural history (in 1773): 'There are no foxes; no serpents, toads, or frogs, nor any venomous creature. They have otters and mice here; but had no rats till lately that an American vessel brought them. There is a rabbit-warren on the north-east of the island, belonging to the Duke of Argyle. Young Coll (the laird) intends to get some hares, of which there are none at present. There are no black-cock, moor-fowl, nor partridges; but there are snipe, wild-duck, wild-geese, and swans, in winter; wild pigeons, plover, and great number of starlings; of which I shot some, and found them pretty good eating. Woodcocks come hither, though there is not a tree upon the island.' He also mentions the great variety of fish in the brooks and trout and eel in the lochs. Coll has no stoat or weasel and today the Duke of Argyll's rabbits have become a serious pest.

Little lochans scattered over the north end of the island, covered with white water-lilies in the summer months, are the home of red-throated divers and the heather conceals red grouse.

* * *

Most of **COLL** is bleak with gnarled lumps of rock protruding through a thin skin of grass and heather. But the trim whitewashed cottages of **Arinagour** (G. *airigh na gobhar* – shieling of the goats), lying beneath two churches on the hill, are welcoming. They were built by Maclean, laird of Coll, about 1800 in an attempt to modernise the island. They are now mainly holiday cottages with most of the 'Collachs' (the local inhabitants) occupying the council houses. Arinagour is alongside Loch **Eatharna** (G. – loch of the small fishing boats). There is an old stone pier and a ferry pier which was built in 1969. The Isle of Coll Hotel overlooks the loch. It is a pleasant building with a 'Flavour of Scotland' award; it has bicycles and mopeds for hire and is the most useful information centre on the island.

Across the island from Arinagour is **Arnabost** where the ruined school was built over a medieval earth house with the entrance under the school porch [NM209600]. The islanders had used this as a hiding place during Viking raids and a gold brooch was found there in 1855.

East of Arnabost the land is virtually empty – low-lying, rocky, and peppered with lochans but the road runs up the northern coastal strip which was the most densely populated part of the island in the 19th century. The area was deserted by choice, not by forced clearance and the old township of **Bousd** is there to be seen. **Sorisdale**, at the northern tip, is a lovely crofting settlement of thatched buildings by a pleasant beach. Along this northern coast, the machair is so rich and fertile that there was an experiment to grow tulips in competition with the Dutch. The climate is mild, Coll is one of the sunniest spots in Britain, and the flowers were a great success but the cost and difficulty of transportation defeated the project. The road passes a cemetery and the remnants of a medieval chapel – **Cille Ionnaig** – where Young Coll, host to Dr Johnson and Boswell, lies buried [NM221618]. He was drowned the year following the visit when sailing from Inch Kenneth to Mull.

Off the northern extremity of Coll are some dangerous rocks and islets although the space beside **Eilean Mór** is known as Acairseid Mhór (G. – big anchorage). **Eag na Maoile** (G. – cleft bare rock) is north of Eilean Mór and **Sùil Gorm** (G. – blue eye) with a light tower on it.

Turning south-west at Arnabost the road passes **Grishipoll**. In the 15th century MacNeill of Barra set up a garrison at this farm when he chose to annex Coll. But Iain Garbh, his stepson and hereditary owner of the land, raised the Collachs, took the garrison and regained his inheritance. His descendants have owned part of Coll until the present time. The road turns into a track beside **Ben Hogh** (104m), Coll's highest hill. On it is a huge boulder balanced on three small ones which according to folklore was placed there by a giant. It is worth following Boswell's footsteps up this hill as the views south are worthwhile. (Dr Johnson chose instead to sit down and read a book).

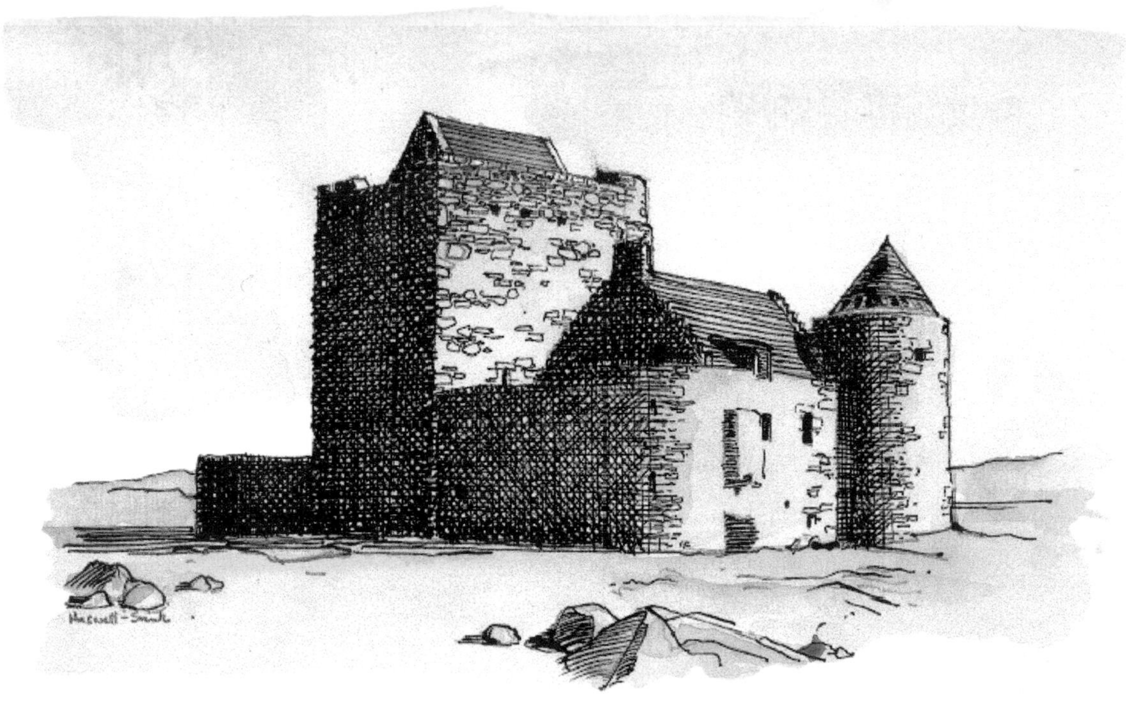

BREACHACHA – WHERE MACLEAN FOUGHT MACLEAN

From Arinagour there is a pleasant road leading to an airstrip on the sand dunes and **Breachacha** (G. – the field speckled with wild flowers). Here, on the shore of the loch, stands ancient Breachacha Castle, which dates back to the 15th century and probably earlier. It has been carefully restored by the Project Trust, a training scheme for young people to give voluntary service in underdeveloped countries. Near it is the attractive new castle, recently renamed Breachacha House, built in 1750 by Hector Maclean and visited in October 1773 by Boswell and Dr Johnson. The irascible Johnson 'relished it much at first, but soon remarked... that... it was a mere tradesman's box.' It was later enlarged and somewhat mutilated by a Victorian owner. It has been renovated recently and is now a private residence.

When the MacLeans of Duart invaded Coll in 1593 they were mown down by the Macleans of Coll and the burn that flows into Loch Breachacha was choked with the heads of the Duart clansmen. It has been called ever since Struthan nan Ceann (G. – the stream of the heads).

There are a number of prehistoric remains in this southern area – standing stones, cairns, traces of brochs and crannogs, and **Dùn an Achaidh**, an ancient fort beside the road from Arinagour [NM183546]. West of Loch Breachacha there are two large attractive bays, Crossapol Bay, with the off-shore islet of **Soa** almost linked to **Eilean Iomallach**, and Feall Bay, separated by marram dunes. The neglected shell of the 13th Maclean's Mausoleum is on the peninsula between the southerly bays [NM149524].

* * *

Access: Vehicle ferry: Oban/ Coll/ Tiree, every day, 08000-66-5000. Bicycles for hire, Coll Hotel, 01879-230334. Tourist information, 01631-563122.

Anchorages: These anchorages are only suitable in favourable conditions and are all open to any directional swell.

1. Loch Eatharna (Arinagour). Popular but exposed to S'lies. Head dries out about ¾M. Divided into two parts by Eilean Eatharna 13.4m high. W part most used but open to S and only suitable for occasional anchorage in summer. Bottom sand. There are visitors' moorings (pay). E anchorage very restricted with narrow entrance and many moorings but less swell.
2. Sorisdale Bay. Temp anchorage in 3m, sand, off concrete block and close to N side.
3. Acairseid Mhór, SSW of Eilean Mor. Claimed to be best anchorage on Coll. Approach from E until N of Glas Eileanan. Requires great care.
4. Hogh Bay on N coast. Occasional anchorage. Sheltered NE-E-S. Approach from N, head for break in sand-dunes. Anchor in 3m, firm sand.
5. Feall Bay on N coast. Occasional anchorage. Sheltered NE-E-S. Approach from N, slightly E of centre line, and anchor in 2–6m, sand and rock patches (usually visible).
6. Loch Breachacha. Many rocks. Head shoals gradually.
7. Loch Gorton. Narrow sandy cove 1M E of Breachacha. Anchor in 3m, sand.

3.14 Carna

(G. càrn – cairn, heap of stones, rocky mound, ON -øy – island).

O.S.Maps: 1:50000 Sheet 49 1:25000 Sheet 383
Admiralty Chart: 1:25000 No.2394

Area: 213ha (526 acres)
Height: 169m (554 ft)

Owners: Tim and Sue Milward and Mr Milward's sisters, Vanessa Towers and Frances Milward.

Population: 1881–7. 1891–10 (2 houses). 1931–3. 1961–2. 1971–3. 1981–0. 1991–4. 2001–0.

Geology: Mainly a Moine schist bedrock of quartz-felspar constitution, except for the west coastal strip which is mixed schists and mica-schist.

Wildlife: An interesting variety of habitat for, among others, willow warblers, redstarts, wheatears, whinchats, twites, ravens and kestrels. A rare protected coral-like serpulid reef in upper Loch Teacuis is found in only three other places in the world.

* * *

The dinosaur back of **CARNA** rears up behind the tidal island of Oronsay. It straddles the mouth of remote Loch Teacuis, one of the most interesting lochs on the West Coast, dividing the entrance into two narrow kyles. **Eilean nan Gabhar** (G. – goat island), usually covered with basking seals and not a goat in sight, is in the

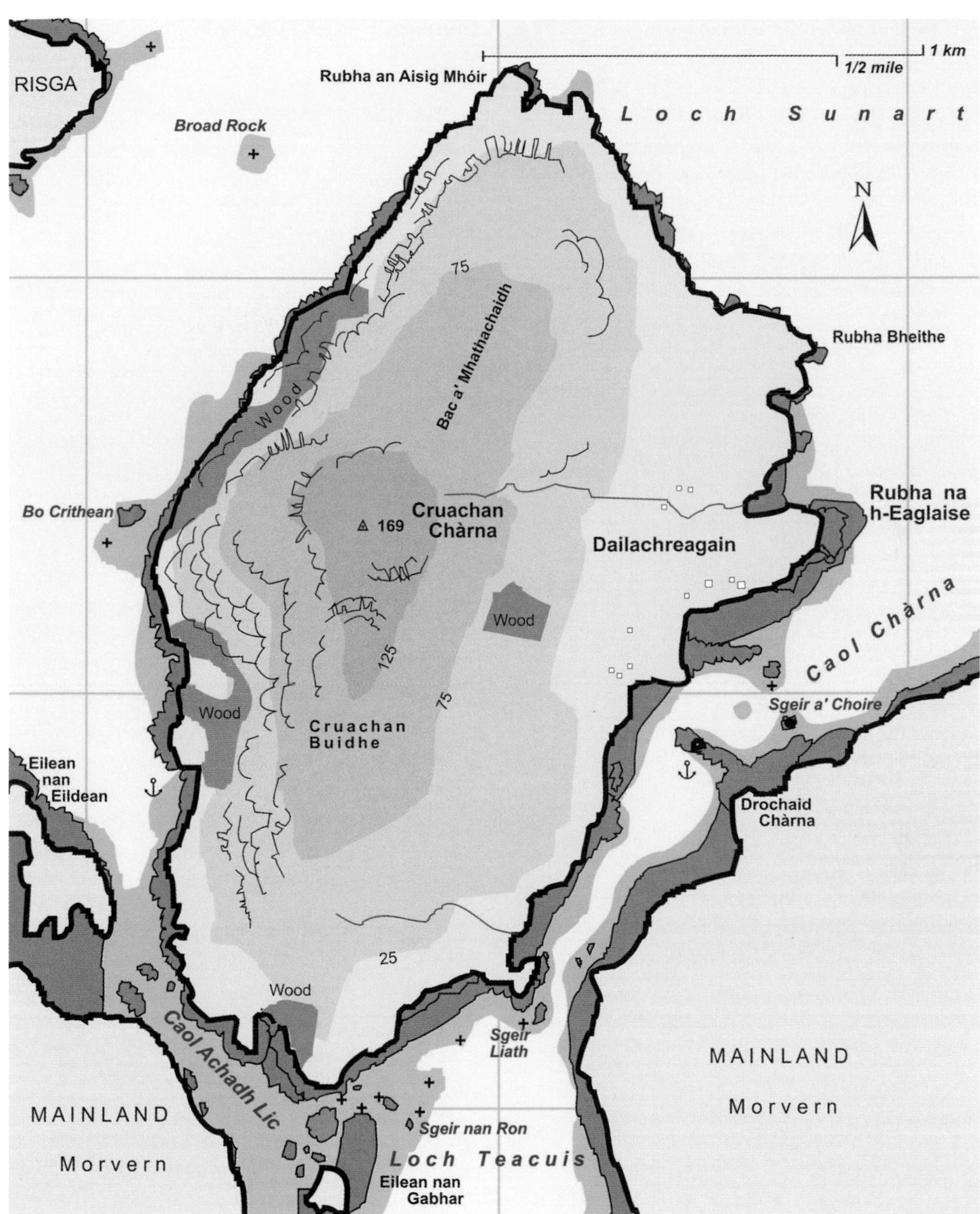

loch just south of Carna's southern headland.

For those approaching by land, Rahoy on Loch Teacuis is a beautiful spot in the heart of Morvern reached by a very minor road from Loch Aline. A walk up the east lochside towards Carna passes an excellent example of a vitrified fort set in oak woodland on a hill above the narrows [NM633564].

The west side of Carna is steep and unwelcoming. Wet, slippy and boggy with abrupt rocky slopes covered in a profusion of flag irises, tufts of sphagnum moss, bracken, grass and scrub birch.

There is a central peak, **Cruachan Chàrna** (G. – the conical hill of Carna), which is the highest part of the knobbly north-south ridge dividing the island. South of it is Cruachan Buidhe (G. – the yellow stack). The eastern slopes are sheltered from the prevailing winds and are much gentler than the west side. As on neighbouring **Oronsay**, the inevitable lonely little ruined cottages are scattered south of a stream which trickles down the mountain and into Caol Chàrna at Rubha na h-Eaglaise (G. – headland of the church). But at least Carna still has a token population with three occupied houses and one being renovated at the time of writing. There is not much in the way of level ground but there is a mellowness in the landscape with a stand of conifers and a small copse of deciduous woodland. A few rowan and birch trees are sprinkled over the higher ground. In 1845 Carna was considered to be more fertile and productive than the larger and less mountainous Oronsay, although there is a fish trap on Oronsay, which must have made a big contribution to its larder. Interestingly, the northern part of Carna is called **Bac à Mhathachaidh** (G. – the cultivated bank).

In the centre of Loch Sunart between Oronsay and Carna there is the steep little island of **Risga** with **Eilean a' Chuilinn** and **Garbh Eilean** further up the loch.

* * *

Access: Ardnamurchan Charters, Laga Bay, 01972-500208 run two holiday cottages on Carna and a passenger ferry from Tobermory on Mondays and Fridays.

Anchorages:
1. Temporary anchorage on W side, immediately N of narrow entrance to Loch Teacuis, off the bay opposite Eilean nan Eildean. 6–8m, sand with some mud and weed. Sheltered except NW-N.
2. E side, in the channel leading to Loch Teacuis in the pool immediately S of Drochaid Chàrna (G – Carna's bridge). Rather awkward entrance needing sailing directions but good shelter.

3–Appendix Staffa

(ON stafi-øy – stave or pillar island) The basalt columns resembled the vertical log staves used by the Norse for house construction.

The town of Stäfa on Lake Zurich in Switzerland was named after this little island by a monk from Iona.

O.S.Maps: 1:50000 Sheet 48 1:25000 Sheet 373
Admiralty Charts: 1:25000 No.2652 or No.2771

Area: 33ha (82 acres)
Height: 42m (138 ft)

Owner: Originally part of the Ulva Estate of the MacQuarries but sold in 1777. After a few years bought by Colin MacDonald of Loch Boisdale. Sold by Ranald MacDonald in 1816 to trustees. Bought in 1966 by a retired army padre, Gerald Newall who sold it to Alastair de Watteville, a direct descendant of the Boisdale MacDonalds. He sold it to the Langs in 1978 who held it until it was bought and donated to the National Trust for Scotland in 1986 by Mr Jock Elliott Jr of New York as a sixtieth birthday present for his wife Elly. She was appointed 'Steward of Staffa' by the Trust.

Population: 1772–1. 1784–16. Uninhabited since 1800.

Geology: Cliffs over 40m high are riddled with caves and the regularity of the basalt columns is such that it is sometimes difficult to realise that these are natural formations. At parts the columns have been twisted into dramatic and contorted shapes. This is a result of the same volcanic activity which created the Giant's Causeway in Ulster. The rock is an almost-black fine-grained Tertiary basalt surmounted by amorphous lava. Slow cooling caused the lava to split in a columnar pattern which then formed regular hexagons or, occasionally, pentagons after lateral compression. This is said to be the only sea-cave in the world formed entirely out of columnar basalt.

History: In the 3rd century Fionn MacCool, the Irish hero who was known to the Scots as Fingal (G. *fionn na ghal* – chief of valour) is said to have defended the Hebrides against early raids by the Vikings and to have died in battle in Ulster in 283. It is not known whether he ever visited Staffa but the beautiful cave on the island is now named in his honour.

On 13 August 1772, Sir Joseph Banks, President of the Royal Society, not long returned from the famous voyage with Captain James Cook and en route to Iceland, 'discovered' Fingal's Cave. His ship had been driven by bad weather into the Sound of Mull. There he met an Englishman, a Mr Leach, who told him of this extraordinary island and he went to see it for himself. In spite of spending the night in the house of the island's sole inhabitants and becoming infested with lice as a result (his companions used a tent), Banks waxed lyrical about Staffa and following his report when back in London, tourists started to appear in droves. Among them in subsequent years were Sir Walter Scott, John Keats, Felix Mendelssohn, J W M Turner, William Wordsworth, Queen Victoria and Prince Albert, Jules Verne, Dr David Livingstone and Robert Louis Stevenson.

Staffa was made a Site of Special Scientific Interest in 1973.

Wildlife: In 1788 barley, oats, flax and potatoes were grown and in 1800 there were three red deer on the island. In 1801 one deer became dangerous and had to be shot and the other deer started following boats which left the island and on one occasion went too far and drowned. Goats replaced the deer and were followed by a small herd of black cattle which were resident for many years. These in turn gave way to sheep. Seabirds nest on the island but not in any great number.

We anchored off **STAFFA** very early on a morning in May. The sea lay like molten lead and it was warm in the sun. We were exceptionally lucky to have such favourable conditions and we had the island to ourselves. The landing place, which was constructed in 1991, is beside **Am Buachaille** (G. – the herdsman), a dramatic tidal islet composed of gracefully bent stone columns in a curious pyramid about 10m high [NM326351]. Nearby, across a narrow channel is **Clamshell Cave,** which has an entrance portico of twisted columns resembling a giant scallop. Shags give eery warnings from their nests in the shadows.

A path across the natural hexagonal paving, called The Causeway, leads along the beautiful colonnaded cliff-face and round the corner to **Fingal's Cave** which is spectacular and quite unique. It is lined with glossy black

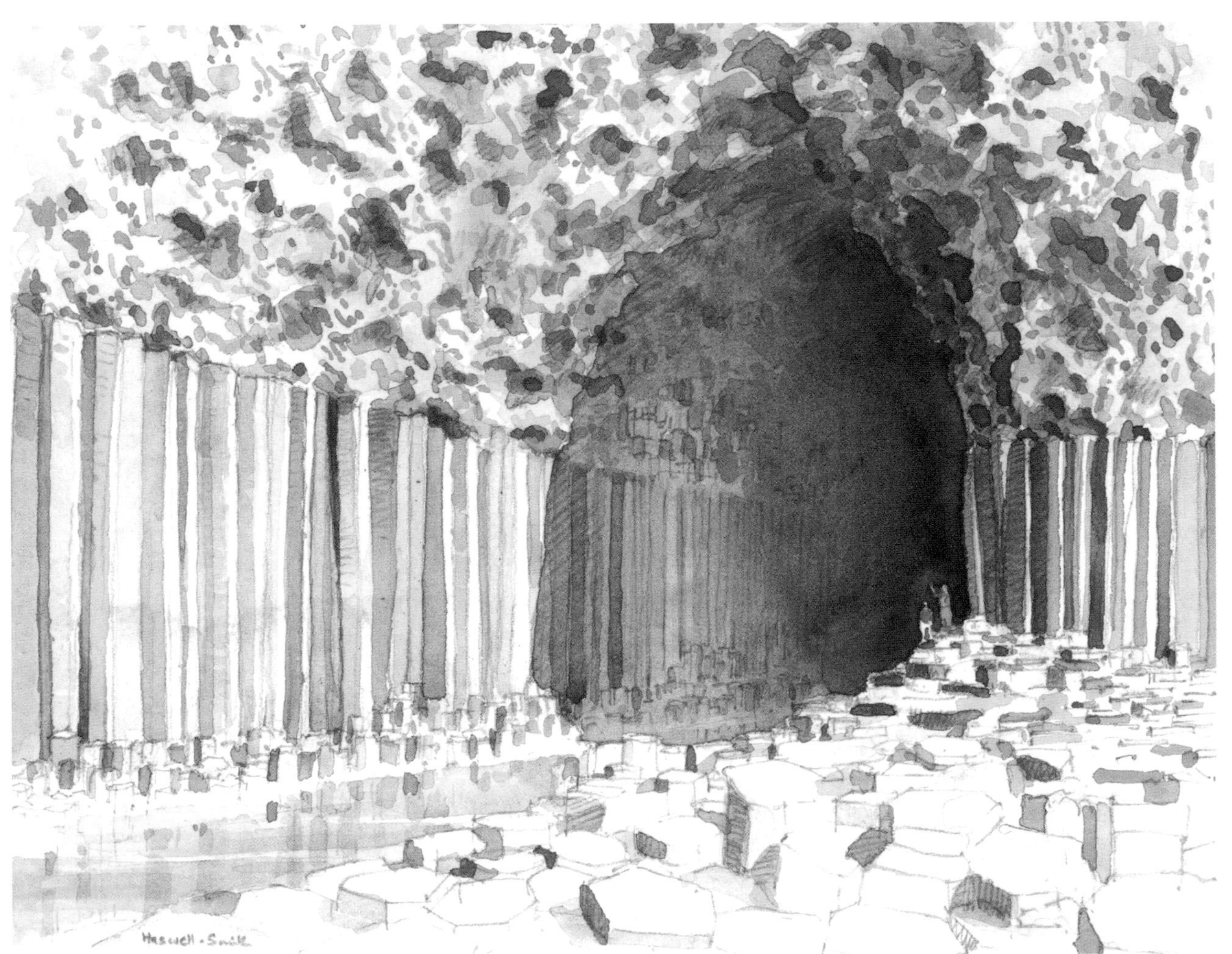

FINGAL'S CAVE

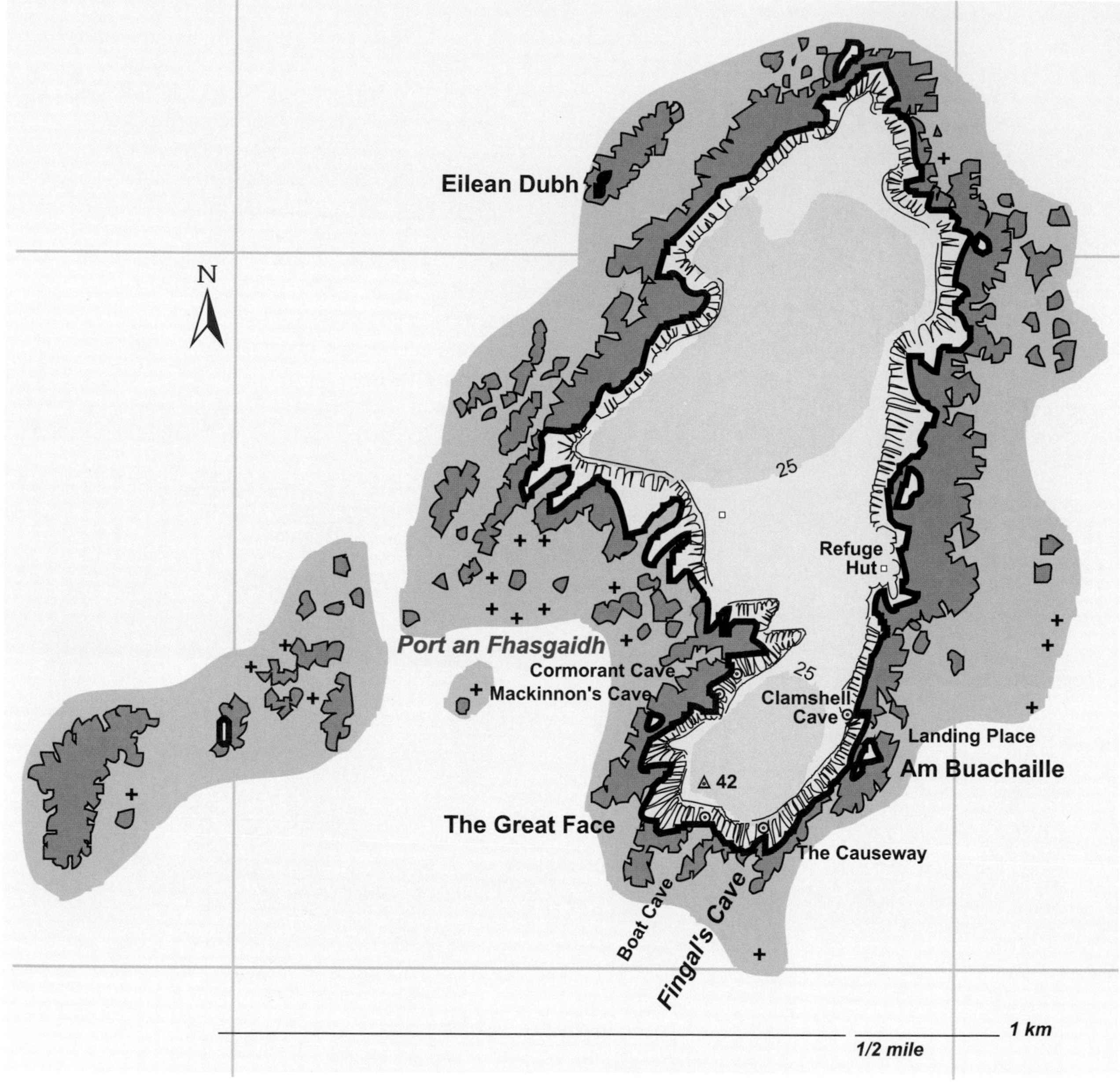

hexagonal columns which on the west side rise symmetrically 12m out of the sea: the roof, like a complicated Gothic vault, is 20m high and the cave is 75m long. A rough path runs among stumps of column to the back of the cave (a torch is needed) and below it is a 20m deep arm of seawater which sighs with the swell. This gives the cave its Gaelic name, An Uamh Bhin (G. – the melodious cave).

It is possible to reach the back of the cave by dinghy.

Mendelssohn visited the island in 1829 and was inspired to write his Hebrides Overture (Die Fingalshöhle). If conditions allow you to visit the island, and only if you can avoid disturbing other visitors, then for an experience that you will remember for the rest of your life play a recording of the Overture inside the cave and afterwards sit in silence and listen to the music of the sea.

Crowds can destroy the magic so try to visit the island out of season. May and June are the best months. Wordsworth was disgusted at being accompanied by too large a crowd of fellow travellers in 1833:

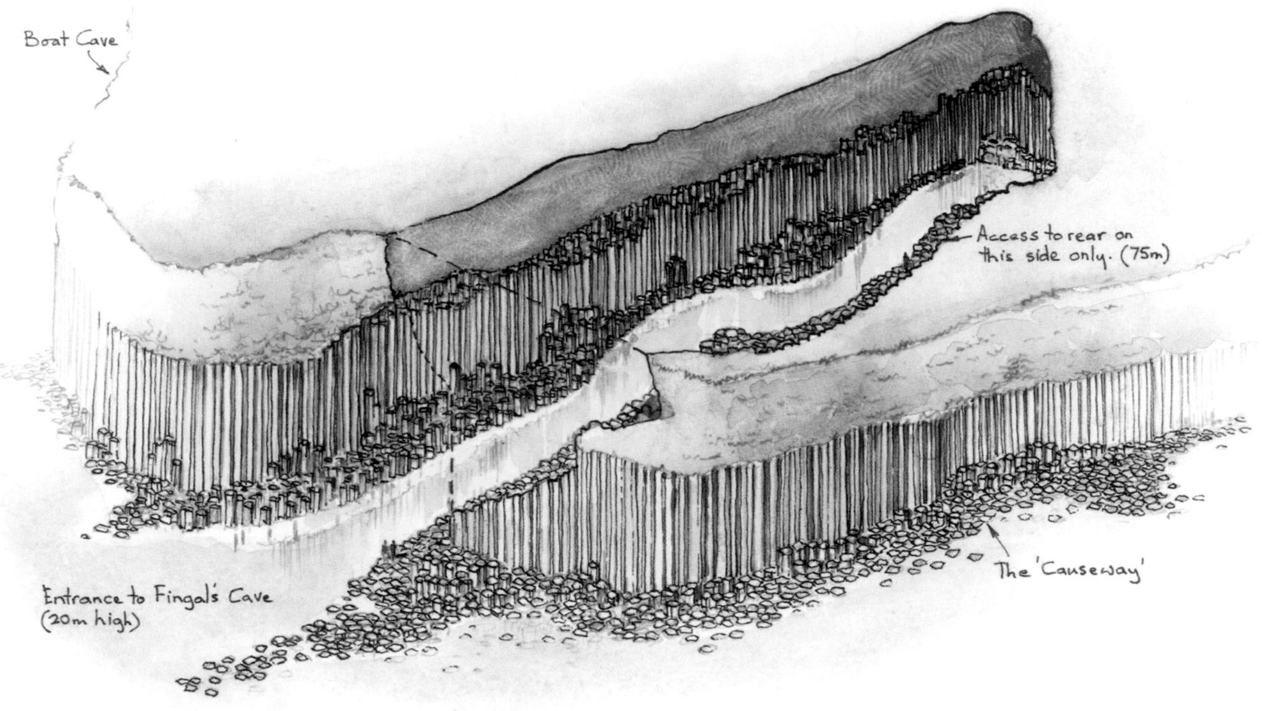

THE ANATOMY OF FINGAL'S CAVE

We saw, but surely in the motley crowd
Not one of us has felt, the far-famed sight;
How could we feel it? Each the others blight,
Hurried and hurrying volatile and loud.

Round the southern end of the island and west of Fingal's Cave is the Colonnade, otherwise known as The Great Face, – a vast expanse of columns reaching up 17m towards the sky with **Boat Cave** below them. In May 1945 a vagrant mine exploded here and the marks can be seen on the cliff-face. Opposite this southern tip is a strange formation known as the Wishing Chair. Further round on the west side **Mackinnon's Cave** (named after Abbot MacKinnon of Iona, who died in 1500) is almost as grand as Fingal's and has a tunnel connection through to **Cormorant Cave**. These caves can be reached at low water from the bay on the west side, which is fully exposed to the wild Atlantic and is called, strangely, Port an Fhasgaidh (G. – the port to clean off vermin) though a slightly different emphasis makes it the more probable, Port of Refuge. Access is not easy.

Access: Frequent summer trips, often combined with Lunga (weather permitting): Gordon Grant Marine, Fionnphort, Mull, 01681-700338: Turus Mara, Dervaig, Mull, 0800-085-8786: or Ardnamurchan Charters, 01972-500208.

Anchorages:
No adequate anchorage and landing only possible in settled conditions.
1. At least 1c SE of the landing-place in 6–12m, bottom rock and weed. Use tripping line. Many unmarked rocks so approach carefully from SE with Erisgeir astern.
2. Small beach at NE end suitable for dinghy landing but no anchorage.

SECTION 4

The Small Isles

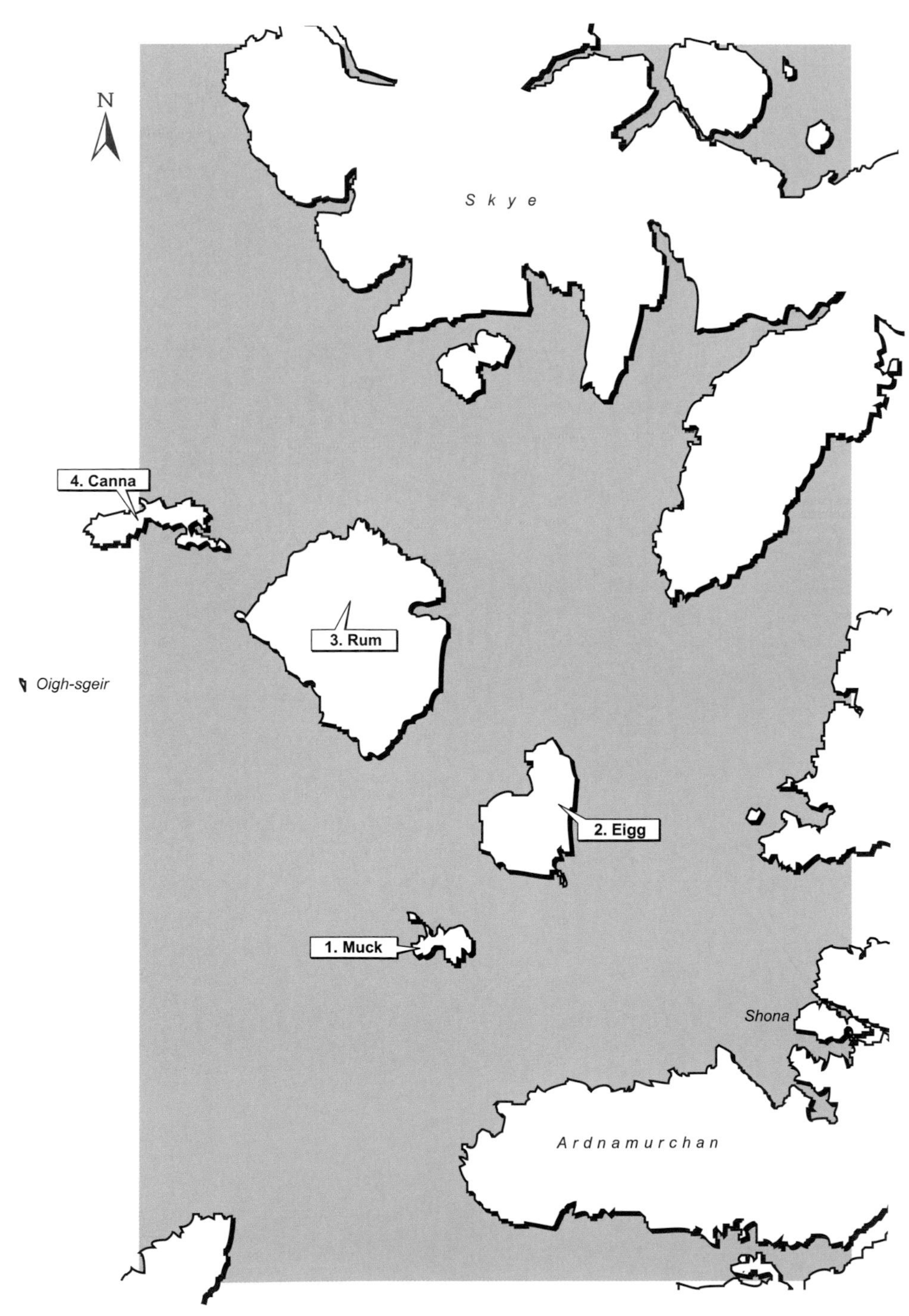

SECTION 4, Table 1: Arranged according to geographical position

No.	Name	Latitude	Longitude	Table 2* No.	Table 3** No.	Area in Acres	Area in Hectares	
4.1	Muck	56° 50N	06° 15W	54	48	1381		559
4.2	Eigg	56° 54N	06° 10W	24	14	7534		3049
4.3	Rum	57° 00N	06° 20W	13	3	25854		10463
4.4	Canna	57° 04N	06° 33W	36	32	2792	1130	
	Sanday	*57° 03N*	*06° 29W*			455	184	1314

*Table 2: The islands arranged in order of magnitude
**Table 3: The islands arranged in order of height

Introduction

The four islands in this section are not particularly small but they are generally known as the Small Isles, or Sma' Isles, because that is the name of their parish. The total number of parishioners in 1755 was 943 and in 1794 it was 1339. Unfortunately these early statistics do not give separate figures for each island.

When sailing 'over the sea to Skye' from Ardnamurchan each island shows a very distinctive profile – the long stretch of Canna, the high cloud-wreathed mountains of Rum, the almost-primeval Sgurr of Eigg, and Muck creeping past like a grey-green submarine.

Some miles to the west lies lonely **Oigh-Sgeir** (G. – maiden or virgin rock), maybe better known by its Norse name, **Hyskeir**. **Garbh Sgeir** (G. – rough rock) lies alongside with a neat little mooring in between. These rocks are only about four hectares (10 acres) in area, formed of hexagonal basalt columns – like Staffa, and rising to only 11m above sea-level. The lighthouse on Oigh-Sgeir was built in 1902–04 and, until it became automatic, the keepers grew vegetables and flowers in a walled garden and played golf on a miniature golf course. As always, these random skerries claimed the lives of many ships – the last on record was a Fleetwood trawler, the *Wyre Victory*, which sank about 4½ miles south-east of Oigh-Sgeir on 14 January 1976.

I am indebted to Malcolm MacGregor for the map information. He is the great-grandson of Robert Thom, one-time owner of both Canna and Oigh-Sgeir (see No.4.4). In the 19th and early 20th centuries sheep from Canna were regularly taken to Oigh-Sgeir to graze on the lush grass. The main islet is in three parts linked by a footpath. The largest part on the east is called Cnoc na h-Airigh (G. – knoll of the summer pasture) and the western part with the lighthouse and quay is called Cnoc nan Uibhean (G. – the lumpy knoll). In settled weather it is possible to lie alongside the quay.

On the north side, Camas na Cloiche Ruaidhe (G. – bay of the rose-coloured stone) almost looks like part of the rim of a submerged volcanic crater – and maybe it is, while the area to the south of the lighthouse has many dangerous rocks and reefs including Sgeir nan Cuag (G. – the twisted skerry) and, more ominously, A' Ghruagach (G. – the brownie).

Tucked away in the corner of the Ardnamurchan peninsula, Loch Moidart is split in two by tidal **Eilean Shona** which was leased by J M Barrie in the 1920s as a peaceful place to write the screenplay for *Peter Pan*. This lovely island of 525ha was sold in 1995 by Richard and Anna Stead to Robert Devereux of London for a price believed to be about £1.3m. It has high and precipitous hills, natural woodland, exotic trees and a large house and grounds. The house overlooks South Loch Moidart with a densely wooded islet called **Riska**, and romantic Castle Tioram (G. *tioram* – dry, or fair) on its own drying islet, the home of Ranald, son of Somerled, Lord of the Isles.

Shona's old schoolhouse, now occasionally occupied as a holiday home, is on the opposite side of the island from the main house. It is reached by walking nearly two miles along a well-constructed track which follows the beautiful shore of North Loch Moidart. In the last century, I was told, the lady of the house ordered the school to be built as far from the house as possible so that she would not be disturbed by the children's voices! The schoolmaster's house, renovated by a professor from the USA, has a stunning view over the Small Isles with sunsets that have the sort of magic no photograph can ever capture. Otters frequent this lonely place, herons pose on the shores of the loch, golden eagles nest in the heights, and civilisation is light-years away.

The entrance to North Loch Moidart from the sea is fairly straightforward once the skerries beside **An Glas Eilean** (G. – the grey island) and **Eilean Coille** (G. – wooded isle) have been located. **Eilean a' Choire** (G. – corrie isle) lies below the mountain slopes of Shona. The South Loch Moidart entrance is more devious and entails crawling past **Eilean Raonuill** (G. – Ranald's island) and then slipping round a rock pimple called **Eilean Corra** (G. – peaked island) with a few skerries in between providing interesting diversions.

North of Moidart the Sound of Arisaig is divided into Loch Ailort and Loch nan Uamh (G. – loch of the caves). **Eilean nan Gobhar** (G. – goat island) and **Eilean a' Chaolais** (G. – channel island) are at the entrance to Loch Ailort. Halfway along the loch are **Eilean nam Bairneach** (G. – isle of the limpets), **Eilean Buidhe** (G. – yellow isle) and **Eilean Allasaigh** (G. – tilted isle) and at the head of the loch are some very tiny islets – the Black Islands or **Eileanan Dubha**.

On the north shore of Loch nan Uamh the **Borrodale Islands**, a string of skerries, give partial shelter for a yacht to anchor in attractive surroundings. The best spot is north of **Eilean nan Cabar** (G. – island of the rafters or poles). **Eileanan Sgurra** (G. – rocky isles), **Am Fraoch Eilean** (G. – the heather isle) and **An Glas Eilean** are to the south-west surrounded by rocks. At the head of the loch there is another anchorage to the east of **Eilean Gobhlach** (G. – forked island), an islet with a cleft between two hillocks.

At the entrance to the Sound of Arisaig a treacherous group of skerries, **Eilean an t-Snidhe**, can be a hazard in poor visibility. By the coast to the north **Eilean a' Ghaill** (G. – stranger's isle) has the remains of a fort on it.

Virtually all the off-shore hazards here are tidal,

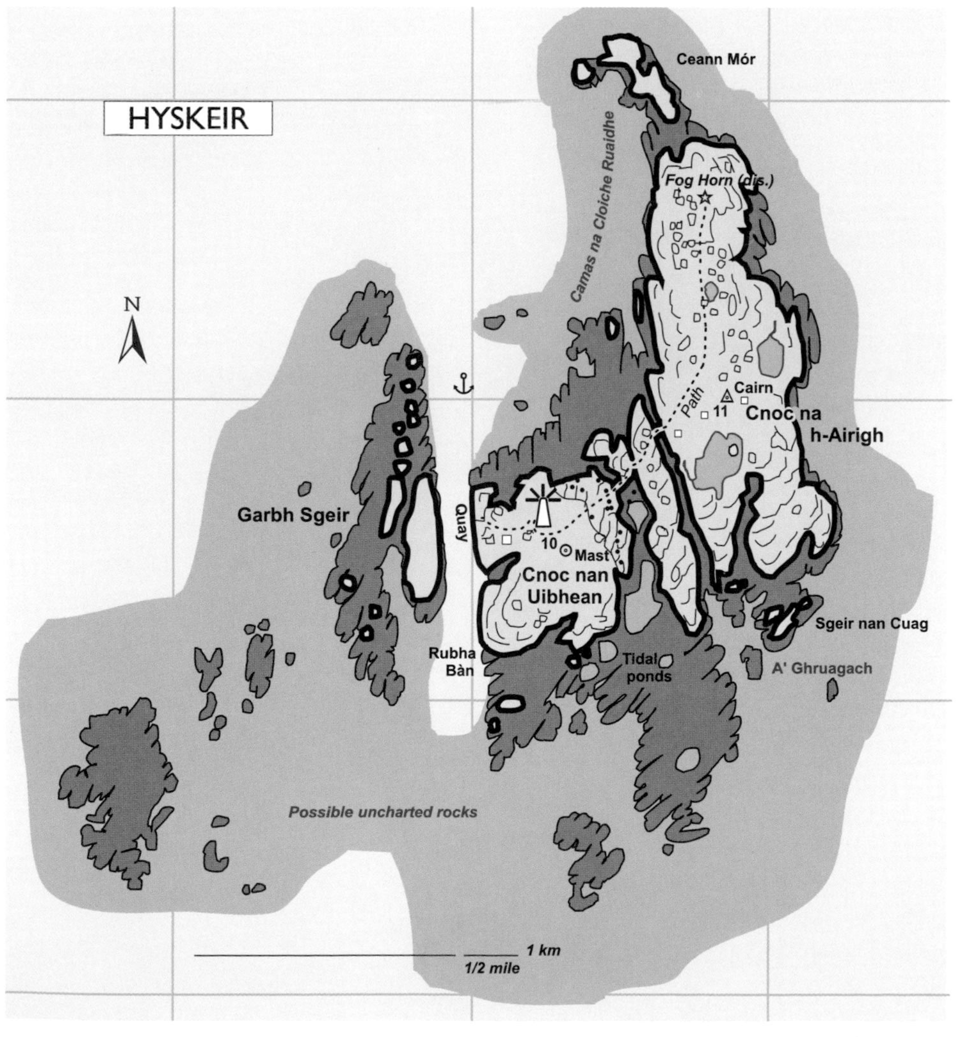

with **Luinga Mhór** and **Eilean Ighe** being the largest. Loch nan Ceall, which is the harbour for Arisaig, is guarded by a minefield of rocks, islets and skerries. There are perches to mark the passage through these but yachtsmen used to claim that the perches often swam about or the rocks did. This is no longer true as all the perches have now been renewed and painted and the passage is fairly easy. If nothing else, a visit by sea to Arisaig is a memorable experience and there is the benefit of a large selection of buoys provided for visiting craft.

A rather shabby little islet, **Eilean na h-Acairseid** (G. – harbour island), lies off Mallaig near the entrance to the harbour.

4.1 Muck

(G. eilean nam muc – isle of pigs.) Fordun called it Helantmok – isle of swine. (G. muc-mhara – whale) is a kind but improbable option. In 1582 Buchanan referred to it as insula porcorum. When Dr Samuel Johnson met the Laird of Muck he was told that 'Muck' (Lord Muck) was the incorrect title. With a touch of wishful thinking the Laird asked to be called 'Monk' as he claimed that his property's original owner was a hermit from Iona.

OS Maps: 1:50000 Sheet 39 1:25000 Sheets 390 or 397
Admiralty Charts: 1:100000 No.1796 1:50000 No.2207

Area: 559ha (1381 acres)
Height: 137m (449 ft)

Owner: Purchased by the MacEwens in 1896. Lawrence and Ewen MacEwen are the principal owners.

Population: Early 1800s–280. 1841–68. 1861–58. 1881–51. 1891–48. 1931–48. 1961–29. 1971–24. 1981–20. 1991–24. 2004 – 35. The MacEwens advertise at intervals for young families to settle on the island as it is essential to maintain a viable primary school.

Geology: Mostly Tertiary sheet basalt with typical terraced cliffs, grassy ledges and flattened crowns. Dolerite dykes run NW to SE. Very fertile soil composed of glacial drift and sea-blown shell-sand which produces appetising potatoes as early as May.

History: In 1588 when a Spanish galleon was wrecked in Tobermory Bay, Sir Lachlan Maclean of Mull, encouraged by the Campbells, employed the surviving Spanish sailors as mercenaries and let them loose on several islands belonging to the MacDonalds. Consequently Muck was burned, plundered and left in a desolate state.

By 1773 when Boswell and Dr Johnson were passing by the island it was again reasonably prosperous, thanks to a considerate laird and the production of kelp (which was used to make potash). Boswell reported that the Laird had 'seven score of souls' on Muck. 'Last year he had eighty persons inoculated, mostly children, but some of them eighteen years of age. He agreed with the surgeon to come and do it, at half a crown a head. – It is very fertile in corn, of which they export some; and its coasts abound in fish. A taylor comes there six times in a year.' Almost Utopian, but some fifty years later, in 1828, the kelp market collapsed and 150 islanders were shipped off to Nova Scotia. Then in 1854 Muck was purchased by Captain Thomas Swinburne RN, who started a fishing industry but also rented the land for sheep farming, causing further depopulation. Only today is the island recovering once again – or at least surviving – thanks to the enlightened and benevolent policy of the owners.

Wildlife: Some alpine plants grow here 600m below their usual altitude – dwarf juniper, crowberry, club moss, rose root sedum, mountain cats-paw and pyramidal bugle. In early summer the fields are covered with the flowers of marigold, iris, cornflower and bluebell. The only heather

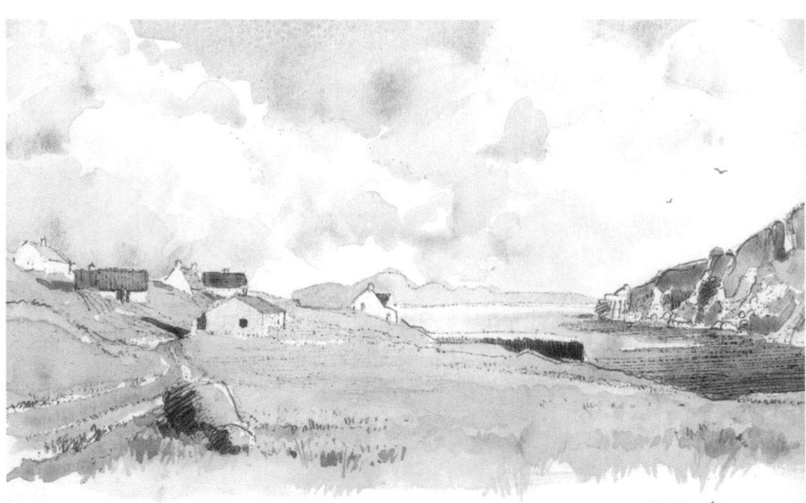

PORT MÓR

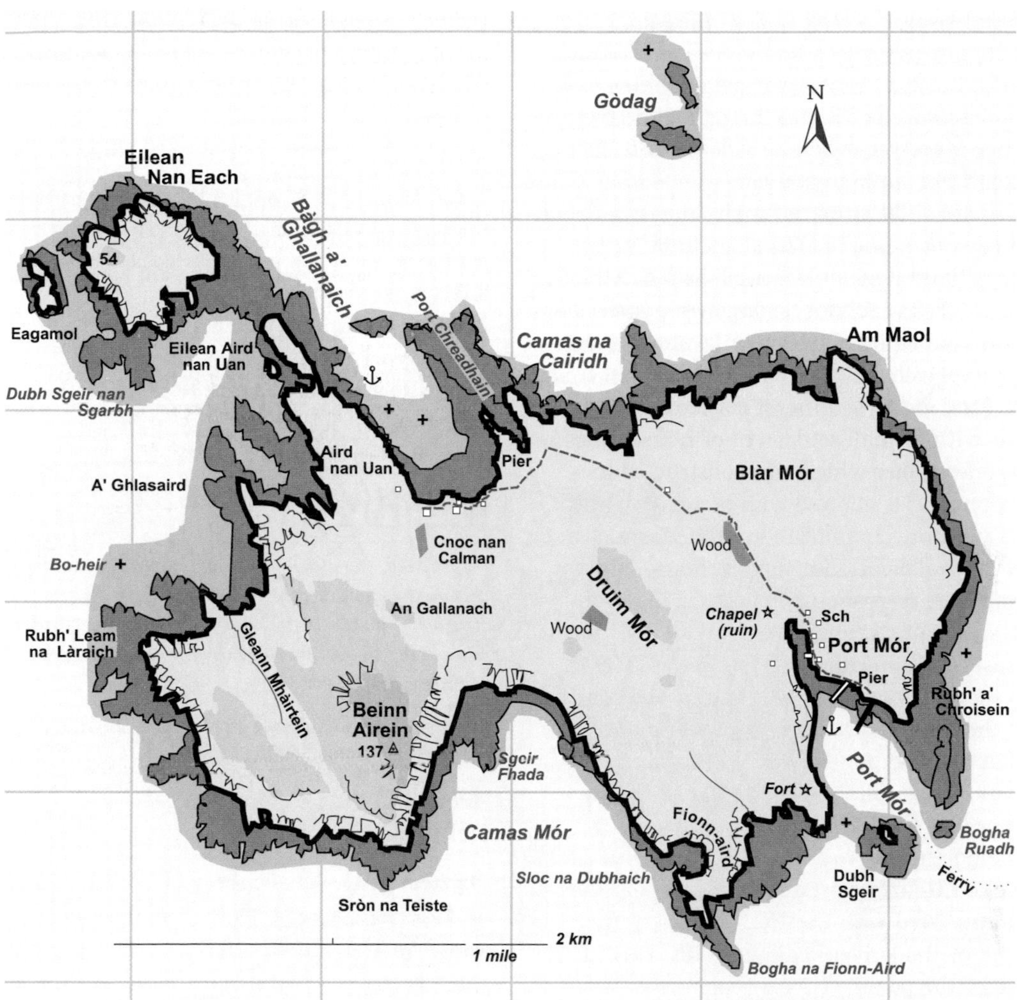

is in Glen Martin. There are a few acres of woodland mostly planted in 1922 but there are plans to plant more trees.

Some Rum ponies are bred on the island and as there used to be no stallion the mares were occasionally ferried over to Rum. Otters can be seen in Gallanach Bay and there are a number of small rodents but, luckily, no rabbits.

Gallanach Bay is also a popular playground for porpoises, which may have been a factor in the naming of the island as they are called 'sea-pigs' in Gaelic.

Over eighty species of birds nest here with the sea-birds favouring isolated Eilean nan Each. There are also many visiting species.

MUCK is a peaceful, low-lying island with attractive beaches but exposed to the Atlantic gales. This brings in the shell sand which keeps the basalt soil fertile. Most of the coast is rocky and near the west end are cliffs 15m to 18m high. There are some springs of good water.

This is the most fertile of the Small Isles and Lawrence MacEwen, the laird, runs the main farm at **Gallanach** (G. – full of young trees), with his wife Jenny and some additional help. It is a mixed farm with cattle, sheep, a small dairy herd, and crops of potatoes, oats and root crops. There are also two small tenant farms and the island is self-sufficient in milk, eggs and vegetables with the islanders having a communal vagetable patch for their own use. Cars are of limited use as there are only two kilometres of road and the farm tractor is still an important means of powered transport. There is no peat so all fuel, apart from driftwood, has to be imported. Electricity is provided by two wind-powered generators installed in 2000.

Jenny's father was in the colonial service in

paddle-shaped legs and a long neck and tail, were found on Eigg. In 1992 a similar fossil was found on Skye.

History: St Donan or Donnan, who had been trained at Whithorn and may have stayed for a time at Loch Alsh (Eilean Donan), eventually set up a sizeable monastery on Eigg but was murdered together with fifty-two of his monks in 617 according to the Irish annals.

The island was part of the Norse empire but was seized by the MacDonalds, Lords of the Isles. Robert the Bruce granted official title to MacDonald of Clanranald in 1309.

The earliest recorded meeting of island chiefs seems to suggest that it took place on Eigg – although Islay may be the correct interpretation: '...at Kildonnan in Eigg, where the staff of Lordship of Clanranald was given to one who was nominated Macdonnall and Donald of Isla...'

One story runs that in the winter of 1577 some MacLeods from Skye were sent home castrated after being caught raping MacDonald girls on Eigg. When the MacLeods, led by Alasdair Crotach (Hunchback Alasdair) from Rodel on Harris (see No.8.14), retaliated in force, 395 MacDonald islanders hid in Uamh Fhraing (G. – St Francis Cave) but were eventually discovered by the MacLeods who tried to smoke them out by lighting a brushwood fire in the entrance. Every MacDonald is said to have suffocated in the smoke and the cave is still known as 'Massacre Cave'. Some bones were removed from the cave for burial in the 19th century.

The population seems to have recovered quickly for eleven years after this incident Sir Lachlan Maclean and his Spanish mercenaries burnt and plundered the island.

The Reformation had left the islanders uncertain which religion it was safe to follow. At that time they were part of the Protestant parish of Sleat in Skye but their minister, Reverend Mackinnon, never visited them. A missionary priest, Father Ward, landed in 1625 and soon renewed their Catholic faith. Mackinnon was furious and sent soldiers to seize the priest but the people refused to yield. Mackinnon retreated and was looking for additional support when MacDonald of Clanranald (a Catholic) offered to pay Mackinnon one-third of the island's tithes if he left the islanders in peace. Mackinnon readily accepted.

The MacDonalds of Eigg supported the Catholic Jacobites in the 1745 rebellion so Captain John Ferguson of the King's ship, *Furnace*, was sent to arrest the leader John MacDonald. He surrendered and handed over all arms on the promise that there would be no reprisals against his clansmen but as soon as he was in custody Ferguson sacked the island and deported the young men.

In 1829 the MacDonalds sold Eigg to Dr Hugh MacPherson, Professor of Greek at Aberdeen University, for £15,000 and several minor clearances followed. The next owner, Robert Thompson, a wealthy shipbuilder, bought the island in 1893 and spent a lot of money on improvements including the construction of a large house which he called the White Lodge. It was a time of comparative prosperity for the crofters. Thompson died in 1913 and his grave is on Eilean Chathastail. A Danish shipping magnate, Sir William Petersen, was the next owner. When he was in residence his flag flew at the Lodge and his luxury yacht, *White Eagle*, would anchor near the pier but in 1924 a fire destroyed the White Lodge and a year later Petersen died in debt.

One of his creditors, Lord Walter Runciman, a shipowner, and his brother James, a writer, then took over the island. They built the present lodge, created the home farm, planted a semi-tropical garden of palms, bamboo and lush woodland and ploughed back profits. Relative prosperity was regained until a Shropshire farmer, Robert Evans, bought the island in 1966 for £82,000 and resold it for £120,000 in 1971 to a Christian charity, the Anglyn Trust, which had dreams of using the island for the treatment of mentally handicapped children.

This came to nothing and it was something of a relief for the islanders when the Schellenbergs took over in 1975.

Wildlife: Campion, golden rod, a variety of heathers, thyme, willow, remnant hazel scrub, and even some imported eucalyptus trees grow in the mild, damp climate which also encourages a wealth of saxifrages. A number of wild goats frequent the heights.

The island is managed as a wildlife reserve supervised and part-owned by the Scottish Wildlife Trust. There are a few rare species of butterfly.

A fairly large and noisy colony of Manx

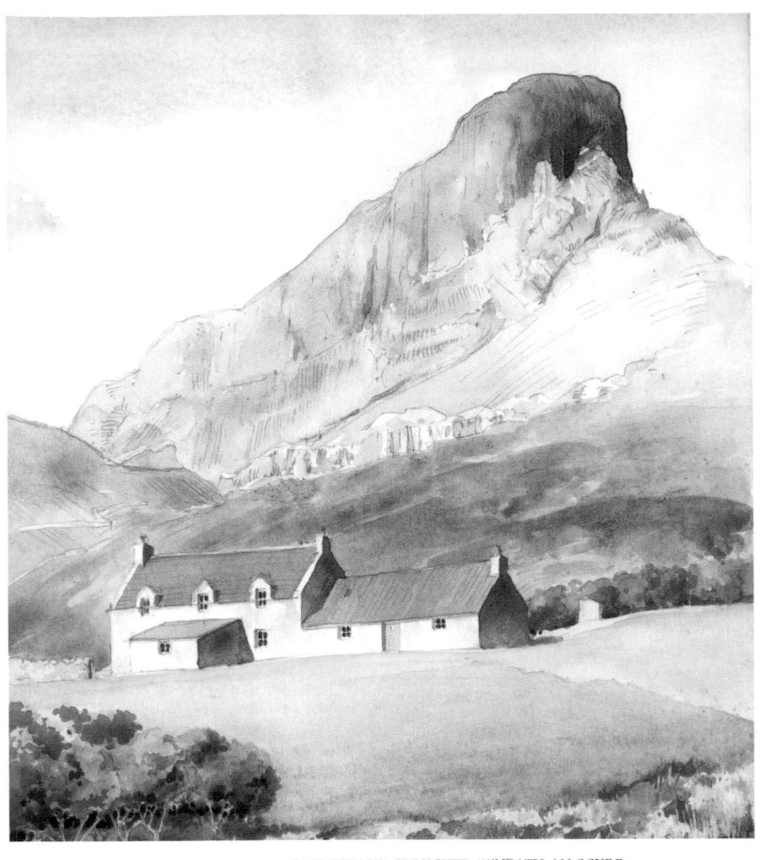

GALMISDALE, CROUCHED BENEATH AN SGURR

shearwater burrows into the soil on An Sgurr, and there are some colonies of puffins on the sea-cliffs. Until about 1900 white-tailed sea-eagles had eyries on the cliffs of Eigg before disappearing from the list of native British birds.

* * *

For an island the size of **EIGG** it is unfortunate to have no harbour, and no bays or inlets which give satisfactory shelter, but a new ro-ro ferry pier was completed in 2004 at a cost of £7.8 million and passengers and goods no longer have to disembark from the ferry by flit-boat. Although most of the population lives at **Cleadale** in the north-west the ferry has always called at **Galmisdale** in the south-east, where rocky **Eilean Chathastail** (G. – castle island) gives some protection from the ocean swell. Although cars will be able to reach Eigg without difficulty only islanders' cars will be allowed to land – to maintain 'the peace and tranquility of the island'. However Eigg is a fairly large island and other forms of transport have been provided as it is a long walk to Cleadale and back.

Above Galmisdale is 'The Lodge' – the laird's house – a white Italian-style (15-room) residence once set in a garden of crazy-paving, catmint and carnations. It was in very serious disrepair but a couple of ecologists with a young family bought it in 2004 and are gradually restoring it and running courses on sustainable technologies. Meanwhile in 2008 a £1.5m development of hydroelectric, wind and solar electricity fed through 7 miles of underground cables has provided 'green' power for all.

At **Kildonnan**, (G. – Donan's cell) an ancient Celtic cross-slab is set near the ruins of a 14th-century church which was built on the site of a monastery founded by St Donan in the 7th century [NM489854]. The saint and his fifty-two monks were massacred in 617, some say by pirates, others by a band of warrior women who lived on a crannog in **Loch nam Ban Móra** (G. – loch of the mighty women) [NM455852]. The loch and several little lochans are in a sheltered hollow high in the hills behind the Sgurr. The women apparently disliked missionaries but it was Norsemen who destroyed the monastery buildings.

Macdonald's Cave and **St Francis Cave**, both of them worth a visit, lie half a mile southwest of the old pier. Walk up the road towards An Sgurr and climb the first stile on the left. Follow the path to the cottage, then a sheep track to the cliff fence. Follow the fence to a zig-zag track leading down to the shore beside a small burn. Turn left to Massacre Cave (St Francis Cave) [NM476834] and right to Cathedral Cave (Macdonald's Cave). Cathedral Cave is still sometimes used for Catholic services, a custom dating from the persecution following the 1745 rebellion. A stone wall in the cave may have been an altar.

A strip at the extreme north end of the island is low-lying but ½km in from the shore steep cliffs rise to about 250m clearly marking, there and on the east coast, the change in sea-level since the Ice Age. Cliffs nearly encircle the island with the dramatic hump of the **Sgurr of Eigg** rising a further sheer 150m above the plateau. When the clouds are low, there is a touch of mystery; when the sky is blue, throw in some imaginary palm trees (there are real ones at the Lodge) and it could be Tahiti.

Kenneth MacLeod, composer of many beautiful songs including the 'Road to the Isles' was born on Eigg in 1872.

There are many enjoyable exploits for experienced climbers. On The Sgurr there is Collie's Cleft in the South Wall rated as severe; Eagle Chimney – hard severe; The Flue – very severe and Botterill's Crack – severe. The latter has a fossilised coniferous tree trunk at the foot. On the cliffs overlooking Cleadale, called the Cleadale Face, there is Laig Buttress – severe, and the Pod – very severe.

Less dangerous, but equally thrilling, is the fine hillwalk from An Cruachan (G. – the rounded hill) to Bein Bhuidhe (G. – pleasant mountain) with the sight of Rum's dark mountains, Ainshval and Askival, towering into the clouds beyond the windswept sound. JRR Tolkien holidayed here and this view is said to have been the inspiration for his mystical *Lord of the Rings*. He lived in Howlin croft house.

* * *

Access: Ro-ro ferry from Mallaig, Mon., Tues., Thur., Fri., and Sat., 01687-462403/011. (Vehicles not encouraged and permit required, 01397-709000). Arisaig Marine, every day except Thur., 01687-450224. Tourist Information, East Bay, Mallaig, 01687-462170.

Anchorages: There are no sheltered anchorages.

1. South of Galmisdale Point. Approach from SSW well clear of En Chathastail. Anchor in the NW part at least 1c off-shore and out of the tidal channel in 3–6m, sand. Exposed to SW and swell.
2. SE of N extremity of En Chathastail. Beware 1½c reef just S of this. Anchor ¾c off the island. Exposed to E'lies and can be uncomfortable.
3. NE of Galmisdale Point. Approach through the narrows or from NE between the perches – with care. Very restricted anchorage in moderate weather NE of the end of the old pier avoiding moorings, reef and ferry. Bottom foul. Subject to swell. Shoal-draught boats may snug-in N of old pier.
4. Poll nam Partan, tidal pool within Rubha na Crannaig. Avoid S access. Approach from SE (2.3m depth at LW) on leading line. Anchor in sand with weed patches.
5. N of Rubha na Crannaig, off Kildonnan. Depths shallow enough for anchorage up to 2c from shore of Eigg but very exposed. Useful in perfect conditions or in emergencies.
6. Bay of Laig. Occasional anchorage in quiet weather or E'lies. Keep about 2c off S shore on approach.

4.3 Rum

[room, or rum] Probably pre-Celtic but possibly (ON röm-øy – wide island) or maybe (G. i-dhruim – isle of the ridge).

(Note: Sir George Bullough changed the spelling to Rhum to avoid the alcoholic association. 'Rh' is not a Gaelic form and in 1991 the Nature Conservancy Council of Scotland after consultation with the School of Scottish Studies at Edinburgh University asked for the spelling to be corrected.)

O S Maps: 1:50000 Sheet 39 1:25000 Sheet 397
Admiralty Charts: 1:100000 No.1796 1:50000 Nos.2207 and 2208

Area: 10463ha (25854 acres)
Height: 812m (2663 ft)

Owner: A Lancashire family, Bullough, were owners from 1888 to 1957. The Government purchased the island on behalf of the Nature Conservancy Council from Sir George Bullough's widow, Monica Lady Bullough, in 1957 for £26,000. The castle contents were donated to the nation by Lady Bullough. Later, control was transferred to Scottish Natural Heritage (SNH).

Population: 1794– over 400. 1831–134. 1841–124. 1881–89. 1891–53. 1931–32. 1961–40. 1971–40. 1981–17. 1991–26. 2001–22. The population is mostly made up of employees and families of Scottish Natural Heritage and a schoolteacher but the aim now is to encourage newcomers to settle.

Geology: A square platform of purple-red Torridonian sandstone, 150m to 300m high, fringed with sea-cliffs, some of the formations on Rum are geologically unique. The range south of the Kinloch-Harris divide is called the Cuillin and includes the peaks, **Askival** (812m) (ON – mountain of the ash trees), **Hallival** (723m) and **Trollaval** (702m) (ON – mountain of the trolls) composed of rock allied to gabbro but with fewer basalt dykes than usual. Hallival has escarpments of allivalite, its own pale variety of gabbro and the slopes between are of peridotite, a dark variety which weathers to orange-brown. Small platinum deposits were reported in 1999. **Ainshval** (781m) (ON – hill of the strongholds) and **Sgurr nan Gillean** (764m) are capped by quartz-felsite overlying Torridonian sandstone. On

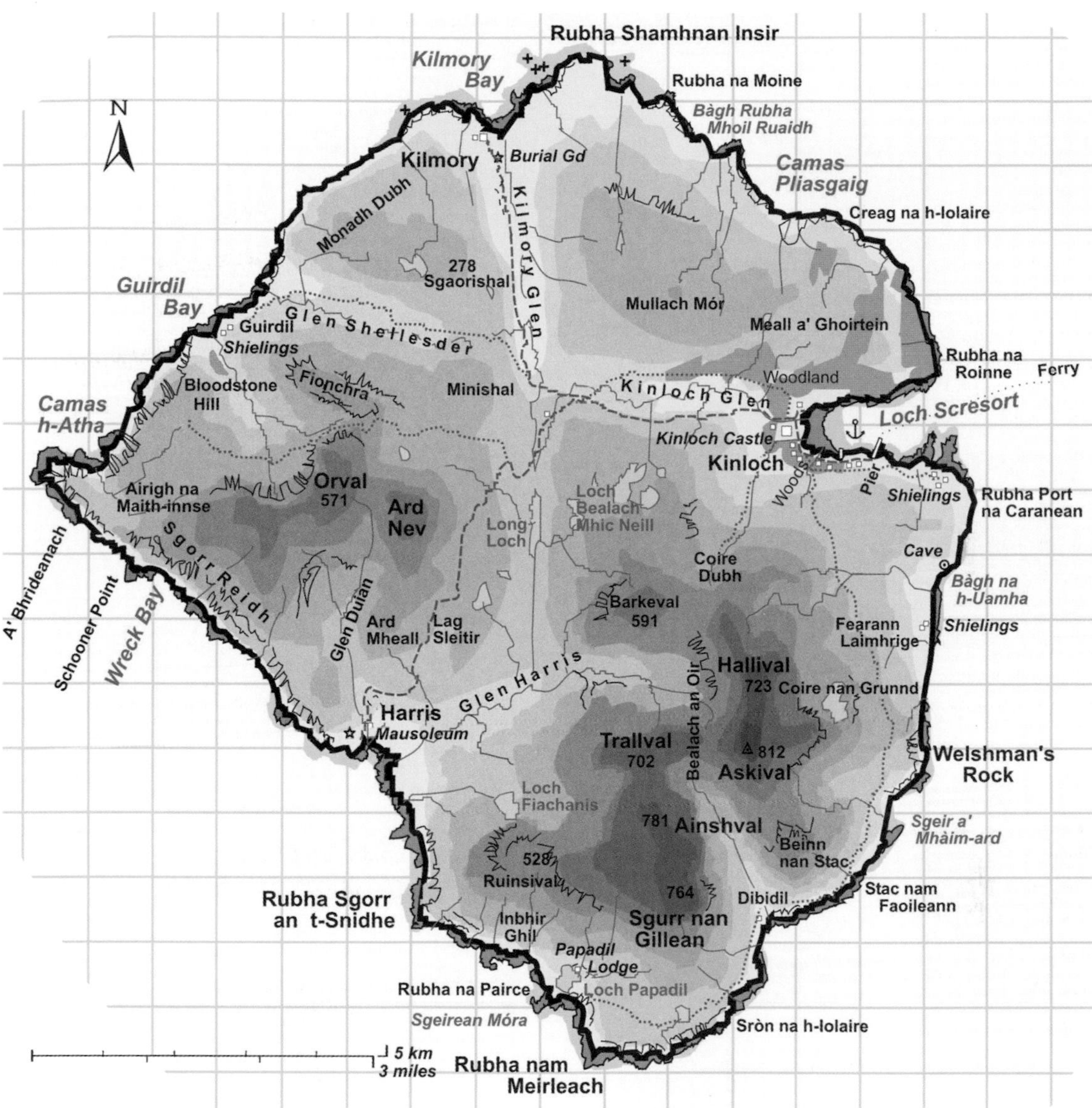

the south and western cliffs there is granite. The strongest gravitational pull in the British Isles has been recorded below Ard Mheall.

Rum was a centre of violent volcanic activity some sixty million years ago. During the last ice age it had its own independent glaciers, one of which carved out Kinloch Glen. There is a raised beach at Harris and long raised terraces cut by the sea into the spectacular western precipice which is now being carved by the Atlantic breakers at a lower level.

Only a few patches of arable land exist – at Harris, Kilmory and Kinloch.

History: In spite of its somewhat inhospitable climate today, Rum was one of the earliest places of human settlement in Scotland although little is known of its early prehistory. Its interest for Mesolithic man was probably the availability of rare bloodstone from Bloodstone Hill – an attractive substitute for flint.

Various topological features have Norse names but there is little conclusive evidence of Norse settlement except for a carved narwhal ivory gaming piece found at Bàgh na h-Uamha in the 1940s.

Rum passed from the Norwegian to the Scottish Crown in 1266 and early records show that Rum was chartered to John of Islay in 1346. It was attacked and plundered by Sir Lachlan MacLean and his mercenaries in 1588, and in 1695 became part of the lands of the Macleans of Coll. The main industry – fishing – was

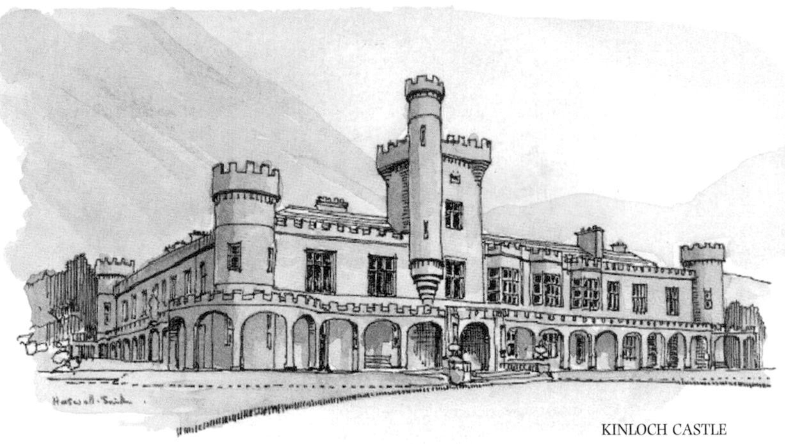

KINLOCH CASTLE

damaged by the Salt Tax, and yet in spite of the difficult conditions the population steadily increased. By the beginning of the 19th century there was overcrowding and extreme poverty. A clearance was arranged and over 300 islanders were 'persuaded' to emigrate to Canada and the United States, leaving less than fifty inhabitants behind. Maclean leased the island for sheep-farming and 8000 sheep were introduced and some shepherds. They were joined by some families of crofters who emigrated from Skye and settled at Port nan Caranean in 1827. By 1831 the population had risen to 134 but eventually stabilised at about ninety. In 1845 Maclean sold the island to the Marquis of Salisbury as the sheep-farming was unprofitable. The Marquis converted Rum to a sporting estate by stocking the burns with trout and bringing in red deer before he too sold out.

There was a further unsuccessful attempt at sheep-farming by the Campbells of Oronsay and then in 1888 a Lancastrian MP, John Bullough of Oswaldtwistle, stepped in. He had made a fortune from the design and production of milling machinery. Rum became his holiday retreat and sporting estate and according to his widow he wrote poetry when out shooting while enjoying his after-luncheon cigar 'by some bonnie burn'.

His wealthy and eccentric son, George Bullough, aged twenty-one, took over in 1891. After sailing round the world he built Kinloch Castle in 1900–02. He imported London architects (Leeming & Leeming), red Arran sandstone, and Lancashire stonemasons to build a home on the island fit for a laird. The workmen were paid extra to wear kilts and tuppence a day for tobacco (midge money). Even the garden soil was imported from Ayrshire. This was a prime example of extravagant Edwardian opulence – live turtles and alligators in heated tanks; birds of paradise and humming-birds in the conservatory; a large mechanical 'orchestrian' with brass, woodwinds and drums for military marches and operettas; central heating, double-glazed stained glass, a baronial hall, a billiard room with air-conditioning (to remove the cigar smoke), and a Victorian 'jacuzzi' bath. Guests were brought to Mallaig by a private train, taken by steam yacht to Scresort and met by Albion motor cars which were kept on the island. Grapes, figs, peaches and nectarines were grown in the glasshouses.

Sir George was married on Rum and stayed there for three weeks every year.

Wildlife: In 1957 Rum was declared a National Nature Reserve and has since been declared a National Scenic Area, a Special Site of Scientific Interest, a Biosphere Reserve, and a Specially Protected Area.

The entire ecology is being managed by Scottish Natural Heritage (SNH) to conserve the natural and cultural history of the island. The existing mixed woodland at Loch Scresort was mainly planted by the Bulloughs about 1900. Over one million native trees and shrubs have now been planted as part of an extensive woodland regeneration project and open heathland preserved for study and conservation of the natural flora and fauna in a unique environment. An excellent SNH booklet is on sale at the post-office.

Plant life is prolific and some is undisturbed since the last ice age. Rare arctic sandwort and penny-cress can be found, the spotted orchids, *Dactylorhiza maculata*, are of a sub-species unique to Rum, and there are three unique micro-species of eyebright. The moors are studded with blue heath milkwort, sundew, tormentil, butterwort, black bog-rush and bog asphodel, and thrift, roseroot and Scots lovage grow on the cliffs. Nineteen species of butterfly have been recorded.

Rum ponies are sometimes claimed to be descended from ponies saved from a wrecked Spanish galleon, or the offspring of Eriskay ponies. The current herd originate from a cross between an Arab sire and a West Highland mare but stand only 14 hands high (1.4m). Sir George introduced a pure white Arab stallion to improve the bloodstock.

Highland cattle are kept to maintain, by controlled feeding, the herb-rich pastures of Glen Harris and a small herd of feral goats favour the south-western cliffs. The biology and habits of the red deer are closely studied. One surprising discovery was that they are occasionally carnivorous – eating live young seabird nestlings, presumably to compensate for mineral deficiencies. (See Foula No.11.6 for carnivorous sheep). Rum ponies are used to bring the deer carcasses in during the annual cull by professional stalkers.

The peak season for ornithologists is April to October, with many varieties of upland species. In all, over 150 species of bird have been recorded. Corncrakes breed on the farm at Kinloch and there are sea-bird colonies on the south and north-east coasts – mainly kittiwake, puffin, razorbill and guillemot. About 61,000 pairs of Manx shearwater breed in mountain top burrows. Their ghostly sounds in the night probably gave Trollaval its name (a midnight ascent in May is unforgettable). Golden eagles are to be seen over the glens. One of Rum's great success stories has been the reintroduction of the white-tailed sea eagle during the 1970s and 80s using chicks taken from Norwegian nests. The last Scottish bird was seen on Skye in 1916.

RUM is by far the largest island in the Small Isles group but because it is so mountainous and its climate is less mild it has never been able to support a population relative to its size. The average annual rainfall at Kinloch is 240cm but in the mountains above it is over 300cm. Before the 15th century most of the island was cloaked in native woodland but slashing and burning by man destroyed it all except for a few stray trees on rocky cliffs. The present bleak moorland slopes are a direct result of this, followed by overgrazing of sheep and deer.

A roadway connects the three 'settlements' of Kinloch, Harris and Kilmory and there is also a rough track running south from Kinloch to Dibidil and on to Papadil.

Kinloch on Loch Scresort is the main settlement centred round **Kinloch Castle**, which is filled with remarkable 'objets d'art' collected by Sir George in the Far East. (Sadly, if understandably, this unique monument is deteriorating but there are, at last, some proposals under review which give grounds for hope. SNH is probably doing its best but obviously does not have the resources or interest of a benevolent landlord.) The **Post Office** is the oldest inhabited building on Rum. It used to house the kitchen for Kinloch House – the original laird's house which was near the site of the present Castle. The beech and sycamore trees behind the Post Office were planted about 1830 when Kinloch House was being built.

Until the ferry pier was completed in 2001 everything was normally trans-shipped ashore to the old stone pier at **Loch Scresort** which is only accessible at high water. Electricity is provided by a small hydro-electric turbine but coal was formerly delivered only once a year and stored in a store by the jetty.

A prehistoric site at Kinloch was discovered during ploughing in the summer of 1983.

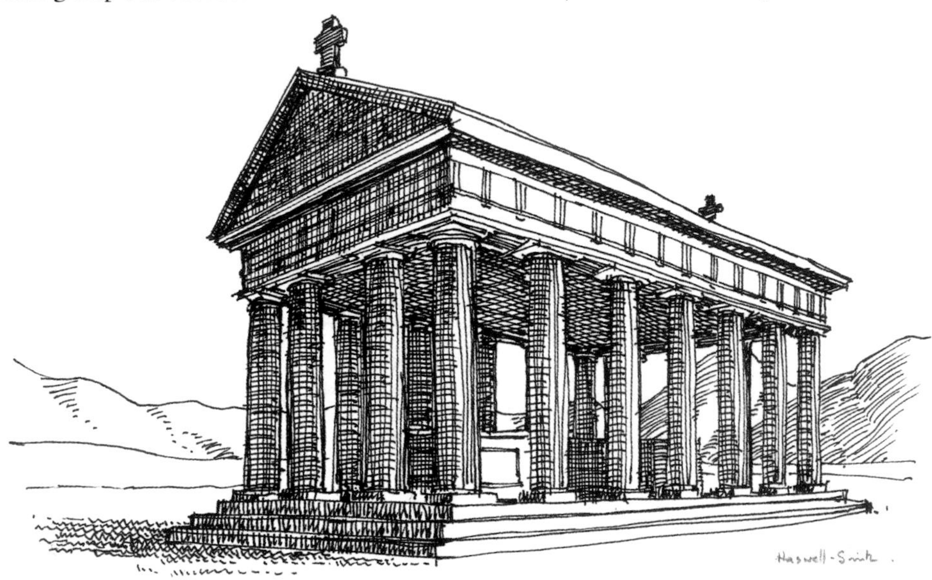

THE BULLOUGH MAUSOLEUM – A GREEK TEMPLE IN REMOTE GLEN HARRIS

Excavations were carried out between 1984 and 1986 which revealed extensive Mesolithic and later activity dating from 7000BC providing the best evidence to date of the early settlement of Scotland. A vast number of artefacts were recovered, mainly stone tools made of Rum bloodstone and flint.

On the south side of Loch Scresort is the schoolhouse, built in 1962 in front of the previous schoolhouse, and further east on the headland are the remains of an old village, **Port na Caranean**. It lies across Gleann Carn nan Dobhran (G. – glen of the cairn of the otters) and otters can still be seen here in the early morning. The village population was twenty-seven in 1841 but by 1861 it was abandoned.

Harris in the south-west has the lowest rainfall on Rum (140cm). The main feature there is the Bullough mausoleum – as eccentric as everything else – built in the style of a Greek temple [NM336957]. It contains the tombs of John, George and Monica. John (Sir George's father) was first laid to rest in a tiled burial vault but a friend said it looked like a public lavatory for London Underground so Sir George built a new mausoleum and blew up the vault with dynamite.

The track from Kinloch to **Dibidil** (ON *djup-dalr* – deep valley) on the south-east coastline passes Creag a' Wealishech (G. – Welshman's rock). Some Welsh slate quarriers widened a precipitous path near here. The track leads on round the southern extremity to **Papadil** (ON *papa-dalr* – valley of the hermit), romantically lonely and attractive with a loch backed by a small wood of mixed trees. The Lodge was built by Sir George but Lady Bullough disliked it and let it fall into ruin [NM366922]. There is a climbers' bothy there now.

At the opposite extreme in the far north **Kilmory** has a very fine beach, the remains of quite a large village settlement, an old burial ground [NG361036], one inhabited cottage and the original Kinloch Castle laundry. The area is sometimes closed to the public (for deer research).

For the mountaineering fraternity, both Askival and Ainshval are classed as 'Corbetts' but climbers and hill-walkers on Rum should always remember that there are no facilities for rescue. Many interesting climbs have been listed – easy, moderate, difficult and severe. Allivalite is similar to the black gabbro of the Cuillin on Skye, rough, but firm. A traverse of the main ridge involves little actual climbing yet is a classic expedition, and walking the ridges of Hallival, Trollaval and Sgurr nan Gillean, down Glen Dibidil, and back along the coast to Loch Scresort is a memorable experience.

There is also spectacular hill-walking (first contact the Reserve Office). For one long and strenuous walk, take the Dibidil track starting close to the pier at Loch Scresort, 8½km over a 230m ridge (easier than crossing the tussocky moor) to Dibidil then an indistinct 4km to Papadil. From Papadil and across Glen Harris, 6km, keeping roughly to the 200m contour to avoid the sea-cliffs.

The west coast may be reached from the road junction point. From there a stalker's path goes to the 370m bealach at the top of Glen Guirdil, then under the basalt summit cliff on Orval, across to 388m Bloodstone Hill and the fine sea-cliffs of Sgòrr Mhór. An alternative track leads down Glen Shellesder past waterfalls to the shielings at Guirdil. Both these walks are 6km there (and 6km back) and only the man-eating midges can spoil one's pleasure; but remember also that this is a big rough island, hard-going at places and distances are misleading.

Fishing may be purchased at the Reserve Office but there are no boats and all catches must be reported. Deer stalking can also be arranged (for a price). The only vehicles permitted are SNH's own jeeps.

* * *

Access: Ro-ro ferry from Mallaig, Mon., Wed., Fri., Sat., calls twice a day giving stopover time, 01687-462403. (Vehicles not encouraged and permit required, 01687-462026). Accommodation at Kinloch Castle Hostel, 01687-462037. For use of campsite first contact the SNH Reserve Office, Isle of Rum PH43 4RR, 01687-462026. Arisaig Marine, Arisaig, every day in summer, 01687-450224. AquaXplore, Elgol, Skye, full day trips by RIB., 0800-731-3089. Tourist Information, East Bay, Mallaig, 01687-462170.

Anchorages:

Generally, the bottom is rock off S and W sides, mud off E side with irregular depths, and sand off N side. There are no landing restrictions.

1. Loch Scresort affords good anchorage but subject to squalls in W'lies and swell from E'lies. It is shallow, and the

head dries out about 2c. S shore moderately steep-to, except for reef extending 2c N from Rubha Port na Caranean. Old pier dries and concrete slip has a least depth of 0.6m at outer end. Anchor well off the slip or NE of the old pier in sufficient depth, stiff mud and thick kelp.

2. Bay W of Rubha na Moine near N extremity of the island. Temp. anchorage in suitable conditions.

3. Kilmory Bay, near N extremity, has possible spots to anchor in depths of 2.5–5.5m, sand, but requires great care and suitable weather. Several rocks on both sides of bay.

4. Camas na h Atha, on NE side of A' Bhrideanach, the W extremity, is a small sandy bay with a rock off each entrance point. Temp. anchorage only when conditions ideal.

4.4 Canna

(EI cana – wolf-whelp) island, or (ON kne-øy – knee-shaped island), or possibly (G. cana – little whale or porpoise) island.

Sanday

(ON sand-øy – island with a conspicuous sandy beach)

O S Maps: 1:50000 Sheet 39 1:25000 Sheet 397
Admiralty Charts: 1:100000 Nos.1795 or 1796 1:50000 main anchorage and western part No.2208

Area: 1314ha (3247 acres)
Height: 210m (689 ft)

Owner: Ownership donated in 1981 to the National Trust for Scotland (NTS) by the late Dr John Lorne Campbell (1906–96) who had owned it since 1938.

Population:

	1841	1881	1891	1931	1961	1981	1991	2001
C'na		57	40	40	24	11	20	6
S'day		62	62	20	0	7	0	6
	255	119	102	60	24	18	20	12

(In 2006 the Trust successfully advertised for two more families to settle)

Geology: A lava platform of terraced Tertiary basaltic rock has formed a generally rich and fertile soil. The basalt columns on the south coast are up to 6m in height. Compass Hill (139m) at the north-eastern corner is undifferentiated tuff with a sufficiently high iron content to distort ships' compasses helped by a vein of iron ore which continues under the sea to the north.

History: Canna belonged to the Benedictine Monastery of Iona followed by Norwegian suzerainty although the monks continued to cultivate it until the Reformation. Piracy was such a problem however that the Abbot of Iona appealed to the Pope to threaten excommunication if the raids did not cease. Canna became part of the Kingdom of Scotland

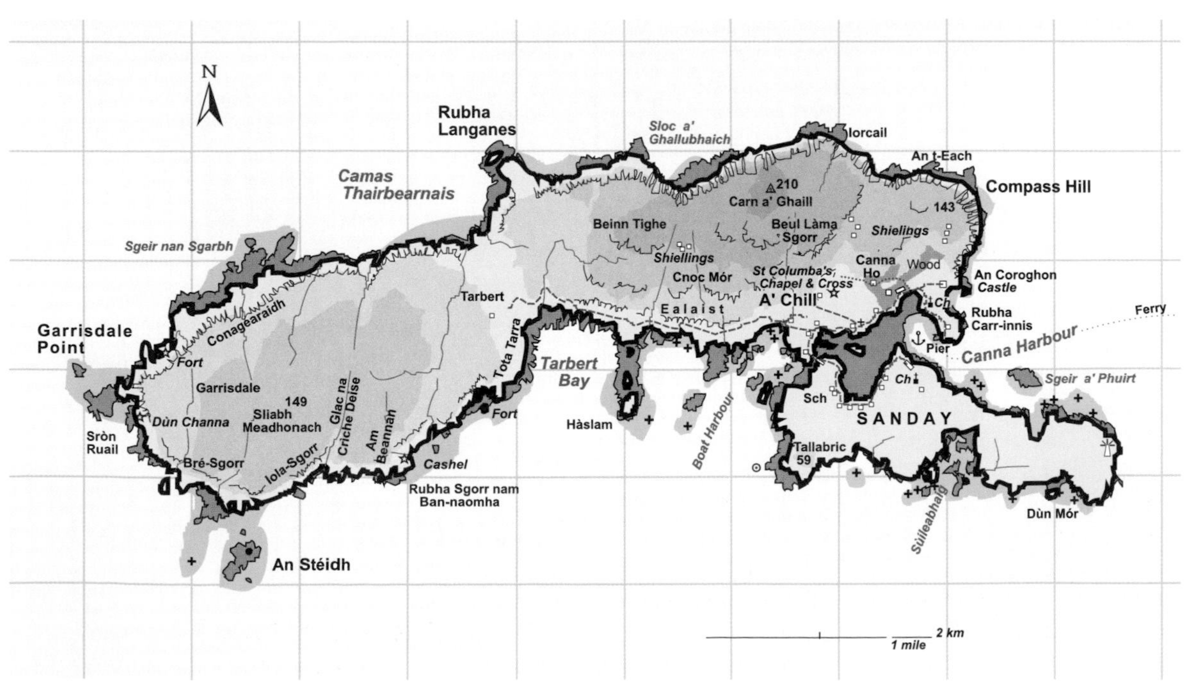

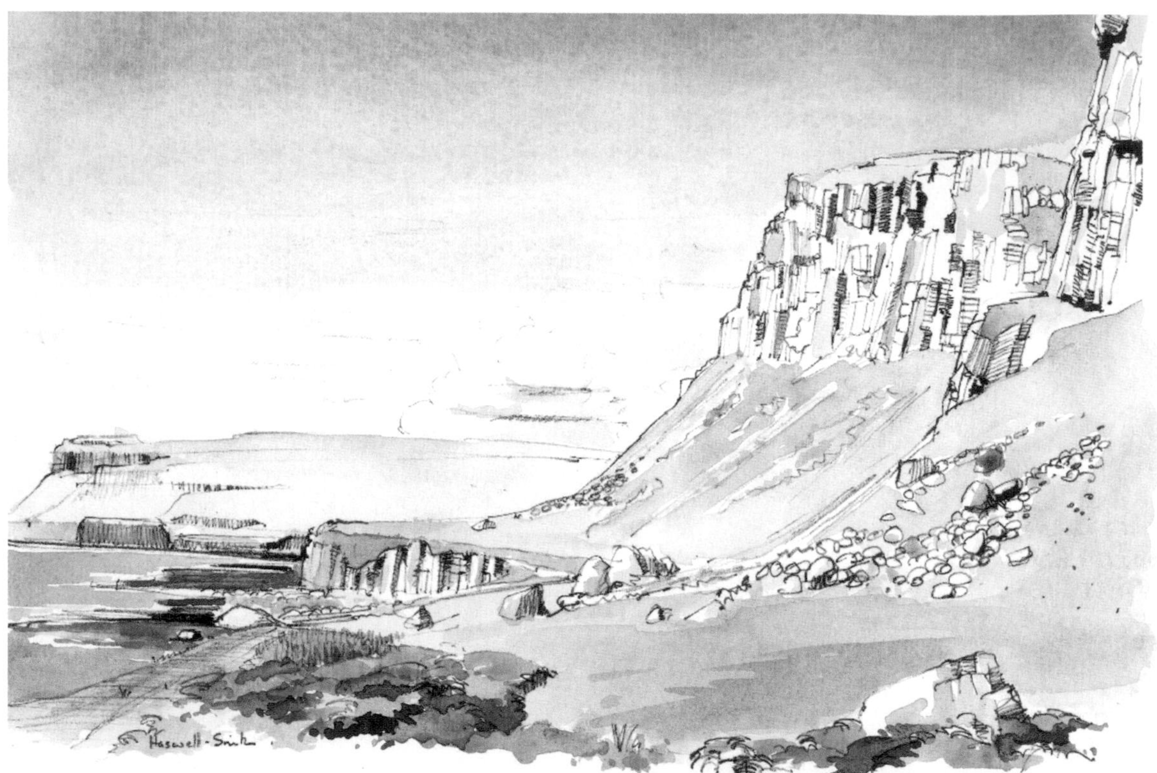

ESCARPMENT NEAR TARBERT BAY

in 1266 under the nominal rule of the Lord of the Isles which passed to the Macdonalds of Clanranald. As with the other Small Isles, Canna was subjected to fire and plunder by Sir Lachlan Maclean's mercenaries in 1588.

Macdonald of Clanranald found himself short of income when the kelp boom collapsed so he sold Canna in 1827 to Donald MacNeil.

Severe clearance followed the death of MacNeil in 1848. His natural son, Donald, was still a minor at the time and therefore not responsible. In 1881 he sold the island to Robert Thom, a Glasgow shipowner, for £23,000. Thom brought in a much more benevolent regime which continued until 1938 when his family took the trouble to look privately for the right sort of understanding purchaser. This they found in the Gaelic scholar, Dr John Lorne Campbell, historian, folklorist, farmer and 'bonny fechter', who was sold Canna for just £9000 and took up residence on the island with his American wife. Campbell had founded the 'Sea League' with Sir Compton Mackenzie when they both lived on Barra in the 1930s – a pressure group to try to protect the West Coast fishing industry from external incursions. He worked for most of his life on the preservation and encouragement of Gaelic culture and collected in Canna House the world's biggest library of Celtic language and literature. He also fought to keep Canna as a viable community although, 'I'm not a laird,' he said, 'I'm an owner-occupying farmer.' In 1981, when he gave Canna to the National Trust for Scotland, he also gave them his large and invaluable library and collections of Gaelic songs for safe-keeping. The hope of this conscientious custodian was that the Trust would fully understand the needs of this small community and not allow it to become depopulated and a mere tourist attraction.

Wildlife: Woodland of natural rowan and hazel interspersed with introduced sycamore, ash, elm, oak, birch, willow, elder, beech and some Sitka spruce, Corsican pine, Austrian pine and Japanese larch on the hillsides above the harbour with bluebells and wild garlic for ground cover. Hedgehogs were introduced by the Campbells – for better or for worse – and thistles are encouraged to support several species of butterfly and moth.

This is a superb bird sanctuary. It was being invaded by rats but these were (hopefully) eradicated in 2006 and Manx shearwater and puffins are returning. Occasionally white-tailed sea-eagles fly over from Rum – they were once indigenous here.

* * *

Viewed from due north or south, each end of **CANNA** appears to terminate in a bluff with the middle sinking to a low neck or saddle. Compass Hill is at the eastern extremity and the highest point **Carn a' Ghaill**, (G. – rocky hill of the storm) about 1km west of it, is 210m high.

SANDAY, close south, joined by a footbridge and a drying reef, rises to 44m height at its east end where there are several detached rocks in the sea. Two of these lie close to the cliff – a small one like a steeple and the other like a large tower (31m). They are Dun Mor and Dun Beag and they are known as the puffin stacks.

The space between Canna and Sanday forms a very well protected harbour with a ferry pier which was upgraded in 1992. The harbour is entered by rounding a graffiti-covered rockface – originally the names of fishing boats and early traders from the Baltic States, but now also those of day-trippers seeking immortality. There is a small restaurant which was granted a licence in 2003.

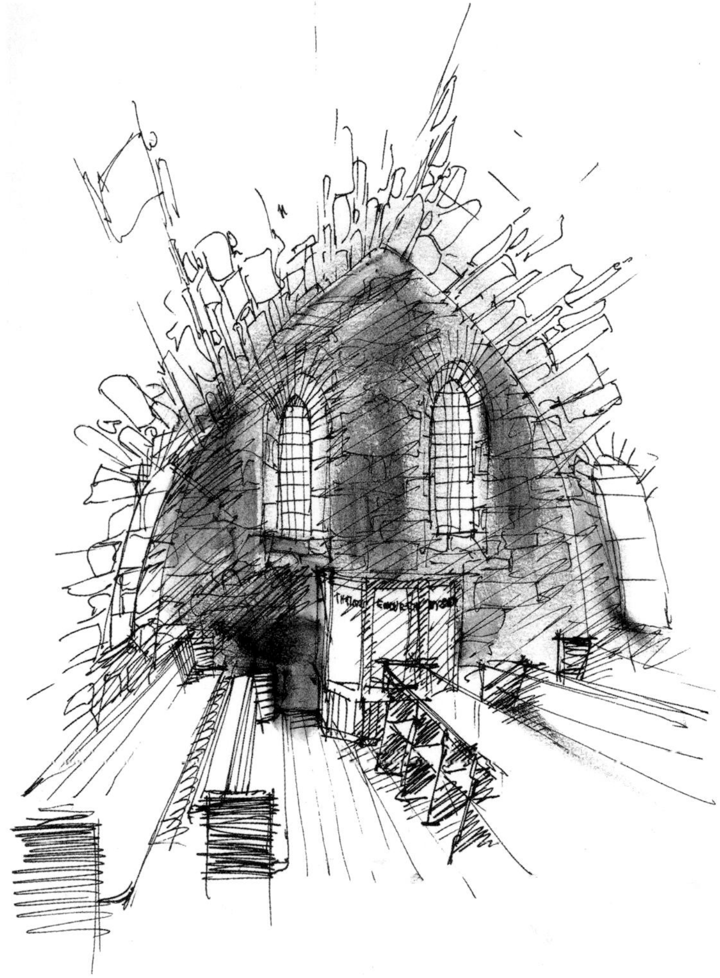

IN THE SCOTS KIRK

The principal house on this idyllic island is **Canna House** [NG273056], surrounded by thick woodland and overlooking the harbour. It was built about 1865 and was the home of the late Dr Campbell (1906–1996) and his wife, the American scholar, Margaret Fay Shaw (1903–2004). Above Canna House and partly concealed by the trees is **Tighard**, the house built in 1905 by Robert Thom. Close by is the main farm – The Square. With no high mountains to south or west, the clouds usually slip past Canna and the climate is pleasant and sunny. The fertile soil gives a rich and unusually early yield with particularly delicious early potatoes. Fields lying fallow are cropped by pedigree Highland cattle and Cheviot sheep.

The islanders are Catholic but there is a carefully maintained and charming little **Protestant Church**, built like early Celtic churches with a conical bell tower, on the east side of the harbour [NG277054]. This was constructed in 1914 as a memorial to Robert Thom. On Sanday and facing it is the much more ornate Catholic Church designed by William Frame and built by Lady Bute in memory of her father [NG275048]. This has now been tastefully converted to a Gaelic Study Centre – the **St Edward's Centre** – where scholars have the benefit of access to Dr Campbell's extensive library. The islanders now worship in a less elaborate building near the main farm. The proud title of **Post Office** is given to a tiny creosoted wooden shed with an adjacent telephone box – painted blue when I first saw it. It is beside Canna's oldest inhabited house, the Changehouse, which usually has resident collies. Canna is permitted to issue its own postage stamps.

A' Chill (G. – the cell or chapel), north-west of the harbour and above the main farm, was the site of the original township, cleared by MacNeil in 1851. Here there is a broken but beautifully carved Celtic cross [NG270055] but no sign of the remnants of the early 7th-century St Columba's Chapel. An adjacent standing stone probably proves that this is another case of the Early Christian policy of building on important pagan sites, although a small hole at head height in which an offender's thumb was supposed to be jammed has led to this being called Clach a' Pheannais – the pillory stone.

An Coroghon, on the coast east of the harbour [NG280055], is a medieval prison tower on top of an isolated stack built by John MacLeod of Dunvegan in 1666. Some say he used it to imprison his daughter, Mor MacLeod, but others say that an 18th-century laird imprisoned his beautiful daughter there to keep her from her lover, Iain Ban Og of Skye, but Iain rescued her and carried her off to his home. Sir Walter Scott wrote a sensible warning:

Seek not the giddy crag to climb
To view the turret scathed by time:
It is a task of doubt and fear
To aught but goat or mountain deer.

Tarbert Bay is almost central on the south coast, defined by the islet Hàslam like a punctuation mark. A ruined fort is on the bay's western shore and the remains of a very ancient nunnery or 'cashel' are on a grassy terrace beyond the bay, 4km along the road from the harbour [NG230043]. The site overlooks **Sgòrr nam Ban-naomha** (G. – sharp rock of the holy women) and, 5km away to the south-west, the isolated basalt rock of **Humla.**

A very well-preserved Viking ship burial was uncovered near Rubha Langanes (ON – the long ness) in **Camas Thairbearnais** on the north side of the central neck. Signs of reputed Viking graves can still be seen and a rectangular outline of boulders is known as **Uaigh Righ Lochlainn** (G. – the grave of the King of Norway). On adjoining Sanday signs of Norse burials have also been discovered but unfortunately the graves had been rifled in the distant past.

A fairly long, but interesting, hill-walk to Garrisdale Point at the western extremity brings you to Dùn Channa (G. – Canna's fort). Garrisdale farm was abandoned in 1881 and there is another Pillory Stone at the deserted Conagearaidh farmstead. This distant end of Canna was fortified by a wall and there is another fort about ½km to the north-east.

* * *

Access: Ro-ro ferry (No vehicles allowed) from Mallaig, Mon., Wed., Fri., and Sat., 01687-462403. For cottage accommodation or permission to camp contact NTS., 01463-232034. Arisaig Marine, Arisaig, trips from Arisaig daily in summer, 01687-450224. AquaXplore, Elgol, Skye, full day trips by RIB, 0800-731-3089.

Anchorages:

1. Canna harbour. One of the best and most popular anchorages on the west coast. Beware reef N of Sanday on the approach and rocks alongside pier. Bottom is prolific kelp on thick mud – good holding, but only if anchor is well bedded-in.
2. Tarbert bay. W of Sanday and SE of the central dip on Canna. Approach W side of bay keeping well clear of the islet called Hàslam then anchor in NE side 2c off-shore, 4.6m. Worthwhile in fair weather. Exposed S and subject to swell.
3. Boat harbour. Temp. anchorage between S side of Canna and W end of Sanday in settled weather. Many rocks to be avoided. Anchor in 3.7m N of Sgeirean Dubha with landing on sandy beach in SE corner.

SECTION 5

Islands Surrounding Skye

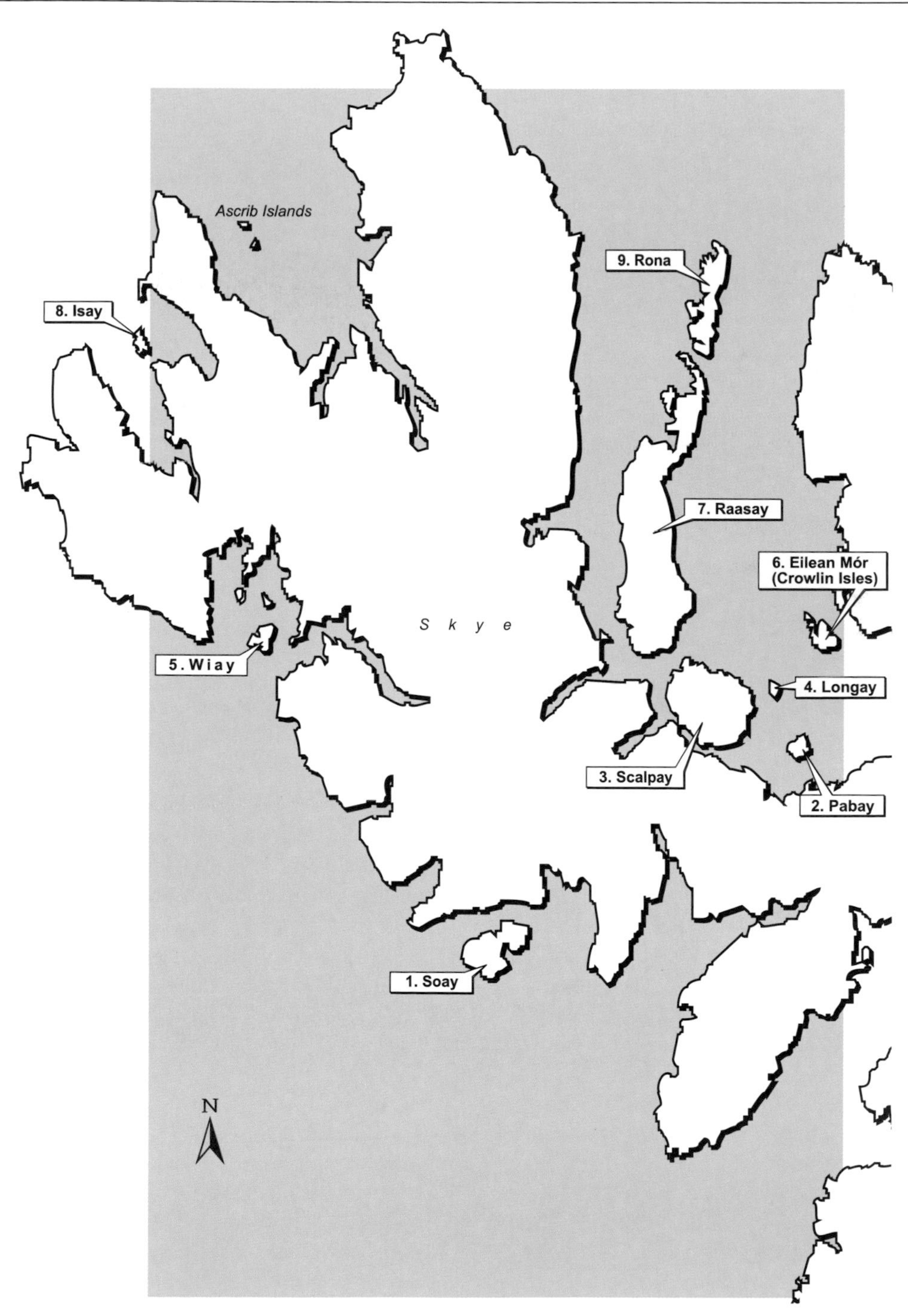

SECTION 5, Table 1: Arranged according to geographic location

No.	Name	Latitude	Longitude	Table 2* No.	Table 3** No.	Area in Acres	Area in Hectares	
5.1	Soay	57° 09N	06° 13W	41	47	2560		1036
5.2	Pabay	57° 16N	05° 52W	104	154	301		122
5.3	Scalpay	57° 18N	05° 58W	28	15	6135		2483
5.4	Longay	57° 19N	05° 53W	146	95	124		50
5.5	Wiay	57° 20N	06° 30W	94	103	366		148
5.6	Eilean Mór (Crowlin I)	57° 20N	05° 50W	72	59	477	193	
	Eilean Meadhonach	*57° 21N*	*05° 51W*			190	77	270
5.7	Raasay	57° 25N	06° 03W	17	11	15397	6231	
	Eilean Fladday	*57° 29N*	*06° 02W*			297	120	
	Eilean Tigh	*57° 31N*	*06° 00W*			133	54	6405
5.8	Isay	57° 31N	06° 39W	137	152	148		60
5.9	Rona	57° 33N	05° 59W	42	51	2298		930
5.A	*Skye*	*57° 22N*	*06° 11W*			*409259*		*165625*

*Table 2: The islands arranged in order of magnitute
**Table 3: The islands arranged in order of height

Introduction

I must admit to having misgivings about omitting Skye from a comprehensive book on the Scottish islands. But rules are rules and, having decided that a bridge destroys insularity, there was no other option. So, by my definition, Skye, which has always been the very essence of a Scottish island, no longer qualifies for inclusion. With the construction of a bridge it has now joined the mainland. Just as Seil took the same step many years ago.

To fend off criticism, however, I have compromised and included Skye as an appendix to this section. As with all the large islands, the description is necessarily brief. There are, after all, many excellent guides and books about Skye already available and my interest here is to pay more attention to the somewhat smaller islands which are given inadequate coverage elsewhere.

Apart from the nine classified islands in the vicinity of Skye, each of which has its own unique story and its collection of satellite islets, there are the other tiny islands hugging the mainland coast which at least deserve a mention.

North of Mallaig, at the entrance to sombre Loch Nevis, **Glas Eilean** (G. – green island) and **Eilean Dearg** (G. – red island) add an imaginative touch of colour and, further north, **Airor Island** shelters the small bay by the village of Airor in Knoydart.

Loch Hourn is a lovely loch to explore, stretching deep into mountain wilderness. **Eilean Ràrsaidh** with adjoining **Eilean a' Chuilinn**, just within the entrance of the loch and by the north bank, provide a delightful anchorage under the wooded crags of Beinn Mhialairigh. There is another anchorage south of **Eilean a' Phìobaire** (G. – the piper's island), on the south-west bank where there is a navigable channel between the island and the shore. At the first narrows a wide shoal and several tidal islets are beyond **Corr Eileanan** at Barrisdale Bay and beyond the second narrows – Caolas Mór – a central islet, **Eilean Mhogh-sgeir**, supports some twisted pines.

Eilean Chlamail is just north of the entrance to Loch Hourn, and projecting into the Sound of Sleat are the **Sandaig Islands**. These are all tidal with the exception of the largest, Eilean Mór, which has a light beacon on it.

Sailing through Kyle Rhea at mid-tide is like having a jet-engine attached to the hull. In the middle of Loch Alsh (which is a millpond compared to Kyle Rhea) **Glas Eilean** is little more than a permanent shoal covered with grass – a large flat expanse of grazing land. **Eilean Tioram** (G. – drying island) is tied to the land by a muddy tidal isthmus and beyond it another tidal island, **Eilean Donan**, linked by a bridge to the mainland, is the site of one of Scotland's most photographed castles.

The entrance to Loch Alsh is named after King Haakon, Kyle Akin. Some islets off Kyle of Lochalsh, **Eileanan Dubha**, lie in the navigable channel. Beyond is the site of the newsworthy or notorious, depending on your viewpoint, Skye Bridge which makes use of Eilean Bàn (G. – white or unused island), a National Trust for Scotland property, for support. **Eilean Bàn** is a double islet with a drying channel between and there are lighthouse-keepers' houses beside the lighthouse on the western half. It was one of these houses that Gavin Maxwell occupied after writing his best-selling novel, *Ring of Bright Water*. Otters are resident on many of the islets in this area, most of which belong to the National Trust for Scotland. The larger of these islands are **Eilean a' Mhal**, **Black Islands** and round the corner by Duirinish – still all Trust property – **Eilean Dubh Dhurinish**, **A' Ghlas-leac**, **Eilean na Bà Mór** (G. – isle of the big cow) and **Eilean Dubh**.

Eilean a' Chait (G. – cat island) has a disused light beacon on it at the entrance to Loch Carron. The largest of the Strome Islands in the loch is **Eilean an-t-Sratha**. Plockton – that little gem of a Highland village – snuggles into a corner of the bay on the southern shore wrapped in its own private Mediterranean climate. **Ulluva** is the name of the little island which appears in every photograph of Plockton – a few lone pines standing to attention on warm-grey rocks covered with orange and yellow lichen. A similar island near the shore, **Eilean na Creig Duibhe**, is tidal.

Off the peninsula dividing Loch Carron from Loch Kishorn are a number of rocks and skerries dominated by **Kishorn Island** and **An Garbh-eilean**.

Very much further north, there is a tiny islet of no particular significance, **Eilean Chuaig** (G. – twisted island), where the mainland turns away to make room for Loch Torridon.

On the south side of Outer Loch Torridon, **Eilean Mór** shields a deep pool which is a pleasant but limited anchorage as the bottom drops away fairly steeply. Loch Torridon divides into three distinct parts but the middle section has a change of name – Loch Shieldaig. There are two little islets in this part, **Eilean an Inbhire Bhain** and **Eilean Dùghaill**, and one distinctive larger island of about thirteen hectares, **Shieldaig Island**, which sits in tree-covered splendour opposite the sleepy whitewashed village of Shieldaig. Shieldaig Island was bought by the National Trust for Scotland in 1970 as it represents a small surviving sample of the ancient Caledonian Forest which used to spread over this entire region. The Scots pine regenerate because there are no sheep or deer to destroy them and they provide a refuge for many species of bird. There is a heronry at the north end of the island. In 1974 the cost to the NTS was reimbursed in full by Mr and Mrs Armistead Peter III of Washington DC who 'adopted' the island.

5.1 Soay

[so-ay or soy] (ON so-øy – sheep island)

O S Maps: 1:50000 Sheet 32 1:25000 Sheet 411
Admiralty Chart: 1:50000 No.2208

Area: 1036ha (2560 acres)
Height: 141m (462 ft)

Owner: The author, Gavin Maxwell, bought Soay in 1944 from Dame Flora MacLeod of MacLeod for £900. In 1946 he set up a shark-fishing venture with his wartime comrade, Joseph 'Tex' Geddes, as his harpooner. Maxwell eventually abandoned the project but Geddes continued it for a time and acquired crofting rights on the island. A Kent doctor, Nicholas Martin, bought the island for £100 in 1980 but he thought this included the crofting rights and there were long and expensive Land Court hearings. Dr Martin had a home on Soay. In 1993 'Tex' Geddes at last bought the island from him for an undisclosed sum but, sadly, died in 1997. His son Duncan is also known as 'Tex'. The island was put up for sale in 2003 for £280,000.

Population: 1821– one family. 1841–113. 1851–158 (the peak). 1861–129. 1881–102. 1891–78. 1931–64. 1953– most of the population moved voluntarily to Mull. 1961–11. 1981–8. 1991–14. 2001–7. 2003–2.

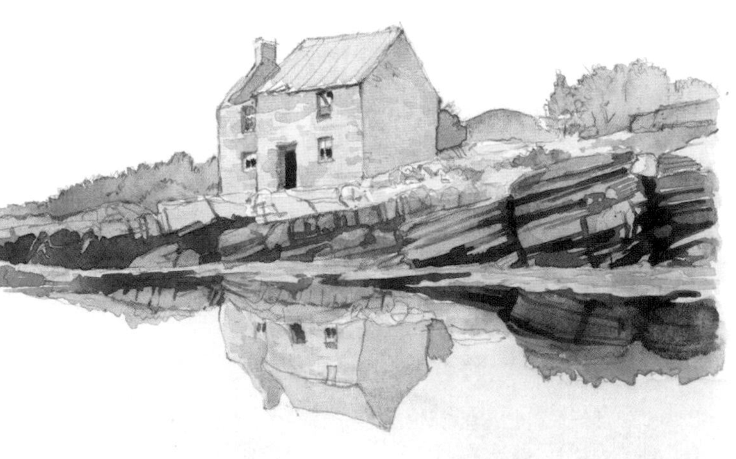

MAXWELL'S DELELICT SHARK-OIL FACTORY

Geology: Mainly Torridonian sandstone alternating with greywacke traversed by a fine-grained igneous rock.

History: Soay was the property of the MacLeods of Dunvegan from the 13th century. They sold it to Gavin Maxwell in 1944. The island was very lightly populated until the Clearances on Skye in the mid-1800s when more than one hundred of the dispossessed crofters chose to settle on this infertile little island rather than go to America.

After the Second World War, the islanders petitioned the government for evacuation, mainly because communications were so poor. So on 20 June 1953, with a great deal of publicity and a lone piper playing a lament the *SS Hebrides* evacuated the 27 islanders and took them to Mull, where land had been purchased for them by the government at Java Lodge, Craignure. Only one family refused to leave – that of Mr Geddes who had bought some of the island's crofting rights from Maxwell in 1951 and the rest from the departing crofters. The affair had some overtones of the sad evacuation of St Kilda (No.9.1) in 1930. The purchase bankrupted Geddes and he had to sell the island on to Dr Michael Gilbertson in 1963 for £2500 but the doctor kindly gave a farm to the Geddeses with secure tenure and eventually they regained possession of the island. Recently the population has seriously dwindled. Mail and stores are landed on a fortnightly basis

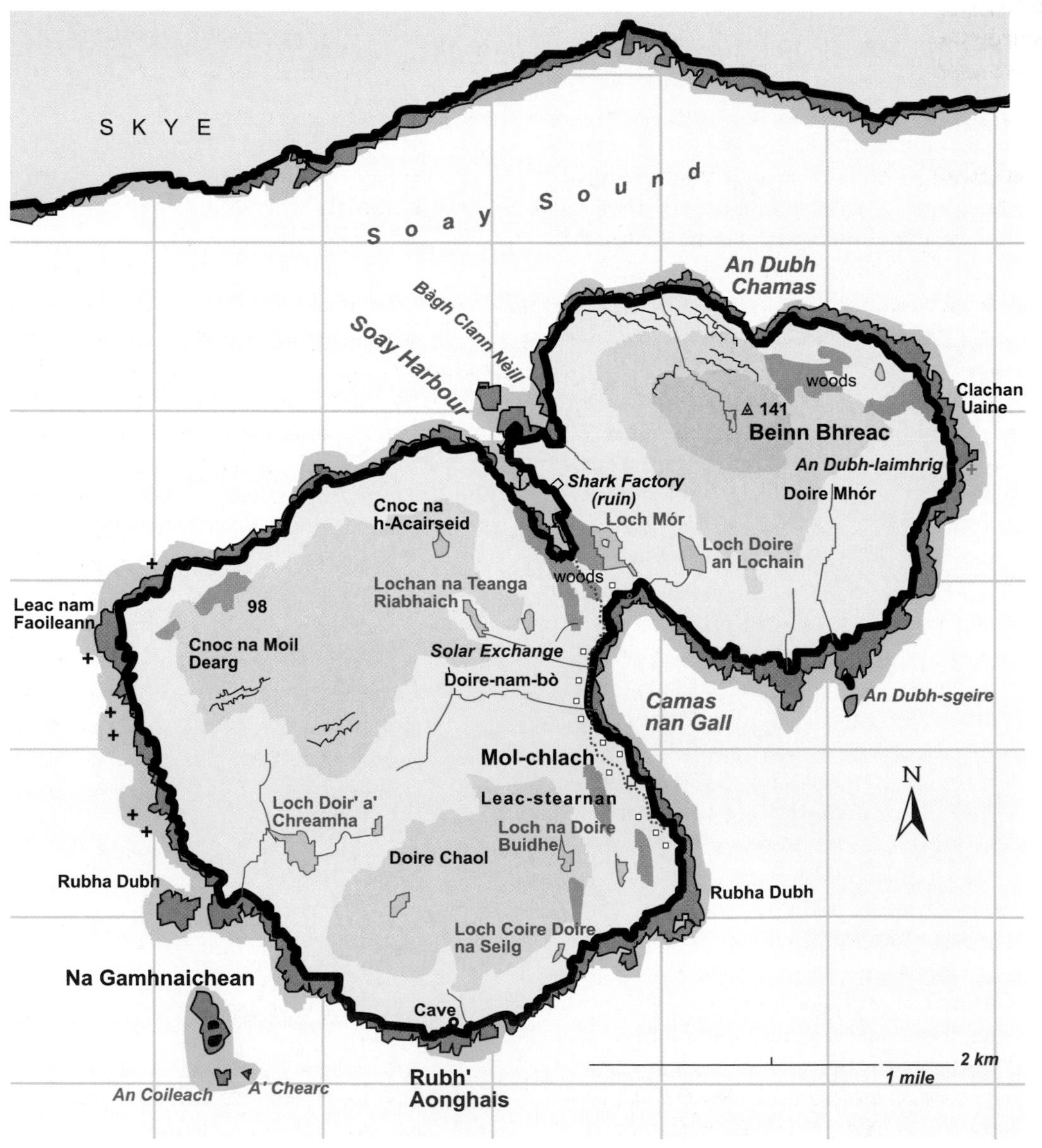

from Elgol on Skye and library books from Portree are transported in boxes with flotation buoys.

Wildlife: Not very fertile land but there is a profusion of deciduous bushes and trees such as birch, oak and rowan in the low saddle near the centre with a consequent variety of birdlife. Herons nest near the harbour and ravens cross the sound from Skye.

Unfortunately, in spite of his espousal of the cause of conservation, Maxwell's shark-oil venture on Soay contributed to a serious reduction in the numbers of basking sharks in West Coast waters. These inoffensive and harmless creatures may have been saved by the drop in value of shark oil in 1949 but they have never really recovered from the onslaught and are rarely seen. Maxwell wrote a book about his experiences – *Harpoon at a Venture.*

* * *

A dumbbell-shaped island with a narrow isthmus almost cutting it in half, **SOAY** is dwarfed by the Cuillin mountains which tower over it. **Acarsaid Soa** (G. – Soay harbour) is the northern part of the central gut.

When Maxwell bought Soay at the end of the Second World War he founded the Island of Soay Shark Fisheries Ltd and built a 'factory' for processing shark oil beside the harbour. But the venture only ran for three years and, although there is still a small community on Soay, the harbour today has a deserted aspect. One or two fishing boats are moored or beached but there are abandoned fish cages and the old shark-oil factory buildings now form an attractive group of derelict structures [NG451151]. Blackbirds nest in the broken boiler stoke-hole, the generator base is covered in rust and the original two-storey house (built about 1849) has only part of its slated roof remaining. It was first constructed to help the fishing industry with curing facilities at ground floor level and accommodation for visiting fishermen upstairs. At least some of Maxwell's corrugated-asbestos-roofed buildings are still in use as stores for fishing gear. A dry 'mill lade' runs from a brick and concrete tank to an 'oven' by the house. The area was littered with the brass cases of rifle cartridges when I first saw it, presumably used to scare the herring gulls away.

A well-constructed cobbled pathway, constructed in the early 1900s with government funding, runs through birch, rowan and alder woodland in the central cleft and on past the solar 'telephone exchange' [NG453144]. This was the first in the world of its kind and powers nine telephones. The path leads on down to a settlement of pleasant, well-maintained houses, **Mol-chlach** (G. – village by the pebble beach), on the west shore of **Camas nan Gall** (G. – bay of the strangers, or Norsemen), a deep indentation on the southern side of the central isthmus. When the islanders were evacuated to Mull in 1953 only Tex Geddes, Maxwell's harpooner, and his family stayed on. The settlement grew again to a tiny community which has remained ever since on the verge of viability.

Two bright, fresh-faced and well-spoken boys (eleven or twelve years old when we met them) were the only pupils at the island school. They had a full-time schoolmaster who was, they said, 'really quite good'. But they soon left to attend high school and sadly, but inevitably, with no further intakes the teacher had to go and the school was 'mothballed'.

The north-eastern part of the island is smaller and higher than the south-western area. It contains **Beinn Bhreac** (G. – speckled hill), almost central, 141m high and with wooded patches on its eastern slopes. It was more thickly wooded in the past and the area on its south side is still known as Doire Mhór (G. – the big oak wood). Two small lochs nestle directly north of Camas nan Gall – Loch Doire an Lochain, and Loch Mór which contains a small islet.

In October 1868 a schooner, *Woodman of Berwick on Tweed*, with a cargo of slate from Easdale, foundered on the east coast of Soay. Her skipper, Thomas Weatherhead, and his wife were drowned but the crew of two men and a boy were swept ashore and rescued by the islanders. The off-lying rocks have always been a hazard in this area, particularly off the south-west side of the island.

South of Mol-Chlach is rough hilly ground with a number of lochans. Once again the names recall ancient woodland – Loch na Doire Buidhe (G. – loch of the pleasant copse), Loch Coire Doire na Seilg (G. – corrie loch of the hunting thicket) and the whole area is called Doire Chaol (G. – thin woodland).

Access: By arrangement with Bella Jane Boat Trips, Elgol, Skye, 0800-731-3089.

Anchorages: The tidal stream in Soay Sound appears to run continuously W.

1. An Dubh Chamas (G. – the black bay), a small bay on the N side of Soay, about 8c ENE of Soay harbour. Good shelter in S'lies. Anchor in centre, 4–8m, good holding.
2. Soay Harbour is a narrow creek with a shingle bar drying 0.6m at the entrance. Access after half flood along inconspicuous leading line. Anchor W of pier, 3–4m, black mud, good holding and good shelter.
3. Harbour entrance, temp. anchorage in light S'lies, outside the entrance, 8–10m, but beware drying reef.
4. Camas nan Gall on S coast. Exposed S-SE. Poor holding on shingle.

5.2 Pabay

(N pap-øy – hermit or priest island).

OS Maps: 1:50000 Sheet 32 1:25000 Sheet 412
Admiralty Charts: 1:50000 No.2209 1:25000 Nos.2498 or 2534

Area: 122ha (301 acres)
Height: 28m (92 feet)

Owner: A resident farmer. For sale 1996 for £395,000.

Population: 1841–21. 1881–10. 1891–7.

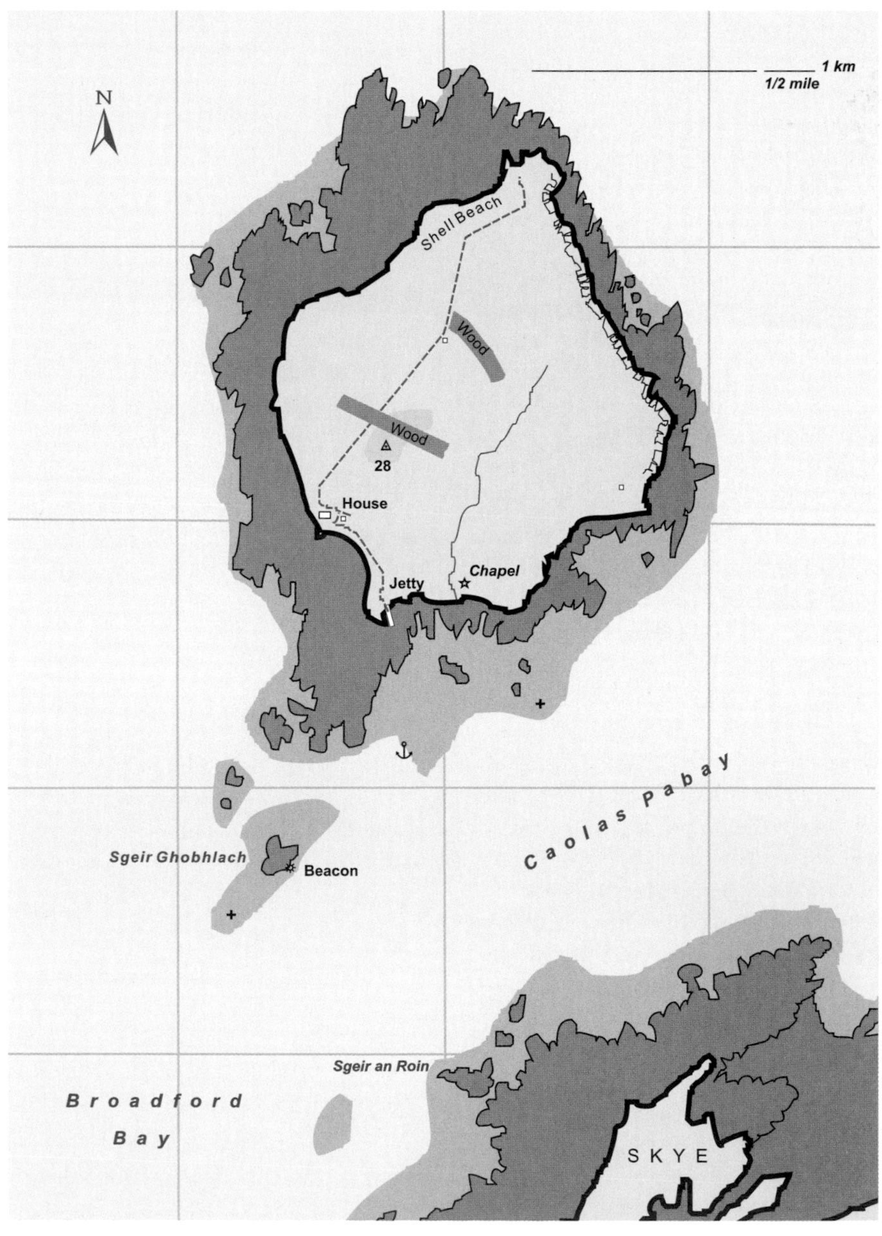

1931–3. 1961–7. 1971–5. 1981–3. 1991–0. 2001–0.

Geology: The island is mainly Lower Jurassic limestone with many fossils and a fertile soil. It is interspersed with shales (Pabay Shales) and intersected by dark fine-grained igneous dykes.

History: Possibly the holy man who originally occupied this island was never canonised because his name is not on record. But in the early days of Christianity Pabay obviously had some significance.

However, in the 16th century, pirates and so-called 'broken men' were using Pabay, which was then well wooded, as a base for their nefarious activities. Dean Monro in 1549 described it as 'full of woods, good for fishing, and a main shelter for thieves and cutthroats'.

A century and a half later much of the woodland must have been cleared because Martin Martin wrote: 'It excells in Pasturage, the Cows in it afford near double the Milk that they yield in Skie. In the Dog-Days there's a big Fly in this isle, which infests the cows, makes them run up and down, and discomposes them exceedingly.'

Wildlife: 75 acres of woodland have been planted with seventeen native species. There are many resident otters.

* * *

The island plateau of **PABAY** with its neat fields of agriculture draped over it like a brightly coloured tablecloth lies almost straight ahead as one sails through the Kyle of Lochalsh. At low water the island grows before your eyes as extensive drying reefs appear from beneath the surface of the sea.

The east and west coasts rise steeply to about 12m and there is then a very gradual slope to the highest point (28m) near the west coast. A road runs across the island from the concrete jetty in the south west to Shell Beach in the north. The main farmhouse is not far from the jetty and looks south across Caolas Pabay to Broadford Bay on Skye. An ancient ruined chapel and burial ground are east of the jetty [NG674265].

The owner in the 1990s, who was a working farmer, had planted large areas of mixed native deciduous woodland and also extended some of the small existing stands of timber. There were some holiday cottages to let.

Pabay is one of the few islands which is licensed to issue its own postage stamps. This is because it is uneconomic for the post-office to provide a boat. Deliveries are left at Broadford for collection.

* * *

Access: No regular access but ask Pabay island, 07787-565401.

Anchorages: There are extensive drying rocks 2½c on W side, 3c on NW side, 1½c on E side and 2c from S side and foul ground extends 6½c to the SSW so it is important to study the charts carefully.

1. The landing place is a concrete jetty at the SW extremity of the island, the outer end of which is marked by an iron perch. Anchor 1c S of the perch, sand with weedy patches, 4–6m.

5.3 Scalpay

(ON skalpr-øy – scallop island) for its shape? Or possibly (ON – cave island). Although there is no notable cave there are many small ones on the coast.

O S Maps: 1:50000 Sheet 32 1:25000 Sheet 409
Admiralty Charts: 1:50000 No.2209 or 1:25000 No.2498

Area: 2483ha (6135 acres)
Height: 392m (1286 ft)

Owner: The island is owned by a merchant banker and farmed by his sons.

Population: 1841–90. 1881–37. 1891–49. 1931–27. 1961–2. 1971–5. 1981–6. 1991–7. 2001–10.

Geology: Almost entirely of Torridonian rocks – red and grey sandstones, conglomerates, siltstones and shales which were deposited about 800 million years ago. Part of the west coast is granite but the ground by Scalpay House is on a patch of fertile lias of the same type as Pabay.

History: Dr Johnson, in 1773, wanted to buy the island and to 'found a good school, and an episcopal church, ... and have a printing-press, where he would print all the Erse that could be found' but thought better of it after discovering that ownership carried an obligation to spend at least three months every year on the island.

In the 19th century Sir Donald Currie constructed the first roads and planted trees.

Wildlife: The hill slopes are covered with heather,

mainly *Calluna vulgaris*, *Erica carnea* and *Erica tetralix*.

The island's herd of red deer is carefully managed and there are good trout in the mountain lochs.

* * *

SCALPAY rises abruptly from its south and west coasts to **Mullach na Càrn** (G. – cairn hill), its highest peak of slightly more than 392m. It is rough and hilly, other main peaks being **Beinn Loch a' Mhuilinn** (G. – mountain of the mill loch), 291m, and **Beinn Reireag Bheag**, 225m. Mullach na Càrn stretches in a ridge across the centre of the island with a lochan-studded plateau and two mini-mountains, An Ailldunn (G. – the castle rock) and Sithean Glac an Ime (G. – the fairy hill in the butter bowl). Below lie the Mill Loch, the Black Loch, and the much-larger **Loch an Leòid**. The north-east coast is rocky and fringed by a reef but the mountain slopes here are more gradual.

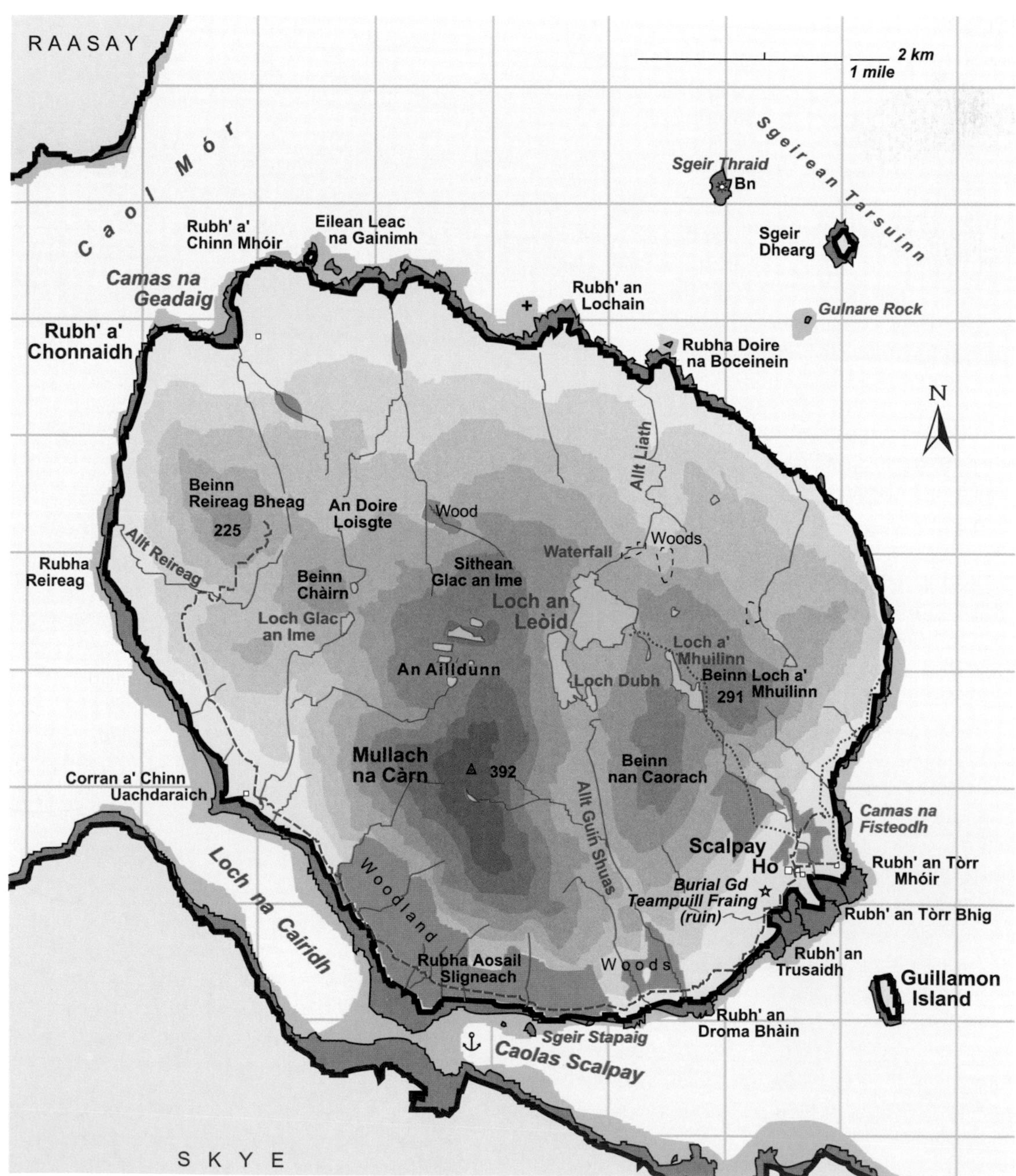

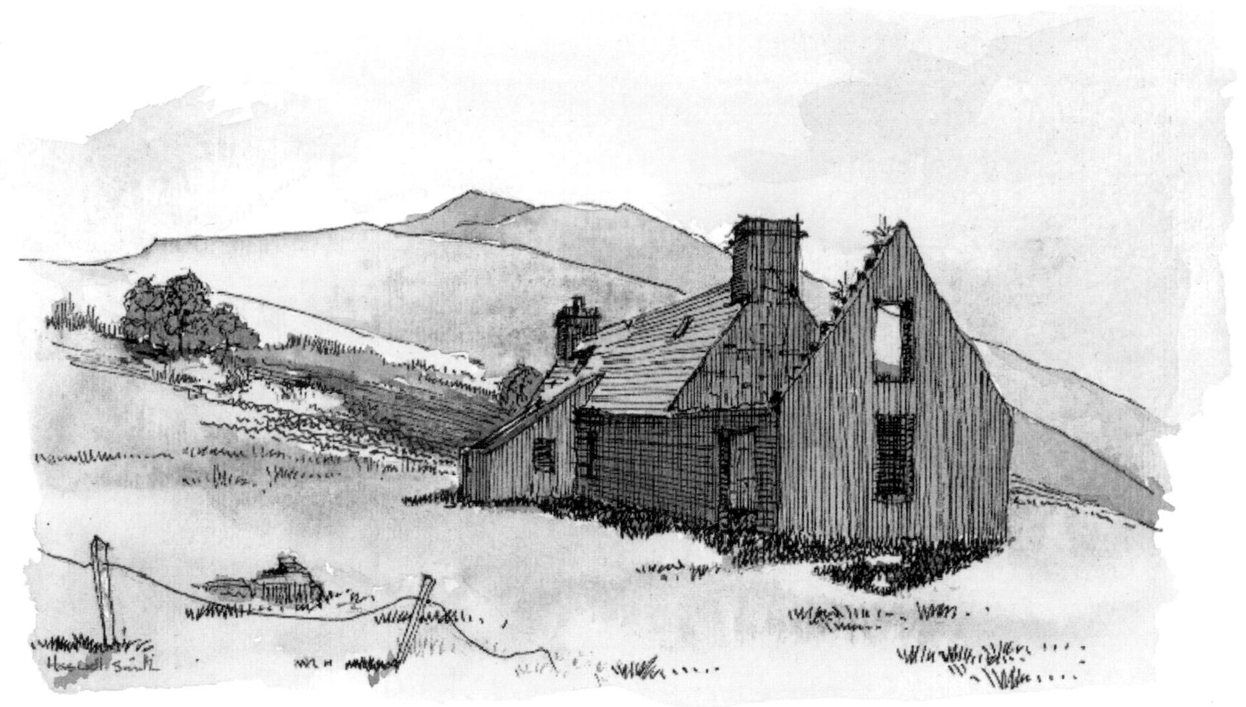

RUINED CROFT AT CAMAS NA GEADAIG

Scalpay is separated from Skye by the narrow and shallow Caolas Scalpay. **Scalpay House** in the south-east corner of the island looks over a small tidal harbour with, beyond it, **Guillamon Island**, 24m-high, rocky and speckled with sea-birds. To the west of Scalpay House are the remains of a chapel, **Teampuill fraing** (G. – St Francis' Chapel), built on the site of an ancient Celtic cell [NG628281]. The area around Scalpay House is well cultivated and there are patches of woodland.

A road runs from the harbour along the west coast, through extensive conifer plantations to a holiday cottage at **Corran a Chinn Uachdaraich** (G. – the upper projection), facing Skye. The track leads on from there up towards the summit of Beinn Reireag Bheag.

Some 1600ha is fenced off in this north-east area for red-deer farming which was developed with the support of the Highlands and Islands Development Board (now Highlands and Islands Enterprise). Venison was successfully exported to Germany where it is a very popular meat, but, unfortunately, with access to Eastern European venison this is no longer such a profitable enterprise.

A recently ruined croft in the north of the island is beside the aptly named **Camas na Geadaig** (G. – bay at the patch of lazybeds) because the lazybeds beside it can still be clearly seen beneath a layer of buttercups.

The heathery hillsides provide pleasant walking as, being sheltered by Skye from the wettest winds, the ground is not too boggy, but from whatever direction you approach you can still expect rough going to reach the bouldered summit of Mullach na Carn. However, the views from the top make the exercise worthwhile, and be sure to rest for a while by Loch Dubh where you can see the waterfall tumbling down the hill behind Loch an Leòid and listen to the skylarks.

Scalpay offers good camping and fishing but it is important first to obtain permission from Scalpay House.

* * *

Access: No regular access but try Peter Urquhart, Portree, 01478-613718 or Dan Corrigall, Portree, 01478-612333.

Anchorages:

1. Camas na Geadaig, at NW extremity. The head of the bay dries out about 1¼c. Beware reefs both sides of entrance. Occasional anchorage in the centre, 5–7m, sand. Sheltered

from S'lies but squally in strong winds.
2. Loch na Cairidh (G. – weir loch). NW of the narrows. Anchor anywhere in suitable depth.
3. Caolas Scalpay. E of narrows, midway between narrows and Sgeir Stapaig. Can be squally.

5.4 Longay

(ON long-øy – longship island). Note also (G. long spùinnidh – pirate ship).

O S Maps: 1:50000 Sheet 32 1:25000 Sheet 409
Admiralty Charts: 1:50000 No.2209 1:25000 No.2498

Area: 50ha (124 acres)
Height: 67m (220 ft)

Population: Uninhabited and no Census records.

Geology: Longay is the southern end of a reef, Sgeirean Tarsuinn (G. – the traverse or oblique reef), running parallel with the east side of Scalpay. It is formed of large slabs of volcanic rock but with a considerable area of red sandstone.

History: Longay is one of the group of islands in this area which was frequented by pirates in the 16th century. It would have been covered

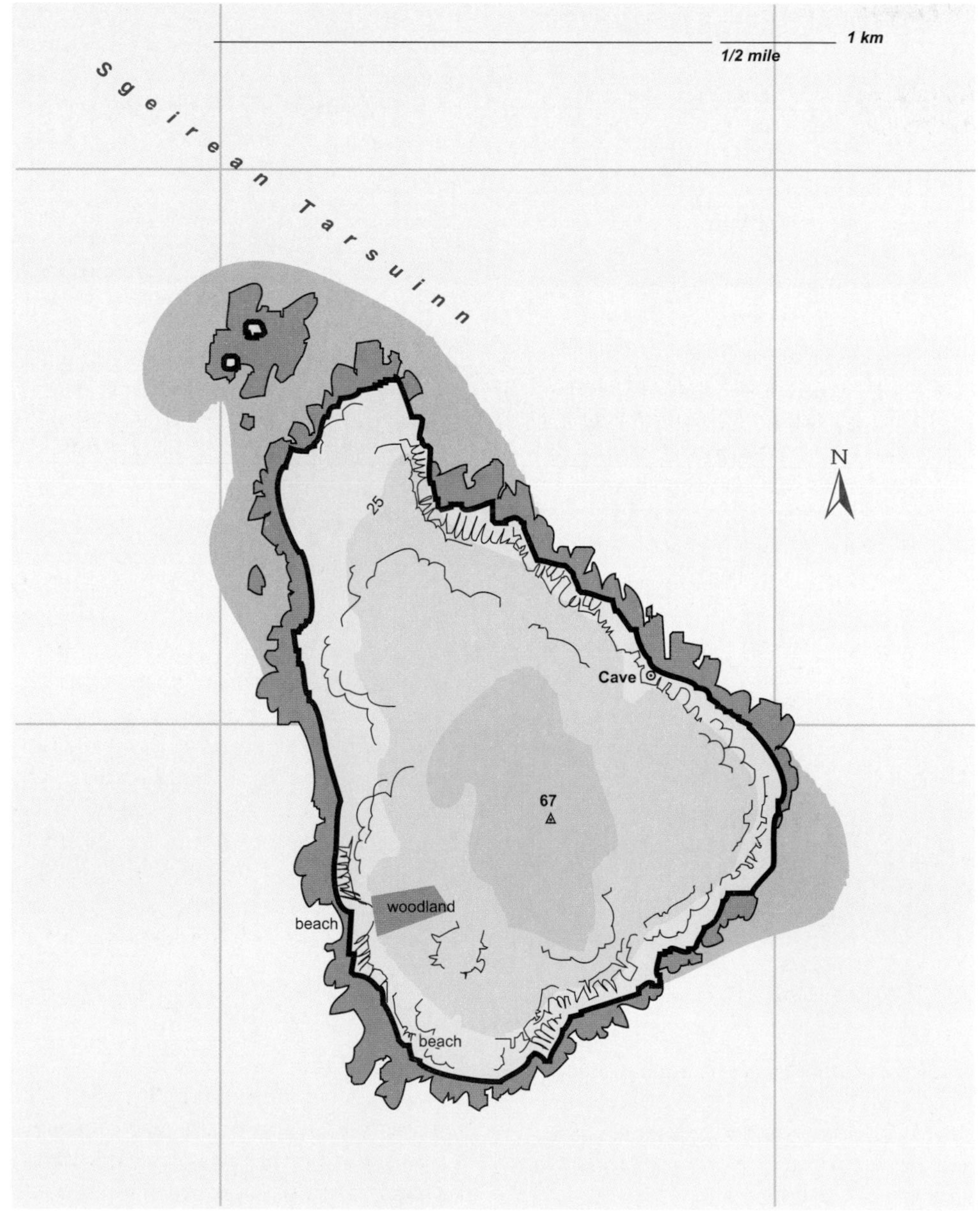

with Caledonian Forest trees at that time giving added cover. The thieves and cut-throats, with no clan or territorial attachments, must have concentrated their attacks only on 'foreign' ships – Dutch, Lowland Scottish, Flemish and English commercial and fishing craft which ventured into the Inner Minch; otherwise the local clan chiefs would certainly have suppressed them. They had ample power to do so. The pirates probably paid insurance to MacLeod of Raasay in the form of a proportion of the plunder but in any case their depredations helped to protect the local fishing grounds.

Wildlife: Sheep are occasionally pastured here. A fair number of nesting sea-birds take advantage of the lack of human habitation.

There is little of note to report about the compact little island of **LONGAY**. It could be considered a good example of a desert island, but not an ideal one on which to be marooned.

We found no adequate anchorage. The chart shows a possible area of suitable depth on the east coast but we were unable to find less than a dubious 15m of possibly boulder-strewn bottom so we landed by dinghy while *Jandara* stood off. The island is covered with rough scrub making walking uncomfortable. It rises to a single central ridge with its peak 67m above sea-level. Crossing the ridge, the west slope has scattered patches of rowan and alder but the terrain is mainly heather, bracken and coarse boggy turf. In the extreme south-west corner a patch of beach made up of red sandstone pebbles lies above tongues of semi-submerged rock. Further north there is the impression of a wide cleft or cove with a copse above a narrow gravel beach. This may be a suitable spot for temporary anchorage but I have had no opportunity to test it.

At our landing place on the east coast directly below the crest of the hill there was a narrow rocky beach of tumbled volcanic slabs and a small cave [NG660313] with fresh water trickling down the back of it – a useful pirates' den.

Access: No regular access but try Dan Corrigall, Portree, 01478-612333 or Calum, Plockton, 01599-544306.

Anchorage: There is no recommended anchorage but temp. anchorage may be possible in depths of 12–15m clear of the reef on the S or E sides, or in less depth off the small beached 'cove' on the W side near the S corner. Be sure to use a tripping line.

5.5 Wiay

(G. bhuidhe – yellow or pleasant, ON -øy – island). Sometimes written in the past as 'Vuiay', or 'Buia' (Martin Martin).

OS Maps: 1:50000 Sheet 32 1:25000 Sheet 410
Admiralty Chart: 1:100000 No.1795

Area: 148ha (366 acres)
Height: 60m (197 ft)

Owner: MacLeod Estates.

Population: 1841–6. 1881–4. 1891–0. Uninhabited since 1890.

Geology: Basaltic lava.

History: One might assume that Boswell and Johnson visited the island of Wiay since Boswell reported:

'In the afternoon, Ullinish carried us in his boat to an island possessed by him, where we saw an immense cave... It is one hundred and eighty feet long, about thirty feet broad, and at least thirty feet high. This cave we were told had a remarkable echo; but we found none. They said it was owing to the great rains having made it damp. Such are the excuses by which the exaggeration of Highland narratives is palliated.'

Wildlife: Two large colonies of herring gulls nest on the cliff-tops near the lochans above Geodha nan Faochag.

* * *

WIAY is the largest island in Loch Bracadale. Most of the coastline consists of vertical cliffs and the southern bluff is a striking overhanging cliff 59m high and covered with yellow lichens and sea-bird droppings. There is a large sea-cave [NG296356] at its base which amplifies the sound of the surf breaking in it and another large cave on the north-east side of the island [NG301370]. I have been unable to establish if either of these caves was the one referred to by Boswell but it seems probable as there are no other prominent island caves close to Ullinish where they were staying. Johnson's account was written from memory in London. He too mentions visiting a sea-cave by boat at low water but he could be describing a cave on Idrigill Point.

The beach in **Camas na Cille** (G. – church bay) is composed of round pebbles many of which are so large that they are better described as boulders. A pleasant green valley stippled with

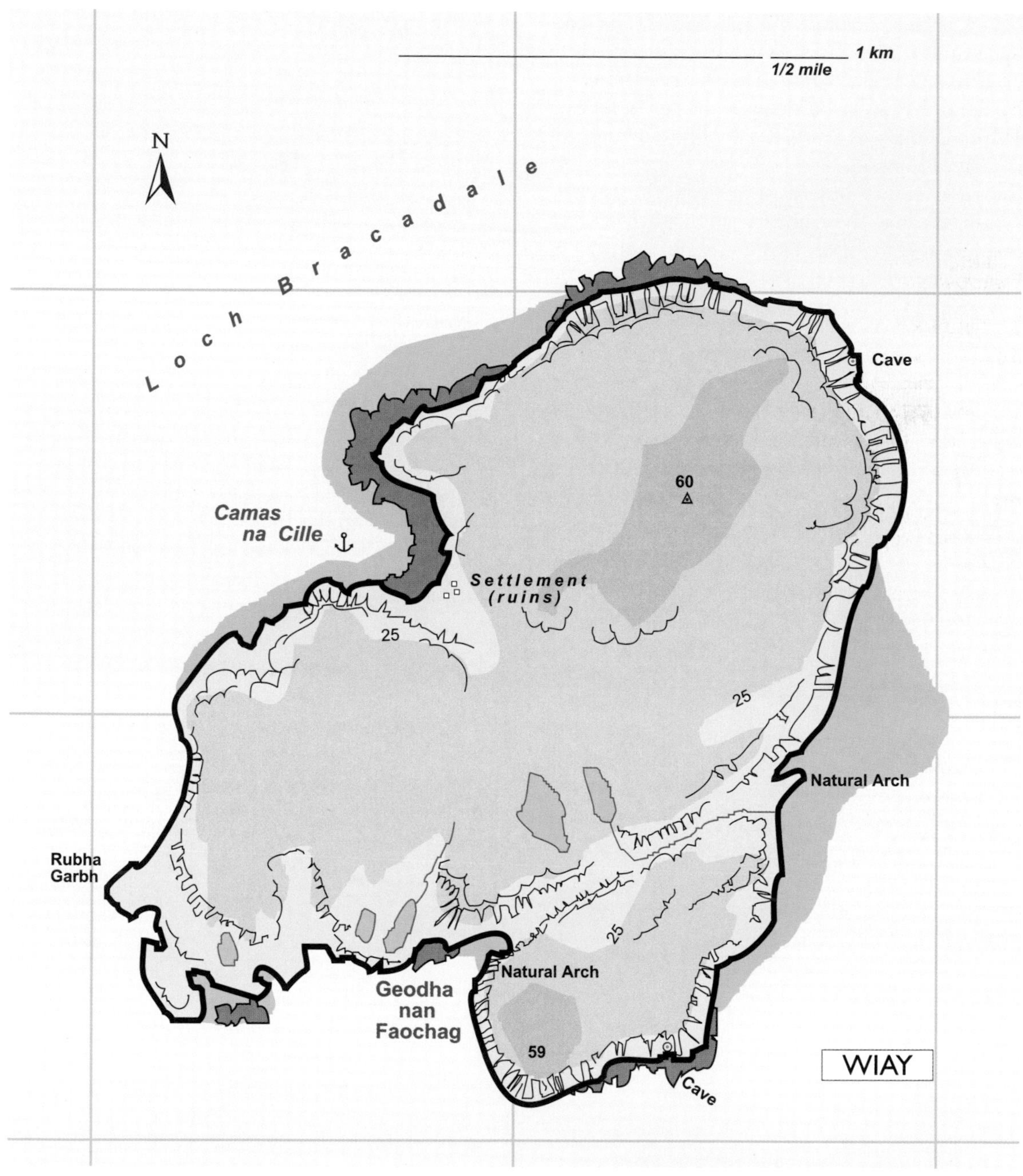

yellow irises, reeds and patches of bracken leads up from the bay to a plateau area of rough bog and coarse grazing for sheep. The derelict remains of at least three dwellings are near the beach, one of which was a black house [NG292366]. There was also a church in this area in bygone times although we saw no obvious trace of it. Flax was once grown here, and Seton Gordon mentions that Donald MacLeod of Ose had a tablecloth spun of Wiay flax, but the arable land has long since disappeared. The central summit (60m) is almost at the geometric centre of Loch Bracadale and the view is all-encompassing. To the east is the dramatic 'castle' of tidal **Oronsay**, great cliffs rising abruptly from the sea like a fortress. To the north are the lesser cliffs of **Tarner Island** and **Harlosh Island**, but **Macleod's Maidens** – three large rock stacks realistically sculpted by the sea – can only be seen from the southern part of the island as they are concealed by Idrigill Point.

In this area there are several tiny lochans and the entire south-western portion is almost isolated by a very deep cleft forming the **Geodha nan Faochag** (G. – narrow creek of the periwinkles). The cliffs here are the steepest and most cave-riddled on the island.

* * *

Access: No regular access. Enquire at Portnalong, Loch Harport.

Anchorage: Admiralty Pilot says landing only possible in two places, one being the small bay on NW side. Shores clean to within 1½c.

1. Camas na Cille. Temp. anchorage. Rocks on NE side but clear in middle and towards SW side of bay. Approach centrally and anchor off the pebble beach in a suitable depth, shingle.

5.6 Crowlin Islands

*[**kroa**-lin] Probably (G. crò linne – eye-of-a-needle channel).*

Eilean Mór

(G. – big island).

Eilean Meadhonach

[meeoo-unuch] (G. – middle island).

Eilean Beag

(G. – little island)

OS Maps: 1:50000 Sheet 24 or 32 1:25000 Sheet 428
Admiralty Charts: 1:50000 No.2209 1:25000 No.2498

Area: 270ha (567 acres)
Height: 114m (374 ft)

Population: 1841–40. 1881–9. 1891–9. 1931–0. Uninhabited since.

Geology: This is a group of three eroded chunks of Torridonian sandstone with volcanic rock intrusions.

Wildlife: Common seals seem to be particularly fond of Eilean Beag

* * *

The largest island in this tight-knit group is **EILEAN MOR**. It is 170ha in area and rises to a height of 114m. There are some ruined cottages in the north-east corner near **Camas**

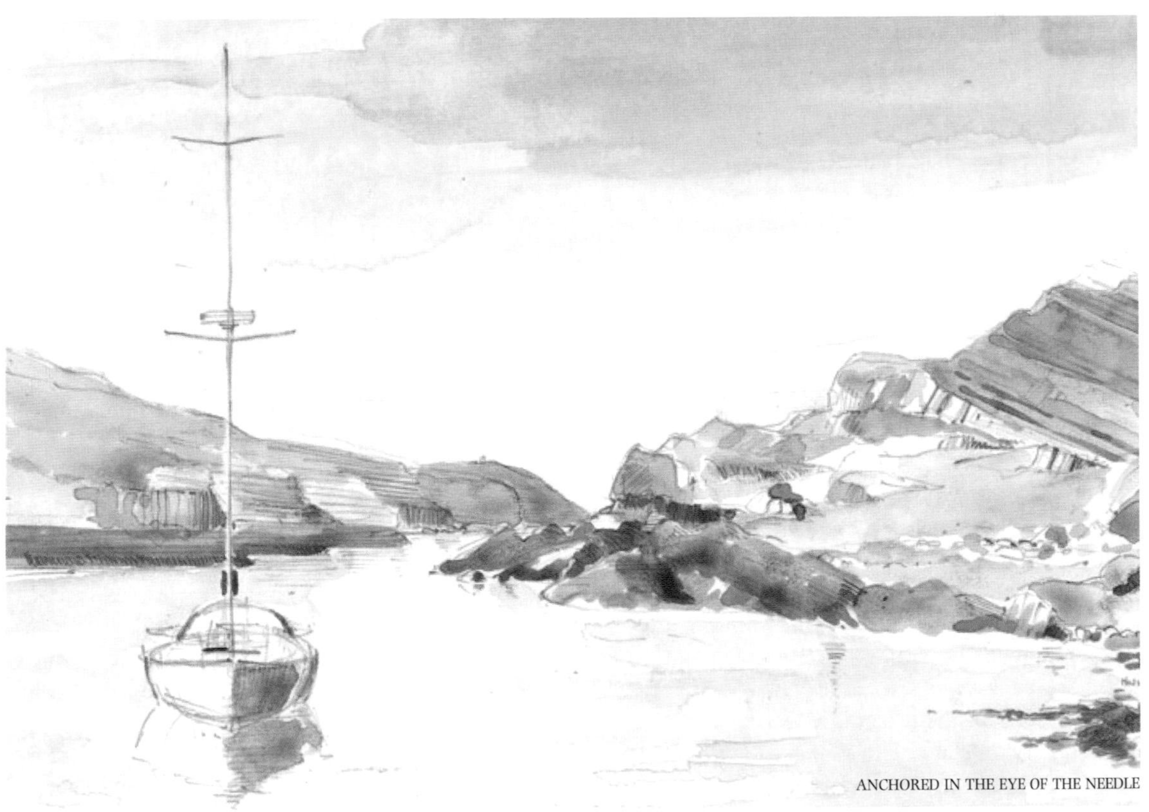

ANCHORED IN THE EYE OF THE NEEDLE

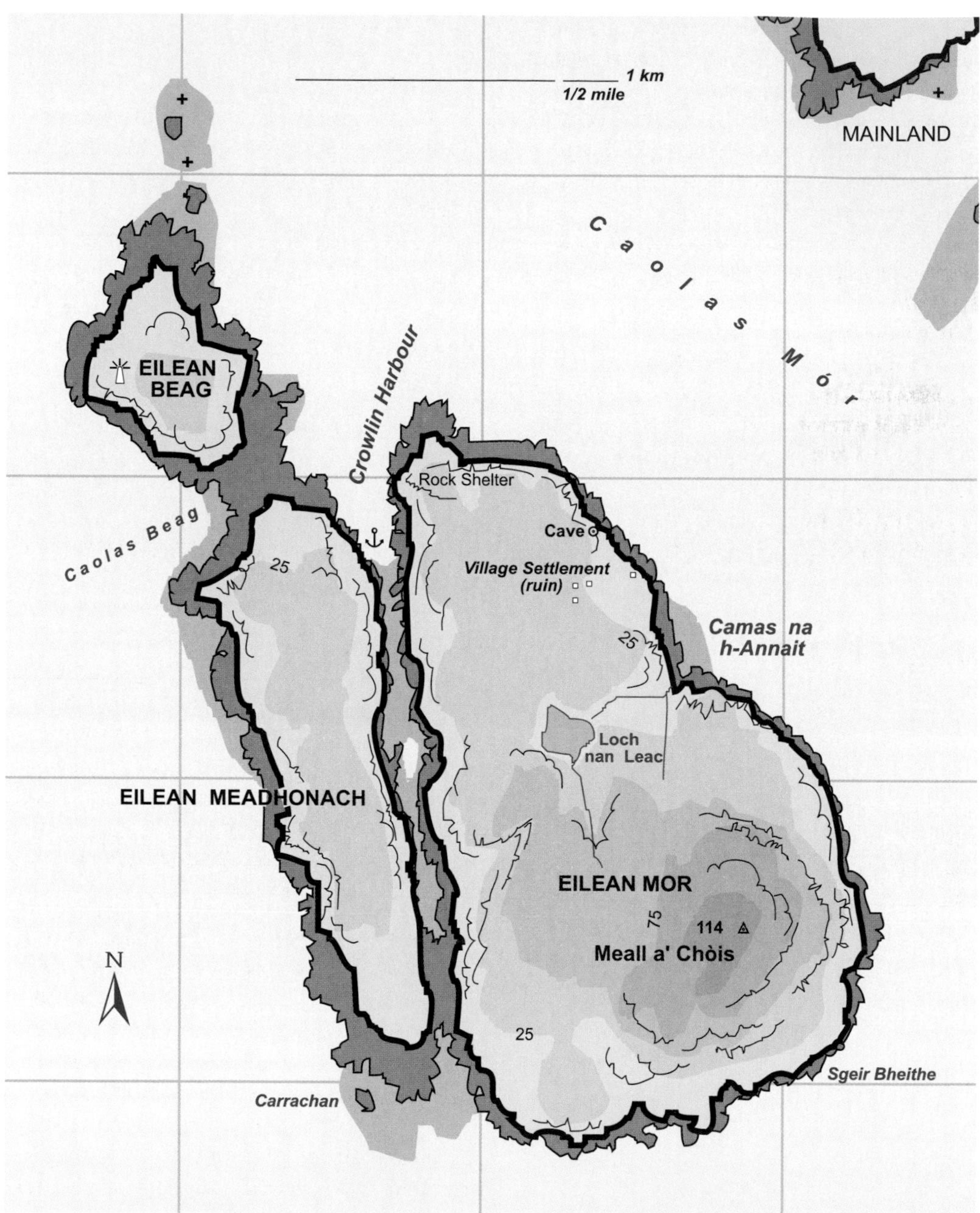

na h-Annait (G. – bay of the church-land). In the north-west corner by the anchorage a rock shelter has provided storage for visiting fishermen [NG690353] and on the east coast there is an interesting cave [NG695352]. The islands have been denuded of trees and grazing sheep prevent regeneration. A small loch, Loch nan Leac (G. – tombstone loch), in the undulating central plateau of Eilean Mór overflows into a small burn leading down to Camas na h-Annait. On the south side a shallow cave was excavated recently and found to have evidence of human settlement from 8000 years ago.

Eilean Mór is separated from Eilean Meadhonach (50ha) by a narrow cleft which is only about 50m wide. Boats can enter from the north at a suitable state of the tide, and there is a pool in the centre which forms a snug little harbour, but reaching it can be a bit like threading a needle. A reef fringes the south coasts of both Eilean Mór and Eilean Meadhonach.

When approaching or leaving the anchorage at

high water it is important not to cut the corners. To the west is a submerged reef and on the east a narrow rocky beach which covers, as one poor man discovered when he grounded his hired yacht on it. We arrived at low water to find him high and dry but unhurt. His blushes shone like a beacon in the driving rain.

The smallest island, Eilean Beag (3ha) has a light beacon on its summit and there are many small caves on the rocky shoreline. A reef extends northwards from this islet.

North of the Crowlin Islands is the grassy expanse of **Eilean na Bà** (G. – island of the cattle) and, north again, sheltering the anchorage of Poll Creadha is **Eilean nan Naomh** (G. – island of the saints), which has a lot of seaweed-covered rock, but hardly enough dry land to support a single saint.

* * *

Access: No regular access but try Calum, Plockton, 01599-544306 or Dan Corrigall, Portree, 01478-612333.

Anchorages: Give S coast a wide berth and, similarly, N coast of Eilean Beag.

1. North entrance to harbour. Occasional anchorage just within the mouth of the gut between the two larger islands, 6–8m.

2. Harbour. Access above half flood through narrows for 1.5m max. draft. Safe anchorage in N of first pool. Reef projects from W shore at centre of pool.

5.7 Raasay

Possibly (ON raa-s -øy – roe-deer island) or (ON ross-øy – horse island)

OS Maps: 1:50000 Sheet 24 1:25000 Sheet 409
Admiralty Charts: 1:50000 Nos.2209 and 2210

Area: 6,405ha (15,827 acres)
Height: 443m (1453 ft)

Owner: The entire island was purchased by the Government in 1922. Raasay House and some other key properties on the island were sold for a low price in the 1960s to Dr John Green – a Sussex pathologist – who visited the island once and never returned. After considerable pressure over many years and the payment of a high price he was eventually 'persuaded' to sell out to the Highland and Islands Development Board in 1979. Highlands and Islands Enterprise (the successor to HIDB) still owns farmland, a hotel and other property on the island which is rented out at commercial rates. Some years ago the Government offered to transfer all the crofts it owns to a local trust but the crofters did not favour change.

Population: Figures include the tidal island of Eilean Fladday. 1780– over 400. 1803– over 900. 1841–676. 1881–532. 1891–489. 1931–377. 1961–223. 1976– ferry service introduced. 1981–152. 1991–163. Raasay has the lowest proportion of children of all the populated Scottish islands (10.4%). 2001–194.

Geology: The south is mainly Torridonian sandstone and shale but with two large areas of granite. Iron ore was mined here by Baird & Co using the labour of German prisoners-of-war during the First World War, but it became uneconomic and was closed in 1919. Some of the Torridonian shales on Raasay contain the oldest fossilised plant remains yet found. There is unique loam at the Glam in the centre of the island at the 200–300m level which is evidence that this part of Raasay for some reason probably escaped glaciation and therefore still has its rare and ancient living flora. The extreme north of the island is Archaean gneiss.

History: The first MacLeod on Raasay was Calum Garbh, younger son of Calum, the 9th Chief of Lewis. In 1518 he was granted title to Raasay, Rona and some estates on Skye and he had a lucrative line in piracy which he master-minded from Brochel Castle. He founded the cadet branch of Mac Gille Chaluim which survived mainly by avoiding involvement with his relatives, the Macleods of Lewis and Dunvegan. In fact the MacLeods of Raasay often preferred to support the MacDonalds of Sleat. Calum son of Gille Chaluim was a poet who was awarded a further charter to his estates by James VI. The next Calum, the 4th Chief, accepted the feudal superiority of Mackenzie of Kintail after Mackenzie had wrested Lewis from the Macleod Clan but there was family tragedy when his son, the much-loved Iain Garbh, met his death by drowning.

Although the MacLeods were Protestants and the Skye Macleods supported the Government, the MacLeods of Raasay, in their usual contrary way, chose to support the Catholic Jacobites, possibly for purely chivalrous reasons. The islanders followed their Chief wholeheartedly and thus tiny Raasay provided one hundred men and twenty-six pipers at Culloden. Later, when Skye was being searched, they secretly rowed the Young Pretender over from Portree at dead of night. Government troops had already burned down the Laird's house and almost every dwelling on the island in reprisal for their Jacobite sympathies but Prince Charles was nevertheless hidden in a shepherd's hut and fed oat-bread and whisky. He was then smuggled over to Loch Broom where he hoped to

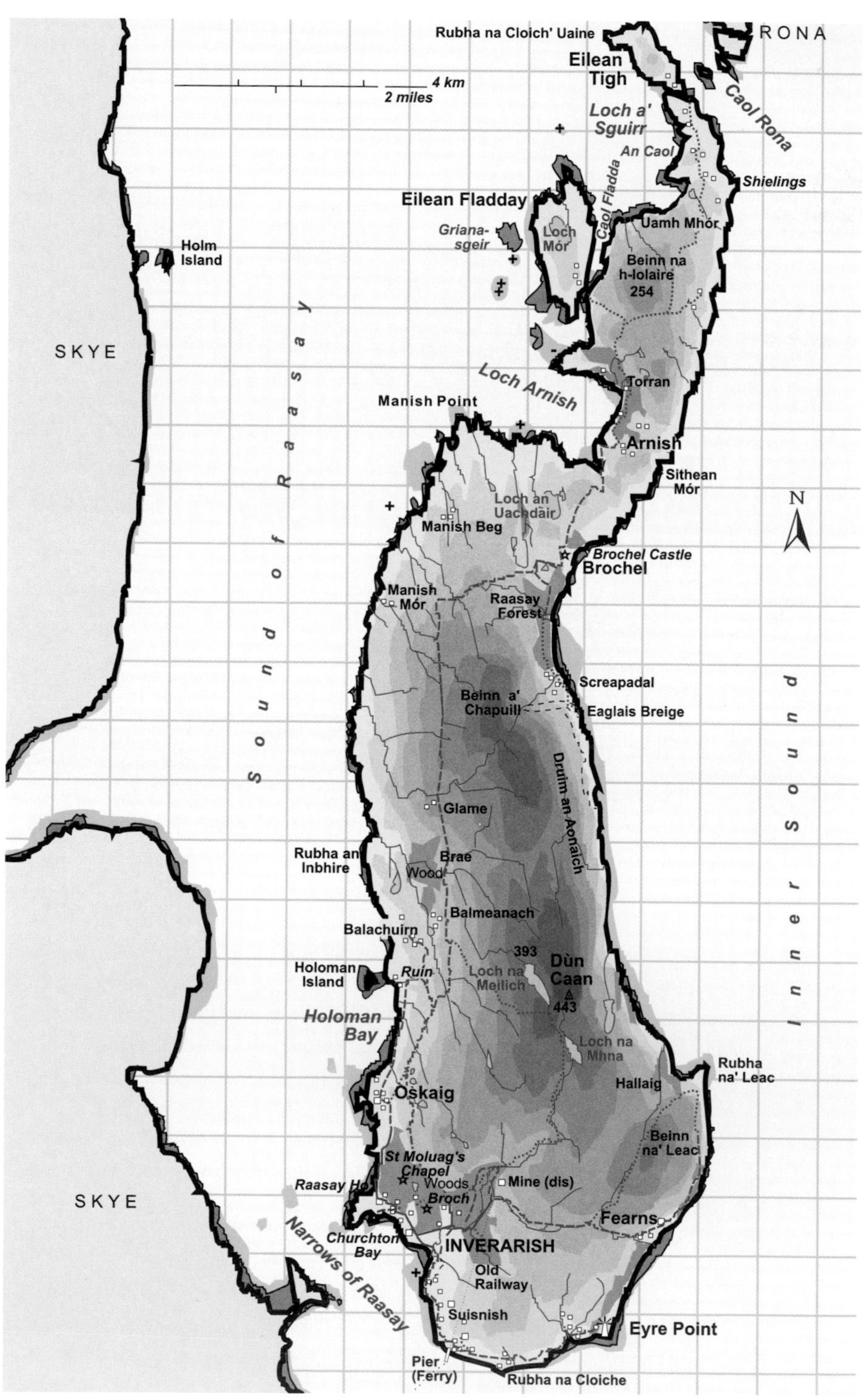

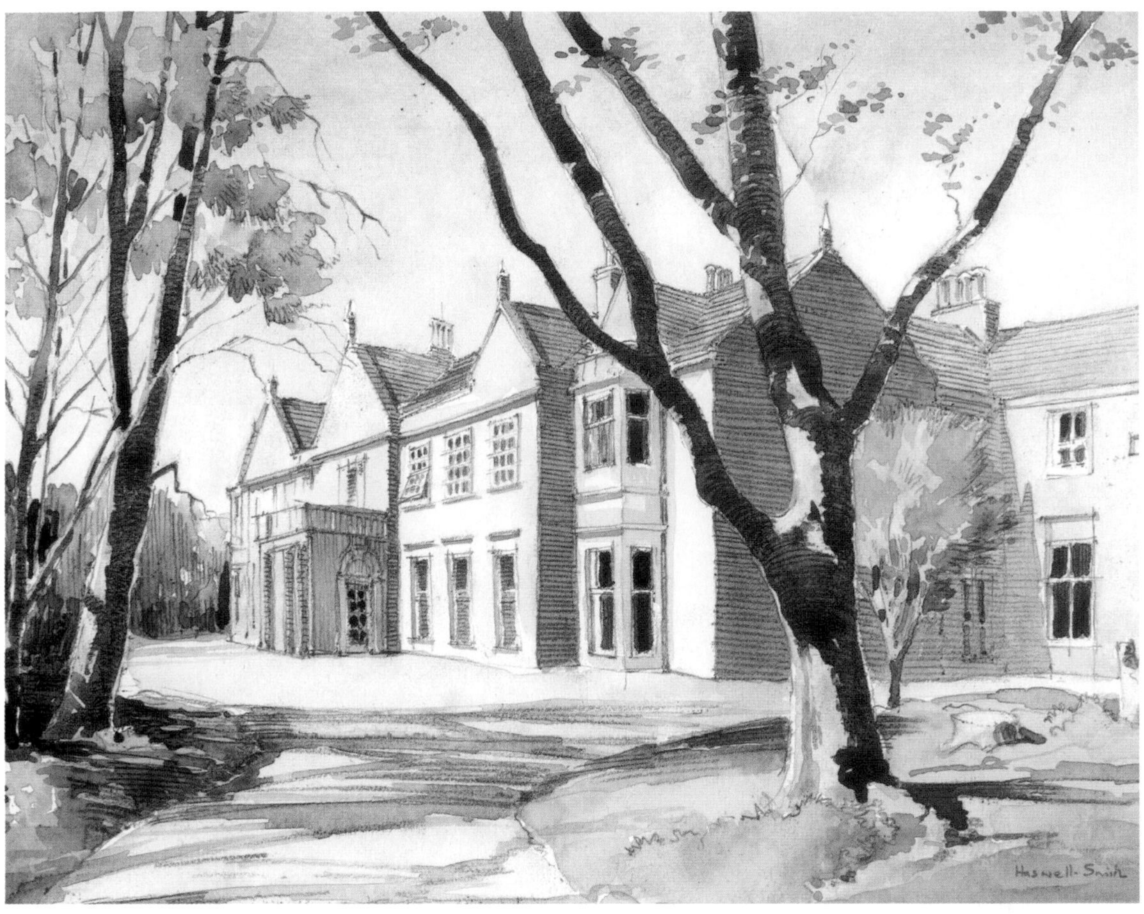

RAASAY HOUSE (WHERE DR JOHNSON STAYED)

be rescued by a French ship.

Raasay's support of the Stuarts proved catastrophic. Homes and boats were destroyed, men murdered, women raped, and 'there was not left in the whole island a four-footed beast, a hen or a chicken.'

The MacLeods spent their family fortune on reconstruction and consequently within thirty years the island appeared to have made a remarkable recovery.

By the early 1800s, however, the population was increasing rapidly and poverty became widespread. Emigration began and the Laird, John MacLeod, did what he could to help but by 1843 he was so deeply in debt that he had to sell the island before he too emigrated (to Australia). George Rainy of Edinburgh bought Raasay for 35,000 guineas and genuinely tried to improve conditions on the island for a time, but having failed he turned to sheep-farming which resulted in the inevitable eviction of over one hundred families. Raasay's world-renowned Gaelic poet, Sorley MacLean, has immortalised in haunting verse this sad period in Raasay's history.

After Rainy's twenty-seven-year-old son and heir died in 1872 there was a succession of unsympathetic owners until a commercial mining company, Baird & Co, bought the island in 1912 to extract iron ore. This brought jobs and housing until mining ceased in 1919. The Government eventually bought the island in 1922 for £37,000 after the episode of the Rona Raiders (See Rona, No.5.9).

Raasay is famous for its pipers, the finest being John MacKay (b.1767) who was sent as a child to Skye to study. He and his son Angus – first piper to Queen Victoria – are remembered for their exceptional talent and for recording and preserving much pipe music which would otherwise have been lost.

But the sound of music died in 1893 when Raasay became the centre for a strict and repressive sect of the Free Church introduced by a Mr Macfarlane. All pleasure was frowned upon

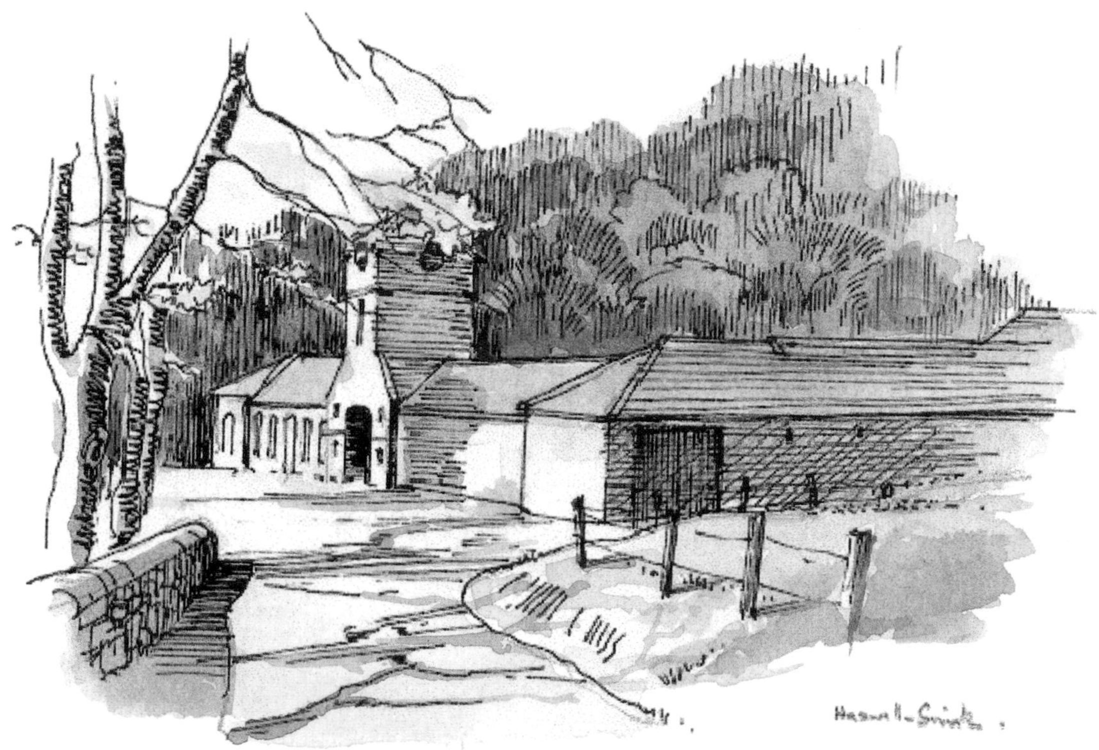

THE STABLES WHERE THE CLOCK STOPPED. . .

and music, dancing and poetry were banned. Although there has been some adjustment of attitudes with the passing years, religious observance on the island, and particularly on the Sabbath, is still very strict. Raasay folk are friendly but they expect their beliefs to be respected.

Wildlife: Since Raasay partially escaped glaciation, extensive rare and ancient flora can be found on the steep grassy slopes of the east coast, particularly below the long Druim an Aonich (G. – steep sloping ridge) escarpment. There are many varieties of alpines, saxifrages, orchids, ferns and mosses. Sea aster and bog asphodel flourish beneath Dùn Caan. It is worth going to Hallaig in the south or Screapadal in the north to see the variety of the wildflowers and the island also has several areas of pleasant mixed woodland and some remarkable tree species.

Animal life includes red deer, alpine hare, otter, water shrew and a unique sub-species of bank vole, darker and twice the weight of the mainland vole; this may not in fact be a sub-species, but an ancient survivor of an original Scandinavian species. Raasay is the only Hebridean island on which the pine marten still survives.

Rabbits were introduced by a thoughtless proprietor, Herbert Wood, in the 19th century and they almost destroyed the agricultural economy.

Birdlife is more varied than usual and golden eagles can be seen circling over the rocky landscape in the north.

* * *

The long stretch of **RAASAY** is separated from Skye by a narrow sound and sheltered by it from the prevailing winds. Its east coast is steep with **Dùn Caan** near the centre, 443m high and very conspicuous – like a truncated Fujiyama – with the same appearance from all sides except the north-east. The view from the top is one of the most inspiring in the Western Isles. The southern half of the island is mountainous, with gentle gradients to the west and cliffs to the east while the northern portion is comparatively low except for **Beinn na h-Iolaire** (G. – hill of the eagle) about 3km from the northern extremity.

The main village is **Inverarish**, 2km north of the ferry terminal at Suisnish where the remains of Baird & Co's ore trans-shipment station are still to be seen. Inverarish was also partly built by the mining company. A roadway leads from it to the east coast bypassing the disused mine [NG567367], then on past a 3½km track leading to a waterfall by the shore at Hallaig, before reaching **Fearns** where the Rona Raiders seized land in 1919. Inverarish is set in pleasant woodland which is best experienced by taking a forest walk up the Inverarish Burn.

Dùn Borodale is an ancient broch with part of the walls and galleries remaining, in woodland just north of the village [NG555363].

Churchton Bay, overlooked by Inverarish, is named after the 13th-century chapel [NG548367] dedicated to St Moluag (who founded the monastery on Lismore. See No.3.9). **St Moluag's Chapel** ruins stand in an ancient wooded burial ground north-east of Raasay House, together with two other buildings, the smaller of which may be 11th century. Boswell considered there was 'something comfortable in the thought of being so near a piece of consecrated ground', when he and Dr Johnson were guests at Raasay House. A Celtic cross to commemorate the saint's landing place is in a small gated woodland enclosure off the lane behind Raasay House and overlooking the bay is **The Battery** [NG545363], a cannon emplacement on a knoll, built in 1807 and guarded by two busty stone mermaids. A shallow tidal harbour behind the knoll is not obvious from the sea.

Raasay House standing above the Battery and looking towards the mountains of Skye is on the site of the family home of the MacLeods. The original house was burned down by Government troops in reprisal for the help given to the Young Pretender during the Jacobite Rebellion. All the cottages on the island were also destroyed. Raasay House was rebuilt a few years later by the MacLeods but the Regency frontage was added in the early 1800s by John MacLeod and there have been subsequent additions since Dr Johnson stayed there. Raasay House was run as a hotel between 1937 and 1960 when it was bought by Dr Green. He allowed both it and the land to fall into serious disrepair but refused to sell it, even when vandals wrecked the house and stole the contents including the library books. Nor would he sell a small piece of land needed for a ferry pier to serve the island. After years of acrimony and Government inaction the property was eventually purchased for a high price by the Highland and Islands Development Board. The Board converted Borodale House into the Isle of Raasay Hotel but failed to restore Raasay House or build a new pier. For 23 years the House was used as an outdoor centre but in 2007 the Raasay community bought it and started renovations. The wooded grounds are still derelict but with delightful surprises – mossy pieces of sculpture and an overgrown fountain. In 2008 the Council commenced work on a new ferry terminal

The road passes beneath the clocktower of the **Raasay House Stables**. In 1914 the thirty-six able-bodied men of Raasay assembled here to go to war and only fourteen returned. The day they left the clock stopped and it has never been satisfactorily repaired. Beyond lies **Temptation Hill** with an incised Pictish Ogam-stone, possibly dating from the 7th century. Temptation Hill is supposed to have been named by the MacLeod who was first tempted by the magnificent outlook to become the island's owner.

Another Pictish stone in front of Raasay House has a cross of unique design incised on it and these stones may have been part of a number historically marking an area of sanctuary.

To the south of the flat summit of Dùn Caan, on which James Boswell danced a reel 'in sheer exuberance', is **Loch na Mhna** (G. – the loch of the woman). A water-horse which haunted this loch devoured the daughter of a local smithy according to legend. The father trapped and killed the monster and found to his surprise that it was made of jelly. **Loch Storab** to the west is named after a Norwegian prince whose grave is beside it.

The tarmac road overlooks **Holoman Island** in Holoman Bay on the west coast – it is tidal and connected to the shore by a pebble strand – before it ends in the north at **Brochel Castle**, built by the MacSwans in the 15th century and then the pirate stronghold of the MacLeods of Lewis. Iain Garbh who died in 1671 was the last inhabitant. The fantastic fairy-tale ruin sits on a pinnacle of sheer rock – a volcanic plug – and originally stood three storeys high. A track runs 2km south through east coast woodland to the shielings of Screapadal, scene of the George Rainy clearances. This area has been immortalised in the poems of Sorley McLean (1911–1996), a Raasay man and one of Gaeldom's greatest poets.

The road running 2½km north from Brochel to **Arnish** was built by Calum MacLeod, a postman. His entire Arnish community of eight families was proposing to leave because there was no road access but the council refused to help. So in 1966, armed with a four-shilling book on roadbuilding,

Calum constructed the road himself with a pick, shovel and wheelbarrow. He was awarded the BEM when he eventually completed the work but by then he and his wife were the last remaining inhabitants and he died soon after in 1988.

A track leads on round the shore of Loch Arnish through Torran, where the school was closed in 1960, and branches off to the tidal island of **Eilean Fladday** which used to accommodate four families with their own school. The houses there are now holiday homes. Continuing to the northern tip of Raasay is more than an hour's further walk. Remote **Eilean Tigh** (G. – home island) can be reached by crossing a rock ledge which is exposed at low water.

* * *

Access: Vehicle ferry from Sconser, Skye to East Suisnish, Raasay, 08000-66-5000. Several crossings daily and two on Sunday. 20 minutes crossing time. Note that there is no petrol for sale on Raasay. Summer boat excursions from Portree, 01478-612333.

Anchorages:

1. Churchton bay, SE of Eilean Aird nan Gobhar. Anchor either side of Perch Rocks, holding good. Head dries off one cable and SE of bay is foul. 4 visitors' moorings available. Pier on NW side of the knoll affords good shelter but it dries.
2. Oskaig Point. Some shelter during E winds, S of point.
3. Fladday harbour, on E side of S end of Eilean Fladday, is a narrow inlet. Secure anchorage in 5–10m but bottom foul. Approach from SW between Ard an Torrain and Fraoch Eilean following sailing directions carefully.
4. Caol Fladday, on E side of Eilean Fladday with easy approach from N avoiding Bo na Faochag. Holding can be poor due to kelp.

5.8 Isay

*[**ee**shĕ] (ON ise-øy – porpoise island)*

OS Maps: 1:50000 Sheet 23 1:25000 Sheet 407
Admiralty Charts: 1:100000 No.1795 1:25000 No.2533

Area: 60ha (148 acres)
Height: 28m (92 ft)

Owner: The three islands were owned for a time by Donovan, the folk singer, but sold in the early 1980s. In 2002 the present owner, Moneyedge, an English company, started selling one-square-foot 'unspecific' plots of the smallest island, Clett, through the Internet (Clett.com) for £22.50 each. Many Americans and Canadians, and a few Britons, are reported to have already bought plots giving them the right to an 'undivided' share of the 7½-acre island – i.e. the freedom to visit and explore.

Population: 1841–90. There was a final clearance of the last twelve crofter families in 1860. 1881–0. Uninhabited since.

Geology: Basaltic lava with shale and quartzite covered with a reasonably fertile soil.

History: Olave the Black, a Norwegian warlord, is understood to have been the earliest recorded owner of Isay, Mingay and Clett.

In the early 16th century Roderick MacLeod of Lewis, whose daughter had married twice, decided to eliminate two entire families so that his own grandson should inherit the island of Raasay (See No.5.7) and the lands of Gairloch. He invited the families to a banquet on Isay promising that they would hear something to their advantage. They all turned up and during the meal Roderick said he wanted the private and personal views of everyone present on a matter of great importance. He left the room and each guest was summoned in turn to a room where Roderick had them stabbed to death.

Wildlife: On a June visit there were dozens of pairs of nesting wrens around the ruins and near the headland south-west of the laird's house a large colony of gulls were nesting on the grass. Eider and shelduck paddled along the shores with their young. Wildflowers were in bloom everywhere – marsh marigold, campion, thrift, common spotted orchids, and forget-me-not to name a few – but the many grazing sheep have obviously taken their toll.

* * *

Grass-covered **ISAY** with its two lesser companions, **Mingay** and **Clett**, lies peacefully in Loch Dunvegan. The south-western headland forms a vertical bluff over 20m high but the rest of the coast is generally low.

'. . .There is a beautiful little island in the Loch of Dunvegan, called Isa,' recalled Boswell in 1773. 'M'Leod said he would give it to Dr Johnson, on condition of his residing on it three months in the year; nay one month. Dr Johnson was

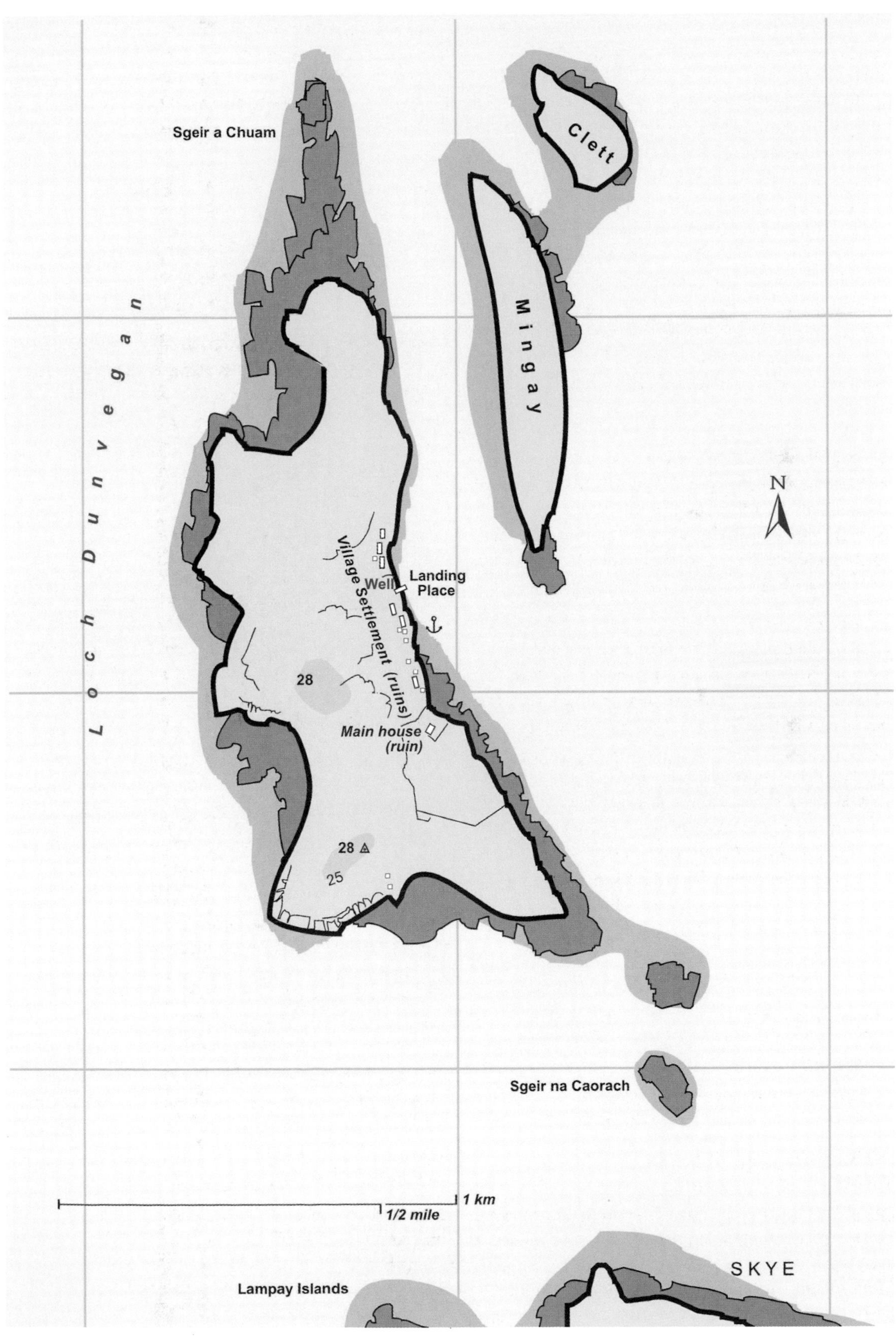
Sgeir a Chuam
Clett
Mingay
Loch Dunvegan
N
Village Settlement (ruins)
Well
Landing Place
28
Main house (ruin)
28
25
Sgeir na Caorach
1 km
1/2 mile
SKYE
Lampay Islands

highly amused with the fancy. I have seen him please himself with little things, even with mere ideas like the present. He talked a great deal of this island; – how he would build a house there, – how he would fortify it, – how he would have cannon, – how he would plant, – how he would sally out and take the isle of Muck; – and then he laughed with uncommon glee, and could hardly leave off... M'Leod encouraged the fancy of Dr Johnson's becoming owner of an island; told him that it was the practice in this country to name every man by his lands; and begged leave to drink to him in that mode: "Island Isa, your health!"'

At that time Isay was a populous and industrious island and by the early 1800s it was a big fishing station with its own general store. The evidence of human activity is still there but the people have long since gone.

A 'street' of more than eighteen cottages and black house ruins lines the east shore where there are also the remnants of a crude stone jetty. At the south end of this village is the main house [NG220567]. Its west gable has a large 'arched' opening like the west gable of a church. This is evidently where the fireplace for the main hall on the first floor used to be. The main entrance to this hall is from the higher ground level on the south side by way of a fine stone staircase with splayed stone balusters. The ground floor appears to have been divided into three rooms and there is an outhouse on the east gable – possibly the kitchen. One of these ground-floor rooms was presumably the site of the notorious 16th-century murders.

The soil is fertile but the land is now only used for grazing sheep.

South of Isay at the head of Loch Dunvegan the famous MacLeod castle is sheltered by **Gairbh Eilean**. **Eilean Grianal** and **Garay Island** are two tiny reefs or skerries alongside a double island, **Eilean Dubh** and **Eilean Mór**, linked by a drying channel.

On the other side of the Waternish Peninsula in Loch Snizort are the basalt **Ascrib Islands**, – **Eilean Iosal**, **Eilean Creagach**, **Eilean Garave** and **South Ascrib**. These were purchased in 1985 by Peter Palumbo, property developer and past Chairman of the Arts Council, as a site to build a subterranean residence for himself. 'There are already traces of underground 18th-century monks' cells and being below ground will cause the least disturbance to a beautiful environment,' he said at the time. However his family was not so enthusiastic and the islands, including a newly built traditional house, were up for sale in 1996 for offers over £200,000.

* * *

Access: Summer excursions from Dunvegan Castle slip, 01470-531500.

Anchorages:

1. Anywhere in the S part of the narrow channel between Isay and Mingay island. Well sheltered from all winds, but winds from the E and SE can sometimes raise an unpleasant sea. Best anchorage possibly in 6m opposite the village ruins S of the S extremity of Mingay Island but well-N of the chapel-like ruin of the main house, weed and mud. Bottom shelves steeply.
2. About the centre of the E side of Isay there is an iron stepladder giving access to a landing platform.

5.9 Rona

Probably (ON hraun-øy – rough island), but possibly (G. ròn – seal, ON -øy – island)

O S Maps: 1:50000 Sheet 24 1:25000 Sheet 409
Admiralty Chart: 1:500000 No.2210

Area: 930ha (2298 acres)
Height: 125m (410 ft)

Owner: Owned by the Department of Agriculture and Fisheries until 1992 then sold on the open market to Mrs Dorte Mette Jensen of Denmark for a price of, possibly, £250,000.

She also has right of pre-emption over 142 acres at the north extremity owned by the Ministry of Defence.

Population: (In 1763 the Laird of Raasay kept a cowman and 160 head of cattle on the island.) 1841–165. 1851–115. 1861–147. 1881–176. 1891–181. 1922–14 tenants and their families. 1931–16. 1971–3. 1981–3: these were all Royal Navy personnel at the NATO station at the north end. 1991–0. 2001–2. A caretaker is now resident at the Lodge throughout most of the year.

Geology: The rocks, some of the oldest in Scotland (and western Europe), are of glaciated Archaean gneiss which is loosely described as Lewisian gneiss. This is a complex group containing dark masses of amphibolite and crystalline veins of pink pegmatite. The earliest metamorphosis – the Scourian – took place about 2500 million years ago.

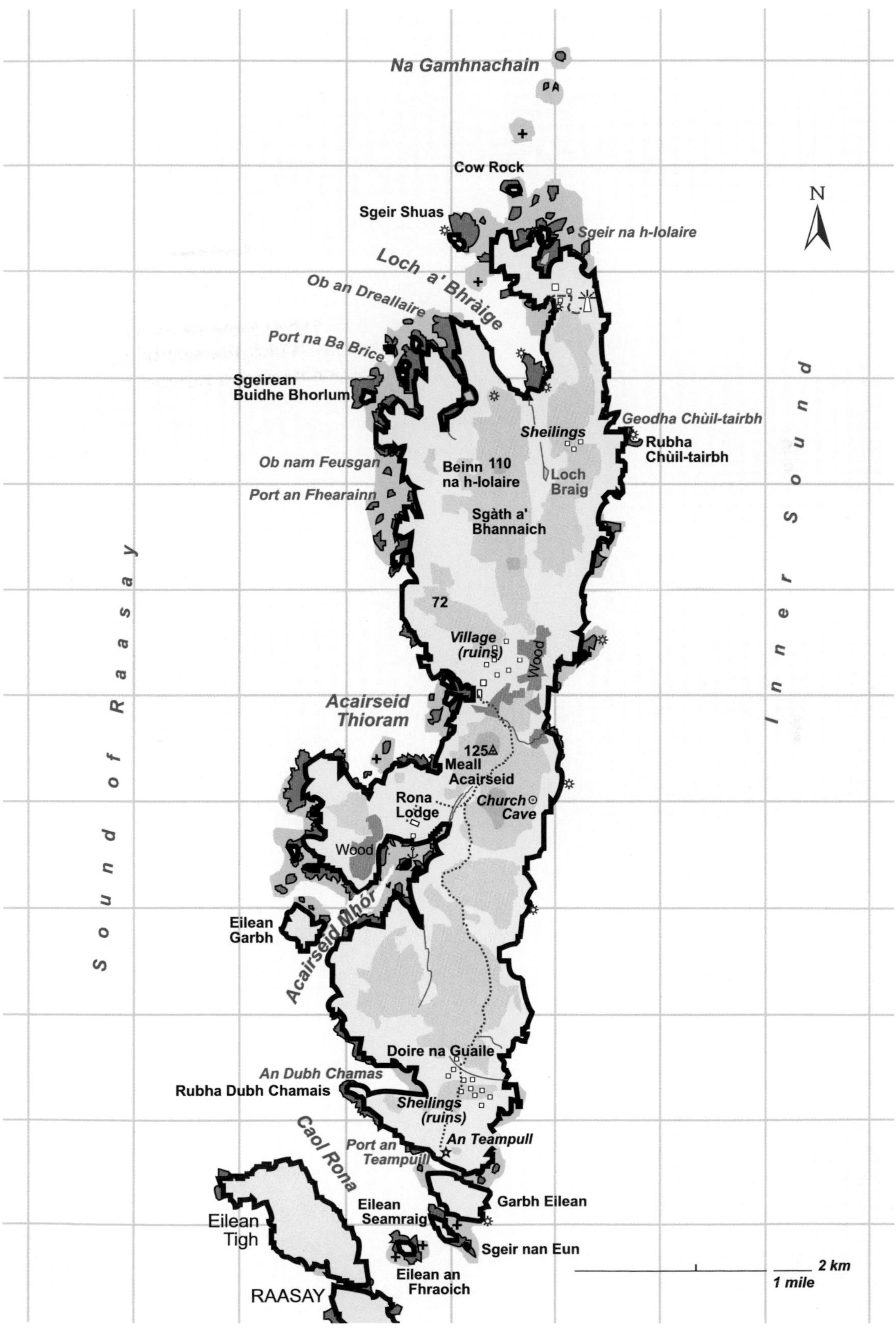
Na Gamhnachain
Cow Rock
Sgeir Shuas
Sgeir na h-Iolaire
Loch a' Bhràige
Ob an Dreallaire
Port na Ba Brice
Sgeirean Buidhe Bhorlum
Geodha Chùil-tairbh
Rubha Chùil-tairbh
Sheilings
Ob nam Feusgan
Beinn na h-Iolaire
110
Loch Braig
Port an Fhearainn
Sgàth a' Bhannaich
72
Village (ruins)
Wood
Acairseid Thioram
125
Meall Acairseid
Rona Lodge
Church Cave
Wood
Acairseid Mhór
Eilean Garbh
Sound of Raasay
Inner Sound
N
Doire na Guaile
An Dubh Chamas
Rubha Dubh Chamais
Sheilings (ruins)
Caol Rona
Port an Teampuill
An Teampull
Garbh Eilean
Eilean Seamraig
Eilean Tigh
Sgeir nan Eun
Eilean an Fhraoich
RAASAY
2 km
1 mile

History: In 1518 the first MacLeod to have taken up residence in Brochel on Raasay, Calum Garbh (Lusty Malcolm), younger son of Calum, the 9th Chief of Lewis, established the line of Mac Gille Chaluim, with the lands of Raasay, Rona and parts of Trotternish, Vaternish and Assynt. He came to an arrangement with the pirates and so-called 'broken men' hiding on the islands and raiding ships as they passed through the Sound of Raasay and the Inner Sound. Rona's perfectly concealed natural harbour of Acairseid Mhór (G. – big harbour) was known at that time as Port nan Robaireann (G. – the robbers' port) because it was the centre for piracy in the area. So, like that other island chieftain, MacNeil of Barra, who carried out piracy on a much bigger scale, MacLeod and his descendants prospered. But in 1745 they made a grave misjudgement by backing the Jacobites and for this they paid dearly.

Although MacLeod entertained Boswell and Johnson royally, he was deeply in debt. So when the Duke of Argyll, Governor of the new British Fisheries Society which was planning the construction of a number of fishing stations (see Nos.6.4 and 6.7), sent a questionnaire to him in 1787, MacLeod speedily replied:

'There is a part of my property (an island called Rona) which is allowed by the best judges to be one of the most advantageous places on this coast for a fishing station. It is surrounded with numbers of banks which are daily discovered by the country people who come to fish from the mainland, which makes me think there is an inexhaustible fund of them about the island. It is likewise supplied with the best harbours at every creek, both for large vessels and small boats.'

But finance was not forthcoming and in the end the imposition by Whitehall of a salt tax stopped the enterprise and crippled the Hebridean fishing industry. Salt was needed to preserve the fish on the way to market.

By 1843 the MacLeod debts were so great that Raasay and Rona had to be sold. They were bought by George Rainy who was something of a philanthropist and in 1850 he did his best to negate the effects of the potato famine. But the population of Raasay had been rising and instead of turning to fishing the people tended to spread on to the more unproductive land such as on Rona. Rainy then started the inevitable sheep-farming and evicted over one hundred families. Some of these also settled on Rona – an island already much less able to support them than Raasay. Rainy died in 1863 and his eighteen-year-old son and heir took over. He did his best for the islanders but died only ten years later. The next owner George Mackay was a ruthless Gael who forced up the rents and within three years sold the two islands for a handsome profit to an Englishman, William Armitage. He in turn sold them on after eighteen months to another Englishman, Herbert Wood, whose only interest was sport. He imported deer, pheasants and rabbits and cleared the best agricultural land on Raasay which put even more pressure on Rona.

Throughout the Western Isles islanders were at last provoked into retaliation and there was the episode of the 'battle of Braes' on Skye in 1882, just across the water from Raasay House. Parliament responded with the Crofter Act, which was passed in 1886, and which protected the crofters' existing holdings although it failed to return their dispossessed land.

Meanwhile the struggle for survival continued among dwindling numbers on rocky Rona. The small settlement in the north at Braig was abandoned in 1889. Then the Great War gave the chance to travel and see new horizons. In May 1921 seven of Rona's demobilised ex-servicemen and their families staked a claim to their own ancestral land at Fearns on Raasay. They built homes and had prepared ground for planting when they were arrested and given prison sentences. This created a public outcry which resulted in Raasay and Rona being purchased by the Government (Scottish Board of Agriculture) in 1922.

At this time there were fourteen tenants and their families still remaining on Rona at Doire na Guaile, Acairseid Mhór, and Acairseid Thioram, but by 1930 the numbers had dwindled to only two tenant families. The last of these, the Macrae family, left the island in 1943.

The Department of Agriculture stocked the island with fifty-five Highland cows and 150 Blackface ewes and let it as a grazing farm in 1946. There were a number of different tenants until 1987 when the livestock was removed and the island was put up for sale in 1992. The owner, Mrs Jensen, must be given great credit for sensibly renovating the house by the big harbour, converting the 'mission house' at Acairseid Thioram into two holiday homes, planting native trees, introducing a small herd of Highland cattle, improving the main track/road and installing a water supply without, thankfully, destroying Rona's wonderful ambience. All this has cost a very large sum of money paid from a Trust set up by her late father 'to promote worldwide conservation'. As a result of this work (and the lack of sheep) the native woodland is steadily regenerating and wildflowers are recolonising the area. Rental of the holiday homes will help to bring in a small income.

Wildlife: At one time there were some wild goats on Rona but these have been absent for many years. There are no rabbits. A small herd of pedigree Highland cattle (from the Ardbhan Fold of North Uist) was introduced in 1996 and these now roam freely over the island and in 2002 six red deer hinds were brought in – much to the delight of a stag on neighbouring Raasay.

The small mature patches of mixed woodland with some fine Scots pines provide cover for a variety of bird species.

* * *

RONA, which is sometimes called South Rona to distinguish it from its namesake which lies well north of Cape Wrath (No.9.4), has a bare, rugged appearance from the sea. There are several hills of 60–90m in height which form a broken ridge and most of the eastern side of the island falls steeply to the sea. The highest hill, **Meall Acairseid** (G. – harbour hill), is 125m high and roughly central.

Rona has been part of the Raasay Estate (See No.5.7) for over 600 years. Martin Martin described it as '..the most unequal rocky piece of ground to be seen anywhere'. and the description in the Gazetteer of 1844 is also graphic as it shows the changing perception of beauty:

'...To an ordinary observer its aspect is quite repulsive; presenting no picturesque features and but little verdure to chequer its grey and sterile surface... Nearly all its arable ground lies round a scattered village which is situated at the head of a bay and contains most of the population.'

Unlike so many of the islands there is a small area of mature native woodland on Rona but at one time it was entirely covered with trees and was used as a source of timber for neighbouring islands. One remaining patch of about two or three hectares, which is on the north side of **Acairseid Mhór** (G. – big harbour), is mainly oak, birch, and hazel but interspersed with some fine Scots pine. Another patch to the north is mainly alder.

A stony road runs from the renovated house known as Rona Lodge at Acairseid Mhór, round Meall Acairseid which has a triangulation beacon on it, to the settlement at **Acairseid Thioram** (G. – dry anchorage). A track carries on to the lighthouse in the extreme north passing between Sgath a' Bhannaich (110m) and the long rib of gneiss to the east of it and then meandering by little Loch Braig. A track also runs south from Acairseid Mhór to the remains of the southernmost village, **Doire na Guaile**, and the ruins of An Teampull at the southern tip.

In the days when the lighthouse was manned, Callum MacLeod BEM, of Arnish on Raasay (See No.5.7), was for a time the Rona postman (this was before he built his famous road from Brochel to Arnish). He used to collect the mail at Arnish twice a week, walk to Eilean Tigh, row across Caol Rona, and then walk the entire length of Rona to the lighthouse, deliver the mail and retrace his steps, a total distance of 30km! Only when you have tried to follow in his footsteps for a few tortuous kilometres can you start to appreciate his dedication.

The lighthouse is now automatic but 142 acres next **Loch a' Bhràige** at the north tip of the island are used as a deep-sea listening post by the Ministry of Defence. To the west of it is **Ob an Dreallaire** (G. – the loiterer's creek) and a tidal pond which was probably used as a fish trap.

The three settlements on Rona boasted two schools and a church. The largest settlement was at **Acairseid Thioram**. The old schoolhouse [NG622580] is still there near the renovated (2002) and sub-divided single-storey Mission House. Islanders worshipped there after it was built in 1878. It is now two holiday cottages. To the north are many ruined cottages which the owner plans to clear and repoint some of the stonework. This will reveal the island settlement as it once was – a sort of living museum. Some of the crofters evicted from Raasay in the 19th century settled at **Doire na Guaile** in the south-east of the island. This is fairly close to the ecclesiastical site known as **An Teampull** (G. – the temple) [NG617544], which is thought to have been an early Christian monk's cell. A stone wall surrounds the ruin of a small chapel and there is one gravestone for a man called Graham. He is reputed to be the only person actually buried in Rona's stony ground, everyone else being buried on Raasay.

Caol Rona is a relatively narrow stretch of water dividing Rona from Raasay and the tide can run through briskly past **Eilean an Fraoich** (G. – heather island) in the centre of the kyle. **Eilean Seamraig** (G. – shamrock island) is a narrow islet on the north side of the kyle beside tidal **Garbh Eilean**.

On the east coast almost directly across the island from Acairseid Mhór is Giant's Cave [NG626572] now known as **Church Cave**. Before the island had a church the islanders worshipped in this cavern and the tradition continued of having babies baptised in the cave. The entrance is like a large Gothic arch and there is a large rock which was used as a pulpit. Beside it is a depression in some stones fed by drips of water from the cave roof and this served as a font. Rows of stones were used as pews by the congregation. A service was held in 1970 attended by thirty members from the Portree Parish Church and another service at Easter 2003 with sixty-four worshippers.

This cave is well worth a visit but it is not marked on the Ordnance Survey maps. Take the road from Acairseid Mhór, follow it north from the junction with the south-going path and at the head of the rise there is a discreet sign at the verge. Follow this across a flat boggy patch, over a small ridge and further boggy patch. The next ridge has a small cairn on its rocky top – cross it and carry on down the hill through thick heather (approx. SE direction). There is a flat depression with four birch trees (and a narrow cleft running down towards the sea). Turn right (approx. S) up a rise into a shallow valley with old peat cuttings. This leads down and round the side of a cliff in which the cave is located. Tough going, but even grannies used to do it!

In 1840 the tiny cottage by the slipway (now renovated with four bunk beds for visitors) was occupied by the Mackenzie family, the only residents of Big Harbour at the time. That summer Kenneth Mackenzie was lost at sea but his widow, Janet, would not believe it so she kept a light burning in the cottage window to guide his boat back into harbour. This was of such great assistance to other vessels that after some years the Navy gave her a £20 award and the Commissioners of Northern Lights also gave her a small sum to purchase lamp-oil. She kept the light burning for twelve long years but her husband never appeared and in 1852 she gave up and emigrated to Australia.

* * *

Access: Visitors welcome but should make a courtesy call at the lodge first; Bill Cowie, 07831-293963. Bill also runs a Rona–Raasay ferry

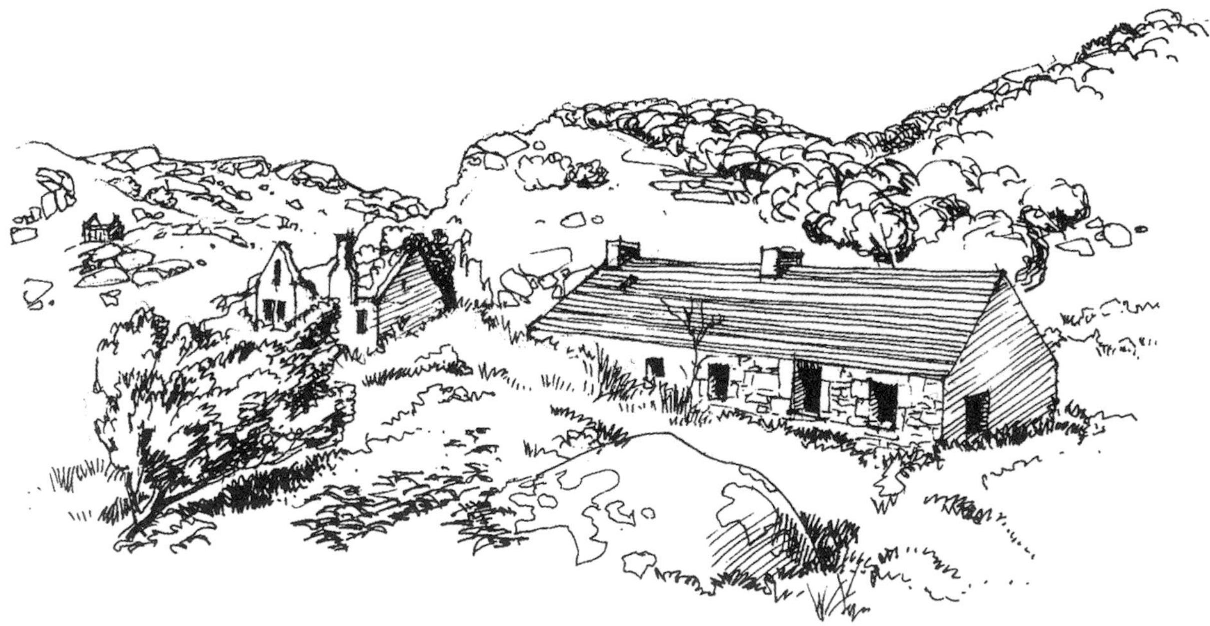

THE OLD SCHOOLHOUSE AND THE MISSION HOUSE (NOW RENOVATED) AT ACAIRSEID THIORAM

service. Regular Sat. ferry from Portree, Dan Corrigal, 01478-612333.

Anchorages:
1. Acairseid Mhór. Popular sheltered anchorage. Entrance concealed by Eilean Garbh and care needed in the approach. Shingle or mud, holding varies. Pontoon for dinghy access. One mooring by pontoon (pay at cottage).
2. Loch a' Bhraige. Anchorage used by MOD. Well lit, good shelter but unattractive and entry discouraged.

5–Appendix Skye

[sky] Probably (Early Celtic skitis, or G. sgiath – winged) isle. Interpreted by Norse as ?(ON skuy – misty) isle.

OS maps: 1:50000 Sheets 23, 32 and 33 1:25000 sheets 407, 408, 410, 411 and 412.
Admiralty Charts: 1:100000 No.1795 1:50000 Nos.2208, 2209 and 2210.

Area: 165,625ha (409259 acres)
Height: 993m (3257 ft)

Owner: Multiple ownership but the Scottish Office (Government) has sizeable holdings.

Population: 1755–11252. 1794–14470. 1821–20827. 1841–23082 (peak).
1881–16889. 1891–15705. 1931–9908. 1951–8537. 1961–7479. 1971–7183.
1981–7276. 1991–8847. 2001–9232.

Geology: The dramatic Cuillin mountains in the south were formed by volcanic activity some fifty million years ago. Narrow tilted strata of brittle rock run through the iron-hard gabbro, which has been shaped by ice into great jagged and irregular teeth. The Red Cuillin on the other hand are of granite (gabbro which flowed out of the ground and cooled quickly) and this by comparison is soft enough to have eroded into more rounded shapes. The oldest rock on Skye, gneiss, is found south of Isle-ornsay on the Sleat [slayt] peninsula.

There is a wealth of geological variety on Skye. Marble is quarried near Torrin, there are coral beaches on Loch Dunvegan, and north of Trotternish there is a beach of green sand (due to the presence of olivine). Gold has also been found on the island.

History: St Columba visited Skye in 585AD. From the 8th century until 1266 – three years after King Haakon's defeat at the Battle of Largs – the Norse were in control. Later the land was divided between the MacDonalds, the Mackinnons and the MacLeods who were constantly feuding and fighting.

In 1745 twenty-four-year-old Flora MacDonald helped Bonnie Prince Charlie, with a price of £30,000 on his head, to escape capture. With the Prince disguised as a maid and called Betty Burke, Edinburgh-educated Flora brought him by boat from Benbecula 'over the sea to Skye', landing at Kilbride Bay, where he hid in caves and cattle byres. Then he crossed to Raasay (See No.5.7) by night and arrived there just after the staunchly Jacobite island had been sacked by government troops from *HMS Furnace*. His French rescue ship failed to appear so he returned to Skye and then crossed over to Knoydart on the mainland. On the 19 September 1746 he was picked up from Loch nam Uamh by the French and escaped to France. He died in Rome in 1778. Flora was arrested and taken to London but she was freed in 1747 after the passing of the Indemnity Act by Parliament and became very popular with London society.

Many families were forced to leave Skye after the unsuccessful Jacobite Rising and between 1840 and 1880 a further 30,000 people were evicted from their crofts by landlords and forced to emigrate to the New World. Yet more left when bad harvests struck the island in 1881–85. The ruined houses and empty glens can still be seen as testimony of this misery.

Wildlife: Skye has a rich diversity of flora with a number of rare species. On the east side of the Trotternish ridge a relative of the sorrels which are native to Iceland was discovered in 1934. Mountain avens, guelder-rose and helleborine can be found in the birchwoods behind Broadford and rock whitebeam and red broomrape flourish on the cliffs and slopes above the sea.

'There are in Skye neither rats nor mice; but the weasel is so frequent that he is heard in houses rattling behind chests or beds as rats in England,' according to Dr Johnson, whose natural history was not always accurate.

The white-tailed sea-eagles nested on Skye until 1907, and the last sighting was recorded in 1916.

* * *

The 'capital' of **SKYE** is **Portree**. It was called Kiltragleann (G. – the church of St Talarican in the glen) until the 16th century or thereabouts.

It is said to have been renamed in honour of a visit in 1540 by King James V (G. *port-rìgh* – King's port) but some say the derivation is (G. *portrigheadh* – port on the hillside). The Royal Hotel is on the site of McNab's Inn where Bonnie Prince Charlie bade fond farewell to Flora MacDonald but there is little of historical interest. The building which used to be the courthouse and jail for the whole island now houses the tourist office. Highlighting Skye's recent insularity it is noteworthy that until 1949 the only electricity on the island was produced by a diesel generator in the Portree Hotel.

The road north to Trotternish passes by the **Storr** (G. – buck tooth) 719m high, with its conspicuous 50m-high rock-needle called **The Old Man of Storr** – first climbed in 1955. **Holm Island** lies off-shore to the south-east.

On the beach north of **Rigg** a church-shaped rock – **Eaglais Bhreagach** marks the place where the Clan MacQueen is said to have raised the devil using an ancient ritual which involved roasting live cats. A small carpark at **Lealt** is the start of an interesting climb down a ravine with a view of several spectacular waterfalls and further on, at **Lonfearn**, are the remains of early Christian beehive cells [NG526626]. These are known as druids' houses in Gaelic. High on the ridge above, near the summit of Beinn Edra (611m), a Flying Fortress bomber crashed in 1945.

Beyond Kilt Rock [NG507665], a piece of natural black basalt with folded strata, is **Staffin**, scene of the alleged wreck of a galleon of the Spanish Armada. This is where the small but intriguing **Staffin Museum** holds a collection of the dinosaur fossils and footprints from the mid-Jurassic period which have been discovered on the Trotternish Peninsula. Off-shore are **Staffin Island** and **Eilean Flodigarry**, where according to local tradition the owner once had his corn harvested for him in two nights by 150 fairies. Above Staffin is the **Quiraing**, a fantastic group of awesome rock formations. A short walk north-east from the highest point of the Staffin-to-Uig road [NG443682] leads to The Table, The Prison, and the 36m-high Needle.

As the road turns west at the head of the peninsula there is a striking viewpoint at **Bàgh nan Gunnaichean** (G. – bay of the cannons). To the north is **Eilean Trodday** (G. and ON – island of the trolls) which once supported a settlement and a chapel. At the extreme north-west of Trotternish the ruin of 15th-century **Duntulm Castle** [NG410743], last occupied in 1732, overlooks **Tulm Island**. Further out to sea are a group of slab-shaped basalt islands owned by Torquil Johnson-Ferguson since 1983 (see No.2.11), – **Lord Macdonald's Table** (G – *Am Bord*), **Gearran Island**, **Gaeilavore Island**, **The Cleats**, and **Fladda-chùain** with a ruined chapel in which, it is said, Sir Donald MacDonald of the Isles hid his title deeds before the 1715 Rising. The cell was founded in Columba's time by a giant of a monk called O'Gorgon and, strangely, the last man to live on the island was also of huge stature and known as Muileach Mór (G. – the big man from Mull).

About 2km south is a **Cottage Museum** in a reconstructed black house, and the burial place of Flora MacDonald. The original MacDonald mausoleum was slowly dismantled by souvenir-hunting tourists and the present memorial replaced it [NG400719]. West of **Balgown** a marshy loch with beehive dwellings and a nunnery on its islands was drained in 1824 [NG377689].

The ferry terminal of **Uig** (ON *vik* – a bay), with services to Harris and North Uist, is in a large cove sheltered by basaltic cliffs.

Travelling south to Loch Snizort Beag, ruined **Caisteal Uisdean** (G. – Hugh's castle) overlooks **Eileanan Mór** and **Beag**. It was built about 1580 by Hugh MacDonald of Sleat with stone quarried from the Ascrib Islands (See No.5.8). Hugh's clan chief found that he had been plotting against him so he entombed him alive in Duntulm Castle with a piece of salt beef and an empty water jug [NG381583].

A broad valley runs from Portree to Loch Snizort containing the village of **Skeabost**. A tiny island in the river below the Skeabost bridge has associations with St Columba [NG418485] and it was in this village that the poet Mairi Mhor Nan Oran (Mary MacPherson) was born. Above **Clachamish** are the remains of **Dùn Suladale** [NG374526], one of the best-preserved brochs on Skye.

The village of **Stein** on the Vaternish peninsula nestles on the side of Loch Bay overlooking the islands of Isay (No.5.8), Mingay and Clett. Further on, at the end of the road, the windswept ruin of **Trumpan Church** [NG225612] above Ardmore Bay was the scene of one of the bloodiest episodes in Scottish history. In 1578, while the MacLeods

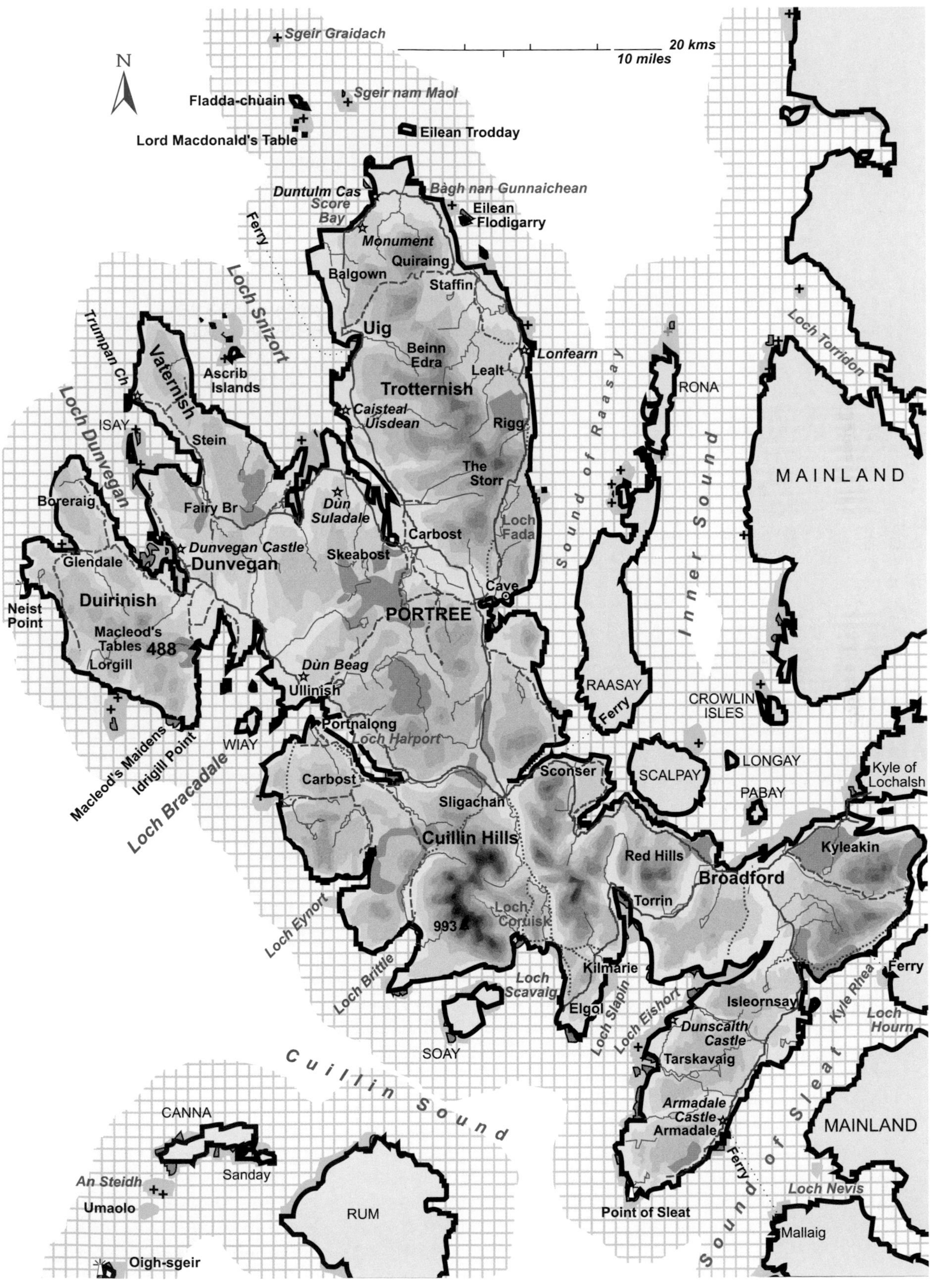

Sgeir Graidach
20 kms
10 miles
N
Fladda-chùain
Sgeir nam Maol
Eilean Trodday
Lord Macdonald's Table
Duntulm Cas
Bàgh nan Gunnaichean
Score Bay
Eilean Flodigarry
Ferry
Monument
Quiraing
Balgown
Staffin
Loch Snizort
Trumpan Ch
Uig
Lonfearn
Vaternish
Beinn Edra
Ascrib Islands
Lealt
Loch Torridon
RONA
Trotternish
Loch Dunvegan
Caisteal Uisdean
Rigg
ISAY
Stein
Sound of Raasay
Inner Sound
The Storr
MAINLAND
Boreraig
Dùn Suladale
Fairy Br
Loch Fada
Carbost
Dunvegan Castle
Glendale
Skeabost
Dunvegan
Cave
Neist Point
Duirinish
PORTREE
Macleod's Tables 488
Lorgill
Dùn Beag
Ullinish
RAASAY
CROWLIN ISLES
Ferry
Portnalong
Loch Harport
WIAY
Macleod's Maidens
Idrigill Point
LONGAY
Sconser
SCALPAY
Kyle of Lochalsh
Carbost
PABAY
Loch Bracadale
Sligachan
Cuillin Hills
Kyleakin
Red Hills
Broadford
Torrin
Loch Eynort
Loch Coruisk
993
Ferry
Kilmarie
Loch Brittle
Loch Scavaig
Kyle Rhea
Isleornsay
Elgol
Loch Slapin
Loch Eishort
Loch Hourn
Dunscaith Castle
SOAY
Tarskavaig
Cuillin Sound
CANNA
Armadale Castle
Armadale
MAINLAND
Sound of Sleat
Sanday
Ferry
An Steidh
Umaolo
RUM
Loch Nevis
Point of Sleat
Mallaig
Oigh-sgeir

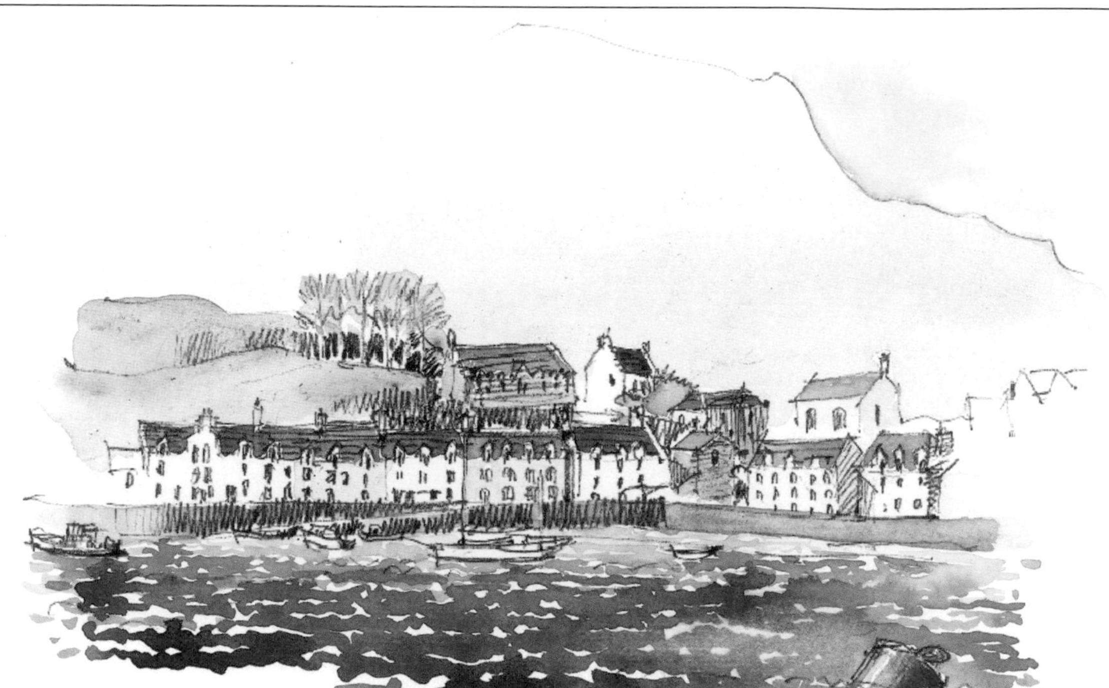

PORTREE

were at worship, the MacDonalds of Uist decided to avenge the massacre of Eigg (See No.4.2) so they barred the door and set fire to the church. One young girl escaped, although she severed one of her breasts while struggling through a small window, but all the rest were burned to death. The girl raised the alarm and the MacLeods quickly gathered a force together. Carrying their famous Fairy Flag they rushed down on the MacDonalds as they were leaving in their galleys. Every MacDonald was slaughtered and the bodies were buried in a dyke. The battle has been remembered ever since as the 'spoiling of the dyke'.

The grave of Lady Grant is in the churchyard. She was exiled to St Kilda (No.9.1) for eight years by her husband and died in 1742, three years after returning to Skye.

By the **Fairy Bridge** [NG278513] on Bay River the road travels south to **Dunvegan Castle** [NG247491], seat of the Clan MacLeod since 1200. This is the longest continuous occupation of any Scottish castle although much of the present castle was built in the 19th century. On Skye, by the way, the *sìthiche* [shee-huch], the fairies or little people, have often played a prominent part in clan history. They were said to live in the rounded grassy mounds called *sìthean* [shee-hen] and enjoy many mischievous pranks.

Duirinish, the area west of Dunvegan, is dominated by twin peaks called **Macleod's Tables**, **Healabhal Bheag** which is the highest (488m) and **Healabhal More**, larger but lower (469m). Much of this area is wild moorland, but there are several villages in the north including **Boreraig**, home of the hereditary pipers to the MacLeod chiefs, the world-renowned MacCrimmons. The Piper's Cave is in the cliffs below the reputed site of their piping college. The MacArthurs founded the first piping school on Skye but they moved to Islay (No.2.4) as hereditary pipers to the Lords of the Isles.

Through the valley to the west is **Glendale** with its restored 200-year-old dry-stone grain mill. Further west still there is a well-made path running out to the lighthouse on Neist Point where the view is panoramic. For memorable scenery try the bumpy road to Ramasaig, followed by a walk down the track to **Lorgill**. On 4 August 1830 every crofter in Lorgill was ordered to board the *Midlothian* in Loch Snizort or go to prison. (Those over the age of seventy were sent to the poorhouse instead). Experienced hill-walkers could take the cliff-top route from here to Idrigill Point but a safer bet is to drive to Loch Bharcasaig at Orbost and take the 6km track from there. Idrigill Point overlooks Loch Bracadale and **Macleod's Maidens**, three dramatic stacks like Victorian statues standing in the sea. They were named to commemorate the drowning of the wife and two daughters of a MacLeod chief.

Loch Bracadale is an interesting loch with many inlets and small islands. Dr Johnson stayed at Ullinish and visited **Dùn Beag**, an interesting ruined broch beside the road at Struan [NG339386]. At the entrance to Loch Harport, which opens off the southern end of Bracadale there is the small fishing village of **Portnalong** which was founded by crofters from Lewis and Harris in 1921, and the famous Talisker Whisky distillery is further south at **Carbost**. A narrow road connects Carbost to **Loch Brittle** in the south-west of Skye with its sandy beach, a campsite for climbers, and the cruel but beautiful spiked ridges of the Cuillin Hills towering above the glen.

The road south from Portree meets the junction at **Sligachan**. There is a track from here [NG487298] which climbs over the mountains to **Loch Coruisk** (G. *coire uisge* – cauldron of water). The approach to Loch Coruisk by sea is from Loch Scavaig into Loch Cuilce (G. – reedy loch). The anchorage behind **Eilean Glas** and beneath a high cliff with a waterfall is one of the most dramatic on the West Coast. There is not much swinging room but there is an alternative spot by **Eilean Reamhar** (G. – fat island). Loch Coruisk – fresh water, only 10m above sea level, and one of the most awe-inspiring places on earth – is only a short walk away. The deep dark loch, 30m deeper than sea-loch Scavaig, is set in a giant amphitheatre of lonely, primaeval mist-shrouded mountains. It was painted by Turner and visited by Sir Walter Scott.

Sgurr Alasdair, on the west side of Loch Coruisk, is Skye's highest peak at 993m (3257ft), while one of the longest rock climbs in Britain is the ascent of Sgurr a' Ghreadaidh (G. – peak of torment) from the head of Loch Coruisk.

The road from Sligachan runs through **Sconser**, ferry terminal for Raasay, round Loch Ainort with a folk museum at Luib and on to Broadford Bay. **Broadford** lies under Beinn na Caillich (732m) and its eastward continuation is called Waterloo because many of the veterans of the 1815 battle made their homes here. The road to Elgol, a little settlement which overlooks Soay (No.5.1) by Loch Scavaig, runs through a broad valley south of Beinn na Caillich. On the way it passes close to **Coire-chatachan** [NG621227] where Mackinnon entertained Dr Johnson and Boswell during their tour of the Hebrides in 1773. Just beyond are the ruins of Cille Chrìosd (G. – Christ's church) and further on, past the **Torrin** marble quarry by Loch Slapin, the village of **Kilmarie** was once the home of the Mackinnon chiefs. A track from here leads over the hills to Loch Coruisk via 'Bad Step' while the view to the east is up lovely Loch Eishort with **Eilean Gaineamhach Boreraig** and **Eilean Dubh** dotted on either side of the narrows like the Morse code.

Sitting on the headland at **Suidhe Biorach** (G. – pointed seat) south of Elgol is reputed to make childless women fertile. There is a marvellous walk along the rocky shore at **Elgol** with its strange honeycomb cliffs facing gloomy Loch Scavaig. The east side of the Strathaird promontory has equally fine views of Sleat and, at Glasnakille, Spar Cave with its stalactites is worth a visit [NG538128].

The **Sleat** [slayt] peninsula between Loch Eishort and the Sound of Sleat is served by a road from Broadford. Opposite dour Loch Hourn on the mainland, lies the pretty little village and anchorage of Isleornsay. Unfortunately, the bottom is thick with weed and anchors easily drag. On the tidal island **Ornsay** (ON *örfiris-øy* – ebb island) there is a ruined chapel and an automatic lighthouse beside Eilean an Eòin (G. – isle of birds).

Further south the pier at **Armadale** for the Mallaig ferry shelters the Skye Yacht Club's anchorage. Above the road stands Armadale Castle [NG640047], which was built in 1815–19 for the second Lord MacDonald. It is surrounded by tree specimens from all over the world and is now the **Clan Donald Centre**. There are estimated to be three million MacDonalds in the world.

The southernmost tip of Sleat – the lighthouse at Point of Sleat with **Eilean Sgorach** (G. – scollop isle) beneath it – can be reached on foot by a track. On the west side of the peninsula ruined **Dunscaith Castle** [NG595120] is between the villages of Tokavaig and Tarskavaig. According to legend this was the home of the Queen of Skye who taught the art of war to Cuchulainn, an Irish hero. It was last occupied in 1570. **Eilean Ruaridh** (G. – Rory's island) is off-shore.

Kyle Rhea, north of the Sound of Sleat, with its privately-operated ferry from Glenelg is the traditional ferry crossing to Skye, although until

1906 cattle bound for market were tied nose to tail and made to swim across the narrows. The modern ferry terminal was at Kyleakin (King Haakon's kyle, commemorating his visit in 1263) until it was replaced by the bridge. Four miles west is the Skye airstrip and at the end of the runway a row of graves contain the dead from the cruiser *HMS Curaçao*, which was cut in two by the *Queen Mary* when she was escorting her in 1942.

Access: Road access (A87) by bridge at Kyle of Lochalsh linking Skye and the mainland. Frequent vehicle ferry service, 1) Glenelg to Kylerhea, crossing 5 minutes, 01599-522273, and 2) Mallaig to Armadale, crossing 30 minutes, 08000-66-5000.

Anchorages:

1. Camas Daraich, at Point of Sleat. Keep in centre. Occasional anchorage more than 1c off-shore in 6–10m. Exposed S and subject to swell.
2. Port na Long, Sound of Sleat. Temp. anchorage well off-shore.
3. Port a' Chuil, Sound of Sleat. Temp. anchorage well off-shore.
4. Armadale Ardvasar. Beware rocks S of Armadale. Restricted space but good holding in sand. Exposed N and E. Subject to swell from S. All moorings managed by Skye Yachts.
5. Knock Bay, Sound of Sleat. Anchor 1½c SE of castle ruin. Protected from NE swell but holding poor. W side of bay is foul. Beware sudden change of depth.
6. Loch Camas Croise. Temp anchorage, N side and not too far in, clay.
7. Isleornsay harbour. Easy access, good shelter except NE, but head dries out a long way and holding poor due to weed. Best holding due W of N beacon on Isleornsay.
8. Camas nam Mult, opposite Duisdale Hotel. Better holding than Isleornsay, and nearer shore.
9. Loch na Dal. Head dries nearly 5c. Open SE but better than Isleornsay in N'lies.
10. Bagh Dunan Ruadh, S of Kyle Rhea. Occasional anchorage 2c S of river mouth, 2c off shore, good holding. Squally in NW'lies. Beware 2c drying bank at river mouth.
11. Sgeir na Caillich, N of Kyle Rhea. Anchor 2c WNW of the beacon, or closer to shore if using large-scale chart.
12. Loch na Béiste. Foul with old moorings, wreckage, fish farm, deep and weedy. Suitable small area near burn at head in 3–6m. Exposed E.
13. Ob na Partan. Probably foul with cables but sheltered anchorage ½c from W side in 7m. Use tripping line.
14. Kyleakin. 60m length of pontoon on N side of sheltered inlet (pay). Depths 3m outside, 2.5m inside.
15. North of Kyleakin village, off King's Arms Hotel. Beware cables E of hotel. Occasional anchorage, blue clay. Subject to swell from traffic and N'lies. Visitors' moorings available.
16. Corry Pier, Broadford. Anchor off pier on W side of bay clear of moorings and drying rock SE of pier or temp. alongside pier. Exposed N.
17. Caolas Scalpay, E of narrows. Anchor where convenient. Can be squally. Beware Sgeir Stapaig off Scalpay.
18. Loch na Cairidh, W of narrows. Anchor where convenient. Can be squally.
19. Loch Ainort. Anchor off Luib or in either corner at head. Can be very squally.
20. Loch Sligachan. Narrow entrance with several hazards. Anchor off W side of ferry slip at Sconser or less than ½c W of ruined slip at Peinchorran or towards head of loch in not less than 5m. Can be very squally.
21. Balmeanach Bay, S of Raasay narrows. Anchor clear of cables. Holding good.
22. Camas a' Mhór-bheòil, N of Raasay narrows. Beware drying rock in middle of bay. Uncomfortable in N'lies.
23. Tianavaig Bay. Sheltered SW to NNE. Anchor in 5–10m sand. Can be squally.
24. Portree. Restricted by moorings. Anchor NE of pier in 7–10m, soft mud, doubtful holding. Visitors' buoys available (pay) but uncomfortable in S'lies. Temp stay alongside pier when tide and space suitable, but be ready to move off. Alternative anchorage at Camas Bàn, but subject to 'whirlies' in S'lies.
25. Staffin Bay. Enter from NE. Bay is clean but exposed NE and squally in W'lies. Anchor on W side of Staffin Island or SW corner of bay.
26. Kilmaluag Bay. Beware drying reef at entrance and submerged rock off N shore. Fierce squalls in strong W'lies. Exposed E. Anchor in 5–10m, sand and pebbles, good holding.
27. Duntulm Bay. Approach mid-channel by S entrance. Anchor close to NE side of Tulm Island but N of mid-point, or under cliffs at NE of bay. Some swell at turn of tide, but sheltered.
28. Uig Bay. Restricted space behind pier but bottom foul and most of the bay dries. Temp lie alongside pier may be possible in daylight. Camas Beag on S side of bay suitable in S'lies but deep until close to shore.
29. Poll na h'-Ealaidh (Port na Ella). Beware drying rocks N of entrance. Anchor close E of Dùn Maraig islet on S side. Sheltered except W'lies.
30. Loch Snizort Beag. Keep mid-channel on approach up the loch. Anchor just within the middle arm, SW of Skerinish Quay, 4m, mud, good holding and good shelter.

31. Loch Treaslane on W side of Loch Snizort Beag. Keep mid-channel. Head dries off for 4c. Good shelter.
32. Clachamish Bay, first bay on W side of Loch Snizort Beag. Suitable anchorage.
33. Loch Greshornish. Approach and enter loch on course midway between Eilean Mór and Greshornish Point and keep mid-channel up loch. Anchor SW of Borve. Excellent shelter.
34. Loch Diubaig. Head dries off 3c. Occasional anchorage. Exposed N.
35. Aros Bay. Clean and open. Occasional anchorage.
36. Ardmore Bay. W side shoal. Shelter from N'lies but holding doubtful.
37. Stein. Visitors' moorings but usually occupied by local fishing boats. Uncomfortable in S and W winds.
38. Dunvegan Castle. Anchor between Gairbh Eilean and castle, clear of rocks or anchor beyond pier as depths allow. Four yellow visitors' moorings at hotel. (*Visit Dunvegan Castle*).
39. Loch Erghallan. Follow approach directions with care. Anchor ¾c from S of Eilean Mor.
40. Loch Mór. Follow approach directions and anchor in centre of basin or, for best shelter, ESE of Colbost slip.
41. Leinish Bay. Anchor in centre. Exposed N and E.
42. Loch Pooltiel. Occasional anchorage near head which dries off several cables, 3–5m, mud, good holding. Exposed NW but small boats might gain shelter between pier and Sgeir Mór, bottom stony.
43. Loch Bharcasaig, Loch Bracadale. Best anchorage in this area other than Loch Harport. Anchor in SW corner in 4m.
44. Loch Vatten. Anchor near bay in NW corner. Fair shelter but exposed to SW swell. Beware Harlosh Skerry on approach. Shallow-draught boats can enter Poll Roag at HW but not recommended.
45. Loch Caroy. Occasional anchorage exposed to S'ly swell with various hazards on approach. Anchor near jetty on E side.
46. Tarner Island. Approach from S and anchor close to NE side of island in 9m. Reasonable shelter.
47. Oronsay, bay on NW side. Clean and good holding in 4m, sand. Sheltered NE to SW, but some swell at HW.
48. Loch Beag, Loch Harport. Occasional anchorage but exposed SW. Holding poor, dries out halfway and obstructed by moorings.
49. Gesto Bay. Fair anchorage except in SW'-W'lies.
50. Carbost. Visitors' moorings or anchor near shore between pier and distillery. Beware extensive shoal at burn. Head of loch dries. Two visitors' moorings. (*Visit Talisker distillery*).
51. Port na Long. Anchor off jetty, good holding and fair shelter except from E. Bay obstructed with moorings and fish cages.
52. Fiskavaig Bay. Temp anchorage off burn on W side, 7m.
53. Loch Eynort. Occasional anchorage. Exposed W but some shelter beyond bend. Holding uncertain. Head dries 8c. Subject to squalls.
54. Loch Brittle. Temp anchorage if no swell.
55. Loch Scavaig, Eilean Reamhar. Care needed on approach. Anchor NW of Eilean Reamhar, 10m, mud and weed. Reasonable shelter but subject to squalls.
56. Loch na Cuilce, Eilean Glas. Follow sailing directions carefully for approach to anchorage on NW side of Eilean Glas. Good holding in mud and sand but subject to violent squalls. (Access to Loch Coruisk).
57. Loch Slapin. Follow directions for the approach. Best anchorage near W shore beyond the narrows, 4–6m, mud. Head dries off 5c. Fish cages and occasional swell.
58. Loch Eishort, Heast Island. Follow sailing directions carefully for difficult approach. Anchor E of island, clear of moorings and N of fish cages, mud, good holding.
59. Bagh an Dubh Ard, SW of Loch Eishort narrows. Follow directions for approach. Occasional anchorage in suitable weather. Bottom shelves steeply.
60. Tokavaig (Ob Gauscavaig). Temp. anchorage in clean sand. (*Visit Dun Scaich*).
61. Tarskavaig. Occasional anchorage in settled weather, clean sand.
62. Acairseid an Rubha, on W side of Point of Sleat has a jetty for servicing the lighthouse. Not recommended.

SECTION 6

Gairloch and the North Coast

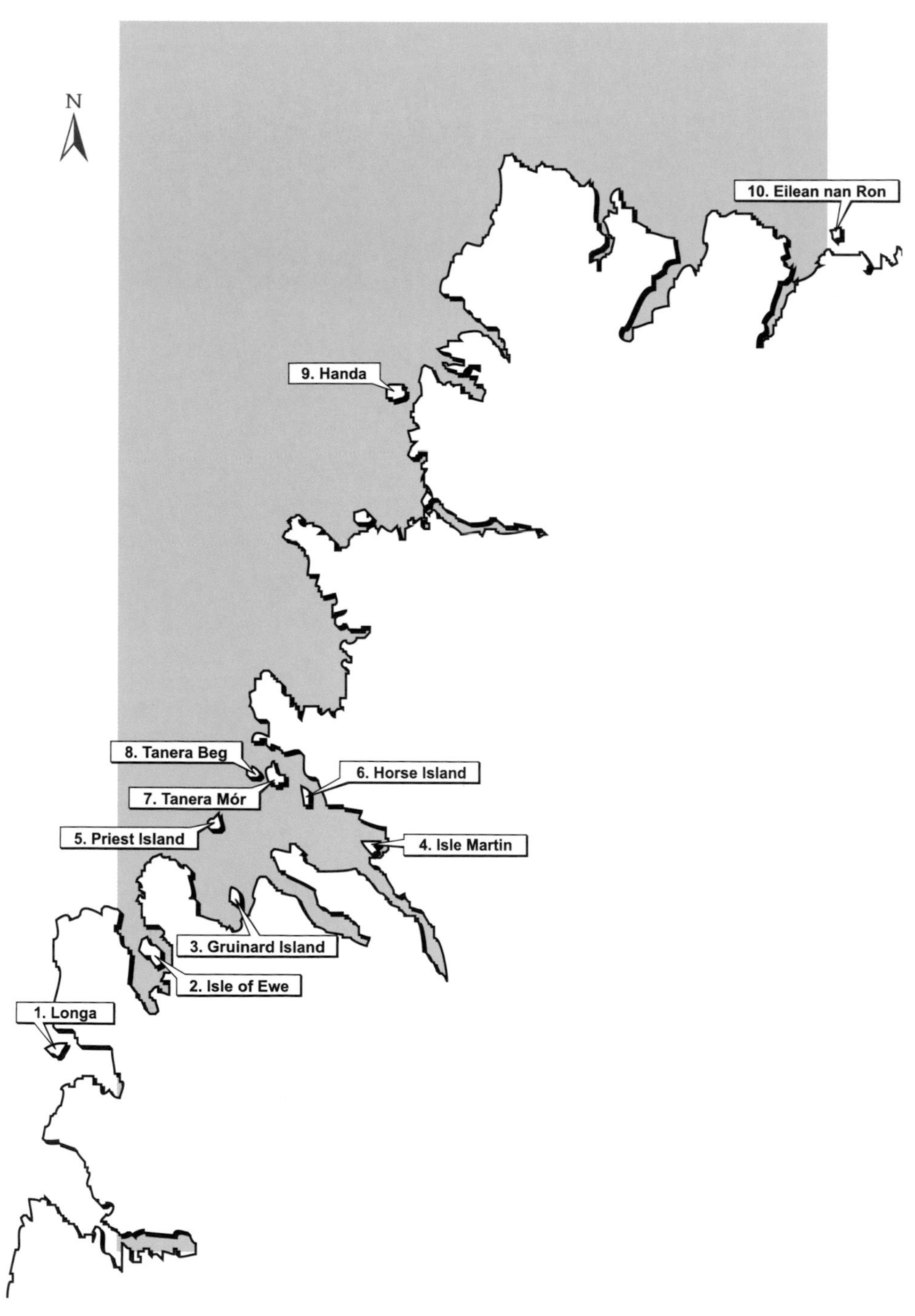

SECTION 6, Table 1: Arranged according to geographic position

No.	Name	Latitute	Longitude	Table 2* No.	Tab 3** No.	Area in Acres	Area in Hectares
6.1	Longa	57° 44N	05° 48W	100	91	311	126
6.2	Isle of Ewe	57° 50N	05° 37W	68	89	764	309
6.3	Gruinard Island	57° 53N	05° 28W	86	63	484	196
6.4	Isle Martin	57° 57N	05° 13W	91	56	388	157
6.5	Priest Island	57° 58N	05° 30W	105	85	301	122
6.6	Horse Island	57° 59N	05° 20W	144	105	131	53
6.7	Tanera Mór	58° 01N	05° 24W	66	55	766	310
6.8	Tanera Beg	58° 01N	05° 27W	133	80	163	66
6.9	Handa	58° 23N	05° 12W	67	52	764	309
6.10	Eilean nan Ron	58° 34N	04° 20W	98	87	341	138

*Table 2: The islands arranged in order of magnitude
**Table 3: The islands arranged in order of height

Introduction

There are no large islands off the north-west coast of Scotland from Skye to Cape Wrath but there is a surfeit of little ones.

What is the collective noun which best represents a collection of small islands? A cluster, a scatter, an accumulation, an agglomeration? How about a swarm or an assembly? A clutter or a hotchpotch? Anyway, some such term is badly needed for the medley of assorted islets scattered in patches along this coastline.

Seen as part of a vast primeval landscape with its reedy pools, patches of heather, and enormous expanses of smooth pink rock, the islets are almost indistinguishable in the random mix of land and water. The land dominates. The sea is a mere intrusion.

That is the view from the land but, as always, the view from the sea is very different. Now the islets create a patchwork of fascinating channels, each one different, each turn revealing new vistas and tempting further exploration. The scale is more human and immediate, each discovery more exciting, possibly because speed is limited and distances are restricted by a sea-level viewpoint. The sea is in control and there are no hill-top views of distant horizons to give a foretaste of things to come.

The region prospered during the herring boom of the late 18th century. **Isle Ristol**, a tidal island near the **Summer Isles**, was the site of a fishing station founded in the later 18th century by Morison and Mackenzie. Close beside it is **Eilean Mullagrach** while **Eilean Ghlais** gives its name to a bay to the north. The Summer Isles, by the way, were so named because they were, and still are, used for summer grazing.

The huge Inverpolly Nature Reserve abuts Enard Bay with the islets of **Eilean Mór**, **Eilean Mòineseach** (G. – diffident isle), **Fraochlan** (G. – heather island) and **Green Island** immediately off-shore. There are anchorages in Lochan Sàl and Loch an Eisg-brachaidh east of these islets. The busy fishing harbour of Lochinver is a few miles to the north with **Soyea** (ON – sheep island) marking its entrance and **A' Chleit** (G. – the reef) nearby.

In the next huge bay to the north, Eddrachillis Bay, there are many islets. **Oldany Island** is larger than Isle Ristol but is also linked to the mainland by a drying channel. **Eilean Chrona** (G. – faulty island) is to the west of it and **Eilean nan Uan** (G. – lamb island), **Eilean an Achaidh** (G. – field island), and **Cùl Eilean** (G. – island at the back) are the larger of the tight group of islets to the east.

The islets in the centre of Eddrachillis Bay, **Meall Mór** (G. – big lump) and **Meall Beag** are almost a continuation of the line of a proto-peninsula formed by Calbha Mór which is part of the mainland, and **Calbha Beag** (G. – little headland), an independent island in spite of its name. They are at the entrance to Loch a' Chàirn Bhàin which is spanned by the beautiful Kylesku Bridge. **Eilean a' Ghamhna** (G. – isle of the stirks) is west of the bridge and **Eilean na Rainich** below the bridge on the east side. The bridge itself is built on the tidal islet of Garbh Eilean.

There is another **Eilean na Rainich** (G. – isle of the ferns) in the **Badcall Islands**. If any group of islets needs a suitable collective noun, this is it. A 'school' is too orderly, a 'gaggle' sounds better.

The larger islets are **Eilean a' Bhreitheimh**, **Ceannamhór** (G. – bighead), **Ox Rock**, **Eilean na Bearachd** (G. – island with the pointed snout) – the largest of the gaggle, **Glas Leac**, **Eilean Riabhach** (G. – grizzled island), and **Eilean Garbh** (G. – rough island).

Lochs Laxford and Dùghaill, between Handa Island and Kinlochbervie also have their share of 'wee ones.' **Eilean Ard** (G. – high island) is the largest. And there are also **Eilean a' Mhadaidh** (G. – isle of the dog), the inevitable **Eileanan Dubha**, **Eilean an Sithein** (G. – isle of the fairy mound), Eilean Meall a' Chaorainn (G. – island hillock of the rowan tree) and **Eilean Port a' Choit** (G. – isle of the small boat harbour) beside Weaver's Bay.

Loch a' Chadh-Fin which opens off Loch Laxford, and which is the magnificent setting for John Ridgeway's adventure school, has **Eilean an Eireannaich** at the entrance and **Eilean a' Chadh-fi** in the centre.

At Loch Clash by Kinlochbervie, barren **Eilean a' Chonnaidh** (G. – island of the faggot of firewood) has a thought-provoking name. Could this have referred to driftwood or was there a shipwreck there in some bygone age? About one and a half miles away two islands **Eilean an Ròin Mór** and **Beag** (G. – large and small seal island) are linked together with only a narrow channel separating them from the mainland. From the sea they look like a peninsula and as with so many of the islets in this part of the world, they have little vegetation and the rock faces are worn into smooth, rounded shapes.

With the exception of one tiny group of rocks a mile off the remote and beautiful Sandwood Beach, the biggest descriptively named **Am Balg** (G. – the belly), the coast is now devoid of islands all the way to wild Cape Wrath (ON *hvarf* – turning point).

Cape Wrath itself is a Ministry of Defence base which is full of activity in the summer months. Apart from firing practice and testing of explosives, tourists at Durness take great interest in the air-launched missiles and bombing runs which use tiny **Garvie Island** (G *An Garbh-eilean* – the rough island) midway between Cape Wrath and Faraid Head as the target.

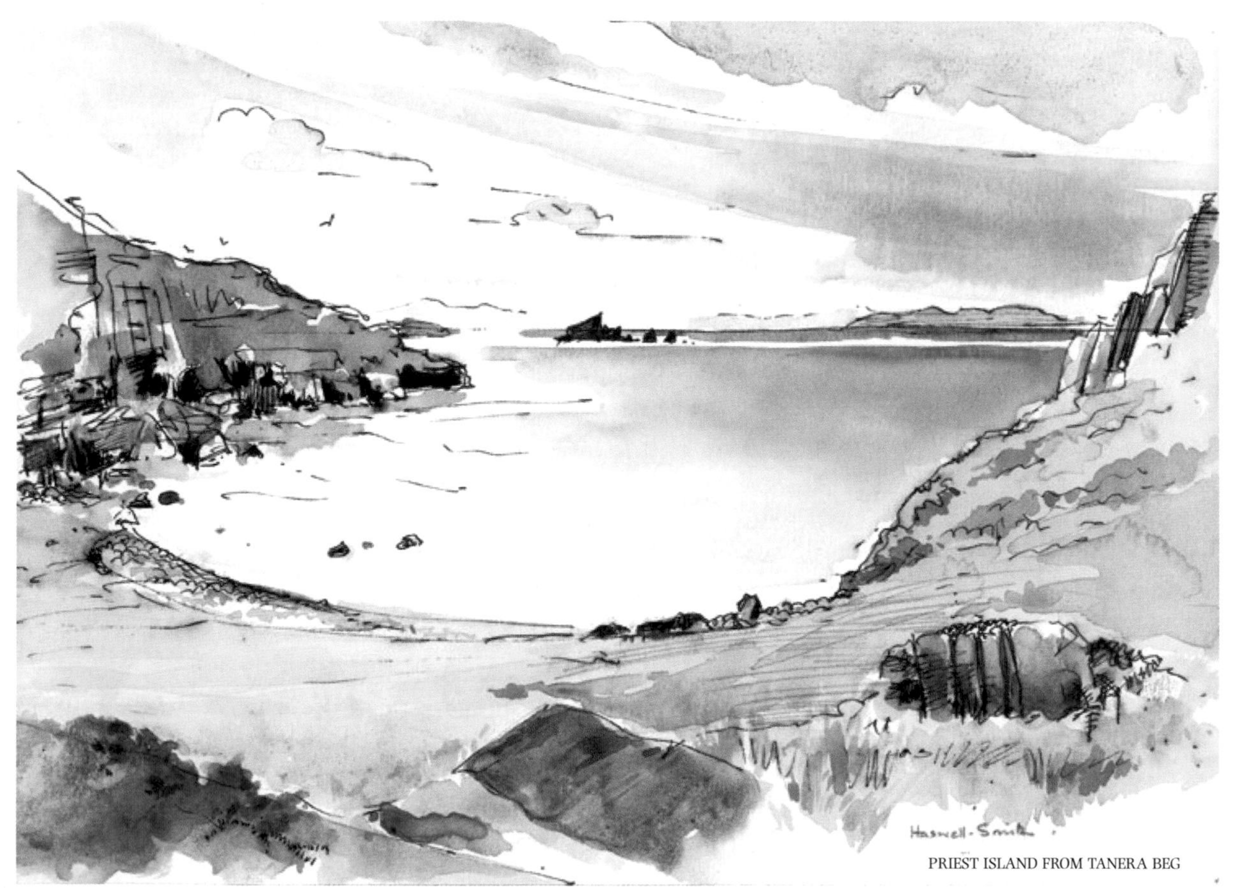

PRIEST ISLAND FROM TANERA BEG

6.1 Longa

(G. long, ON -øy – ship island).

O S Maps: 1:50000 Sheet 19 1:25000 Sheet 434
Admiralty Charts: 1:50000 No.2210 1:15000 No.2528

Area: 126ha (311 acres)
Height: 70m (230 ft)

Owner: William and Moira Cameron of Big Sands.

Population: 1841–35 (6 houses) 1881–0. Uninhabited since then.

Geology: Mainly sandstone.

Wildlife: Many otter familes.

LONGA is covered with grass and heather and attains a height of 70m at **Druim an Eilein** (G. – the island ridge). The west side, which has its own mini-peak called Carr Mór (G. – the big pap) and inlet, Camas nam Faochag (G. – bay of the whirlpools), is almost divided from the rest by a low neck of land between two bays. The north bay, **Camas na Rainich** (G. – bracken bay), has a small sandy beach backed by a bracken-covered slope. It is the favourite place to anchor provided the wind is not in the north. The south bay, which is rockier, is called **Eag Mhór** (G. – the big notch). Longa is separated from the beach and village of Big Sand on the mainland by Caolas Beag (G. – little channel).

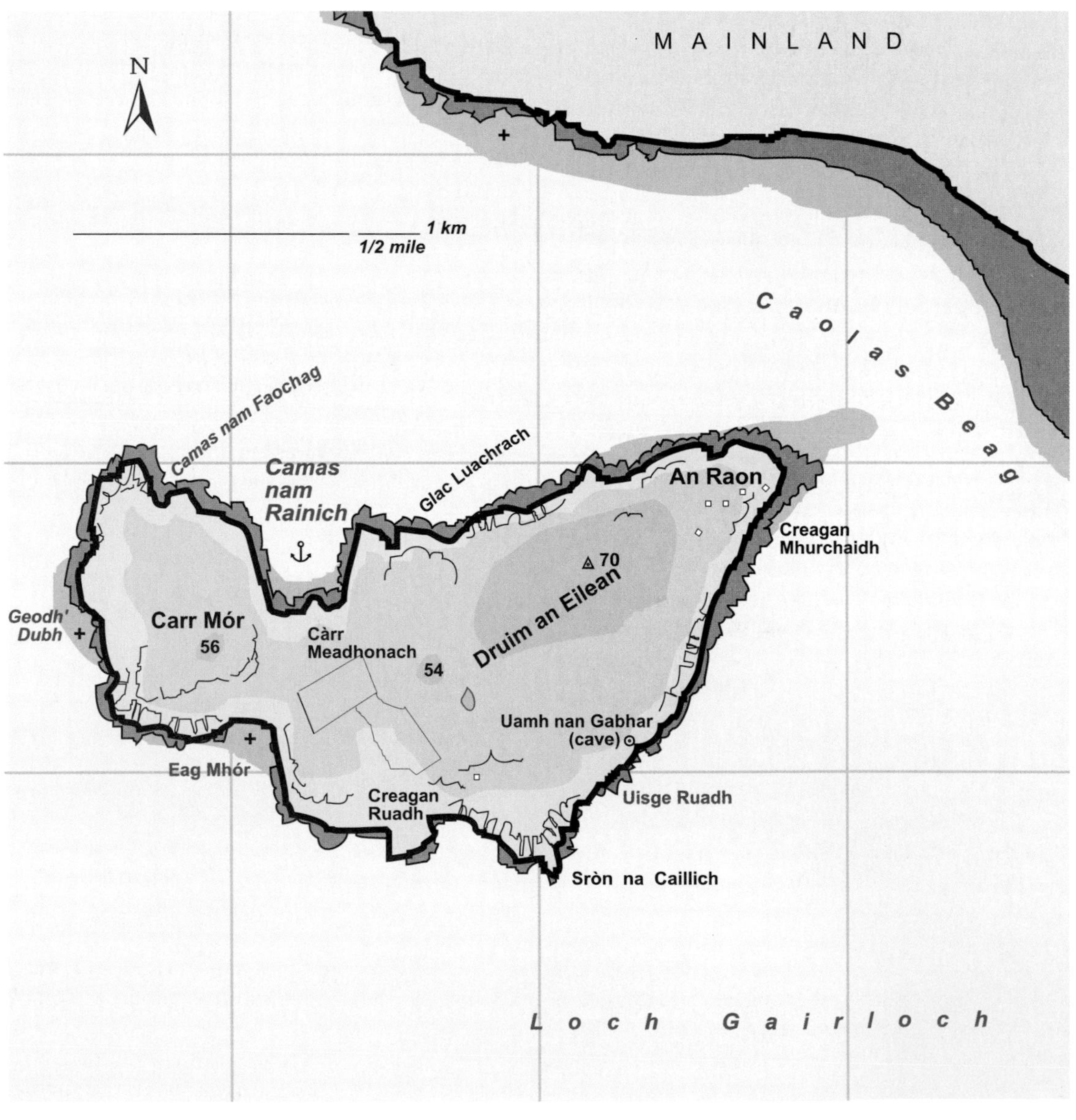

There is one tiny lochan almost in the centre of the island and directly south of it a rocky promontory with a hooked silhouette descriptively called **Sròn na Caillich** (G. – the old woman's nose). Further along the coast is Uamh nan Gabhar (G. – cave of the nanny-goats).

On the south side of Loch Gairloch and opposite Longa the small and crowded harbour of Badachro is sheltered by **Eilean Horrisdale**. Although unkempt with wild irises and bracken, the centrally-situated owner's house creates the impression from a distance that the island is an informal private garden. This tiny islet, less than one-third the area of Longa, supported twenty-seven people in four houses in 1841 and the population had risen to thirty-one islanders in five houses by the end of the 19th century. This was surely overcrowding, but they would be fishing folk so the area of land would be of little consequence.

Glas Eilean is a useful sea-mark when sailing up the loch to the pier by Charlestown and **Fraoch-eilean** (G. – heather isle) marks the entrance to Gairloch's Loch Shieldaig, which is a pleasant anchorage when you want to avoid being crushed by fishing boats at the pier.

* * *

Access: Try Gairloch Cruises, 01445-712636 or Hebridean Whale Cruises, Gairloch, 01445-712458.

Anchorages: The W coast of the island is foul for about ¾c off-shore and a reef fringes the island. Note that the mainland shore dries for 2c at Caolas Beag and there is a fairly shallow spit NE of the island.

1. Occasional anchorage in centre of bay on N coast, 5–8m, sand.

6.2 Isle of Ewe

Island of Loch Ewe. (EI eo – yew tree) but Watson thinks (G. eubh – echo) from place-name on adjoining mainland.

O S Maps: 1:50000 Sheet 19 1:25000 Sheet 434
Admiralty Charts: 1:100000 No.1794 1:12500 No.3146

Area: 309ha (764 acres)
Height: 72m (236 ft)

Owner: J I H Macdonald-Buchanan and leased to the two families of Grant. The Grant family have lived on the Isle of Ewe since the middle of the 19th century.

Population: 1841–34. 1881–43. 1891–39. 1931–37. 1961–10. 1981–11. 1991–12. 2001–12.

Geology: Torridonian sandstone with acidic soil in the north and a more fertile soil on New Red Sandstone (Permian or Triassic) in the south.

History: Loch Ewe was an important naval anchorage during the Second World War and is occasionally still a scene of NATO activity.

Wildlife: Dean Munro recorded in 1549 that the island was wooded. Nowadays, most of the island is a working farm with the type of flora and fauna to be expected in such an environment but a visit to Loch Ewe provides the added bonus of access to the world-famous Inverewe Gardens – more than 2000 acres of magnificent landscaping and plant life now under the care of the National Trust for Scotland. Loch Ewe may be remote and at the same latitude as Hudson Bay or Siberia but these Gardens are visited every year by more than 100,000 people who revel in their subtropical splendour.

* * *

The **ISLE OF EWE** looks steep and rocky when approaching by sea from the north but from Aultbea (G. – the birch-lined stream), the nearby village on the mainland, it can be seen that much of the island is gently undulating farmland. The highest point (72m) is in the north-west above a cliff, **Creag Streap** (G. – climbing cliff), which has a large rock, Sgeir a' Bhuich (G. – rock of the roe-buck), in the sea below. North of it is Uamhag nan Gobhar (G. – rock shelters of the goats). The high ground (68m) on the north-east peninsula is called **Sitheanan Dubha** (G. – the black fairy hillocks) and the soil here is peaty with a thick cover of coarse grass, heather and sphagnum moss.

The anchorage at **Camas Angus** is echoed by a bay on the opposite side of the island, **Camas Beithe** (G. – birch-tree bay). A hummock between the bays called **Cnoc na Gaoithe** (G. – windy knoll) shelters the anchorage from the prevailing wind.

A small copse of trees on **Druim nam Freumh** (G. – ridge of roots) defines the northern limit of the arable land.

The Families: Roddy Grant is a fisherman. He was born on the island and his family has lived

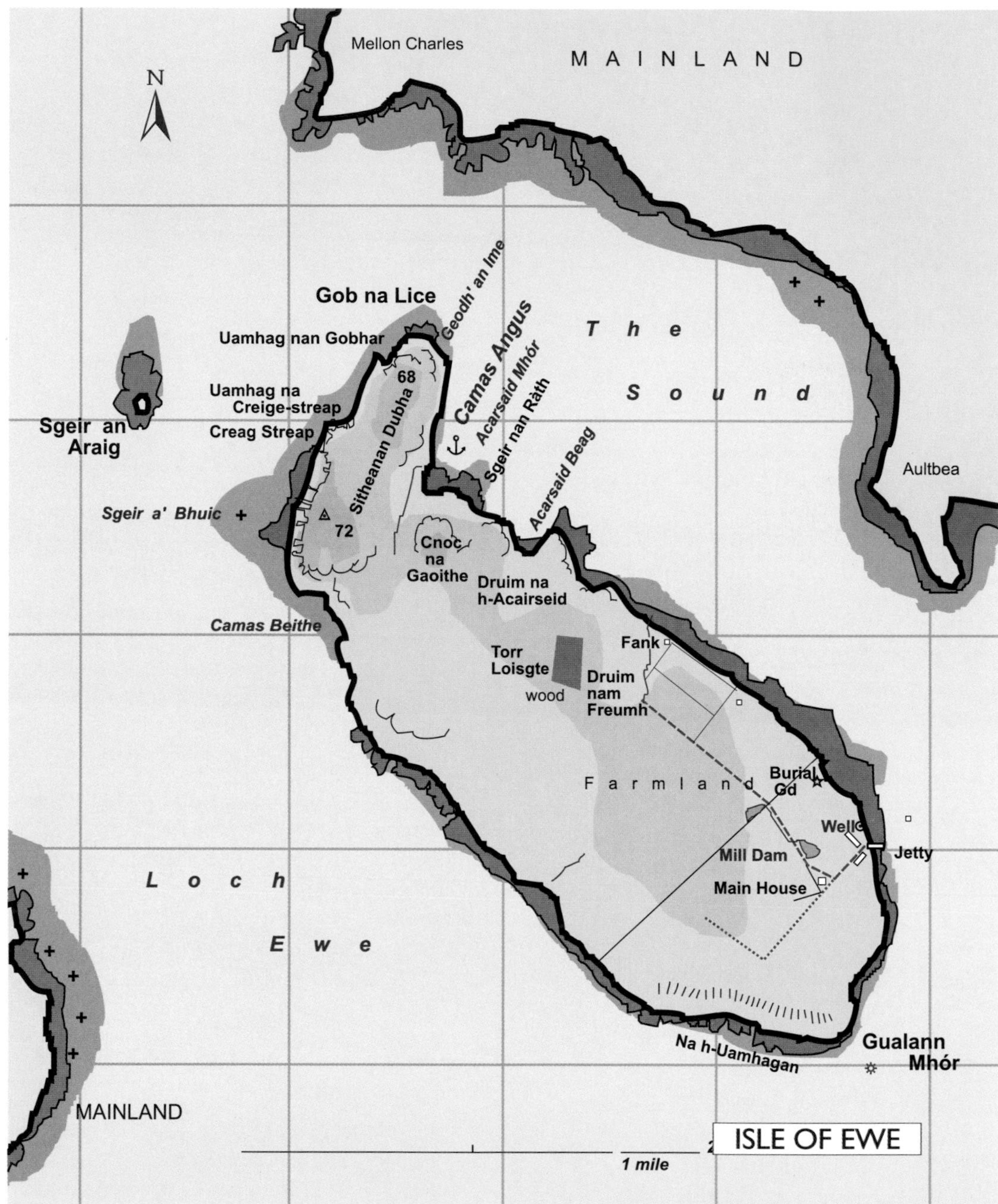

here since the middle of the 19th century. He is married to Marion and their life revolves round work, family and church. Their two children enjoyed a carefree childhood. Neil, the elder, was born in 1987.

Roddy's cousin Willie is married to Jane, a Somerset girl who met him when she was a ship's engineer in the Merchant Navy. For ten years they sailed the world together but now Willie farms the island croft. Jane built a landing stage, helped Willie build their house, and cared for their children when they were young – but she would probably have preferred to strip diesels instead. She dives for scallops as recreation.

There were more families living on the island in the past but they left during the Second World War.

Schooling for the children meant sailing across to the mainland each day followed by a thirteen-mile bus trip; and the same return journey each evening. The education authority wanted the children to board at school but both mothers insisted that island life was an essential part of their education in spite of the difficulties of daily transport. There is no doubt that children given a mainland education will rarely settle for island life when they are adults.

There is a direct telephone link to the island. Its installation was agreed by British Telecom before the company realised that the connection had to cross the sea and would cost a fortune! (That, of course, was long before the advent of mobile phones.)

Access: Enquire at Aultbea or try Creag Ard Charters, Ullapool, 01854-633380. Ullapool Tourist Information, 08452-255121.

Anchorages:
1. Camas Angus (Acarsaid Mhór), in NE, 3c S of N extremity. Beware unlit buoys, and partly submerged reef to SE. Good shelter in W'lies.
2. The Sound. Off the island's SE jetty in 7m or more, good holding but exposed.
3. Acarsaid Beag, 2c SE of Acarsaid Mhór. Poor holding on kelp.

6.3 Gruinard Island

(ON groenn fjordr – green firth) island.

O S Maps: 1:50000 Sheet 19 1:25000 Sheet 435
Admiralty Charts: 1:100000 No.1794 1:25000 Nos.2500 or 2509

Area: 196ha (484 acres)
Height: 106m (348 ft)

Owner: Bought by the Government in 1947 for £500 from the Eilean Darach estate and resold to them for the same sum in 1993 (N & M Scobie, Highland Coastal Trading Co.).

Population: 1881–6. 1891–0. Uninhabited since the 1920s.

Geology: Mainly Torridonian sandstone with laminated shales and micaceous sandstone in the north-east.

History: Gruinard Island has a notorious recent history.

In 1941, during the Second World War, some scientists decided to use this 'useless' uninhabited Scottish island as a test ground for biological warfare and bombed sixty penned sheep with anthrax spores. The sheep duly died and their bodies were buried in a cave on the island under tons of rock. Even so, one of the carcasses floated over to the mainland and infected some livestock but, as there was a war on, the affair was quickly hushed up and the owners compensated.

As there was no satisfactory antidote known at the time, anthrax was rather a foolhardy choice, but it was suspected that the Germans were carrying out similar experiments. Anthrax is a particularly deadly and indestructible bacillus. Even forty years after it was sprayed over Gruinard, up to 385 viable spores per gram of soil were found when the Chemical Defence Establishment carried out one of its periodic tests. In 1986, after many protests from environmentalists, the Ministry of Defence decided to disinfect the island by soaking the entire surface area in formaldehyde and sea-water. Sheep and rabbits were then introduced to test whether the result was satisfactory.

In April 1990 Gruinard Island was declared free of anthrax. It was opened to press and public and returned to its pre-war owners with a 150 year Government indemnity. However Dr Brian Moffat, an archaeologist involved in the investigation of a medieval hospital at Soutra, claimed in a radio broadcast that anthrax spores had survived for 500 years on that particular site. Vegetation he claimed brings them up to the surface of the soil and certainly nothing on earth would persuade him to risk landing on Gruinard! The Ministry of Defence replied that this was an unfair comparison. Soil samples had shown that the island was clear of danger although no one could say there may not still be a few spores around; the sheep were fit and healthy and so were the wild rabbits.

Wildlife: In 1549 Dean Munro recorded that the island was wooded. The peak sea-bird season in Gruinard Bay is October to May. This is a prime area to see the great northern diver.

* * *

GRUINARD ISLAND rises gently to a rough rounded summit (106m) which is called simply **An Eilid** (G. – the hind). The island is covered with rough grazing – grass, heather and bracken and fringed by a rocky shore and occasional pebbly beach.

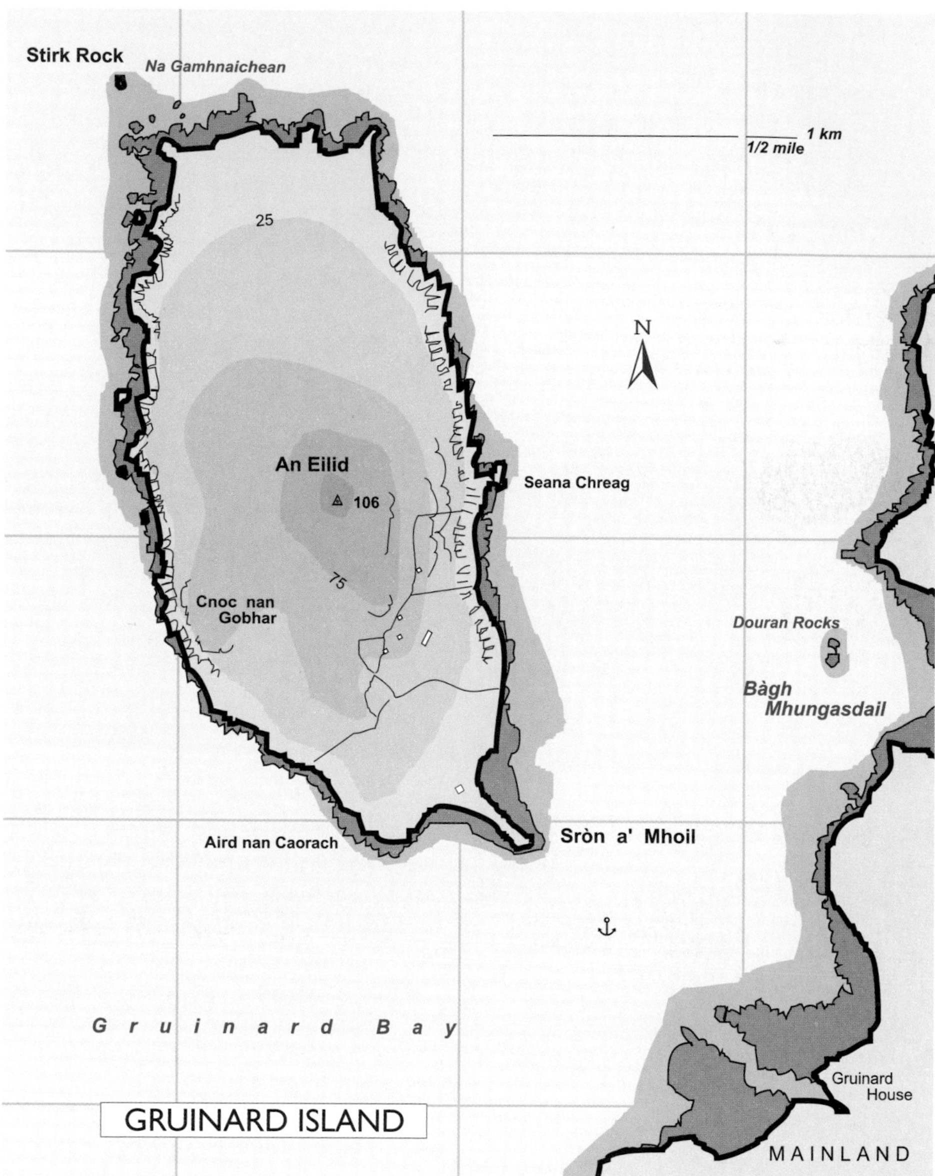

One good result of the Microbiological Research Establishment's unfortunate experiment on Gruinard was the development of an effective vaccine against anthrax for both animals and humans. But it is a pity that animals had to be introduced so quickly after the clean-up, as it would have been an excellent opportunity for botanists (wearing suitable clothing, of course!) to study the effect of forty-five years of sheep- and rabbit-free existence.

For the committed island-hopper keeping below the high-water mark should present no danger. Going above it is a matter of personal choice!

It is probable that historically the island has always provided useful pasturage, the flocks and herds being swum across the narrow kyle to a point near Gruinard House on the mainland. Certainly the headland beside the long spit at the southern extremity is called **Aird nan Caorach** (G. – sheep or livestock point).

Access: Try Creag Ard Charters, Ullapool, 01854-633380.

Anchorages: Reefs extend up to 1c off the island at places and the bottom is generally rocky. There are no regular anchorages but there are moderate depths SE and E of the island with some mud and sand.

6.4 Isle Martin

Named after Saint Martin to whom the island chapel was dedicated.

OS Maps: 1:50000 Sheet 19 1:25000 Sheet 439
Admiralty Charts: 1:100000 No.1794 1:25000 No.2500

Area: 157ha (388 acres)
Height: 120m (394 ft)

Owner: In 1965 Mrs Monica Goldsmith bought Isle Martin. She presented it to the RSPB in 1981, having carefully renovated four houses. In May 1999 the RSPB, in turn, gave it in trust to the community of Lochbroom and Ullapool (after, unfortunately, letting the houses fall into disrepair).

Population: 1841–45. 1881–42. 1891–47 (8 houses). In 1901–33. 1931–3. 1961–0. 1971–0. 1981–1. 1991–1. 2001–0. Occasional summer occupation of one house.

Geology: The island is a rounded hill of Torridonian sandstone.

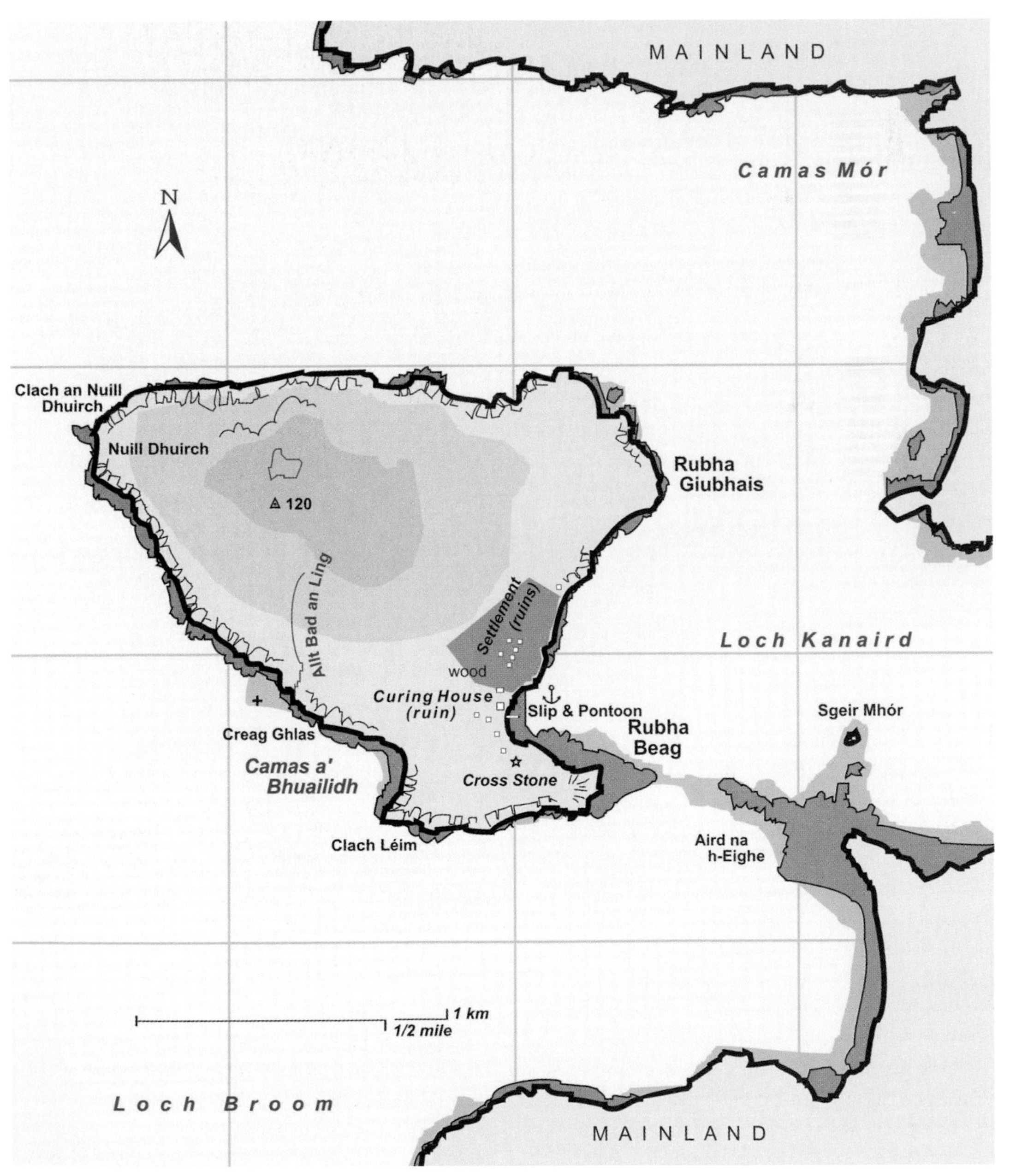

History: In 1775 the British Fisheries Society built a curing station which prospered until the industry collapsed in 1813. In the 1930s, as the last islanders had left, the owner, Commander C G Vyner created employment by converting the ruined building into a flour mill and a school hut was built. Several families returned. But by 1949 the mill was losing money, the islanders moved elsewhere and the school closed. Vyner decided to build a causeway to the mainland to encourage repopulation of the island but planning permission was refused and, as he was being charged rates for the empty mill, he dynamited it in 1952.

Wildlife: Bird sanctuary.

Peak viewing November to May for wintering divers and gulls, especially Glaucous and Iceland. Otherwise, of particular interest are the red-breasted merganser, oystercatcher, ringed plover, heron, tern and eider. Corncrakes can be heard in June.

Two ecology graduates from Edinburgh University ran a tree nursery at Scourie (near Handa. No.6.9) and between 1982 and 1998, under the auspices of the RSPB, they reintroduced native trees to Isle Martin – willow, oak, ash, hazel, rowan and pine. This has already created a young forest which has its own micro-climate and is a larder for native wildlife. They have, in fact, turned the clock back to the island's traditional landscape before it was denuded of trees many centuries ago.

* * *

Close to, but separate from, the Summer Isles group, **ISLE MARTIN** lies beside the entrance to Loch Broom. From the sea it often merges with the background hills. It consists of a single rounded hill 120m high with rocky cliffs on the west and north coasts. The slope is gentle on the sheltered east side where there is a small bay. It is here that the restored houses and the remains of the old fish-curing station [NH096990] can be found but the scant remains of St Martin's chapel are further west. A fairly large settlement of ruined houses lies among the trees and beautifully constructed dry-stane dykes cross the hillside above the bay. The small valley on the west coast is called **Bad an Ling** (G. & ON – tuft of heather).

The British Fisheries Society, with ample funds from the south, built the port of Ullapool in 1788, and several curing stations on key island sites such as Isle Martin. This was to take advantage of the vast herring shoals for which Loch Broom was renowned. These swept into the loch between the months of May and September every year. For hundreds of years the local boats had enjoyed a bonanza as the shoals were so dense that it was possible to scoop the fish out of the sea by hand. The Society curtailed the activities of the local boats, and netted fish for themselves in vast quantities. The boom lasted for fifty years and then this depredation took effect. By 1830 the shoals had thinned and by 1880 they had disappeared. They have never recovered. The curing stations were abandoned and the local fishermen were left to search for alternative catches.

Isle Martin has its local legend. According to this a cooper once worked for the fish curing station and was ordered to cut brooms one evening. The little people took pity on him and miraculously transported him to the woodland on South Rona (No.5.9). In the morning he was back at work with all the brooms that were required.

Access: Landing is permitted by the Isle Martin Trust (01854-612937) but voluntary donations would be appreciated. For the Trust's island ferry contact Ullapool Tourist Information, 01854-612135.

Anchorage:

1. Good anchorage E of island in Loch Kanaird. Anchor N side of bight, bottom gravel and stones, or use the Trust pontoon (pay), 2.7m depth at MLWS.

6.5 Priest Island

(G. Eilean a' Chléirich – island of the Priest or Cleric)

O S Maps: 1:50000 Sheet 15 1:25000 Sheet 439
Admiralty Charts: 1:100000 No.1794 1:25000 No.2509

Area: 122ha (301 acres)
Height: 78m (256 ft)

Owner: Royal Society for the Protection of Birds.

Population: No Census records and uninhabited.

Geology: The island consists of two main masses of Torridonian sandstone cut by a glen running from south-west to north-east. The southern mass is a ridge in which the strata have tilted to form rugged cliffs of fluted columns facing the glen to the north. The southern slope is less steep. The sandstone is smoother and redder than that on the mainland.

History: Three prehistoric stone circles are proof of early human interest and the name shows that this was a retreat or hermitage in the early Christian era, possibly associated with the monastery on Isle Martin (No.6.4). In the 18th century an outlaw banished from the mainland settled here and founded three generations of crofters but his descendants abandoned the island in the 1850s.

Dr Frank Fraser Darling stayed here during the late 1930s and wrote about it in his book, *Island Years*.

Wildlife: Heather is dominant south of the glen, but in the north and west apart from erica and calluna there are plantain and thrift, bog asphodel, bog cotton, crowberry, sheep's fescue and buckthorn.

Aspen, poplar, royal fern, honeysuckle, willow and the inevitable flag irises are widespread around Lochan Fada.

As with all the Summer Isles there are many birds. Shelduck, fulmar, heron, snipe and eider are common and merganser breed along the banks. Twenty-nine species of bird are known to breed here, the most notable being greylag geese and storm petrel, but according to Fraser Darling, forty-three species of bird which breed on Tanera Mór (No.6.7) do not breed on Priest Island – probably due to the wind.

Grey seal, pigmy shrew (to be found near the caves in the south according to Fraser Darling) and otter can all be seen. In particular the two lochans in the main glen are much frequented by otters. All the eight lochans are reputed to have excellent fishing.

* * *

The most westerly of the Summer Isles, 4 miles or 7km south-west of Tanera Mór, **PRIEST ISLAND** has no proper landing place and with its exposed position and a persistent heavy swell getting ashore at its one and only 'anchorage', a bay in the centre of the east coast, can be difficult. Getting off again can be harder still! The alternative landing places depend on wind direction but none is comfortable or easy.

Approaching from due south the island appears to be smooth-topped with two summits near its east end, but from elsewhere its outline is rugged. As there are several small lochs providing a plentiful water supply this could account for the fact that in spite of its inaccessibility it has been inhabited off and on since pre-history.

The highest point (78m) is south of the anchorage at **Moll na h-Uamh** (G. – cave point). This particular cave [NB930017] is on the south-east coast below the ridge and is the

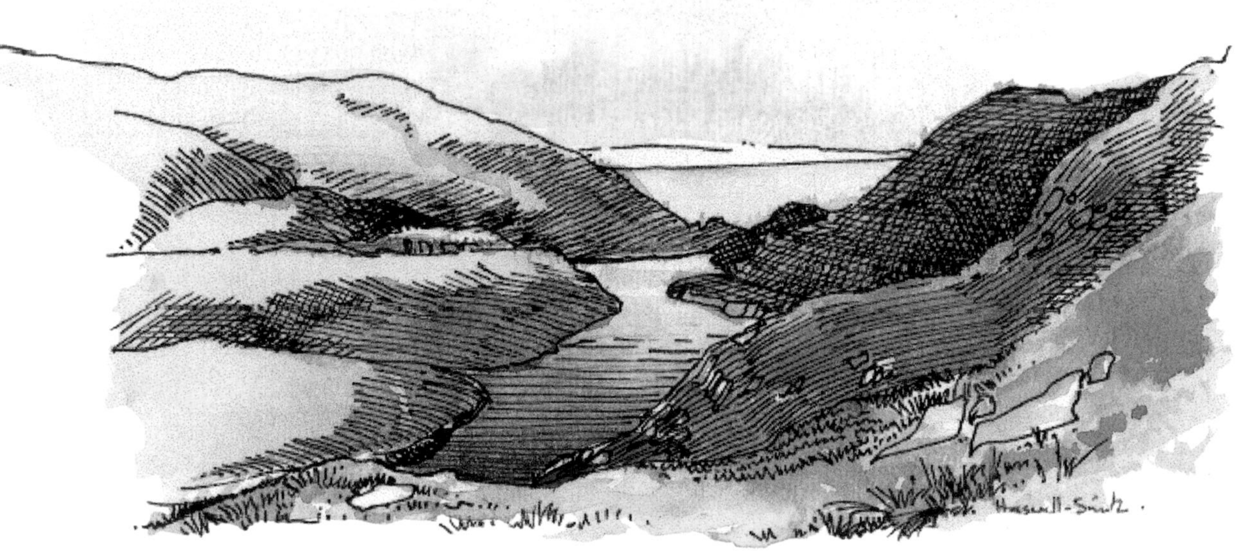

LOCH FADA ON EILEAN A' CHLÉIRICH

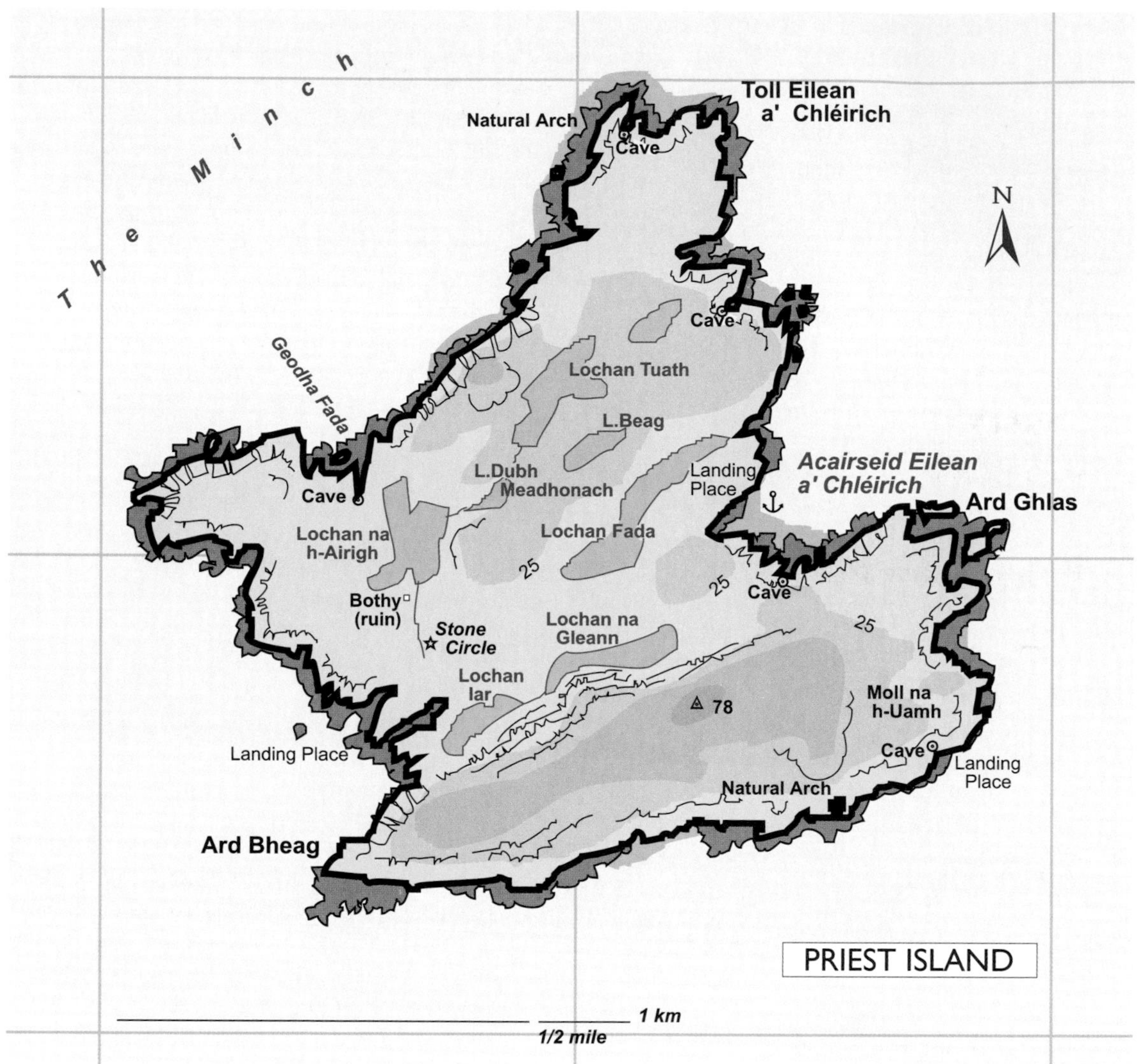

one in which Fraser Darling dug up bones of pig, ox, deer, guillemot and fulmar petrel. Further interesting and fairly deep caves are to the north of the anchorage. One, at a little boulder beach, has signs of human habitation and was probably used by smugglers [NB927026]. Part of a whisky still was found near **Lochan na h-Airigh** (G. – shieling loch). The sea booms eerily as it enters **Toll Eilean a' Chléirich** (G. – Priest's Hole) in the north-east corner – a sea-cave with a fallen roof [NB927029].

The main glen runs right across the island from the anchorage to the west coast and contains two lochans. To the north of the glen there is a tumbled landscape with more lochans, several pools and patches of bog ending abruptly at the steep cliffs and fissures of the north-west coast.

Evidence of an ancient chapel has been uncovered on level ground on the south side of Lochan na h-Airigh [NB920021] which is also the site of the 19th-century ruined bothy. The ground here has been cultivated in the past. A prehistoric stone circle is beside the burn which flows out of the loch. This was originally on the west side of the burn but the Victorian yachtsman and naturalist, Harvie-Brown, found after several visits that it had sunk into the boggy ground and disappeared so he dug it up and transferred it to the dry ground on the other side of the burn!

Between Priest Island and Tanera Beg is the small island (11ha) of **Glas-leac Beag** (G. – little green slab). It is, as described, narrow and flat-topped, about 29m high, and on a fine day its covering of grass, gloriously fertilised by a colony of black-backed gulls, makes it appear bright green.

Access: Landing is prohibited without prior permission from the RSPB, 0131-311 6500. Summer Isles Cruises, Achiltibuie, 01854-622200 or Creag Ard Charters, Dundonnell, 01854-633380. Achiltibuie Tourist Information, 01854-622200.

Anchorages: All are subject to considerable swell.
1. Acairseid Eilean a' Chléirich, bay on E side. Occasional anchorage in settled weather, clean but bottom mainly boulders. Landing best on or near 'pier rock' on NW side of bay.
2. Landing point at cleft in bay on W side of island. Temp. anchorage possible in settled weather ½c off-shore in 15–20m.
3. Landing point at cave on SE side of island. Temp. anchorage possible in settled weather in 15–18m.

6.6 Horse Island

O S Maps: 1:50000 Sheet 15 1:25000 Sheet 439
Admiralty Charts: 1:100000 No.1794 1:25000 No.2501

Area: 53ha (131 acres)
Height: 60m (197 ft)

Population: Uninhabited and without Census records but is reputed to have been inhabited in the 19th century.

Geology: Torridonian sandstone.

History: Treasure from a ship of the Spanish Armada is said to have been hidden here in 1588. The story is reinforced by a local record that a shepherd in the 19th century found a gold doubloon in his boot-top after stumbling in the heather. He rushed to the mainland and told his friends, who immediately organised a treasure hunt but when they were on the island they could find nothing. One piece of heather looks much like another and the shepherd then wondered if he had remembered the correct spot where he tripped. The dejected group returned empty-handed. Unlike so many local legends, the unsatisfactory ending makes this story ring true!

Wildlife: Multi-coloured lichens, thrift, sea campion, lovage and scurvy grass grow on the ledges of the cliffs.

Only wild goats inhabit Horse Island nowadays but no one is sure how they came to be on the island. The first official record of their presence was in 1837. But there seem to have been resident goats in earlier times as the drying islet at the north end is called Meall nan Gabhar (G. – hillock of the she-goats).

* * *

HORSE ISLAND is separated from the mainland by a deep channel called Horse Sound. The highest point (60m) is **Sgùrr nan Uan** (G. – conical hill of the lambs) – near the south-east coast. **Meall nan Gabhar** (13ha) is at the northern extremity and connected to the main part by a reef which dries at low water. The opposite hill on the main island is **Meall an Fhithich** (G. – raven's hill). **Iolla Mór** (G. – big drying rock), lying off the south coast, is a flat rock which is extensive at low water.

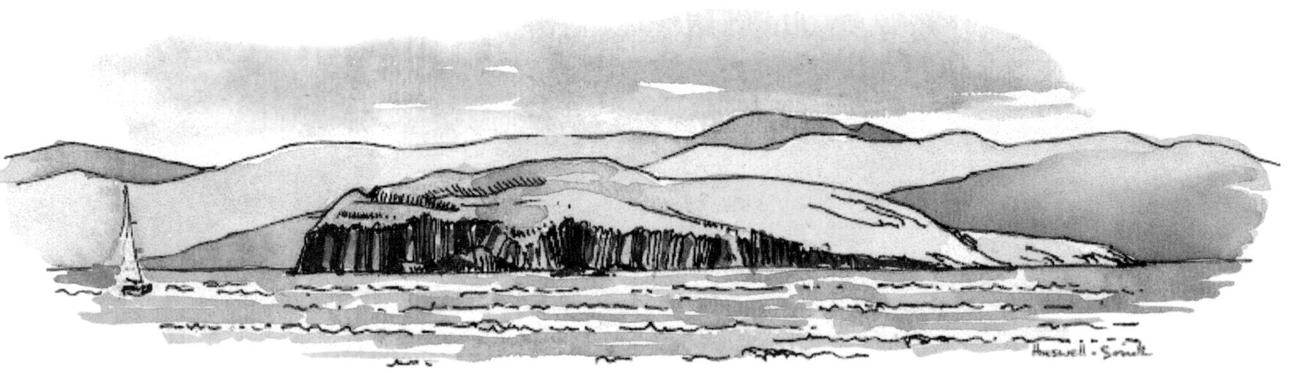

HORSE ISLAND FROM THE SOUTH WITH ACHILTIBUIE BEYOND

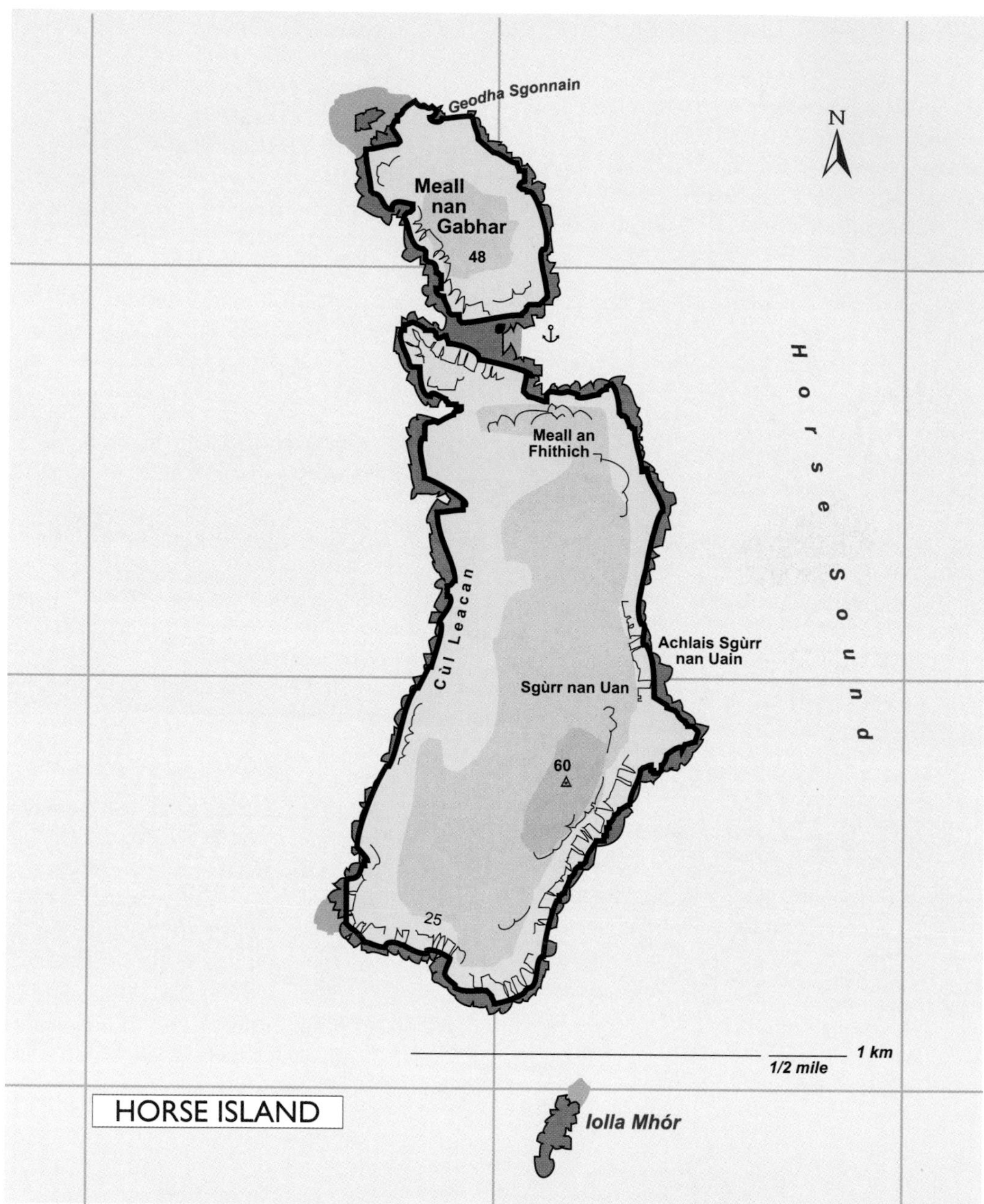

Similar plants to those on Horse Island are to be found on **Carn nan Sgeir** – two small islands separated by a shingle spit which lie to the south but, unlike the rest of the Summer Isles which are of Torridonian sandstone, these islets are of Hebridean gneiss.

It is natural that in this animal-farm region of horses and goats another nearby islet should be called **Meall nan Caorach** (G. – sheep hump).

Access: Summer Isles Cruises, Achiltibuie, 01854-622200, or Creag Ard Charters, Dundonnell, 01854-633380. Achiltibuie Tourist Information, 01854-622200.

Anchorage:

1. Good anchorage in bight SE of Meall nan Gabhar but keep in N half as there is an uncharted reef in the S half, 3m, sand and some weed. Exposed to E.

6.7 Tanera Mór

(ON hawnar-øy – island of the haven, pasture, G. – large) or (ON taren-øy – the kelp island).

OS Maps: 1:50000 Sheet 15 1:25000 Sheet 439
Admiralty Charts: 1:100000 No.1794 1:25000 No.2501

Area: 310ha (766 acres)
Height: 122m (400 ft)

Owner: Sold by Summer Isles Estate in 1991. Bought in 1996 by a family of Wiltshire farmers for about £700,000.

Population: 1745–21 families. 1841–99. 1881–119. 1891–95 (19 houses). 1901–70. The population had fallen to zero by 1931. 1961–6. 1971–2. 1981–8. 1991–0. 2001–5.

Geology: Torridonian sandstone mostly covered with peat, pasture and heather.

History: In 1784 Murdoch Morrison of

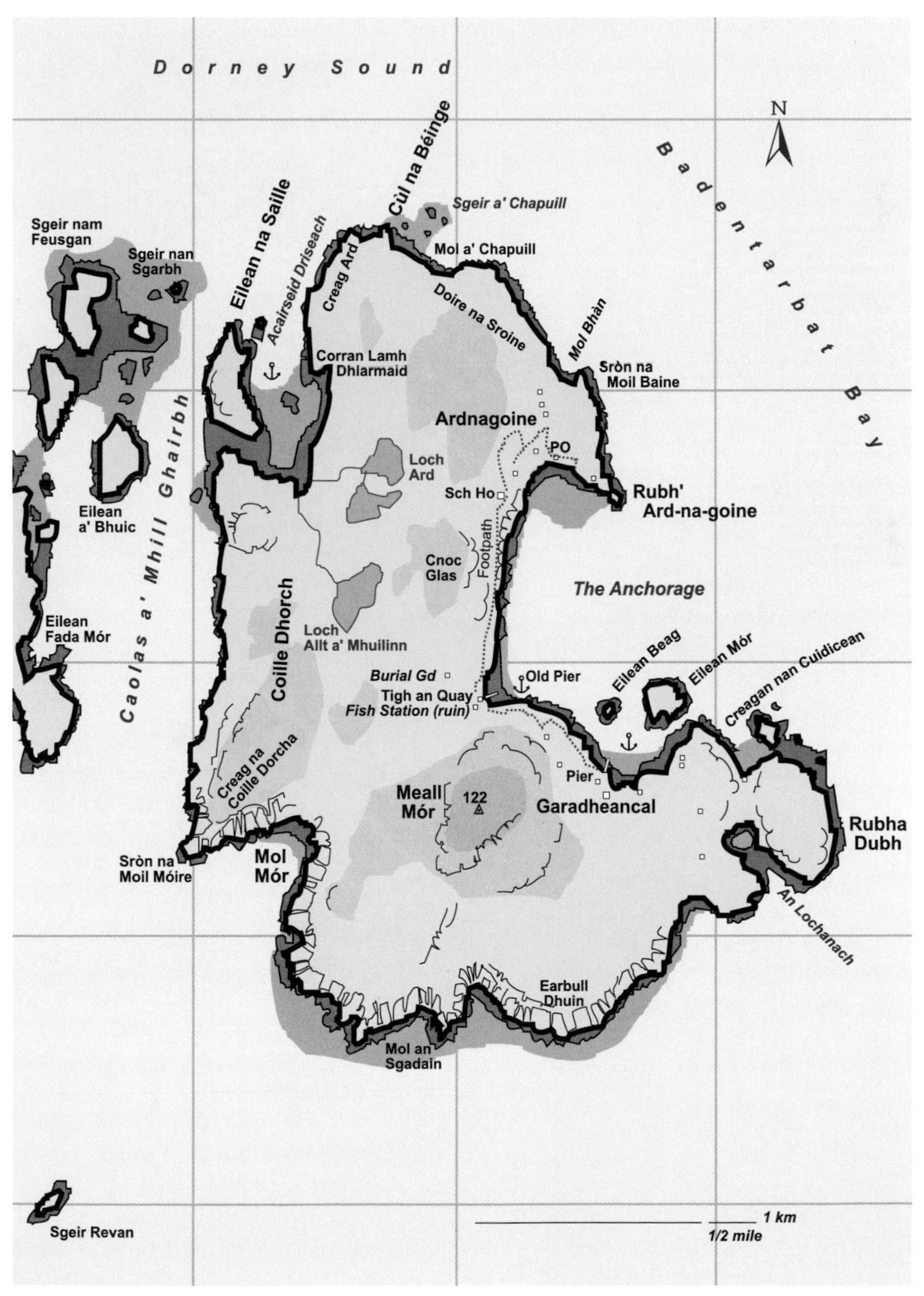

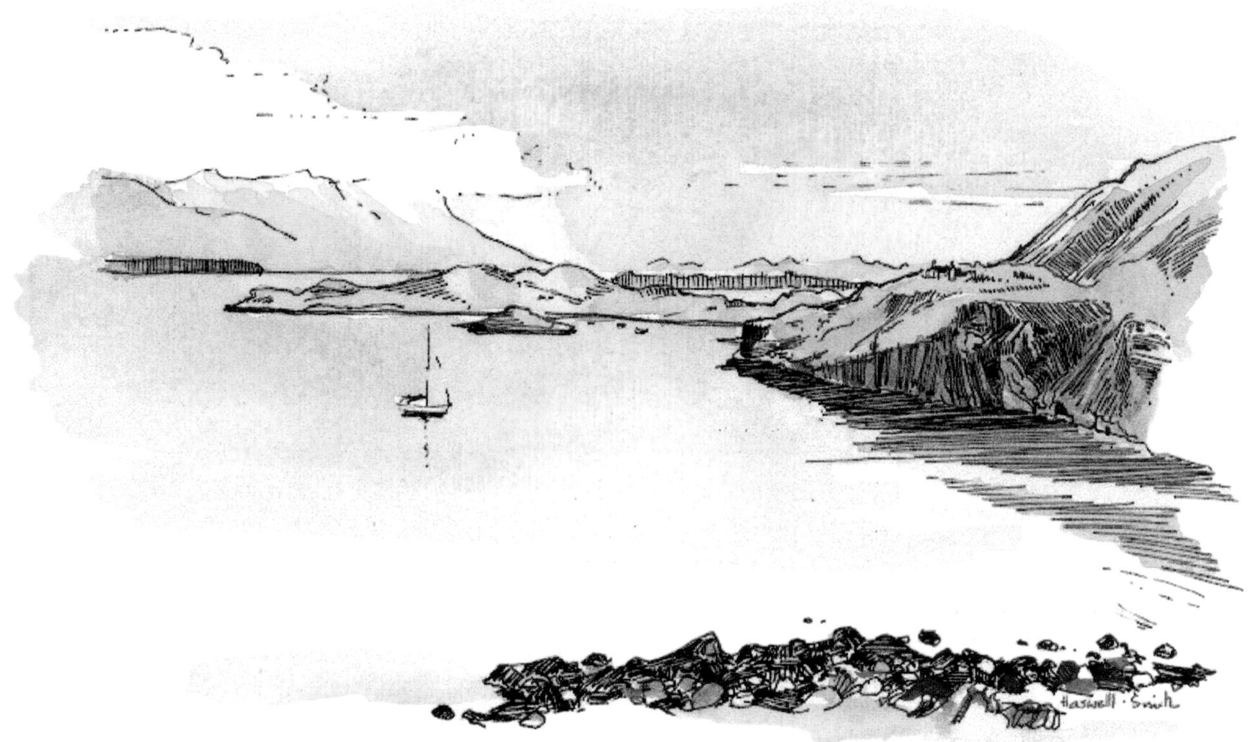

'THE CABBAGE PATCH' BEYOND THE ANCHORAGE

Stornoway was installed as manager of the newly founded fishing station at Tigh-an-Quay (between Ardnagoine and Garadheancal). As with the stations on Isle Martin (No.6.4) and Isle Ristol, this was built by the London-based British Fishery Society. It was a very prosperous enterprise while the herring stocks lasted. Up to 200 vessels at a time would anchor in the bay and salted herring was even exported to the West Indian colonies.

After the fishing spree was over in 1820, and the company was bankrupted, there followed a period of many changes of ownership and greedy tacksmen demanding high rents. So the resourceful islanders took up the distillation of illicit whisky. In 1900 another lucrative sideline was introduced when the island was acquired by Captain MacDonald, a local smuggler. There is a rumour that a cargo of rum was buried at Tigh-an-Quay and another story of buried treasure in the 'big park' between Tigh-an-Quay and Mol Mór.

Wildlife: The climate is mild and there are wild flowers everywhere – heather galore, common orchids, forget-me-not, foxgloves, dandelions, clover and burnet rose. Near An Lochanich there are flag irises, honeysuckle, willow and aspen poplars which grow to 3–4m in height. Bluebells and primroses are sheltered by rowan and birch which grow on the slopes. Unlike Priest Island (No.6.5) the lochs here are almost lifeless except for tadpoles.

Gulls and arctic terns are common but few other sea-birds are to be seen. There is, however, a wide variety of general birdlife including breeding heron, shelduck, buzzard and red grouse.

* * *

TANERA MOR is the largest of the Summer Isles, a small group of a dozen or so islands lying close to the mainland which were used for summer grazing. The highest hill, **Meall Mór**, (122m) has a flat summit when viewed from the south and below it is one of the best natural harbours in the north-west. It is known as **The Anchorage** and was a great favourite with the Vikings but they would not recognise it today as it is now usually packed with fish-farming cages.

The last permanent inhabitants left in 1931 but from 1938 to 1944, Frank Fraser Darling, the naturalist, farmed on the island and wrote his book *Island Farm*. There followed another period when the island was uninhabited and then in 1963 the new owners, Summer Isles Estate, restored and let many of the cottages and the schoolhouse as holiday accommodation and provided facilities for boating, sailing and fishing. (All the houses have drainage, water, and electricity and many are centrally heated.) This created the need for a small population to service the enterprise, and a few more connected with the fish-farm. Not only is there now a Summer Isles Post Office – situated in a tea room which opens when a boatload of tourists arrive – but it is officially permitted to issue its own postage stamps. These are most attractive and popular with collectors.

Rock shapes on the coasts of Tanera Mór and Tanera Beg can take on exquisite colours in the changing light. There are two tiny islands in The Anchorage – **Eilean Mór** and **Eilean Beag** – and a drying island, **Eilean na Saille** (G. – salt island), on the north-west coast sheltering **Acairseid Driseach** (G. – anchorage of thorns). Burns feed into this anchorage from three small lochs. In the south-west there is another cove, Mol Mór (G. – the big pebble-beach) while the north extremity of the island is called Cùl na Béinge (G. – the back of the bed-board or bench)

Between the two settlements, **Ardnagoine** and **Garadheancal** (G. – the cabbage-patch or kail-yard), are the remains of the herring fishing station at **Tigh-an-Quay**. The old building is now partly used for fish-farm storage purposes and also houses an electricity generator. Close north of it is a new house with a beautifully maintained garden – the work of an enthusiast – beside the level area above the quay known as the 'Planestones'.

When Fraser Darling first purchased Tigh-an-Quay the ruin was much more extensive. The northern part of the stone structure was a three-storey building with an attic and slate roof – part of which was still intact. An alleyway had divided this building from the fish factory on the south side but an arcaded wall between the alley and the factory had collapsed in the 1870s leaving an enclosed unroofed area with two gables still standing. He called it the 'Walled Garden', removed much of the rubble, and demolished the top of the gables which were in a dangerous state. He also demolished the roof and upper floor of the residential buiding as the timbers were rotten and the wind turned the slates into dangerous missiles. He rebuilt some of the lower walls and reconstructed the quay to its original design.

The walled field between Tigh-an-Quay and the hill to the north, **Cnoc Glas** (G. – green knoll), is called 'Little Irish Park' because much of the soil came from Ireland as ships' ballast. The large field west of Tigh-an-Quay is the 'Big Park' with a rocky hillock in it called Cnoc an-t-Sidhe (G. – fairy knoll). Using coral sand from Tanera Beag (lime), and seaweed and boiler slag (potash), Fraser Darling reinstated this field as productive arable land. Clover provided the nitrogen content.

* * *

Access: Annette McKay, Ullapool, 01854-612472. Summer Isle Cruises, Achiltibuie, 01854-622200. Ferry, Achiltibuie, 01854-622272. Ullapool Tourist Information, 01854-612135.

Anchorages:

1. The Cabbage Patch. Between, and S of, the two small islands on the S side of The Anchorage; best shelter and good holding but cluttered with moorings.
2. The Anchorage. Anchor between fish-cages and old pier in SW corner of bay, or between fish-cages and beach at N of bay.
3. Acairseid Driseach (at NW corner of Tanera Mór). Enter from N and anchor between Eilean na Saille and Tanera Mór, but not further S than mid-island, 4m sand.

6.8 Tanera Beg

(ON hawnar-øy – island of the haven, pasture, G. Beag – little) or (ON taren-øy – the kelp island).

OS Maps: 1:50000 Sheet 15 1:25000 Sheet 439
Admiralty Charts: 1:100000 No.1794 1:25000 No.2501

Area: 66ha (163 acres)
Height: 83m (272 ft)

Owner: (?) Summer Isles Estate.

Population: No Census records and uninhabited.

Geology: Torridonian sandstone, mostly covered with peat, pasture and heather. There is a bank of coral sand and on the shores unusual displays of pink coral can be seen at low water. Nearby Eilean Fada Mor which lies between Tanera Beg and Tanera Mór has similar coral.

Wildlife: Honeysuckle, irises, dwarf willow and aspen poplars flourish.

Merganser ducks breed along the water edge and gulls nest among the pink thrift on the shoreline rocks Wheatears and pipits frequent the heathland and many other mainland varieties thrive.

Seals breed here but not in any great number.

TANERA BEG is separated from Tanera Mór (No.6.7) by a fairly narrow but easily navigable channel, Caolas a' Mhill Ghairbh (G. – channel of broken pieces).

Its coastline is very irregular with delightful little pebble coves sheltered between low cliffs overhung by green terraces. Beneath the summit of the central hill (83m) is a tiny pool, the only one on the island, and from there the heather-clad slope runs down to a bluff above a shallow valley with a large cave at sea level.

Tanera Beg's main claim to fame must surely be its bank of fine coral sand – something which is quite uncommon in this part of the world. It lies close to the best anchorages in the corner

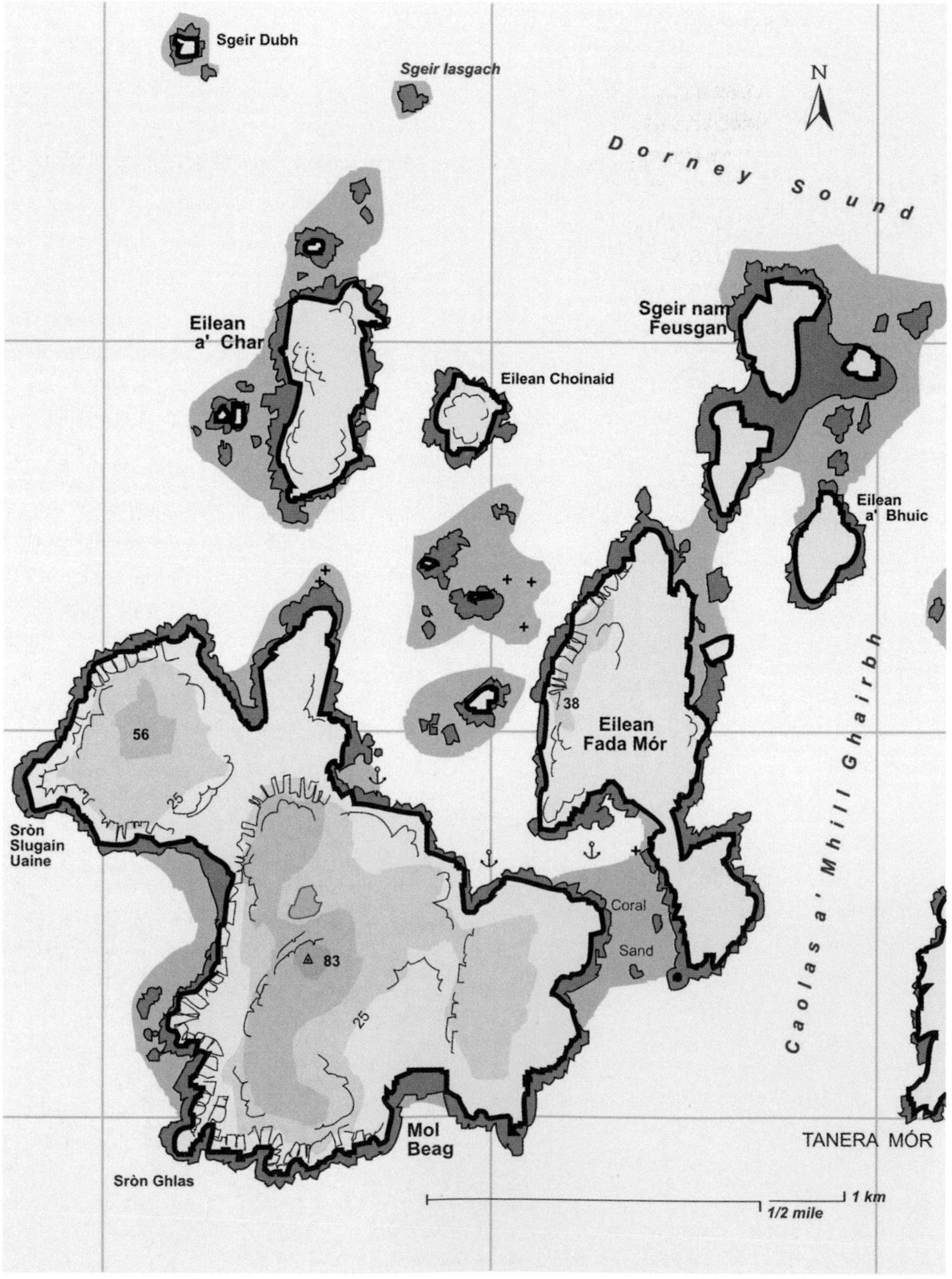

of the 'lagoon' but it is only visible at low water [NB972074]. Luckily it was not entirely destroyed by Fraser Darling (see No.6.7).

The anchorages to the north are protected by several islets and many rocks and skerries. **Eilean Fada Mór** (G. – big long island) hides little **Eilean a' Bhuic** (G. – buck island) behind it and the larger **Sgeir nam Feusgan** (G. – skerry of the mussels). And directly north is **Eilean a' Chàr** (G. – island of seal-flesh) and **Eilean Choinaid** (G. – rabbit island). **Glas-leac Mór** (G. – big green slab), a fair-sized islet to the north-west with heather slopes and a small lochan, is almost part of the same group.

About two miles south of Tanera Beg there is an island, **Eilean Dubh**, which only just fails to meet my 40-hectare minimum size limit. It has probably never been permanently inhabited and there is no safe anchorage but its American owners, Dr Van Arman and his wife, have built a substantial log house in the cove on the north-east side. Eilean Dubh is one of a group of islets and skerries. Two of these, **Carn Iar** (uninhabited, but which has the unlikely distinction of being allowed to produce its own postage stamps) and **Carn Deas** (G. – west and south rockpiles), are linked by drying rocks, and another islet has the suggestive name of **Bottle Island**.

* * *

Access: Summer Isles Cruises, Achiltibuie, 01854-622200, or Creag Ard Charters, Dundonnell, 01854-633380. Achiltibuie Tourist Information, 01854-622200.

Anchorages:

1. S side of Eilean Fada Mor. Good anchorage in bight, north of shoal, 4m, sand. Strong tide at springs.
2. Pool SW of Eilean Fada Mor. Anchor in 10m, sand.
3. Inlet in centre of NE side of Tanera Beg, 3m, sand. Beware reef of drying rocks N of the inlet.

6.9 Handa

(ON hund-øy – dog island) or (ON sand-øy – sand isle).

OS Maps: 1:50000 Sheet 9 1:25000 Sheet 445
Admiralty Charts: 1:100000 No.1785 1:25000 No.2503

Area: 309ha (764 acres)
Height: 123m (403 ft)

Owner: Major and Dr Jean Balfour of Scourie Estate, the owners, gave the RSPB a twenty-five-year lease in 1961 to run the island as a nature reserve. They extended the lease in 1986 for five years. However in 1991 Dr Balfour did not renew the lease as she felt that it was appropriate that a solely Scottish conservation body should run the island. The Scottish Wildlife Trust now manage the island, a body which did not exist when the original lease was signed. Dr Balfour is a founding member of the Trust and she is also a former chairman of the Countryside Commission for Scotland.
Handa is a Site of Special Scientific Interest.

Population: 1841–65 (11 houses). 1851–onwards, uninhabited. 1991– no permanent inhabitants but about 5000 visitors each summer.

Geology: An outcrop of Torridonian sandstone separated by the Sound of Handa from the mainland of Lewisian gneiss.

History: In early times the island was used as a burial ground by people on the mainland so that wolves would be unable to scavenge the corpses. Later, seven families settled and started cultivating the rough pastureland. They were self-sufficient, living on a staple diet of oats, potatoes, fish and sea-birds. The population grew, they had their own 'queen' – the oldest widow – and the men held a daily parliament to decide the allocation of work. It was, in fact, a very similar form of society to that on St Kilda (See No.9.1).

But then in 1848 the potato famine struck and the islanders emigrated to America. Handa has been uninhabited since that time but the old cottages and lazy-beds can still be seen.

Wildlife: Handa is renowned for its birdlife.

Best bird-watching is from early-May to mid-July, by August the cliffs are deserted. Over 170 species have been recorded, with thirty regular breeders. Twelve species of nesting seabirds include large populations of guillemot (100,000 strong – the largest colony in Britain), razorbill, fulmar and kittiwake. There are also four other gull species, shag, puffin, black guillemot and small numbers of Arctic and great skua.

No raptors breed here at present, but golden eagle, buzzard, peregrine falcon, sparrowhawk and merlin may be seen. White-tailed sea-eagles last nested here in 1864.

Other interesting species include great northern

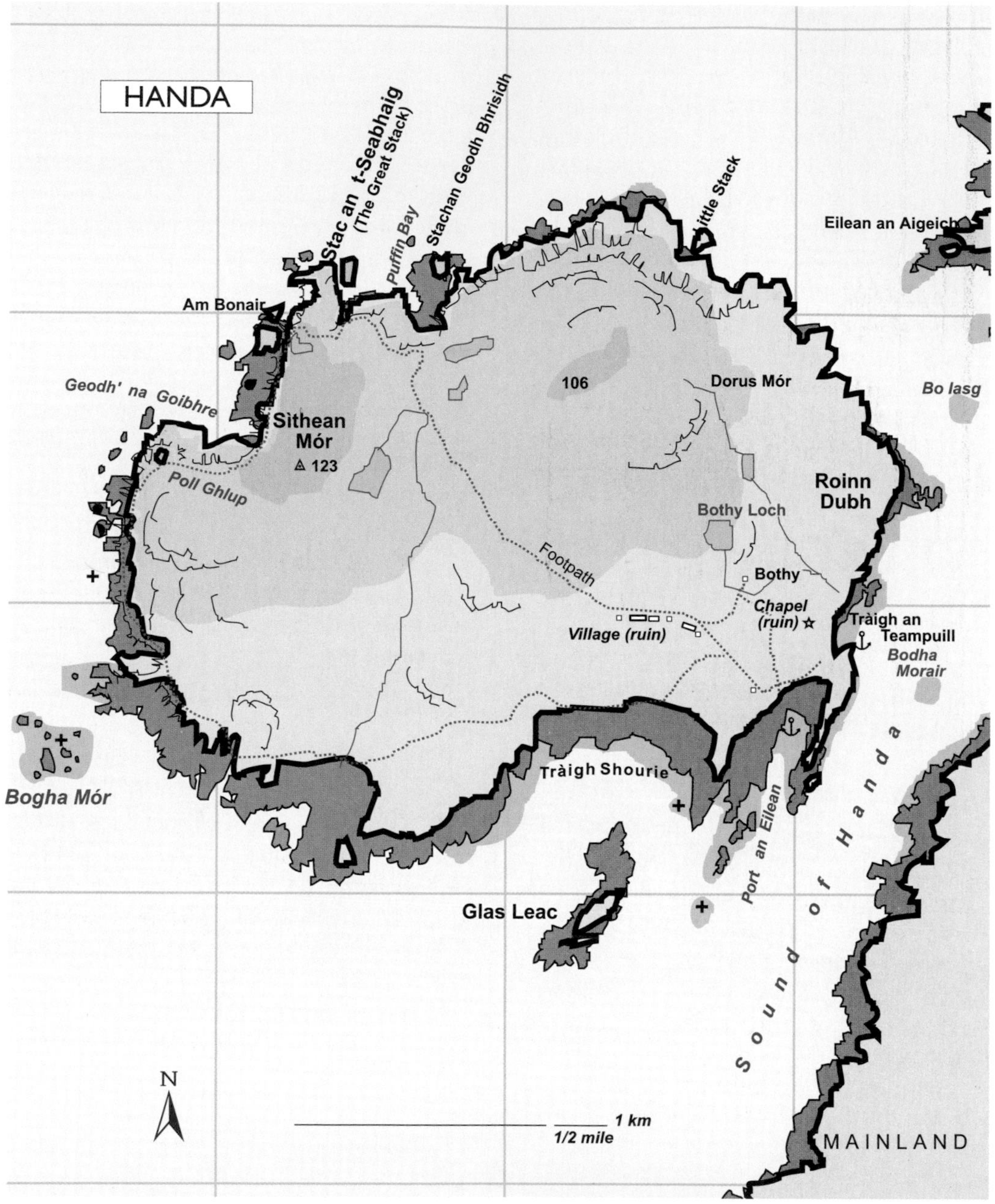

diver, red- and black-throated diver, eider and shelduck, oystercatcher, ringed plover, common and Arctic tern and rock dove. Inland breeders include snipe, wheatear, stonechat and sometimes, red grouse, golden plover and reed bunting. Migrants include pink-footed and greylag geese, dunlin, greenshank, turnstone, sanderling, whimbrel, Pomarine skua and Manx and sooty shearwater. A few barnacle geese turn up in winter.

Rats had become a serious problem, particularly to the puffin and Manx shearwater populations, but they were eliminated by the same method as that used on Ailsa Craig (No.1.1).

216 species of plants have been recorded and more than 100 species of mosses. The only trees are small plantations of lodgepole pine and alder. The island is home to thousands of rabbits.

Whales are fairly frequent visitors in this area and sometimes swim through the Sound.

HANDA is mostly heather, peat-bog and

rough pasture on top of a large tilted block of Torridonian sandstone which rears sharply out of the sea to a height of over 100m on the precipitous north and west sides. Here the cliffs are dark-red and brown with horizontal strata sharply outlined in white by sea-bird droppings. In the north-west and close to the cliffs is the higher of the two hills, Sithean Mór [shee-hen moar] (G. – the big fairy-hill). From the top the view stretches almost to Cape Wrath with the tall thin figure of the Old Man of Stoer on the far point of Eddrachillis Bay. Directly north of Sithean Mór the cliffs form an amphitheatre, Am Bonair, with a natural arch [NC130488]. On the east side of this bluff in an inlet or 'geo' and separated by a gap only 24m wide, stands the **Great Stack**, a gigantic rock 115m high and balanced on three legs [NC132488].

The first recorded crossing from the cliff-top on Handa to the flat top of the Stack was in 1876 by Donald MacDonald of Lewis swinging hand-over-hand from a rope. This terrifying narrow chasm has a sheer drop of over 100m down the wet sandstone face to turbulent ocean surf pounding the rocks far below.

In 1967 the original crossing was re-enacted by Dr Tom Patey of Ullapool except that on this occasion the traverse was made by a 180m nylon rope stretched from one side of the geo to the other and lying over the Stack. 'A thought-provoking experience,' he said afterwards.

For a different experience details of the route up the 'very severe' north face can be obtained from the Scottish Mountaineering Club.

Close to the east of the Great Stack is another stack, **Stachan Geodh Bhrisidh** (G. – stack of the broken chasm) in a cove which is usually referred to as Puffin Bay.

The Trust's hut is between **Bothy Loch**, one of Handa's six lochs all of which provide ample water but contain no fish, and the ruined chapel [NC147477] beside **Traigh am Teampull** (G. – temple beach) with its view south over the distant **Badcall Islands** and **Eilean a' Bhuic** off Scourie Bay.

From the landing place by the south-east promontory and **Port an Eilean** (G. – island port) a path runs along the south coast beaches, climbs slowly to the top of the high cliffs, chasms, stacks and natural arches of the west coast, and then turns south-eastwards across the centre of the island, sloping gradually down towards the Sound of Handa – the ocean channel separating Handa from the mainland. The path is partly paved with duckboarding to try to protect the fragile machair from the effect of 5000 pairs of tramping feet each year. A few shells of the old cottages are alongside the pathway before it reaches the burial ground. This has no walled boundary as on St Kilda or Tanera Mór but merely some rough weathered headstones in the grass. This clockwise walk (6km), on an island that combines startling topography with a deep sense of history and an astonishing variety of birdlife, is a 'must'. And a fitting climax is to circumnavigate the island by boat and see the drama on the cliffs from sea-level. Dorus Mór – the big door – is on the north-east side facing the narrow horse-back ridge of **Eilean an Aigeich** (G. – stallion island).

* * *

Access: There is a small charge for visiting (10am–4.30pm. ex-Sundays). Information or permission to camp from Scottish Wildlife Trust, 01463-714746, or from the warden (resident April–August). Overnight accommodation in a bothy occasionally available. A private ferry operates from Tarbert (unclassified road off A894 3M N of Scourie), S MacLeod, Scouriemore, 01971-502347.

Anchorages:

1. Port an Eilean. Approach from S. Avoid reef of drying rocks on west side. Good holding in sand, but some swell from S.
2. Traigh an Teampull. Beware Bo Morair in centre of Sound. Anchor off ruined chapel in 3m weed. Beware dragging in strong current.

6.10 Eilean nan Ron

(G. – island of the seals)

OS Maps: 1:50000 Sheet 10 1:25000 Sheet 447 or 448
Admiralty Charts: 1:200000 No.1954

Area: 138ha (341 acres)
Height: 76m (244 ft)

Owner: Sutherland Estates. (Countess of Sutherland.)

Population: 1841 42 (7 houses).
1881–73. 1891–63 (8 houses). 1931–30. Now uninhabited.

Geology: Undifferentiated Permian or Triassic sandstone.

Wildlife: This is a Site of Special Scientific Interest (SSSI). Hundreds of grey seals gather here in the autumn to pup and about 350 calves are born annually.

EILEAN NAN RON was well populated for much of its history but, like so many of the Scottish islands, is now only populated with ghosts.

The main island has an abrupt rocky shoreline, an irregular grassy surface and two similar hills in the northern part of almost identical height, **Cnoc an Loisgein** (76m) and **Cnoc na Caillich** (75m) (G. – hag's knoll). There are steep cliffs on the east side, north of a natural arch at **Leathad Ballach** (G.– spotted slope) and these continue round to the north coast. Here many broken inlets, another rock arch and a cave have been carved out by the sea.

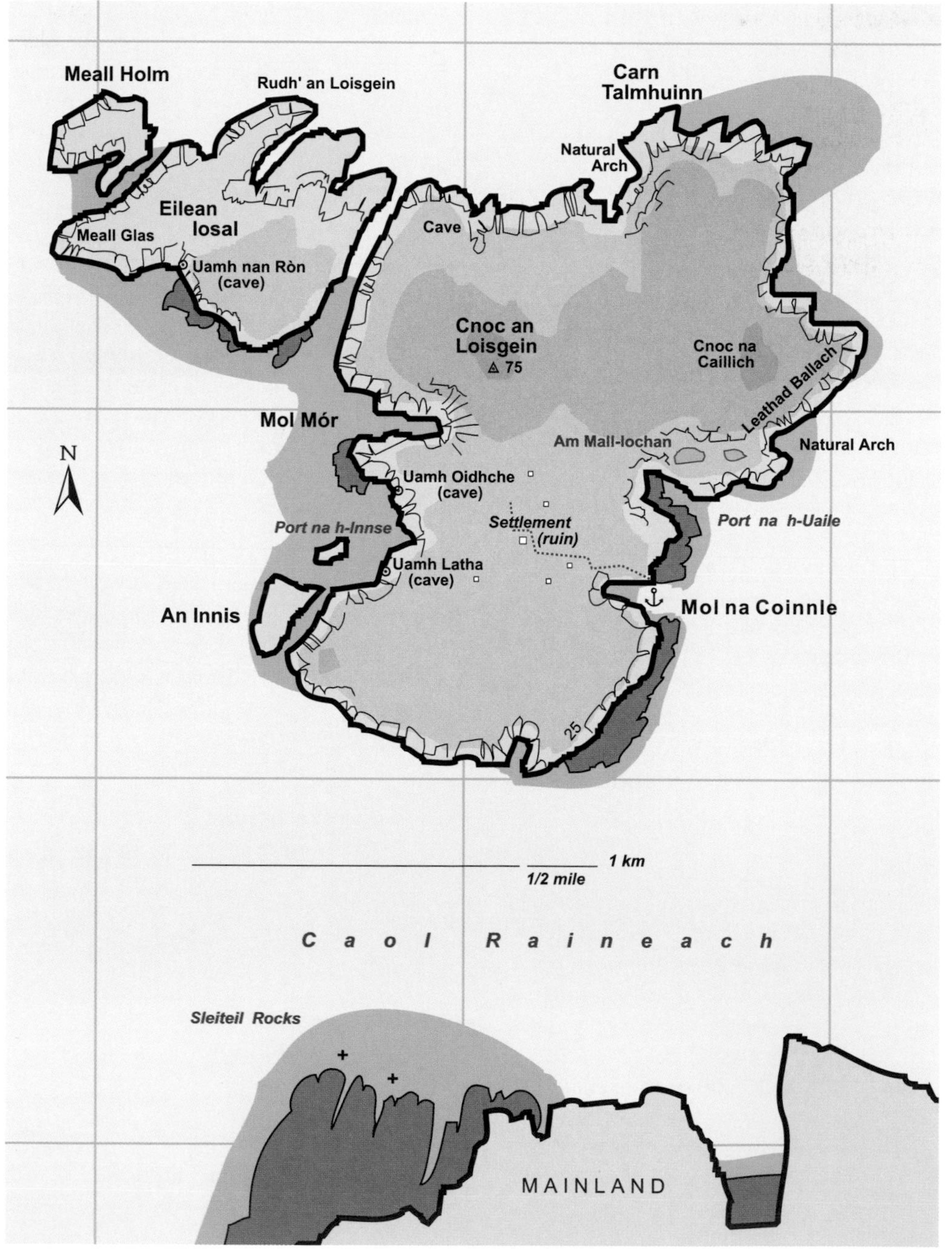

Eilean Iosal (G. – low or humble island) is a drying island connected at a narrow channel on the north-west side. It is steep – just over 50m in height – with a cave, **Uamh nan Ròn** (G. – the seals' cave) on its south side. Beyond lies a smaller islet called Meall Thailm (G. – sling shot) according to the Ordnance Survey, or Meall Holm according to the Admiralty (G. and ON – blob of an islet).

The settlement of houses and ruins is in the waist of the island. To the west is **Mol Mór** (G. – big pebble beach) and a rock-strewn bay. **Port na h-Innse** (G. – island port) is adjacent with a cave on either side – Night Cave to the north and Day Cave to the south.

The **Rabbit Islands** in Tongue Bay can be seen from here. They are aptly named and worth a visit. A partly sheltered anchorage is off the beach on the south side of the larger island.

Port na h-Uaille (G. – false port), well-named – with a gravel beach and many hidden rocks, and **Mol na Coinnle** (G. – oily-surfaced pebble beach) are east of the old settlement.

The island is separated from the mainland by Caol Raineach. East of it, lying just off the coastline, is **Neave Island** (G. *naomha* – holy), also known as **Coomb Island**.

West of the Kyle of Tongue **Eilean Hoan** (G. & ON – haven island) and **Eilean Clùimhrig** lie at the mouth of Loch Eriboll. Deep within the loch, **Eilean Choraidh**, otherwise known as Horse Island, was taken to represent the German battleship *Tirpitz* when it was used for target practice by wartime Mosquito bombers. The Census of 1931 recorded a population of one lonely male on Eilean Choraidh and one hopes he didn't stay on.

Beyond Faraid Head and near Cape Wrath is the very insignificant **An Garbh-eilean** (G. – the rough island).

* * *

Access: No regular access but local boatmen usually arrange visits in the summer months.

Anchorage: Beware below-water rock off NE extremity of island and W coast is foul. E and S sides clean to within ½c.
1. Mol na Coinnle. The most southerly small bight on SE side. Shelter from W and NW winds. Anchor opposite corrugated-iron roofed hut near shore. There are steps up the cliff.

SECTION 7

The Outer Hebrides – South of the Sound of Harris

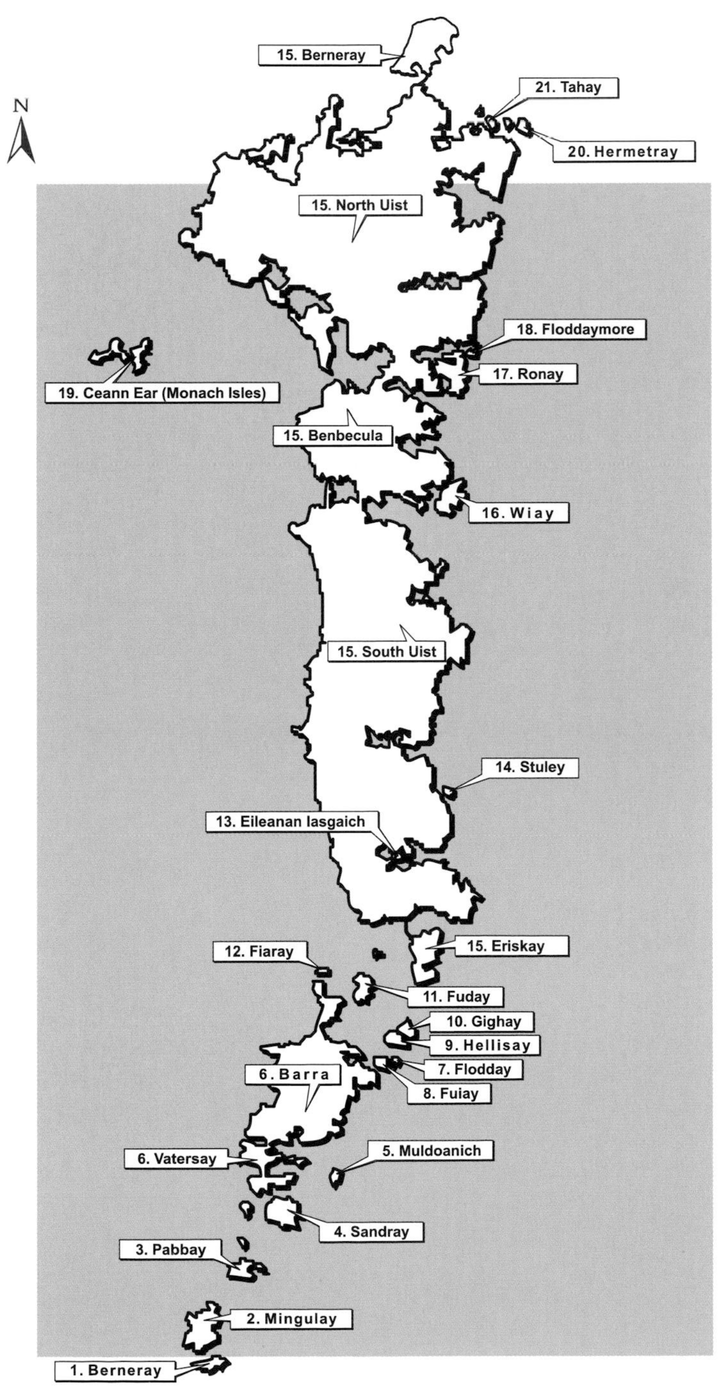

SECTION 7, Table 1: Arranged according to geographic position

No.	Name	Latitude	Longitude	Table 2* No.	Table 3** No.	Area in Acres	Area in Hectares	
7.1	Berneray	56° 47N	07° 38W	84	36	504		204
7.2	Mingulay	56° 49N	07° 38W	52	25	1581		640
7.3	Pabbay	56° 51N	07° 35W	76	39	618		250
7.4	Sandray	56° 54N	07° 31W	57	33	951		385
7.5	Muldoanich	56° 55N	07° 26W	122	44	193		78
7.6	Barra	56° 59N	07° 28W	16	17	14517	5875	
	Vatersay	*56° 56N*	*07° 32W*			2372	960	6835
7.7	Flodday (E Barra)	56° 60N	07° 21W	161	128	98		40
7.8	Fuiay	56° 60N	07° 22W	119	62	208		84
7.9	Hellisay	57° 01N	07° 21W	96	84	351		142
7.10	Gighay	57° 01N	07° 20W	113	74	237		96
7.11	Fuday	57° 03N	07° 23W	79	78	573		232
7.12	Fiaray	57° 04N	07° 26W	159	148	101		41
7.13	Eileanan Iasgaich	57° 09N	07° 19W	147	157	124		50
7.14	Stuley	57° 12N	07° 15W	155	132	111		45
7.15	South Uist	57° 17N	07° 20W	4	6	79136	32026	
	North Uist	*57° 36N*	*07° 19W*			74884	30305	
	Benbecula	*57° 27N*	*07° 19W*			20270	8203	
	Berneray	*57° 43N*	*07° 11W*			2496	1010	
	Baleshare	*57° 32N*	*07° 23W*			2249	910	
	Grimsay	*57° 29N*	*07° 14W*			2058	833	
	Eriskay	*57° 05N*	*07° 17W*			1737	703	
	Vallay	*57° 40N*	*07° 25W*			642	260	
	Kirkibost Island	*57° 33N*	*07° 25W*			507	205	
	Oronsay	*57° 40N*	*07° 18W*			210	85	74540
7.16	Wiay	57° 24N	07° 12W	58	66	927		375
7.17	Ronay	57° 29N	07° 11W	53	58	1391		563
7.18	Floddaymore	57° 30N	07° 09W	140	153	143		58
7.19	Ceann Ear (Monach Isles)	57° 31N	07° 37W	61	159	502	203	
	Ceann Iar	*57° 31N*	*07° 39W*			381	154	357
7.20	Hermetray	57° 39N	07° 03W	129	139	178		72
7.21	Tahay	57° 40N	07° 06W	145	98	131		53

*Table 2: The islands arranged in order of magnitude
** Table 3: The islands arranged in order of height

Introduction

Like Australia's Great Barrier Reef the chain of Outer Hebridean islands parallels and protects the mainland coast from ocean storms. The side facing the Atlantic is an almost continuous strand of sand-dunes and machair while the east coast is savagely indented and irregular with sea-lochs which disintegrate into a maze of inlets between reefs and tidal islets. For the yachtsman, all these lochs are a wonderland and there are anchorages to suit most conditions.

Loch Eynort, near the centre of South Uist, presents a navigational challenge where the wide outer loch suddenly channels through the dog-leg of Sruthan Beag (G. – little tidal streamlet). The tide tumbles through at seven knots with eddies and overfalls but with care it is possible to sneak through at slack water. Once through, the islet **Risgay** and a rocky patch are straight ahead, and to left and right there are many bays and secret inlets in which to anchor (some free of fish cages!).

Although few fish-farms are locally owned there is no doubt that fish-farming has brought limited, but welcome, employment to Scottish islands. Yachtsmen are aware of this and have accepted that some of the finest and safest anchorages are now filled with fish-cages. Their only plea is that when fish-farming ceases the cages should be removed. Some are being abandoned and left to disintegrate on the sea bottom, thus creating a hazard and effectively denying use of that anchorage for a century or more.

At the north end of South Uist where it meets Benbecula the land shatters into fragments. **Corr-eileanan, Eilean an Fhraoich Mia, Glas-eileanan, Eilean a' Bhogha, Glas-eilean na**

Creige, **Eilean a' Mhadaidh** (G. – dog isle) and **Gasay** (G. – swept isle) are only some of the many islets and skerries in the area.

The east shore of Benbecula continues this broken landscape. North of the island of Wiay (No.7.17). **Greanamul Deas** (G. – south Greanamul) and **Greanamul** (ON – green hump) itself act as eastern markers. **Maaey Riabhach** (ON & G. – grizzled seagull island), **Maragay Mór** (G. – big pudding isle) and **Maragay Beag** stand guard at each side of Loch Uiskevagh. **Bearran** islet is in the centre of the loch.

In the channel between Benbecula and Grimsay two islets **Calavay** and **Eilean Leathan** are linked by a long tidal strand.

Loch Eport, in North Uist, is another lengthy sea-loch. Shallow Loch Langass which connects with it near the head can be explored for miles by dinghy and is an alternative route to see the chambered cairn on Ben Langass. Most of the islets in Loch Eport are tidal except possibly **Treanay** at Bay Sponish and **Eilean nam Mult** (G. – island of the castrated rams) in the centre of the loch.

7.1 Berneray

(ON – Bjorn's island.) As the southernmost island of the Outer Hebrides Berneray is often referred to as Barra Head.

OS Maps: 1:50000 Sheet 31 1:25000 Sheet 452
Admiralty Charts: 1:100000 No.1796 1:30000 No.2769

Area: 204ha (504 acres)
Height: 193m (633ft)

Owner: National Trust for Scotland. Acquired in April 2000 from the Barrahead Isles Sheep Stock Club, a syndicate of Barra crofters and owners since 1955.

Population: In the 18th century the population was over fifty. 1841–30. 1881–56. 1891–36 (9 houses). The three lighthouse-keepers and their wives were the only occupants of the island from 1931 until the lighthouse became automatic and, therefore, uninhabited in the late 1970s.

Geology: The granite to build the island's own (Barra Head) lighthouse in 1833 was quarried on the island. Most of Berneray consists of gneiss.

History: In 1992, sponsored by Historic Scotland, Berneray was surveyed by archaeologists from Sheffield University and Prague and eighty-three sites and monuments were noted and recorded. Less than forty were thought to be of post-medieval date.

Wildlife: Designated a Site of Special Scientific Interest in 1993 and a special bird protection area, in early May the hillside is a riot of colour with primroses, celandine, wild violets and yellow flag iris.

Grey seals frequent the cove by the landing place and the island supports 15 species of sea-bird including large numbers of kittiwake, guillemot, auk and some puffins.

Martin Martin (1695) recorded that Berneray 'excels other islands of the same extent for cultivation and fishing. The natives never go a-fishing while Macneil or his steward is in the island, lest seeing their plenty of fish, perhaps they might take occasion to raise their rents.'

* * *

BERNERAY has a wedge-shaped appearance when approaching from the north-east or south-west. The south coast consists of rugged cliffs which have a least height of about 40m at the east end. Barra Head lighthouse is a white stone

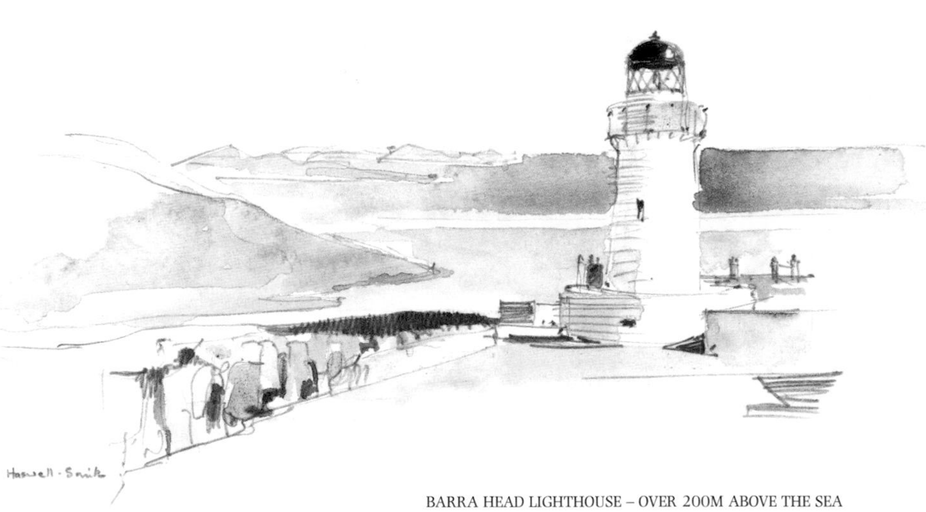

BARRA HEAD LIGHTHOUSE – OVER 200M ABOVE THE SEA

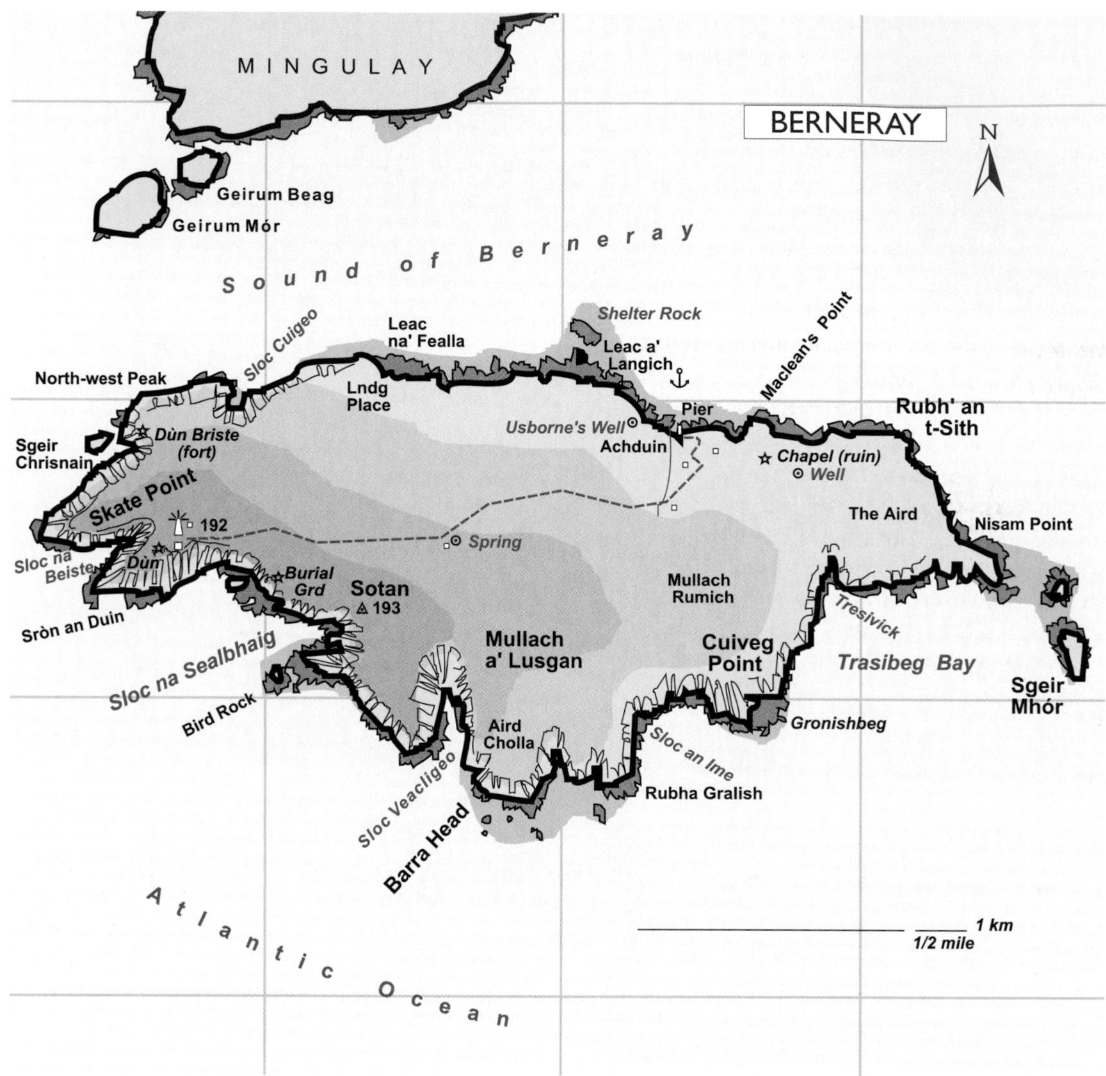

tower on top of **Sròn an Dùin** (G. – fortress promontory) above the western cliffs.

This is the most southerly point of the Outer Hebrides. The magnificent cliffs of 190m height (623ft) on the west side at Skate Point take the full force of gigantic seas because there is no shallow water to impede them. Small fish are often found in the grass at the top of the high cliffs after severe gales. Even if one might suspect that sea gulls dropped them the lighthouse-keepers said that this was not so and as proof of the ferocity of the gales it was reliably reported in 1836 that a forty-two ton rock was moved five feet (almost two metres) during a violent storm.

A vehicle track climbs up the hill from the landing place to the lighthouse at the summit. A 'chalybeate spring' (water with traces of iron in it) is about halfway up, at the side of the track, with a pumphouse to provide water for the lighthouse. A helicopter pad near the top allows maintenance teams to service the lighthouse now that it is automatic.

Two duns or fortified mounds are situated near the summit of the island. One is called **Dùn Briste** (G. – the broken fort) [NL549805]. Unfortunately, the other one, a galleried dun of the Iron Age, was largely destroyed when the lighthouse was constructed. This will be the fort that Martin noted – 'having a vacuity round the walls, divided in little apartments'. A gateway now leads through the ancient wall from the lighthouse yard onto a cliff-top area completely surrounded by a parapet of natural stone slabs and boulders. From here the cliff drops vertically to the surging waves 200m below. Alongside, there is a great chasm – **Sloc na Beiste** (G. – ravine of the monster) – 100m long by 200m deep leading to a cave, but to explore it would require considerable expertise in mountaineering. The roar of the sea breaking into the chasm far below forms a bass chorus to the cries of thousands of sea-birds wheeling past the cliffs.

Apart from the site of a chapel (near the landing place) [NL567803], Berneray has five cists, five suspected burial cairns and four megalithic chamber tombs so the island appears to have been well occupied in the Neolithic/Bronze Age, possibly less intensively settled in the Iron Age but followed by renewed activity in the Christian and medieval period.

Fresh water can be scarce, and in dry summers the islanders had to ship water over from Mingulay.

* * *

Access: Barra Fishing Charters, 01871-890384. Island Adventures, Castlebay, 01871-810284. Tourist Information, Castlebay, Barra, 01871-810336.

Anchorage: Landing on the slippery jetty from an inflatable dinghy can be difficult and potentially dangerous due to the swell.

1. On N side, except in heavy seas, anchor off the concrete jetty and storehouse, 7–8m, good firm sand. This is out of the tidal stream and sheltered from S through W to N. Very heavy squalls sometimes during S and SW gales and very exposed to the E.

7.2 Mingulay

(ON mikil-øy – big island).

O S Maps: 1:50000 Sheet 31 1:25000 Sheet 452
Admiralty Charts: 1:100000 No.1796 1:30000 No.2769

Area: 640ha (1581 acres)
Height: 273m (895 ft)

Owner: National Trust for Scotland. Acquired in April 2000 from the Barrahead Isles Sheep Stock Club, a syndicate of Barra crofters and owners since 1955.

Population: 1841–113 (18 houses). 1881–150. 1891–142 (29 houses). 1901–135. In 1908 many of the islanders claimed land on neighbouring islands, some becoming known as the Vatersay Raiders (See No.7.6) and after this the remaining population dwindled rapidly. The last inhabitants left in 1912.

Geology: Almost entirely of gneiss but with some granite.

History: Mingulay must have been first settled long ago as the island has several potential archaeological sites. Crois an t-Suidheachain (G. – cross of the sitting-place), was a structure on a level area of ground above the road at Aneir. Nothing remains but it has been variously described as a standing stone, a stone circle, or a group of three 'cells or chests'. There may be some Viking graves but the record of Viking influence is in the topographical names such as Hecla, Skipisdale and, for that matter, Mingulay.

When the MacNeils of Barra owned Mingulay they took a paternal interest in their tenants, arranging new husbands and wives for widows and widowers, helping to feed the children, or making good the loss of a milking cow. The community thrived. The laird's annual rent was mainly *fachaich* – shearwater chicks collected from the precipices. As on St Kilda, life here depended on the sea-birds, although fishing also played its part. The famous 'Mingulay Boat Song' was never sung on Mingulay. It is a West Highland air with words written in 1938 by Hugh Roberton for his famous Glasgow Orpheus Choir to sing.

Wildlife: Sorrel and wild celery grow on the hillsides and nettles frame the village ruins. This is a place of annual pilgrimage for ornithologists as it is a principal breeding station for guillemot and kittiwake. A boat trip around the awe-inspiring western cliffs, virtually inaccessible and covered with sea-birds, is an unforgettable experience. A really close approach is difficult except on the rare days of calm water. In the breeding season the granite stacks and very high cliffs are festooned with nesting kittiwakes, razorbills and guillemots and there are also large colonies of puffins and black-backed gulls.

Mingulay was designated a Site of Special Scientific Interest in 1993 and a European bird protection area.

* * *

The islands south of Barra and Vatersay used to be known as the Bishop's Isles and **MINGULAY** is the largest of the group. It is almost an in-shore Hirta (No.9.1) with its St Kilda-like stacks, its towering cliffs and even its village bay. It shows several rounded summits when viewed from the sea, **Carnan** the highest at 273m, **Hecla** (219m) (ON – hooded shroud) close south-west of it and **Macphee's Hill** (224m) in the north. Between them is **Tom a' Mhaide** (G. – hillock of the stick), a smaller peak of over 150m. The west coast has precipitous cliffs but the south and east coasts slope gradually down to a rugged foreshore. Mingulay Bay (or Village Bay) is centrally situated on the east coast with a half kilometre of sandy beach and the extensive remains of the deserted village above it.

The **Schoolhouse** [NL568825], at the south end by the track to the landing place, was built in 1881 for the sum of £494. It replaced the

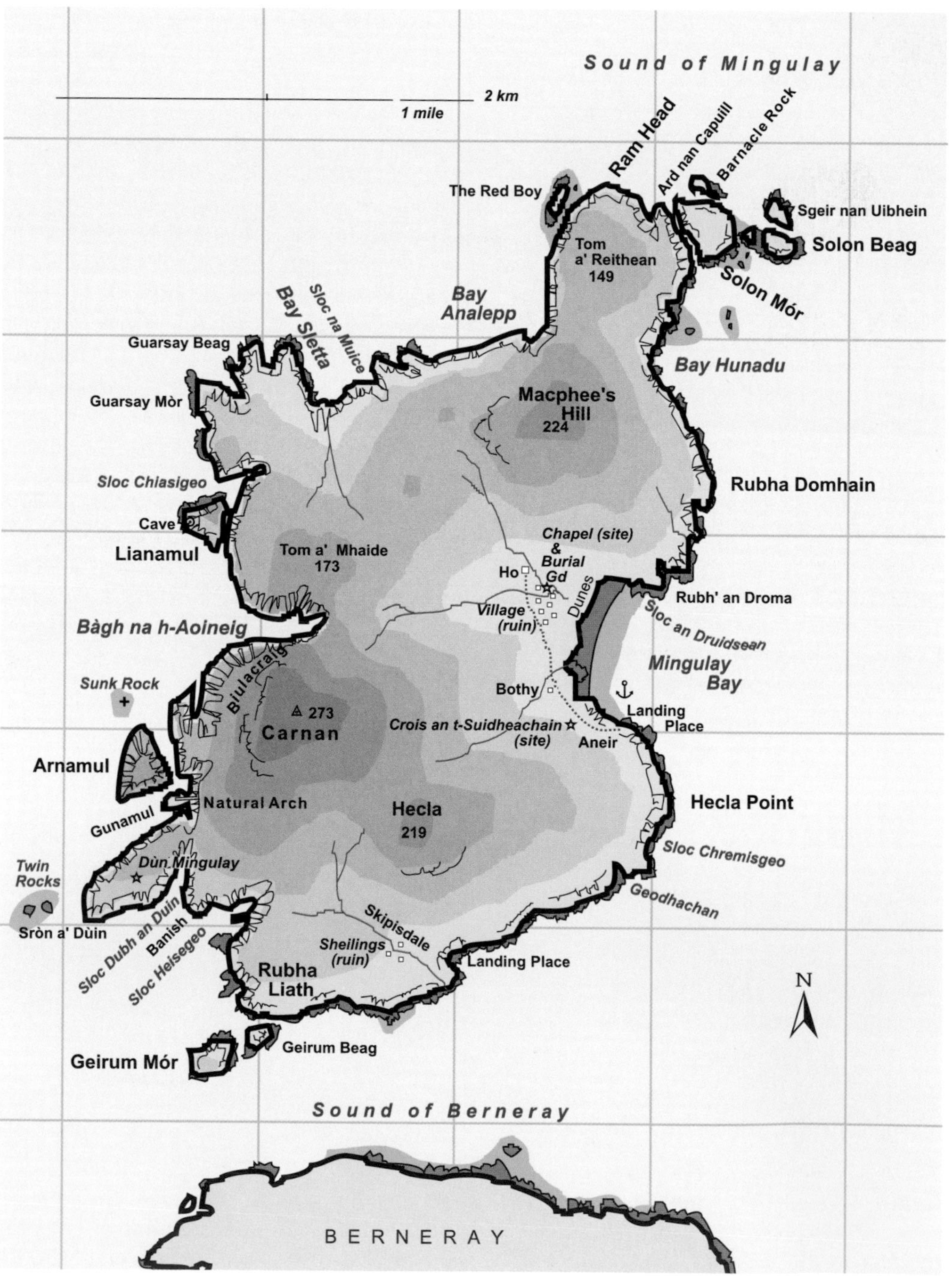

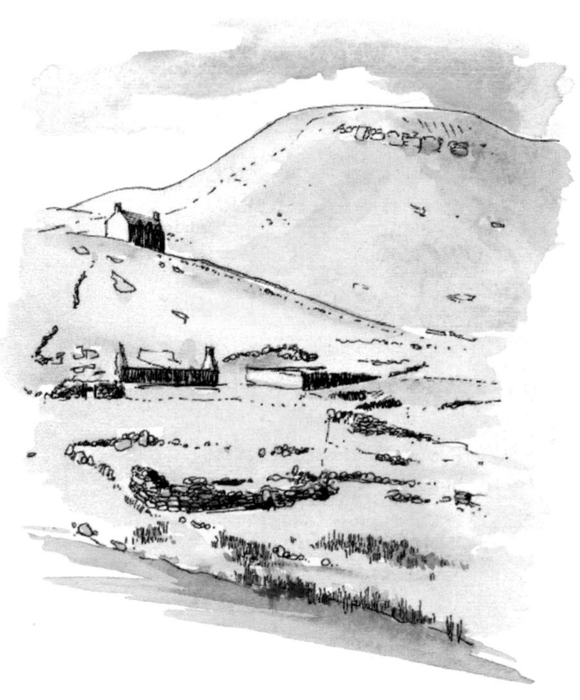

THE CHAPEL HOUSE AND MACPHEE'S HILL

traditional thatched structure established by the Free Church Ladies' Association in 1859. The building was used as a bothy and sheep-fank since sheep-farming took over in 1912 and was reroofed with corrugated iron in 1986 to allow the shepherds to use it on their annual visits. The Catholic priest's house, at the north end beyond the ruined village, was built in 1898. With a chapel on the upper floor [NL564834] it was known as the **Chapel House** but it collapsed in late 1996.

One island story relates how, in the time of MacNeil of Barra's ownership, a rent collector, Macphee, was landed on the island and found everyone dead. He rushed back to the boat and called to the men to take him off quickly as there was 'plague' on the island. On hearing this the men rowed away and left him to his fate. For a whole year he had only the corpses for company. Every day he would climb the hill to the north of the village and signal frantically to passing ships but they would wave back and pass on. He survived and eventually MacNeil decided it was safe to have the island resettled. He made a special grant of land to Macphee by way of compensation and since then the hill has always been known as Macphee's Hill.

This north part of the island has an additional promontory with a small hill on it called **Tom a' Reithean** (G. – hillock of the ram). It has a number of large detached rocks and islets clustered round it including the remarkable stack, **Red Boy**, on the north-west side and on the opposite side, **Solon Mór** (G. – big gannet) which is almost detached by a deep cleft. The Big Gannet has a fledgling called **Solon Beag**.

The sea-cliffs on the west side towering up to 215m in height are among the most dramatic in the British Isles and have many fantastic rock formations. The greatest sheer drop is at **Biulacraig**, below Carnan. ('Biulacraig' is the MacNeils of Barra' war-cry). There are large colonies of seabirds on the treacherous cliffs and the islanders used to scale them to collect the eggs and young birds.

Normally these great rock-faces can only be seen clearly from the sea but an interesting and not too demanding walk westwards up the valley from the derelict village arrives at a point above **Bàgh na h-Aoineig** (G. – bay of the steep promontory), a gigantic cleft cutting deep into the island. From here it is possible to look across the cleft towards Carnan and see the utterly breath-taking height of the precipice rising straight out of the sea and soaring towards the sky. Near the top it leans further and further out in a great rock cornice which looks as though it might overbalance at any moment. Every little horizontal crack, ledge and crevice is stippled white – each insignificant dot another nesting bird.

Sheep were grazed on the grassy tops of the two famous stacks, **Arnamul** (ON – erne mound) and **Lianamul** (ON – flax mound), which stand close to the cliffs on either side of Bàgh na h-Aoineig. For many years Lianamul, which has a sea-cave, was reached by a rope bridge spanning the chasm but this had disappeared by 1871. Before the bridge was constructed the *Statistical Account* of 1794 described how the people would climb to the top of Lianamul 'at the risk of their lives, and by means of a rope carry up their wedders to fatten'.

A huge natural arch at **Gunamul** is on the southern side of Arnamul where the cliffs are over 150m in height [NL547824]. It is possible to sail a small boat through it on the very rare occasions when conditions are suitable. South again there is an island-like promontory called **Dùn Mingulay** [NL545821], which was the site of an Iron Age fort.

Two rocky islets, **Geirum Mór** and **Geirum Beag** break into the Sound of Berneray and further east a burn runs down the south side of Hecla through **Skipisdale** (ON – ship valley) and discharges into the sound. This is sometimes the best spot to land from a dinghy and it was so used by the people of nearby Berneray when collecting water in times of drought.

* * *

Access: Barra Fishing Charters, 01871-890384. Island Adventures, Castlebay, 01871-810284. Tourist Information, Castlebay, Barra, 01871-810336.

Anchorages:

1. Mingulay Bay. Occasional anchorage off middle of beach, sheltered from W and NW winds. There is usually a considerable swell which can make landing – and leaving! – difficult. Usually easier to land at rocks at Aneir – S end of beach.
2. Skipisdale. Occasional landing place but no anchorage.

7.3 Pabbay

(ON papa-øy – priest or hermit island)

OS Maps: 1:50000 Sheet 31 1:25000 Sheet 452
Admiralty Charts: 1:100000 No.1796 1:30000 No.2769

Area: 250ha (618 acres)
Height: 171m (561 ft)

Owner: National Trust for Scotland. Acquired in April 2000 from the Barrahead Isles Sheep Stock Club, a syndicate of Barra crofters and owners since 1955.

Population: 1764–16. 1794– three farming families, about 20 people altogether. 1841–25 (3 houses). 1881–16. 1891–13 (3 houses). 1901–11. 1911–5. Uninhabited since.

Geology: The shell-sand is extremely rich in lime and frequent rains have broken this down to produce beds of impure limestone. Otherwise the island mainly consists of gneiss.

History: In early Christian times Pabbay, as its name would infer, had a hermitage or cell located on it and there is an ancient symbol stone and cross slabs on the slope above Bàgh Bàn.

Martin Martin wrote in the early 18th century: 'the natives observe that if six sheep are put a-grazing in the little island of Pabbay, five of them still appear fat, but the sixth a poor skeleton, but any number in this island not exceeding five are always very fat.' This possibly refers to Lingay (N of Pabbay). Martin's map shows Pabbay and Mingulay interchanged. Today, Pabbay supports about 100 breeding ewes.

On 1 May 1897 every able-bodied man was lost in a fierce storm at sea while out fishing. The Mingulay boat survived the same storm. The island never fully recovered from this disaster and the population dwindled. Within fifteen years no one remained.

Wildlife: Heather is scarce, possibly due to the areas of alkaline soil but the rough grazing is full of daisies and celandine, and sundew and flag irises grow in the damper areas.

There are many rabbits and ground-nesting seabirds. Cliff-nesters are almost absent.

* * *

PABBAY is another member of the Bishop's Isles (recently called the 'Barrahead Isles') and another 'Priest's Isle'.

The summit, **The Hoe**, rises to a height of 171m at the south-west extremity where there are steep sea-cliffs and a massive arched overhang. The settlement which reached a peak population of twenty-six in 1881 was on the eastern side above the blinding-white shell-sand beach in **Bàgh Bàn** (G. – white bay). A cottage still stands on the small central promontory of Sumula. Between Bàgh Bàn and the ruined settlement is an artificial-looking mound about 5m high. The mound may be a burial ground as human bones have been uncovered by the drifting sands. Three cross-marked stones may be gravestones and a fourth marked with a crescent, a cross and a lily is probably Pictish as it is of a design quite different in style to the interlacing Celtic patterns usually found in the Outer Hebrides [NL607874]. Visible traces of an ancient chapel were reported in 1915 beside the nearby rivulet.

Sloc Glansich, said to be named after an Irishman called Glancy, is a steep cleft which concealed the local centre for illicit whisky distillation.

The **Rosinish** peninsula, really a drying island, forms the east side of Bàgh Bàn and rises to 43m

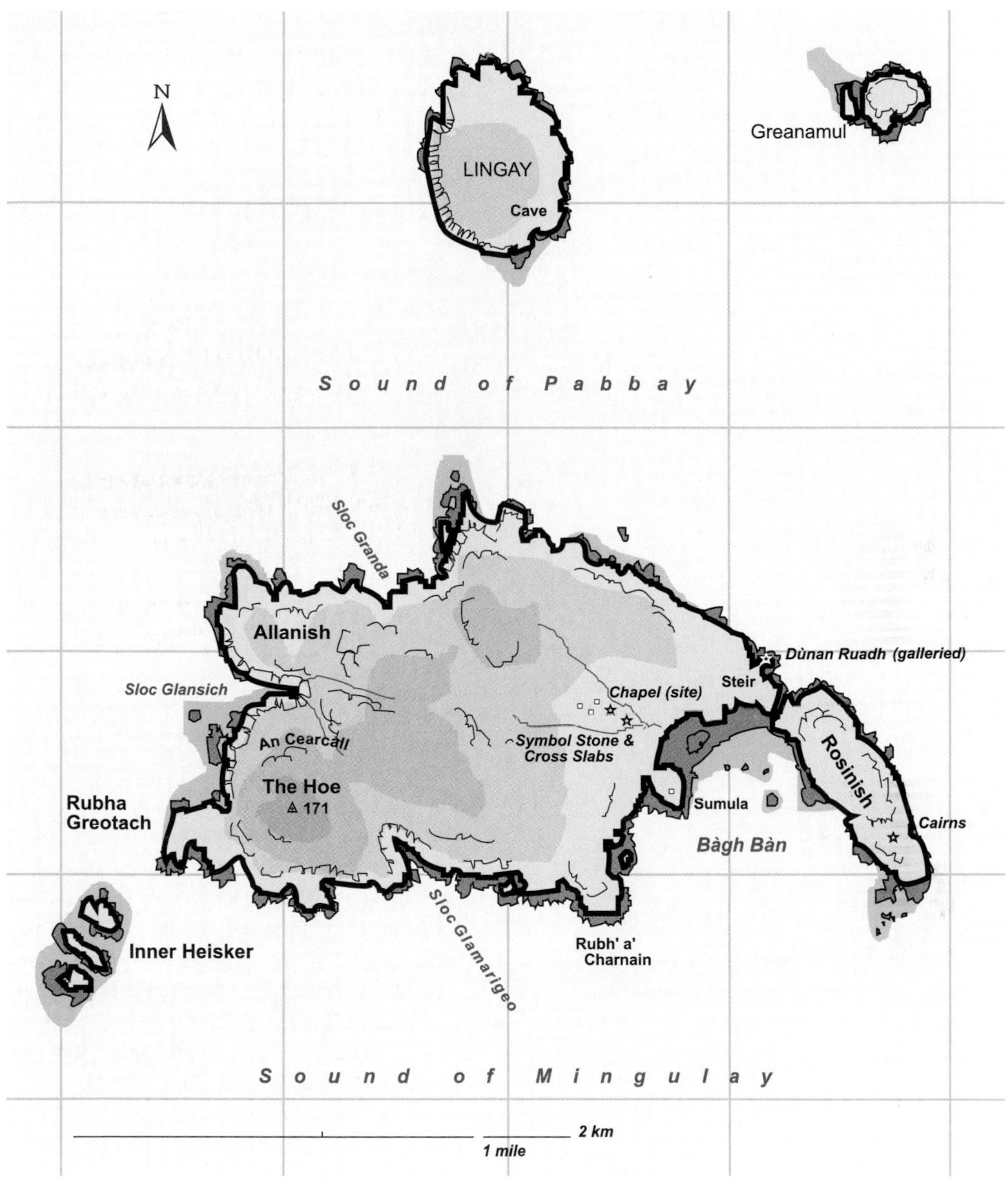

where it juts into the waters of the Minch. Near the junction – a narrow cleft – is **Dùnan Ruadh** (G. – the red fort) [NL613876], a ruined galleried broch which looks across the Sound of Pabbay to its opposite number on Sandray (No.7.4).

Dark, narrow vertical fissures intersect the cliffs on the south-west coast by The Hoe where they tower over the islets of Inner and Outer Heisker. These lie in the Sound of Mingulay. To the north is the Sound of Pabbay with the small hump of **Greanamul** (ON – green mound) in it and the larger island of **Lingay** (ON – heather isle). Lingay is steep but is occasionally used for grazing sheep. It has a cave in its south-east side.

Access: Barra Fishing Charters, 01871-890384. Island Adventures, Castlebay, 01871-810284. Tourist Information, Castlebay, Barra, 01871-810336.

Anchorage: There is no recommended anchorage.
1. Bàgh Bàn is mainly rocky but there is a 4.1m charted sounding off the small headland called Sumula which is sand and affords temp. anchorage in calm conditions. Approach with caution.

7.4 Sandray

(ON sandr-øy – sand island). Old charts have it as Soundray, Sanderay or Sandera.

O S Maps: 1:50000 Sheet 31 1:25000 Sheet 452
Admiralty Charts: 1:100000 No.1769 1:30000 No.2769

Area: 385ha (951 acres)
Height: 207m (679 ft)

Owner: Government owned (Department of Agriculture).

Population: 1835–population cleared for sheep. 1841–14 (2 houses occupied by shepherds' families). 1861–9. 1881–10.
1891–4. 1901–3 shepherds. Temporary influx of evicted people from Mingulay in 1908.
1911–0. Uninhabited since.

Geology: Mainly gneiss bedrock.

History: Neolithic settlements and tombs were identified by Sheffield University archaeologists in 1991. The Iron Age dun which is still some 2m in height is prominent above a steep ridge on the west side of Cairn Galtar [NL638913] facing Dùnan Ruadh on Pabbay. The ruin of another dun was reported on the east coast, and various Iron Age dwellings.

Faint traces of the old chapel site, Cille Bhride (G. – Bride's or Bridget's cell) were reported in 1915 to be partly covered by a sheep dip [NL650918]. The chapel served the nine crofts into which the island was divided in the early 18th century.

The *SS Fair Branch* from Sunderland was wrecked on Sandray in 1882.

Wildlife: According to Dean Monro, who visited it in 1549, Sandray was 'inhabit and manurit, guid for corne and fishing', and Martin Martin in 1695 claimed that 'it is designed for pasturage and cultivation... fruitful in corn and grass'. Today, this is no longer true as the landscape is deserted and fairly barren but in the windbeaten grass there are many wildflowers and a profusion of orchids.

There are no trees, although hazels have been recorded in the past, and the commonest mammals on Sandray are, without doubt, rabbits.

* * *

SANDRAY is a fairly circular island with a central peak, **Cairn Galtar** (207m). A lesser hill to the east of Cairn Galtar is called Carnach (179m) (G. – heap of stones) and, again, to the east of Carnach there is a huge sand-dune 52m high. This has always been a well-known sea-mark as it clearly identifies Sandray's east coast. MacCulloch said: 'At a distance the island appears as if covered with a coating of snow.' My own impression is that the sand is possibly no longer as striking as it once was. Maybe there is more marram grass covering it nowadays.

The grazing rights on this island are held by an association of Barra crofters. There is a reasonable supply of fresh water from two good streams, one in the big glen, Gleann-Mór, and one flowing from a small loch, **Loch na Cuilce** (G. – loch of the reeds). Large, relatively flat rock plates make walking on parts of this island a pleasure.

A Gaelic tale recorded in Barra in 1859 told how the wife of a herdsman on Sandray had her

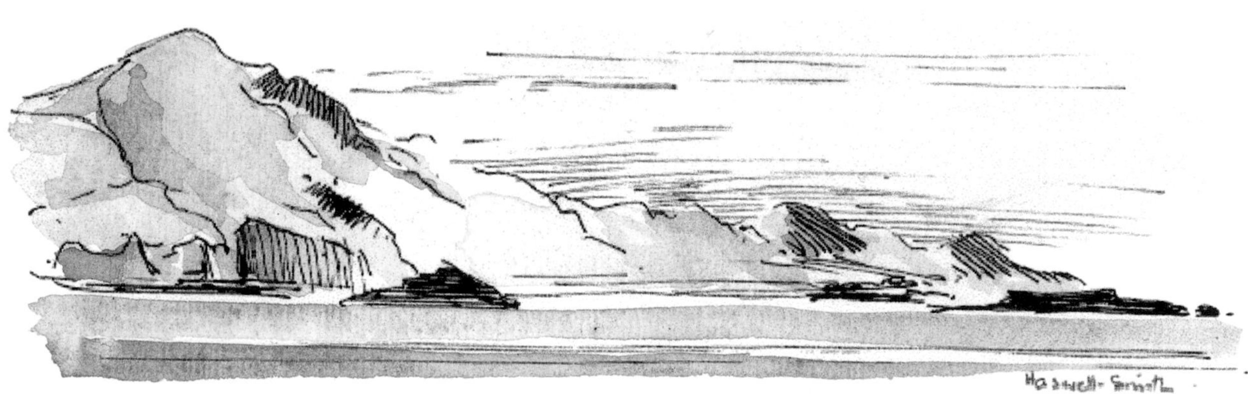

SANDRAY FROM THE SOUTH-EAST

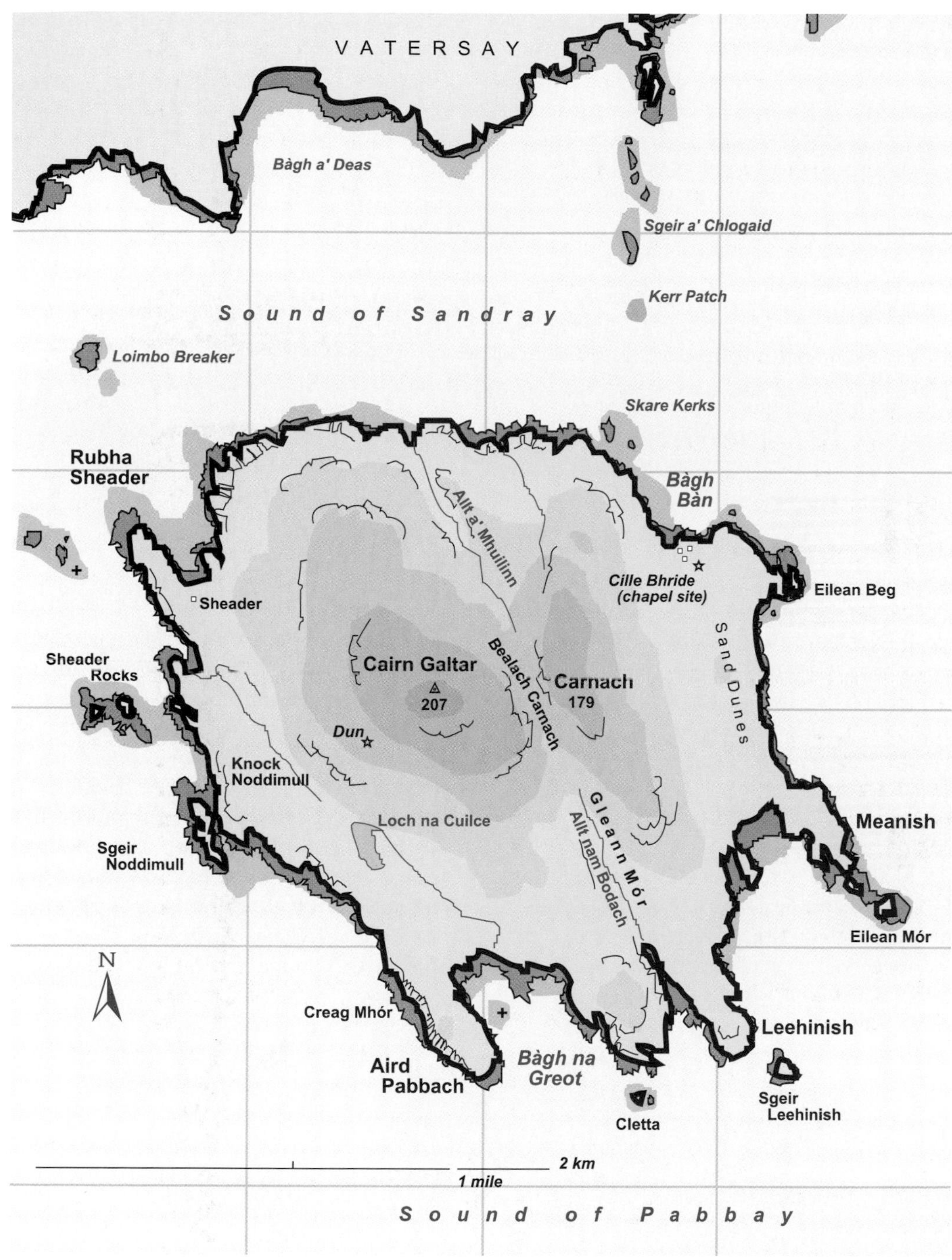

kettle borrowed every day by a woman of peace (a fairy). Before she would let go the kettle the wife would say: 'A smith is able to make cold iron hot with coal. The due of a kettle is bones, so bring it back again whole.' The kettle was returned every day with fresh meat and soup bones in it.

One day, as the wife was leaving by boat to visit Castlebay on Barra, she warned her husband to say the same words when the fairy came to borrow the kettle. But when the woman of peace came to the door the husband took fright and refused to open it. Then the kettle started jumping and it jumped right through the smoke hole in the roof. When the housewife returned the husband confessed that he had lost the kettle.

So the housewife went to the fairy hill and

found her kettle there with flesh and bones in it. She had just picked it up when two vicious fairy dogs started chasing her. She held them at bay by throwing them the contents of the kettle and managed to reach her home unharmed. But the fairy never returned to borrow the kettle.

This story is a fairly typical fireside tale. According to tradition fairies always feared iron and it is of course particularly mentioned in the wife's rhyme. Some scholars suppose that these fairy stories originated in the time when the new Iron Age immigrants met the wild and shy Neolithic settlers.

About one nautical mile west of Sandray the interesting little island of **Flodday** is 43m high, with black cliffs on its west coast and a natural rock arch in the centre. This is a small, but popular, grey seal nursery. There is no shelter whatsoever and the island is constantly windswept by Atlantic gales yet, remarkably, Flodday has its own unique subspecies of butterfly – a tiny pale-coloured form of the dark green fritillary *Argynnis aglaia scotica*.

* * *

Access: Barra Fishing Charters, 01871-890384. Island Adventures, Castlebay, 01871-810284. Tourist Information, Castlebay, Barra, 01871-810336.

Anchorages: There are no recommended anchorages but, proceeding cautiously, temp. anchorage in suitable conditions is possible at the following locations:

1. Small bay directly SW of Meanish. Occasional anchorage off centre of sandy beach in 4–5m, sand. Subject to swell.
2. Wide bay in E between Meanish and Eilean Beg. Temp. anchorage in 7–8m, sand. Avoid N end of bay. Subject to swell.

7.5 Muldoanich

(G. – Duncan's mound) or (G. mul Domhnach – Sunday island.) Dean Munro in 1549 seems to refer to it as Scarp and it is Scarpa on Blaeu's 1654 map (ON scarfr – cormorant) – island, or (ON – sharp, stony, hilly terrain) but in 1695 Martin Martin called it 'Muldonish'.

O S Maps: 1:50000 Sheet 31 1:25000 Sheet 452
Admiralty Charts: 1:100000 No.1796 1:30000 No.2769

Area: 78ha (193 acres)
Height: 153m (502 ft)

Population: No Census records. Uninhabited.

Geology: A hill of gneiss with a light covering of soil.

History: The island was part of the domain of the MacNeils of Barra. Dean Monro claimed in 1549 that 'Scarp' once had a chapel on it and that it was 'full of pastures and very guid for fishing'.

Wildlife: In 1695 Martin Martin said that, 'Muldonish is high in the middle, covered over with heath and grass, and is the only forest here for maintaining the deer, being commonly about seventy or eighty in number'. (A deer forest, of course, does not require trees.) I presume in Dean Munro's time it was cattle that were pastured on the island but that MacNeil of Barra had at some stage stocked it with deer to provide his family with a regular source of venison.

Botanists have found the pyramidal bugle growing on Muldoanich.

The sea-eagle nested here before it was exterminated in the early 20th century.

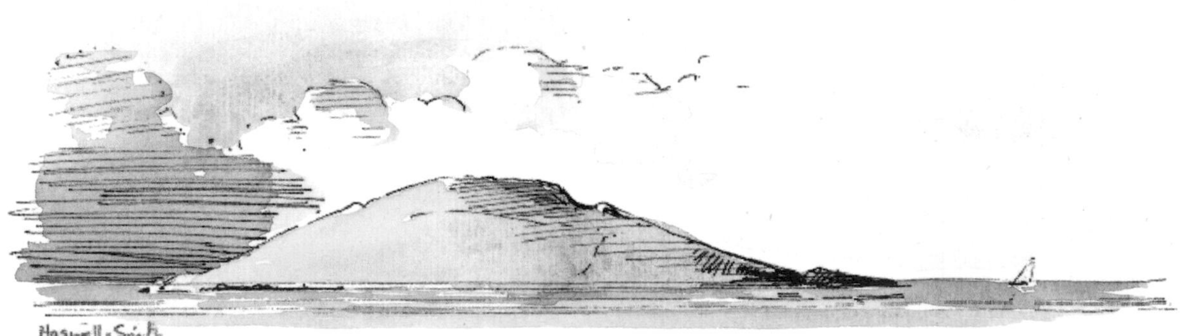

MULDOANICH FROM THE SOUTH-EAST

* * *

This distinctive dark hump of an island lies two miles east of Vatersay and clearly marks the entrance to Castlebay on Barra.

It was MacCulloch who suggested that the name **MULDOANICH** came from St Duncan. The chapel, if it ever existed, may have been dedicated to this important saint but MacCulloch's idea is generally considered to be incorrect.

Muldoanich has no level ground and rises fairly steeply on all sides to a central rounded summit of 153m – **Cruachan na h-àin** (G. – midday hill).

As there is no regular water supply, if anyone ever did live on the island life would have been difficult. A small two-roomed ruin was possibly a bothy (but is reputed to have been a jail!). The east side has the highest cliffs with two deep clefts defining **Creag na h-Iolaire** (G. – eagle crag). This probably referred to the once-common white-tailed sea-eagle which became extinct in Scotland but has now been reintroduced (See Rum No.4.3). The rudimentary inlets on this coast are **Sloc an Lus a' Chorrain** (G. – spleenwort hole), **Sloc na Uillean** |oylun| (G. – honeysuckle hole), and **Sloc na Calaman** (G. – pigeon hole).

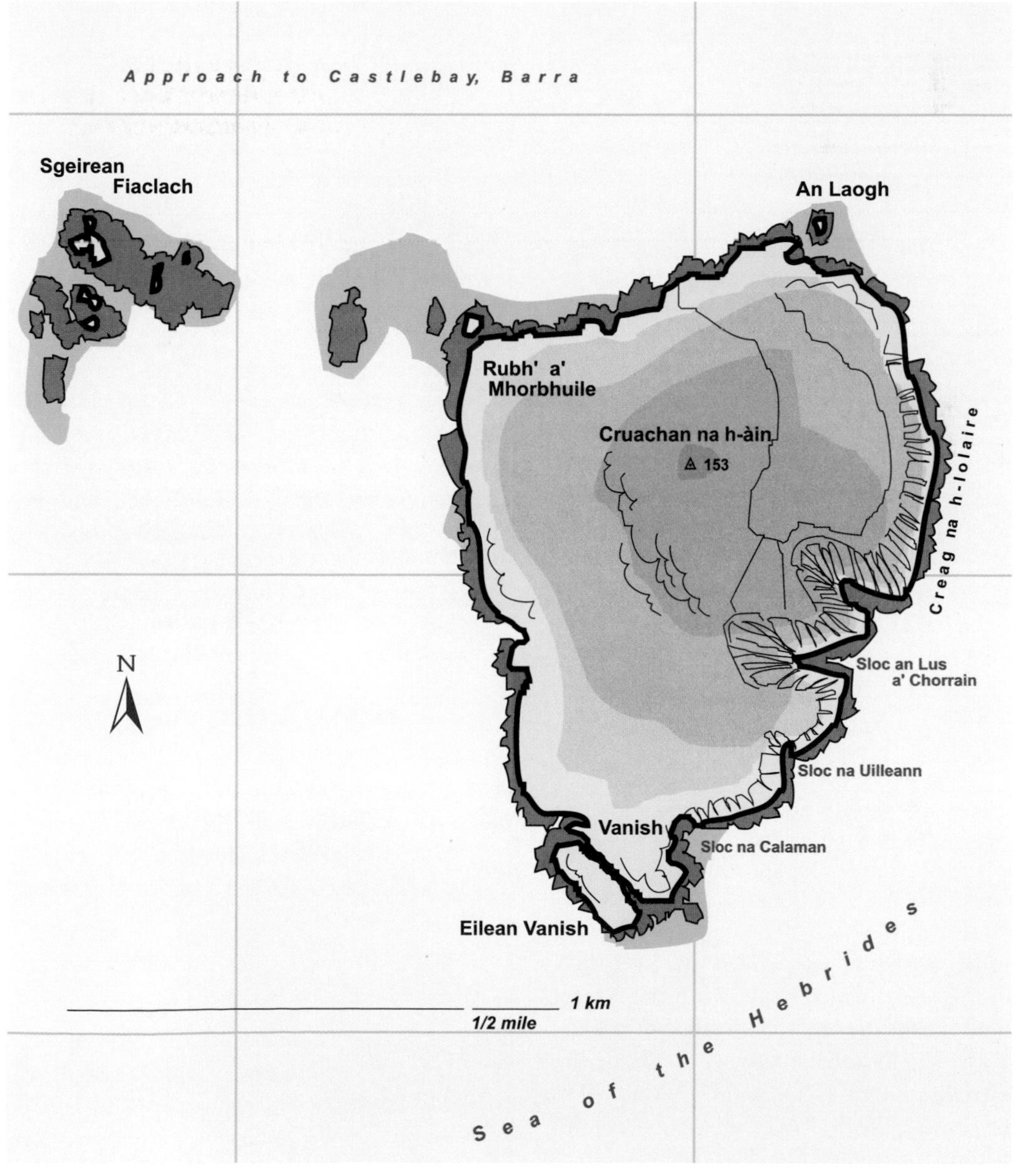

On the north side there is a detached rock called **An Laogh** (G. – the calf) and on the north-west is another detached rock off **Rubh' a' Mhorbhuile** (G. – miracle point).

The southern headland called **Vanish** [vay-neesh] (ON – headland of the house or sacred place) may indicate past habitation of some kind.

* * *

Access: Barra Fishing Charters, 01871-890384. Island Adventures, Castlebay, 01871-810284. Tourist Information, Castlebay, Barra, 01871-810336.

Anchorage: No recommended anchorages.

1. Temp. anchorage is possible in suitable conditions NE of Rubh' a' Mhorbhuile but beware foul ground north and west of this headland.

7.6 Barra

(ON Barr-øy – Barr's island). Barr was a 6th-century saint (G. Finbar – St Barr). He was an Irish missionary and disciple of St Columba who is reputed to have been sent to Barra because his predecessor had been eaten by the inhabitants.

Vatersay

Probably (ON – fathers' island), priest island. (ON vottr-øy – glove island), from the finger-shaped peninsulas? or (ON vatr-øy – wavy island), have also been suggested.

O S Maps: 1:50000 Sheet 31 1:25000 Sheet 452
Admiralty Charts: 1:100000 No.1796 1:30000 Nos 2769 and 2770

Area: 6,835ha (16,889 acres)
Height: 383m (1,256 ft)

Owner: About 9000 acres of Barra was owned by the 46th clan chief, the MacNeil of Barra – Ian MacNeil, an American law professor of Northwestern University, Chicago, who now lives in Edinburgh. In 2003 he gifted nearly all the land, including fishing and mineral rights, to the Scottish Executive who will manage it until the community wishes to take it over. The Scottish Executive already owned the crofts in the north of the island so this made a total holding of some 440 crofts. The MacNeil family will continue their long association with Barra and Clan MacNeil by visits to Kisimul Castle, their home at Garrygall, and meeting their many friends and acquaintances.

The Scottish Office owns Vatersay which the Scottish Board of Agriculture bought in 1909 for £6250.

Population: Barra only:1755–1150. 1794–1604.

	1841	1881	1891	1931	1961	1981	1991	2001
Barra	1977	1869	2131	2001	1369	1264	1244	1078
V'say	84	19	32	240	95	107	72	94
	2061	1888	2163	2241	1464	1371	1316	1172

Geology: The island, of heavily glaciated gneiss, has a rocky and broken east coast and fine, sandy bays on the west coast backed by machair. East of the central fault line the gneiss has been sheared to give a belt of mylonite, or flinty crush. A mile-long coral reef lies at a depth of 100m off Barra's coast.

History: Following the centuries of Norse domination Alexander, Lord of the Isles, granted a charter to Gilleonan MacNeil in 1427, and this was confirmed by James IV in 1495. Some say that MacNeil ownership actually goes back to 1030. The family is reputed to be descended from Niall of the Nine Hostages, the 4th-century High King of Ireland. By the 16th century the MacNeils were using Castlebay on the island as a pirate base for raids on the ships of the English Queen Elizabeth. MacNeil explained to James VI (James I) that his actions were merely because 'that woman' had killed his mother (Mary Queen of Scots). The comment saved his life. The MacNeils were keen sailors and it is said by some that an invitation from Noah to a MacNeil of Barra to sail with him on his ark was turned down by MacNeil because he had a boat of his own.

Martin Martin in the 18th century said that when the islanders were too old to work the MacNeil chief would take them into his household and provide for them. Boswell recounts the Earl of Argyll's comment on receiving a letter from MacNeil of Barra – 'His style of letter runs as if he were of another kingdom.'

By 1838 the 21st chief General Roderick MacNeil was so heavily in debt that he had to sell the island. It went for £38,050 to Colonel Gordon of Cluny who had also bought Benbecula, South Uist and Eriskay. Without any consideration for the islanders the colonel offered Barra to the Government for use as a penal settlement – an offer which was not accepted. Then in 1851 on the grounds of receiving insufficient rent he imported

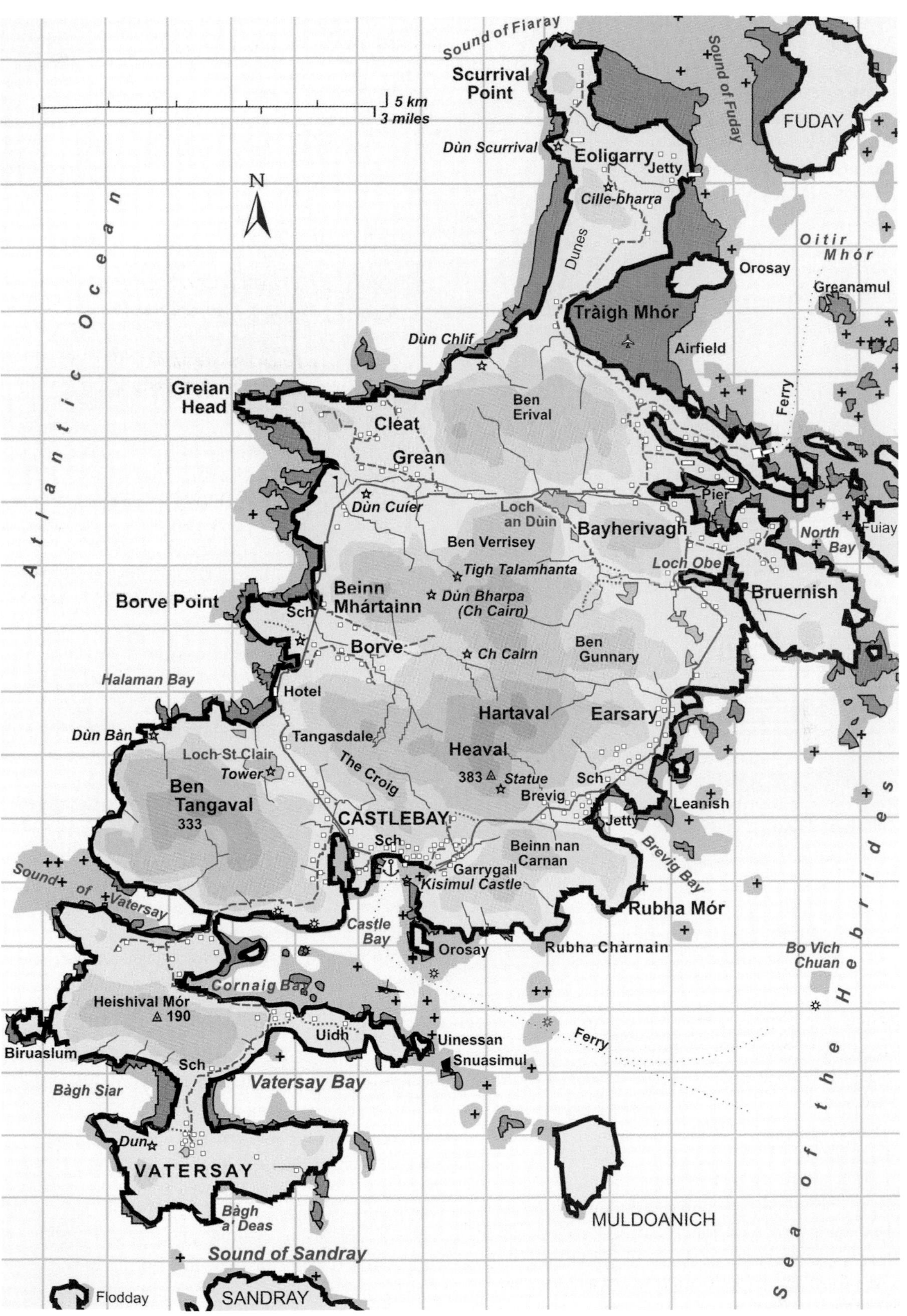
Sound of Fiaray
Scurrival Point
5 km
3 miles
Dùn Scurrival
Eoligarry
Jetty
Cille-bharra
Sound of Fuday
FUDAY
N
Atlantic Ocean
Dunes
Orosay
Oitir Mhór
Greanamul
Tràigh Mhór
Airfield
Dùn Chlif
Ferry
Greian Head
Cleat
Grean
Ben Erival
Dùn Cuíer
Loch an Dùin
Pier
Bayherivagh
North Bay
Fuiay
Ben Verrisey
Loch Obe
Tigh Talamhanta
Bruernish
Borve Point
Beinn Mhártainn
Sch
Dùn Bharpa (Ch Cairn)
Borve
Ch Cairn
Ben Gunnary
Halaman Bay
Hotel
Hartaval
Earsary
Dùn Bàn
Tangasdale
Heaval
Loch St Clair
Tower
The Croig
383
Statue
Sch
Ben Tangaval
333
Brevig
Leanish
CASTLEBAY
Jetty
Sch
Beinn nan Carnan
Brevig Bay
Sound of Vatersay
Garrygall
Kisimul Castle
Rubha Mór
Castle Bay
Orosay
Rubha Chàrnain
Bo Vich Chuan
Cornaig Bay
Heishival Mór
190
Uidh
Uinessan
Ferry
Biruaslum
Snuasimul
Sch
Bàgh Siar
Vatersay Bay
Sea of the Hebrides
Dun
VATERSAY
Bàgh a' Deas
MULDOANICH
Sound of Sandray
Flodday
SANDRAY

policemen to clear the island of its crofters, confiscate their stock and belongings, and send them penniless to the New World. These were some of the most cruel and shameful cases of inhumanity ever seen on the West Coast. In 1858 when the colonel died he was said to be the richest commoner in Scotland. Barra and its few survivors then passed to Lady Gordon Cathcart and her husband, who, in their dealings with both Barra and Vatersay, followed in the unlamented colonel's footsteps.

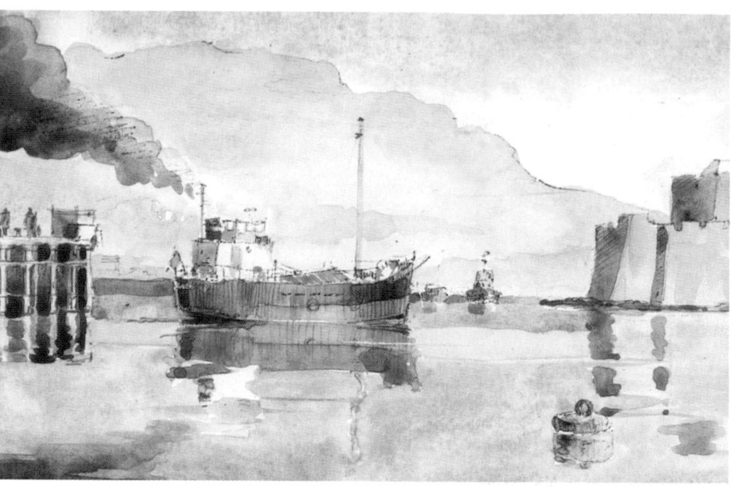

PUFFER IN CASTLEBAY

Most of Barra was bought back in 1937 from the Cathcart estate by Robert Lister MacNeil, who had been recognised by the Lyon King of Arms as the Clan's 45th chieftain. In 1979 the laird offered to transfer the freehold of all the crofting land to the crofters for only £30,000 but the crofters for various reasons preferred to keep to the traditional arrangement.

Wildlife: Over 150 bird species and 400 plant species have been recorded. This is comparable with the rest of the Outer Hebrides but the island is particularly noted for the profuseness of both its wildflowers and its butterflies.

* * *

There are spectacular views from both of the highest hills on **BARRA**, **Heaval** (383m) and **Ben Tangaval** (333m). Little idea of the island's size can be gained at Castlebay but from the top of Heaval one can see great rolling hills to the north and the wide sweep of the Borve Valley dropping down to the sandy west coast. But take care when walking in these hills for the mists and sudden climatic changes have given rise to many ghost stories and mysterious disappearances. There are enjoyable walks from Garrygall to Brevig, Ben Tangaval to Tangasdale and Glen Dorcha to Northbay. **Northbay** is a second harbour for the island. It is beyond the **Black Islands**, which are south of **Lamalum** islet, and in a sheltered corner but it is a rather rocky, bleak, and uninspiring area.

A pleasantly energetic 18km hill-walk from Castlebay can include climbing the five highest summits (1040m or 3400ft of total ascent). Heaval – 396m ascent, Hartaval – 60m, Greanan and Corrabheinn – 76m, then west by **Dùn Bharpa** chambered cairn [NF672019] to Beinn Mhártainn – 122m, down to sea-level and 4km along the coast road before climbing Ben Tangaval, over the top, and back down to Castlebay.

Another interesting walk is from Cleat past Ardmhor with its seals and bird life to **Vaslane Sands**. There is reputed to be an underground passage running from Cleat to **Uaimh an Oir** (G. – cave of gold) on the east coast. Two hairless mad dogs which emerged from Uaimh an Oir were reported to have entered the Cleat cave with their masters several days before but the men were never seen again. (This is another example of the standard Hebridean cave tale.)

In the late 19th century, **Castlebay**, the principal town, was a very active and prosperous herring port with a fleet of over 400 boats using the harbour. This was started by James Methuen in 1869 with associated curing and packing industries to take advantage of the herring boom. Castlebay has shops, a post-office, tourist office, schools, hotels, a bank and a cottage hospital and its residents are cheerful and good-natured. In fact, Barra is full of friendly people.

The medieval fortress of **Kisimul Castle** (?ON – tax or tribute mound) which includes a keep, hall and castle is built below the town on a rocky island outcrop in the bay. The first fortifications were built in the 11th century but the present building dates from the 15th century. Beneath the castle there is a very convenient geological pipe which provides a supply of fresh water to a well. A herald used to proclaim from the Great Tower: 'Hear ye people and listen ye nations. The great MacNeil of Barra having finished his meal, the princes of the earth may dine.' The castle was burned down in 1795. The MacNeils had to sell Barra in 1838 due to debt but the 45th Chief of the Clan MacNeil, Robert Lister MacNeil, an American architect, bought back the ancestral home in 1937 together with almost half of Barra. He restored the castle which had been uninhabited for more than 200 years and turned it into a place of pilgrimage for MacNeils from all over the world. He died in 1970 and is buried in the castle chapel. In 2000 his son leased the castle to Historic Scotland for £1 and a bottle of Talisker whisky a year to ensure its upkeep for the MacNeil clan and as a visitor attraction.

Cars can be hired in Castlebay but it is possible to have a strenuous walk round the island in an afternoon. One of the world's most exciting airfields, a great sweep of beach in the north of the island called **Tràigh Mhór** or the Cockle Strand is covered at every tide. In the 18th century as many as 200 cartloads of live cockles were collected from this famous beach every day during times of famine. There is talk of building a hard airstrip here as few aircraft are now suitable for beach landings, but opinions are, naturally, divided on the consequences. Worse still, there is the threat of closure of this vital lifeline.

The 1745 Jacobite rebellion led to the chief of the Clan MacNeil being imprisoned for implication in the revolt although he had taken no active part. Two years later the clan moved its headquarters from Castlebay to **Eoligarry** in the extreme north of the island. A small cemetery here, **Cille-bharraidh** [NF705074], is the burial ground of the MacNeils. The only Hebridean example of a Norse sculpted stone (which is now in the National Museum of Antiquities in Edinburgh) was found here among the three ancient chapels and interesting tombstones dating back to the 14th century. Sir Compton Mackenzie, the famous novelist who made Barra his home, is also buried here in sight of Eriskay (See No.7.13) – the setting for his novel *Whisky Galore*. It was at *Suidheachan*, his home by Tràigh Mhór, that Sir Compton and John Lorne Campbell formed the Sea League in the 1930s to try to persuade the Government to protect local fishermen.

A prehistoric galleried fort, **Dùn Scurrival** [NF695080], is beside a cave near Eoligarry.

A hotel set in striking scenery with an outlook over the wild Atlantic at **Halaman Bay** on the west coast was used as a hideout by the children of the Shah in the lead-up to the Iranian Revolution. Their nurse came from Barra. Across the sand dunes from it is fresh-water **Loch St Clair**, stocked with trout and with Castle Sinclair perched on an islet [NL648996]. Nearby is

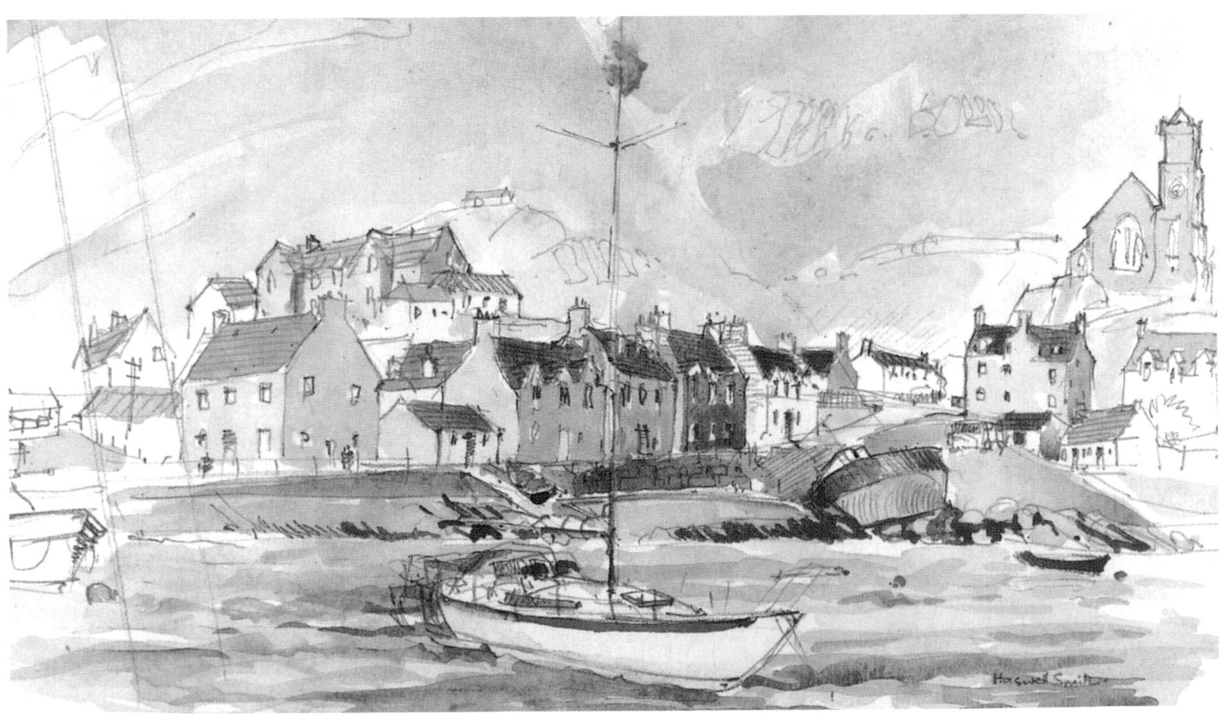

CASTLEBAY

Barra's perfumery where visitors are welcome.

The island is predominantly Catholic and on the slopes of **Heaval** is a white Carrara marble statue of the Madonna and Child [NL679992].

The remains of a fine chambered cairn [NF677012] are further north on the west slope of Grianan, and there are a pair of standing stones [NF653015], said to mark the grave of a Norse warrior killed by a local champion, on the way to Borve Point. An old burial ground and black houses are nearby.

* * *

VATERSAY, whose economy is based on sheep – and cattle – farming, and fishing, is linked to Barra by a long-awaited causeway which was completed in 1990 at a cost of £3.8m. To send the cattle to market they traditionally swam across the Sound of Vatersay to Barra to meet the ferry but when a prize bull, Bernie, drowned in 1986 the resulting publicity at last helped to persuade the Government to build the causeway.

In 1853 off the west coast of Vatersay the *Annie Jane* ran aground and capsized. The bodies of 450 emigrants bound for the New World were washed ashore.

Lady Gordon Cathcart owned Vatersay for a period of fifty-four years but only visited it once. Her tenant ran the island as a single farm. At the turn of the century the demand for land by the crofters of Barra was so great that pressure was put on her to sell land for crofting. She refused, so, in 1906, an ambitious crofter landed on Vatersay and laid claim to some land. Others copied him and these men became known as the **Vatersay Raiders**. They were brought to trial and imprisoned for a time. There was a public outcry and in 1909 a Government Board bought the island and divided it into fifty-eight crofts.

The highest hill on Vatersay is **Heishival Mór** at 190m. Entering the Sound of Vatersay by sea from the east you pass a small tidal island called **Uinessan** with the remains of a church on it [NL665956]. This is known as the Chapel of Mary of the Heads. (Apparently Mary was a short-tempered islander who beheaded anyone who upset her.) **Snuasimul** islet east of Uinessan marks a narrow but navigable shortcut between Vatersay Bay and Castle Bay. Avoid all other shortcuts.

* * *

Access: Vehicle ferry (summer) from: Oban to Castlebay, every day; return every day except Sat.: Lochboisdale to Castlebay, Mon., Tues., and Thur.; return, Wed., Fri., Sun., 08000-66-5000. Vehicle ferry: Eriskay/ Barra, frequent daily service, 08000-66-5000. Island post bus circuit includes airport and ferry terminals, 01871-810312. Scheduled air service: Glasgow/ Barra, and Benbecula/ Barra daily except Sun., 0870-850-9850. Hotel accommodation. Bicycle hire. Fishing permits from Post Office. Tourist Information, 01871-810336.

Anchorages:

1. Bagh Beag, Castlebay. Good shelter but tricky narrow channel with only 1.3m at half-tide and inadequate information on chart. Risky.
2. Castle Bay, NW of castle. 12 visitors' moorings, or anchor in 6m, mud, holding poor unless well bedded-in. Avoid obstructing ferry pier. Reasonable shelter except S'lies.
3. Castle Bay, NE of castle. Good shelter but very limited space between drying rocks and moored craft, 3.5–5m or close W of the castle in 7m mud.
4. North Bay on E coast affords good shelter. Anchor in Bruernish Bay, in inlet W of the Black Isles or continue into N side of Bagh Hirivagh and anchor 2c W of the jetty if there is room. Not the most attractive anchorage. There are other options among the islets NW of Fuiay.
5. Oitir Mór in the Sound of Barra. Best approach N of Gighay and pass 5c N of Greanamul midway between the beacons. Anchor SE of freshwater stream on Fuday in clay and sand, with some weed. Unpleasant in E'lies. Beware rock in bay.
6. Eoligarry Jetty, about 6¼c NNW of N side of Orosay is a tidal harbour with pier where small craft might find shelter.
7. Sound of Fiaray is a possible anchorage but the approach is difficult and potentially dangerous.
8. W coast of Barra has no anchorages but the Admiralty Pilot records one landing place amongst the rocks 1M S of Greian Head.
9. Sound of Vatersay. Some useful shelter may be found in the the Sound where it is blocked by the causeway. Beware rocks at entrance.
10. W coast of Vatersay has no anchorages. Bagh Siar has moderate depth and sandy bottom but no shelter.
11. Vatersay Bay – good anchorage. Enter passing 2–3c S of Muldoanich and then steer centrally for the bay. Anchor W of Sgeir Vichalea in suitable depth, sand.
12. Cornaig Bay, S of causeway and Orosay. Pipeline, cable and rocks to be avoided but well sheltered from SW.
13. Causeway bay, between causeway and Orosay is a useful anchorage but pipeline and cable must be avoided.

7.7 Flodday

(ON floti – a raft or flat island) This island is east of Barra. There is another smaller Flodday south-west of Barra which does not appear to have ever been inhabited.

O S Maps: 1:50000 Sheet 31 1:25000 Sheet 452
Admiralty Charts: 1:100000 No.1796 1:30000 No.2770

Area: 40ha (99 acres)
Height: 42m (138 ft)

Population: 1841–7 (1 house). The island was cleared in the mid-19th century and has been uninhabited since then.

Geology: The bulk of the island is made up of gneiss with a sufficient covering of soil to provide good grazing.

Wildlife: The low-lying nature of the island gives encouragement to only a few seabirds but rock-pipit and twite can be seen and may even be resident.

FLODDAY rises gradually to a height of 42m and is covered with grass and heather, but Rubh' a' Chaolais (G. – the kyle headland) in the south-west is bare and rocky. Opposite it in the south-east is the equally barren Grey Rock. It is an easy island to explore but has few features of any particular interest.

The 1991 Census quotes Flodday as having

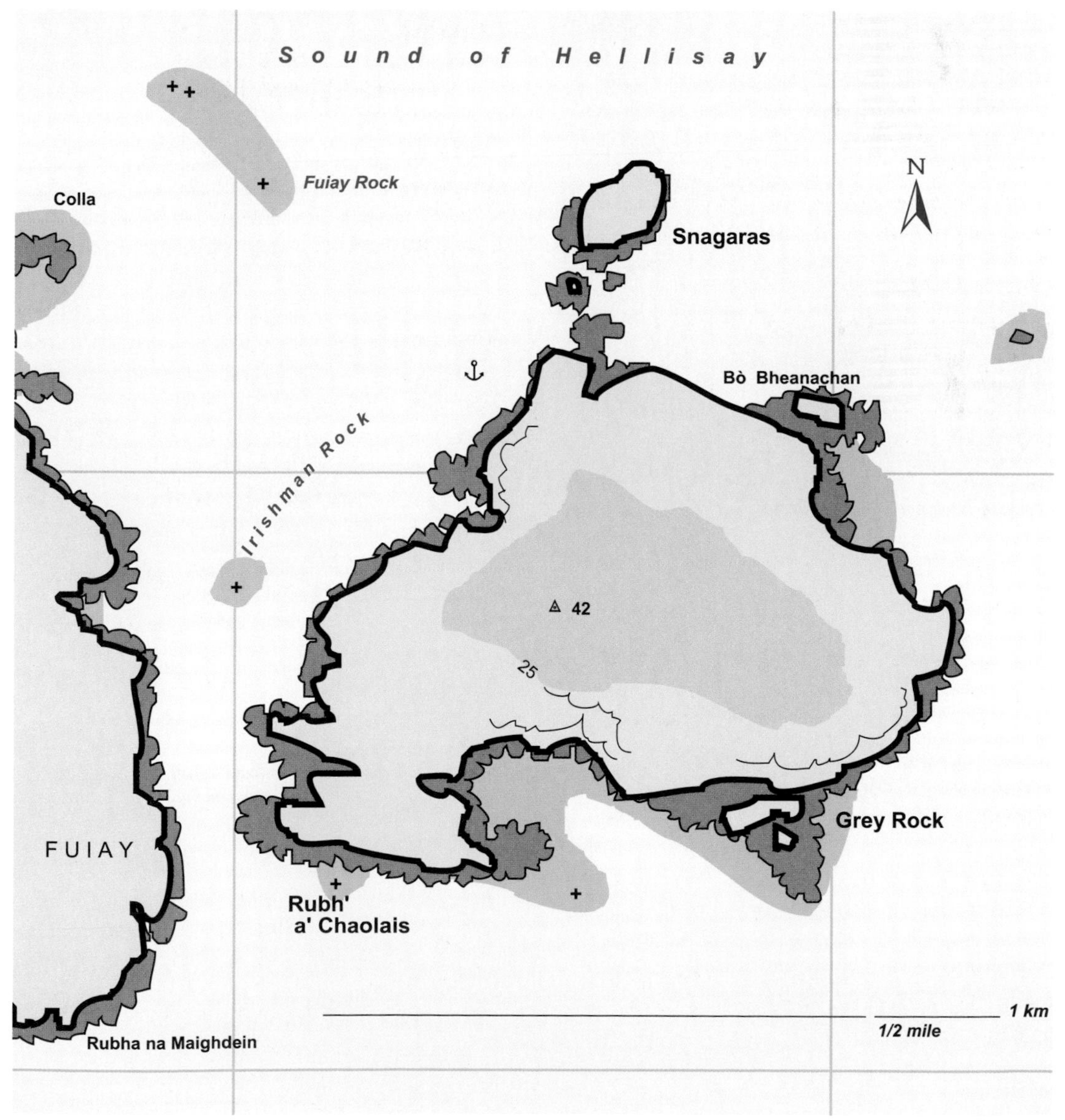

a population of eight but this refers in fact to the tidal island which is part of Benbecula in the Civil Parish of South Uist and should not be confused with this Flodday. The name was very popular and applied freely to any flat island.

Flodday never appears to have supported more than one family and it was cleared for sheep by Colonel Gordon of Cluny in 1851. It has no reliable source of fresh water so water would have had to be brought in by boat when there were long dry spells.

A small, drying islet off the north extremity called **Snagaras** lies at the end of a reef.

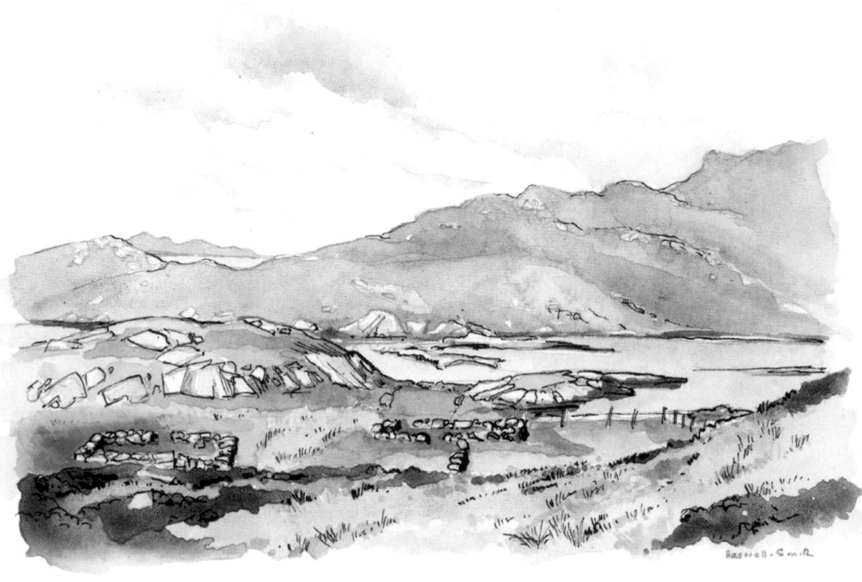

RUINED HOUSES BY THE TIDAL LOCH, FUIAY

* * *

Access: Barra Fishing Charters, 01871-890384. Island Adventures, Castlebay, 01871-810284. Tourist Information, Castlebay, Barra, 01871-810336.

Anchorage:

1. The only recommended occasional anchorage is NE of Irishman Rock, W of the N extremity of Flodday, in 13–14m, mud. It may be possible to find a shallower spot (5–6m) in the channel S of Irishman Rock but the bottom is uncertain.

7.8 Fuiay

Probably (G. bhuidhe, ON -øy – yellow or pleasant island).

O S Maps: 1:50000 Sheet 31 1:25000 Sheet 452
Admiralty Charts: 1:100000 No.1796 1:30000 No.2770

Area: 84ha (208 acres)
Height: 107m (351 ft)

Population: The island was populated with at least six households during the 19th century, possibly until about 1850, but I have found no Census records. Uninhabited since.

Geology: Gneiss generally, but large dark slabs of volcanic rock with pronounced cleavage planes.

Wildlife: Rabbits, bracken and heather.

FUIAY is a bit of a puzzle.

Firstly, I have found no record of any population. And yet, **Rubh' an Aiseig** [ash-ug] (G. – ferry headland), has the ruins of a neat village 'street' [NF737027] laid out along the side of the tidal inlet. There were at least six cottages and by comparison with similar ruins elsewhere they were probably occupied until the mid-19th century and possibly later. Of course, the ten-yearly census only started in 1831, and it was fairly sketchy to begin with, so the odds are that Fuiay's inhabitants were included somewhere but not specifically mentioned.

The second mystery, if such it is, is at the tidal inlet. We visited the island at high water and the sea was flowing downhill *into* the inlet. A stony shelf or bar crosses the entrance opposite the ruined cottages and there was about 300mm, or one foot, difference between the two water-levels. The inlet is like a miniature sea-loch when full but is shallow and dries out at low water. Our conclusion was that when the tide ebbs and the outside sea-level falls below the 'floor-level' of the inlet the water in the inlet drains out through the rock strata, but when the tide rises the water cannot seep in fast enough to fill the inlet: the sea therefore floods over the 'bar' when it reaches the required level. This would seem to create a natural fish trap at the spring tides which the islanders must have found very convenient.

Fuiay has a prominent peak (107m) which is almost at the exact centre of the oval-shaped island. The headland in the south-east is called **Rubha na Maighdein** [myjun] (G. – maiden's headland) – a name which begs another intriguing question.

The sea to the north and north-west of Fuiay is littered with islets, skerries, and rocks. The nearest islets are **Eilean Sheumais**, **Colla** (G. – hazel island), and **Sgeirislum**. Beyond these lie **Garbh Lingay** and **Lingay-fhada** (G. – rough heather-isle and long heather-isle).

To the south there are more rocks off Barra's Bruernish peninsula gathered around an islet called **Heilem**. The large lone rock, **Curachan**, is prominent in the south-west with patches of sea-grass on it.

Access: Barra Fishing Charters, 01871-890384. Island Adventures, Castlebay, 01871-810284. Tourist Information, Castlebay, Barra, 01871-810336.

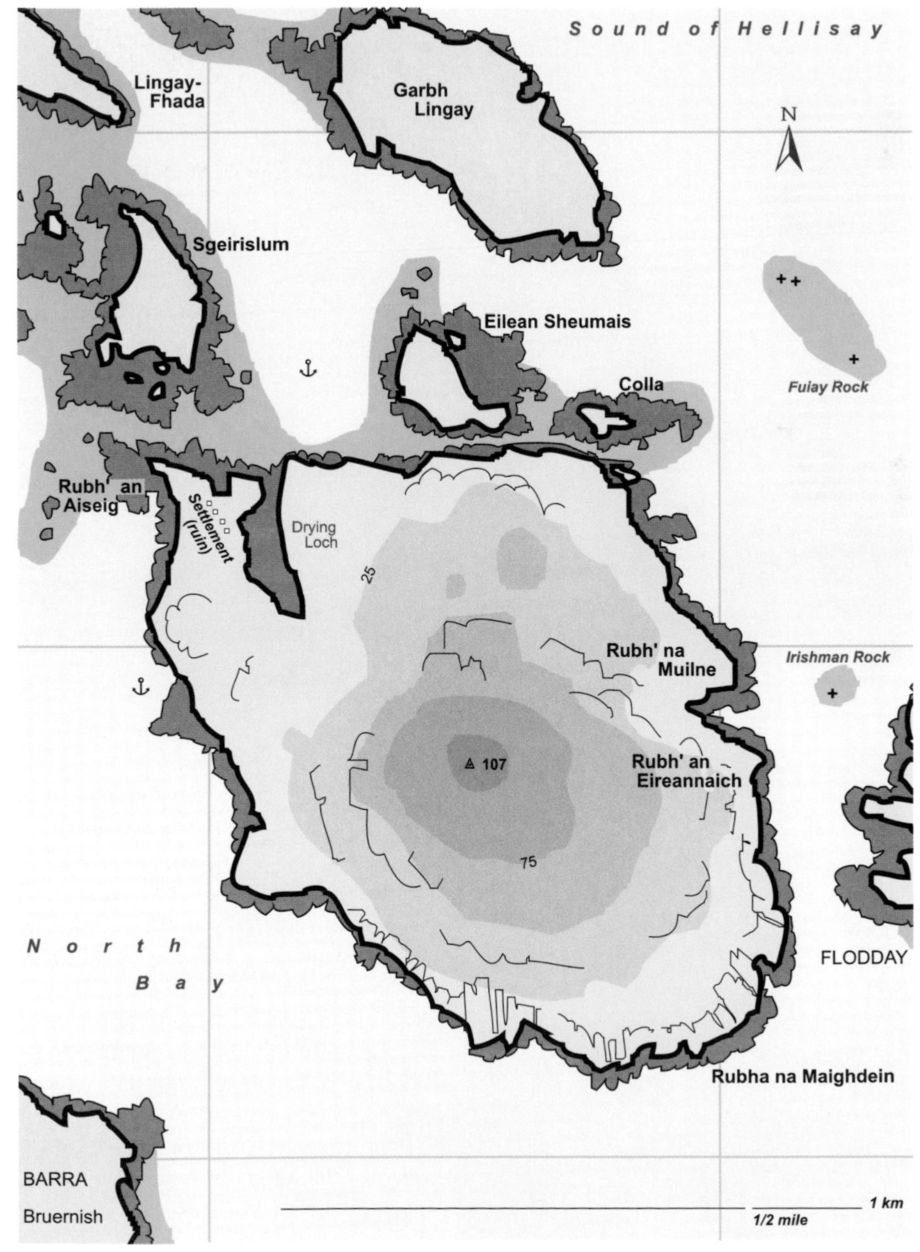

Anchorages: There is a tricky navigable channel through the reefs between Sgeirislum and Fuiay, except possibly at LW.

1. Off N coast. Anchor midway between Sgeirislum and Eilean Sheumais, 5m mud. Good anchorage but partly obstructed by fish-cages. If approaching from E keep close S of Garbh Lingay to avoid rocks N of En Sheumais.

2. W of Rubh' an Aiseig. Occasional anchorage about ½c off-shore and about 3c S of the N extremity of the headland opposite some rocks which form a natural 'jetty', 5–6m mud.

7.9 Hellisay

(ON – island of caves) but Blaeu's map of 1654 uses 'Hildesay' (ON – Hilda's island), which may be more acceptable as the number of caves is not excessive.

OS Maps: 1:50000 Sheet 31 1:25000 Sheet 452
Admiralty Charts: 1:100000 No.1796 1:30000 No.2770

Area: 142ha (351 acres)
Height: 79m (259 ft)

Population: 1764–56. 1841–108. 1851–7.

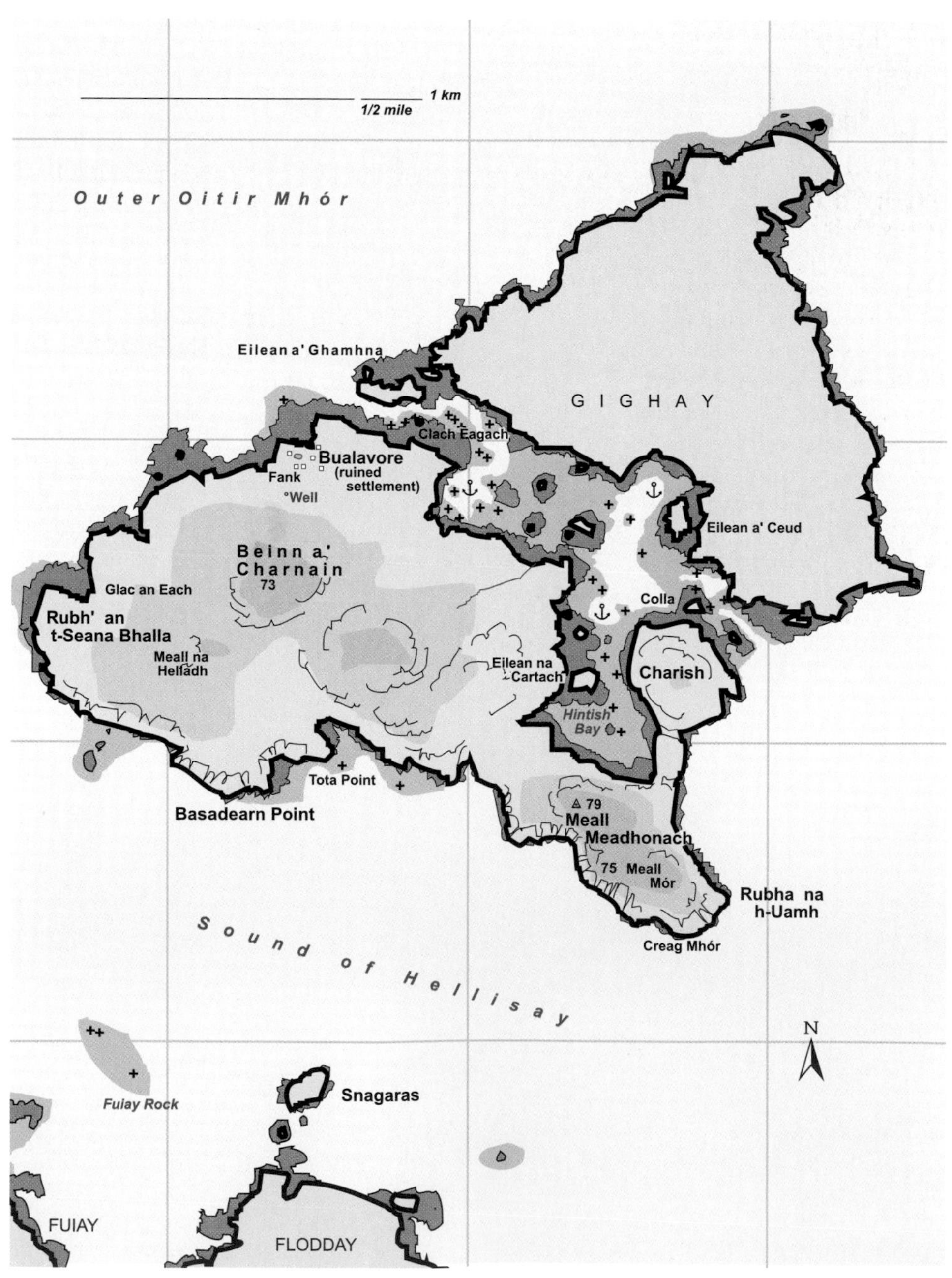

1861–20. 1881–9. Uninhabited since 1890.

Geology: Mainly gneiss with occasional quartz veins.

History: Clearances on the adjoining islands led to an influx of population in the early 1800s. Then in the 1840s the people of Hellisay were themselves evicted and by 1851 there were only seven inhabitants left. Most of the families cleared from Hellisay found refuge on Eriskay.

Wildlife: Every pocket in the rocks above sea-level is filled with sea-thrift. There are many grey seals and apart from sea-birds we saw falcon and a pair of golden eagles.

* * *

There are two distinct peaks on **HELLISAY**, **Meall Meadhonach** (G. – middle mound), in the south-east (79m) and **Beinn a' Charnain** (G. – cairn hill), in the north-west (73m). Meall Meadhonach has a vertical face over 60m high on its west side with distinctive orange lichen near the top. It is on a peninsula which finishes steeply at **Rubha na h-Uamh** (G. – cave headland). **Meall Mór** (G. – big mound) is on this peninsula and is virtually an extension of Meall Meadhonach [meeoo-unuch]. At 75m it is not as high, but its position is more prominent.

The most westerly part of the island is **Rubh' an t-Seana Bhalla** (G. – headland of the ancient wall). Most of the island is rocky and uneven and it is difficult to see how it could have supported over 100 inhabitants at one time, even with the advantage of good fishing in the Sound of Barra. The main settlement was on the lower ground at **Bualavore** [NF754046].

The easiest landing place by dinghy in Hintish Bay is in the south-east corner. On the outside of the neck of land the sea surges into a narrow rock cleft with a noise like severe indigestion. From here there is a pleasant scramble up Meall Mór and Meadhonach with extensive views from the top.

Hellisay is an island rich in fairy tales and myths. The stories of Alasdair Alpin MacGregor tell of a magic land of strange happenings remembered by the old folk on winter nights by the peat fire.

Access: Barra Fishing Charters, 01871-890384. Island Adventures, Castlebay, 01871-810284. Tourist Information, Castlebay, Barra, 01871-810336.

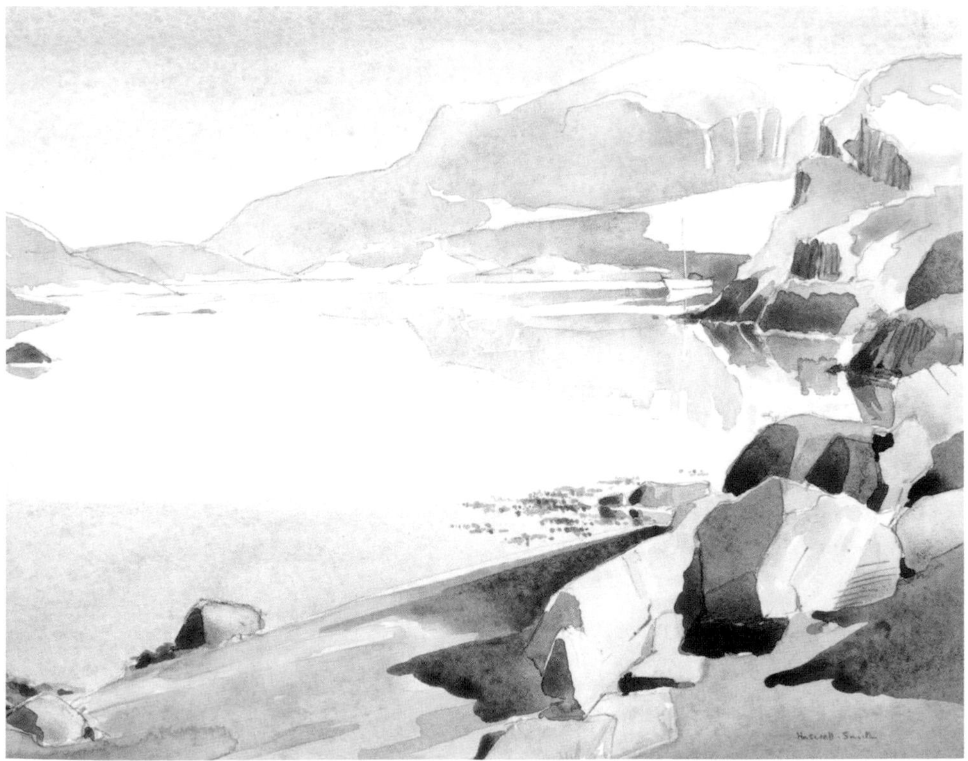

THE SECRET ANCHORAGE BETWEEN GIGHAY AND HELLISAY

Anchorages: The anchorages are in the sound between the two islands. Entrance to the sound is tricky and there may be uncharted rocks.

1. Hintish Bay. In the SE part of the sound, anchor NW of Charish. Excellent shelter, good holding, sand and mud.
2. Pool in W part of the sound, ENE of Beinn a' Charnain. Many submerged rocks.

7.10 Gighay

(ON – Gydha's island) Gydha was a woman's name in Old Norse.

O S Maps: 1:50000 Sheet 31 1:25000 Sheet 452
Admiralty Charts: 1:100000 No.1796 1:30000 No.2770

Area: 96ha (237 acres)
Height: 95m (312 ft)

Population: Dean Monro recorded that Gighay

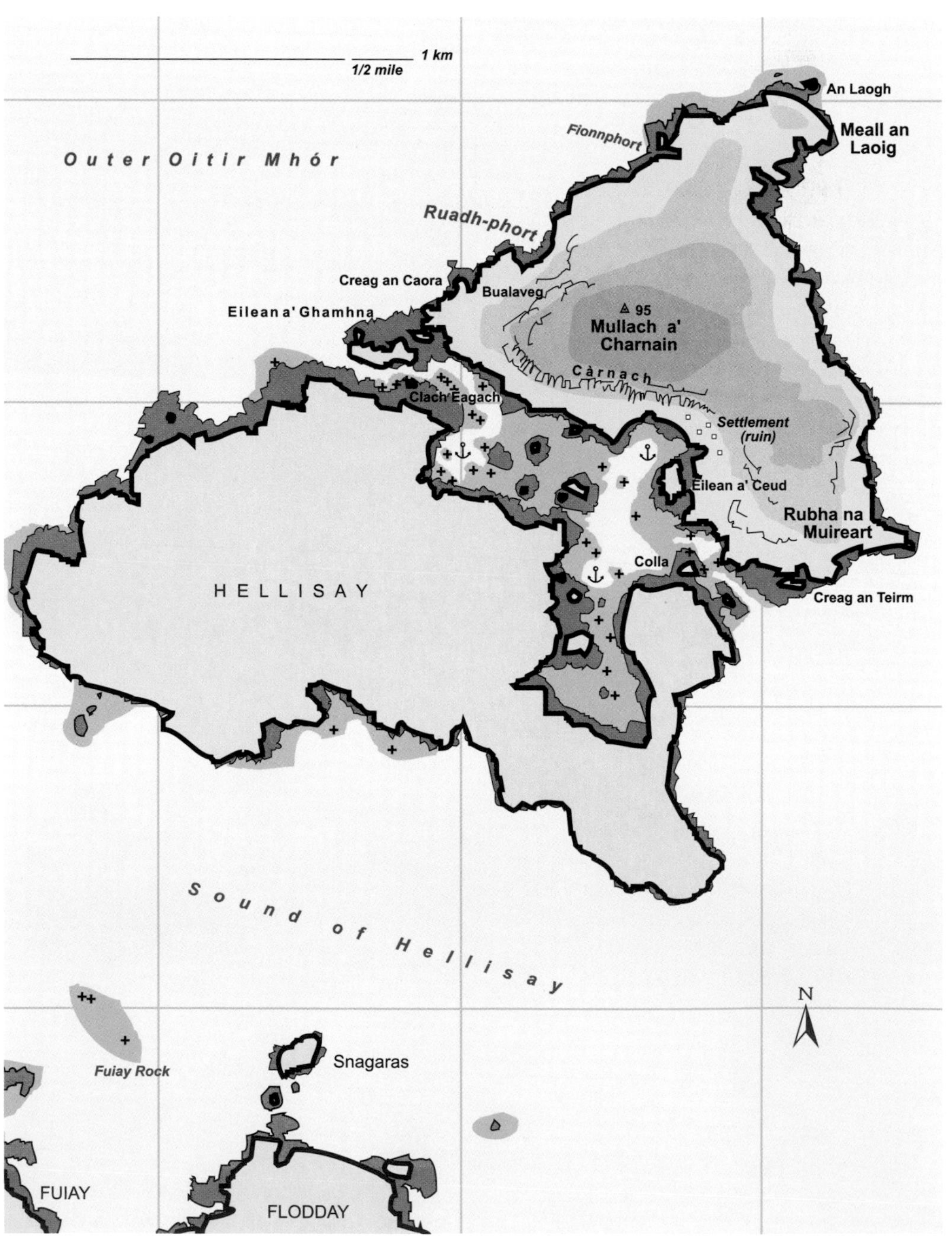

was inhabited in 1549, but there is no other information. The island was known to be inhabited at the end of the 18th century but it has been deserted for a long time and there are no Census records.

Geology: Mainly gneiss. The Hebridean Fault Line runs approximately NE–SW at Eilean a' Ceud and Hintish Bay.

History: It is probable that the increase in population recorded for Hellisay during the Clearances in the mid-19th century overflowed on to neighbouring Gighay.

Wildlife: Heather is fairly widespread – mainly calluna with very little erica. Banks of nettles surround the areas of former human habitation. The wet areas have marsh marigolds and yellow flag among the reeds and there are daisies and wild violets on the slopes.

Rats frequent the area near the sheep-dip.

When we visited Gighay it was the month of May. Oystercatchers were busy on the shore, skylarks larking in the sky, and an eagle was being mobbed by falcons above Mullach a' Charnain's cliffs.

* * *

Like its sister island, Hellisay, **GIGHAY** is another magical place, no doubt given additional charm by the fairly difficult entry into its secret anchorage. Because *Jandara*, having achieved entry, was trapped until the tide rose again the feeling of isolation was exaggerated. We were marooned.

The easiest landing place was in the bay behind **Eilean a' Ceud** [ked] (G. – hundred island). Only the sheep and sheep pens beneath the bluff destroyed the impression that man had not set foot on the island for many years.

This is the area that was once inhabited because among the reeds, nettles and bracken there are still signs of the old habitations. Over a dozen are easily discovered – small, rude, stone dwellings giving an impression of desperate poverty; and on the opposite slope of the bay, to the northwest, there are the regular striations of old lazybeds.

A short visit here is delightful, particularly in fine spring weather but the islanders' existence must have been finely balanced. Gighay is barren enough in late spring – what must it be like during the long winter months? Only the inland sea, the Sound of Gighay, sheltered between the islands, could tip the scales by providing all-weather fishing with nothing but seals for competition.

The highest peak **Mullach a' Charnain** (G. – cairn summit), 95m high, has a steep cliff on its south-west side above the anchorage. There is also a high flat point in the extreme north-east ending in a hummock called **Meall an Laoigh** (G. – calf hill). The calf itself, **An Laogh**, is a miniature stack at the end of this promontory. Round the corner, on the exposed north-west coast there is an indentation with enough space to draw small boats ashore called **Ruadh-phort** (G. – red port).

Although the anchorage beside Eilean a' Ceud is excellent, if the wind is in the north or north-west squally gusts can come tumbling over the cliff. In that case it is better to cross the sound to the Hellisay side, but remember that at high water a large reef crossing most of Hintish Bay is not visible.

* * *

Access: Barra Fishing Charters, 01871-890384. Island Adventures, Castlebay, 01871-810284. Tourist Information, Castlebay, Barra, 01871-810336.

Anchorages: The anchorages are in the sound between Gighay and Hellisay. Entrance to the sound can be tricky, depends on the state of the sea and the tide, and there may be uncharted rocks.

1. In the small bay NW of Eilean a' Ceud, thick mud.
2. Pool in W part of the sound just S of the line between Mullach a' Charnain on Gighay and Beinn a' Charnain on Hellisay. Many submerged rocks.

7.11 Fuday

Possibly (ON fut-øy – bailiwick or bailiff's island) or (ON ut-øy – outside isle).

O S Maps: 1:50000 Sheet 31 1:25000 Sheet 452
Admiralty Charts: 1:100000 No.1796 1:30000 No.2770

Area: 232ha (573 acres)
Height: 89m (292 ft)

Population: Walker's list for 1764 gives a population of 56 for 'Fuda' but doesn't mention the island of Hellisay (No.7.9). Yet in 1841 Hellisay had 108 and Fuday only 5. Francis

Thompson says that Hellisay was sometimes known in Gaelic as 'An t-eilean Fuideach' which may be the cause of confusion. 1841–5 (1 house). 1861–7. 1881–6. 1891–7 (1 house). 1901–4. Uninhabited since.

Geology: The island is covered with grass on a core of Archaean gneiss and with a wide sand-based shelf on the west side.

History: Fuday is supposed to have been the last retreat of those Norsemen, a small section of King Haakon's defeated forces, who remained in the Hebrides after the Battle of Largs in 1263. According to tradition, an illegitimate son of MacNeil of Barra wished to ingratiate himself with his family. He managed to attract the attention of one of the Norse maidens and courted her assiduously. She fell in love with him and through her he gained detailed information about the Norse defences. He then led a raid on the island and wiped out the entire population.

Wildlife: Seabirds nest on the southern headland, Rubha nan Eun (G. – headland of the birds) and

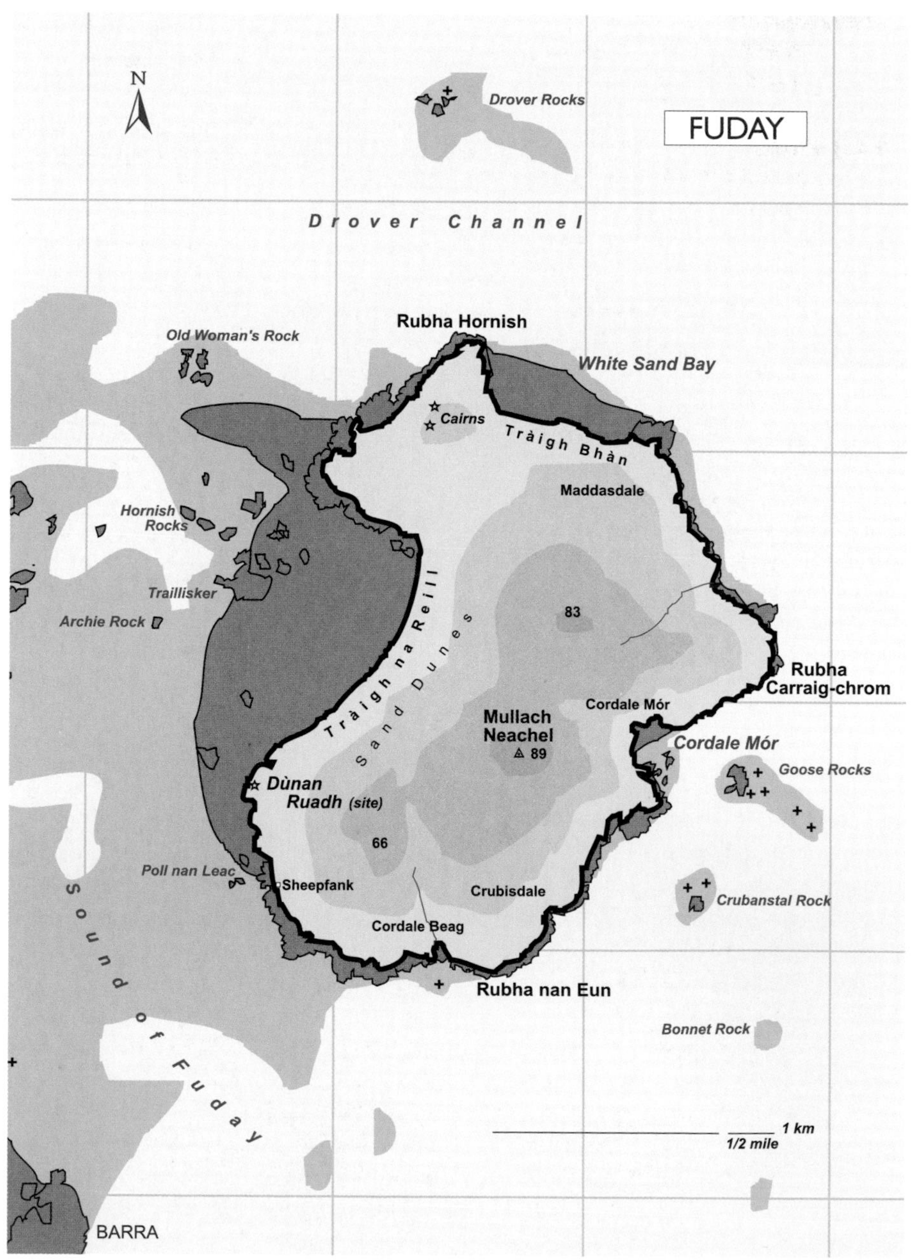

among the sand dunes on the west coast. Otters have also been seen here.

Tradition says that **FUDAY** was a Norse burial ground. Certainly graves can still be seen in the sand, built of rounded stones. The Norse liked to have a quiet island for the dead to rest in peace although, if the MacNeil massacre actually took place, it is uncertain who buried the dead. At the north end of the island, **Ru Hornish**, there are two cairns which are evidence that the Norse were not the first inhabitants.

The Sound of Fuday which separates the island from the Eoligarry peninsula of Barra is full of rocks and shifting sandbanks and at low water it is sometimes only a few centimetres deep but it can be navigated with care at the right state of the tide.

The island rises to three rather flat hills. The central hill, **Mullach Neachel** (G. – lone summit) is 89m high with a slightly lower hill to the north. The westward slope runs down to a wide expanse of high sand-dunes and a great stretch of beach, **Tràigh na Reill**, exposed by the low tide. South-west of Mullach Neachel and joined to it is a small hill called **Dùnan Ruadh** (G. – the red heap). A crystal clear burn runs from the saddle of this hill down to Cordale Beag on the south coast where it discharges into the sea. On the east side a rock-strewn sandy cove, **Cordale Mór** (G. and ON – the big tapering valley) is sheltered from the north by Rubha Carraig-chrom (G. – cliff-ridge point) and on the north coast there is a wide attractive beach, **Tràigh Bhàn**, or White Sand – a white chalk-mark on a blue ground when seen from across the Sound of Barra.

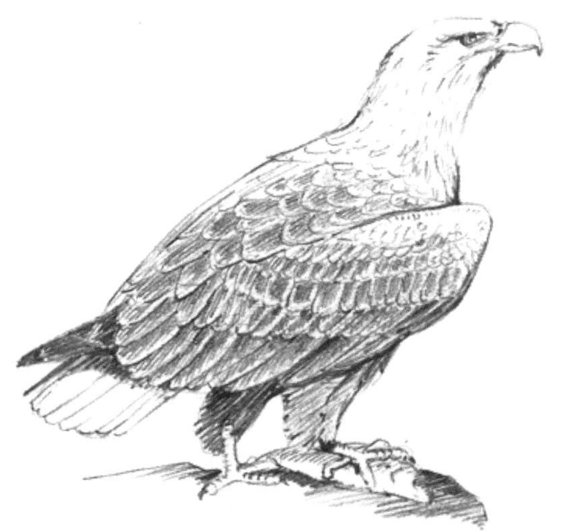

WHITE-TAILED SEA EAGLE

Greanamul is an islet which provides a useful point of reference when approaching Fuday from the south because navigating in this area of skerries and shifting sand-banks requires care.

* * *

Access: Barra Fishing Charters, 01871-890384. Island Adventures, Castlebay, 01871-810284. Tourist Information, Castlebay, Barra, 01871-810336.

Anchorages: No recommended anchorages.

1. Cordale Beag. Best approach N of Gighay and pass 5c N of Greanamul midway between the beacons. Anchor SE of freshwater stream by Rubha nan Eun. Clay and sand, with some weed. Unpleasant in E'lies. Beware rock in bay.
2. Cordale Mór. Temporary anchorage NW Goose Rocks, outside the bay, 4–6m, sand. Very careful navigation required. Goose Rocks cover so best to approach near LW.

7.12 Fiaray

(G. feur – grass or pasture, ON -øy – island).

O S Maps: 1:50000 Sheet 31 1:25000 Sheet 452
Admiralty Charts: 1:100000 No.1796 1:30000 No.2770

Area: 41ha (101 acres)
Height: 30m (98 ft)

Population: No Census records and uninhabited.

Geology: Archaean gneiss with a sandy soil.

Wildlife: A favourite staging-post for barnacle geese.

* * *

Except for two small hillocks on the west side, **FIARAY** is a flat and featureless island. The most northerly hill is the highest at 30m. There is a distinctive sandy promontory at the east side called **Corran Bàn** (G. – white sickle-shaped tapering point) and a seaweed-covered headland on the other side of the island facing the Atlantic called **Gruagach** (G. – beautiful head of hair). The original shielings were at **Port a' Tuim Bàn** (G. – port of the white knoll) near Corran Bàn.

Fiaray boasts, which is remarkable for such a tiny island, two little lochans and it is entirely surrounded by a drying reef. Some local fishermen would swear that this is the home of a fairy woman, often seen by passing boats.

In a collection of folk stories the Rev. Fr. Allan

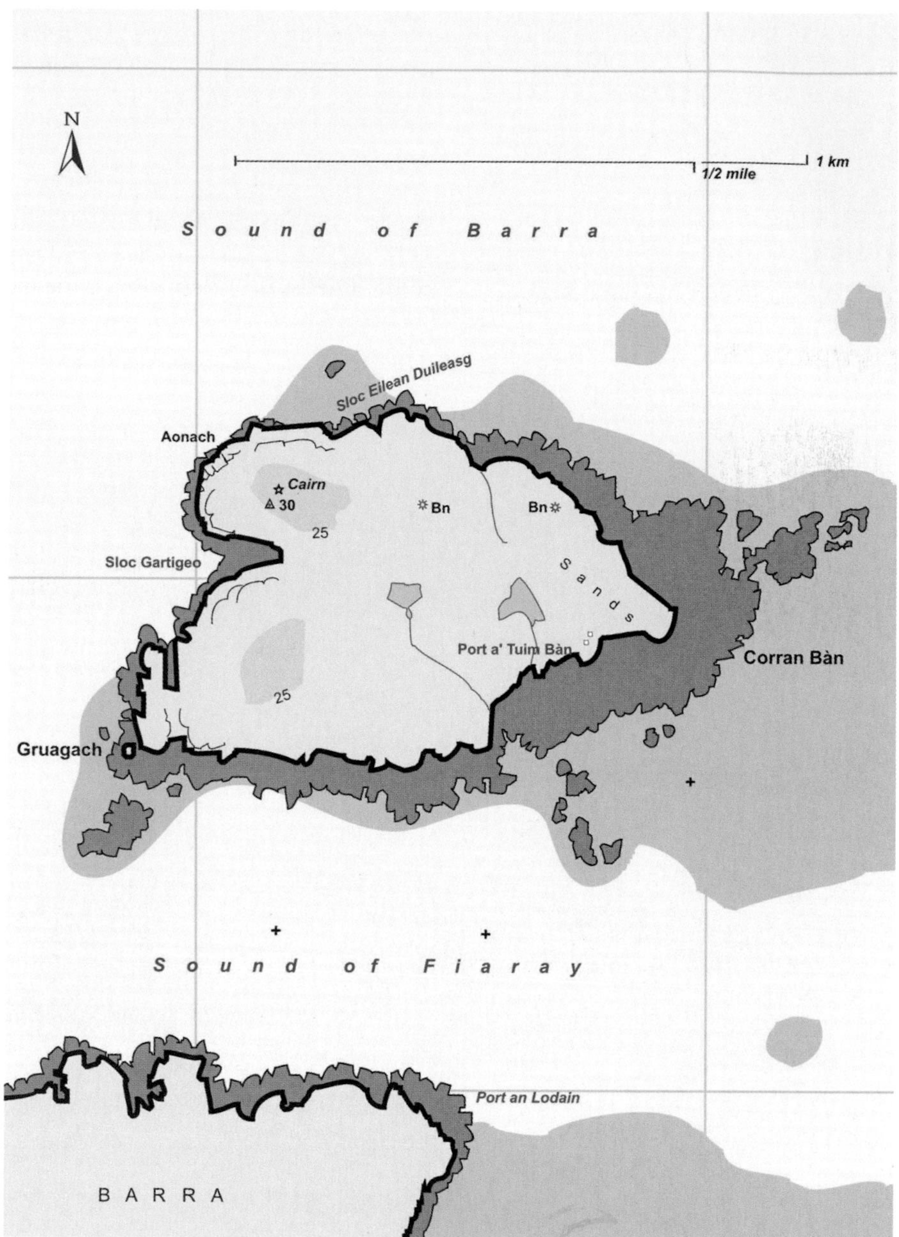

McDonald (d.1905) recorded that towards the end of 1890 people on the shore of South Uist heard dreadful cries coming from **Lingay** (ON – heather isle). Lingay is the little islet in the middle of the Sound of Barra, east of Fiaray. A rescue boat put out for the island as it was assumed that sailors were drowning. The screaming suddenly stopped when they were close to Lingay and although they searched the area they could find nothing to account for the cries. Almost exactly eight years later, in October 1898, a boat from Eriskay was wrecked on Lingay and the sailors cries brought help from South Uist. All were saved but the first incident was claimed by the islanders to have been a forewarning. (Nowadays it would be called, in science-fiction terms, a 'time-warp'.)

Access: Barra Fishing Charters, 01871-890384. Island Adventures, Castlebay, 01871-810284. Tourist Information, Castlebay, Barra, 01871-810336.

Anchorage: No recommended anchorage.

1. Temp anchorage in Sound of Fiaray in settled weather but carefully follow sailing directions.

7.13 Eileanan Iasgaich

(G. – the fish, or fishing, islands).

O S Maps: 1:50000 Sheet 31 1:25000 Sheet 453
Admiralty Charts: 1:100000 No.1795 1:12500 No.2770

Area: 50ha (124 acres)
Height: 23m (75 ft)

Population: No Census records and uninhabited.

Geology: Gneiss bedrock with scanty areas of soil.

Wildlife: The many pockets and cracks in the rocks provide a home for prawns and lobsters and shelter for fish.

* * *

EILEANAN IASGAICH is an ill-defined group of low-lying islands in Loch Boisdale linked by reefs and skerries at low water. The largest of the group, **Eilean Iasgaich Mór**, is the most easterly and it rises to a central hummock which is just 23m high. Vegetation is sparse due to the lack of

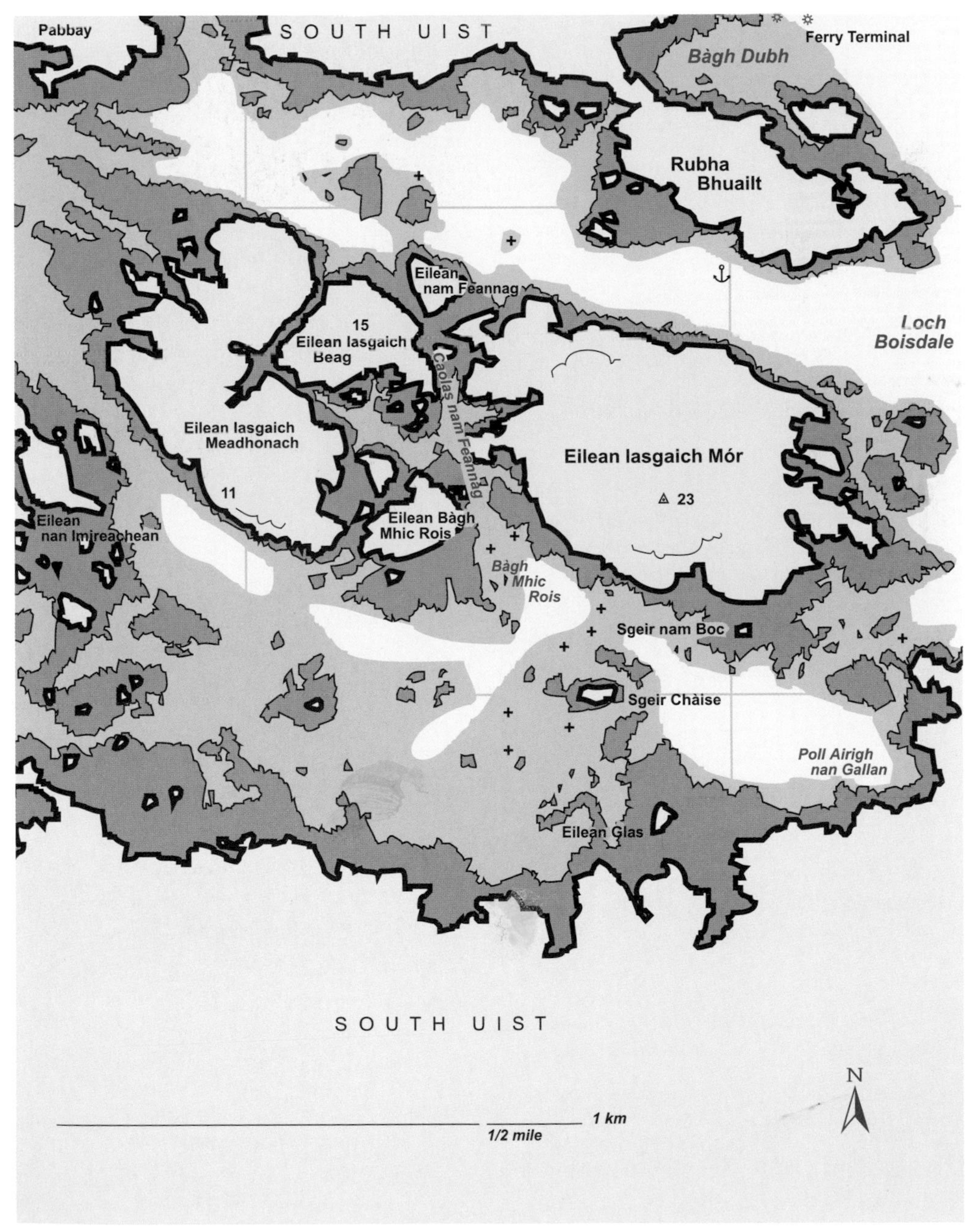

soil and the high salt content. There is a channel in the centre of the group which has a sufficiently narrow entrance to form a natural tidal fish-trap and it is possibly this that gave the islands their name.

Loch Boisdale is generally shallow and studded with tidal islands and rocks. The most conspicuous islets, both of which are in the entrance to the loch, are **Calvay** and **Gasay**. Calvay has a ruined castle on it which guarded the entrance in medieval times and the ubiquitous Prince Charles Edward Stuart spent a night in hiding there. To the west of Eileanan Iasgaich are **Eilean nan Imireachean** (G. – island of the processions), tiny at high water but extensive when the tide is out, **Eilean Mór** (G. – big island), and **Pabbay** to the north-west. These are all tidal islands. It is out of character for a Pabbay, or priest island, to be tidal as it would allow the hermit to interrupt his isolation and walk ashore to meet his friends whenever the tide went out. This was obviously the abode of an extrovert anchorite.

* * *

Access: No regular access. Enquire at Lochboisdale. Landing can be difficult due to seaweed-covered reefs.

Anchorages:

1. Rubha Bhuailt. In channel N of Eileanan Iasgaich. Fish cages block much of the anchorage. Holding reported to be poor.
2. Rubha Arinangallan. Anchor 1c NW of the ruined pier on S shore of Loch Boisdale. Beware drying rock and shoal patch NW of the pier and Hut Shoal N of the pier.

7.14 Stuley

(ON – Stula's island) The peak on South Uist overlooking Stuley is Stulaval (ON – Stula's hill).

O S Maps: 1:50000 Sheet 22 1:25000 Sheet 453
Admiralty Charts: 1:100000 No.1795

Area: 45ha (111 acres)
Height: 40m (131 ft)

Population: No Census records and uninhabited.

Geology: Intermediate and basic Lewisian rock with a distinctly greenish colour.

STULEY is made up of three low grass-covered hills with the highest point (40m) near the centre. Both the island and its grazing sheep have a leisurely unassuming appearance.

We approached the island from the north-east and then rounded the coastline between Stuley and Broad Rocks to enter the Sound. According to both the chart and the Pilot there is a shoal area at the north end of the sound fairly close to **Creag an t-Sagairt** (G. – priest's rock) but we failed to find it. The echo-sounder gave a steady reading of 20m right up to the point where the sound narrows in width although the depth certainly decreases south of this point. The original soundings, of course, were by leadline and date back to 1852. It is not a bad little anchorage, given suitable conditions, and landing is easy on the green, slatelike, slabs of rock.

Although I have found no written record of permanent human habitation the green ridges of old lazybeds and a few scattered shieling ruins show that Stuley was probably yet another place where people who were considered of less importance than sheep fought to survive. The cleft in the north is called **Sloc Duilich** (G. – awkward inlet) and the cliffs facing the Priest's Rock are

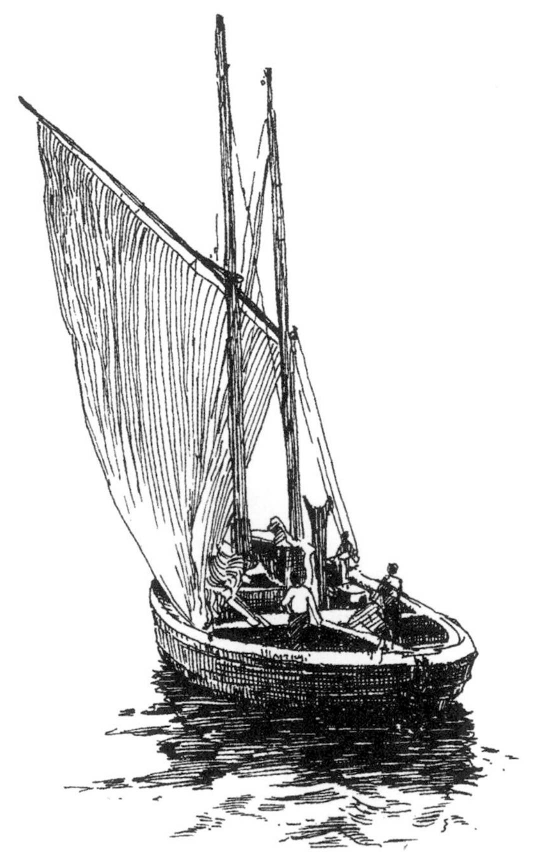

A HERRING DRIFTER IN THE 1930S

– according to one old map – aptly named **Creag na h-Oraíde** (G. – sermon crag).

Glas-eilean Mór (G. – big green island), south-east of Stuley, is, as its name suggests, covered with a sward of bright green grass.

Access: No regular access. Try a Lochboisdale boat-owner.

Anchorage:

1. Stuley Sound between South Uist and Stuley. According to the Admiralty Pilot 'small vessels pass through or use it as an anchorage'. It is about ½c wide at its narrowest and a submerged rock is charted about midway but the channel appears to be clean if a course nearer to Stuley is maintained.

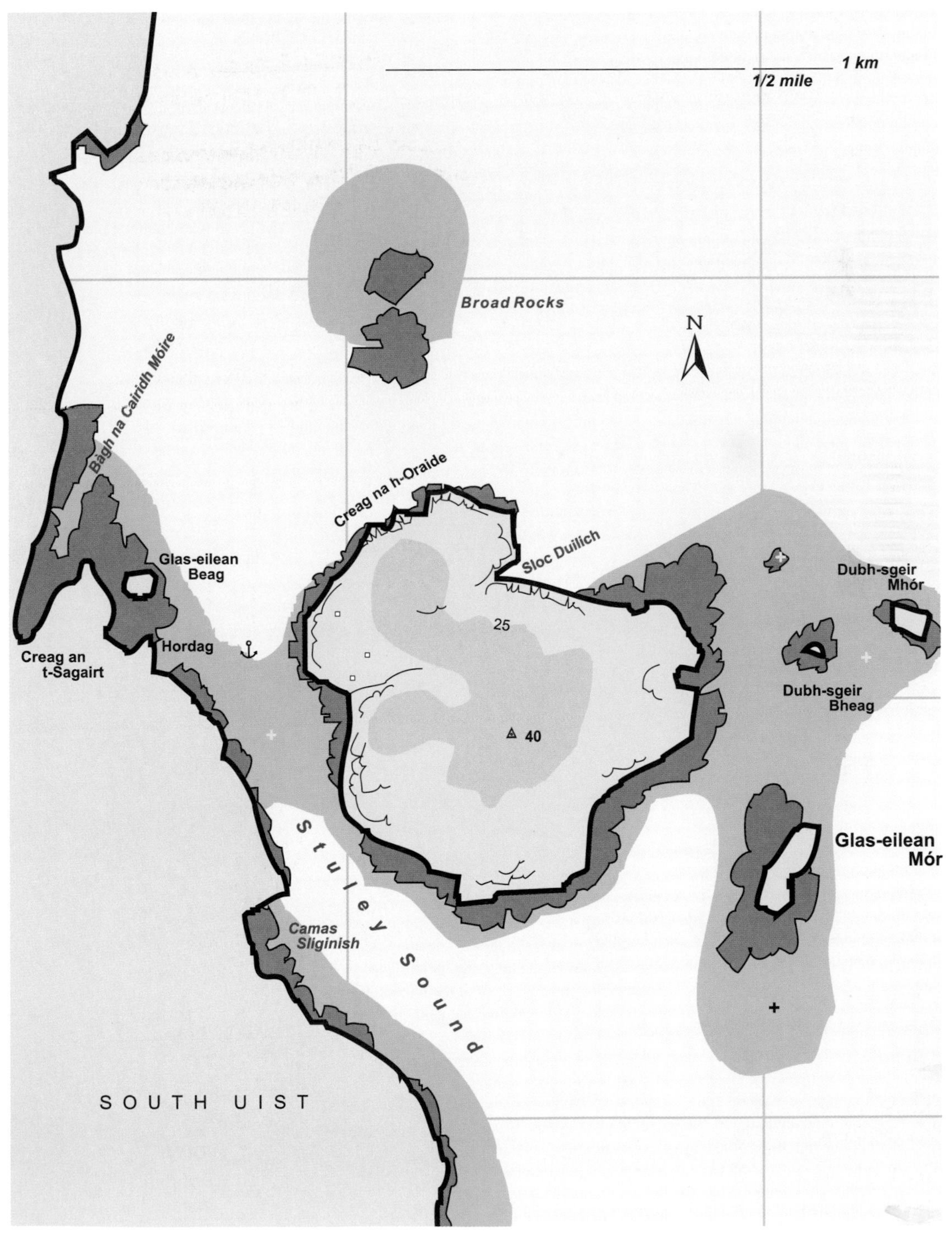

7.15 Uist

[yoo-ist] (ON – west)

Benbecula

(G. beinn bheag a' bh-faodhla – little mountain of the fords) referring to the only means of access before the causeways were built.

Berneray *or* Bernera

(ON bjarnar-øy – bear island) or possibly (ON – Bjorn's island).

Baleshare

(G. baile ear – east town)

Grimsay

(ON – Grim's island)

Eriskay

(G. ùruisg, ON -øy – goblin or water-nymph island). 'Eric's island' is sometimes given as the derivation but this is probably incorrect.

Vallay

(ON – hill island)

Kirkibost Island

(ON – church farm)

Oronsay

(G. – drying or tidal island)

O S Maps: 1:50000 Sheets 18, 22 and 31. 1:25000 Sheets 453 and 454.
Admiralty Charts: 1:200000 No.2722. Complete E coast 1:100000 No.1795. Sd of Barra & Loch Boisdale 1:30000 No.2770. E coast, L Skiport to L Eport 1:25000 No.2904. Berneray (part) 1:20000 No.2642. Lochs on E coast 1: 15000 No.2825.

Area: 74,540ha (184,189 acres)
Height: 620m (2034 ft)

Owner: The MacDonalds of Clanranald held South Uist and Benbecula until 1838. In 1838 Colonel Gordon of Cluny bought Benbecula and his family were owners until 1942. Since 1961 Eriskay and almost all of South Uist and Benbecula were owned by South Uist Estates, the rest is owned by the Scottish Government and the Ministry of Defence. In 2006 the whole of South Uist Estates passed into community ownership for £4.6 million (HIE and the Lottery each contributed £2 million).

The MacDonalds of Sleat owned North Uist. The greater part of it (including Grimsay and Baleshare) is now owned by Lord Granville's family as the North Uist Estate Trust 1990. The RSPB also has a sizeable holding. Berneray was part of the Bays of Harris estate. It was bought in the 1920s for £500 (without crofting rights). The current laird is Rodney Hitchcock, an English businessman.

Population: Approximate pre-Census totals excluding Berneray and Eriskay: 1755–4118. 1794–6668. 1821–11009.

	1841	1881	1891	1931	1961	1981	1991	2001
N.U't	3870	3398	3250	2349	1622	1399	1404	1271
Be'a	2160	1638	1787	1006	1390	1876	1803	1249
Be'y	713	452	501	331	201	133	141	136
S.U't	5093	3831	3708	2810	2376	2231	2106	1818
Ba'e	157	266	318	136	59	67	55	49
Gr'y	269	292	281	259	239	204	215	201
Er'y	80	466	454	420	231	201	179	133
Va'y	59	29	34	19	0	0	0	0
Ki't	25	12	6	6	0	0	0	0
Or'y	102	0	0	0	0	0	0	0
	12528	10384	10339	7336	6118	6111	5903	4857

Geology: North Uist, Berneray, Benbecula and the northern half of South Uist is a 2.5-million-years-old gneiss but the southern half of South Uist and Eriskay is younger gneiss – about 1.5 million years old. On Berneray there are no workable peat deposits. In 1607 a tidal wave removed the sand-bank which at that time almost connected Berneray to Pabbay. During the last ice ages there were minor glaciers on Hecla (whose rocks are mildly magnetic), Beinn Mhór in South Uist and on Eavel in North Uist with the result that the rocks in the bealachs (mountain passes) are ice worn but the summits are not. There was never a heavy all-enveloping ice-sheet as on the mainland. The 'long island' was in fact one long island at this time and it was only in the post-glacial era that the sea-lochs broke through. Ancient peat and the stumps of forest trees can be found below mean sea-level at Borve on Benbecula, at Loch Eynort, Lochboisdale, on the west coast of South

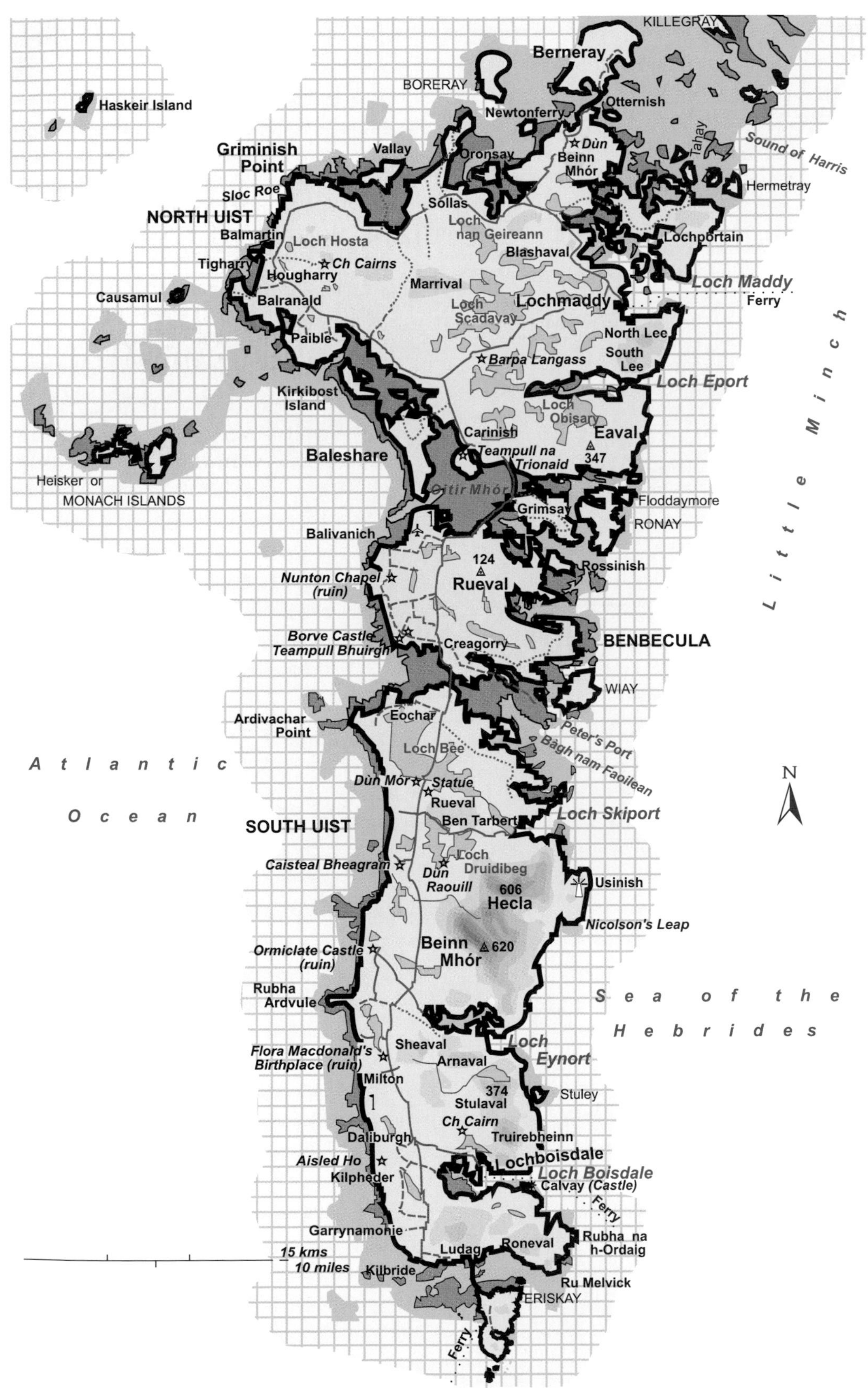
KILLEGRAY
Berneray
BORERAY
Haskeir Island
Otternish
Newtonferry
Tahay
Sound of Harris
Griminish Point
Vallay
Oronsay
Dùn Beinn Mhór
Hermetray
Sloc Roe
Sollas
NORTH UIST
Loch nan Geireann
Balmartin
Loch Hosta
Lochportain
Blashaval
Tigharry
Ch Cairns
Hougharry
Loch Maddy
Marrival
Causamul
Balranald
Lochmaddy
Ferry
Loch Scadavay
Paible
North Lee
South Lee
Barpa Langass
Loch Eport
Kirkibost Island
Loch Obisary
Little Minch
Carinish
Eaval
Baleshare
Teampull na Trionaid
347
Heisker or MONACH ISLANDS
Oitir Mhór
Floddaymore
Grimsay
RONAY
Balivanich
124
Nunton Chapel (ruin)
Rueval
Rossinish
Borve Castle
Teampull Bhuirgh
Creagorry
BENBECULA
WIAY
Ardivachar Point
Eochar
Peter's Port
Loch Bee
Bagh nam Faoilean
Atlantic Ocean
Dùn Mór
Statue
Rueval
N
Ben Tarbert
Loch Skiport
SOUTH UIST
Loch Druidibeg
Caisteal Bheagram
Dùn Raouill
Usinish
606
Hecla
Nicolson's Leap
Beinn Mhór
620
Ormiclate Castle (ruin)
Rubha Ardvule
Sea of the Hebrides
Loch Eynort
Sheaval
Flora Macdonald's Birthplace (ruin)
Arnaval
Milton
Stuley
374
Stulaval
Ch Cairn
Truirebheinn
Daliburgh
Lochboisdale
Aisled Ho
Loch Boisdale
Kilpheder
Calvay (Castle)
Ferry
Garrynamonie
Rubha na h-Ordaig
15 kms
10 miles
Ludag
Roneval
Kilbride
Ru Melvick
ERISKAY
Ferry

Uist and off the Prince's Strand at Eriskay.

History: In 1098 King Magnus III of Norway pillaged the Hebrides, 'gained much gold', and set the Uists on fire.

On 23 July, 1745 on the beach of Coilleag a' Phrionnsa (G. – the Prince's cockle-shell strand) on the west coast of **Eriskay** Prince Charles Edward Stuart was put ashore from the French ship *Du Teillay*. This was the first time he had set foot on Scottish soil. The MacNeils of Barra owned Eriskay at the time and this continued until 1758 when the island passed to the MacDonalds of Clanranald.

South Uist, which had been ruled by the Clanranald chiefs since the Norse occupation, has also many associations with Bonnie Prince Charlie following the collapse of his venture. The Prince landed in Corodale Bay, directly beneath Beinn Mhór, on 14 May 1746 and hid in a forester's hut. From Prince's Cave he watched the navy patrolling the Minch in the search for him. Neil MacEachain MacDonald who was helping him, introduced him to the twenty-three-year-old Flora MacDonald who had arrived from Skye on a visit to her brother, and it was he who suggested that when Flora returned to Skye she should take the Prince with her disguised as her servant girl. The island at the mouth of Loch Boisdale, Calvay, has the ruins of a 13th-century castle on it where the Prince took refuge on 15 June 1746.

During the clearances which followed the purchase of Eriskay, South Uist and **Benbecula** by Colonel Gordon of Cluny in 1838 some crofters were chased into the hills by the police and more than 1000 destitute islanders were shipped from Lochboisdale to America on *The Admiral*. Cluny turned a blind eye when some of the crofters whom he had evicted from Uist settled on Eriskay as he considered the land to be too poor even for sheep to survive. But many crofters preferred destitution in Scotland to forced emigration and they built raised lazybeds of peat and seaweed on the rocky ground and grew meagre crops of barley, oats and potatoes for sustenance.

The MacRuairidhs ruled **North Uist** after the Norse occupation until the MacDonalds of Sleat were given official title by James IV in 1495.

About 1850 Lord Macdonald of Sleat brought police there and ruthlessly evicted many families. This resulted in bloody fights, burned cottages and much misery but it was a pointless exercise as only five years later Macdonald sold the island to Sir John Powlett Ord.

In 1614, when Tormod (G. – Norman), third son of Ruaridh Mór chief of the Clan MacLeod, was five years old he was settled with **Berneray** by his father. The remains of the home that he later built are still to be seen. He received a knighthood after the Restoration for his services to the exiled Charles II. Sir Norman, who died in 1705, was an ardent supporter of Gaelic art and literature and he gave a house on Berneray to Mary MacLeod, the famous Gaelic poet.

At this time the MacLeod Chiefs were reasonably good proprietors and keen to ensure satisfactory communication between the islands. In 1705 a boat was purchased by MacLeod of Harris for use as a ferry. Lauchlan MacLean as ferryman was instructed to maintain a regular service between Harris and Skye and also the islands of Berneray, Ensay, Killegray and Pabbay.

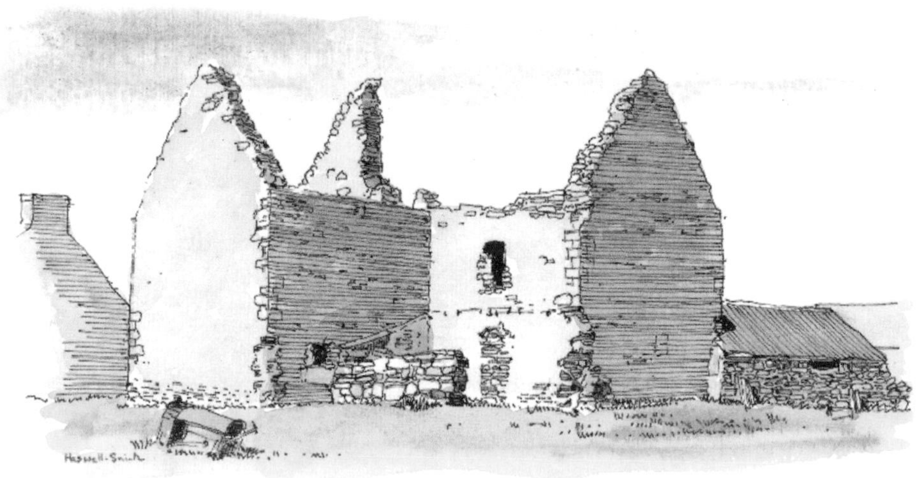

SHORT-LIVED ORMICLATE CASTLE

Wildlife: White and yellow water-lilies dapple the surface of the many fresh-water lochs. These are now scarce on the mainland due to disturbance and plundering by plant collectors. The small islands in these lochs have dense thickets of the native willow, aspen, birch, hazel and rowan growing on them because they are beyond the reach of hungry sheep. Originally these trees were the elements of widespread island afforestation. Martin Martin wrote of Berneray in 1695: 'The west end of this island which looks to St Kilda, is called the wooden harbour, because the sands at low water discover several trees that have formerly grown there. Sir Norman MacLeod told me that he had seen a tree cut there, which was afterwards made into a harrow.' A patch of trees still clings to a heathery rock-wall on Beinn Mhór on South Uist, and a few other sheltered corries in the hills north of Loch Eynort. Here too are several varieties of fern, including the royal fern, *Osmunda regalis*, and many alpine species.

But for sheer profusion and floral display nothing can compare with the machair in the spring and summer months spreading down the entire west coast. About 200 different species of wildflowers have been identified which bloom in sequence giving rolling waves of colour throughout spring and summer. On Berneray there is very little heather and with no peat bogs there are few midges. The soil structure is rich in shell-sand and, fortunately, with no rabbits the machair is particularly beautiful.

It has been claimed that the pink sea-convolvulus (*Calystegia soldanella*) growing above the beach on Eriskay came from seeds dropped by Bonnie Prince Charlie when he stepped ashore. It is however also found at several other places in the Hebrides including Vatersay (No.7-6). It blooms in June with a small heart-shaped leaf and large trumpet.

Nests of the very rare northern *colletes* mining bee have been found in the sand dunes of North Uist.

Mute swans are sometimes seen on South Uist's shallow Loch Bee. The Uists have the highest density of breeding waders in Britain and many rare bird species although these were seriously threatened by hedgehogs which were thoughtlessly introduced in 1974 and mink which have swum over from Harris. Culling of the hedgehogs and mink has gone ahead despite some controversy. Some of the more interesting birds to be seen throughout the year are: corn bunting, reed bunting, twite, raven, wheatear, stonechat, black-headed and common gulls, black guillemot, rock dove, short-eared owl, rock pipit, greenshank, redshank, snipe, golden plover, hen harrier, buzzard, golden eagle, merlin, peregrine, red grouse, red-breasted merganser, eider, shoveller, teal, gadwall, little grebe and heron. Red-necked phalarope arrive mid-May. Also pink-footed goose, pintail, knot and bar-tailed godwit. In summer quail, knot, sanderling and ruff. Later, little stint, curlew sandpiper, dunlin and whimbrel. In winter, turnstone, purple sandpiper, scaup, water rail, jack snipe and woodcock, and many more.

The Loch Druidibeg National Nature Reserve on South Uist, lying astride the main road, is the most important breeding ground of the native British greylag goose; and the Balranald RSPB Nature Reserve in North Uist is an equally outstanding site.

Corncrakes, which can be heard from mid-April, benefit from this being an Environmentally Sensitive Area (ESA), allowing crofters to be paid to manage their land in ways which benefit corncrakes and conservation.

Eriskay ponies stand 12 to 13 hands high and are now proven to be a distinctive Scottish breed. They have a pleasant temperament and were bred for croftwork such as carrying peat and seaweed.

For the local fishermen, the velvet crabs which were once thrown away or used as bait now fetch good prices in southern Europe. The coastline is generally rich in sea-life – a fact appreciated by the numerous grey and common seals.

* * *

Off the southern tip of Eriskay lie the **Stack Islands**, where the ruin of Weaver's Castle can be seen on **Eilean Leathan**, the largest of the group. The castle was the base for a notorious MacNeil pirate and wreck-plunderer. The other islets in the group **Eileanan Dubha** and **Eilean a' Gheòidh** are linked together by drying reefs.

* * *

ERISKAY, which is joined to South Uist by a causeway completed in 2001, is possibly best-known for the lovely 'Eriskay Love Lilt' and several other beautiful Gaelic songs. In a way, the music is more beautiful than the land for this is a barren island, the only soil being rocky moorland. Even so there is a relatively large population.

The main township, **Haun** (ON *havn* – harbour), is on the north coast with another

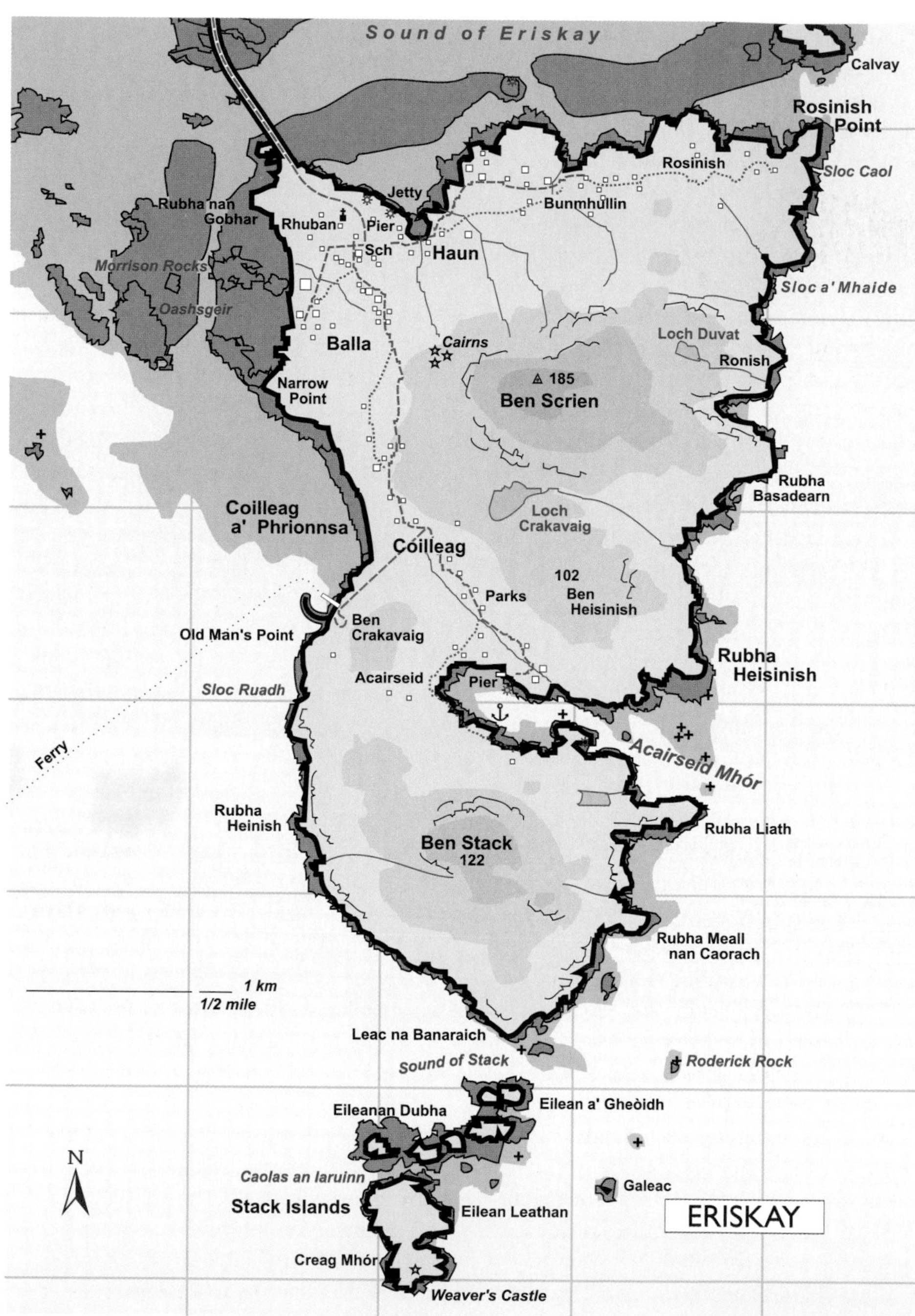

small settlement beside the natural harbour in the east. A number of the men are prawn and lobster fishermen and the women knit fishermen's jerseys and gossamer shawls in distinctive Eriskay patterns.

Almost all are Roman Catholics. A former priest who was born on South Uist, Father Allan McDonald, is remembered for his valuable collections of Gaelic folk-tales (see Fiaray, No.7.12), his dictionary of Gaelic phrases and his poetry. In 1893 he built a new church at Haun. He died in 1905 at the early age of forty-six, a simple man and a dedicated scholar. Unfortunately, much of his literary work was mutilated by Ada Goodrich-Freer, a German woman, who befriended him, persuaded him to hand over his manuscripts and then published much of the material, incorrectly edited, under her own name. Luckily, what was left of Father Allan's work was rescued by John Lorne Campbell of Canna.

Others followed the lead of Father Allan. Hebridean songs and folklore were passed on orally so it was important that they should be recorded before they were lost. Unfortunately, some of these records are now the subject of controversy such as *The Songs of the Hebrides* (which included the famous 'Love Lilt') published by Marjory Kennedy Fraser. She, with the help of the Rev Dr Kenneth MacLeod of Skye, visited Eriskay in 1905 to record Hebridean songs.

The church built by Father Allan, **St Michael's Church**, has a bell which is the ship's bell from the German battle-cruiser *Derfflinger*, scuttled at Scapa Flow (see No.10.7), and the altar base is the bow of a lifeboat from the aircraft-carrier *Hermes*.

The 12,000-ton steamship *The Politician* sailing from Liverpool and bound for New York, avoided striking the lone islet of **Hartamul** east of Eriskay, but foundered in the Sound of Eriskay near the islet of **Calvay** and broke in two. This was on 5 February 1941, at the height of the Battle of the Atlantic when Hitler's U-boats were exacting a terrible toll on merchant shipping. The Harrison Line ship was unaccompanied and trying to avoid attention by sneaking through the Minch but she should not have ventured into the shallow Sound of Eriskay. Among her assorted cargo of plumbing fittings, motorcycle parts, art silks and Jamaican currency were 264,000 bottles of whisky. The story goes that as soon as the crew were safe the islanders naturally turned their attention to the precious cargo. Before long, nearly every living creature on the island, including the ponies, was blind drunk. During the ensuing weeks the cargo was steadily removed from the wreck. Then, to the islanders' surprise, Charles McColl and Ivan Gledhill of H M Customs & Excise appeared on the scene with some police and began searching the crofts. Most of the whisky miraculously disappeared into peat stacks, hot-water bottles and rabbit holes. The local police disliked the affair and withdrew but thirty-six islanders were sent to court by the excisemen, including a fourteen-year-old boy. Nineteen were found guilty of illegal possession and imprisoned at Inverness.

Some years later Sir Compton Mackenzie based his hilarious book *Whisky Galore!* on the incident (but naturally omitted the sad fact that islanders had been prosecuted). The film was made by Ealing Studios on the adjoining island of Barra (No.7.6) in 1948.

In 1989 a company was formed to try to salvage any whisky remaining in the wreck but the whole expensive operation only yielded a few bottles. The stern of the ship, which contained No 5 hold and the whisky cases, can still be seen at low tide where it has drifted some distance north-west of Calvay but much of it is now bedded deep in the sandy bottom.

Strangely enough, Eriskay had always been a 'dry' island until its first public house was opened in 1988. Naturally it was called *Am Politician* and the Eriskay islanders could be found there happily drinking a dram with their friends. I first visited it on a Thursday, mid-afternoon. It was crowded, and the sweet smell of spirit and soft Gaelic voices encouraged dreams of secret treasure troves of golden liquid. Some bottles still occasionally turn up in unlikely hidey-holes. The islanders call them 'polly-pottles' and I was told by John Alan MacNeil of Barra that genuine ones can be recognised because they are stamped – 'No resale without Federal approval.' They were of course originally destined for the United States.

The best anchorage for the island is unfortunately some distance from Haun. **Acairseid Mhór** (G. – big anchorage) is an inlet which cuts deep into the island between the two main peaks, **Ben Scrien** in the north (185m) and **Ben Stack** in the south (122m). Practically all the houses, brightly painted and with a distinctly Scandinavian flavour, are in the north clustered near the anchorage at **Haun**. This is a shallow little bay, but it was the terminal for the vehicle ferry from South Uist, and the lifeline for the community, before the causeway was built. Besides the church there is a well-stocked village store, a primary school (with eighteen pupils in 1997), and a post-office.

* * *

SOUTH UIST has a spine of mountains along its eastern side the highest being **Beinn Mhór** at 620m (2034ft). Hecla is also conspicuous at 606m. The spine is broken by three sea lochs, Boisdale, Eynort, and Sheilavaig; and a fourth, Skiport, which slices right through the island by joining up with Loch Bee on the west coastal plain. The Atlantic coast, which is the populated side, is virtually a continuous stretch of white shell-sand backed by dunes and flower-filled machair. Between the machair and the barren and mountainous east coast is a maze of lochans interspersed with peat moorland and deserted black houses. These lochs are well stocked with trout but angling is strictly controlled.

South Uist is predominantly Catholic. **Lochboisdale** with a population of about 300 is the ferry port, and the only township on the east coast.

A chambered cairn, 26m diameter and 6m high, can be found about 2½km north-west of Lochboisdale and due west near **Kilpheder** on the west coast there is a wheelhouse dating from about 200AD which was excavated in 1952 [NF734203]. It has a circular plan with the hearth at the hub. It was probably a farmhouse. Nearby at Garrynamonie School, as with most of the island schools in the early 1900s, the children were never allowed to speak in their native tongue – Gaelic.

At Cladh Hallan near **Daliburgh** in 2002 the 3000-year-old mummified remains of a family were found under a Bronze Age roundhouse. These are the first deliberately mummified prehistoric bodies to be found in Britain. And nearby at *Askernish* a golf-course designed in 1891 by the world-famous golfer, Tom Morris, was 'rediscovered' in 2005 under the machair sward.

About 5½km north of Daliburgh and just north of **Milton** is the birthplace of Flora MacDonald. It was here, to the family home [NF741269], that she came to visit her brother when her chance meeting with the Young Pretender put her name in the history books. The house is now a ruin. In nearby **Loch Kildonnan** a Norse church and island settlement similar to that at Loch Finlaggan (See No.2–4) were recently investigated. A further 5½km brings one to the ruins of **Ormiclate Castle** built in 1701–8 by a French architect and burned down in 1715 during a boisterous Jacobite party. It was the short-lived residence of the Clanranald Chiefs [NF740318].

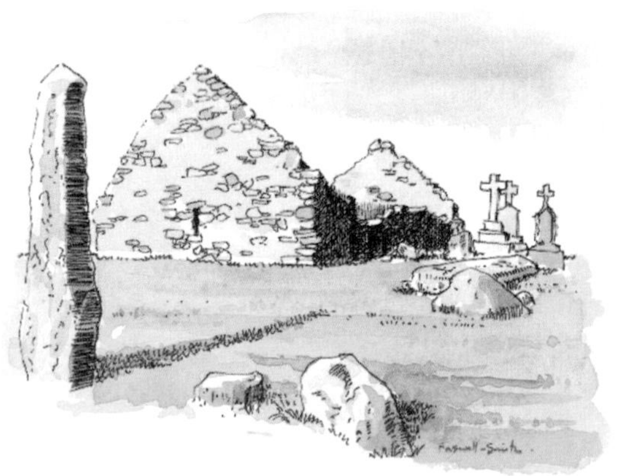

ILL-FATED NUNTON CHAPEL

Off the south shore of Loch Druidibeg and about 1½km from the road is an islet with rectangular **Dùn Roauill** on it [NF778371]. This is perhaps the best dun on South Uist. **Caisteal Bheagram**, the ruin of a small 15th or 16th-century tower, is on the other side of the road on an islet in Loch an Eilean [NF761371].

A road crosses from the **Loch Druidibeg Nature Reserve**, a waterfowl paradise, to Loch Skiport's decayed pier which was built for steamers in 1879 [NF829387]. South of the Usinish peninsula on the east coast is **Nicolson's Leap**. The story goes that Nicolson was found in bed with the wife of the Clanranald Chief. As he escaped he snatched the Chief's baby son as hostage and to escape the clansmen he leapt the 5m chasm on to the rock stack [NF864332]. From there he tried to bargain with his pursuers but ultimately jumped to his death into the sea below with the boy in his arms.

The Royal Artillery Missile Range, which was built in 1961, is in the north-west corner of South Uist. The range is sandwiched between the main road and the Atlantic, and its missiles are tracked from Hirta (St Kilda, No.9.1) which is more than forty miles to the north-west. On the Hill of Miracles, Rueval, just east of the road, stands the great granite statue of **Our Lady of the Isles** sculpted by Hew Lorimer in 1957 [NF776408] and above the statue is 'space city' – the range control installation.

Just south of the causeway across Loch Bee there is a small loch to the west of the road with clear traces of a large dun – **Dùn Mór** [NF775415]. Loch Bee itself, a west coast loch, is like a Panama Canal cutting right through South Uist because it has a long arm with a flood gate which connects with an arm of Loch Skiport, an east coast sea-loch. Loch Skiport has a number of fascinating channels and anchorages just asking to be explored. By **Shillay More** and **Shillay Beag** there are two popular pools, joined by a shallow but navigable channel, known as Wizard Pool and Little Kettle Pool. **Ornish Island** marks the entrance to Loch Skiport with **Luirsay Dubh**

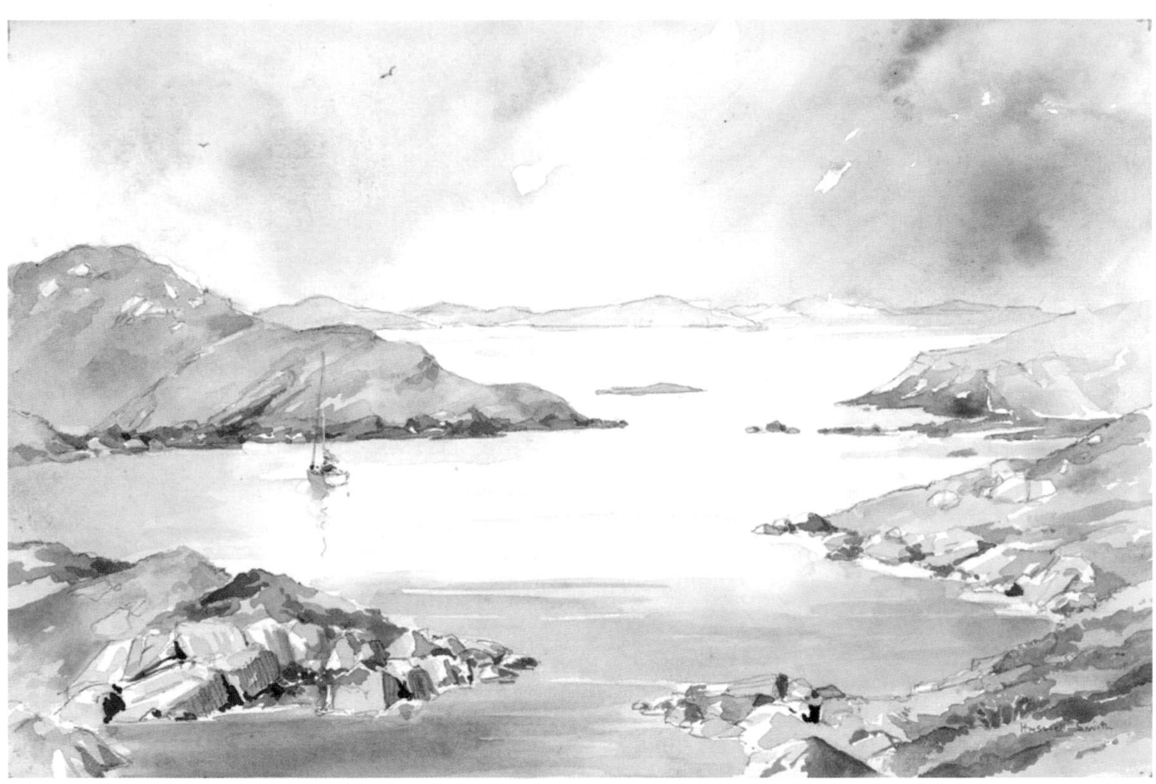

WIZARD POOL – LOCH SKIPORT

and **Luirsay Glas** on the north headland.

South Uist provides some excellent hill-walking and climbing. Ben Tarbert, Hecla, Feaveallach, Beinn Mhor, Ben na Hoe, Sheeval, Arnaval, Stulaval, Triuirebheinn, Roneval and some of the lesser peaks are all recommended. On the south wall of Coire Hellisdale by Beinn Mhór are 260m high cliffs with deep gullies.

* * *

BENBECULA is the stepping stone between the Uists, not only physically but because it is here that the predominant religion changes from the Catholic south to the Protestant north. The island is mainly low and flat but has an almost-central solitary hill of 124m, also called **Rueval** like the adjacent peak on South Uist. There is a magnificent view from the top. The causeway which crosses the sands of South Ford and links South Uist to Benbecula was built in 1983. It replaces a wartime bridge built in 1943 to serve the airfield.

In 1896 a pier was built at **Peter's Port** [NF849457] in the narrows between Benbecula and the island of Wiay (No.7.17). This was a typical Governmental folly as there was no road access and a hazardous approach by sea. A road and causeway were eventually built but the pier has never been of much practical use.

Beside the west coast road is the remnant of **Borve Castle** [NF773506]. This was probably the castle of 'Vynvawle' granted in a royal charter to Ranald, son of John of Islay, in 1372. Opposite it is the ruin of **Teampull Bhuirgh** [NF769503].

Surprisingly for the Atlantic, there is normally little swell on this coast because the water is very shallow for a long distance off-shore. Consequently shipwrecks here have had few fatalities as the crews could often wade ashore.

South-west of the airport is the island's main village, **Balivanich** with the army base built in 1970 to house the men servicing the rocket range on South Uist. This is a transient population which has been a great help to the economy of the island. Just south are the ruins of 14th-century **Nunton Chapel** – a nunnery which was wrecked during the Reformation and the nuns massacred [NF766537]. It was from Lady Clanranald at Nunton House that Bonnie Prince Charlie obtained the clothing with which he disguised himself as Betty Burke, maidservant to Flora MacDonald. Nunton House was built by the MacDonald chieftains after Ormiclate Castle on South Uist was burned down but it has had alterations since.

The east coast has many small coves and rocky islands and it was in April 1746 that the Prince's party landed on the peninsula of Rossinish where they took shelter in an empty boat. It was also from here that he sailed 'over the sea to Skye' with Flora MacDonald.

North Ford causeway over **Oitir Mór** (G. – the big shoal) was opened in 1960. The strand can be crossed on foot in fine weather when the tide is out but the crossing can be dangerous.

* * *

NORTH UIST is low-lying and so sprinkled with lochs that half the total area is under water. The lochs teem with trout and salmon (this is one of the earliest salmon runs in Scotland). Loch Scadavay alone has an area of 8 sq km and a shore line of 83km. The highest hill is **Eavel** (347m) but hills are few and far between and the Atlantic winds blow over the island virtually unchecked. The Rev Cruttwell wrote in 1798 – 'In the warm season of the year, no country in the highlands can exhibit a more delightful prospect but in bad weather when the wind blows the sea swells to a prodigious height and rolls with inexpressible violence against the shores, exhibiting a prospect awfully grand beyond description.'

Most of the crofts in North Uist are large enough to be just-about economically viable.

In the south east the drying island of **GRIMSAY** is linked to North Uist and Benbecula by a causeway which was completed in 1960. This is the centre for North Uist's fishing industry (mainly lobster) and there is an active processing plant. **Baymore** is an attractive spot for artists.

After crossing Oitir Mhór the road cuts straight through the middle of a stone circle with a chambered cairn to be seen to the north-east [NF837603]. Just beyond in the hamlet of Carinish is the Ditch of Blood – where a battle between the MacLeods of Harris and the MacDonalds of Uist took place in 1601. Nearby is a curious ruin, **Teampull na Trionaid** (G. – Trinity Temple) with twin churches founded by Somerled's daughter, Beathag, in about 1200 on an earlier Celtic site [NF816603]. The churches were later rebuilt with a unique vaulted roof and fine carved stonework by Robert II's daughter, the wife of John, first Lord of the Isles. This is said to have been a seat of learning similar to Iona and is one of the most important archaeological sites in the Western Isles. It was attended by Duns Scotus (c1265–1308), who became a renowned teacher at the universities of Oxford, Paris, and Cologne. Because he argued that religion depended on faith and not on reason the establishment called anyone with similarly 'stupid' views a 'dunce'.

The last battle in Scotland fought without firearms was between the MacDonalds and the MacLeods at Carinish in 1601.

The main road circles the island. At Ben Langass there is a chambered cairn, **Barpa Langass** (NF837657), 5½m high and 22m wide which is entered through a tunnel. After crossing a desolate central stretch of loch-strewn moorland the road then reaches **Lochmaddy**, the main ferry terminal and administrative centre for North Uist. Here there is a court house and jail, a cottage hospital, a bank, a garage and a comfortable hotel which particularly caters for the needs of anglers and sailors. Loch Maddy or **Loch nam Madadh** (G. – loch of the dogs) is named after the two dog-shaped rocks, **Madadh Beag** and **Madadh Mór,** standing guard on each side of the entrance to the loch with a further one to the south called **Madadh Gruamach** (G. – the surly dog). In the 16th century this was a favourite pirate rendezvous but a century later it was hosting a fleet of 400 fishing vessels and by the 18th century the port was frequented by many ships trading from Ireland, the west coasts of the English and Scottish mainlands, and as far afield as the Baltic. Sponish is the site of one of the local industries, a factory to process seaweed for alginates.

Loch Maddy is full of islands, many tidal or little more than skerries. It is worth mentioning **Glas Eilean Mór**, **Faihore**, **Ruigh Liath**, **An Glais-eilean Meadhonach**, **Hamersay**, **Flodday**, **Ferramas**, **Cliasay More** and **Beg**, and **Keallasay More** and **Beg**.

North-west of Lochmaddy the road skirts the hill of **Blashaval**. On its western slope are three standing stones called Na Fir Bhreige (G. – the false men) [NF887717]. They are reputed to mark the graves of three traitors who were buried alive although another story claims that they are three men from Skye who were turned to stone for having deserted their wives.

Near here a minor road wanders eastwards

through the broken land to the north of Loch Maddy. It passes through **Lochportain** with its small fishing pier and ends up at Cheese Bay in the furthest north-east corner.

After the main road has skirted Crogary Beag hill a secondary road runs north by **Newtonferry** to the jetty for a car ferry at **Otternish** which sails to Leverburgh (An t-Obbe) on Harris (No.8.14). Here also is the causeway (opened 1998) to Berneray. The latter ferry route passes close to **Torogay**, a large islet with extensive reefs which shelter the ferry jetty in **Loch nam Ban**. Near Newtonferry is a lochan with a causeway to the remains of a broch last occupied in 1602 by Hugh MacDonald of Sleat [NF897777]. There is also a white house where W. S. Morrison, later Lord Dunrossil, was brought up. He was a Speaker in the House of Commons who became Governor General of Australia. A scramble up **Beinn Mhór** (190m) is rewarded by a superb view of the Sound of Harris and the fragmented landscape.

The main road crosses Loch nan Geireann where, on **Eilean-an-Tighe**, are the remains of the earliest Neolithic potter's workshop yet found in Western Europe. The drying island of **ORONSAY** lies to the north in Vallaquie Strand – uninhabited since the Clearances – and further west the road passes **Sollas**, forever remembered as the centre of one of the most inhumane Clearances. The culprit was Lord MacDonald of Sleat.

Evidence of a Norse settlement has been found on the low sandy peninsula to the north of here.

The road now skirts Vallay Strand. **VALLAY**, another drying island, is like a long breakwater so that the Strand is virtually an enclosed sea-loch when the tide is in. When it is out a track fords the huge expanse of sand and stone to reach ruined Vallay House which was built on the island by Erskine Beveridge, owner of linen mills in Fife. He wrote an authoritative book on the archaeology of the area. Vallay is crowded with antiquities – duns, standing stones, and chapel ruins. The family of the 5th Lord Granville, who was the benign landlord for much of North Uist and undertook valuable experiments in land improvement, stayed at Griminish overlooking Vallay. His son, the present Earl and his wife, Countess Granville, inherited the estate but bought a smokehouse at Clachan where they fillet, smoke and sell salmon and sea trout. 'We are determined to stay in North Uist and we're not quite as rich as some people assume,' he says.

Loch Olabhat is near the road. Its tiny island, **Eilean Domhnuill**, is a crannog built nearly 5000 years ago – predating Ireland's earliest-known crannogs by 2000 years [NF747753].

A 9m-high natural rock arch is at **Griminish Point** at the north-west corner of North Uist. **Sloc Roe** (G. – the pit passage) is a cave with an entrance from both sides of the point and two holes opening to the surface. During gales, the water spouts through these to such a height that it can be seen from ten miles away at sea [NF727765].

Turning south through **Balmartin**, Loch Hosta is said to cover a drowned village, and across the road in the cliffs of Tigharry (G. – house on the rock) is another spouting cave, the Kettle Spout. A track leads east up South Clettraval where there are two chambered cairns and an impressive view of the loch-strewn landscape [NF749714]. The RSPB's **Balranald Nature Reserve** juts into the Atlantic at the next headland and includes the tiny off-shore islet of **Causamul**. An even smaller islet, **Deasker** (G. – south skerry), lies nearly three miles south. The churchyard of **Hougharry** holds the graves of many of the island's 'nobility' [NF708706].

Off the wide white sand beaches lie the drying islands of **KIRKIBOST** and **BALESHARE**. Kirkibost Island is now uninhabited whereas Baleshare (G. – east town), the first Hebridean island to gather kelp, has a small but thriving population. Baleshare's sister island, Baile-siar (G. – west town) and nearby Husabost township were swept away in the 1607 tsunami (see Monach Islands No.7.19).

North of the road at this point a prominent hill stands alone among the moorland lochans. A 2½-km cross-country trek leads to **Unival** chambered cairn or barrow – a large New Stone Age tomb [NF801669] – near a 3m-high standing stone on the barren hillside.

There are many interesting walks among the hundreds of lochs, and some of the best fishing in the Western Isles, but always take a good map and a compass.

* * *

The two hills on **BERNERAY** are both on the east side. The west is a wide stretch of low-lying machair, rough grazing and sand dunes and one of the loveliest stretches of white shell-sand beach in Britain – about 4km of perfection. **Beinn**

Shléibhe (G. – mountainous hill), also known as Moor Hill, is 93m high and south of it is **Borve Hill** (ON – fort hill), 85m high. Between these two hills is a wide freshwater loch, **Loch Bhruist**, and a reef-ridden sea-loch, **Bays Loch**, forming a deep indentation on the south-east coast.

Although Berneray lies close to North Uist it was traditionally part of the parish of Harris. All the habitation is on the south-east side. The village of Borve lies south of Borve Hill but the road which runs almost the full length of the east coast links this settlement with its northerly neighbour, **Ruisgarry**. In between, on Bays Loch, is the post-office, the harbour, the shop, and the church and manse (a rare example of church and manse under one roof). At one time there were three churches on Berneray.

It is a good little harbour, well sheltered, built with EC funds in the late 1980s. Fuel and water are available although the nearest water tap sometimes produces more peat than water.

The harbour is particularly appreciated by visiting sailors after successfully dodging the rocks in Bays Loch. For years there was no reliable guide to the position of these rocks which the locals navigate entirely by instinct. One old

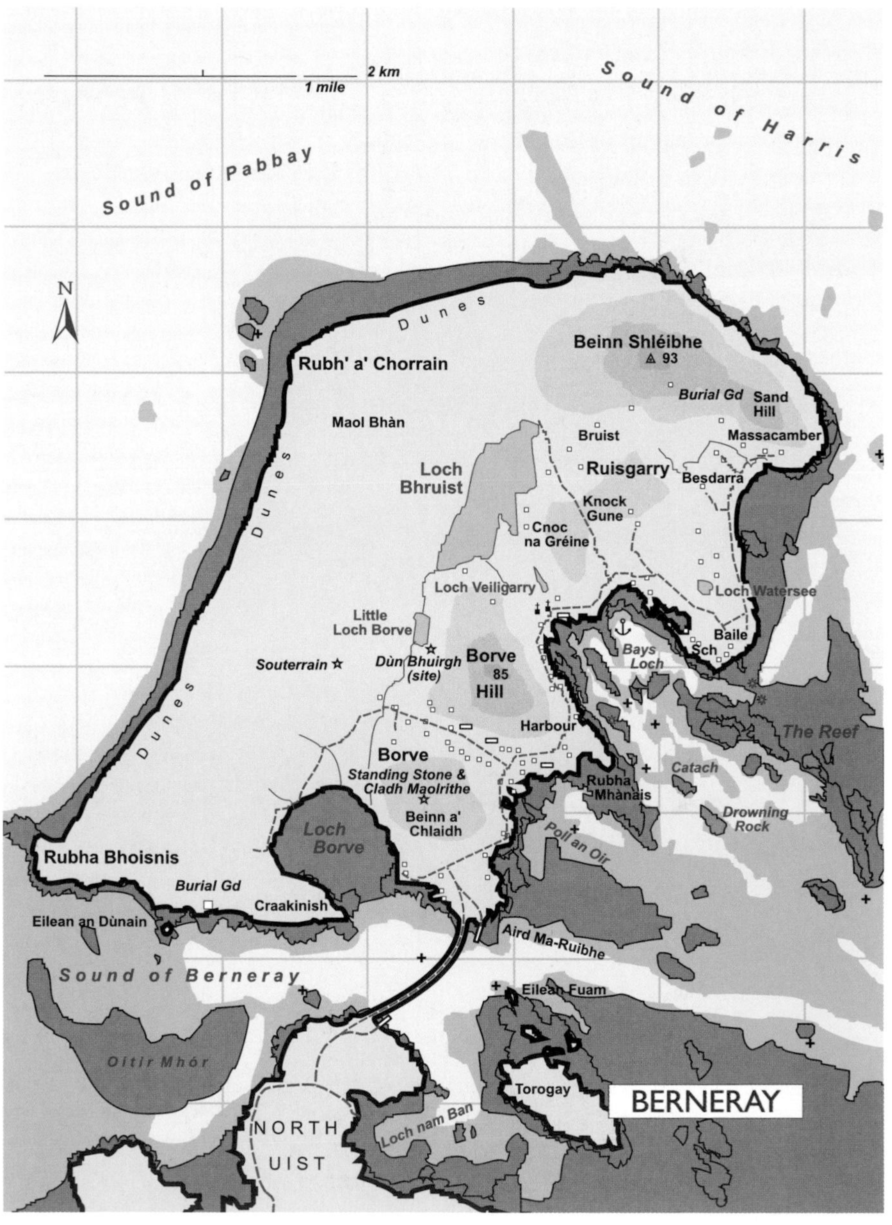

islander bringing a visitor across from Harris ran his boat on to the rocks. 'But I thought you knew all the rocks!' cried the visitor. 'Aye,' said the old man, 'I do. And that is one of them.'

Even when the kelp boom was over Berneray survived on its potatoes. The light sandy soil, still manured with kelp, grows a generous and tasty crop and for many years most of the potatoes eaten on Harris were imported from Berneray. Nowadays, sheep farming and fishing are the main industries although potatoes are still grown. The fishing is for prawns, lobsters and velvet crabs. Berneray is a good example of how years of decline have been replaced by hope and a belief in a viable future. Trim new suburban bungalows, however incongruous in such a beautiful setting, are appearing among the deserted black houses.

In the late 1980s the Prince of Wales wanted to 'get away from it all' and experience life among these gentle and friendly people. He arranged to spend some time on Berneray, lodging in a typical household. The home of 'Splash' McKillop and his wife was chosen. It says much for Hebridean loyalty and respect for privacy that both during his stay and thereafter not a single man, woman or child breathed a word about their famous guest to the media. It was the Prince himself who revealed the facts four years later.

While there the Prince went lobster fishing, helped gather potatoes and dip the sheep. He planted some trees of which only a few have survived the gales but these have since been replaced and some are becoming established.

There are few prehistoric remains here but part of a stone circle [NF912807] stands on a hillock, **Beinn a' Chlaidh** (G. – hill of the churchyard), beside Loch Borve – a large shallow and circular sea-loch. And there is a souterrain west of Borve Hill [NF907816] near Little Loch Borve – a freshwater lochan.

Berneray was the birthplace of the 'Cape Breton Giant' – one of the world's tallest and strongest men. Angus MacAskill (1825-1863) was a well-proportioned 2.36m (7ft 9ins) in height and weighed 425lbs. He died in Canada.

* * *

Access: For all ferry information, 08000-66-5000. South Uist ro-ro ferry: Lochboisdale/ Oban, Mon., Wed., Fri., Sat.; Oban/ Lochboisdale, Tue., Thu., Sat., Sun; Ro-ro ferry: Eriskay/Barra and return, frequent daily service.

North Uist ro-ro ferry: Uig(Skye)/ Lochmaddy, daily return service. Ro-ro ferry: Berneray, North Uist/ Leverburgh, Harris, several daily return sailings.

Benbecula; scheduled daily return air service from Glasgow, Barra and Stornoway, 0870-850-9850

Post bus services cover most of the island including Benbecula airport; Lochmaddy, 01876-500337; Lochboisdale, 01878-700288. There are also a number of private bus services and hire cars. Hotel and bed & breakfast accommodation available. Western Isles Tourist information, 01851-703088 (Lochboisdale 01878-700286, Lochmaddy 01876-500321).

Anchorages:

1. Acairseid Mhór, Eriskay. Well sheltered. Follow sailing directions to avoid drying rocks at entrance. There are 2 visitors' moorings or anchor S of the pier. W of pier is foul with old moorings.
2. Bàgh Hartavagh. Some shelter not more than 2c within entrance except from NE.
3. South Loch Boisdale. Ruined pier on south shore. Beware drying rock and shoal patch NW of the pier and Hut Shoal N of pier. Anchor E of the ruined pier, SE of the fish cages.
4. South Loch Boisdale. Anchor close S of Gasay. Poor in W'lies or SW'lies.
5. Loch Boisdale, in channel W of Ru Bhuailt. Fish cages block much of anchorage but quieter in SE gales.
6. Lochboisdale. 4 visitors' moorings NE of pier, or anchor in Bàgh Dubh SW of pier. Many moorings, very restricted, poor holding, soft mud. Swell in SE gales.
7. Stuley Sound, about ½c wide. Submerged rock is charted about midway, position uncertain.
8. Cearcdal Bay, Loch Eynort, SW corner of outer loch, NW of Eilean Eallan, sand. Clean and easy access but exposed E and SE swell. Or, occasional anchorage N side of loch due N of Eilean Eallan in 10m, mud. Holding good but open SE.
9. Poll Craigavaig, Loch Eynort, W of first narrows. Entrance difficult and subject to tides. Restricted by fish cages.
10. Upper Loch Eynort. Plenty of room for anchorage clear of rocks and fish cages, 2–10m, mud. Dramatic scenery, good shelter but seldom visited due to difficult entrance.
11. Mol a Tuath, bay on NW side of Usinish promontory, temp. anchorage with moderately good holding.
12. Loch Skiport, enter N of Ornish Island. Anchor S of Shillay Beag in Wizard Pool – squally in S'lies; or, in Caolas Mór (Little Kettle Pool); or Bagh Charmaig – not so good; or Poll na Cairidh – excellent shelter in S'lies; or Linne Arm – holding poor.
13. Caolas Luirsay just N of Loch Skiport entrance. Narrow,

shallow, entrance behind Luirsay Dubh. Affected by swell in N'lies. Anchor in settled weather in 7–11m mud.

14. Loch Sheilavaig, N of Loch Skiport. Fish farms and featureless but rocky challenge. Anchor SW of Canmore Island, 4m rock. Inner loch obstructed by fish nets.

15. Loch Carnan, approach S of Steisay and along marked channel. Jetty for Uist power station and oil terminal is 55m long with 2.5m depth. One visitors' mooring, or anchor clear of fairway and moorings NW of quay, or 3c further NW beyond Direy. Beware rocks and shoals.

16. Peter's Port, 3¼c W of SW extremity of Wiay, approach round N side of Lingay. Slipway at SE extremity of Eilean na Cille has depth 2.4m, rocky bottom. Alongside it and only 15m away is a parallel reef. If anchoring, keep clear of approach to slip.

17. Loch a' Laip. Enter between Wiay and Bo Carrach keeping ½c off Wiay until Bàgh a Bhràoige opens, then cross to N side and follow right through into NW arm beyond Keiravagh Islands. Anchor E of 0.6m drying rock. Good shelter.

18. Loch Keiravagh. Enter with caution and anchor anywhere suitable.

19. Loch Meanervagh. Approach with caution. Good, but very restricted by fish farm.

20. Loch Uskavagh, between Maaey Riabhach and Greanamul. Intricate navigation required but well-protected anchorage. Anchor anywhere suitable. Neavag Bay is very soft mud. Scarilode Bay has many rocks.

21. Caolas Wiay Beag, W of Maragay Mór and Beag. Enter with caution. Anchor N of Ballagary or further in.

22. St Michael's Point, opposite Sugar Bay on W side of Ronay. Anchor 1½c W to NW of Ru na Monach in 4–7m, sand. In summer there is seldom any swell. Or, 2c NNW of Ru na Monach and ¾c from W side of Ronay. Or small craft can anchor in bay surrounded by drying reefs N of islet N of St Michael's Point. Pass 20m NE of islet.

23. Kallin Harbour, 2.5m depth inside but 1.7m at entrance, very restricted temp. space. Approach with care by Vallastrome W of Garbh Eilean Mór. Anchorage difficult as fairway narrow, rocks at the sides and strong tide. There is one visitors' mooring.

24. Acairseid Fhalaich in Flodday sound between Ronay and Floddaymore. Tight entrance to restricted anchorage. Metric chart of rocks considered incorrect (see Martin Lawrence's Pilot).

25. Upper Flodday Sound. Beware mid-channel rocks SE of Haunaray if near LW. Anchor in pool SE of E end of Haunaray, or W of Floddaybeg, or in W side of Poll nan Gall.

26. Moireaig Bay or Harbour. Concealed and awkward entrance about 3c N of Floddaybeg, but good, interesting anchorage. Follow directions carefully.

27. Loch Eport. Follow sailing directions carefully for entrance to loch then possible anchorage E shore of Acairseid Lee or either side of Deer Island. Holding poor due to weed and soft mud, and subject to squalls. Better anchorage in Bàgh a' Bhiorain but narrow entrance to bay between reefs. Other anchorages can be found from Chart 2825 or anchor at head of loch (tricky approach) E of pier, 2m mud, or N of Eilean a Cairidh, 4m mud.

28. Loch Maddy, Ardmaddy Bay, on S shore 6c WSW of Rubha nam Pleac. Anchor off SE shore, 3–5m, no swell. Squally in SW'lies. Exposed NE. 2 visitors' moorings.

29. Loch Maddy, Ferry Terminal. 5 visitors' moorings or anchor SW of pier and well clear of ferry approach. There is a narrow slot, 2m depth, on N side of the pier which can be useful in emergencies.

30. Loch Maddy, south basin or Vallaquie, in SW corner of Loch. Anchor between old mooring buoy and wreck but beware reef and squalls can be heavy. Fish cages.

31. Loch Maddy, Charles Harbour, W of Hamersay, space confined, rocks, fish cages, and bottom soft mud or rock. Best E of Eilean Fear Vallay where there is 1 visitors' mooring or, if any space, in small pool by Oronsay.

32. Loch Maddy, Sponish Harbour, cleaner than Charles Harbour but poor holding. Anchor at head or in pool E of Ferramas.

33. Loch Portain (Partan), off Loch Maddy. Well-sheltered but holding uncertain in soft mud. All sides shoal. Careful approach required. Anchor where suitable but not more than 2c beyond islet.

34. Bàgh Chaise (Cheese Bay), W of Groatay. Best holding in the area but care necessary. Anchor W of Righe nam Ban.

35. The Caddy, W of Orasay. Approach S of Righe nam Ban and beware Strome Rock. Anchor off concrete slip, WNW of Orasay or try tricky Calm Bay, E of Orasay.

36. Berneray causeway – east side. Good anchorage sheltered from the W by the causeway.

37. Berneray Harbour. Excellent shelter but very restricted. Follow buoyed ferry passage into Bays Loch. (See Martin Lawrence's pilot or CCC for instructions).

38. Berneray by Cope Passage (remember that navigation in these waters is not a science but an art). Temporary anchorage in settled weather off the sandy beach 2–3c N of the Reef beacons. Turn S from Buoy 12 and pass 1c off Massacamber.

39. Bays Loch. Pass through the narrow gap in the Reef keeping 5m E of both beacons, ease round to starboard and follow the deeper water about ½c off the shore. 3 Visitors' moorings W of school, or anchor in N corner of bay, 3–4m, mud. Sheltered except from SE. No swell.

40. Lingay, in large bay between Sound of Berneray and Caolas a' Mhòrain. Anchor close off the island's SW side

in 5.5m, sand. Open to NW but very little swell. Note that Lingay strand connects E side of Lingay to the shore. Beware shoaling sandbanks in this area.

41. Vallay, a drying island midway between Griminish point and Aird a' Mhòrain. Anchorage in Vallay Sound is rock encumbered and difficult to enter. Depth inside 1.8m, sand, and protected from swell. Anchorage S of E side of Vallay has a bar to cross (0.6m depth at LW). Pool inside is 1.5–2.7m deep and sheltered from swell. Avoid shoals ¾c S of Vallay.

42. West coast of N Uist, Benbecula and S Uist has no shelter or safe landing places. Nor are there any sheltered anchorages on the S coast of S Uist.

7.16 Wiay

(G. bhuidhe – yellow or pleasant, ON -øy – island.) Sometimes written in the past as 'Vuiay', or 'Buia' (Martin Martin).

O S Maps: 1:50000 Sheet 22 1:25000 Sheet 453
Admiralty Charts: 1:100000 No.1795 or 1:25000 No.2904

Area: 375ha (927 acres)
Height: 102m (335 ft)

Population: 1861–6. 1881–5. 1891–10 (2 houses). 1901–4. Since then, uninhabited.

Geology: Lewisian gneiss, similar to the west side of Benbecula.

Wildlife: Wiay is a bird sanctuary and home to a number of species of raptors together with a good selection of marsh and shoreline species.

* * *

WIAY is the largest of the many rocky islands lying to the east of Benbecula. Although it lies closer to South Uist it belongs to the Parish of North Uist.

The rounded summit of **Beinn a' Tuath** (G. – north peak) near the centre of the island is the highest point at 102m with **Beinn a' Deas** (G. – south peak) considerably lower at 56m. The island is thickly covered with heather and pasturage on fairly gentle slopes and has only a few rocky outcrops but quite a number of lochans. The largest of these is **Loch na Béiste** (G. – loch of the beast) which was once believed to shelter a monster. It has three small islands in it, one of which may be a crannog. North-west of the loch, in the valley between the two hills and overlooking Sruth a' Chomhraig are the remains of a small settlement. Although this is a relatively large island it never appears to have been densely populated.

In the south, **Meall an t-Sruith** (G. – the hillock by the tidal channel) shelters a shallow rock-strewn bay, **Bàgh na Haun** (ON *havn* – harbour) with a narrow channel through which the tides rush. The islets, **Lingay** and **Steisay** are to the south-west.

The north of Wiay is bounded by rocky Loch a' Laip (G. – spoon-shaped loch) with the tidal **Keiravagh Islands** to the north. The entrance to the loch is guarded by Rubha Cam nan Gall (G. – crooked headland of the strangers). On our first entrance into this loch, creeping tentatively between the reefs and islets we were hit by a violent squall which flattened the water and covered the rocks with spume. **Bagh na Creige** was too restricted for shelter and **Bàgh a' Bhràoige** cluttered with fish cages. The squall was so strong that we left on a reciprocal course but, needless to say, as soon as we reached the open sea the wind dropped, the rain stopped and the sun appeared.

The western half of Wiay is puddled with lochans in the wide stretch between two small hills with **Lochan nan Lachan** (G. – little loch of the reeds) the most central.

Peter's Port on **Eilean na Cille** [NF849457] to the west of Wiay was completed in 1896 at a cost of £2000 in response to a demand for a new Hebridean port. Parliament wanted to be helpful, and the County Council gave assistance, but the result was a typical bureaucratic blunder. Not only was access by sea difficult but there was not even any access by land. Nevertheless the pier was built and extra expenditure of another £100 approved for the removal of a large rock which blocked access to the end of the pier. Although the sea approach was still considered hazardous, without a road the pier was, in any case, unusable.

At last a further grant of £1800 was obtained to construct a road which, if nothing else, helped communication between the local crofts. The 1931 edition of the *West Coast Pilot* dryly remarked '. . . the approach is so difficult, and there is so little room to turn, that it is not used by the local steamers. The port should not be entered without local knowledge . . .'

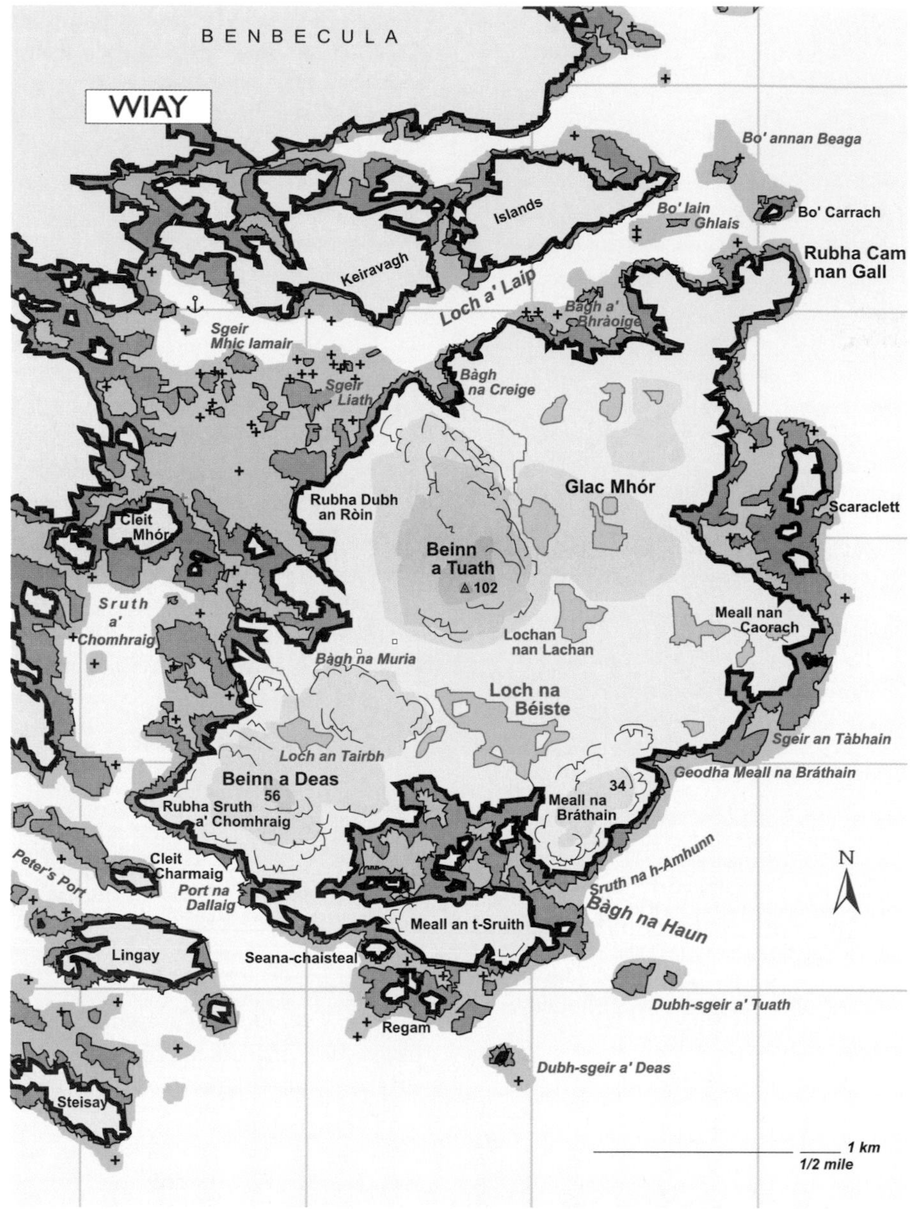

Access: Try Uist Outdoor Centre, Lochmaddy, 01876-500480 or Sea Trek, Uig, Lewis, 01851-672464.

Anchorages:

1. Bàgh a' Bhràoige, Loch a' Laip. Enter Loch between Wiay and Bo Carrach keeping ½c off Wiay until Bàgh a' Bhràoige opens. Formerly best anchorage behind drying rock, now probably no room due to fish cages.
2. Bàgh na Creige, Loch a' Laip. Cross over to N side of Loch when Bàgh a' Bhràoige opens, then SW course for Bàgh ne Creige. Just enough room at bay entrance for smaller craft.
3. Loch a' Laip. Best anchorage is in far NW corner, N or S of 0.6m drying rock. Good shelter but ½M distance from Wiay.
4. Sruth a' Chomhraig, W side of Wiay, approached from S. Not now suitable as fish cages obstruct W side and too many rocks on E side.
5. Peter's Port approach. Beware drying rocks SSW of Wiay. Approach round N side of Lingay and anchor in 4m, sand on rock, leaving clear approach to slipway. Awkward anchorage, about 4c from Wiay.
6. It may be possible to find a temp. anchorage in suitable conditions N or W of Cleit Charmaig in 6–8m but the bottom is mainly rock.

7.17 Ronay

(ON hraun-øy – rough island) or (G. ròn, N -øy – seal island).

O S Maps: 1:50000 Sheet 22 1:25000 Sheet 453
Admiralty Charts: 1:100000 No.1795 1:25000 No.2904

Area: 563ha (1391 acres)
Height: 115m (377 ft)

Owner: Let to a North Uist farmer as grazing for some 300 sheep. In 1974 the Spanish Ambassador in London had a house here.

Population: 1826–180 (Gaelic School Society *Moral Statistics Report*). Cleared in 1831, many settling on the neighbouring tidal island of Grimsay. 1841–9. 1861–4. 1881–6. 1891–6. 1931–6. Uninhabited since then.

Geology: Lewisian gneiss with some flinty crush and a peaty soil.

History: Ronay appears to have had a number of religious associations in its past. It has a

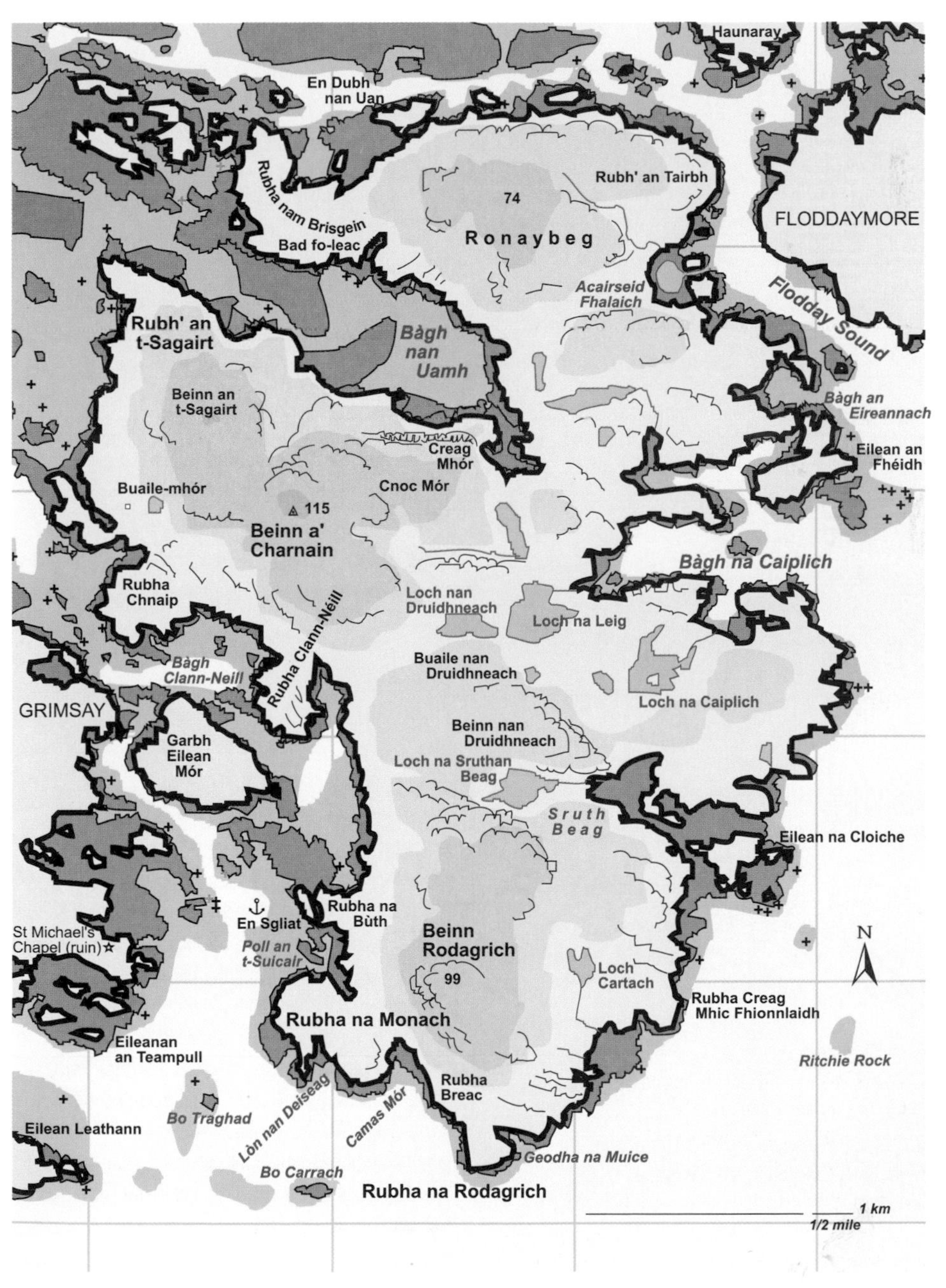

priest's hill, a monk's headland, a Druid's hill, and it had a chapel according to Martin Martin. Archaeological investigation may prove interesting.

Wildlife: One of the few islands in the area which is home to the Atlantic grey seal – protected by a special Act of Parliament in 1921.

* * *

RONAY is a fairly large rugged island with an extremely indented coastline. It has a series of hills which are bare to the north but heather clad to the south. The northern peninsula, Ronaybeg, is joined to the rest of the island by an isthmus and encloses a large and very shallow bay in the north-west called **Bàgh nan Uamh** (G. – bay of the caves). South of this bay are the two highest hills, Beinn an t-Sagairt (G. – the priest's hill) at 104m and **Beinn a' Charnain** (G. – the cairn hill) at 115m.

Ronay is divided from North Uist by a channel on the west side, which is an impenetrable morass of rocks and reefs although the island could be circumnavigated by an inflatable dinghy in suitable weather and at the right state of the tide (distance almost nine miles). **Garbh Eilean Mór** (G. – big rough island) is in the middle of the channel with **Eilean a' Ghobha** (G. – island of the dipper) to the north.

Martin Martin noted that there was 'a little Chappel in the Island Rona, called the Low-landers Chappel, because Seamen who dye in time of Fishing, are buried in that place.' This apparently refers to a pre-Reformation chapel. Fishermen from Ronay may have been buried at St Michael's Chapel on Grimsay [NF882548]. The ruins are clearly visible only just across the water from **Rubha na Monach** (G. – headland of the monks), Ronay's south-western tip, and Martin may have confused the geography. On the other hand there is a small rocky knoll near the west side of Ronay known as Cnoc nan Gall which can be translated as (G. – knoll of the Lowlanders) so maybe there was a 'Lowlander's chapel' actually on Ronay.

The hill in the centre of Ronay is called **Beinn nan Druidhneach** [drooi-niach] (G. – hill of the sorcerers). There was a Gaelic tendency to attribute anything ancient, like a Neolithic ruin for instance, to Druids or sorcerers but the hill may well have been the site of pagan rites.

Access: Try Uist Outdoor Centre, Lochmaddy, 01876-500480, or Sea Trek, Uig, Lewis, 01851-672464.

Anchorages:
1. Off St Michael's Point, on W side of Ronay. Anchor 1½c W to NW of Ru na Monach in 4–7m, sand. In summer there is seldom any swell. Or 2c NNW of Ru na Monach and ¾c from W side of Ronay.
2. Acairseid Fhalaich in Flodday Sound. Very tight entrance between two islets to restricted but snug anchorage. Metric chart of rocks may be incorrect (see Martin Lawrence's Pilot) as channel depth may be 4m.
3. Haunaray. Restricted temp. anchorage between Haunaray and Rubh' an Tairbh. Bottom mud but depth increases rapidly when clear of drying rocks.

7.18 Floddaymore

(ON floti, G. mór – big raft).

O S Maps: 1:50000 Sheet 22 1:25000 Sheet 453
Admiralty Charts: 1:100000 No.1795 1:25000 No.2904

Area: 58ha (143 acres)
Height: 28m (92 ft)

Population: No Census records and uninhabited.

Geology: A low-lying slab of Lewisian gneiss.

Wildlife: Barnacle and greylag geese stop off here in winter.

* * *

FLODDAYMORE, or Flodday Mór, lies close off the north-east side of Ronay. **Floddaybeg**, or Flodday Beag, lies to the north of it.

It is a low and fairly barren island but it is not short of fresh water as it contains one large central loch with its own islets and two other lochans connected to a stream in the south. The western headland, which is almost disconnected, is called **Rubha nan Caorach** (G. – the headland of the sheep or cattle). This may still be a landing place for stock. In the north continuous skerries join up a number of small islets and only a very narrow channel separates Floddaybeg.

All these small islands such as Floddaymore offer rather poor-quality grazing but they are popular with sheep-farmers and crofters because no fencing is required. This largely compensates for the fewer sheep per acre and the difficulty of access.

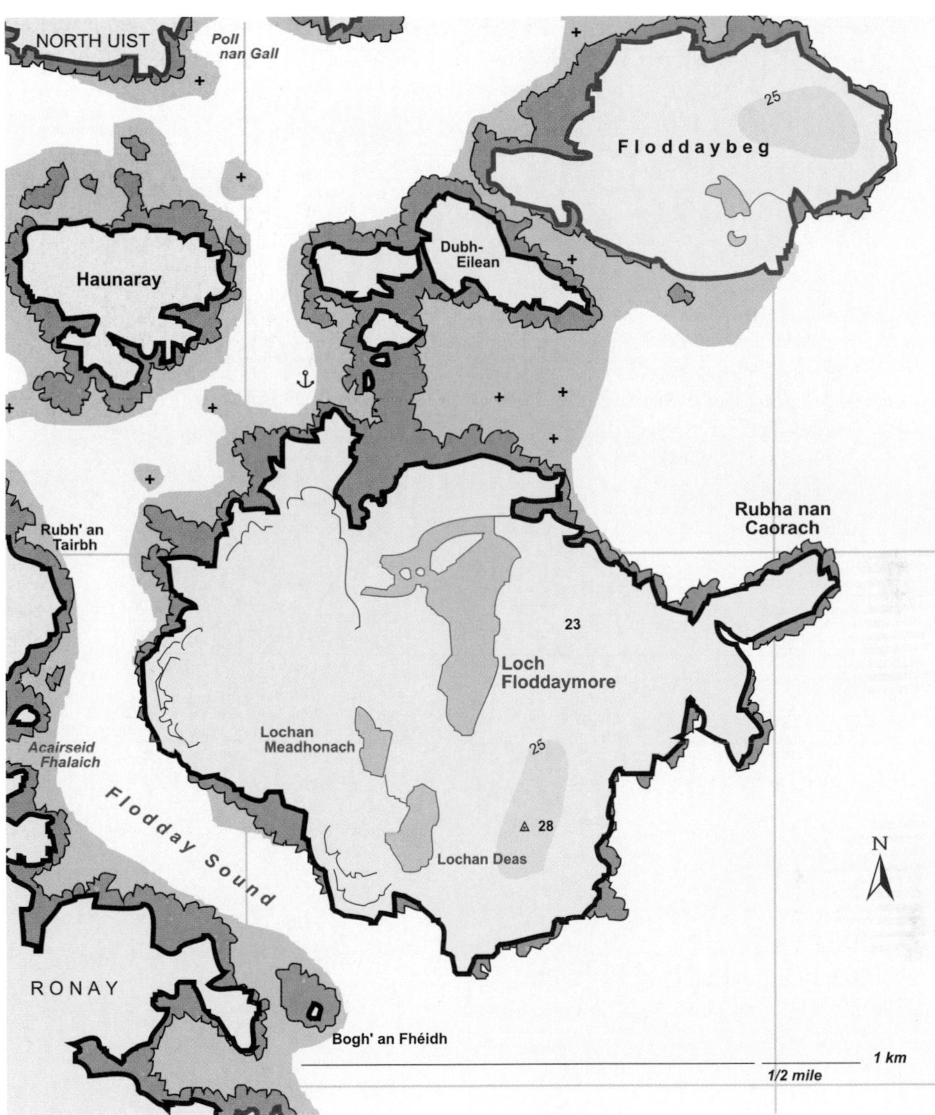

To the north-west the definitive hump of **Haunaray** divides the channel between Floddaymore and Ronay at a deep pool. Among the shallows beyond here is **Eilean nan Gearr** (G. – isle of the hares).

Our landing on Floddaymore was abrupt. *Jandara* was temporarily anchored south of Haunaray and near the Ronay shore. Two of us had no sooner cast off the dinghy than the outboard cut out. The gusty west wind immediately caught us and as we blew clear of Ronay's shelter we were thrown across the channel with almost hurricane force. Oars were useless and in a different situation there could have been nasty consequences. As it was we came to a comfortable stop at our intended destination cushioned on a heap of Floddaymore kelp.

Access: Try Uist Outdoor Centre, Lochmaddy, 01876-500480.

Anchorages:

1. Acairseid Fhalaich in Flodday Sound. Very tight entrance channel between two islets to a restricted but snug anchorage. Metric chart of rocks may be incorrect (see Martin Lawrence's Pilot) as channel depth may be 4m.
2. Haunaray. Restricted temporary anchorage between Haunaray and Ronay, N of Rubh' an Tairbh (G. – bull point). Bottom mud but depth increases rapidly when clear of drying rocks.
3. Upper Flodday Sound. Beware mid-channel rocks SE of Haunaray if near LW. Anchor in pool SE of E end of Haunaray (off N point of Floddaymore), or W of

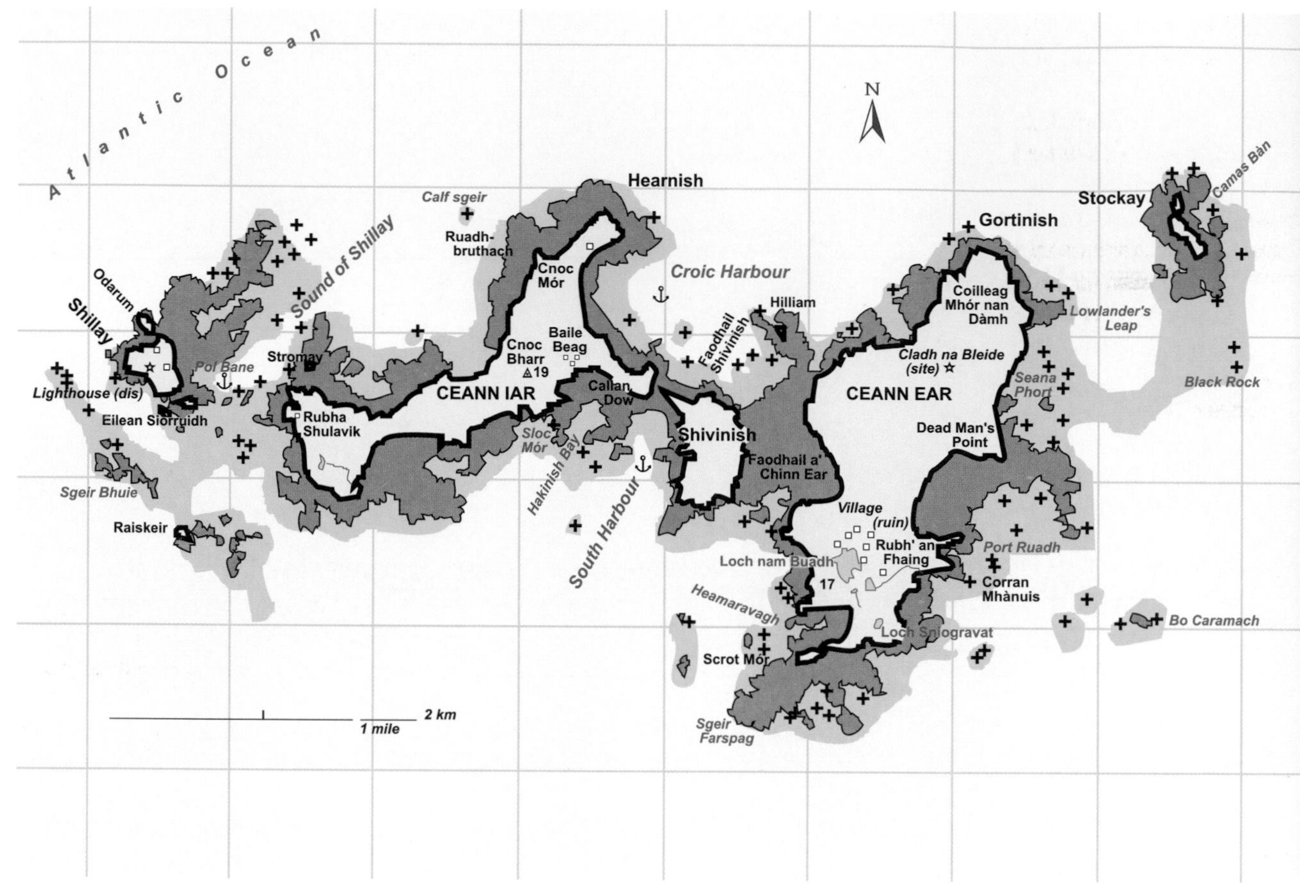

7.19 Monach Islands

(G. and E. – monk islands) Also known as Heisker.

Ceann Ear

[er] (G. – east head)

Ceann Iar

[eeur] (G. – west head)

O S Maps: 1:50000 Sheet 22 1:25000 Sheet 454
Admiralty Charts: 1:200000 No.2722

Area: 357ha (883 acres)
Height: 19m (62 ft)

Owner: North Uist Estate Trust 1990 (Lord Granville). Schoolhouse owned by Franklyn Perring (leased to Scottish Natural Heritage).

Population: In 1595 the islands were said to be able to raise twenty men of military age suggesting a population of about one hundred. 1764–70. In 1810 the population left because of the failure of the soil due to overgrazing which had exposed large areas of sand. Before the ground could recover there was a great storm which tore up the remaining turf and covered the islands with sand. By 1841 39 people had returned (4 houses). Later, marram grass was planted to stabilise the soil and by 1861 the population had risen to 127. 1881–24. 1891–140 (17 houses). 1914–80. 1921–66. 1931–33. Everyone then moved to North Uist except the lighthouse-keepers who were there until 1942. One family returned 1943–1947. Since uninhabited.

Geology: Schistose and granite bedrock covered with fine shell-sand and uncultivated machair, but great changes in the surface take place from Atlantic storms acting upon such a light soil.

History: Human settlement goes back to before 1000AD. In about the 13th century a nunnery or convent having connections with Iona was established on Ceann Ear, and the now-deserted lighthouse on Shillay marks the site of a monastery in which part of the monks' duties was to maintain a light as a guide for mariners. The religious associations of the Monachs however failed to survive the Reformation although the islands continued to be well populated until the 20th century.

Lady Grange (see Hirta No.9.1) was held prisoner here for two years (1732–34) by MacDonald of Sleat before being transferred to St Kilda by MacLeod of Dunvegan. She had hidden behind a sofa and overheard a Jacobite plot at her house in Edinburgh. Stupidly, she threatened to denounce the conspirators so, with her husband's agreement, she was sent to the Western Isles while Edinburgh society attended her 'funeral' at Greyfriars Church.

Wildlife: The Monachs are a National Nature Reserve and permission to land is required from Scottish Natural Heritage, 0131-447 4784.

There are no trees but there is good machair consisting of very little grass but a great deal of buttercup, red and white clover, dandelion, eyebright, blue speedwell, daisy, harebell, hop and birdsfoot trefoil, pansy, silverweed and wild thyme.

Fulmars which normally prefer high cliffs nest here in the sand dunes and herons nest in an empty house as there are no trees. Favoured for wintering by barnacle geese and frequented by common, Arctic and little terns.

The grey seal was one of the world's rarest seals with two-thirds of the total population of about 160,000 animals in the British Isles, and more than half that number in the Hebrides. Recently, however, numbers have been increasing rapidly. About 4000 pups a year come from the Monachs and the reefs of Stockay are a favoured breeding location in the last four months of each year. This is a comparatively recent phenomenon as the area was only colonised after the islanders had left. Grey seals are more cautious of man than the common seal. In the past, islanders found seals useful for food and clothing. They were easily killed when breeding, so depopulation of the islands has been of some benefit to the species.

* * *

Five small islands and several drying rocks form the **MONACH ISLANDS** group which lie about five miles west of North Uist and Benbecula. The group is also known by the old Norse name of **HEISKER** (bright skerry). The three central islands are all interconnected at low water.

Ceann Ear is the largest of the group (231ha), connected to **Shivinish** (28ha) which, in turn, is almost a part of **Ceann Iar** (134ha). There are difficult waters round about but these low-lying islands – little more than sand-banks – have wide sandy beaches and high dunes which offer shelter from the worst of the westerlies. Several sandy hillocks near **Gortinish**, in the north-east of Ceann Ear, reach their highest point of 18m at **Coilleag Mhór nan Dàmh**. To the east there is an islet called **Stockay**, and to the west one called **Shillay**.

It is said that there was once a great five-mile stretch of sand which was exposed at low water and which linked the entire group to North Uist. But in 1607 an enormous tidal wave – the same titanic tsunami which formed the Sound of Pabbay (See No.8.4) – swept away the sand-banks. The Monach Islands and their inhabitants have been isolated ever since. History does not record how many of the islanders, if any, survived this disaster.

The remains of some patches of grazing and cultivated land can still be seen in the vicinity of the small village in the south-west of Ceann Ear. This village is visible from Croic harbour and lies between **Port Ruadh** (G. – red port) and **Loch nam Buadh** (G. – loch of virtues). The village had good amenities, a post-office and a school which was maintained by the Church until 1874 and thereafter by the School Board. There were no shops – but there was a resident missionary. Sadly, the deserted village is disintegrating although the old schoolhouse is still kept weatherfast for the accommodation of visiting lobster fishermen from time to time. The village houses were unusual for the Hebrides as they had grain-drying kilns built inside them instead of in out-houses. This arrangement is common to Shetland.

Port Ruadh is south of **Rubh' a' nam Marbh** (G. – dead man's point). To the north is the probable site of the old monastery and churchyard, **Cladh na Bleide** [NF644624].

As one of the duties of the ancient monastery and convent on Ceann Ear the monks were expected to maintain a fire on the small western island of **Shillay** to help ships avoid the many rocks in the area. Eventually a red brick lighthouse was built in 1864. This was abandoned in 1942 but there is now a solar-powered replacement. A dressed stone from the old lighthouse is now built in to the church wall at Paible. On it the lighthouse-keeper had carved – 'Eternity oh eternity.'

Although by the 1930s the last of the islanders had left the Monachs this was no St Kilda type of evacuation. It was merely that, as with so many of these isolated settlements, the young people had travelled 'abroad' and failed to return and numbers steadily dwindled away.

Hebridean sailors believed, and maybe still do, that if they drown the sea will always carry their body home. A cairn on Ceann Iar marks the grave of Lieut Wm A McNeill RN, who drowned off Northern Ireland when his ship, *Laurentic*, struck a mine in 1917. His body was washed up on Ceann Iar which is part of the clan lands of the McNeills.

* * *

Access: By arrangement; try Kilda Cruises, Leverburgh, Harris, 01859-502060, or Seatrek, Uig, Lewis, 01851-672464.

Anchorages: Navigation around the Monach Isles requires great care as there are many hazards.

1. Croic Harbour. Good shelter except from NE, but uncomfortable swell in W to N winds. Good holding in sand or clay, 6m. Anchor middle of W side of bay, or in SE corner, clear of drying rocks.
2. Port Ruadh, on E side of Ceann Ear was the boat harbour for the village but it almost dries and has many reefs. It is well protected by high rocks and has very little swell but is rather open to SE winds.
3. South Harbour. Good shelter in N'lies, but scend may be uncomfortable. Beware drying rocks.
4. Shillay. Only approach from N, with stone beacons on Eilean Sìorruidh [shioorooi] (G. – eternal island) in line. Anchor off lighthouse jetty, 5m. This is the best anchorage but ill-positioned for easy exploration of the islands.

7.20 Hermetray

(ON Hermundr-øy – Hermundr's isle). Hermundr was a man's personal name.

O S Maps: 1:50000 Sheet 18 1:25000 Sheet 454
Admiralty Charts: 1:100000 No.1795 1:20000 No.2642

Area: 72ha (178 acres)
Height: 35m (115 ft)

Owner: Government-owned (Scottish Office).

Population: 1841–8 (1 house). Uninhabited since mid-19th century.

Geology: Lewisian gneiss.

History: In 1633 Charles I founded a 'Company of the General Fishery of Great Britain and Ireland' with its 'registered offices' in Lewis. (He already had proposals afoot for the purchase of Lewis by the Crown.) Lord Seaforth, who was owner of Lewis at the time, was invited to join the board so that his influence would 'keep the islanders in awe'. The corporation set up one of its fishing stations on Hermetray but the scheme collapsed in 1640 due to the start of the troubles which eventually led to the civil war. Charles II tried to revive it but it was seriously under-capitalised. In 1695 Martin Martin wrote that when he visited Hermetray he saw 'the foundation of a house built by the English in King Charles the First's time, for one of their magazines to lay up the cask, salt, etc, for carrying on the fishery, which was then begun in the Western Islands; but this design miscarried because of the civil wars which then broke out.'

In 1921, on the 16 March, following a savage storm, Alexander (Alex Beag) MacDonald was out checking his lobster pots when he saw two men waving on Compass Knoll, Hermetray. He found a ship broken apart on the rocks and three survivors in poor condition. Among the wreckage was a case of whisky so he first tried to persuade them to drink some but they refused. They were Norwegian and spoke neither English nor Gaelic. MacDonald had dry clothing aboard and after making them as comfortable as possible he took them home to Berneray where his wife and a neighbour fed them well and put them to bed. The following day, arrangements were made by the islanders for the men to travel to the mainland and thence to Scandinavia. Strangely, at no time did the men give any indication of gratitude or thanks to their rescuers and they were never heard of again. The name of the ship was the *Puritan* and to this day the islanders consider this must account for the men's inexplicable behaviour – their refusal to drink good whisky!

Wildlife: Some strange humps near the shores like large goose-pimples have been created by generations of gulls' nests. The rough grass, scattered with ragged robin and bog cotton, provides good grazing. Adder's tongue fern and flag iris grow in the wet turf and white clover where the soil is drier.

Buzzards sometimes make their home in the low

cliffs and help to control the rat population. There are no fish in Loch Hermetray.

HERMETRAY is the southernmost island of a group which lies close to North Uist in the Sound of Harris. **Cnoc a' Chombaiste** (G. – compass knoll), the highest point, is only a mere 35m above sea-level. It is in the north-east opposite Acairseid Mór (G. – big harbour), which is a shallow and weedy inlet with a rocky shore. It is formed by a neck of land with a rectangle of dry-stone walls (now used as a sheep-fank) and some ruined shielings. The sheep fank is probably the remains of the single house mentioned in the 1841 census and it might in fact cover the site of the original fish station. The east coast is moderately steep but Loch Hermetray in the centre of the island is low-lying. It contained fresh, clean and drinkable water when I tested it but it might occasionally pick up sea-spray when the wind is in the east.

The irrepressible Martin Martin reported that

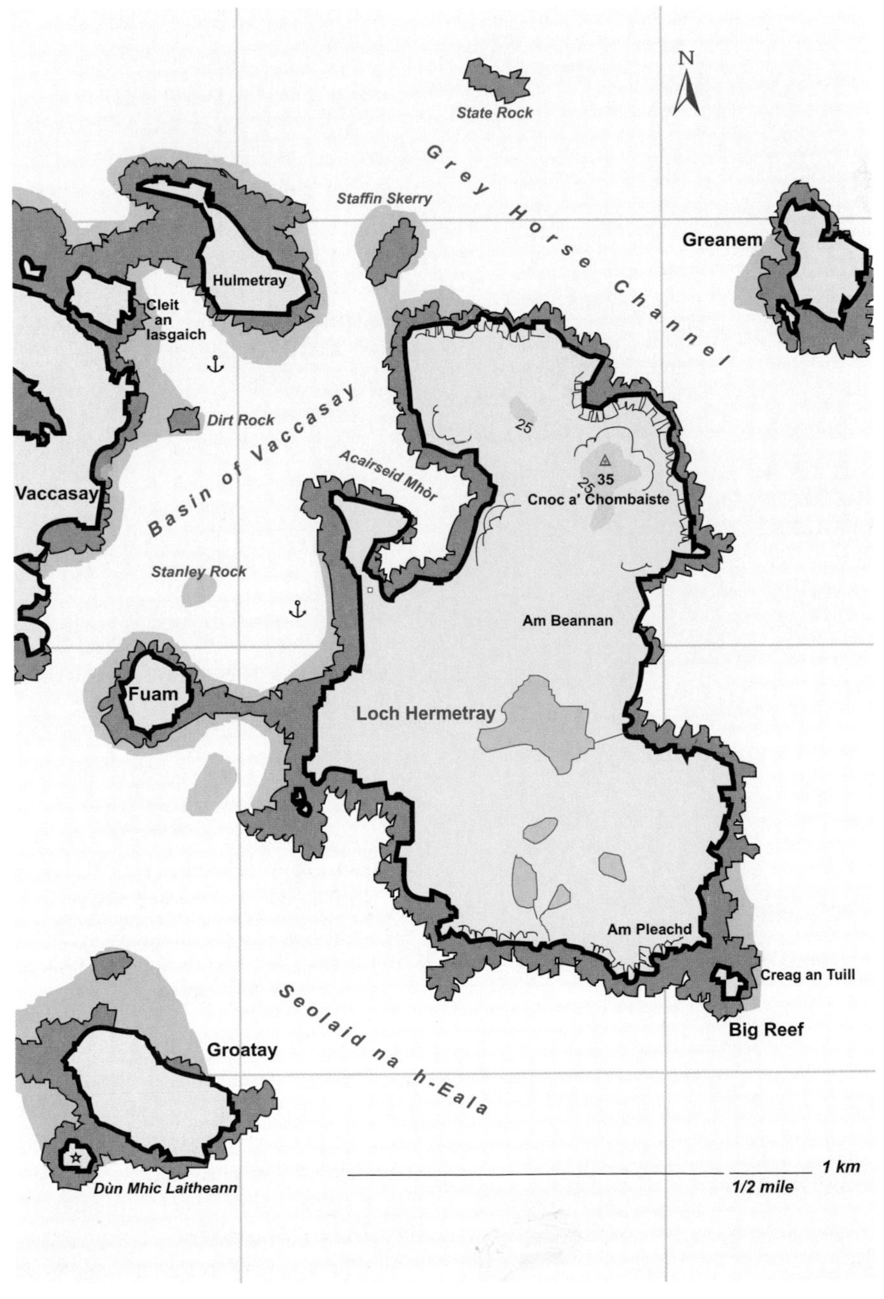

Hermetray had '...a moorish soil, covered all over almost with heath, except here and there a few piles of grass and the plant milkwort. Yet, notwithstanding this disadvantage, it is certainly the best spot of its extent for pasturage among these isles, and affords great plenty of milk in January and February beyond what can be seen in the other islands'. Hermetray still provides good all-year-round pasturage, but for sheep – not cattle, and peats were cut here until quite recently. The island is on the North Uist/Harris boundary and officially is part of Harris.

There are many small islands and skerries surrounding Hermetray, with **Greanem** (ON – green holm) to the north-east. Site Rock lies due north of State Rock and both cover at high water. About a century ago two Berneray men, with their guns and a dog were landed on Site Rock at low water to shoot sea-birds. A strong wind blew up and the boatman lost an oar when returning to take them off the rock. The wind and tide carried his boat away but, luckily, he landed back on Berneray. He immediately roused a rescue party. By then it was blowing a gale and night had fallen but in pitch darkness the rescuers managed to navigate through the reefs and reach Site Rock. The tide was still rising and by the time they reached the rock the fowlers only had their shoulders above water with the dog on one man's back.

Groatay [groa-ay], to the south-west, has a small drying islet between it and the North Uist coast on which can be seen the ancient ruins of **Dùn Mhic Laitheann** (G. – MacLean's fort). The fort was used as a herring magazine in the 17th century and has an artesian well for its water supply. The seaway between Groatay and Hermetray is part of the **Seolaid na h-Eala** (G. – channel of the Swan), named after a famous 17th-century Skye-built birlinn called *White Swan*.

Vaccasay (ON *vagr-øy* – island with a bay) lies immediately west of Hermetray and with extensive reefs linking it to **Hulmetray** provides valuable shelter for the Vaccasay basin. Martin referred to an island 'in Loch Maddy' called 'Vacksay' on which there 'is still to be seen the foundation of a house, built by the English, for a magazine, etc., for carrying on a great fishery.' It would seem likely that he was referring to Vaccasay (and not Loch Maddy) as the Hermetray fishery project would have used the Vaccasay basin for its anchorage. The full name for the drying islet forming the south barrier to the basin is **Fuam an Aon Fhoid** (G. – far-out isle of the one peat). It has shallow soil which only allowed a cutting depth of one peat.

To the north of Vaccasay is the large, almost circular 'Cabbage Patch' group which contains the Grey Horse reef, **Opsay**, and two islets, **Sarstay** and **Narstay**, sounding like the ugly sisters in a pantomime.

* * *

Access: Try Uist Outdoor Centre, Lochmaddy, 01876-500480 or Free Spirit, Leverburgh, 01859-520251.

Anchorages:

1. NE of Fuam in Vaccasay Basin. Beware fish-farm, Stanley Rock 1c NNE of Fuam, and drying reef between Fuam and Hermetray. Good anchorage NE of Fuam off pebble beach on Hermetray.
2. Acairseid Mór, narrow inlet on NW side of Hermetray. Except for the entrance only really suitable for shallow draught boats and very restricted space. Bottom mainly weed.
3. Between Vaccasay and Hulmetray, Vaccasay Basin. Beware Dirt Rock 1c E of Vaccasay. Anchor N of Dirt Rock. Distance to Hermetray 3–4c.

7.21 Tahay

(ON tagg-øy – island with a prominent hill).

O S Maps: 1:50000 Sheet 18 1:25000 Sheet 454
Admiralty Charts: 1:100000 No.1795 1:20000 No.2642

Area: 53ha (131 acres)
Height: 65m (213 ft)

Owner: Scottish Office.

Population: 1841–0. 1851–34 (6 households). Uninhabited since 1855. Although close to North Uist, Tahay is part of the administrative district of Harris.

Geology: Lewisian gneiss.

History: Six families (five MacLeods, one MacAskill) – evicted from Pabbay in 1846 tried to make a home for themselves on Tahay. Although there is virtually no arable land they hoped to survive by fishing. They constructed houses and a boat harbour; the ruins are still visible and one of the old houses has been converted to a sheep-fank. Several children were born on the island but conditions were appalling and in the mid-1850s the families gave up the struggle and emigrated to Australia with financial assistance from the Highlands and Islands Emigration Society.

Wildlife: A few small stunted rowan trees less than a metre in height support the only heronry in the Sound of Harris. A number of families of the birds like to group together for protection with their young of differing ages.

TAHAY is 65m high, easily the highest and most conspicuous island in the surrounding group. It has a regular – almost rectangular – shape and a central peak. There is a very narrow and shallow channel between tidal **Trollaman** and Tahay which is all that separates it from North Uist. Tahay has small inland cliffs and hilly tracts of heath and peat bog; the latter has always

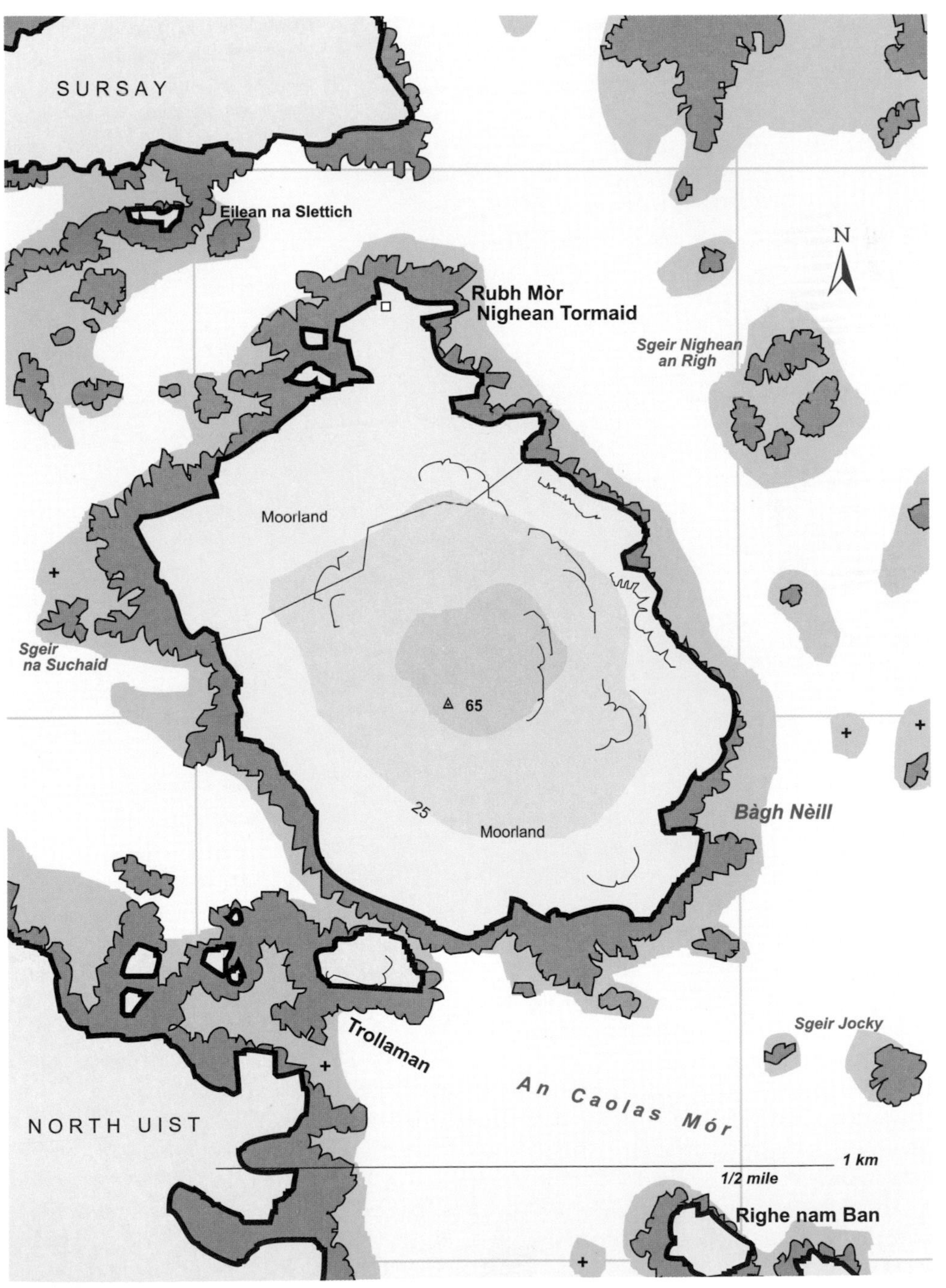

been a useful source of fuel for the Berneray islanders. The normal landing place for the peat boats was at **Rubha Mòr Nighean Tormaid** (G. – promontory of Morag, daughter of Norman).

To the north and north-west are **Sursay** and **Votersay**. The ruined shieling on the south side of Sursay is called Airigh na h-Aon Oidhche (G. – one-night shieling) because in the late 19th century a lone shepherd had to stay overnight on the island but was awakened by screeching seagulls and his terrified dog. He rushed outside and saw with horror what he described as an enormous cartwheel in the sky making a strange noise. As frightened as his dog, he ran to his boat, and beat all records to reach North Uist. He never returned to Sursay.

To the south of Tahay there is a group of three islets with the curious name of **Righe nam Ban** (G. – ?shieling of the women) although they are better known locally as Eileanan na Yacht.

Access: Try Uist Outdoor Centre, Lochmaddy, 01876-500480 or Free Spirit, Leverburgh, 01859-520251.

Anchorages: There are no recommended anchorages for Tahay.

1. Temp. anchorage is possible in suitable conditions due S of Tahay hill and ESE of Trollaman in 7m sand and shingle. Approach with care ½c N of Righe nam Ban.
2. The Caddy. Off concrete slip on N Uist, 5c S of Tahay and WNW of Orasay, 3–4m, subject to weed. Approach S of Righe nam Ban keeping closer to Orasay. Beware Strome Rock and other rocks W of Righe nam Ban.
3. Bàgh Chaise (Cheese Bay) on North Uist is ¾M SE of Tahay but is the best available anchorage in the vicinity. Anchor SW of central islet but beware drying rocks.

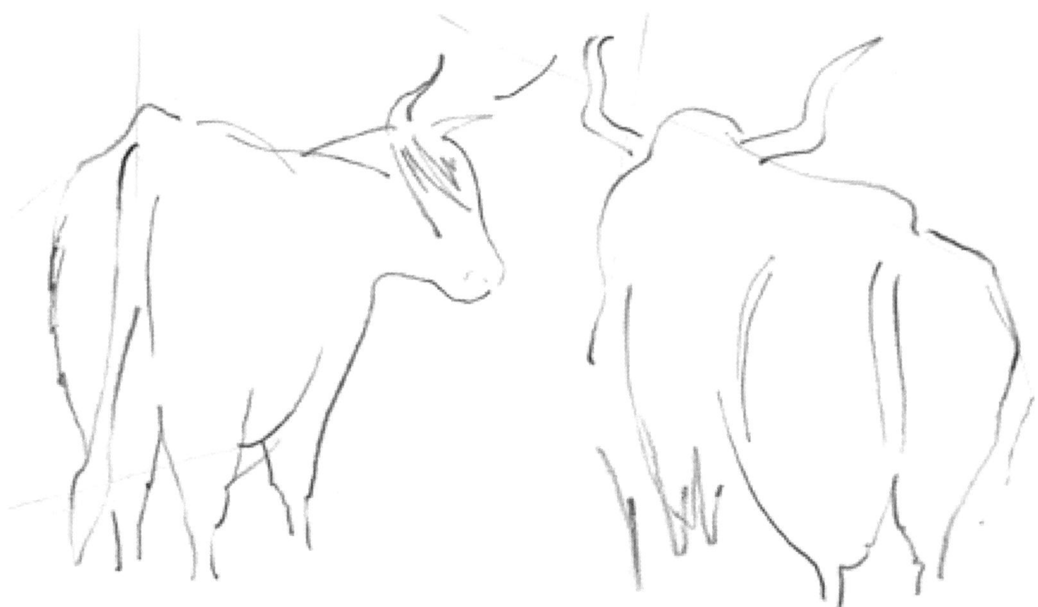

SECTION 8

The Outer Hebrides – The Sound of Harris and North

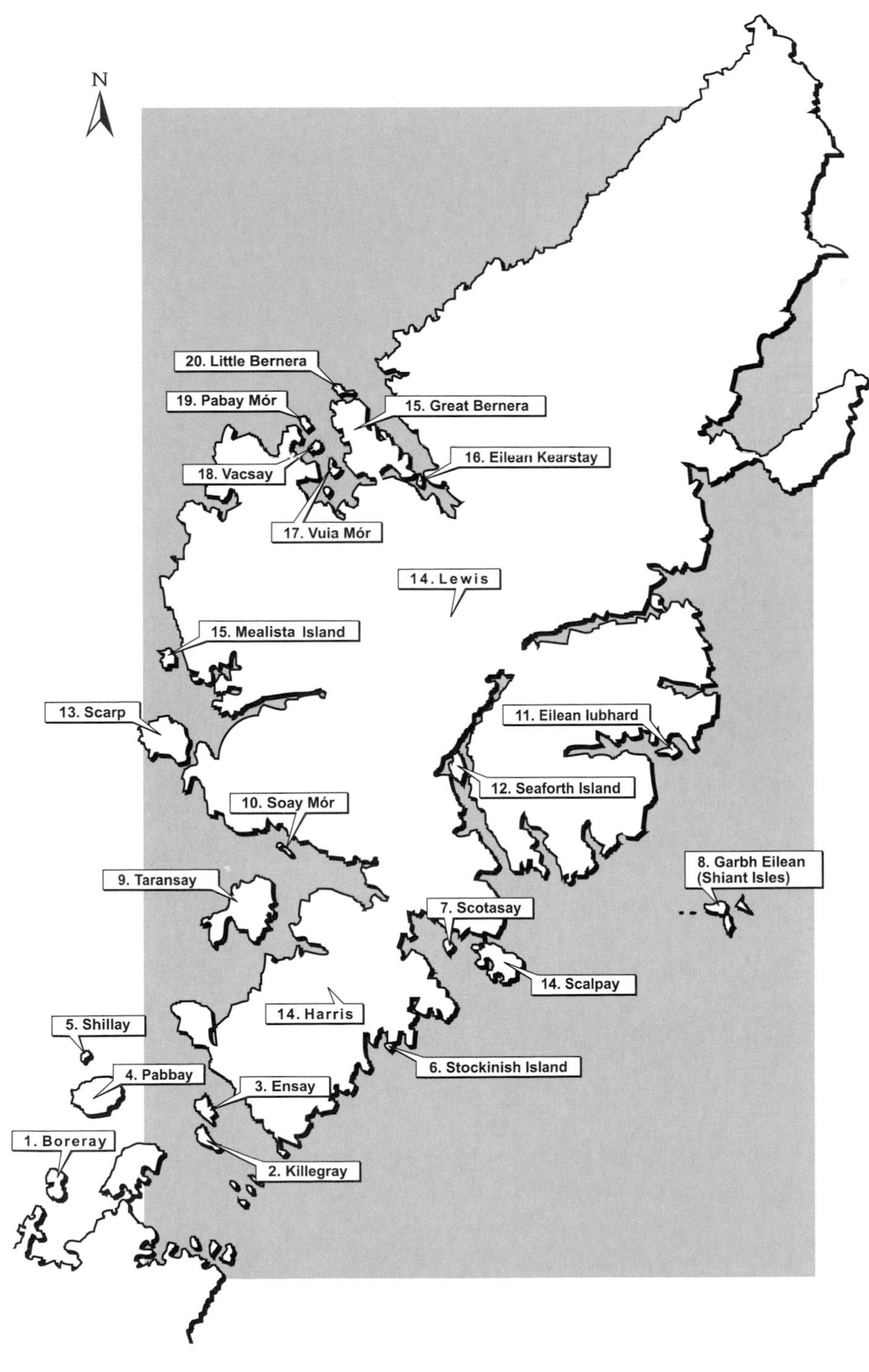

SECTION 8, Table 1: Arranged according to Geographical Position

No.	Name	Latitude	Longitude	Table 2* No.	Table 3** No.	Area in Acres	Area in Hectares
8.1	Boreray	57° 43N	07° 18W	85	108	489	198
8.2	Killegray	57° 45N	07° 05W	90	123	435	176
8.3	Ensay	57° 46N	07° 05W	87	119	460	186
8.4	Pabbay	57° 46N	07° 14W	46	35	2026	820
8.5	Shillay	57° 48N	07° 15W	152	83	116	47
8.6	Stockinish Island	57° 49N	06° 49W	150	126	121	49
8.7	Scotasay	57° 53N	06° 45W	149	107	121	49
8.8	Garbh Eilean (Shiant I.)	57° 54N	06° 22W	95	42	217	88
	Eilean an Tighe	*57° 54N*	*06° 20W*			136	55 143
8.9	Taransay	57° 54N	07° 02W	33	27	3645	1475
8.10	Soay Mór	57° 56N	06° 58W	153	135	111	45
8.11	Eilean Iubhard	58° 00N	06° 26W	102	88	309	125
8.12	Seaforth Island	58° 00N	06° 44W	71	31	675	273
8.13	Scarp	58° 01N	07° 08W	40	22	2582	1045
8.14	Lewis/Harris	58° 03N	06° 40W	1	4	5384126	217898
	Great Bernera	*58° 13N*	*06° 51W*			5243	2122
	Scalpay	*57° 52N*	*06° 40W*			1614	653 220673
8.15	Mealista Island	58° 05N	07° 07W	103	86	306	124
8.16	Eilean Kearstay	58° 12N	06° 46W	125	134	190	77
8.17	Vuia Mór	58° 13N	06° 53W	118	94	208	84
8.18	Vacsay	58° 14N	06° 55W	160	141	101	41
8.19	Pabay Mór	58° 14N	06° 56W	110	93	250	101
8.20	Little Bernera	58° 16N	06° 52W	99	131	341	138

*Table 2: The islands arranged in order of magnitude
**Table 3: The islands arranged in order of height

Introduction

The Hebrides are said to derive their name from the Norse word, *Havbrødøy* – meaning islands on the edge of the sea. On the other hand, long before the Norse era, Pliny called them the Hebudes – inhabited by the Ebudae tribe – and Ptolemy in the 2nd century wrote of the Eboudai islands above Ivernia (Ireland).

The great archipelago of the Outer Hebrides can look like a single island and is often spoken of as the 'Long Island'. Geologically it was, in fact, one long island in the distant past but, as the ground level changed in relation to the sea several shallow but distinctive interruptions were formed. The most significant of these is the Sound of Harris. Lewis and Harris, north of the Sound of Harris, combine to form the largest off-shore island of mainland Britain and Ireland. For comparison, it is more than twice the area of the next largest island – mainland Shetland – and one-third larger in area than Skye. The Isle of Man is not much bigger than Harris alone and the Isle of Wight does not even enter the lists.

It is hard for the modern city-dweller to realise the importance of water transport in early ages. Without roads, or even satisfactory tracks, and with forests, bogs, rocky escarpments, wild animals, and possibly hostile tribes, the sea was the main thoroughfare. The smaller islands were every bit as important then as our townships are today and, by the standards of the time, island access was relatively simple.

From this viewpoint it is easy to see why Lewis and Harris were thought of as separate islands. They are divided by a forbidding mountain barrier and to get from one to the other required a long boat ride round an irregular coastline. Mankind has farmed this land for some 5000 years yet the sheer size of the land-mass meant that, for centuries, human settlements clung only to the coastline. Inland was a large area of forest wilderness and swamp. Peat was scarce as the climate was warmer so timber was the primary fuel. Steadily the forests were cleared for fuel and to gain more land for subsistence farming. Such were the conditions 4000 years ago when the stones of Callanish on the west side of Lewis were erected on open meadowland. A thin layer of fine soil lay over the ashes and pollen grains of ancient forest.

Within a few more centuries only scattered patches of scrub birch, hazel and rowan remained and it was about this critical time that the climate turned colder. Tundra-type vegetation now took over the barren, treeless land. Heathers, sphagnum and other mosses, bog cotton and coarse grasses failed to decompose in the cold atmosphere and peat started to build up. When Callanish was excavated in 1856 the peat had reached a thickness of five feet (1½ metres) and in some areas it is as much as twenty feet deep (6 metres).

Magnus Barelegs, the Norse marauder, is usually blamed for burning down the forests in Lewis in 1098 but although he caused devastation virtually all the woodland had been destroyed by the islanders themselves long before Norsemen arrived in the area.

8.1 Boreray

*[**baw**-rë-ray or **baw**-rë-rë] (ON borve, or burgh, -øy – fort island)*

O S Maps: 1:50000 Sheet 18 1:25000 Sheet 454
Admiralty Charts: 1:200000 Nos.2721 or 2722

Area: 198ha (489 acres)
Height: 56m (184 ft)

Owner: Owned by the Scottish Government and leased to Borve Township, Berneray (except for one croft in the NE).

Population: 1841–181. 1881–137. 1891–152 (37 houses). Evacuated by request in 1923 but one family stayed on with a land-holding of 87 acres. 1931–8. 1961–5. Uninhabited since late 1960s to 1999. Since then – 1.

Geology: Lewisian gneiss with a light sandy soil.

History: Boreray has been inhabited since prehistoric times. Coins dating from the reign of James IV have been found in its sands.

Boreray was MacLean territory and the MacLeans of Boreray – up to the 13th laird who died in 1821 – are buried in the family graveyard on the east side of Aird a' Mhòrain, North Uist.

Wildlife: Eels breed in Loch Mór. Barnacle geese fly in each winter from Greenland to its shores and common seals collect round the coasts in high summer. Huge flocks of starlings can be seen and Boreray is at the southern limit of the range of the purple sandpiper.

* * *

BORERAY's highest point is **Mullach Mór** (G. – big top) which is 56m high and has a flattish summit. It is in the larger northern part of the island which is connected to the flat southern part by a strip of rocks and a low neck of land with sand dunes. The dunes continue on to the south-eastern shore while the north and west coasts are shelving cliffs.

The sand dunes curve round a wide bay bounded by **Tràigh na Lùibe** (G. – the bay beach). Ruins of an abandoned village are scattered on the flank of Mullach Mór and near a small burn which babbles down to the sea at Breivik (ON – broad bay). An archaeological site known as the **Nuns' Burial Chamber** lies north of the village [NF857816]. The old schoolhouse is now occupied by the sole island resident and the nearby crofthouse is holiday accommodation. South of the dunes there are more black-house ruins by the shore and below the chapel and churchyard site with its cup-marked stones [NF856805] a lone standing stone marks the edge of the rocks. **Cladh Manach** (G. – the monks' churchyard) was renowned in Martin Martin's time (1695) – 'for all the Monks that dyed in the Islands that lye Northward from Egg were buried in this little plot'.

In the centre of Boreray and almost cutting it in two is **Loch Mór**. The loch has its east side protected by the line of sand dunes but the Atlantic, when the mood takes it, breaks over the steep rocky reef closing the west side – there was also a submarine passage in Martin's day – and consequently the water is brackish. The rocky point beside the reef is aptly called **Sròn Fhuar** (G. – cold nose). Just south of Loch Mór is Loch Beag – a mere puddle by comparison – but fresh water.

Late in the 19th century, in an attempt to increase the area of fertile land, Loch Mór was drained for a time. It was proudly recorded that this action created '47 Scotch acres of good alluvial soil at a cost of only £125'.

A large vessel of the Spanish Armada (over 30m length) is said to have sunk in the area between Berneray's Rubha Bhoisnis and Boreray during a severe Atlantic storm. A collection of small boats brought survivors ashore at Port nan Long on North Uist but the dead were buried near the south-east corner of Boreray.

* * *

Access: Ask the sole resident, Mr Cox, 07733-065382; Sea Trek, Uig, Lewis, 01851-672464; or

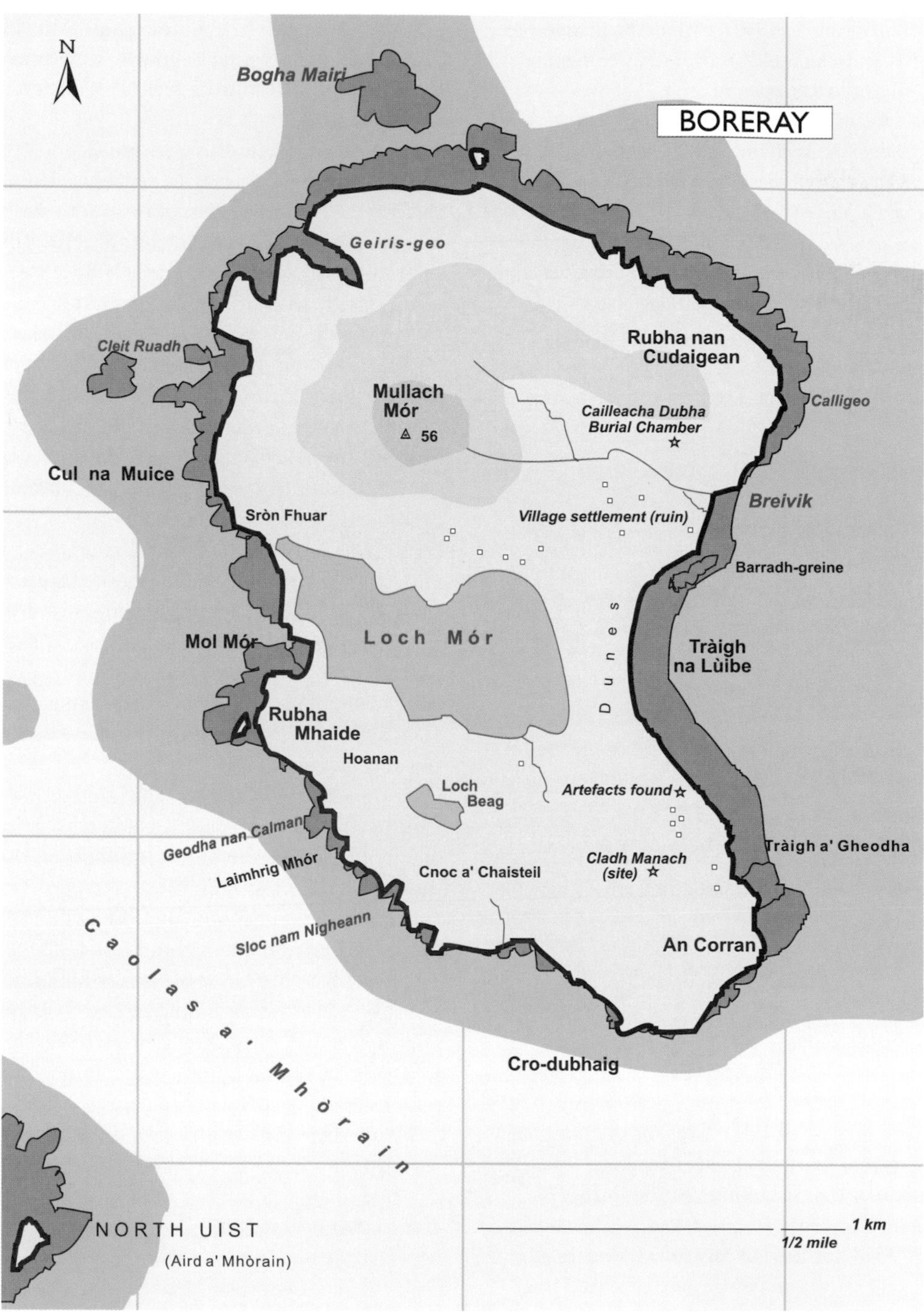

Uist Outdoor Centre, Lochmaddy, 01876-500480.
Anchorage: There is no safe anchorage near Boreray and no large-scale charts available (Imray's C66 is 1:150000, only slightly better than the Admiralty Chart). The deeper water has a rocky bottom and where there is sand it is either shoal or exposed to swell, but on a rising tide and in quiet weather it is possible to find temporary anchorage among the sand-banks to the east of Boreray.

8.2 Killegray

(ON kjallard-øy – graveyard island).

OS Maps: 1:50000 Sheet 18 1:25000 Sheet 455
Admiralty Charts: 1:50000 No.2841 1:20000 No.2642

Area: 176ha (435 acres)
Height: 45m (148 ft)

Owner: Bought by Sir Harry Wolfe in September 1985 from the Campbell brothers of Leverburgh.

Population: 1841–7 (2 houses). 1861–5. 1881–6. 1891–8 (1 house). 1911–3. 1921–3. 1931–5. 1951–0. 1961–0. 1971–2. 1981–0. House was being renovated in 1991. 1991–0. 2001–0.

Geology: As there is no suitable building stone in Leverburgh on Harris many of the black stone lintels used there have been brought over from Killegray.

History: This was one of the group of islands in the Sound of Harris served by ferryman Lauchlan MacLean in 1705 on the instructions of MacLeod of Harris.

The most expensive gravestone in the Rodel cemetery on Harris, apart from the MacLeod mausoleum, is in memory of John MacDonald, the MacLeod estate factor and former Army officer, who died on Killegray, his personal domain, after thirty-one years of service.

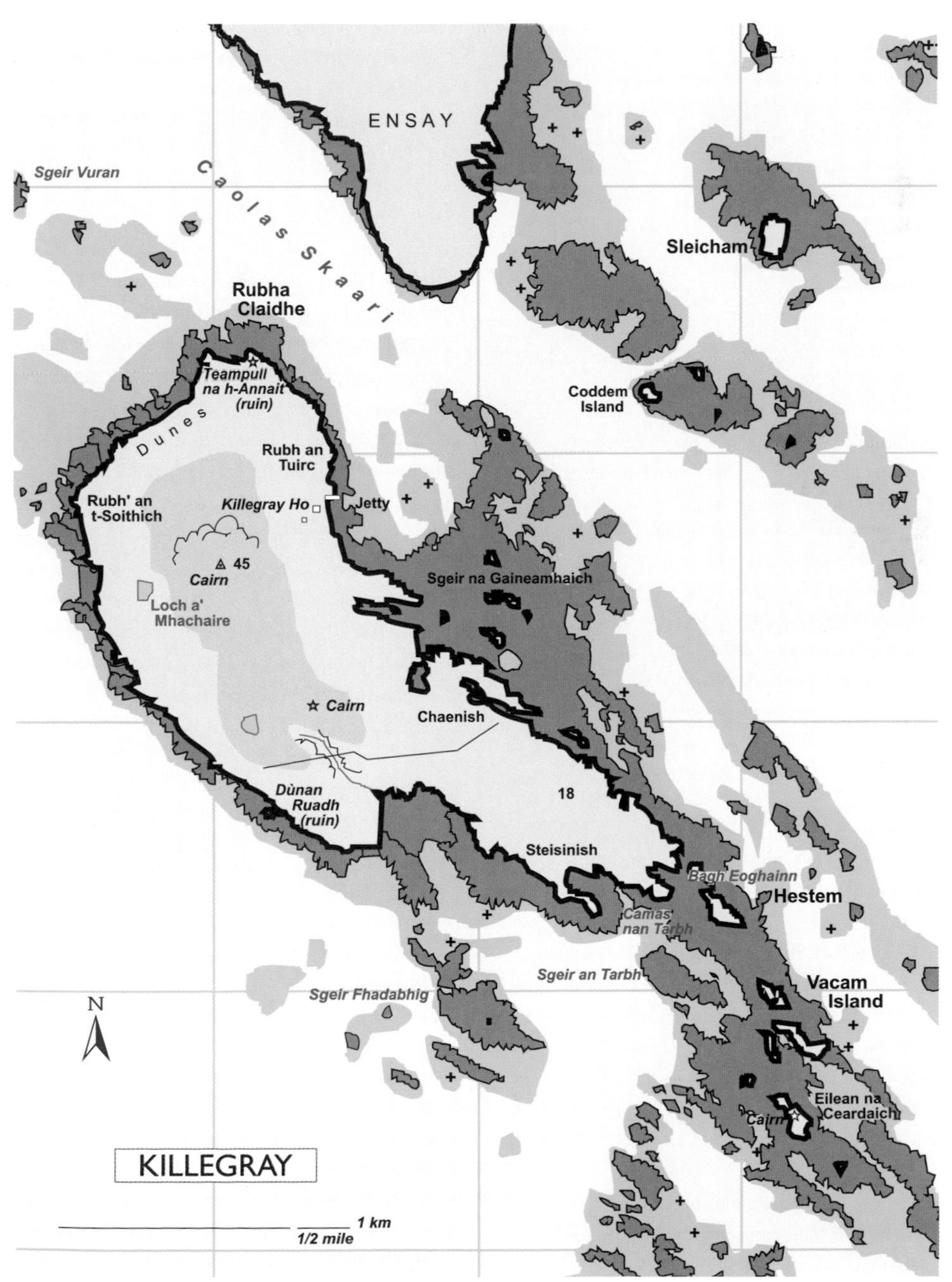

Wildlife: The shallow waters and many reefs in this area are a rich breeding ground for velvet crabs and lobsters.

* * *

KILLEGRAY is the most southerly of the two larger islands which lie opposite Leverburgh (An t-Obbe) – the small ferry-port on the south coast of Harris. **Killegray House** overlooks a shallow reef-rimmed bay on the north-east side with a pleasant beach and a small stone jetty. Behind the house a grassy hill 45m high has a conspicuous cairn on its summit. In 1991 the house, which is the only one on the island, was being renovated.

The island provides rich grazing for sheep in the summer months. On the north coast there are sand dunes between **Rubh' an t-Soithich** (G. – ship headland) and **Rubha Claidhe** (G. – churchyard headland) – the site of a ruined chapel, **Teampull na h-Annait** [NF975846]. This could be the churchyard site that gave its name to the island. Two tiny lochans sparkle in the machair on the west coast guarded by a small ruined fort to the south [NF975831]. Here, a small burn runs through a cleft which divides off the southern peninsula. An old dyke spans the island at this point and the ground south of it is uncultivated deep moss and a good source of peat which was worked for a time. There is an attractive sandy cove near Steisinish on the south coast, but the south-eastern extremity deteriorates into a confused group of drying islands, **Hestem**, **Vacam**, and **Eilean na Ceardaich** (G. – the tinker's island), and weed-covered skerries.

Both Killegray and Ensay were visited occasionally by the Royal Family in the past when cruising in the royal yacht.

To the south-east a group of tiny green islands guard the northern side of the Sound of Harris, **Groay**, **Gousman**, **Gilsay**, **Lingay** and **Scaravay** with an even tinier group beside them – **Langay**, **Gumersam Mhór** and **Bheag**, and **Dùn-aarin**. To explore these islets it is possible to anchor on the east side of Groay (north-west of Lingay). This is a sheltered spot but can be uncomfortable sometimes due to the swell.

* * *

Access: Try Free Spirit, Leverburgh, 01859-520251 or Hamish Taylor Scenic Cruises, 01859-530310.

Anchorage: There are no recommended anchorages.
1. Caolas Skaari between Ensay and Killegray can be reached by a narrow channel extending to the Groay group of islands. This requires considerable navigational care and is best attempted near low water when most dangers are visible. Occasional anchorage due NE of Killegray House but beware central shoal patch.

8.3 Ensay

(ON – John's island).

OS Maps: 1:50000 Sheet 18 1:25000 Sheet 455
Admiralty Charts: 1:100000 No.1795 1:50000 No.2841 1:20000 No.2642

Area: 186ha (460 acres)
Height: 49m (161 ft)

Owner: Archibald Stewart bought Ensay in 1856 and rebuilt Ensay House. In 1931 the chapel (restored in 1910) was bequeathed to the Episcopalian Church. Simon Mackenzie of Leverburgh bought the island from the Stewart family in 1933 and in 1957 the Mackenzies sold Ensay House to John David, a surgeon. The Mackenzies put Ensay on the market in 1999 for offers over £500,000 but the David family still own Ensay House.

Population: 1841–16 (2 houses). 1861–15. 1881–6. 1891–11 (1 house). 1931–8. 1951–2. 1961–2. 1971–2 (seasonal shepherds). 1981–0. 1991–0. 2001–0.

Geology: Gneiss bedrock.

History: A standing stone in the north proves that Ensay was of interest to prehistoric man. There are also two cup-marks on a small rock ridge lying parallel to the shore and about 100m north of the pier. The island, which is said to have been well wooded up to that time, was raided by Norsemen about one thousand years ago. They slew the inhabitants and slashed and burned the woodland. It never recovered and much of the soil was lost. The islanders had to resort to 'lazybeds' to make up for the deficient soil and the overgrown ridges are still clear to see.

Ensay was linked by the ferry service paid for by MacLeod in 1705 with Berneray, Killegray, Pabbay and Obbe (Leverburgh) on Harris.

In 1779 MacLeod of Harris' factor, Donald Stewart, bought Ensay from him together with some other properties when the MacLeod was facing bankruptcy. Donald is said to have ruthlessly evicted the tenants and his son John Stewart of Ensay followed in his father's footsteps. But it is also said that the Stewarts were good farmers who, for instance, introduced a horse-drawn precision seeder on Ensay when dibbers were still being used elsewhere. In due course the Stewarts sold Ensay and it changed hands several times before Archibald Stewart bought it in 1856.

Wildlife: Stunted elder, fuchsia, and sycamore – almost laid flat by the wind – struggle with beaten veronica bushes to survive by the main house.

In summer sheep are grazed on **ENSAY** which is very similar in appearance to neighbouring Killegray. The ground rises to a maximum height of 49m. A small stone jetty juts into a cove near

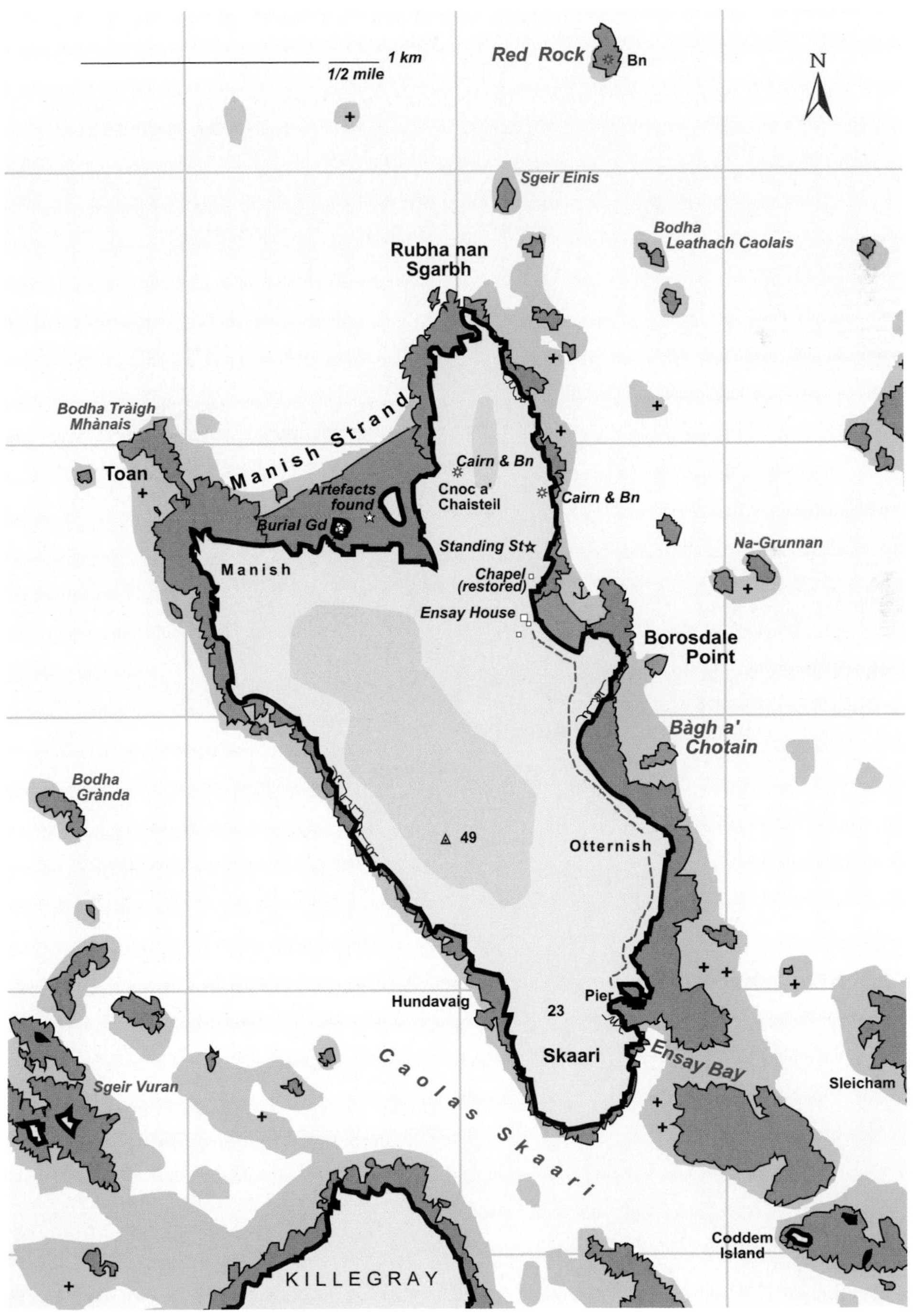

the south-east end of the island, and **Ensay House** overlooks a more attractive bay on the east side with a gateway and steps leading down to a crescent beach of white sand. The restored chapel near Ensay House [NF982866] has a fine carved oak door and a stone piscina.

Toan, the north-west extremity and **Rubha nan Sgarbh** in the north are steep dark-coloured rocky points with a beautiful shell-sand beach, **Manish Strand**, between them. One of the tidal islands on the beach is the site of an old burial ground. A 12th-century chapel [NF975868] possibly buried by the great storm of 1697 or the earlier tsunami, lies beneath three metres of sand. There may well be much earlier remains at a lower level. A Stewart grave has also been exposed and Viking relics have been found nearby. Martin recorded in 1695 – 'there is an old chapel here, for the use of the natives; and there was lately discovered a grave in the west end of the island in which was found a pair of scales made of brass, and a little hammer, both which were finely polished.'

It was from Ensay that Martin set off on his later voyage to St Kilda, on 'the 29th of May, at Six in the Afternoon, 1697, the wind at S.E...'

As with Killegray, Ensay is surrounded by rocks and skerries. The only ones which might justify the title of islets are **Stromay** in the north-east, **Saghay More**, **Saghay Beg**, and **Suem** to the east, and **Sleicham** and **Coddem Island** to the south-east. **Sùnam** is beside the entrance to An t-Obbe (Leverburgh) harbour but the **Carminish Islands** on the coast of Harris are all tidal.

Access: Try Free Spirit, Leverburgh, 01859-520251 or Hamish Taylor Scenic Cruises, 01859-530310.

Anchorage:
1. In bay on NE side off Ensay House, sand. Approach with caution following sailing instructions carefully. Sheltered except for N'lies and E'lies. Note reef on SE of bay.

8.4 Pabbay

(ON pap-øy – hermit or priest island).

OS Maps: 1:50000 Sheet 18 1:25000 Sheet 455
Admiralty Charts: 1:200000 Nos.2721 or 2722 1:50000 No.2841 1:20000 No.2642

Area: 820ha (2026 acres)
Height: 196m (643 ft)

Owner: Bought from the Stewarts by the Campbells of Rodel (Harris) at a London auction in March 1934. Sold in 1974 to Mr David Plunkett – a Lloyd's broker. North Uist Estates Trust (Lord Granville's family) own the crofting rights and these are managed by Mr Kenny Campbell of Leverburgh.

Population: In the early 19th century there were twenty-six families (about 100 people) living in comparative comfort. 1841–338 (61 houses). The island was cleared for sheep in 1846. 1861–21. By 1868 only a single shepherd's family remained. 1871–8. 1881–2. 1891–3 (1 house). 1931–3. 1961–2. 1971–4. 1981–0. 1991–0. 2001–0.

Geology: Gneiss bedrock with a fertile sandy soil and very little peat.

History: It is not known which priest or hermit settled on Pabbay and gave it its name. Columba never crossed the Minch and although the small chapel was dedicated to St Moluag it is doubtful if he ever landed here.

In the early 15th century the MacLeods of Pabbay spotted a raiding party of MacDonalds approaching. All the islanders took cover so when the MacDonalds landed they found the village deserted and set about looting and burning the houses. The MacLeods meanwhile set the MacDonald boats adrift and then rowed over to Berneray to summon help. A large party returned to Pabbay and found

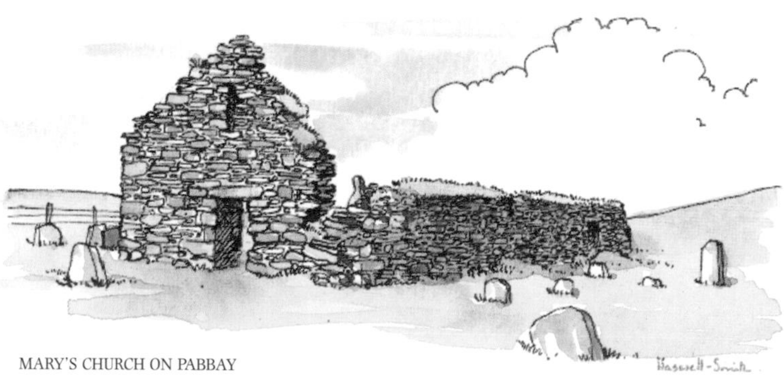

MARY'S CHURCH ON PABBAY

the MacDonalds now intent on dividing the spoils and rounding up the cattle. They hid by the shore and when the MacDonalds tried to escape to their boats they were trapped and slaughtered. The final battle probably took place between Seana-Chaisteal and the river, Abhainn Lingay, but the whole area has now been covered with sand dunes.

Pabbay was a favourite island of the MacLeod chiefs and some years after the Norsemen left they built a castle which, at the time, was equal in importance to Dunvegan in Skye. It was not until the 16th century that their interest concentrated on Dunvegan and the castle on Pabbay lapsed into disrepair. In 1467, Iain Borb, Chief of the MacLeods, died at the castle while fencing with his cousin. He apparently lost his temper and an old battle wound on his forehead could not be staunched when it started bleeding profusely.

It is recorded that in 1680 there were four 'townships' on Pabbay – Baile fo Thuath, Baile Meadhonach, Baile Lingay, and Baile na Cille – but in 1697 a violent storm destroyed Baile Meadhonach, stripped off the topsoil and buried the wrecked village in sand.

Pabbay once had a considerable population and most of the Stewards of St Kilda were Pabbay men. In 1705 a boat was purchased by MacLeod for use as a ferry to serve Pabbay, Berneray, Ensay, Killegray, Harris and Skye. Unlike the MacLeods of Berneray who had Jacobite sympathies, the MacLeods of Pabbay supported the Government in the 1745 rebellion.

There was a population of about one hundred at the start of the 19th century living in comparative comfort and producing, and even exporting, corn, barley and illicit whisky. Pabbay was then part of the 'quod sacra Parish of Bernera'. Numbers had risen to over 300 by 1841 before the island was cleared for sheep. It is known that there were still a few cattle because three of these won a prize for the heaviest Highland cattle at Smithfield – proof of the richness of the island machair. Some of the displaced population went to Canada and Australia, but many settled on Scalpay, Berneray and in the Bays area of Harris. But with the island clearance in 1846 the value of centuries of careful husbandry was lost to coarse grazing.

The island is now run as a single sheep-farm.

Wildlife: Ancient birch tree trunks, roots and peat deposits are sometimes exposed by the wind and sea, particularly during abnormal spring tides, in the intertidal zone at the north end of the Quinish reef and on the shore opposite. Marram-grass on the dunes struggles to hold down the windblown sand. It is also found in patches by the ruined main homestead at Baile fo Thuath – probably originally seeded from the thatched roofs.

A small resident herd of red deer, introduced in 1880, graze on Beinn a' Charnain. Shag and fulmar nest on the low north-coast cliffs but gulls and eider prefer the tidal reef at Quinish. Barnacle geese winter on Pabbay in large numbers.

* * *

The island of **PABBAY** was once rich and green and known as 'the granary of Harris'. But since clearance in the mid-19th century, drift, sea spray and lack of care have destroyed much of its former fertility and sheep now graze on the wildflowers of the machair. Nevertheless, it is still one of the most beautiful islands in the Hebrides with its white sands, rich machair and aquamarine sea. **Beinn a' Charnain** (G. – cairn hill), a sharp-peaked hill in the north is the highest point at 196m.

A pointed sandy hillock between two beaches on the south-west coast still shows traces of the walls of **Seana-Chaisteal** (G. – ancient castle). This is the site of the old MacLeod castle or dun [NF902871]. The wide beaches below the castle are backed by sand dunes.

West of the castle site and beyond Abhainn Lingay (ON and G. – heather burn) is the landing place of Haltois below **Bailenacille** (G. – Kirktown). A small cottage which is used by visiting shepherds faces the sea with a burn behind it dividing it from the ruin of **Teampull Mhóire** (G. – Mary's Church) in its old kirkyard [NF890870]. One gable and part of the walls remain. The age of the building is uncertain but it may be early 16th century. Only four metres to the west are the remains of an earlier chapel which was probably dedicated to St Moluag and between these ruins and the Lingay Burn is an old corn-drying kiln.

The stone from many of the old houses has been used to build a wall enclosing a Pairc Mhor (G. – big park) for the sheep at lambing time and within this area is a ruined Iron Age dun.

The lost village of **Baile Meadhonach** (G. – Midtown) lay to the north of Seana-Chaisteal but

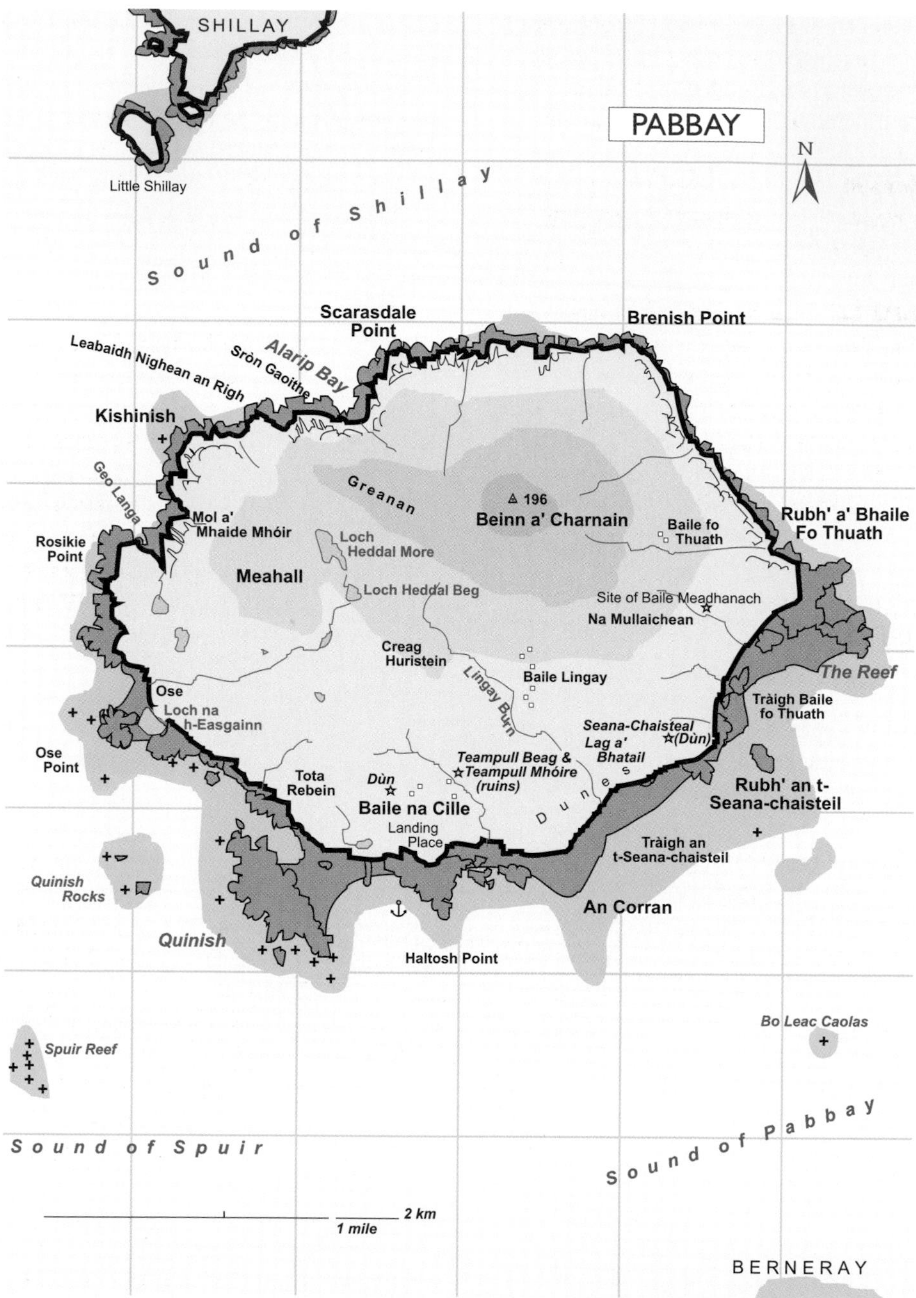

the houses of **Baile Lingay** are clearly visible beside the Lingay Burn. These form two groups – the MacNeill farm buildings, and the workers' houses higher up the hillside and above the arable land. West of the workers' houses is Creag Huristein – an odd collection of eroded erratic boulders likes pieces of imaginative modern sculpture.

Baile fo Thuath (G. – Northtown) is high on the western hillside with a T-shaped main farmhouse and a circular ruin behind it. Looking across the Sound of Harris from here the **Druim na Beisde** (G. – the ridge of the beast) can be seen as a pale shape across the water. This three-mile long sand-bank shifts its position frequently and sometimes cuts off the passage to Pabbay.

The north coast consists of rugged cliffs which stand against the tide that sweeps through the Sound of Shillay. In the cliff-face at **Sròn Gaoith** (G. – nose of the wind) is a cave known as Carn mhic an t-Sronaich after a notorious murderer who is said to have hidden there and the small plateau to the west of it is called, strangely, **Leabaidh Nighean an Righ** (G. – the king's daughter's bed).

The lochs in this remote western side of the island have a few peat deposits near them and were probably, therefore, the site of the old illicit whisky stills.

Although there are the ancient remains of sacred buildings on Pabbay, in recent centuries folk usually crossed the Sound (weather permitting) to attend church on Berneray. The sand spit from Berneray was once said to be so close to Pabbay that a wife could throw her washboard across the channel between them.

* * *

Access: Try Free Spirit, Leverburgh, 01859-520251 or Hamish Taylor Scenic Cruises, 01859-530310.

Anchorage: Avoid the N coast as local fishermen say there are uncharted in-shore rocks, the W coast is too exposed and the SW foul with skerries. On the E side the shoals and sand-banks move and must be navigated carefully.
1. Temp. anchorage on S coast near Haltois Point, E of drying reef in 4m, sand. Land, and re-embark, at or above half-tide, swell permitting.

8.5 Shillay

(ON selr-øy – seal island).

OS Maps: 1:50000 Sheet 18 1:25000 Sheet 455
Admiralty Charts: 1:50000 No.2841 1:20000 No.2642

Area: 47ha (116 acres)
Height: 79m (259 ft)

Owner: Scottish Office (Department of Agriculture). Borve Township, Berneray has the grazing rights.

Population: No Census records and no signs of past habitation.

Geology: Gneiss with a light sandy soil.

Wildlife: In 1695 Martin Martin said that he had found sheep on Shillay with the biggest horns he had ever seen.

Both storm and Leach's petrel breed among the boulders on Shillay and probably also the Arctic tern, *Sterna paradisaea*.

Hundreds of grey seals, once one of the world's rarer species, also breed here producing between 150 and 200 calves per year. They collect in huge numbers on the foreshore during the pupping season. When the weather is particularly bad seals which normally give birth on Haskeir join those on Shillay. The seals on Shillay were studied in detail when a special camp was set up in October 1961. Juveniles were branded to track their movements but as a consequence some of the seals moved over to Coppay to give birth.

The Sound of Shillay yields reasonable quantities of the edible crab, *Cancer pagarus* and some of the tastiest lobsters in the Hebrides. Donald MacKillop of Berneray records that in 1946 a lobster found under a rock on the North Uist shore was 35ins long, 15½ins in circumference, with 7½ins of cutting edge on the scissors claw and an empty shell weight of 10¾lbs.

* * *

The water lapped gently under our hulls as *Jandara* lay alongside *Berneray Isle* in the Sound of Shillay. We had stopped for a chat with Angus MacAskill and his nephew Roddy who were out lobster fishing. The sunlight glinted off the wet seaweed on the rocks of Shillay. *Berneray Isle* is the boat in which Prince Charles, Lord of the Isles and Prince of Wales, went lobster fishing with all the long experience of Angus to assist him (and it was Angus's wife, Mary, who cooked the Prince his favourite clootie dumpling).

SHILLAY has dark-coloured vertical cliffs at its northern end beneath a round-topped hill of 79m height. Vegetation is sparse but offers grazing for sheep. The southern part of the island slopes towards the **Sound of Shillay**, the channel between Pabbay and Shillay, and has a small bay with a sand and boulder beach on its south-east side where the grey seals gather in the autumn sheltered by **Aird an Laoigh** (G. – headland of the seal-calf). Although the gentle slopes make it easier for the seals to come ashore it also means greater infant mortality when there are storms and high seas. These sweep the young ones into the water before they can fend for themselves.

Little Shillay, lying south-west of Shillay, is a rocky outcrop that rises to a height of 30m. And some distance away in the opposite direction,

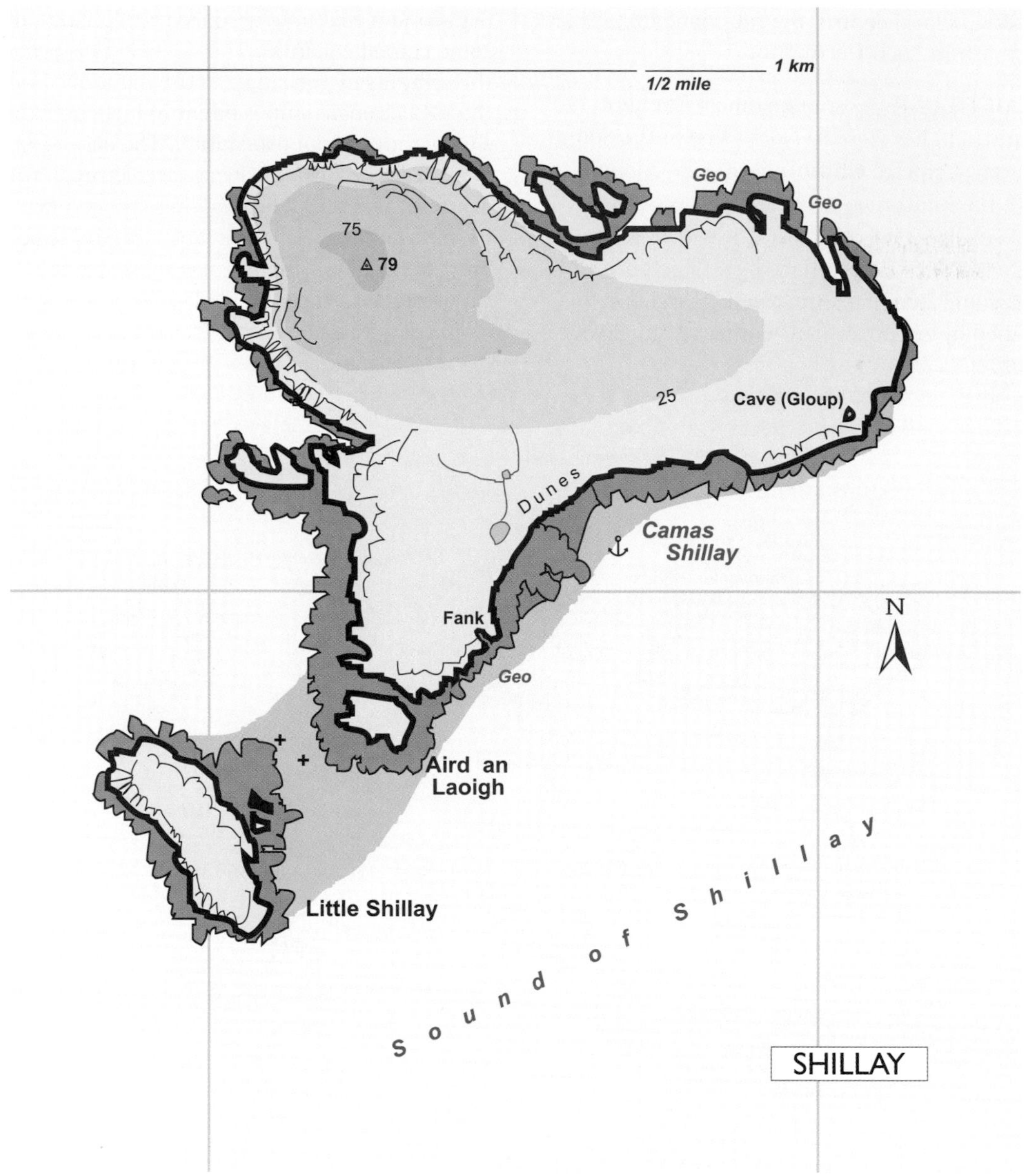

guarding the north-west entrance to the Sound of Harris is the steep little island of **Coppay** (ON – cup-shaped island).

* * *

Access: Try Free Spirit, Leverburgh, 01859-520251 or Hamish Taylor Scenic Cruises, 01859-530310, or ask on Berneray.

Anchorage: Temporary anchorage when winds between NW and NNE off the centre of the sandy beach on the SE side in suitable depth. Bottom chiefly sand with patches of rock and kelp which can normally be seen and avoided.

8.6 Stockinish Island

(ON stakkr – stack, ON nes – promontory.) Rock stacks guard the seaward approach.

OS Maps. 1:50000 Sheet 14 1:25000 Sheet 455
Admiralty Charts: 1:100000 No.1795 1:50000 No.2841

Area: 49ha (121 acres)
Height: 44m (144 ft)

Owner: Tenancy held by Donald MacLeod, Stockinish. Previously held by the Campbell brothers, Leverburgh.

Population: No Census records and uninhabited

Geology: Lewisian gneiss similar to the geology of neighbouring Harris with small pockets of poor peaty soil.

* * *

Loch Stockinish is another of the many firths penetrating the frayed eastern edge of Harris – dark brown, barren, and beautiful. Where the Golden Road skirts the loch there is a youth hostel and a few houses scattered in the hollows. **STOCKINISH ISLAND** at the entrance to the loch is separated from the 'mainland' by a long, narrow, but navigable channel – **Caolas Beag** (G. – little channel). In fact, in spite of its narrowness (27m minimum), it is an easier route into the loch than **Caolas Mór** on the west side, which is wide but littered with rocks. A tiny islet, **Eilean Leasait**, snuggles by the west shore of Stockinish Island.

Stockinish has no habitation on it and matches the surrounding landscape – pink and grey glaciated rock with little pockets of dark-umber peat and a tangle of twisted heather. Its main feature is a large shallow central pool, Loch an t-Sàile (G. – saltwater loch), opening off an inlet from Caolas Beag which may once have served

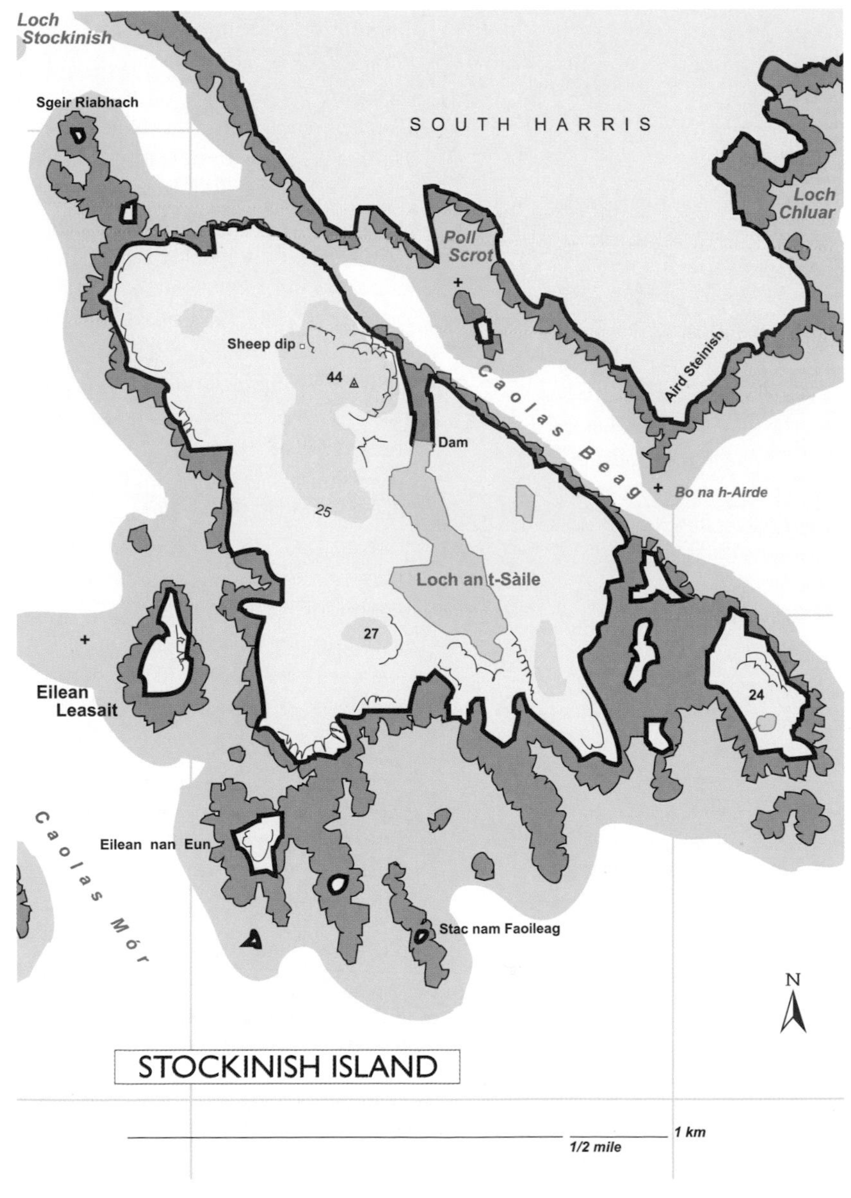

as a fish-trap but which is now permanently dammed and used by the local fishermen as a lobster pond. The island's highest point (44m) is a steep hillock beside this inlet.

At the southern end of the island there is a deep skirt of drying islets, rocks, reefs and stacks.

Access: Try Free Spirit, Leverburgh, 01859-520251, Hamish Taylor Scenic Cruises, Tarbert, 01859-530310 or a boat-owner at Poll Scrot.

Anchorage: No recommended anchorage close to the island. 1. Loch Stockinish. Easiest access to loch is through Caolas Beag, E of Stockinish Island; best before half-tide. Very narrow (only 27m at one point) but clean if close in to Stockinish Island. After passing Stockinish Island keep just NE of mid-channel. Anchor in mouth of westerly arm at head of loch, completely sheltered, 9m sand. Beware rock off Ardvey Point & overhead cable to N (15m? clearance). Distance is slightly over 1M by dinghy to Stockinish Island.

8.7 Scotasay

Probably (ON – Skati's island) but possibly (ON Skot's-øy – Scot's island).

OS Maps: 1:50000 Sheet 14 1:25000 Sheet 455
Admiralty Charts: 1:100000 Nos.1794 or 1795 1:12500 No.2905

Area: 49ha (121 acres)
Height: 57m (187 ft)

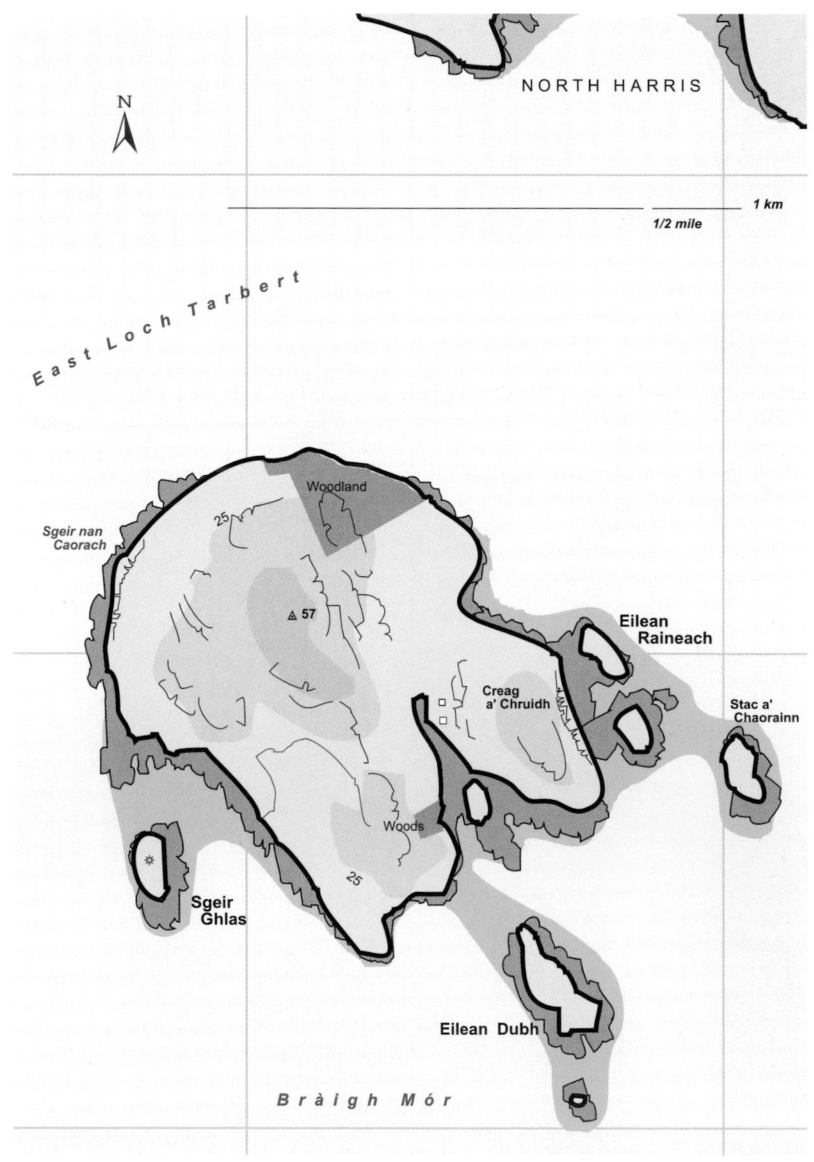

Owner: Mr John Taylor, an English architect, who also owns neighbouring Scalpay.

Population: 1861–14. 1881–0. 1891–18 (2 houses). 1901–15. 1911–20. 1921–19. Uninhabited since, except for summer visits by the owner and his family.

Geology: Banded gneiss bedrock.

* * *

Mainly covered with heather and rough grazing, **SCOTASAY** is in a central position in East Loch Tarbert and together with Scalpay provides valuable shelter for the ferry terminal at Tarbert. The croft house is in the cleft running up from the cove on the south-east side of the island while the highest point of 57m is towards the north. There is a fish-farm on the north-east side.

The owner is well liked by the local people because he 'leaves them alone', I was told by a Scalpay ferryman (before the bridge was built).

The rowan tree on **Stac a' Chaorainn** (G. – stack of the rowan tree) no longer grows there, and **Sgeir Ghlas** (G. – pale grey-green skerry) with its beacon is more of an islet than a skerry. **Eilean Dubh** is part of the underwater reef which extends south of Scotasay while the islets, **Eileanan a' Ghille-bheid** and **Eilean Arderanish**, continue the parallel line of the Gloraigs opposite Scalpay.

* * *

Access: Try Hamish Taylor, 01859-530310 or Kilda Cruises, 01859-502060 or enquire at Harris Hotel, Tarbert.

Anchorages: No recommended anchorages.

1. Occasional anchorage opposite the small bight on the NE side in 10m if not obstructed by fish-farm.
2. Tem. anchorage E of Sgeir Ghlas.

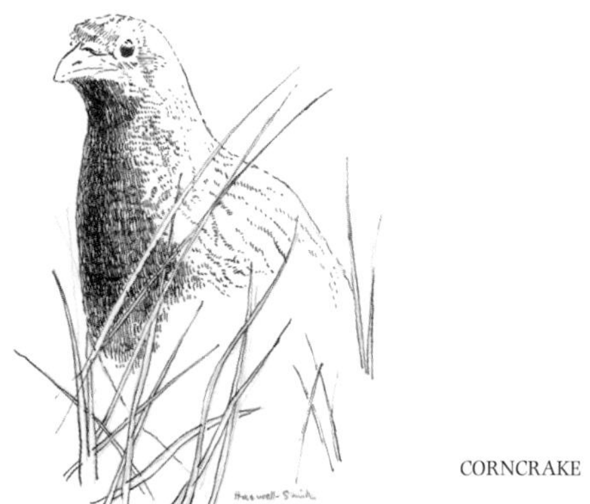

CORNCRAKE

8.8 Shiant Isles

[sh-unt] (G. na h-eileanan seunta – of the enchanted islands).

Garbh Eilean

(G. – rough island)

Eilean an Tigh

(G. – house or home island). Pre-19th century this was called Eilean na Cille (G. – church island)

The largest separate island is **Eilean Mhuire** *(G. – Mary's island).*

The entire group of about a dozen islands and skerries is also known locally as Eileanan Mora.

OS map. 1:50000 Sheet 14 1:25000 Sheet 457
Admiralty Charts: 1:100000 Nos.1794 or 1795

Area: 143ha (353 acres)
Height: 160m (525 ft)

Owner: Sir Compton Mackenzie bought the group at a London auction for £500 in 1925. He renovated the shepherd's derelict cottage on Eilean an Tigh and stayed there very occasionally during the summer months when he wanted solitude for writing. He sold the islands in 1936 to a Colonel Macdonald from Skye who resold them to the publisher Nigel Nicolson in 1937 for £1300. The Nicolson family still own them. The grazing rights are let to a sheep farmer on Scalpay.

Population: There are scattered signs of early settlements on Garbh Eilean at Annat and Bagh, on the plateau of Eilean Mhuire (although these may have been summer shielings), and on two areas of Eilean an Tigh, and it seems that about forty people in five families were still living on Eilean an Tigh in the mid-18th century. By 1770 the Shiants were uninhabited but in the 1820s under the Stewart tenure a shepherd and his wife were again living on Eilean an Tigh. It was at this time that it started to be called 'home island' instead of 'church island' – Eilean na Cille. For twenty years after 1842 there were no inhabitants but in 1862 a shepherd, Donald Campbell, and his wife Catherine Morrison moved in. Their two strikingly beautiful – and accommodating – daughters, Mòr and Catriona, gained widespread renown. The Victorian yachtsman and naturalist, Harvie-Brown, said that Mòr would

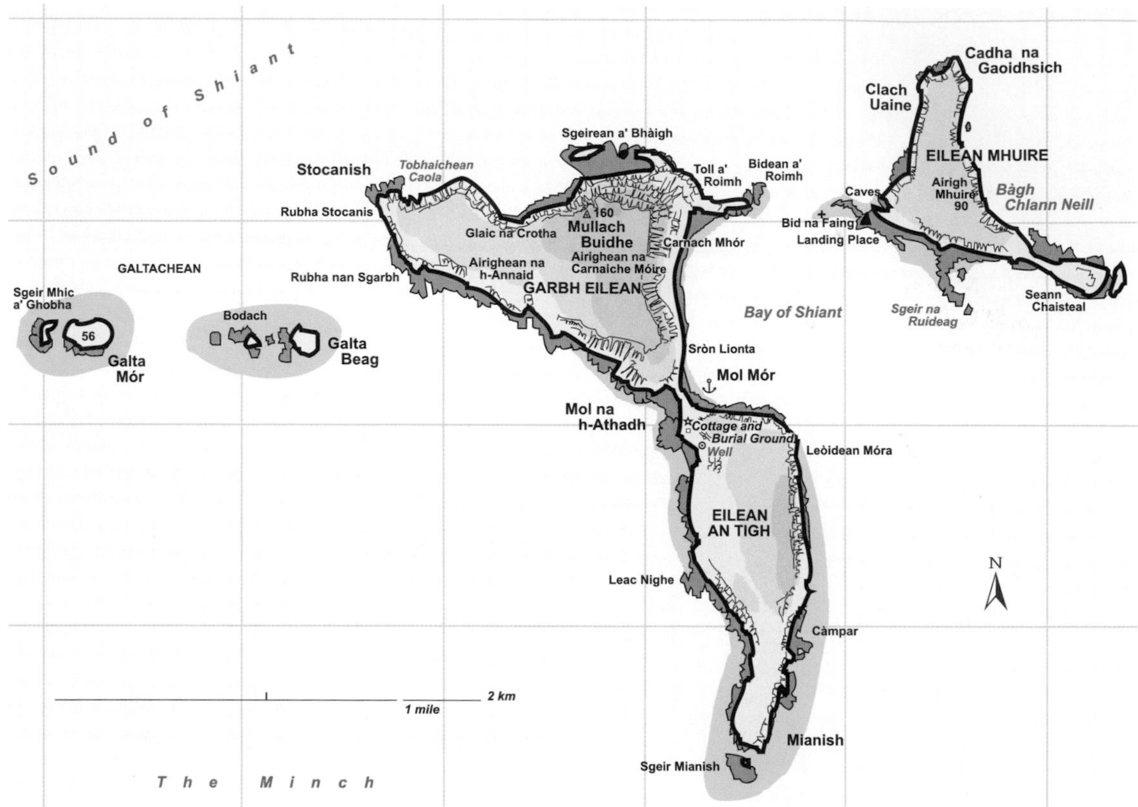

have graced any ballroom – 'one of the very loveliest women I ever beheld', and that they were both 'uncommonly handsome girls', A few years later both girls gave birth to children fathered by visiting fishermen, whom they brought up as part of the family. The Campbells left the island in 1901.

Nigel Nicolson met Mòr Campbell in 1946 on Harris when she was a forlorn 86 years old. The Census shows that in 1881 there were two males and four females in the Shiants. 1891–8 (3m,5f) 1901–1 family (4m,4f) Since then, uninhabited.

Geology: Geologically the Shiants are outliers of Skye, although they are closer to Lewis. The rock formations are similar to Staffa, the Giant's Causeway in Antrim and parts of Mull – columnar (tertiary) basalt, forming spectacular cliffs of over 120m in height. The columns are almost 2m in diameter on Garbh Eilean's north face. This is geologically young rock; not like the ancient weathered gneiss of the 'Long Island'. There are fine natural stone arches on Eilean Mhuire's south-west shore and also a natural arch on Eilean an Tigh. Basalt is not generally a suitable rock for climbing.

Martin Martin said there was a blue stone in the Shiants and that he had seen a set of 'table men' carved from it.

History: In the 1820s two brothers, Alexander and Archibald Stewart of Pairc (Park), Lewis, were notorious and sadistic tacksmen who severely punished any fisherman who landed on the Shiant Islands, even in an emergency. It was always assumed that they were sheep-stealing (and sometimes, no doubt, they were). Their tenure lasted until 1842.
Lord Leverhulme, the Lancashire soap magnate, bought Lewis (which included the Shiants) in 1917 and planned at one stage to breed silver foxes there.

Wildlife: The common seal breeds here and basking shark, dolphin, porpoise, blue shark, and Minke whale often frequent these waters.

There are no rabbits but the islands are rat-infested, probably from a shipwreck, and someone imported cats to try to deal with them. The cats have died out (or been eaten by the rats, which are fearless!) and, as the rats live in the scree below the cliffs and steal the sea-birds' eggs and young, it was planned to eradicate them by the same method as that used on Ailsa Craig (See No.1.1). But it was then realised that these were not common Brown Rats, *Rattus novergicus*, but Black Rats, *Rattus rattus*, the 'plague rats' of old. As they are very rare in the British Isles (much rarer than puffins) it was decided in the interests of conservation that they should be declared – like puffins – a protected species. So we now have puffins and black rats sharing an island habitat and apparently co-existing.

Some 240,000 puffins nest here in the turf at the top of the sea-cliffs – about two per cent of the world population. There is a colony of herring gulls, and oystercatchers, nesting eider, shag, snipe, lark, pipit, wheatear, greater and lesser black-backed gulls, rock dove, turnstone, hooded crow, blackbird, and many other species have been seen.

Thousands of kittiwakes, guillemots, razorbills and fulmars nest among the huge fluted basalt columns on the northern cliffs.

* * *

According to legend the ghostly and menacing Blue Men of the Minch live in the Sound between the **SHIANT ISLANDS**. Some say they are storm kelpies who must be treated with great respect by sailors, and others that they are bad-tempered angels who fell into the sea when they were expelled from Heaven. The minister of Tiree from 1861 to 1891, the Rev John Campbell, claimed that one followed a fisherman's boat when he was sailing in the area – 'a blue-covered man, with a long, grey face, and floating from the waist out of the water', The creature sometimes came so close that he could have touched him.

If you are accosted by a Blue Man it is important to have the Gaelic. One skipper had to answer a Blue Man's questions in rhyming couplets on the threat of being dragged to the bottom of the Minch if his replies were not poetic.

Even if you don't see any Blue Men, the columnar basalt rock formations are every bit as spectacular. This is the back-street Manhattan of the Western Isles. A vast skyscraper city of seabirds, noisy and rank-smelling. In *The Highlands and Isles of Scotland* MacCulloch (1773–1835) claimed that these '. . . form one of the most magnificent colonnades to be found among the Western Islands. But these islands are nowhere more striking than when viewed at a sufficient distance from the northward; the whole of this lofty range of pillars being distinctly seen rising like a long wall out of the sea; varied by the ruder forms of the others which tower above or project beyond them, and contrasted by the wild rocks which skirt the whole group'.

The well-known pillars of Fingal's Cave on Staffa are a mere 10m high, those on the Shiants are over 150m (500 ft). In comparing them MacCulloch said that they 'exceed them in simplicity, in grandeur, in depth of shadow, and in that repose which is essential to the great style in landscape'.

The Shiants are a group of two islands and several islets and outlying rocks. There is pasturage for sheep brought over from Scalpay (No.8.14) but there are no permanent inhabitants nowadays. **Eilean an Tigh** which is the southern part of the largest island of the group is connected with **Garbh Eilean**, the northern part, by a low narrow neck of polished pebbles. This isthmus covers at spring tides or during storms. Garbh Eilean is very steep; Eilean an Tigh is lower but has precipitous cliffs on its eastern side. Eilean Mhuire lies a short distance to the east of Garbh Eilean, so that the group almost forms a bay with a south-eastern exposure.

There is a cottage on the west side of Eilean an Tigh near the shingle link with Eilean Garbh [NG418976]. This is the cottage that was renovated by Sir Compton Mackenzie when he owned these islands. Behind it is the ruin of an older dwelling and on the north side there are the limited remains of a probable graveyard and a small church. This would account for the island's former name of Eilean na Cille (church island). A crystal clear spring of fresh water about one hundred yards from the cottage is hidden by lush green grass and wild flowers. The large scale Ordnance Survey map shows three wells or springs on Eilean an Tigh but only the one near the cottage is reliable.

In the early 19th century only a shepherd and his wife were living on the island. In order to collect seabirds and their eggs he would lower his wife down the cliff-face. When she had caught and killed each bird she would attach it to the rope round her waist to keep her hands free. One day the rope broke and she fell into the sea. She was unable to swim but the collection of dead birds kept her afloat. Her husband could not get down the cliff in time to save her and watched helplessly as, crying for help, the tide carried her away.

Eilean Mhuire, the Virgin Mary's island, has also been inhabited and it is in fact the most fertile island in the group. There are steep cliffs on all sides and access is up a rock 'stair' but the top is like the 'lost world' – a large plateau covered with arable land and ancient lazybeds, and the remains of turf dwellings marked by clumps of nettles – a certain sign of human occupation.

It has always been assumed that the chapel on these holy islands was on the Virgin Mary's island because Martin Martin had recorded that: 'Island-More hath a chapel in it dedicated to the Virgin Mary, and is fruitful in corn and grass; the island joining to it on the west is only for pasturage.'

But Adam Nicolson has suggested that Martin Martin's 'Island-More' was only referring to 'the main island' and not Eilean Mhuire. The island joining to it on the *north-west* would then be Garbh Eilean which is certainly only fit for pasturage while Home Island, or Church Island as it used to be known, was relatively fruitful in corn and grass. This seems to me to be a reasonable assumption. Churches and graveyards are usually linked and whereas there are the apparent signs of a graveyard on Eilean an Tigh, none has yet been found on Eilean Mhuire.

Martin Martin claimed that the cows on the 'Siant' were much fatter than any he saw on Lewis. It must have been a hard life but at least the islanders had the means to be self-sufficient. There would be seafood and seafowl, potatoes, cabbages, milk, eggs, meat, seal-oil, driftwood and some peat, and fresh water: all the essentials for a healthy existence.

* * *

Access: Try Woody, Stornoway, 01851-703908; Kilda Cruises, Tarbert, 01859-502060; or Hebridean Whale Cruises, Gairloch (Mainland), 01445-712458. No visiting April/May during lambing.

Anchorages: Tidal currents are strong in the vicinity of these islands and there are overfalls both N and S. Landing can be hazardous.

1. Approach from N or S for occasional anchorage between the islands in settled weather. Avoid reefs extending 1½c W and 1½c S of Eilean Mhuire. Anchor E of neck of gravel between Garbh Eilean and Eilean an Tigh but the bottom slopes steeply and holding may be uncertain. Exposed NE to SE but sheltered N through W to S. With SW winds a heavy swell sets in. Better holding has been reported in the NW corner of the Bay of Shiant in 10m sand.

2. Temporary anchorage on W side of neck of gravel between Garbh Eilean and Eilean an Tigh. Sheltered N to E.

8.9 Taransay

(ON – Taran's island) or (ON taren-øy – the kelp island).

O S Maps: 1:50000 Sheet 18 1:25000 Sheet 455
Admiralty Charts: 1:200000 No.2721 1:50000 No.2841

Area: 1475ha (3645 acres)
Height: 267m (876 ft)

Owner: Purchased by John Mackay of Horgabost, Harris in 1967, or thereabouts, from Roddy Campbell. Mr Mackay has a transport company – John Mackay & Sons – and farms sheep on the island.

Population: 1841–88 (16 houses). 1881–55. 1891–56 (12 houses). 1911–76. 1931–33. Last family left the island in 1942 but it was later reinhabited. 1961–5. 1971–5. 1974– again abandoned.

Geology: Grey gneiss traversed by veins of granite with a grassy top-soil. The isthmus is mainly sand.

History: Eponymous Taran is an uncertain figure in Celtic history. According to Adomnan he was the son of a noble Pictish family who requested St Columba's protection. Columba agreed and asked Feradach, a rich man on Islay (No.2.4), to accept him in his retinue and treat him as a friend but Feradach chose instead to have him murdered. Columba was naturally outraged and condemned Feradach with a divine judgement.

Some scholars however consider that Taran was the Irish Saint Ternan or Torannan who had great influence on the Pictish mainland. As one of the chapels on Taransay was dedicated to St Taran this may be a more likely candidate.

Prehistoric man was well-established on Taransay and the Vikings may also have settled here judging by the wealth of Norse nomenclature.

In 1544 a raiding party of Morrisons from Ness, Lewis, was slain on the shore at Sgeir a'

Bhuailt, smitten-rock, by the chief of Berneray and his men and in 1549 Dean Munro described Taransay as a place with good barley, corn and fishing, where people delved with spades.

Taransay was chosen by the BBC in 1999 as the site for their 'Castaway 2000' series of programmes and again gained star status as the setting for the film story of Herr Zucher and his rocket mail experiment on Scarp (No.8.13).

Wildlife: The shoreline is magnificent in summer with brilliant white sands and the sea-thrift in bloom.

There is a small herd of red deer.

Unfortunately, mink – which are strong swimmers – have established themselves on the island and are attacking ground-nesting birds, in particular the populations of puffin and shelduck. In 2003 Stirling University started co-ordinating

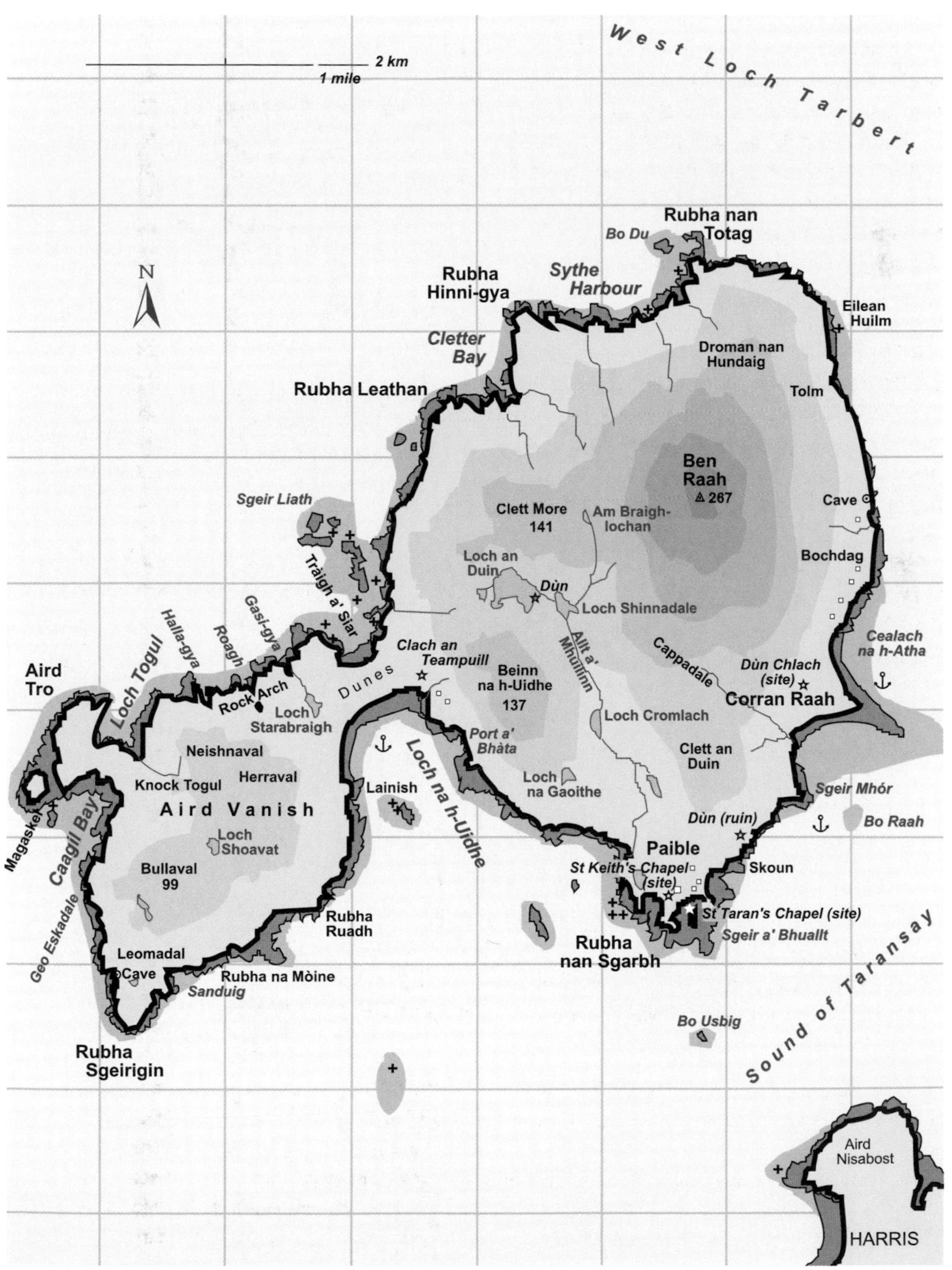

a Taransay research project to radio-track the elusive predators with a view to finding a way of eradicating them.

* * *

TARANSAY is divided into two shapely hills by a low sandy neck of dunes. The village of **Paible** which is on the larger part of the island was the main settlement with a maximum population of seventy-six, but the school (next to the landing) closed in 1935 and numbers gradually dwindled until the last family left in 1942.

Then in 2002, after the BBC left, and after the island had been used for filming *The Rocket Post*, the schoolhouse (The School Chalet) and the Mackay Farmhouse were completely renovated and are now let out for holiday accommodation.

Beinn Raah, 267m high, dominates the northern section with a ridge to the north and lesser peaks to the south-west where there are a number of small lochs. **Loch an Duinn** [NB022013] has a dun and probable crannog near its east shore. It is linked to Loch Shinnadale and then by Allt a' Mhuilinn (G. – the mill burn) to Loch Cromlach. The stream eventually reaches the sea beside Paible. North of Paible is the ruin of another Iron Age dun at **Corran Raah** [NB041005]. Little is known of the history of either of the two duns on Taransay.

The sites of two ancient chapels are at Paible, one dedicated to St Taran where only women were buried and the other to St Keith where only men were interred [NG030991]. This time-honoured method of segregation was upset, it is said, when a mixed burial took place in one of the graveyards. The following morning one of the bodies was found lying on the surface of the ground beside the grave.

Loch na h-Uidhe (G. – loch of the isthmus), the sea-loch which divides the island into two parts, is bounded by a magnificent stretch of shell-sand beach. **Aird Vanish** (ON *ve-nes* or *van-nes* – promontory of the sacred place or of Wane, the fertility god), the south-western part of the island, is a rough and lonely area, riddled with sea-caves. It has twin peaks, Herraval and Bullaval.

Taransay is separated from Harris by the Sound of Taransay. At no point is the sea here deeper than 12m. The sandy spit of Corran Raah projects into the Sound and the bay on its north side is called Cealach na h-Atha (G. – the fireplace of the kiln). This presumably refers to the shape and should not give visitors a misleading impression of the temperature.

* * *

Access: For holiday accommodation or day trip info. ring Norman Ian, 07867-968560. Regular full-day visits from Horgabost Beach, Mon. to Fri., weather permitting.

Anchorages:

1. South of Corran Raah and Bo Raah in Sound of Taransay. Close inshore, sand. Good shelter from NW but beware Bo Raah.
2. Cealach na h-Atha, on N side of Corran Raah. Anchor well in-shore, sand. Sheltered from SW winds by Corran Raah.
3. Loch na h-Uidhe. Beware Old Rocks and Langaraid on approach. Keep nearer E side of bay when entering to avoid rocks on W side. Reasonable shelter, except in S'lies.

8.10 Soay Mór

(ON so-øy – sheep island, G. mór – big).

OS Maps: 1:50000 Sheet 13 1:25000 Sheet 456
Admiralty Charts: 1:200000 No.2721 1:50000 No.2841

Area: 45ha (111 acres)
Height: 37m (121 ft)

Owner: Findlay Campbell (?). The islands are leased by a fish-farming company.

Population: 1841–no census record. 1881–0. 1891–15 (2 houses). No further record of any habitation.

Geology: Lewisian gneiss with some granite and quartz.

The two islands, **SOAY MOR** and its associate **Soay Beag**, reach the same height of 37m and have few features of note. Reefs extend from both sides of the southern extremity of Soay Mór and drying rocks fill the passage between Soay Mór and Soay Beag. The fish-farm is on the north-east side of Soay Mór facing Soay Sound.

West Loch Tarbert lies south-east of Soay Mór with small but steep **Isay island** (ON – porpoise isle) in its centre.

Access: No regular access. Boat excursions by Seatrek, Uig, Lewis, 01851-672464.

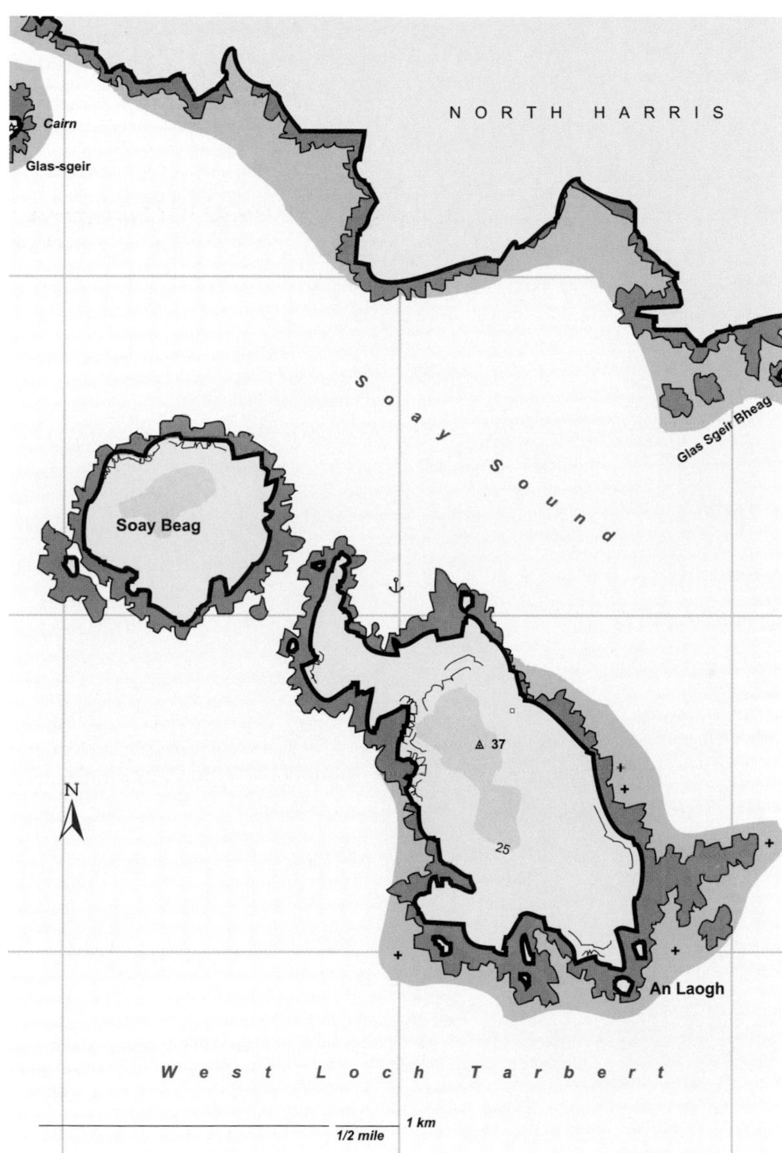

Anchorage:
1. Occasional anchorage near centre of bay at N end of Soay Mór, facing Soay Sound if fish cages permit. An approach from direction of Soay Beag is safest.

8.11 Eilean Iubhard

[elan ***yoo****-urt] (G. – yew-tree island).*

OS Maps. 1:50000 Sheet 14 1:25000 Sheet 456
Admiralty Charts: 1:100000 No.1794

Area: 125ha (309 acres)
Height: 76m (249 ft)

Owner: Part of the Parc Estate owned by Parc Crofters Ltd (Lomas family).

Population: No Census records, uninhabited today and apparently uninhabited in 1746 – see below – but five families lived here in the early 19th century at Seann Bhaile (G. – ancient settlement) and Tigh a' Gheumpail.

Geology: Gneiss bedrock with some basaltic intrusion.

History: On 4 May 1746 Prince Charles Edward Stuart with two companions and a guide landed near the head of Loch Seaforth at Aribruach. They set off across country to Stornoway where

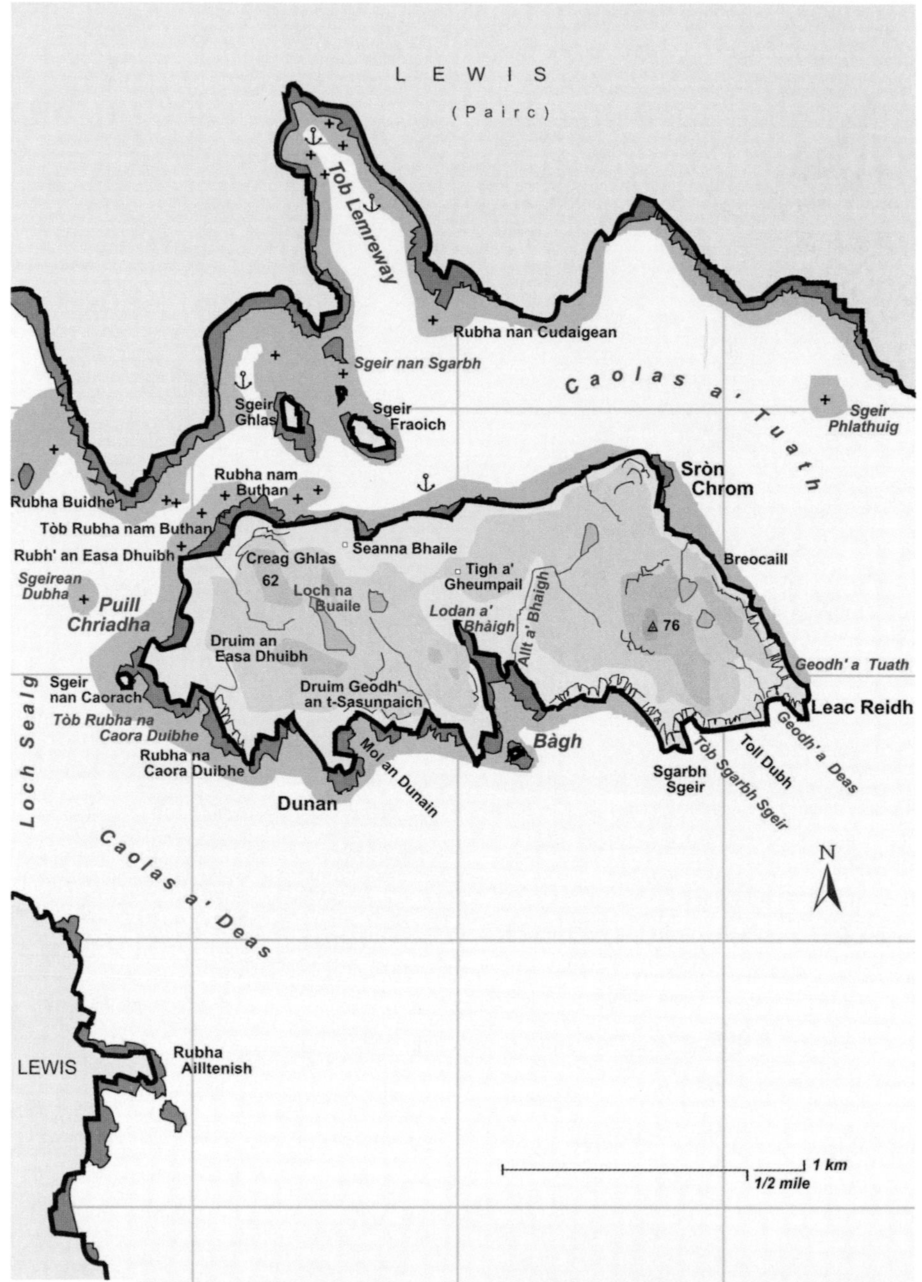

Donald Macleod had arranged for a ship to take the Prince to France. The party lost its way during the night among the bogs of Arnish moor and only reached the outskirts of Stornoway in the late morning very wet and tired. They were sheltering under a rock when Donald Macleod reported to them that news of the Prince's approach had reached Stornoway and the captain of the ship now refused to sail. Mrs Mackenzie, a farmer's wife, provided overnight shelter and food for the party and at 8am on the 6 May the Prince, O'Sullivan, O'Neill, Donald and Murdoch Macleod, Ned Burke and four boatmen set sail in Donald Campbell of Scalpay's boat. They intended to cross the Minch to Poolewe but the wind was against them and ships of the Royal Navy could be seen on patrol. So they chose instead to land the Prince in the bay on the south shore of Eilean Iubhard and, as the boatmen refused to leave, the boat was possibly concealed on the north side of the island.

It was raining heavily and the party stretched

a sail over a 'low pitiful hut' and spent four days there. Local fishermen used the island for drying their catches so Ned and the Prince cooked some of these fish for sustenance.

Wildlife: Dean Munro (1549) reported: '. . .guid to pasture and schielling of store, with faire hunting of ottars out of their bouries.'

* * *

EILEAN UIBHARD lies at the entrance to Loch Shell – or Loch Sealg – on the east coast of Lewis. It shelters an inlet and the village of Lemreway but it lies close to the coast and on approaching from the sea it can be difficult to recognise it as an island at all. It looks much more like a part of Lewis.

There are two minor peaks at opposite ends of the island, the one in the west being 62m high and the other in the east 76m high. The ground is very rough and irregular and there are several lochans and a number of small burns. Most of the coastline drops abruptly into the sea but there is a shallow bay at the west end called **Puill Chriadha** (G. – clay pool) and a cove in the centre of the south coast called merely **Bàgh** (G. – bay).

The eastern half of Eilean Iubhard is separated from Lewis by **Caolas a' Tuath** (G. – north channel) but at the western end this kyle becomes shallow and is obstructed by a number of rocks and islets.

* * *

Access: Try Hamish Taylor Scenic Cruises, 01859-530310 or enquire at Lemreway or Scalpay.

Anchorage:

1. Occasional anchorage on narrow shelf close to N shore of Eilean Iubhard, S of Sgeir Fraoich, but mainly obstructed by fish cages. Sheltered in S'lies. If winds change, move N into Tob Lemreway.

8.12 Seaforth Island

(G. Mulag from ON Múlí – craggy ridge between fiords).

OS Maps: 1:50000 Sheet 13 1:25000 Sheet 456
Admiralty Charts: Only 1:100000 No.1794 covers Loch Seaforth but it is unsatisfactory.

Area: 273ha (675 acres)
Height: 217m (712 ft)

Owner: Heirs of A S Halford-MacLeod, CMG.,CVO. (Bought 1964)

Population: No Census records and uninhabited.

Geology: Lewisian gneiss bedrock covered with poor acid soil supporting rough grazing.

History: Seaforth Island belonged to the MacLeods until they were usurped by the Mackenzies in 1610. Francis Mackenzie, or Lord Seaforth, inherited the island in 1783.

* * *

Loch Seaforth is a long narrow loch wedged between high mountains and towering cliffs. The winds whisper through the peaks, build up their strength, meet in the corries, and then without warning sweep savagely down the mountain sides and flatten the waters of the loch with unpredictable ferocity. **SEAFORTH ISLAND** sits four-square in the centre of Loch Seaforth, six and a half miles from the entrance. It is a great heap of rough heather and bracken-covered slopes reaching up to a height of 217m above the loch with few signs of any human habitation or cultivation. When, in a strong sou'-westerly, the rain is whipped straight up the island's steep face like smoke the locals tell their youngsters that the fearsome witch who lives inside it is cooking a meal of naughty boys and girls.

A couple of miles down the loch on the western shore is Loch Maaruig – where naval craft sometimes anchor near little **Maaruig Island**. The loch here forms the boundary between Harris and Lewis: Harris to the west, Lewis on the precipitous east side.

Seaforth Island (Mulag) lies on the county boundary. Shepherds from the Barvas area in Lewis (Ross & Cromarty county) used to regularly invade Harris (Inverness county) and occupy shielings as far south as the Vigadale river and sometimes beyond while Harris fishermen would often enter Lewis territory to cut kelp and collect

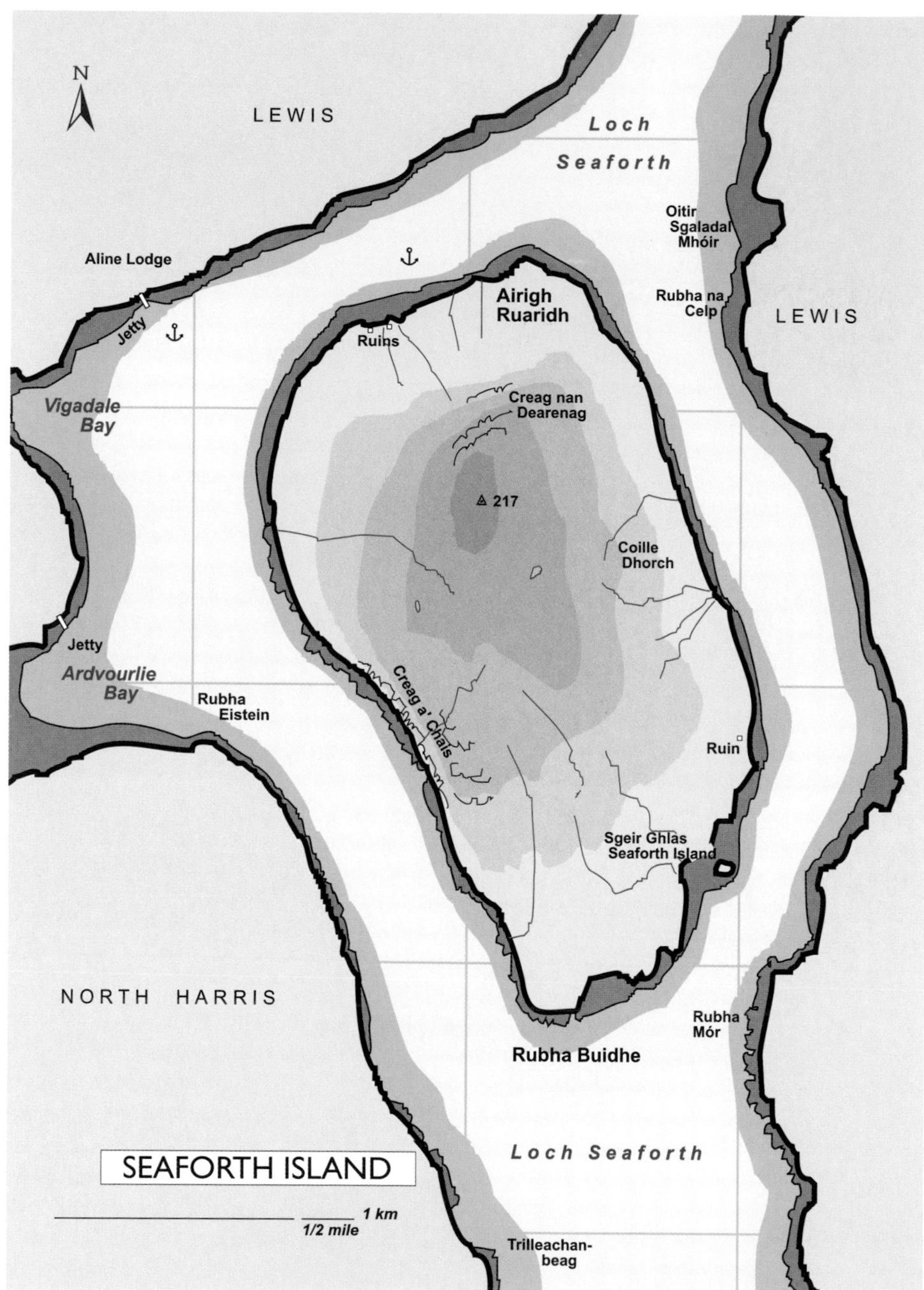

shellfish. This led to many, occasionally violent, disputes. These were at last settled in 1851 when the boundary line was agreed with the unusual decision to allocate the entire, *undivided* island to both counties *equally*.

The loch entrance is guarded by **Rhenigidale Island** on the Harris side and three islets on the Lewis side, **Eilean Mór a' Bhàigh**, **Dubh a' Bhàigh** and **Beag a' Bhàigh** (G. – big, black and little island at the bay).

Access: It may be possible to arrange transport on one of the local boats at the jetties at Aline Lodge or Ardvourlie beside the A849.

Anchorages:

1. Anchor off the N coast of the island ½M NE of Aline Lodge jetty in 7m, or off Aline Lodge jetty itself which is NW of the island. Good shelter and holding but can be subject to violent squalls.
2. Temp. anchorage where suitable depth can be found

in the navigable channels W and E of Seaforth Island but beware squalls.

8.13 Scarp

(ON skarpoe – sharp, stony, mountain terrain).

O S Maps: 1:50000 Sheet 13 1:25000 Sheet 456
Admiralty Charts: 1:200000 No.2721 1:50000 No.2841

Area: 1045ha (2582 acres)
Height: 308m (1010 ft)

Owner: Bought by a Panama company for £100 in 1978. In 1983 sold for £50,000 to LIbco Ltd who resold it to Orbitglen Ltd for £500,000. Both deals were by Nazmudin Virani, a director of BCCI – the bank which held the title. BCCI collapsed and the property was resold in 1995 to Mr Anderson Duke Bakewell of Oxfordshire for £155,055. The present owner is Mr Bert Bakewell.

Population: There were eight crofting tenancies in 1802. About 1823, thirteen villages in Harris between Loch Resort and Bunabhainneadar were cleared and some of the displaced villagers

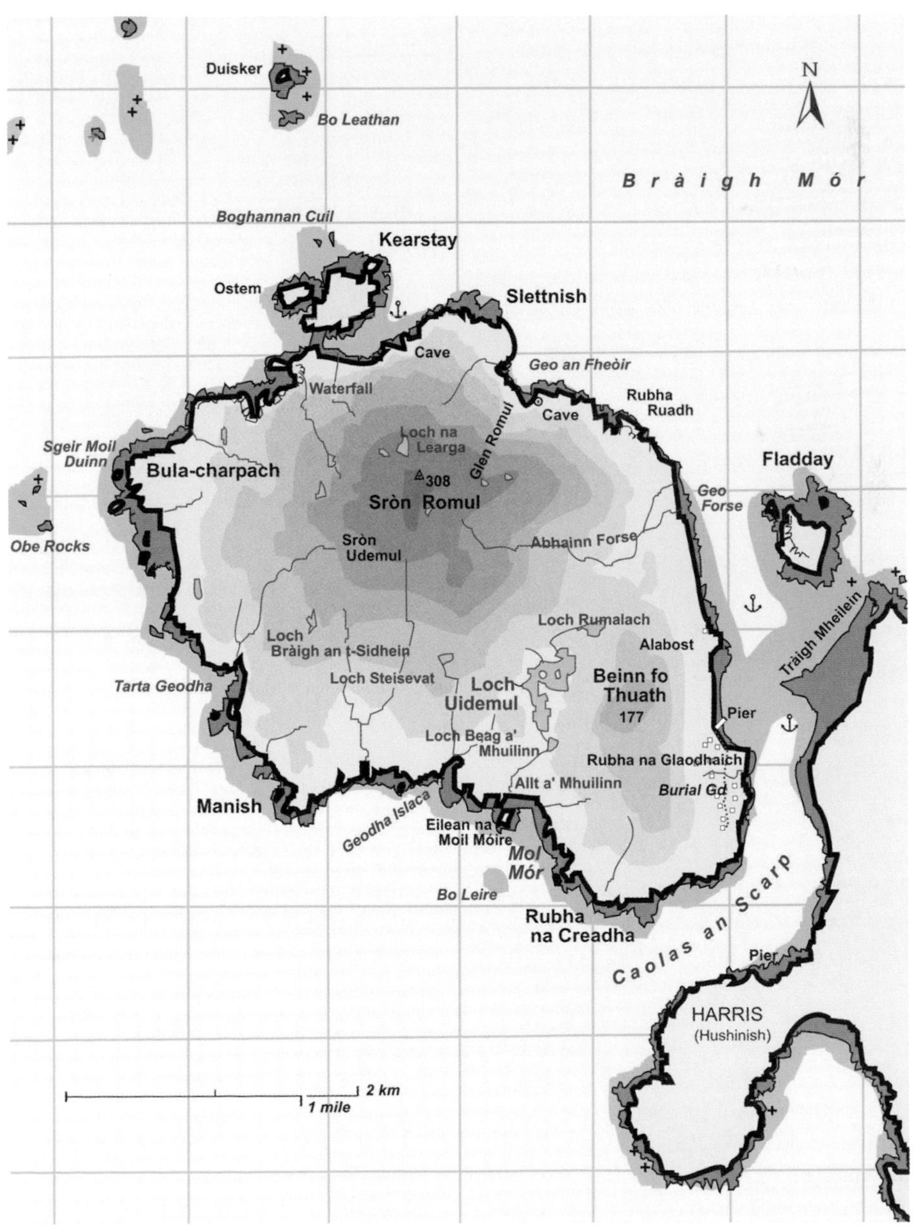

settled on Scarp. 1841–129 (23 houses). In 1850 the original eight crofts were subdivided into sixteen smaller units. 1861–151. 1881–213. 1891–143 (29 houses). 1931–95. 1951–74. 1961–46. 1971–12. The last two resident families, seven people in all, left Scarp in December 1971. 1981–0. 2001–0.

Geology: Chiefly gneiss and gneissose granite but containing some soft asbestos-bearing rock above Tarta Geodha (G. – the noisy creek) which is geologically unique in this region. The asbestos content was noted by geologists in the early 1930s.

History: On 14 January 1934, attended by an eighty-five-year-old midwife in her home on Scarp, Mrs Christina Maclennan gave birth to a child. On the following day her condition was poor and as there was no telephone on Scarp an islander crossed to Hushinish. But the telephone there was out of order so the postman's son was sent to Tarbert to call the doctor. The doctor decided that Mrs Maclennan must go to hospital. The sea was rough but she was taken to Hushinish tied to a stretcher laid across a bouncing open boat. There she was laid on the floor of the local bus for the seventeen miles of bumpy road to Tarbert. She was then taken by car to the hospital at Stornoway where the cause of her distress was discovered. She gave birth to a second healthy child, and felt much better for it! Thus the twins were born on different islands, in different counties and in different weeks.

This story, widely reported in the press at the time, came to the ears of a young German rocket-enthusiast who had dreams of future space travel. He had already built a number of large solid-fuel rockets and become a local celebrity. So on 28 July of the same year – which came to be known as 'Latha na Rocait' (G. – the day of the rocket) – twenty-six-year-old Gerhard Zucher chose to demonstrate his rocket-mail invention on Scarp. Special stamps were printed for the occasion and a letter was written to the King. The one-metre-long solid-fuel rocket weighed 14kg and could carry several thousand letters at 1000 mph but when Gerhard lit the fuse the rocket exploded scattering mail over a wide area. The local postmaster had the letters collected and he stamped each cover with violet ink reading – 'Damaged by first explosion at Scarp – Harris'. A second experiment with the same mail fired from Harris back to Scarp was successful but the project was abandoned, although a few letters addressed to Orkney actually reached their destination having travelled by rocket, ferry, automobile, mail-steamer, railway, and Highland Airways.

When Herr Zucher, unaware that the Nazis were secretly experimenting with rockets, returned to Germany, he was accused by the Gestapo of selling rocket technology to the British, imprisoned for fifteen months, and at one stage transferred to an asylum. He was banned for life from conducting any further rocket experiments. During the war he served in the Luftwaffe but was invalided out in 1944. He died in 1985.

* * *

The population of **SCARP** – one of Britain's most westerly and isolated outposts – was well over one hundred at the start of the 20th century but it was dwindling steadily. The authorities were unconcerned and it was not until the 1930s that they chose to build a small jetty on the island (but without providing an equivalent one on the Harris 'mainland' shore). The Hydro-Electric Board would not provide an electricity supply and in 1966 the Church of Scotland refused to replace the lay preacher. The small island school closed in 1967 and the post-office in 1969 with the cessation of all mail deliveries. Then the single telephone cable was severed in a storm and the GPO refused to repair it. So in December 1971 the seven remaining islanders had little choice but to abandon their homes. Angus Macinnes and his wife Margaret were the last to leave with their son, Donald John, aged twenty-one. Donald John now lives in Dunbartonshire but his brother Murdo still crofts in Harris and visits Scarp frequently to tend the sheep.

The island is rocky and the north part is 308m in height (over 1000ft) with a steep drop to the sea. The village, mainly of well-built stone houses which are now in serious disrepair, is in the south-east corner and partly sheltered from the Atlantic winds by a low hill. The only land capable of cultivation is here on the east coast. It is easy to see how the island could not support a large population and the lack of an all-weather anchorage was also a serious deficiency which must have contributed to the depopulation of the island. The local economy would have been very basic – potatoes, cabbages, oats, turnips, milk, fish; lobster fishing for the Billingsgate market; wool and Harris Tweed; and the sale of a few livestock. There was no electricity and oil lamps were the only means of illumination but there was some piped water. The village had one small shop and the telephone line was installed in 1947.

Scarp has a proud educational record and it is claimed that more professionally qualified people came from the island than from any other island community of similar size. As for its remote situation, the Hebridean writer, Francis Thompson, tells of the Londoner who was amazed at the sheer isolation of Scarp and asked a Scarpach how he ever got the news from London. 'Well,' was the puzzled rejoinder, 'how do you get the news from Scarp?'

Although the **Kyle of Scarp** is a short crossing, landing at the pier can be difficult when there is any swell. The sea here is very shallow.

The drying islet by Slettnish in the north, **Kearstay**, is divided from Scarp by a narrow channel less than 1m deep called the Sound of Kearstay. To the north there is a reef marked by **Duisker** (G – *Dubh Sgeir*, black skerry). Another small island, **Fladday**, lies somewhat further off-shore on the east and there is **Liongam** near the Lewis coast to the north-east. Low-lying **Gasker**, marked by a navigation light, is some five miles south-west of Scarp. In spite of its small size and lack of height it has some fresh-water pools on it. The landing place in suitable conditions is in a cleft on the south side. Gasker is principally noted for its large well-established seal colony.

* * *

Access: No regular access but Seatrek, Uig, Lewis, 01851-672464, provide boat excursions.

Anchorages:

1. Occasional anchorage in suitable weather just S of the bar in Caolas an Scarp, off Rubha na Glaodhaich.
2. Occasional anchorage in suitable weather in N entrance to Caolas an Scarp, N of the bar and SW of Fladday.
3. Sound of Kearstay. Temporary anchorage in E entrance of the sound in 9m, sand. Good shelter from S and NW.

8.14 Lewis

The derivation normally given is (G. leogach [loo-ach] – marshy). The entire area together with its off-shore islands, once MacLeod territory, is referred to as 'The Lews'. (G. Eilean Leodhais [loo-is] – Leod's island). Leod or 'Ljod' is Norse for 'clan'. The Norse occasionally referred to the whole island as (ON Ljodusherad – Lewis Province).

Harris

(ON hearri – hills) or (G. na h-àirdibh – the heights).

Great Bernera

(ON bjarnar-øy – bear island) or (ON – Bjorn's island).

Scalpay

(ON skalpr-øy – scallop island).

OS Maps: 1:50000 Sheets 8, 13, 14, and 18 1:25000 Sheets 456, 457, 458, 459 and 460
Admiralty Charts: 1:500000 No.2635 1:200000 No.2721 west coast 1:100000 Nos.1785, 1794 and 1795 east coast 1:50000 No.2841 south-west coast 1:20000 No.2642 Sound of Harris 1:12500 Nos. 3381 and 3422 Loch Roag 1:12500 No.2905 Loch Tarbert various scales No.2529 Loch Erisort and Stornoway

Area: 220673ha (5390983 acres)
Height: 799m (2621 ft)

Owners: Multiple ownership. The largest landowners are the Stornoway Trust, Scottish Office, Galson Estates, Richard Kershaw, Barvas Estates, Rodney Hitchcock, J N Oppenheim Partnership, Helen Panchaud, and the Lomas family. Jonathan Bulmer, the cider heir, bought North Harris with Amhuinnsuidhe Castle in 1994. In 2003 the Harris islanders (North Harris Trust) bought the 55,000 acre estate with the support of public funds and joined by Mr Ian Scar-Hall, who bought the castle and its 600 acre grounds, for a total £4.5 million. In 2005 the Harris Trust also bought the nearby 7,472 acre Loch Seaforth Estate. Then in 2006 the 53,000 acre Galson Estate in North Lewis was bought out by Lewis crofters under the same Government act.

John Taylor, a London architect, owns Scalpay. He has a cottage there and flies his personal flag (an anchor and lobster) over it when in residence. He bought the island in the early 1980s from North Harris Estate and thus 'gave it its independence'. Most of the island is under crofting tenure.

Great Bernera is owned by Robin Mirrlees, Prince of Coronata, Comte de Lalanne, Freeman of London and Patrician of San Marino. He bought it in 1962 and has his home (and fish farm) there but the islanders have been discussing buying him out using public funds although he is a popular laird and does not wish to sell.

Population: In 1755 Harris had a population of 1969 and Lewis (excluding Bernera) 6386. By 1801 the equivalent figures were 2996 and 9168. The Harris factor settled twenty crofting families on Scalpay about 1843 and five years later added another twenty families – some evicted from Pabbay (No.8.4) in the Sound of Harris.

	1841	1881	1891	1931	1961	1971	1981	1991	2001
L'is	16988[1]	24876	27045	24685	21614	20047	22476[2]	21737[2]	19918[3]
H'is	3058	3463	3681	3357	2493	2175			
Ber'a	596	535	514	317	276	278	262		
Sca'y	31	540	517	636	470	483	455	382	322
Total	20077	29475	31778	29192	24894	22981	23209	22381	20240

[1] includes Bernera, Pabay Mór (No.8.19) & Little Bernera (No.8.20)

[2] Lewis/Harris combined

[3] Lewis/Harris/Bernera combined.

Geology: Almost the entire island is gneiss, both orthogneiss and paragneiss, much of it overlaid with glacially deposited boulder clay; the orthogneiss is predominant. It has been metamorphosed from igneous as opposed to sedimentary rock and although it is complex and highly variable it is loosely known as Lewisian rock. It has a crystalline texture, is pink or grey in colour, and glitters with granules of mica or quartz. It is hard and is short of minerals required to make a good fertile soil.

Exceptions are scarce. Near Stornoway there are a few small areas of New Red Sandstone; in Uig scattered areas of granite (Britain's biggest sapphire was found here in 1995); a few linear basalt dykes; a steeply-angled bed of serpentine traversing a promontory at the eastern end of Scalpay; and, at Lingerbay in Harris and in two spots near the Butt of Lewis, anorthosite predominates. This is the only anorthosite in Scotland – a mineral valued as a road aggregate for its reflective and skid-free properties.

The hills of South Lewis and North Harris have been shaped by relatively lightweight glaciers emanating from a central ice-cap during the last Ice Age.

Central Lewis is a vast dark undulating plain of peat moorland which began to be laid down about 4000 years ago and continues to grow in thickness each year as the cold, wet, and acidic conditions delay decomposition of the previous year's layer of dead plants. In other words Lewis is reducing the 'greenhouse effect' by absorbing excess carbon dioxide! Peat is still an important fuel source for many of the islanders but the rate of growth exceeds the rate of consumption.

History: Marauding Vikings probably started settling in Lewis/Harris in the 9th century and the island appears to have been controlled until the 12th century by the Norwegian Nicolsons. They were wealthy farmers and became known as 'Clan MacNicol of the porridge and barley bannocks'. But Torquill Macleod 'did violently espouse' MacNicol's only daughter and gained possession of the whole of the Lews. The Nicolsons retreated to Skye.

After Norwegian rule had been broken, Bruce's son, David II, granted Angus Og's son, John Macdonald, King of the Isles, many of the Hebridean islands including Lewis and Harris. That was in 1335. Lewis became one of the four regional administrative centres for the island kingdom. Later, having demoted himself to 'Lord of the Isles' in deference to the Scottish king, Macdonald granted Lewis and Harris to the indigenous vassal clan Leod and thereafter the Macleods officially ruled the island.

Lewis/Harris was the last area of the western isles to adopt the Gaelic tongue and even today the spoken language of Lewis has many associations with Norse.

King James VI – the 'wisest fool in Christendom' – had no love of the Gaels. He promoted a company called the Fife Adventurers to plunder Lewis, if need be with 'slauchter, mutilation, fyre-raising, or utheris inconvenieties' and openly recommended genocide. Three raids on Stornoway were mounted – in 1598, 1605 and 1609 – but all were beaten off by Neil Macleod and his Lewismen and the Adventurers eventually went bankrupt. James spitefully withdrew the Macleods' charter and granted title to the Mackenzies of Kintail, who took over control of Lewis in 1610. The Mackenzies developed Stornoway and dominated the Macleod clansmen, but their Chiefs – the Earls of Seaforth – never took up residence in the old Macleod castle in Stornoway harbour. Their main interest in Lewis was deer hunting in Park, otherwise they chose to remain absentee landlords. The Seaforths lost their title following support of the Jacobites in 1715 but they quickly regained it by supporting the Hanoverians in 1745. Even so, Bonnie Prince Charlie stopped off at Scalpay in Seaforth territory in 1746 and Donald Campbell, a local farmer, gave him refuge and the use of his boat. The Free Church manse now stands on the site of Campbell's house.Throughout this period, the Seaforths retained possession of Lewis and from their residence in London supported an oppressive regime. Tacksmen, such as the notorious George Gillanders in the late 18th century, were permitted to charge extortionate rents and run what amounted to 'protection' rackets.

In 1778 the Earl of Seaforth raised a regiment to fight in the American War of Independence – the Seaforth Highlanders – for which he was paid a handsome Government levy but his soldiers received no pay until they mutinied in Edinburgh.

In 1783 a younger son of the Mackenzies inherited Lewis, was created Lord Seaforth, and proved a much more understanding

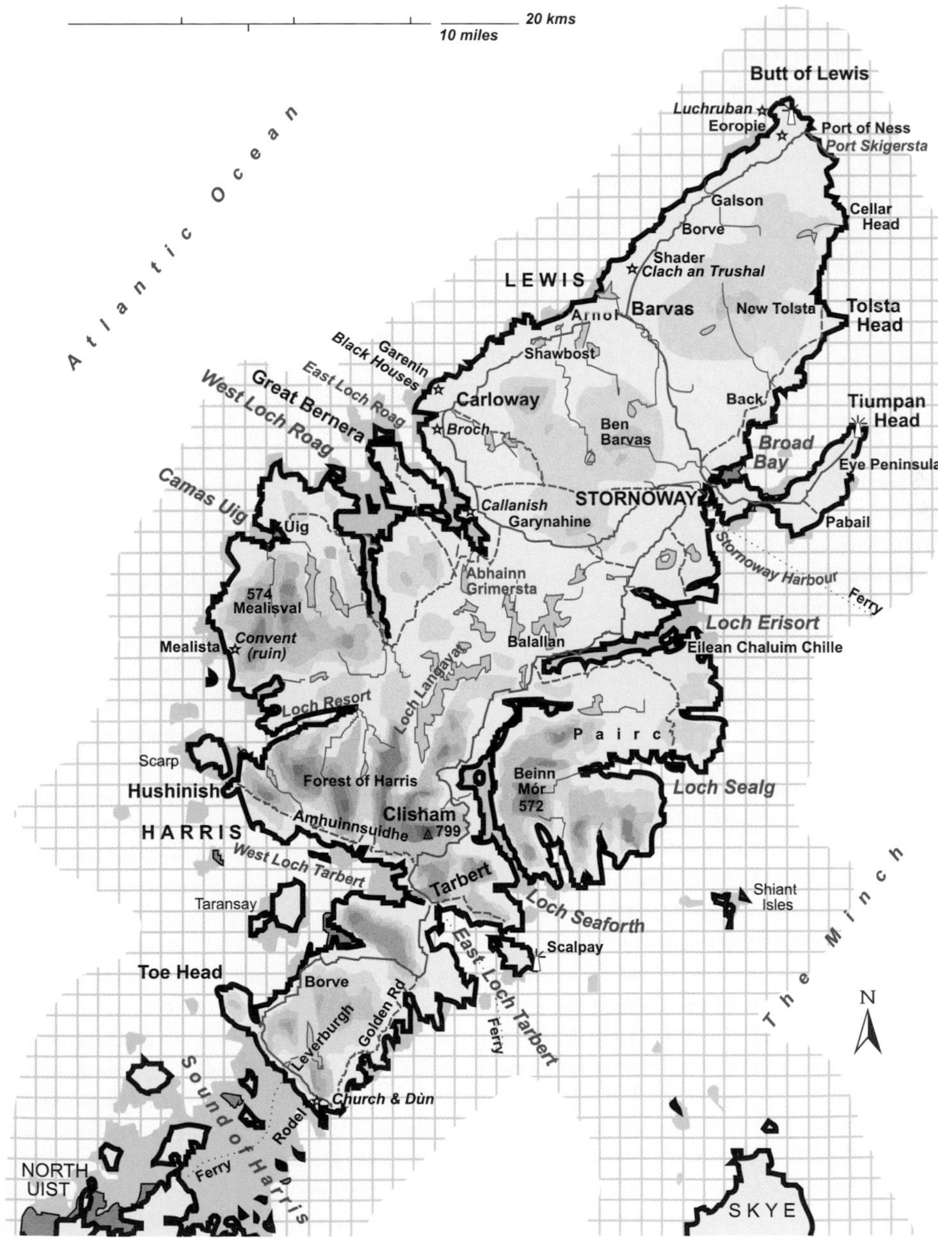

landlord but although he had four sons they all predeceased him.

By the early 1800s Stornoway's fishing industry was booming. Mrs Stewart Mackenzie – Lord Seaforth's daughter – sold Lewis in 1844 to Sir James Matheson for £190,000. He then spent nearly £½m – earned from trade with China – on improvements. He also paid the costs of 1,800 people who wished to emigrate to Canada, for more than half the population had signed on with the Destitution Fund as this was the time of the potato famines.

Matheson's tenure was benevolent and there were no evictions. Nevertheless in 1887 crofters desperate for more land killed 200 deer in the Park area, roasted the venison, and held a feast for journalists in order to attract public attention to their cause. This was one of the last 'uprisings' in what became known as the Crofters' War. The leaders were later charged with mobbing and rioting and tried in court, but they were found not guilty.

In 1918 Lord Leverhulme, the soap magnate, bought the entire island, both Lewis and Harris, and spent nearly a million pounds trying to develop the fishing industry. In 1923 he gifted the 25,000-hectare parish of Stornoway to the people and offered crofts as free gifts although only forty-one tenants accepted. His plans were starting to bear fruit when he died in 1925 but his executors abandoned the project, split the island into several large estates and sold out. Poverty followed and more than 1000 young men emigrated to North America, although some returned during the years of the Depression.

The Macleods of Harris had controlled the southern part of the island until 1779 when it was sold to Captain Macleod of Berneray (No.7.15) who built the harbour at Rodel, constructed roads, restored Rodel church, planted many trees and developed the fishing industry. Unfortunately the Harris population was increasing rapidly and the demand on the land was excessive. As a consequence the islanders were unable to meet their rent obligations.

In 1834 Macleod sold Harris to the Earl of Dunmore, and unlike Sir James Matheson in Lewis he evicted islanders from their west coast crofts in order to lease the land to sheep farmers. However, he did attempt to carry out the evictions in a reasonably humane manner by giving three years' notice to quit. And his wife is to be remembered as the person who first popularised Harris tweed and thus created a new industry. The Earl's heirs sold North Harris to Sir Edward Scott in 1868 and South Harris directly to Lord Leverhulme in

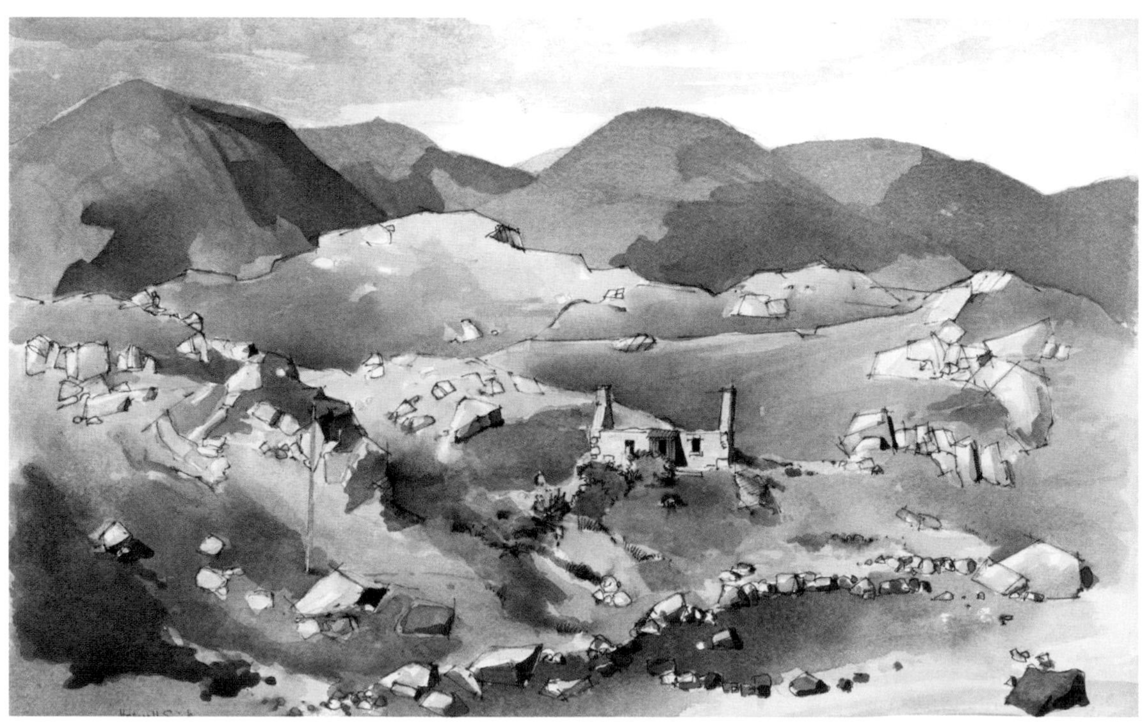

THE EAST SIDE OF HARRIS

1919.

Much of the recent successful development of Lewis and Harris is thanks to the efforts of the Highlands and Islands Development Board (HIDB), now Highland and Islands Enterprise (HIE), and a number of projects funded by grants from the European Community.

Wildlife: Some 4000–5000 years ago Lewis and Harris were covered with stunted forests mainly of alder, oak, pine, ash and elm. But with settlement by man the island was steadily denuded of trees. A change of climatic conditions dealt the final blow.

Lewis has relatively little machair as the west coast has many rocks and cliffs, but the central plain is rich in peat with ling and bell-heather, cross-leaved heath, bog asphodel, sundew, cotton grass, bog-myrtle, blue moor grass, deer's hair grass and sphagnum moss.

Among the Harris mountains there is little heather but wild thyme, saxifrages and violets are everywhere. There are a few alpine willow and roseroot but no *Silene acaulis* and *Azales procumbens*, as these prefer granite. When ferrets were introduced rabbits were almost exterminated and the ferrets also preyed on ptarmigan. But the rabbits, as always, have survived – and multiplied.

Seton Gordon, when writing *A Highland Year*, found Clisham and its environment singularly devoid of animal and birdlife. He mentions grouse and meadow pipits but no golden plover, curlew, buzzards or eagle.

In Stornoway a colony of grey seals inhabit the harbour and the woodland surrounding Lews Castle has been colonised by many species of birds and includes a large rookery.

On the west coast there is a wildfowl refuge at Loch Mór Barvas and corncrakes nest in the undisturbed old burial grounds.

Escapees from the mink farms of the 1950s are now unfortunately established predators threatening the endangered bird populations. They are virtually impossible to eradicate and as they are strong swimmers they are colonising adjoining islands and spreading south to the Uists.

* * *

Although **LEWIS** and **HARRIS** are parts of a single island there is a natural six-mile barrier of high mountains and forbidding moorland between the great sea-lochs of Seaforth and Resort. This so effectively separated the two communities throughout history that they were considered entirely separate islands. Even today, although now connected by road, they speak Gaelic with a distinctly different dialect.

* * *

HARRIS, the southern part of the island, is itself divided into two parts, North and South Harris, where sea-lochs nearly meet at Tarbert (G. *tairbeart* – a narrow isthmus). The west coast has dunes backed by machair which is so thick with wildflowers in early summer that milk from the grazing cattle is said to be perfumed. Here the white shell-sands are blown over the machair by the winds giving it a natural dressing of lime while the islanders spread seaweed as an organic fertiliser. The other traditional farming practice, lazybeds, is reserved for the barren east coast – strips of peat and seaweed built laboriously by hand on top of the rock strata and used for growing oats and potatoes.

At the time of the Clearances the population was larger than the land could support and the standard of living was low. Islanders were turned off their productive west coast crofts and many, loath to leave their homeland, tried to eke out a living on the desolate east coast where the landowners had no interest in such an uneconomic region. To make matters worse families evicted from the neighbouring islands in the Sound of Harris also settled here and lazybeds consequently stretched far up the hillsides amid terrible poverty. In the end depopulation by emigration seemed the only answer.

From the ferry terminal at **Tarbert** there are connections to Skye and North Uist but the town itself, although the largest settlement on Harris, is small, consisting of a few shops, a hotel, post-office, school, small tourist office, churches, and some stores and workshops for the fishermen.

The narrow, winding, road on the east coast south of Tarbert is called the **Golden Road** because it was so expensive to build. In this area, known as Bays, the bare gneiss is pockmarked with tiny lochs, the predominant colours are rich dark browns and greys, and the coastline is a broken conglomerate of inlets and islands. There are mere pockets of sodden charcoal-coloured peat and the ground is so rocky that the dead had to be taken to the west coast for burial. It is difficult to imagine a more desolate, yet awe-inspiring, landscape with human habitation limited to an intermittent smattering of neat little houses near the shoreline.

> The narrow bay
> Has a knuckle of houses and a nail of sand
> By which the sea hangs grimly to the land.
>
> *Norman MacCaig. 'Harris, East side'.*

The Golden Road serves the scattered settlements around the bays. Every turn brings a new picture-postcard scene of white houses in rocky coves, moored boats, lobster pots and nets. There are two islets in Loch Grosebay – **Càiream** and **Eilean Dubh** and at the next firth, Loch Stockinish, a youth hostel overlooks Stockinish Island (No.8.6). Two more islets in bays further to the west are much smaller than Stockinish – **Eilean Mhànais** outside Loch Gheocrab and **Eilean Quidnish** in Loch Finsbay. The road winds and twists past Lingara Bay and **Lingarabay Island**, about which the pros and cons of a gigantic quarrying venture were argued about for years, and arrives at Rodel near Renish Point, the southern extremity of Harris. **Renish Island** is no more than a punctuation mark at the end of Renish Point.

The village of Rodel has an attractive little harbour which was built in the 18th century by Captain Macleod of Berneray. It was here that the Harris ferry would put passengers ashore by tender before the new terminal was built at Tarbert. Above the harbour stands **St Clement's Church** [NG0488832] which was built by Alasdair Crotach (Alasdair the Hunchback), the 8th Macleod in about 1500 using sandstone imported from Carsaig on Mull (No.3.3). Its solid rectangular tower is a distinctive landmark which is unique in the Western Isles, and Macleod's tomb within the church is beautifully carved and well worth a visit. The church was restored in 1787 and again in 1873. If locked, the key can usually be obtained from the nearby hotel.

Leaving Rodel and travelling parallel to the Sound of Harris one arrives at **Leverburgh**, now restored to its original name of **An t-Ob** (G. – the haven). It was named Leverburgh by Lord Leverhulme when he tried to make it a centre for the herring fishing industry after the First World War and spent a considerable sum on providing facilities. But the project languished and he sold out in 1923. The township never really recovered from its growth pains until 1996 when the popular direct vehicle-ferry link across the Sound of Harris to Berneray (and North Uist) breathed new life into the area.

Further to the north-west beyond **Northton** is the distinctive peninsula of **Toe Head**. Its dominant peak is Chaipaval (339m). From its summit on a clear day the St Kilda group (Nos. 9.1/9.2/9.3) can be seen to the west, and the Cuillin of Skye to the east. Between the road and Chaipaval is a vast stretch of perfect Hebridean beach, **Tràigh an Taoibh Thuath** (G. – beach on the north side), which continues on to **Tràigh Scarasta** (G. – beach, ON – the farm in the pass) with its sand dunes below the machair. The road here winds along the Atlantic coast and the scenery is dramatically different from the desolation of the east; wide open meadows, pale pink or cream shell sands, turquoise sea and white surf. At **Borve** (ON – fort) there is a standing stone and an ancient dun and the hills to the south conceal a large loch – Loch Langavat (ON – long water). Borve Lodge, surrounded by woodland planted by the Earl of Dunmore, was Lord Leverhulme's home on Harris. Opposite Taransay (No.8.9) there is another wide stretch of sand – Tràigh Seilebost

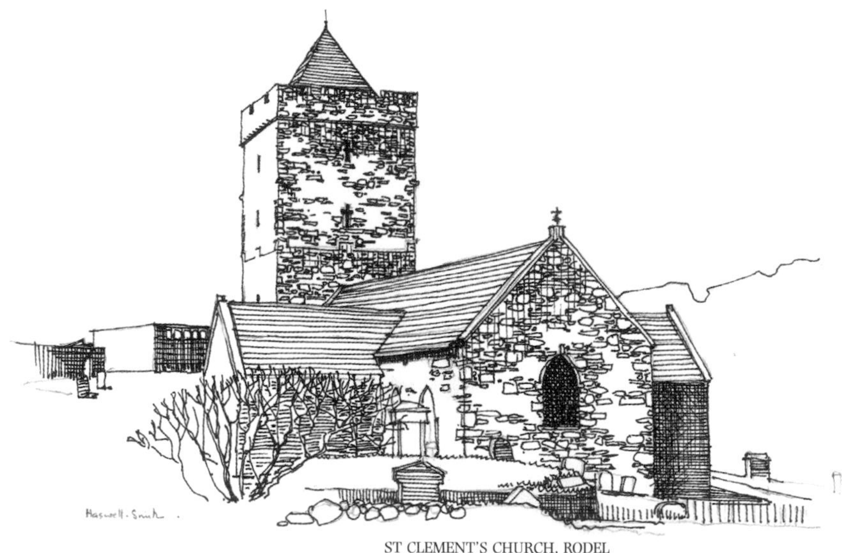

ST CLEMENT'S CHURCH, RODEL

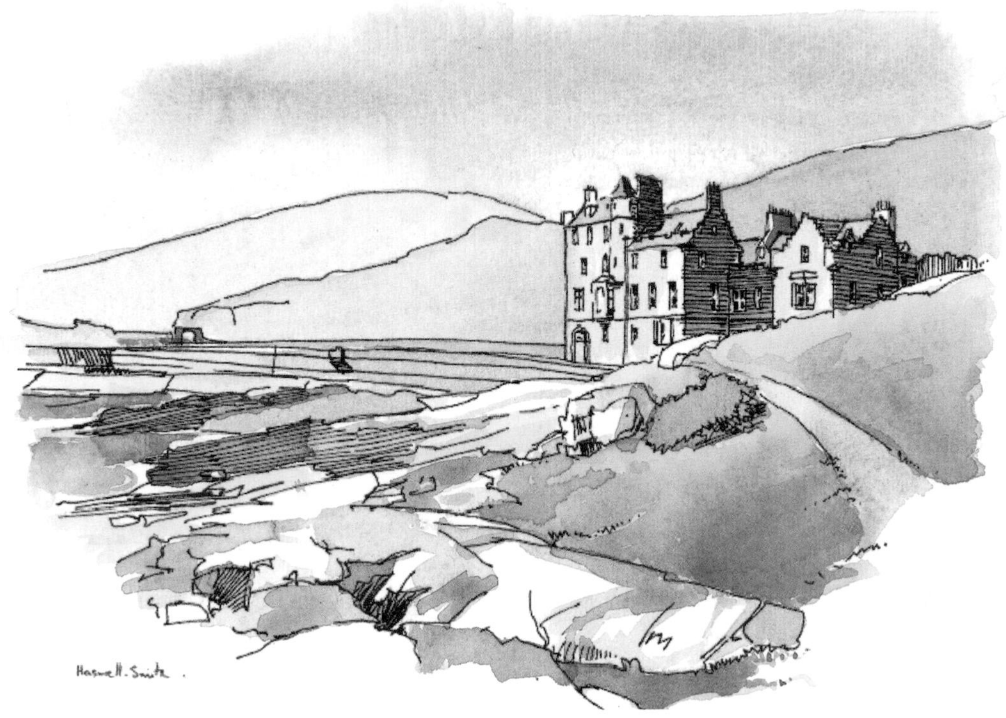

AMHUINNSUIDHE CASTLE IN THE FOREST OF HARRIS

with a spit of sand dunes separating it from the estuarine sands of Tràigh Luskentyre. Here the road turns eastwards through a long valley before returning to Tarbert.

The bare mountains of the Forest of Harris are north of Tarbert; an area with large herds of red deer and lochs rich with salmon and trout. Beneath, on the shore of West Loch Tarbert, the remains of a whaling station built by Norwegians before the First World War and abandoned in 1930, are a reminder of another age. There are dramatic views from the coast road as it runs west round Loch Meavaig and beneath the windows of **Amhuinnsuidhe Castle** [a:vin-soo-ee] (G. – river seat) beside Loch Leosavay [NB043084]. The castle was built by the Earl of Dunmore in 1868 beside stepped falls where the waters of Loch Leosaid tumble over smooth rock slabs and into the sea. Salmon jump these falls in June and July. It was here in 1912 that James Barrie, of *Peter Pan* fame, wrote the drama *Mary Rose*. He was inspired, it is said, by the islets in Loch Voshimid at the head of Glen Meavaig. North of the loch are two medieval beehive huts. A hydro-electric scheme hidden in the hills provides most of the electricity requirements for Harris.

The coast road comes to an end at beautiful **Hushinish Bay** with the island of Scarp (No.8.13) to the north and Taransay (No.8.9) to the south.

For anyone proposing to camp on Harris many sites are boggy and midgy, so be prepared. However, as compensation, there is rock-climbing for enthusiastic climbers on Clisham which is the highest peak in the Outer Hebrides at 799m (a Corbett), or Sgurr Scaladale, Cnoc a Chaisteil, Creag Mò, Glen Scaladale, Gillaval Glas, Sgaoth Ard, Toddun, Craig Stulaval, Oreval, Ullaval, Strone Ulladale and Taran Mor. There are also many fascinating walks along the hill-tracks which are marked on the Ordnance Survey maps; for example, Vigadale Bay on Loch Seaforth to Loch Voshimid, or Aline Lodge to Loch Langavat (a much larger loch than that of the same name in South Harris).

* * *

Travelling in the other direction, east from Tarbert, leads to the island of **SCALPAY**. The ferry was replaced by a bridge in 1998 and Scalpay lost its nominal independence as a separate island.

It is a thriving island with change being the penalty for success. The Scalpachs have always managed to maintain a vigorous community when many other islands have lost theirs.

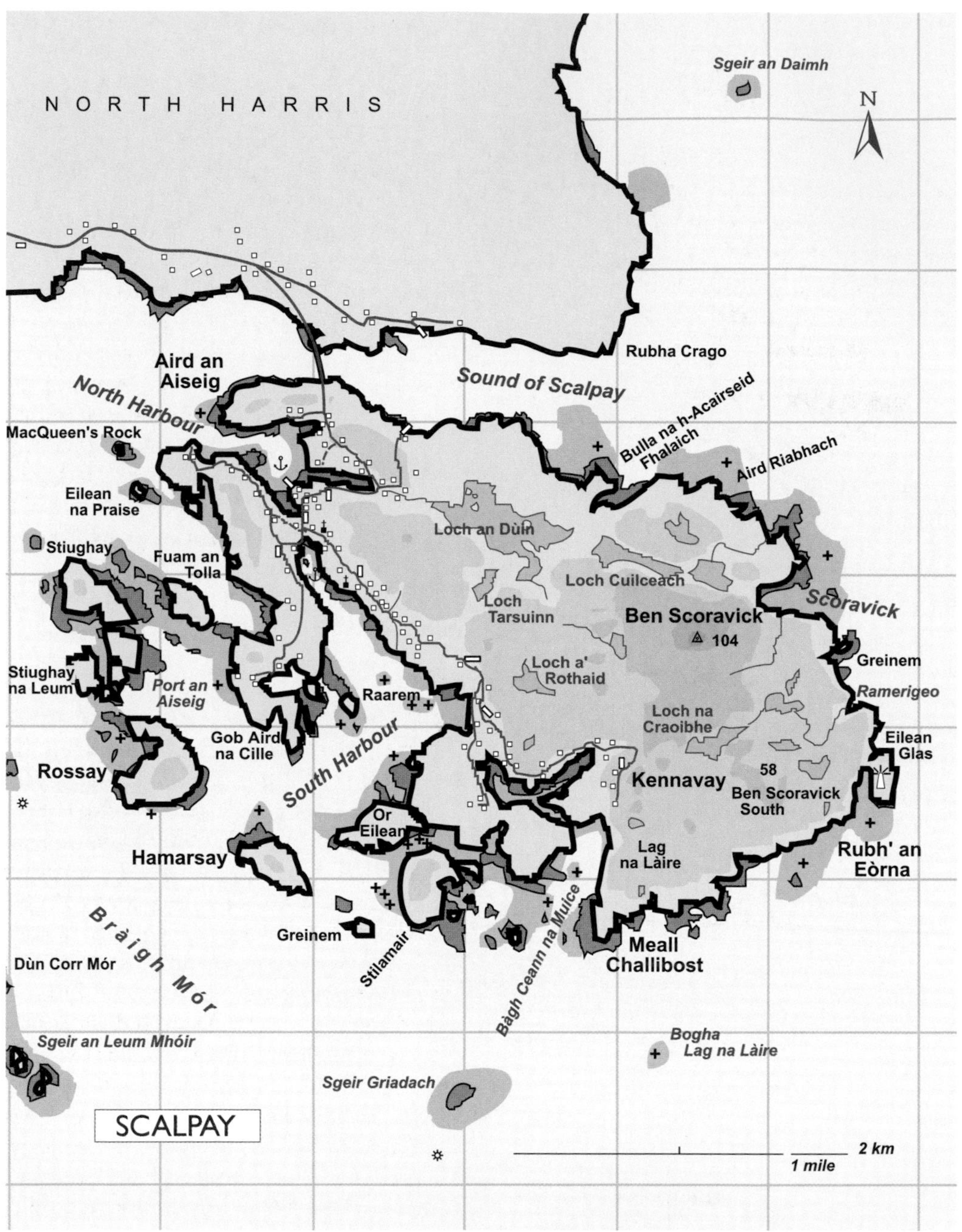

Although there is a reasonable agricultural base, which produces a good crop of oats from forty crofts, the land is poor and the traditional industry is fishing, principally for prawns. Many of the islanders own their own boats and there are also a number of trawlers.

All the settlements are on the south-western seaboard. In the past with a large population having less interest in fishing there was extensive lazybed cultivation. But there were too many mouths to feed and fishing became an essential occupation which eventually led to relative prosperity.

The ferry wades across the kyle. I drive
The car ashore
On to a trim tarred road. A car on Scalpay?
Yes, and a road where never was one before.
The ferrymen's Gaelic wonders who I am
(Not knowing I know it), this man back from the dead,

Who takes the blue-black road (no traffic jam)
From by Craig Lexie over to Bay Head.

A man bows in the North wind, shaping up
His lazybeds,
And through the salt air vagrant peat smells waver
From houses where no house should be. The sheds
At the curing station have been newly tarred.
Aunt Julia's house has vanished. The Red Well
Has been bulldozed away. But sharp and hard
The church still stands, barring the road to Hell.
. . . from 'Return to Scalpay' by Norman MacCaig.

In recent years, such a large number of people on an island of this size has created an almost urban atmosphere and the excellent harbours, surrounded by crisp whitewashed houses, are usually busy.

Scalpay has a very irregular outline with deep indentations. On the east side is **Beinn Scoravich**, 104m high with Loch na Craoibhe (G. – loch of the tree) separating it from 58m-high Ben Scoravich South. The north-west is rough territory of rock and heather-covered slopes, pockets of peat bog, lochs running parallel to the coast – **Loch Cuilceach** (G. – loch of reeds), **Loch an Duin** (G. – loch of the fort) and **Loch Tarsuinn** (G. – the crosswise loch) at right-angles to the others.

Eilean Glas lighthouse, on the east coast, was erected in 1788 by the Commissioners of Northern Lights. It was the first and for a long time the only lighthouse in the Western Isles and was placed strategically on the busy sea lane which existed at that time between Skye, Harris and the Baltic. A new tower was constructed in 1824 with an oil-burning light and this was converted to incandescent in 1907. The lighthouse is now automatic and the keepers' houses are holiday homes. They were built of Aberdeen granite by Robert Louis Stevenson's grandfather.

The road ends by the peat diggings beyond Kennavay but there is an interesting walk around or over Ben Scoravick – down past the east-coast lochans to the lighthouse with its rented accommodation and small restaurant and then along an unmapped south-coast path for the return journey.

The west side of Scalpay shelters behind a line of small islands, **Eilean na Praise** (G. – pot island), **Stiughay**, **Fuam an Tolla**, **Stiughay na Leum**, **Rossay**, **Hamarsay** and **Greinem**: and across the deep channel called Braigh Mór (G. – big neck) is a great cluster of islets and rocks with the largest being **Gloraig a' Chaimbeulich**, **Eilean Mhic Fhionnlaidh**, **Eilean na Gearrabreac** (G. – guillemot isle) and **Eilean na Sgaite** (G. – skate isle).

Scalpachs are renowned throughout the islands for their excellent seamanship. This was proven when, in December 1962, the trawler *Boston Heron* was in difficulties in a full sou'-westerly gale and was driven on to the rocks of **Stilamair** off the south coast of Scalpay. Stilamair is a tidal island near Greinem islet. As there was no time to spare six Scalpay men set out immediately in a small open boat to try to give assistance. In spite of the ferocious seas they managed to rescue three of the trawlermen, one of whom was clinging exhausted to the rocks. They were unable to save the other seven but their heroism was rightfully recognised by the RNLI.

* * *

LEWIS has a mixed economy of weaving, fishing and crofting and occasional construction work for the oil industry. Although Harris tweed, known locally as *clò mór* (G. – big cloth), originated in Harris, the centre of production is now in Lewis, probably because the great majority of the population live there. Until quite recently the tweed was still produced on hand looms and the weavers resisted attempts to introduce power looms although spinning and dyeing were done in a factory. The 650 weavers on the island can produce about 4½ million yards of tweed each year. Unfortunately, with widespread central heating and a preference for light-weight clothing there was an inevitable decline in sales of this fine, warm, water-resistant, and almost indestructible material. But the fashion pendulum swung back for a time in its favour as lighter-weight cloths of broad width are now available.

The road connecting Harris and Lewis runs from Tarbert to Stornoway skirting the shores of Loch Seaforth and Loch Erisort. Loch Seaforth is twelve miles long and the area between it and Loch Erisort is called Park (G. *Pairc*), a 23,000-hectare estate of wild country with many herds of red deer. Much of this area is fairly inaccessible and the simplest method of reaching it is probably by boat from Loch Seaforth. This is a truly remote wilderness just waiting for exploration by hill-walkers although it should be avoided during the hunting season. It was on this sporting estate in 1887 that crofters killed 200 deer to draw attention to their desperate need for land.

At the head of Loch Erisort, another long sea-loch, by **Balallan** (G. – Allan's town) there are roads leading into the north-east of Park, the only area accessible by vehicle. At the loch entrance is a drying-island, **Eilean Chaluim Chille** (G. – island of Columba's church) having, as expected, an ancient ruined church dedicated to St Columba [NB386211] and a small burial ground next to what may have been a monastery. Macleod of Lewis kept an orchard on this island at one time and Murdo Mackenzie, 'Mac Mhic Mhurchaidh,' the first of Lord Seaforth's factors, lived here. **Eilean Cheois** is in the centre of the loch while **Eilean Thòraidh** and **Eilean Rosaidh** are east of the Cromore headland. The **Barkin Isles** are to the north at the entrance to Loch Leurbost; they comprise **Tabhaidh Mhór**, **Tabhaidh Bheag**, **Tannaraidh** and **Bhatarsaidh**.

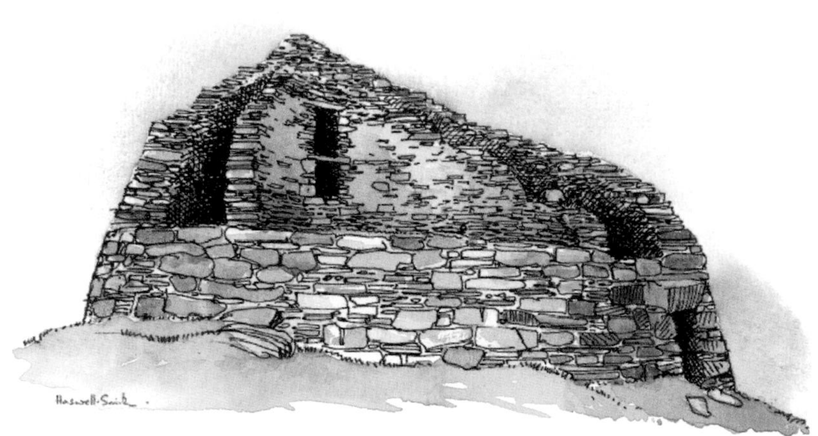

CARLOWAY BROCH

North of Park is the parish of Lochs with its steep and rocky coastline cut deeply by sea-lochs. The dark peat moorland is spattered with lochans like pools of mercury gleaming under a cloudy sky.

STORNOWAY (ON *stjorna* – steering or anchor bay) is the only town of burgh status in the Hebrides and the administrative centre of Comhairle nan Eilean Siar, the Western Isles Council. It has a population of about 8100 and the town is centred on its fine natural harbour. Strangely, it was the Dutch who first recognised the fishing potential of Hebridean waters and during the 17th century their fishing fleets were often to be seen in Stornoway harbour. Although cod and ling were caught, it was herring that proved the great attraction. In 1798 Cruttwell's Gazetteer reported that '...the coast is annually visited by myriads of herrings. So immense are the shoals of dog-fish that pursue the herrings that their dorsal fins are sometimes seen like a thick bush of sedges above water as far as the eye can reach'. By the 19th century Stornoway had become a major fishing port and its architecture reflects the prosperity of this period. The local history is illustrated in the Stornoway Museum in Cromwell Street.

The oldest building still standing is possibly the 18th-century net-loft on **North Beach Quay** while **St Columba's Parish Church** on Lewis Street was erected in 1794. At the upper end of Francis Street is **St Peter's Episcopal Church**, built in 1839, which has an ancient sandstone font brought from the Hermit's Chapel on the remote Flannan Isles (See the appendix to Section 9). Its Tower Bell of 1631 once summoned the burghers of Stornoway to civic meetings and David Livingstone's 1608 Bible which he carried in Africa is kept in the vestry.

Arnish Point, at the entrance to Stornoway Harbour, is the site of a wind-turbine fabricator and a seaweed-processing plant. Nearby is a monument to Prince Charles Edward Stuart and on the opposite side at Holm Point is another monument to the 205 Lewis men who were drowned on New Year's Day, 1919 [NB445305]. They were returning home from service at the end of the First World War when their ship, the *Iolaire*, was wrecked on the Beasts of Holm, the rocks just north of the entrance to the harbour while their waiting families watched helpless from the pier.

Sir Alexander Mackenzie, the explorer who made the first overland crossing of Canada, was born in Stornoway and **Martins Memorial** (1885) stands on the site of the house where he was born. West of the town is Sir James Matheson's **Lews Castle** [NB420332], built in 1856–63, which serves now as a technical college. It is surrounded by spacious grounds and the substantial area of mixed woodland is a unique sight in the Outer Hebrides.

Although Stornoway lies on the periphery of Europe it is a remarkably cosmopolitan place with an unexpected bustle of activity quite unlike the rest of the Outer Isles. Some of the shops are run by Asians who speak fluent Gaelic.

To the east of Stornoway, beyond the airport, is the comparatively densely populated **Eye Peninsula**, known as Point (G. *an rubha*). On the north shore of the narrow isthmus is the 14th-century St Columba's church and graveyard where nineteen Macleod chiefs are buried [NB485322]. The church was last used in 1828.

West of Stornoway a road crosses the island to Loch Roag and another strikes north-west across the moors to Barvas. Much of Lewis is dark peat moorland with hundreds of shallow lochs and intricate patterns created by centuries of peat cutting. In early summer 'going to the peats' is an important social occasion and the peat is still cut for fuel in the traditional way. It has been estimated that there are eighty-five million tons of peat on the island. An average family uses about 15,000 blocks of peat each year, and this takes at least fifteen man-days to cut, dry and stack.

A road runs round **Loch Roag** crossing **Abhainn Grimersta** which is considered one of the best salmon rivers in Europe. The waters come from distant Loch Langavat through a tortuous succession of remote lochs before discharging into Loch Roag. A branch road leads to the large island of **GREAT BERNERA** (G. *Bearnaraidh Mór*) which lies in the centre of the loch. Its access bridge, the first pre-stressed concrete bridge to be built in Europe, was constructed in 1953 after the islanders threatened to dynamite the hillside to form a causeway. Many of the islanders are called MacDonald and are said to be descended from a watchman who was given the island by the MacAulays of Uig as a reward for his services. Great Bernera is a lobster-fishing centre; the processing plant at Kirkibost was built in 1972.

Loch Roag is a fascinating area and one could spend weeks exploring its many islands and inlets. The freshwater lochs which surround it provide excellent brown trout fishing. The beaches and coves near **Valtos** are of particular beauty.

Beyond Loch Roag is **Camas Uig** (G. *camas* – bay, ON *vik* – bay) and the magnificent Sands of Uig. It was here that a 12th-century Norse chess set probably carved from walrus ivory was found in the dunes behind the beach. The Uig sands frame one of the most beautiful views in Scotland – wide, clean, flat and virginal white with an indigo to viridian sea and purple heather-covered Mealisval and Tahaval behind.

The road carries on down the coast from here but it slowly loses importance and dwindles to a track at **Mealista** where there are the remains of an army camp adjoining the ruins of a Benedictine convent called Tigh nan Cailleachan Dubha (G. – house of the old women in black, i.e. nuns) and traces of a 'souterrain' [NA991241].

If spending time by the white sands of Uig or Mangersta Bay try to find the secret cliff-top bothy with its view of Eilean Molach to the north! There are exciting hill walks and many good climbs in this region – Mealisval 574m, Cracaval, Tarain, Tahaval, Teinnasval or Tamanaisval – to name a few.

Back at the head of East Loch Roag the main road from Stornoway reaches one of Britain's most famous landmarks – the ancient standing stones of **Callanish** [NB213330]. It was only in 1857, when the surrounding peat was excavated, that the true height of these stones was realised. This is the second

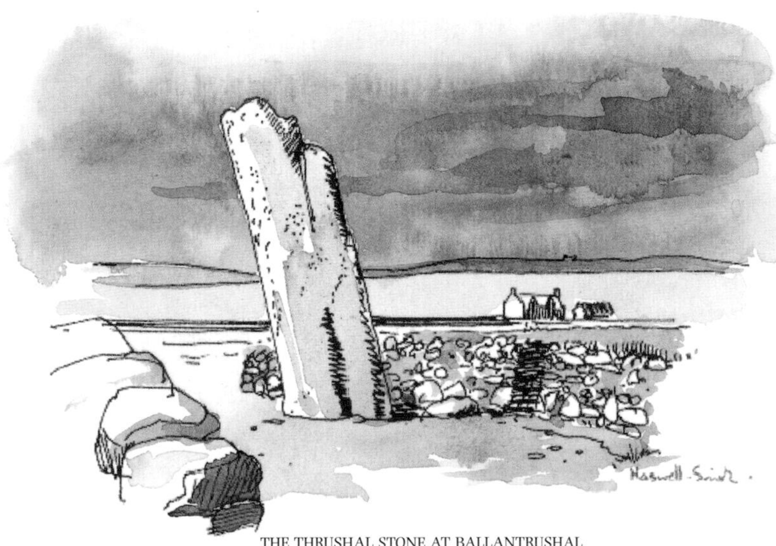
THE THRUSHAL STONE AT BALLANTRUSHAL

greatest prehistoric stone circle in Britain, about 5000 years old – older than both Stonehenge and the Pyramids. The alignment of the stones may relate to observations of the moon, unlike Stonehenge which relates to the sun. The monoliths form an oblique cross, 123m from north to south and 43m east to west with a central circle and cairn in which the remains of a cremation were found. The tallest standing stone is 4½m – nearly 15 feet – high. Many other small stone circles in the vicinity of Callanish are probably related to it. (Calanais Visitor Centre. Mon.–Sat. 10am–7pm.)

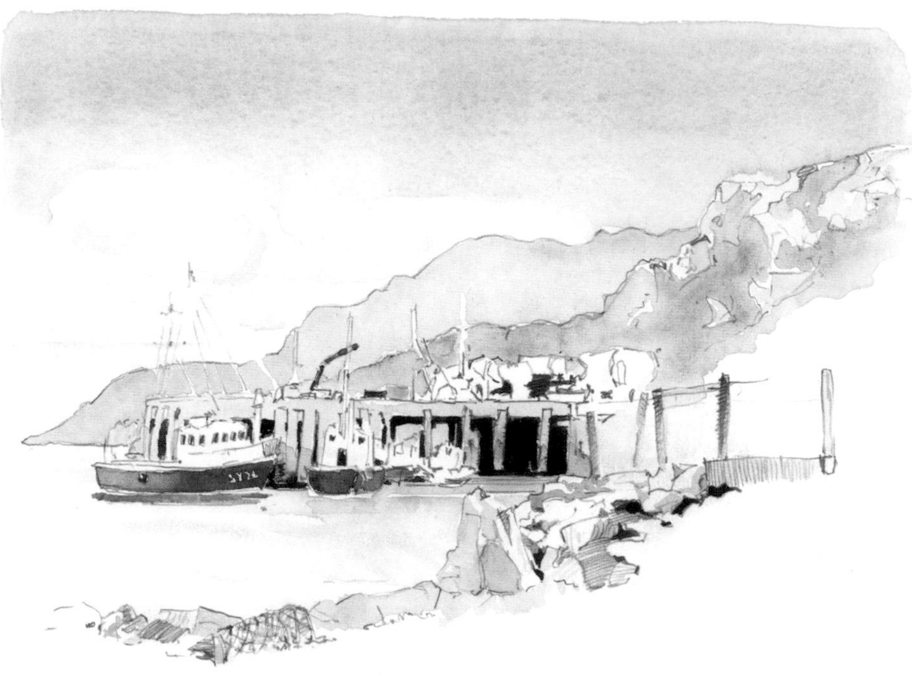

KIRKIBOST PIER, GREAT BERNERA

Local legend claimed that the standing stones of Callanish were giants petrified by St Kieran for refusing to be christened.

About 8km north of Callanish is **Doune Carloway** one of the best-preserved brochs [NB190413]. It is 15m in diameter, parts of the galleries and staircase are still intact, and the quality of the dry-stone masonry is remarkable. The broch is on a height overlooking Loch Carloway. An islet, **Craigeam**, is concealed behind its northern headland.

Just north of the village of Carloway, **Garenin** has the last remaining street of black houses on Lewis. These are clustered above a shingle beach in a sheltered cove [NB193442]. The last inhabitants left in 1973 but the houses are now being restored and re-occupied as part of a far-sighted project to preserve the village in its original state.

This north-west Atlantic coastline is steeped in history. There is a folk museum at **Shawbost**, a 6m high whale-bone arch at **Bragar** with the harpoon which killed the whale suspended from it and a Black House Museum at **Arnol** [NB311493]. This *tigh dubh* was occupied as recently as 1964 and with a peat fire kept burning in the centre it is possible to see an authentic interior with the original straw-lined box beds. It makes one realise how well these houses were suited to the climate. Walls 2m thick and thatch and turf roofs weighted with stones created a warm, dry interior no matter what the state of the weather outside.

At **Barvas** a road cuts across the moors to Stornoway with the rare sight of a petrol station at the junction. There are many prehistoric sites near the coast on the route north. For instance, the tallest standing stone in Scotland (over 6m) is at **Ballantrushal** [NB376537]; a 15m burial cairn and large enclosure is at **Shader** [NB396541]; and there are many brochs, duns and temple ruins.

The main road ends at **Port of Ness**. From here Lewis men sail every August to Sula Sgeir, forty-one miles to the north, to bring back *guga* – young gannet, which is considered a great delicacy but is certainly an acquired taste. Port of Ness is a delightful little harbour although it offers only limited shelter. Just north of it is **Dun Eistean**, a tiny piece of land broken from the coastline with the remains of an old fort on it. This was a place of refuge for the Clan Morrison when the MacAuley's chose to attack and an iron bridge was built over the gorge in 2002 to allow the Morrisons to hold Clan gatherings there.

Near **Eoropie** (ON *eyrar-boe* – beach village), the most northerly settlement, is a natural stone arch and 'pygmy's isle' – **Luchruban** or Eilean nan Daoine Beaga (G. – isle of the little people) [NB508661]. A pygmy race was believed to have lived here and Dean Munro said that they had their 'ane little kirk in it of ther awn handey wark.' The chambered building is on the steep summit of the island. In an excavation many small bones were found which were thought to be human but were later identified as animal bones.

Just north of Eoropie is the restored 12th-century **Teampull Mholuidh** (G. – Church of St Moluag) [NB519653]. The key for access is kept in the local store.

A little more than another kilometre to the north the Outer Hebrides come to a dramatic end at the **Butt of Lewis**. The brick lighthouse overlooks a mist-shrouded tumble of stacks and rocky precipices: the sea boils in the chasms between and the eery sound of the fog-horn sometimes echoes from the cliffs. Apart from Sula Sgeir and Rona there is nothing now but wild sea until one reaches the Faeroes 200 miles to the north.

* * *

Access: Ro-ro ferries, daily except Sundays: Stornoway, Lewis, 01851-702361/ Ullapool, (3hrs) 01854-612358: Tarbert, Harris, 01859-502444/ Uig, Skye, (1¾hrs) 01470-542219; Daily incl. Sundays: Leverburgh, Harris, 01859-502444/ Berneray, North Uist, (70min) 01876-500337.

Stornoway Bus Station, 01851-704327. A good selection of Council and private bus services serves the whole island (and the Uists). Scheduled air services to Stornoway, from Glasgow, Inverness, Benbecula, Edinburgh, and Aberdeen. General enquiries, 01851-702256.

Tourist Information: Stornoway, 01851-703088; Tarbert, 01859-502011.

Anchorages:

1. An t-Obbe (Leverburgh). There is 4.3m depth alongside head of pier but anchor as convenient clear of pier, moorings and ferry. Sheltered and safe in channel 2½c SE of Rubh' an Losaid in 5.5m, very good holding, but very restricted and access difficult.
2. Carminish bay, has some shelter from NW–E in 5m but mostly too shallow.
3. Port Eisgein, Sound of Harris, 1M NW of Renish Point, small inlet noted in Admiralty Pilot. No other information.
4. Loch Rodel, Renish point. Exposed to S'lies but temp. anchorage off boulder beach on NE side, W of church (conspic.). Beware Duncan rock.
5. Poll an Tigh-Mhail, Rodel. Enter from Loch Rodel thro' Bay Channel (which dries 0.5m with large stones). When base of Pillar Rock perch is covered there is 3.4m depth. Pool is deep with perfect shelter. Three visitor's moorings on N side of Vallay. Harbour by hotel dries completely. Anchoring possible but holding poor.
6. Lingara Bay, by Lingarabay island. Good shelter but untenable in E'lies. Anchor just past S side of Eilean Collam in 5m. Go no further in.
7. Loch Finsbay. Little sea, good holding and perfect shelter in all winds. Beware rocks N of Finsbay Island, west of Eilean Quidnish and in loch at Ardvey. Anchor mid-channel N of Ardvey promontory in 4m, mud. Hard to recognise in misty weather but fairly easy entrance if directions followed carefully.
8. Loch Flodabay. Not recommended due to number of rocks but ¾c wide channel along NE shore is charted as clear.
9. Loch Gheocrab. Poor shelter except for pool at head of loch behind a drying reef but obstructed with fish cages.
10. Loch Beacravik, which is the W arm at the head of Loch Gheocrab is well-protected but has fish cages and E side is foul at entrance. Avoid rocky patches on bottom when anchoring.
11. Loch Stockinish. Access best through Caolas Beag, E of Stockinish Island, before half-tide. Very narrow (only 27m at one point) but clean if close-in to Stockinish Island. After passing Stockinish keep just NE of mid-channel. Anchor in mouth of westerly arm at head of loch, completely sheltered, 9m sand. Beware rock off Ardvey point and to N. Poll Scrot off Caolas Beag has 3m depth alongside pontoon.
12. Loch Grosebay. Safe anchorage but poor shelter N of Sgeir a' Chais at head of loch in 9m mud. Several hazards on approach.
13. Loch Scadabay, on N side of entrance to Loch Grosebay. Passage W of Eilean an Duine is shallow and only 30m wide. Keep to E side to avoid drying rocks. Pool depth less than 2m but soft mud. Perfect shelter.
14. Plocrapool, East Loch Tarbert, 57 50.5N 06 45W. Snug but shallow. Approach carefully by sailing directions. Pass W of rock at entrance, steer 210°. and anchor in suitable depth.
15. Ob Meavag, Loch Ceann Dibig, East Loch Tarbert. Many rocks but sheltered. Dries 2c from head. Approach from NW as sailing instructions. Beware fish cages.
16. Bàgh Diraclett, Loch Ceann Dibig. Sheltered but beware drying rocks on approach. Good holding.

17. Eileanan Diraclett, 57 53N 06 47W. N of entrance to Loch Ceann Dibig. Sheltered anchorage but no further than 1c into inlet on W side of islands.
18. East Loch Tarbert. Little space due to moorings and ferry access. Ferry needs space to turn on S side of pier. Anchor W of pier only if space permits.
19. North harbour, Scalpay. A fine natural harbour in a small bight at NW end, with depths of 1.8m to 5.5m but limited space. Beware MacQueens rock and a reef and wreck near the entrance.
20. South harbour, Scalpay. On SW side, enter between Hamarsay and Rossay. Keep midway between south-east shore and Raarem islet. When past Raarem turn north and keep ½c off E side of Raarem and continue close to W shore at the narrows. Anchor SE of islet in inner loch. Beware drying rock ½c SE of islet.
21. Loch Scoravick, Scalpay. Good holding on S side, 5m. Exposed to E'lies.
22. Loch Maaruig, 2½M into Loch Seaforth on W side. Anchor W of Goat Point, mud. Beware rock awash SW of Goat Point. Well sheltered. In places the shore is so steep that it is possible to moor to it and lie afloat.
23. Aline Lodge. Anchor off the jetty, or better, ½M farther NE in 7m. Sheltered but subject to squalls.
24. Loch Claidh. 1M into loch on E side, anchor NE of Eilean Thinngarstaigh (Hingarstay) in 8m, mud and sand. Space just over ½c width. Enter W and N of En Thinngarstaigh. Good holding and shelter and little swell.
25. Tob Smuasavig, inlet on NE side of Loch Claidh. Anchor at head of inlet, bottom stiff clay, shells and stones. Uncomfortable in S winds.
26. Loch Bhalamuis (Valamus). Approach with care only when loch well open and keep W of centre when in the loch. About ½M into loch on E side anchor ½c N of Transit Point if sufficient depth found clear of drying rock and boat mooring.
27. Loch Bhrollum. Tob Bhrollum on NE side of Aird Dhubh is well sheltered but some swell sets in with S'lies. Skirt W and N sides of Aird Dhubh at a distance of 30m until Rubh' a' Bhaird is shut in by Aird Dhubh then anchor as convenient in 4–6m, good holding. This position is east of a sunken rock in the entrance.
28. Loch Bhrollum. Anchor at head of loch on E side of islet. Shallow but soft mud.
29. Loch Shell or Sealg. S side clean but there are rocks W of Eilean Iubhard. Anchor in Tòb na Gile Móire on S side, at head of loch, in Tòb Eishken (beware rock E of entrance) on N side, in Tòb Stiomrabhaigh (Stemervay) or Tòb Orinsay. All areas shoal or shallow, partly exposed and some may be foul with old moorings or obstructed with fish cages. Easy access, good shelter but squalls possible.
30. Tòb Lemrevay (Limervay), Caolas a' Tuath. Follow directions for approach. Anchor off E side of inlet with just enough room to clear shoreline rocks. Good holding but subject to N squalls.
31. Loch Odhairn (Ouirn). Anchor towards the head, opposite N shore jetty, on S shore behind promontory. Bottom good, no sea in any wind, but heavy squalls in SW gales. Loch free from dangers.
32. Loch Mharabhig (Mariveg), 58 05.4N 06 23.5W. Tortuous entrance by Caolas na h-Acarsaid, S of Eilean Rosaidh, or S of Eilean Thòraidh, and several rock obstructions in loch. Best anchorages SE of Sgeir a' Bhuic or in NW corner. Well sheltered.
33. Eilean Thòraidh (Torray), at entrance to Loch Mharabhig. Fairly tricky approach. Anchor between W side of Torray and mussel farm or in opposite bay off Aird Fhalasgair (beware drying rock off S point). Well sheltered.
34. Camas Thormaid (Witches' Bay), SW of Aird Fhalasgair Beware drying rocks at centre of approach. Approach on course 20m from S shore and anchor no further than SW of islet, clay. Well sheltered.
35. Orasaidh. Anchor in the basin, S or SW of Orasaidh.
36. Camas Orasaidh, inlet W of Orasaidh. Keep to W side on entering. Good holding, mud.
37. Tòb Cromore, on SE side of Peacam, near entrance to Loch Erisort. Snug anchorage in 2–4m, clay, shoal near head and foul ground near shores. Note rock off NW shore.
38. Peacam (Cromore) 58 06.5N 06 25W, E of Eilean Chaluim Chille. Anchor S of Sgeir Peacam.
39. Loch Thorasdaidh (Hurista), S of Eilean Chaluim Chille. Sailing directions must be followed with care. Anchor W of Toa peninsula in soft smelly mud. Alternatively pass S and E of the central islets and anchor S of Toa. Some swell in W'lies.
40. Keose, 58 06N 06 29W, on N shore of Loch Erisort. Anchor SW of jetty in 3m mud or N of Garbh Eilean.
41. Loch Erisort. Several bays with good anchorages. Some drying rocks but no serious navigational difficulty.
42. Loch Leurbost on N side of approach to Loch Erisort. Approach S of the Barkin Isles; Tabhaidh Mhór and Bheag, and Bhatarsaidh and beware drying reef 1c SW of Tannaraidh. Anchor in basin W of Risay at S side of loch entrance, 2–3m, soft mud. Enter basin from N.
43. Loch Leurbost, head is shoal for 3c. Anchor off jetty at Aird Feiltanish: or off slip by the Free Church at Crossbost: or in Tòb Shuardail on S side of loch but note Jackal Shoal (1.8m depth) on approach: or near head of loch S of Orasaigh.
44. Loch Grimshader, 58 09N 06 23W. Well protected. Beware Sgeir a' Chaolais mid-channel. Anchor either side of Buaile Mhor at head. Good holding. SW part of loch is soft mud. Beware power cable over Loch Beag.
45. Glumaig harbour, bay SW of Stornoway Harbour, is

best anchorage but far from town and in industrial area. Reefs marked with beacons on W side of entrance and 1c N of Arnish Point. Bottom foul, anchor should be buoyed.
46. Stornoway Harbour. Poll nam Portan opposite commercial quays. Note drying rocks. Crowded with moorings and exposed to S'ly swell. Avoid swinging into fairway if anchored. North Beach quay, N of No 1 pier in Stornoway Harbour has over 2.7m depth on its W side and over 1.8m on its N side but going alongside amid traffic can be hazardous. Pontoon berths (pay, 01851-702688).
47. Bàgh Phabail (Bayble Bay) on Eye Peninsula. Occasional anchorage. Protected from SW winds. Concrete pier at head with 3.7m at HW at outer end.
48. Broad Bay, N of Eye Peninsula. Some shelter from SW at head.
49. Port of Ness (Callicvol), 2M SE of lighthouse. Small open bay free of dangers but subject to swell. Bottom sand, depths moderate. Exposed E'lies. Boat harbour on N side dries; enter after half flood but not in stormy weather.
50. Eoropie bay. Extensive sandy beach can be approached carefully but avoid Aird Dell vicinity. Temp. anchorage in suitable conditions. *(2km walk to Luchruban)*
51. Loch Shawbost, small bay open N and subject to swell. Shoal with sandy bottom. Keep to centre. About 1c swinging room.
52. Loch Carloway. On approach avoid channel between N headland and Craigeam island. In the loch keep nearer N shore and note shoal patch 1 c WSW of Dunan Pier. Anchor SSW of pier, 3–5m, sand and mud. *(Slip on S shore convenient for access to famous Carloway Broch)*. Good holding but heavy swell in W'lies.
53. Port a' Chaoil, 58 14N 06 46.5W, on E shore of East Loch Roag. Sheltered. Several rocks to be noted. After entering mid-channel anchor close to E shore near head of bay.
54. Tòb Breasclete, E of Keava. Anchor S of old jetty which is E of new pier, mud, good holding and no swell.
55. Callanish, 58 11.5N 06 45W. Temp. anchorage in 2–3m NW of Bratanish islands which are drying islets E of Eilean Kearstay (No.8.18). *(Callanish Standing Stones are close-by.)* Submerged rock S of Bratanish Mór, and another off E shore of anchorage. If going further S, beware power cables over Loch Ceann Hulavig entrance (only 5.7m clearance).
56. Dubh Thob, East Loch Roag, 58 13N 06 48W, between Great Bernera and Vacasay. A secure little anchorage but a number of hazards on entry. N entry easiest.
57. Loch Beag Breaclete, W of Loch Risay, narrow inlet in Great Bernera with 2–9m depth. Rocks on both sides at entrance. Too open to N for good shelter.
58. Kyles of Little Bernera (Bernera Harbour), good anchorage. Keep N of mid-channel on entering, then S of Sgeir a' Chaolais (marked with beacon) and anchor off ruin in NW side of inlet or 1c SW of beacon. Beware submerged rock 1c WSW of beacon near fish cages.
59. West Loch Roag. A large selection of interesting anchorages can be found with the aid of Chart 3381. Examples are; Aird Torranish opposite S of Great Bernera; Loch Drovinish; Miavaig Bay between Floday and Carishader; or the bay by Eilean Teinish.
60. Loch Miavaig, snug, little harbour with free pontoons, or anchor in 3.7m to 9m, very soft mud. Shoal beyond power cable. Water at pier.
61. Shiaram Mór, an islet in Kyles Pabay near Valtos pier. Anchor at NW or SE end.
62. Camas Uig. Occasional anchorage in pool behind two small islets off Carnish, 3m sand. Dangerous to enter or leave in NW'lies.
63. Caolas an Eilean – temp. anchorage in settled weather or quiet W'lies off beach on E shore of Mealista Island (No.8.17), sand.
64. Loch Tamanavay (Hamnaway). Remote and scarcely inhabited. Keep close to east shore to avoid Bo Thorcuill in mid-entrance. Good, well-sheltered anchorage at head of loch but depths decrease sharply.
65. Loch Tealasavay. Occasional anchorage at S side of loch head.
66. Loch Resort, 4M length, good and safe anchorage at loch head or about half-way along at Diriscal on S side, black smelly mud.
67. Loch Cravadale. Occasional anchorage at head of bay.
68. Caolas an Scarp. Anchor in settled weather N or S of the sand-bar. Avoid passage between Fladday and Harris.
69. Husinish bay, temp. anchorage in settled weather in 6m, sand.
70. Govick bay, close E of Rubha Bogha Sgeir. Temp. anchorage in 9m.
71. Loch Leosavay (*by Amhuinnsuidhe*), drying rock off NE shore, at steps S of jetty. Keep towards W side of loch and anchor in bay off mansion, 4m, mud. Sheltered.
72. Loch Meavaig, 2¼M ESE of Glas sgeir, in 2m to 9m, soft mud and shells. Anchor half-way up the loch in 4–6m, beyond which shoals rapidly. Subject to swell.
73. Loch Bun Abhainn-eader (Bunaveneader), excellent shelter off whaling station. Anchor clear of fish cages to suit wind direction, mud. Landing can be difficult.
74. West Loch Tarbert. Anchor W of jetty on S side. (There is also a pier on the N side.) No heavy seas, but squalls in S'lies and swell in NW'lies.
75. Traigh Nisabost. Occasional anchorage in sandy bay E of Aird Nisabost in Sound of Taransay. Beach landing can be difficult due to swell.
76. Camas nam Borgh, a sandy bay 2M E of Toe Head. Drying reefs off W shore. Good shelter and holding in S'lies in SW corner of the bay, but beware windshifts to NW or N.

8.15 Mealista Island

(ON muli-staoir-øy – island by the promontory farm).
Also spelt – Mealasta.

OS Maps: 1:50000 Sheet 13 1:25000 Sheet 458
Admiralty Charts: 1:200000 No.2721 1:50000 No.2841

Area: 124ha (306 acres)
Height: 77m (253 ft)

Population: The island has been inhabited but there are no records. In 1861, at the time of the Census, the crew of a fishing boat from Rosehearty near Aberdeen, including a female cook, was living in a tent on Mealista.

Geology: The bedrock is gneiss, some of which contains a reddish quartz.

History: The Celtic saint Catan, who is believed to have lived in the 6th–7th century and to have had a cell on the Eye Peninsula on the east side of Lewis, had a shrine dedicated to him at Mealista in Uig, just north-east of Mealista island. The

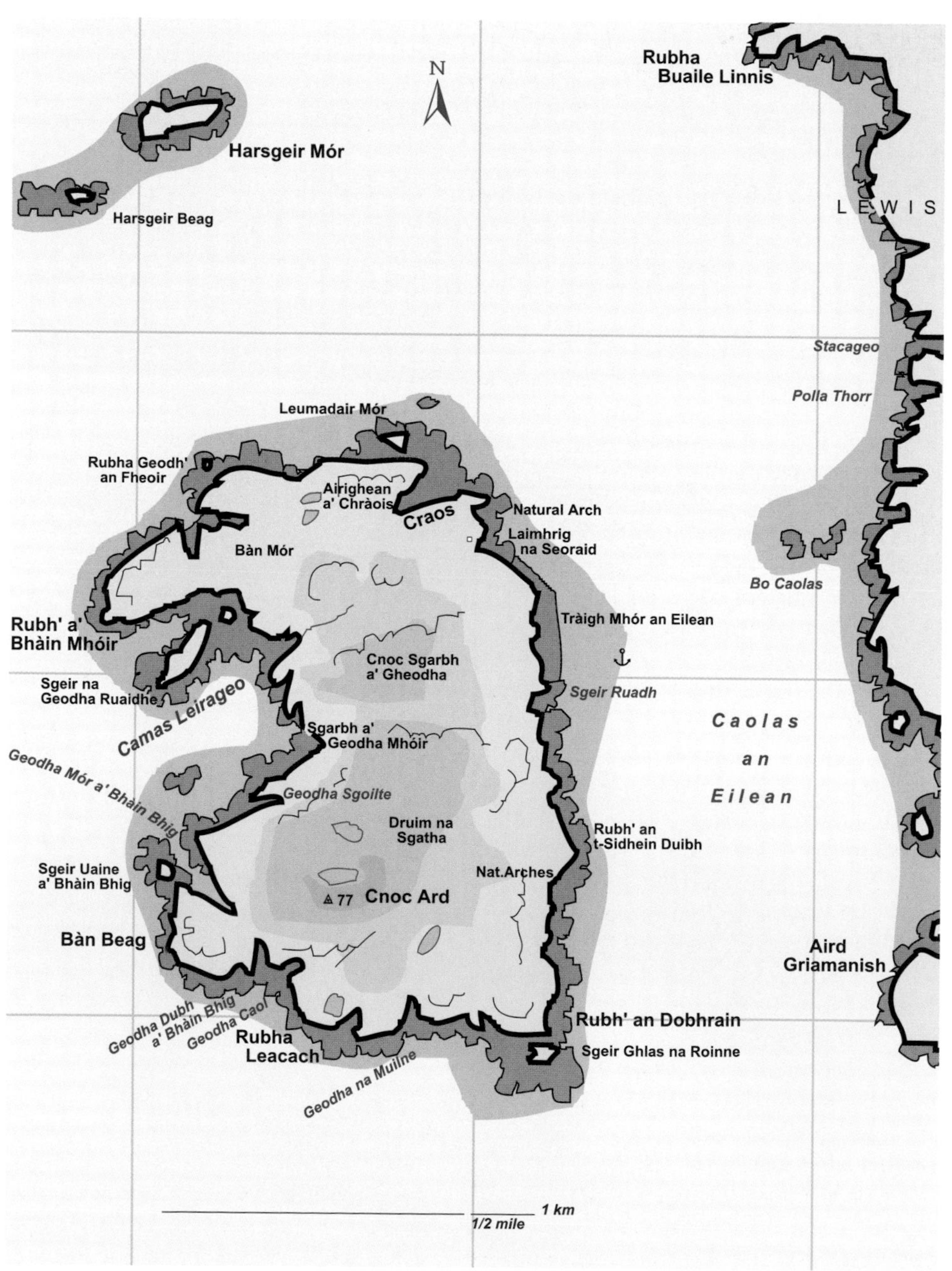

extensive remains of a nunnery – the House of the Old Women in Black – is by the shrine. Knowing the love of isolation of the early Celtic saints, it would be surprising if the island did not feature at some time in the life of St Catan or one of his followers.

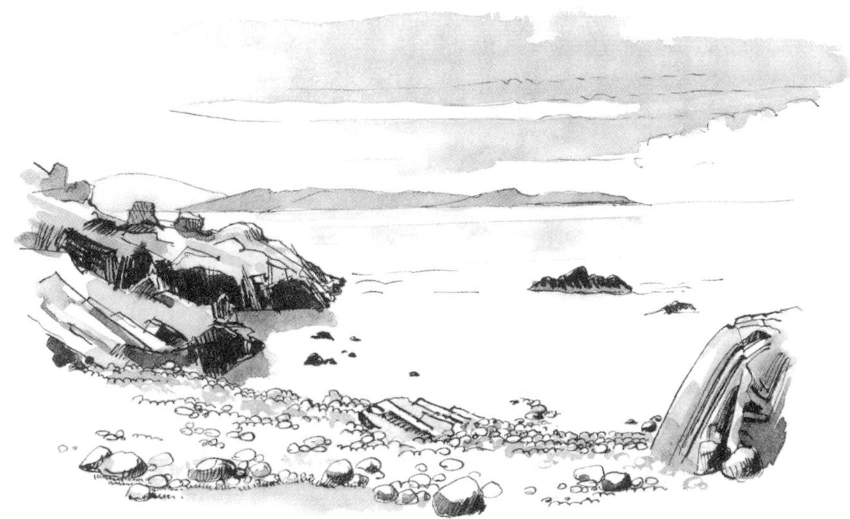

MEALISTA ISLAND FROM THE LEWIS SHORE

Wildlife: Much of the island is covered with grass and grazed by domestic sheep.

* * *

MEALISTA ISLAND is about half a mile off the west coast of Lewis, after the road from Brenish has passed the ancient convent ruins and then disappeared into the confused shoreline where the mountains approach the sea. A clean sandy beach faces on to **Caolas an Eilean** (G. – the island kyle). The island is uncultivated but offers good grazing. The west coast is rocky and unwelcoming.

On the south coast **Sgeir Ghlas na Roinne** (G. – grey rock of the seals) is beside Rubh' an Dobhrain (G. – otter point). The west coast is dominated by a deep bay between rocky headlands called Camas Leirageo (G. – the bay with the obvious cleft). Cnoc Ard (G. – high knoll) is the highest point at 77m. At the northern extremity one can look north from Airighean a' Chràois (G. – shielings by the gaping inlet) to the skerries and scattered rocks near the Lewis coast and see the little island of **Greineim** – 19m high. Another islet, **Eilean Molach**, near the entrance to Uig Bay is hidden from sight by Aird Brenish.

There are some ruined houses on Mealista Island showing that it once supported a small community, but in 1823 the island was incorporated into a sheep farm and, although I have found no record, one could assume that the islanders were encouraged to leave the island at about that time. Certainly there is no record of any population in the 1831 or 1841 census. The small Lewis township of Mealista was itself cleared in 1838 with the majority of the inhabitants being sent to Canada.

Sheep are still grazed on the island and stock is ferried across at Leac na h-Aiseig (G. – ferry ledge) by Rubha Buaile Linnis on the Lewis mainland. This is where the south-going coastal track finally expires. The island collection point is **Laimhrig na Seoraid** (G. – landing place by the primroses).

There was always a desperate need for timber on the islands. Even driftwood was the property of the laird under the old laws and the tacksmen would sometimes ruthlessly enforce this by entering houses and removing driftwood used for roof supports. In 1795 a boat from Mealista was bringing timber back from the Scottish mainland when it ran aground at Bàgh Ciarach in Pairc on the west coast of Lewis. Her crew was murdered for the precious cargo.

It was said at one time that anyone born on Mealista Island would eventually end up as an idiot. Maybe the landlords started the rumour to encourage the islanders to leave.

* * *

Access: No regular access. Boat excursions offered by Seatrek, Uig, Lewis, 01851-672464.

Anchorage:

1. Caolas an Eilean. Temporary anchorage in settled weather, or quiet W'lies, off the central beach on E shore of Mealista, sand. Holding may be unreliable.

8.16 Eilean Kearstay *or* Cearstaidh

Probably (ON garthr-øy – an island with livestock enclosures). Munro called it 'Kertay'. There is another Kearstay north of Scarp.

OS Maps: 1:50000 Sheets 8 or 13 1:25000 Sheet 458
Admiralty Charts: 1:200000 No.2721 1:12500 No.3422

Area: 77ha (190 acres)
Height: 37m (121 ft)

Owner: Sold in 1990 by the laird of Great Bernera, Count Robin Mirrlees to two Australians, Rosemary Nicolson Samois (who has a Lewis family background) and Anne Inglis of Sydney, NSW. Price understood to be £20,000. Since resold to a purchaser who wished to build a house

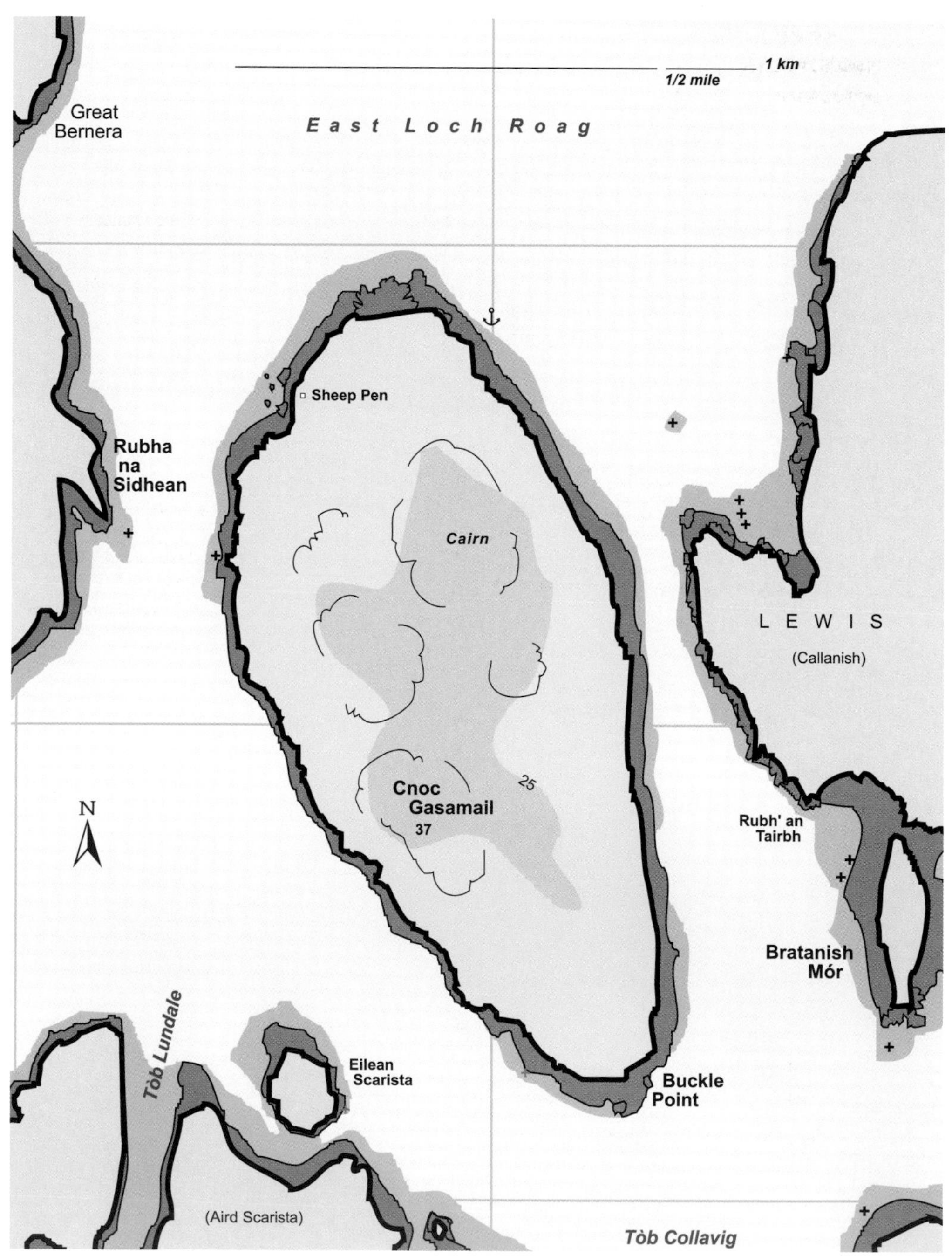

on the island but was refused Council permission in 1994.

Population: No Census records.

Geology: The Admiralty Pilot notes that there is a local magnetic anomaly in this area with the compass needle, unusually, being repelled from the centre of disturbance.

History: A party, attended by many notable Highlanders and Islanders, and the Australian Consul, was held in August 1990 to celebrate the new ownership of the island. An Australian gum tree was planted, supported by Gaelic prayers and classical pipe music. The new owners, who had a shop in Portree on Skye, said they planned to market a specially designed handwoven tweed of local wool which would be called 'Cearstaidh' but by 1993 they had sold the island.

* * *

The seaward approach to **EILEAN KEARSTAY** is southwards through lovely East Loch Roag, between **Vacasay** and **Grèinam** islet and then through Kyles Keava beside the fairly substantial island of **Keava** after which the view of Callanish opens up. There is a narrow channel on each side of Eilean Kearstay, the west one being formed by Rubha na Sidhean (G. – headland of the fairy knoll) projecting from Great Bernera, while the shallow east channel is bounded by the Callanish peninsula.

Eilean Kearstay has few distinctive geographical features but there would seem to be a reasonable chance, in view of its proximity to Callanish, for the discovery of prehistoric associations. The island is smooth and grassy and rises to a low central plateau with a conspicuous cairn at the north end. This is at virtually the same height as **Cnoc Gasamail** (37m) in the south-west, which is the highest point and which overlooks **Eilean Scarista**, an islet tucked into a small bay on the Lewis coastline.

South-east of Eilean Kearstay, Loch Ceann Hulavig shelters **Eilean an Tighe** and **Eilean Trosdam**.

Access: No regular access. Boat excursions offered by Seatrek, Uig, Lewis, 01851-672464.

Anchorage: Temp. anchorage in suitable conditions can be found at several points around the island with the aid of the East Loch Roag chart (No. 3422), e.g. off Rubh' an Tairbh.

1. The nearest overnight anchorage is E of the Bratanish islands, S of Callanish. (*For a visit to Callanish*).

8.17 Vuia Mór

(G bhuidhe, ON -øy, G. mhór – big fair and pleasant island).

OS Maps: 1:50000 Sheet 13 1:25000 Sheet 458
Admiralty Charts: 1:200000 No.2721 1:12500 No.3381

Area: 84ha (208 acres)
Height: 67m (220 ft)

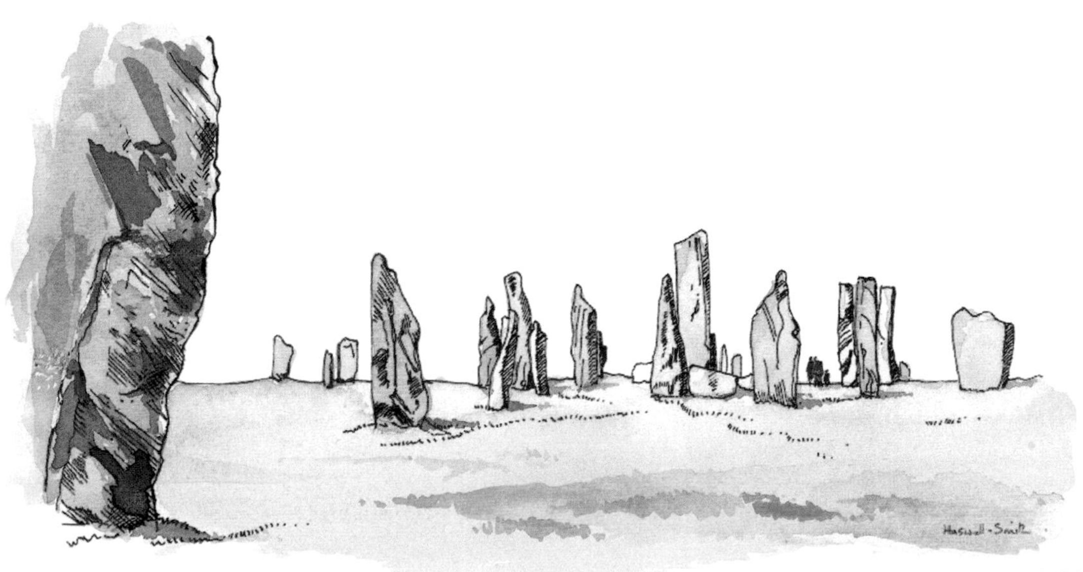

CALLANISH

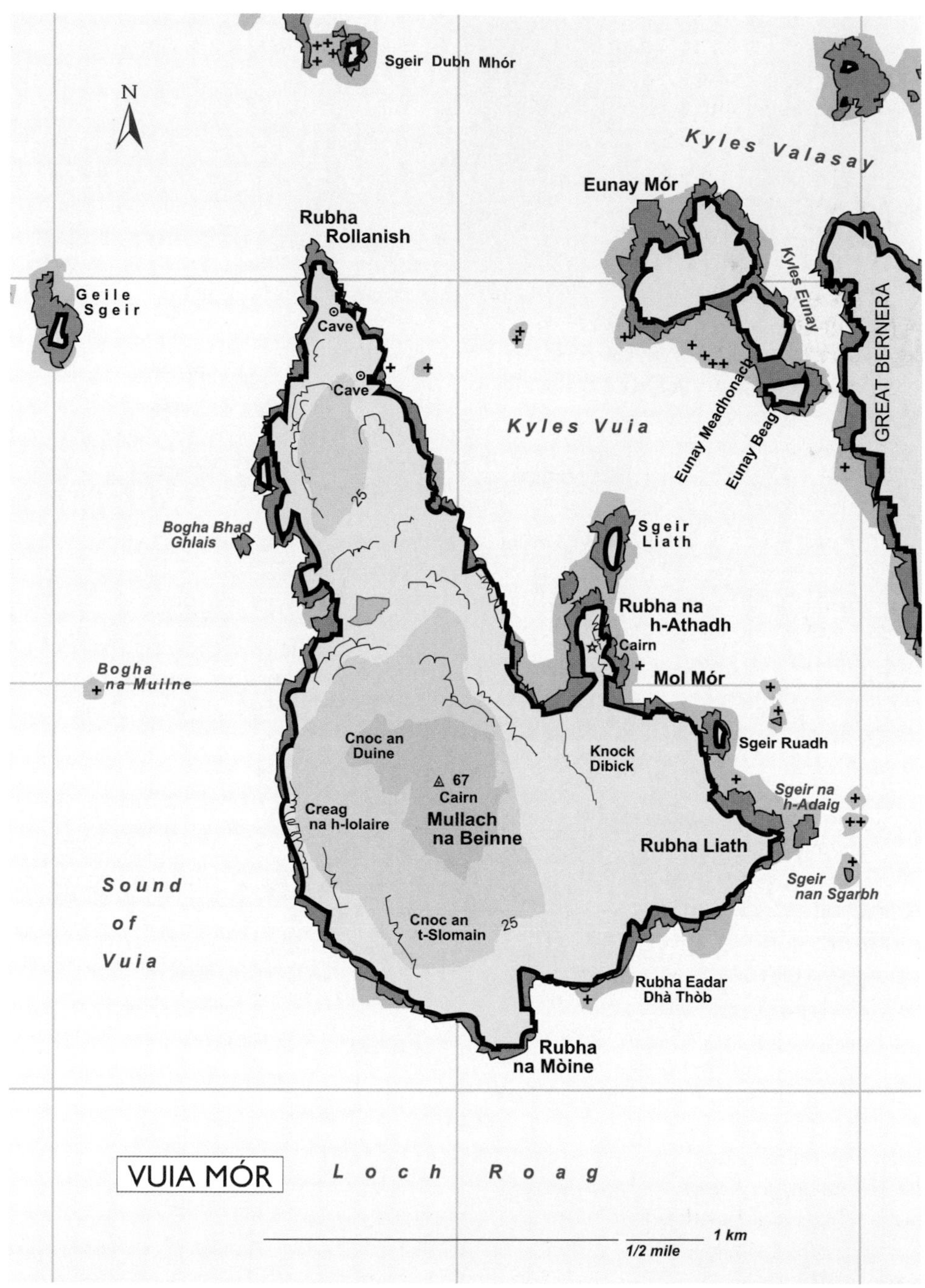

Owner: Uig Crofters Ltd. Part of the Uig (Valtos) grazings.

Population: There were four families in 1807 and in 1841 there were seven houses on the island accommodating forty-six inhabitants. The island was then cleared and there has been no permanent habitation since.

Geology: Mainly Lewisian gneiss.

History: I was told that some of the local people are disinclined to discuss Vuia Mór because of the brutality of the Clearances and that some are even reluctant to land on the island. Others, however, claim that this is a ridiculous notion.

* * *

VUIA MOR is yet another example of an island that once supported a thriving community, was cleared for sheep in the 19th century, and now lies deserted and uncared for. It is almost L-shaped with the northern leg, **Rubha Rollanish**, divided by a shallow valley and rising to a low hill (45m). There are caves in the rocky east coast of this headland. The main part of the island rises to a central hill, **Mullach na Beinne** (G. – top of the hill), with a cairn on the summit (67m). The south-west side of this hill falls abruptly to the sea at **Creag na h-Iolaire** (G. – eagle cliff) and in the words of the Admiralty Pilot this steep cliff '...is very noticeable from the vicinity of **Old Hill** (a remarkable islet about 89.9m high identifying the entrances to East and West Loch Roag)'.

The south coast has three headlands, Rubha na Mòine (G. – mossy headland), Rubha Liath (G. – grey headland) and in the middle, Rubha Eadar Dhà Thòb (G. – the headland between two coves).

Some years ago Mr Norman Buchanan, a nonagenarian resident of Valtos, said he could still remember a neighbour, Mrs Kate Morrison, who was born on Vuia Mór. She died in Valtos in 1908 aged one hundred.

Mr Kenneth Smith, a crofter at Earshader, told me that during the clearances, 'one young married couple were evicted by the Bernera Ground Officer, and they went to Canada. The Ground Officer was later removed from office, and he went to Ontario, Canada, where he died as a tramp. One day he had gone to a certain door to beg for a piece of bread. The lady of the house recognised him at once, but he did not recognise her. She gave him a good piece of bread and never said a word until he had eaten it. She then asked if he was satisfied and he said he was and only then did she tell him that he had evicted her from Vuia Mór'.

There are many small islands in this corner of Loch Roag: **Eilean nam Feannag**, **Linngeam**, **Cliatasay**, **Garbh Eilean** in the entrance to Little Loch Roag, **Vuia Beag** – little sister of Vuia Mór, **Gousam** and **Floday**. Both Vuia Beag and Floday were inhabited until 1827 when they were cleared for sheep and became part of Linshader Farm.

Access: No regular access. Boat excursions offered by Seatrek, Uig, Lewis, 01851-672464.

Anchorages: No recommended anchorage and beware submerged rocks in Kyles Vuia. There is a rough stone jetty of uncertain depth.

1. Occasional anchorage in suitable conditions in N-exposed cove on E side, SSW of Eunay Mór. Anchor in centre of bay, W of the cairn on Rubha na h-Athadh, 4m sand.

2. Temp. anchorage in suitable weather conditions SE of Rubha Liath, the SE extremity, and W of Sgeir nan Sgarbh (dries 1.5m), in 6m.

8.18 Vacsay

(G. Bhacsaidh) (ON vagr-øy – bay island) or (ON bakki-øy – island with a hillock or peat-bank). The present owner tried to change the name to 'Robert Burns Island' although the poet had no historic association with Vacsay.

OS Maps: 1:50000 Sheet 13 1:25000 Sheet 458
Admiralty Charts: 1:200000 No.2721 1:12500 No.3381

Area: 41ha (101 acres)
Height: 34m (112 ft)

Owner: Previously part of the Uig (Valtos) Estate. Sold in 1983 for £9500 to a private buyer but the Uig Estate retained the grazing rights. Resold for £80,000 in 1993 to Sirdar Iqbal Singh, a retired Sikh property dealer from London, now living in Lesmahagow, Strathclyde. Mr Singh purchased the English title 'Lord of Butley Manor' in 1986.

Population: 1861–9. No permanent habitation since then.

Geology: Lewisian gneiss with peaty soil.

History: In 1827 Vacsay became part of Linshader Farm and was partly cleared for sheep.

* * *

VACSAY in West Loch Roag lies off the beautiful white beach of Tràigh na Berie – a popular camping and caravanning spot among the sand dunes.

The island has a very irregular coastline with a confusion of islets and skerries to the north; a small cove between Sionaso and **Liacam** – a drying islet – on the rocky east coast; a larger cove, **Tòb an t-Seann Bhaile** (G. – cove of the old settlement) on the west coast; and a sizeable drying island, **Trathasam**, on the south coast enclosing a shallow pool which forms a natural fish-trap. In between there are a number of irregular hillocks, the highest at 34m in the south-west.

Between Vacsay and the village of Kneep on

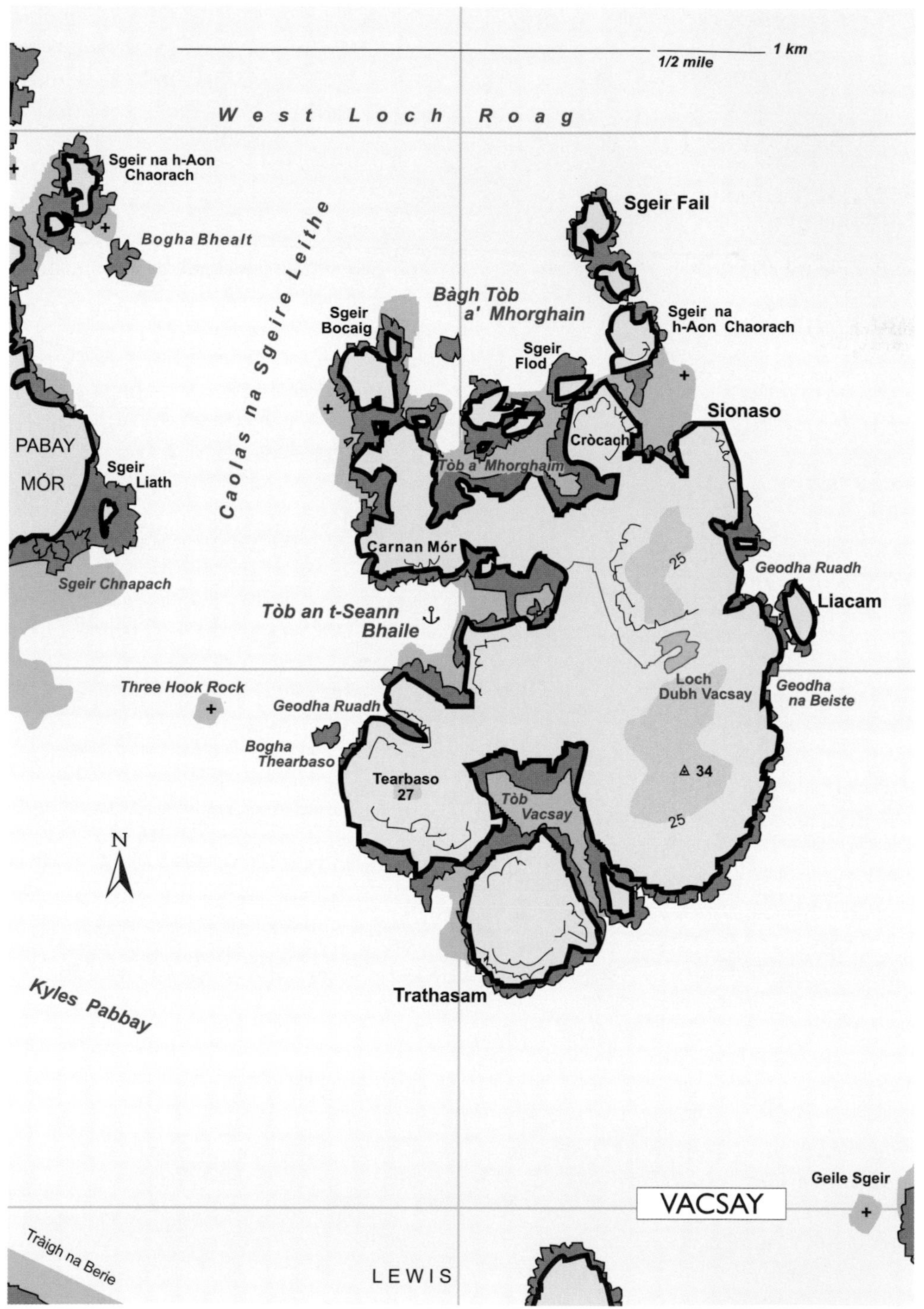

Lewis is the conspicuous islet **Shiaram Mór** and across the loch to the north-east, beside Great Bernera, is another islet, **Grèinam**. Shiaram Mór was bought in 1983 for £11,000 by Mr Sati Gulhati, a London hotelier.

Access: No regular access. Boat excursions offered by Seatrek, Uig, Lewis, 01851-672464.

Anchorage:

1. Occasional anchorage in central bay on W side, 4m, sand. On approach from SW (vicinity of Shiaram Mór) beware Three Hook Rock (covered) and Bogha Thearbaso (dries 1.5m).

8.19 Pabay Mór

(ON pap-øy, G. mór – big island of the priest).

OS Maps: 1:50000 Sheet 13 1:25000 Sheet 458
Admiralty Charts: 1:200000 No.2721 1:12500 No 3381

Area: 101ha (250 acres)
Height: 68m (223 ft)

Owner: Bought for £19000 in 1983 by Mr Hobbs(?), reputed to be either an ornithologist or a surgeon (or both?) and resident in London. He visits Pabay Mór for a month each summer and has restored two of the old black houses. Valtos crofters retain the right to graze sheep on the island as allowed for by the Crofting Act of 1886.

Population: Cleared for sheep in 1827. In 1861 there were two crews totalling fifteen fishermen and two female cooks, all from Banffshire, living

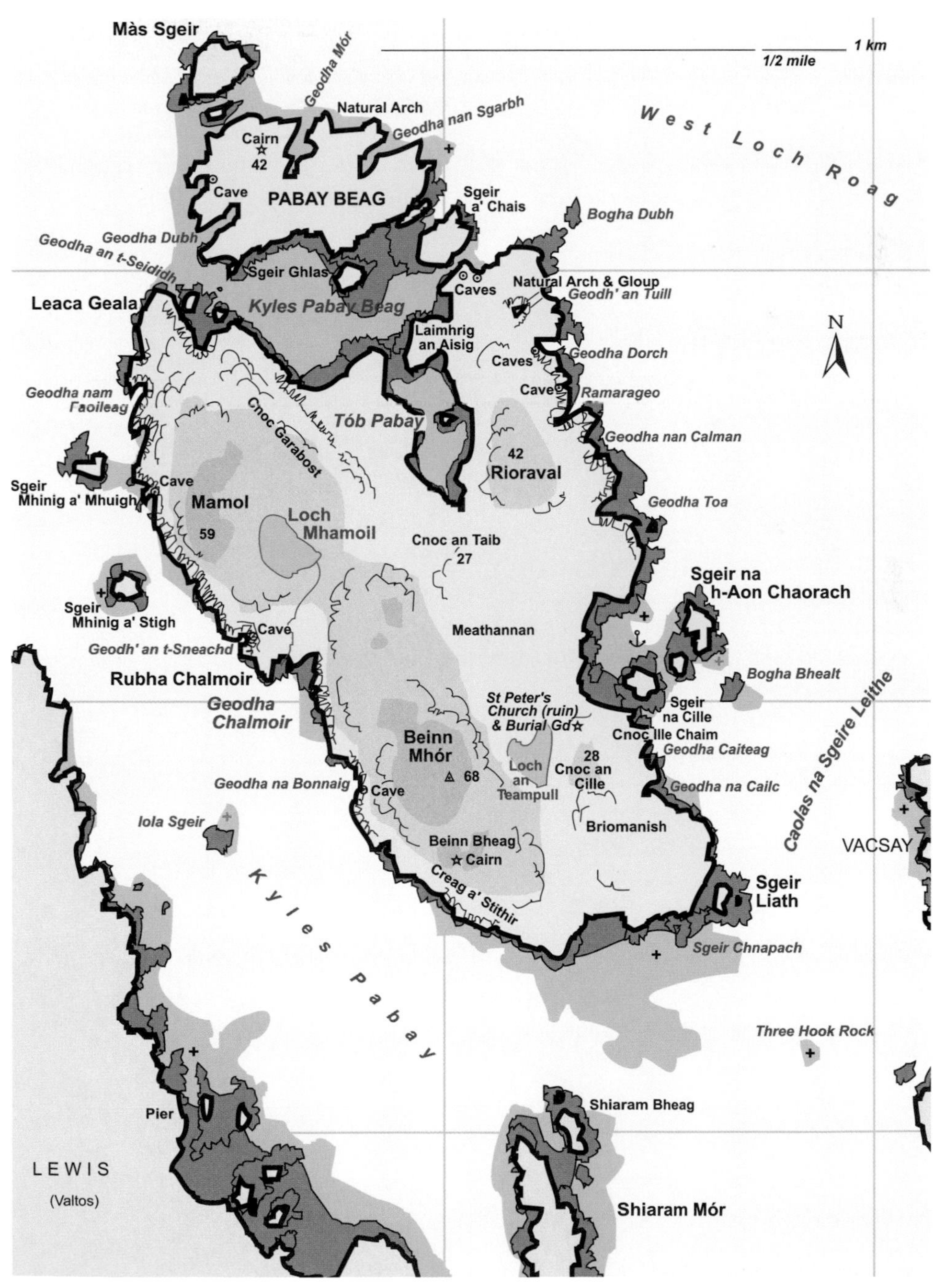

in one of the caves. In 1881 nine Uig men were living in a tent on the island at the time of the Census. Uninhabited since then except for occasional brief visits by fishermen and shepherds.

Geology: Lewisian gneiss with a light soil.

History: Pabay was a MacLeod island and at one time Norman, brother of the last chief, Ruaridh ('Old Rory'), lived there when 'he wald be quyeit, or yet fearit'. But MacLeod power waned and about 1800 the island was given to Sergeant Evander MacIver in lieu of a pension on his retiral from the Seaforth Regiment. The MacIver family settled on the island, but in 1827 or thereabouts they were evicted to provide unimpeded grazing for the sheep of Linshader farm. The family moved to Kneep and their descendants still live in Valtos. Both Valtos and Kneep overlook the Kyles Pabay and Pabay Mór. I was told that when the MacIvers were cleared from the island their youngest child was a little girl aged one. For the rest of her life she was known in Uig as 'Pabay-one-year-old' – 'in the Gaelic, of course'.

* * *

The Lewis coastline opposite **PABAY MOR** has superb shell-sand beaches backed by dunes. The tide runs briskly through the narrow stretch of sea, Kyles Pabay, and in bad weather the surface is broken and dangerous where the Kyle opens out into the Atlantic. But between Pabay Mór and its little brother, **Pabay Beag**, there is a wide and pleasant pool, well sheltered from the weather, which is reputed to have been the haunt of pirates in times long past.

After the First World War some locals claimed that boxes of provisions were found, proving that a German U-boat had visited the island secretly. An even more tenuous claim to fame is that the founder of the Cunard shipping line is thought to have been closely related to the MacIvers of Pabay.

A cairn marks Pabay Beag's highest point (41m) and there is another one near the summit (68m) of **Beinn Mhór** (G. – big hill) on Pabay Mór. East of Beinn Mhór, in a shallow valley beside **Cnoc an Cille** (G. – church knoll), are the ruins of a church and burial ground [NB105377]. A burn runs past the ruin and across a white sandy beach into a sheltered cove. It comes from a heart-shaped lochan, **Loch an Teampull** (G. – temple loch), between Beinn Mhór and Cnoc an Cille. There is another, slightly larger, loch to the north-west, **Loch Mhamoil** (G. – loch by the pap), with its stream discharging into Geodha Chalmoir on the steep-sided west coast.

There are many rocky caverns on Pabay and a natural stone arch in the north-east where the sea sucks and blows through a passage penetrating the hillside before it reaches an inland pool [NB104386]. This is the formation called a 'Gloup' in the Northern Isles.

North of the Pabays is the solitary rock, **Harsgeir**, and a dramatic group of islets and attendant rocky stacks guarding the entrance to Loch Roag, **Bearasay**, **Floday**, and **Old Hill** which rises 90m sheer above the sea like a giant loaf of bread.

* * *

Access: No regular access. Boat excursions offered by Seatrek, Uig, Lewis, 01851-672464.

Anchorages:
1. Tràigh na Cille (Church beach), inlet W of Sgeir na h-Aon Chaorach on E coast. Approach from NNE and keep slightly S of centre of the inlet, 2–3m, sand. *(Church ruins are above the beach)*.
2. The WC Pilot states that the channel between Pabay Mór and Pabay Beag forms an excellent little harbour with depths from 0.4m to 3.2m (the large scale chart shows less depth than this), sand, where boats with local knowledge can lie safely in any weather. Use W entrance after quarter flood owing to rocks that dry. If using the narrow E entrance beware Bogha Dubh.
3. Rubha Caol, S extremity of the island. Occasional anchorage off sandy beach, 3m. Beware Three Hook Rock 2c SE of SE corner and drying rock W of Sgeir Chnapach.
4. S of Tràigh na Cille (S of Sgeir na Cille) giving Bogha Bhealt a wide berth. Anchor off cave in 5m, sand. Some swell at HW.

8.20 Little Bernera

(ON bjarnar-øy – bear island) or possibly (ON – Bjorn's island).

OS Maps: 1:50000 Sheet 13 1:25000 Sheet 458
Admiralty Charts: 1:200000 No.2721 1:12500 No.3381

Area: 138ha (341 acres)
Height: 41m (134 ft)

Owner: Comte Robin de la Lanne Mirrlees has

owned the island since 1962. It was for sale from 1993–96 but has since been withdrawn. He also owns Floday, Kealasay, Old Hill, and Bearasay (See 8.19).

Population: Two inhabitants were recorded in 1807– Neil and Donald Macdonald – (who may have had families) but they later moved to Great Bernera. However by 1831 numbers were sufficient for a school to be established by the Edinburgh Gaelic School Society and nineteen boys, twenty girls, and one adult were enrolled. But in 1832 or 1833 most of the islanders were cleared or 'resettled' at Dun Carloway on the Lewis 'mainland' (including two families called MacAuley) and the school was closed. The last record of any inhabitants was in the 1861 Census.

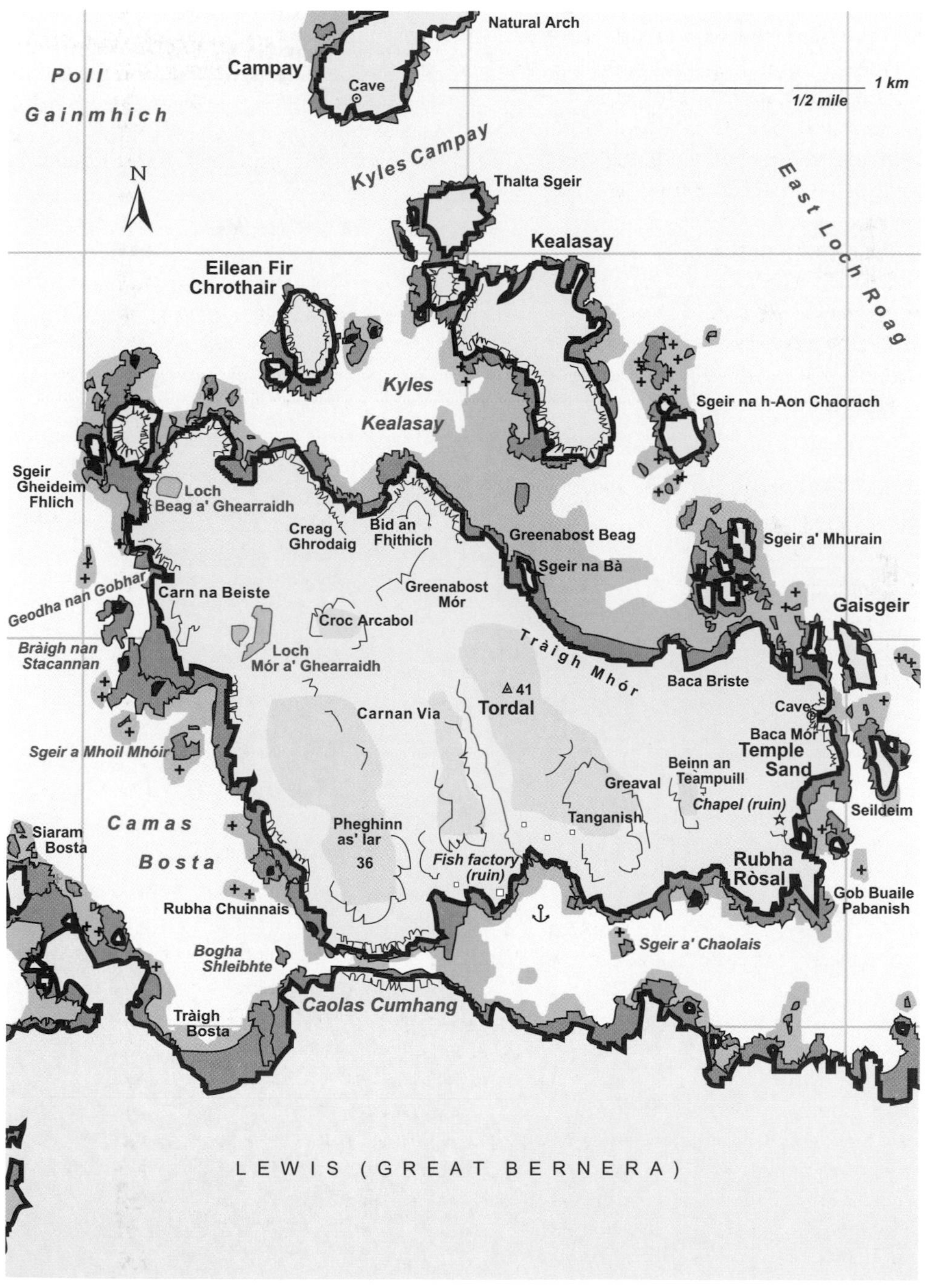

Geology: Lewisian gneiss with a light soil and acidic pockets.

History: Most of the small islands had connections with one or other of the early Celtic saints and in Little Bernera's case it is St Donan who is so honoured. He may have been a Pict and he is noted for his monastic centre on Eigg but the reason for his association with Little Bernera is obscure.

Following the clearance of Little Bernera for sheep-farming, and dissatisfaction with the intolerable demands of Sir James Matheson's factor, crofters on Great Bernera revolted in 1874. It was a relatively minor incident, an altercation with a sheriff officer, but it became known as the Bernera Riot and aroused public sympathy.

Wildlife: Cattle of the Scaliscro estate on Lewis have grazed the island for twenty-five years. A rogue bullock took charge in 1992 and for two years the cattle refused to be rounded up and ran wild.

* * *

LITTLE BERNERA lies immediately north of Great Bernera in Loch Roag on the north-west coast of Lewis. According to that intrepid 16th-century traveller Dean Munro, it was full of rough little craigs with fertile earth between. That description still applies today except that after a century of rough grazing the earth is probably no longer as fertile or 'manurit' as it once was. When Bernera Beag was populated and productive, apart from good pasturage for sheep and black cattle, it had a yield of 200 bolls of barley a year, which is approximately forty-two tonnes.

The ruins, no longer clearly visible, of an old fish-curing building overlook the Kyles of Little Bernera. At its west end the channel becomes very narrow at **Caolas Cumhang** (G. – constricted strait) before reaching the wide, rock-fringed Camas Bosta.

Tordal is Little Bernera's highest hill (41m) but only fractionally so as there are a number of such 'little craigs', all of nearly similar height. Beneath Tordal on the north coast is the beautiful wide sweep of shell-pink sand, **Tràigh Mhór** (G. – big beach). This borders a lagoon, Kyles Kealasay, where the deep blue sea on a sunny day has a touch of South Sea magic, provided one avoids putting a foot in the water! Opposite are **Eilean Fir Crothair** (G. – isle of the shepherd) and **Kealasay**, both surrounded by low cliffs, and **Sgeir na h-Aon Chaorach** (G. – lone sheep rock). Further north and exposed to the full brunt of the Atlantic gales is **Campay**, another steep, rocky, islet with a natural stone arch at its north end and a large sea cave in the south. Màs Sgeir (G. – seagull skerry) is about a mile further north.

East of Tràigh Mhór, by a small bay among the skerries off Little Bernera's east coast is the ruin of **St Donan's chapel**.

Bearasay, the small rocky island to the north-west, was the retreat of Neil MacLeod, the great Lewis patriot, in the 16th century. He assisted in the defeat of the Fife Adventurers – the merchants who were offered Lewis by James VI and who tried to take over the herring fishing industry. James VI had a prejudice against the Gaels and wanted them to be exterminated and replaced by Lowlanders. In his words: 'As for the Highlanders, I shortly comprehend them all in two sorts of people: the one that dwelleth in our mainland that are barbarous, and yet mixed with some show of civility: the other that dwelleth in the Isles and are all utterly barbarous.'

Neil, and forty companions, stayed on Bearasay for three years and defied the attempts of the Mackenzies, who supported the King, to capture him. On one occasion he intercepted a pirate ship, the *Priam*, with a very valuable stolen cargo including silver and jewels and delivered both it and the skipper to the Crown in the hope of obtaining a pardon. He received a pardon but it was worthless for on leaving Bearasay he was captured by a fellow clansman and handed over to the authorities. He was put on trial, found guilty of piracy, and executed in 1613. He died, according to the official report sent to the King, 'verie Christianlie'.

* * *

Access: No regular access. Boat excursions offered by Seatrek, Uig, Lewis, 01851-672464.

Anchorage:

1. Bernera Harbour (Kyles of Little Bernera) between Little and Great Bernera. Approach from E with care following sailing instructions. Anchor WNW of Sgeir a' Chaolais where possible, 4m, mud. Safe anchorage, but may be obstructed by fish cages. Alternative E of Sgeir a' Chaolais in 5–8m, sand. Good holding, no swell.

SECTION 9

The Atlantic Outliers

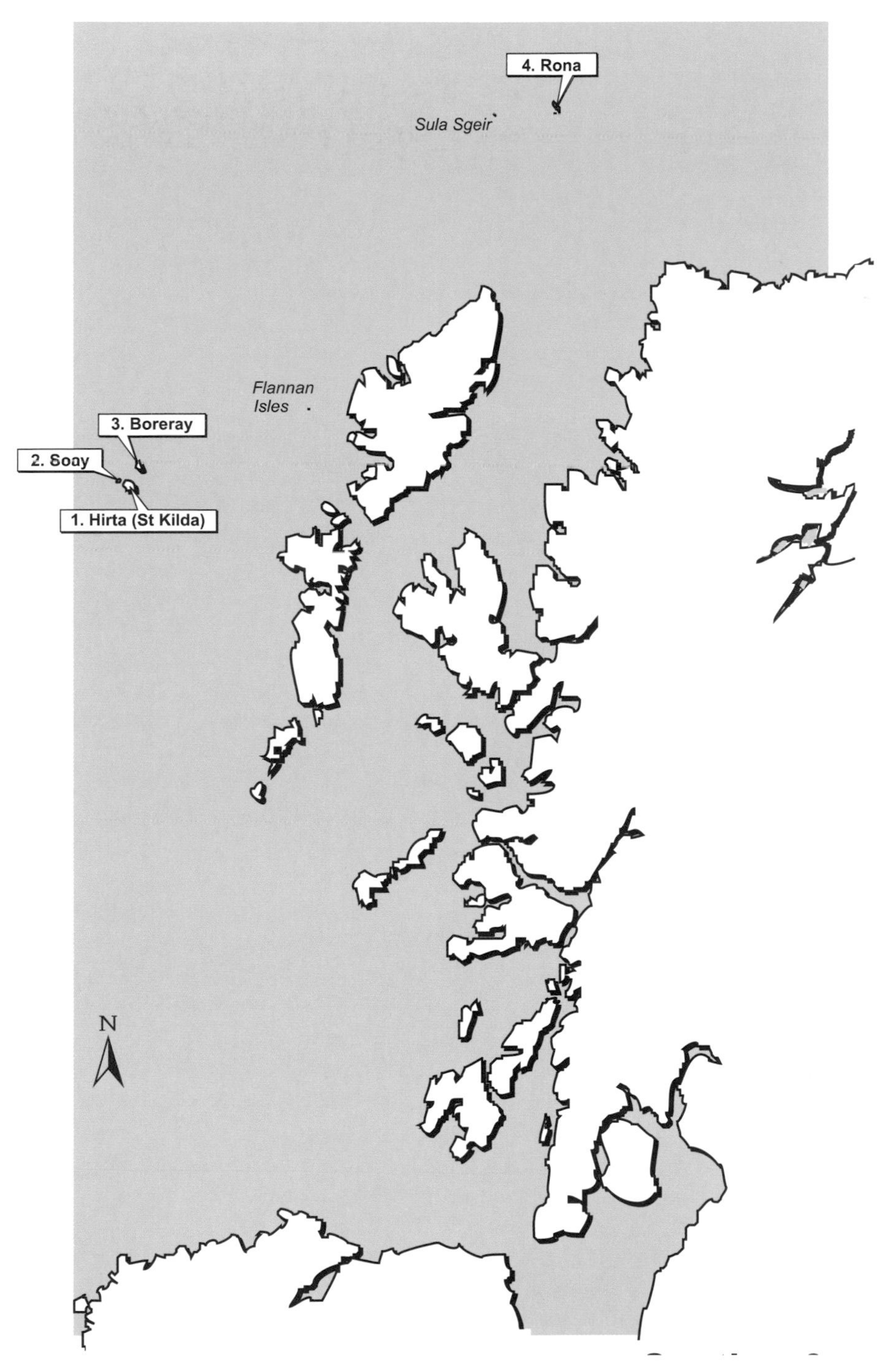

SECTION 9, Table 1: Arranged according to geographical position

No.	Name	Latitude	Longitude	Table 2* No.	Table 3** No.	Area in Acres	Area in Hectares
9.1	Hirta (St Kilda)	57° 49N	08° 35W	50	12	1656	670
9.2	Soay	57° 50N	08° 38W	112	18	245	99
9.3	Boreray	57° 52N	08° 29W	124	16	190	77
9.4	Rona (North Rona)	59° 07N	05° 50W	107	61	269	109
9.A	*Eilean Mór (Flannen Isles)*	*58° 17N*	*07° 35W*			*43*	*17*

*Table 2: The islands arranged in order of magnitude
**Table 3: The islands arranged in order of height

Introduction

In the desert wastes of the North Atlantic a rock stack or a mountain-top breaks the surface. These specks of land represent the outermost regions of the British Isles and at times they are virtually inaccessible. Modern navigational aids locate them with ease but the weather can be so atrocious that landing is often impossible. Yet long ago prehistoric man arrived in his flimsy craft, settled and maintained some sort of intermittent communication with the mainland.

The St Kilda archipelago is the largest island group in this section. It has a mystique all its own and I shall never forget our pleasure when *Jandara* first made landfall there.

The group was declared a National Nature Reserve on the 4 April 1957. It was also designated as both a National Scenic Area and an Ancient Monument by the Secretary of State for Scotland and it is, furthermore, recognised as a Reserve by UNESCO and listed by the International Union for the Conservation of Nature as a World Heritage Site. It deserves all these accolades and one hopes that no visitor will ever introduce a foreign species, whether a plant or an animal such as the domestic cat. This would wreak devastation in such a fragile environment.

The most outlying outlier of all is, of course, **Rockall,** which was only officially annexed by Britain on 18 September 1955 for security reasons when the Benbecula rocket range was opened. A party from *HMS Vidal* landed by helicopter. The first recorded person to set foot on Rockall was Basil Hall, a lieutenant on the forty-gun frigate, *HMS Endymion* on Sunday 8 September 1811. Hall commented: 'The stone of which this curious peak is composed is a dark-coloured granite, but the top being covered with a coating as white as snow, from having been for ages the resting-place of myriads of sea-fowl, it is constantly mistaken for a vessel under sail'.

In 1831, after attaining the rank of Captain, Hall wrote a book called *Fragments of Voyages and Travels,* which is an illuminating record of life in the Navy at that time. Further landings took place, one possibly in 1887–8, and another in 1921. In 1955 it was merely incidental that geologists were talking of the possibility of oil reserves under the Atlantic but the addition of national fishing grounds was recognised. The Union Flag was hoisted on the rock and it was decreed that Rockall should be subject to the law of Scotland and form part of the district of Harris. A navigation beacon was added in 1972. Rockall and neighbouring Hasselwood Rock (57° 36N 13° 41W) are 230 miles west of Manish Point on North Uist so this action effectively made Scotland the same size as England!

The original Gaelic name for Rockall is Sgeir Rocail [rokawl] which could be translated as the sea-rock or skerry which roars hoarsely. No one else worried too much about ownership of this nasty little 21.4m-high obstruction until the possibility of discovering oil became more likely, whereupon the Irish Republic, Iceland and Denmark all laid claim to it. So in the 1980s John Ridgeway, British adventurer and Atlantic rower, volunteered to confirm British ownership by actually living on the rock. He did so by the remarkable feat of lying for the best part of a month in a tiny shelter bolted down on a narrow ledge which is known as Hall's ledge in honour of the first man to land there.

Somewhat nearer home – eight miles west of the Sound of Harris (57° 42N 07° 42W) are two islets – **Great Haskeir** (Haisgeir Mhor), on which there is a lighthouse built in 1997 at the highest point (37.5m), and **Haskeir Eagach** (ON – wild or deep-sea skerry, G. *eagach* – notched) which is about half a mile to the south-west. Their bold geometric silhouettes have an almost classical quality when seen through a pale sunlit summer mist – as though Jason and the Argonauts had just passed by. The main island is studded with vertical rock formations, a high cliff (Castle Cliff) on the north side and several natural rock arches. There is no anchorage or shelter and, if attempting to land, it is difficult to find a purchase on the slippery slabs. The remains of a bothy may have originally been a shelter for fishermen built by the Monach islanders. There is no grass and only a few plants such as sea-pinks, -campion, -plantain and orache bravely survive the continual salt spray. The smaller islet, Haskeir Eagach, is a colonnade of five stumpy rock stacks like the silhouette of a crude Greek temple.

North (59° 06N 06° 08W), in the direction of the Faeroes, the cries of the birds on **Sula Sgeir** (ON – gannet skerry) are carried for long distances by the wind. The Butt of Lewis is forty-one miles south of here and the men of Lewis still traditionally collect their supplies of *guga*, or young gannet, from these rocks every year. It is said that St Ronan's sister, Brianuil, lived with him on Rona until one day Ronan admired her beautiful legs. 'It's time to leave,' she said. She went to Sula Sgeir and died there after several years of solitude.

Rona (No.9.4) with its ancient history lies due east of Sula Sgeir and far beyond Rona are **Sule Stack** (59° 02N 04° 30W), also known as Stack Skerry, a single rock column sticking unexpectedly out of the sea to a height of 37m, and **Sule Skerry** (59° 05N 04° 24W) which is four miles further on and thirty-seven miles from Mainland Orkney. Sule Skerry (ON – lone skerry) is identified by its lighthouse. Both Sule Stack and Sule Skerry are part of Orkney district.

9.1 Hirta

(G. Hiort) Possibly (EI hirt – dangerous, deathlike, ON -øy – island).

St Kilda

The name for the archipelago rather than the island – first appears on a Dutch map of 1666. There was no saint of that name but the derivation may be (ON sunt kelda – sweet wellwater) or that Dutch sailors assumed the popular watering hole above the village, Tobar Childa (G. tobar – well, ON kelda – well) followed the normal practice of dedication to a saint.

Dun

[doon] (G. – castle or fort).

OS Maps: 1:50000 Sheet 18 1:25000 Sheet 460
Admiralty Charts: 1:500000 No.2635 1:200000 No.2721
various scales No.2524 – the outliers

Area: 670ha (1656 acres)
Height: 430m (1410 ft)

Owner: Donated in 1956 to the National Trust for Scotland by the fifth Marquess of Bute. Partly under control of the Ministry of Defence. The nature reserve is managed by Scottish Natural Heritage.

Population: Continuous habitation for at least 2000 years until evacuation in 1930. 1695 – about 180. 1834 – 93 (21 houses). As demand for the island's 'exports' declined (fulmar oil for lamps, feathers, tweed), some of the men had to find work on the mainland. Thirty-six islanders emigrated to Australia in 1852 with State aid. Men were also lost at sea and in accidents on the cliffs, and there was severe infant mortality due to *Tetanus infantus*. 1861–78. 1881–77. 1891–71 (18 houses). 1911–80 (18 houses). 1921–73. 1930–36. 1931–0. 1961–65 (military establishment) 1971–65. 1981–46. 1991–0.

Geology: Hirta is almost entirely composed of two igneous rocks, a light-coloured granite or granophyre and a darker gabbro. The east part of the island is chiefly granite but interspersed with some gabbro. Some of the rock is highly magnetic. The coastline is honeycombed with caves and the sharp jagged skylines are because the ice during the Ice Age failed to reach the St Kilda archipelago and the rocks are unworn.

When marine scientists conducted an underwater survey of the whole archipelago in 2000 they found that the separate islands were peaks of a single large mountain. About 18,000 years ago the sea level was approximately 120 metres lower than now and there is clear evidence of the ancient shoreline.

History: In a study of Hirta on behalf of the National Trust for Scotland an ancient stone building was discovered near the top of a high cliff. The structure, possibly a place of worship or a tomb, is thought to date from the Bronze Age. Archaeologists have still to make a detailed

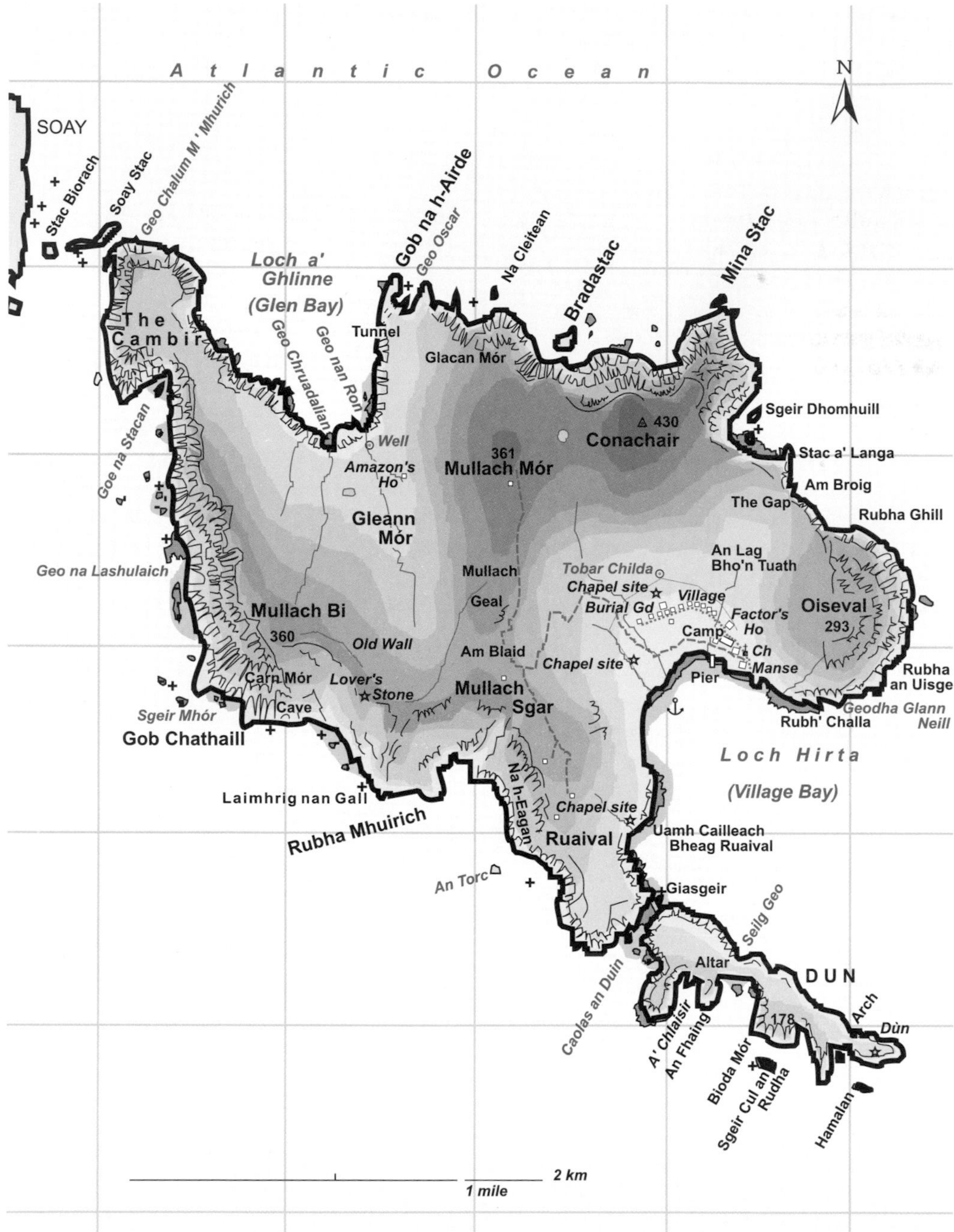

investigation but this may show that Hirta has been inhabited for about 3500 years.

Glen Bay is the site of a pre-Viking settlement but it was not until Dean Monro visited Hirta in 1549 that the first written record appeared. He described a 'simple, poor people, scarce learnit in aney religion'.

Martin Martin, during his visit in 1697 estimated that 180 St Kildans ate about 22,600 birds annually. Stac Lee alone provided about 6000 gannets a year. Rye grass and barley were cut green and stored in the 'cleitean'. Martin found the population – 'happier than the generality of mankind, as being the almost only people in the world who feel the swetness of true liberty'.

One separate dwelling or cleit, south of the main 'street' is known as Lady Grange's house.

She was exiled on the island for eight years to prevent her revealing her husband's Jacobite sympathies. She died in 1745, the year of the Rebellion, and is buried on Skye. (See Section 5–Appendix and No.7.20.)

In the early 18th century there were outbreaks of cholera and smallpox introduced by visiting ships and after 1750 the population possibly never exceeded 70. The islanders paid rent to the owners, the MacLeods of Harris and Dunvegan in Skye, who had been given the islands by a descendant of the Lord of the Isles. The rent was paid in the form of produce such as tweed, wool, feathers or oil from the sea-birds and once a year a steward called from Harris to collect the goods. At this time visitors reported a surprising level of general prosperity among the islanders although they held everything in common ownership and had no personal property. They also had no leadership structure. A 'Parliament' would meet each day to decide what work had to be done. This was by general agreement, but there were occasions when it could take all day to reach a decision!

The *Glenalbyn* was the first tourist ship to call at the island in 1834 and it marked the start of the loss of the islanders' independence and the end of St Kilda. They were almost completely naive and were cheated out of many of their essential possessions by the tourists. They came to rely on modern communications and a post-office was opened on the island in 1899 but this was really to satisfy tourists.

The other vital contribution to the eventual collapse of society on the island was the hell-fire and damnation of crusading Christian ministers. By far the most notorious was the Rev John Mackay who was resident from 1865 to 1889. By the end of his evil ministry the islanders had been browbeaten into so much church attendance every day of the week that there was insufficient time for growing and gathering food.

Apart from imported diseases the islanders were healthy except for 'eight-day sickness' which was 'God's will' and killed 80% of the babies born. In the 1890s it was discovered that the source of the disease was tetanus, now thought to come from the midwife's dirty hands when traditionally anointing the umbilicus with fulmar oil. The new minister, unlike his predecessor, studied midwifery in Glasgow in order to persuade the islanders that God disapproved of this practice.

Because the community was near starvation in 1912, a wireless transmitter was installed by

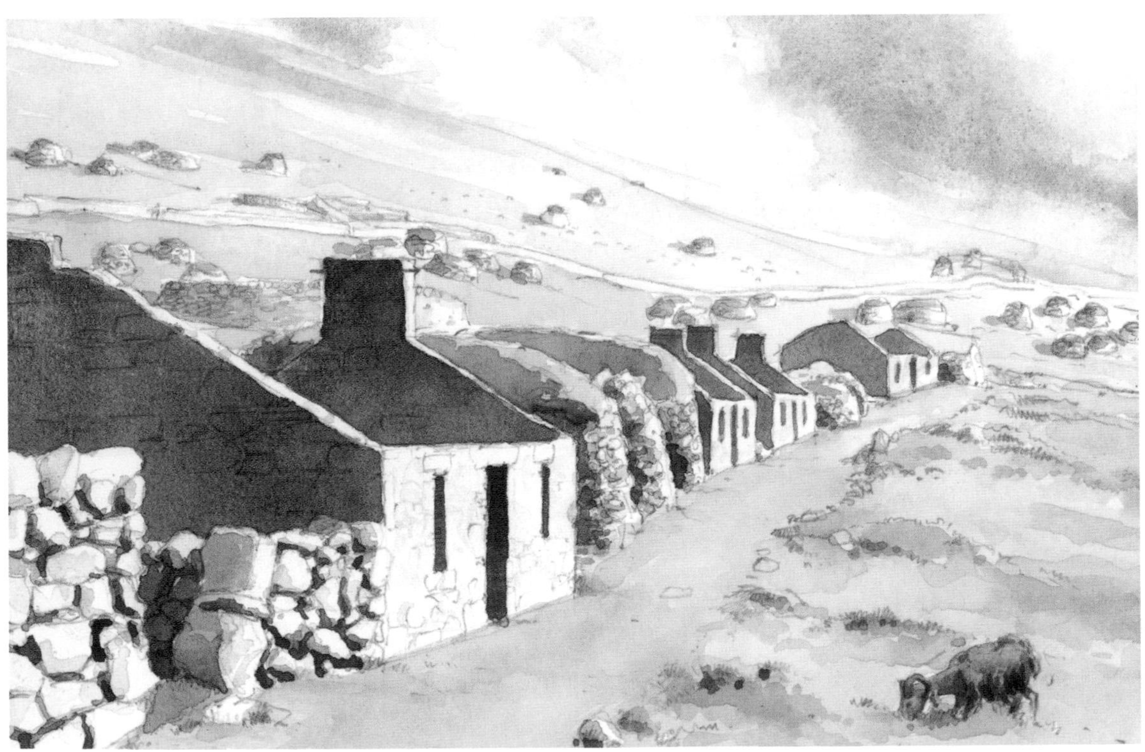

HIRTA'S 'HIGH STREET'

the Government. During the First World War this resulted in a German submarine shelling the island. The church was damaged and a store destroyed but no one was hurt and the submarine was later captured by an armed trawler. A gun was installed south-east of the army camp to stop a repetition of this incident but it has never been fired.

After the war, conditions continued to deteriorate. Many of the active young men emigrated leaving the aged and the very young. Eventually matters became so desperate that the thirty-six remaining St Kildans were more-or-less compelled to agree to evacuation. They were persuaded to do so by Nurse Williamina Barclay who, in 1927, had been sent to assist them.

The sad event took place on the 29th of August 1930. The St Kildans were given jobs and housing near Loch Aline, planting trees for the Forestry Commission, but they never really adjusted to life on the mainland. They were industrious and intelligent but they did not appreciate the use of money, the way of life, the type of diet, and they had never seen piped water, a staircase, or for that matter, a tree.

In 1957 Hirta was resettled with a military base and missile-tracking radar station on Mullach Mór which, since 1998, has been manned by civilians. National Trust volunteers are restoring the village houses and those who have spent twenty-four hours on the island can join the exclusive St Kilda club. But the native St Kildans are no more although, sadly, everything that they needed to provide a viable community is now available on the island.

Wildlife: There are no plants which grow above grass level, but even so there is a wealth of species. Scurvy grass, scentless mayweed, moss campion, plantago sward, and common sorrel are widespread. In the wet ground there are common cotton-grass, tormentil, lousewort, St John's wort, field gentian, bog pimpernel and bog asphodel to name a few. On the hillsides there are primrose, roseroot, heath-spotted orchid, calluna, crowberry, butterwort, heath milkwort, sundew, tiny willow, deer grass and ragged robin. On Dùn can be found lesser celandine, wild angelica, sea campion, red fescue and thrift. In all, more than 130 flowering plants have been recorded and 194 varieties of lichen – including some that are very rare – and beneath the sea here lies one of the world's most colourful marine life sites.

Hirta is noted for some unique forms of wildlife: the St Kilda wren, a sub-species; the mouflon sheep recently introduced from neighbouring Soay; and a species of long-tailed fieldmouse which is twice as heavy as the mainland variety, with larger ears and a very long tail. There was also a St Kilda housemouse, *Mus muralis*, but this poor little creature died out when the islanders left.

On Dùn, the St Kilda wren, puffins, and Leach's petrels nest in large numbers, and the cliffs and peaty turf of Hirta are home to eighteen breeding species of seabirds including the oldest and largest colony of fulmar in Britain. Great skuas are a recent arrival.

The Scottish Seabird Centre in North Berwick near Edinburgh has a direct live video link giving the public a close-up view of the St Kilda wildlife.

* * *

HIRTA is the largest of the spectacular ST KILDA group of lonely Atlantic islands, owned by the National Trust of Scotland. This remote outpost of the British Isles is one of the dream destinations of any committed collector or explorer of islands. All the members of the group are of granite and gabbro forming dramatic jagged stacks and towering cliffs. **Conachair**, the

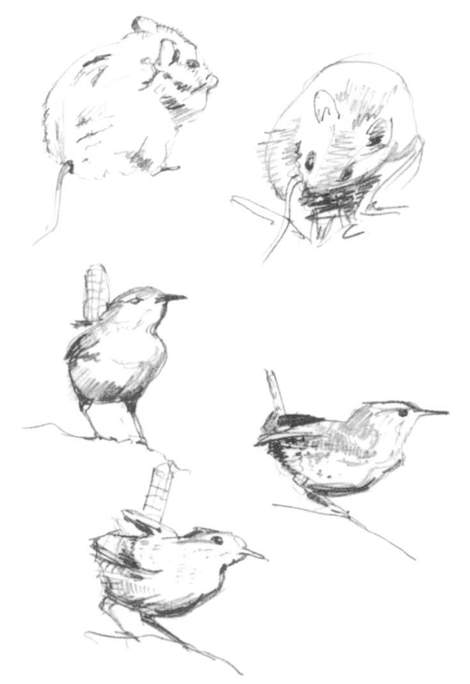

THE ST KILDA FIELD-MOUSE AND THE ST KILDA WREN

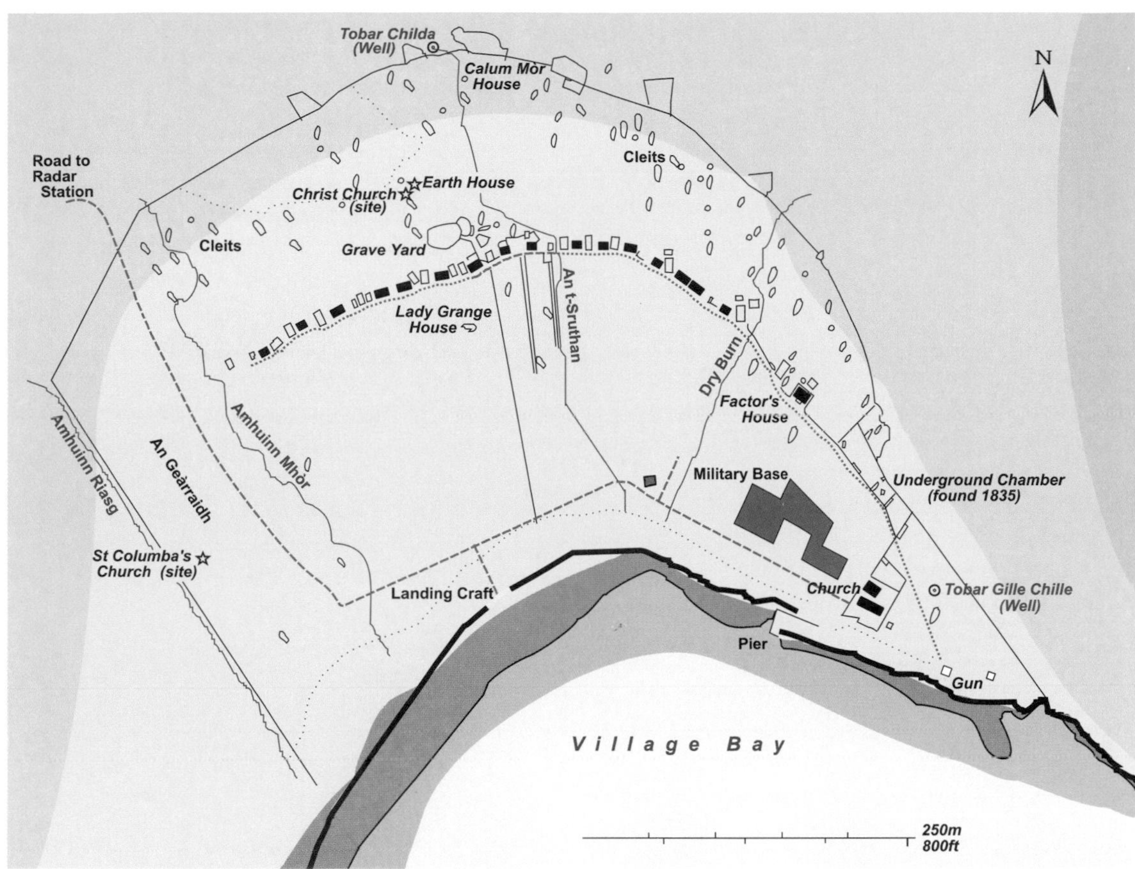

LAYOUT OF THE VILLAGE ON HIRTA

highest peak on Hirta is 430m high (over 1400ft) but there are four other high peaks and the awesome sea-cliffs are over 300m (1000ft) high.

Dean Monro in 1549 wrote that there are '...three grate hills, quhilk are ane pairt of Hirta, quhilk are seen affar off from the fore landis. In this fair ile is fair sheipe, falcon nests and wild fouls biggand, but the streams of the sea are stark, and are verey eivil...'

Village Bay in the south-east shelters the main settlement. Among the cottages and scattered up the mountain side are hundreds of small dry-stone structures with turf roofs called 'cleits' (G. – a stone beehive bothy, water-tight but cross-ventilated). These were mainly used as larders for storing the sea-birds which were the St Kildans' staple diet, but they were also used as general stores for fishing tackle, ropes, etc. Village Bay is an impressive example of a Stone Age culture. The area is covered with dry-stone structures which are the product of centuries of effort.

In 1830 much of the original village was demolished and new black houses were built but most of the present cottages, which are gradually being restored by the National Trust, were built in the 1860s to Victorian standards and using mortar joints. The Army camp is beside the pier and near the church, manse and schoolhouse. It is unsightly, but the island environment is so overpowering that it can be largely disregarded, and the military authorities have in fact been of benefit to the island in many ways. Through the camp and among the village ruins wander primitive Soay sheep, untidily shedding their umber-coloured fleeces in the summer months. The population fluctuations of these evil-eyed, goat-like creatures are being studied with interest by scientists. The native St Kildans only kept domestic sheep on Hirta. They left the Soay sheep on their home territory of Soay (No.9.2).

There are a number of archaeological sites in Village Bay. Less than 40m north-east of **Lady Grange House** [NF101993] stone coffins were discovered in 1835. In the same year an underground chamber was found by the path north of the church. The small stone-walled graveyard is just behind the line of houses [NF100994]. It was too small for the number of burials so older corpses were removed in rotation to make way for new arrivals. Just north of it is the **Earth House**, a souterrain dating from the period 400BC–500AD. A number of artefacts have been found – Hebridean Iron Age pottery, two Christian crosses engraved in stone, Viking brooches and a Viking sword.

Above the village there are fox-holes in the west scree slope which are invisible from below. These were dug by the islanders in case they had to hide from pirates – the great fear of every islander.

Martin mentioned three churches and monkish cells in the 17th century which have now disappeared. One of these, Christ Church, was beside the Earth House, and St Columba's Church was west of Amhuinn Mhór (G. – big river) which is west of the village [NF099991].

At the opposite end of the island is Loch a' Ghlinne or **Glen Bay**. Here there is a ruin called the **Amazon's House** [NA087001] and complexes of small chambers similar to Iron Age settlements. The bay is enclosed by a western peninsula, **The Cambir**, and high cliffs covered with nesting seabirds. On the east side at **Gob na h-Airde** (G. – nose of the point) the sea tumbles through a large deep tunnel which penetrates the rock and frames Boreray beyond [NA088008]. High above, **Mullach Mór** (G. – big top) (361m) broods over the bay with its twin peak **Mullach Bì** (G. – pitch-black top) (360m) on the other side of **Gleann Mór** (G. – big valley). Parts of a Sunderland flying-boat, ML858, are scattered down the glen where it crashed in June 1944. (The gullies below Conachair conceal another wartime wreck – a Beaufighter, LX798). Both crews were lost. The side of Mullach Bì facing the sea is like a cataclysmic land-slip with an abrupt drop from the summit to the sea. Close to the highest point is the **Lover's Stone** [NF085990] where there is a terrifying drop on to the rocks in the surf far below.

St Kilda men were agile climbers and would scale the awesome heights with homemade ropes to collect thousands of sea-birds and their eggs. Fulmars were the most important catch as the body of each bird provides a quarter litre of oil. This oil was used for lamps and also exported. Gannets and fulmars were eaten and puffins were caught for their feathers but nothing was wasted and the entrails were used for manure. Before marriage each suitor had to prove his climbing ability by balancing on one heel right on the edge of the Lover's Stone while holding the other foot with his hands.

These cliffs are only surpassed by Conachair's cliffs on the north-east coast. They are the highest cliffs in the British Isles although Foula's (No.11.6) cliffs are considered more precipitous. Conachair is the highest point of a ridge which runs past Mullach Mór and then curls southwards and descends in two steps, **Mullach Geal** (G. – bright top) and **Mullach Sgar** (G. – the dividing summit). The ridge descends further to **Ruaival**, the south-western arm of Village Bay. **Oiseval** is the opposite arm of the bay.

DUN is almost joined to Hirta at Ruaival but there is a narrow separating channel, **Caolas an Duin**, which is thickly strewn with rocks and reputed to dry during exceptionally low tides. This channel does, however, obstruct invasion by the sheep which roam freely on Hirta with the result that vegetation on Dùn is much more lush. The island is nearly a mile long and looks, with its deeply serrated backbone, like a dragon hanging on to Hirta.

Old maps show the remains of a dun on the headland furthest from Hirta, Gob an Duin (G. – Dùn's beak), but there is little trace of it today [NF109972].

Almost two miles beyond Dùn, the rock ridge which runs through Mullach Sgar, Ruaival and Dùn, and then disappears into the sea, resurfaces at **Levenish**, a lone guano-spattered stack.

* * *

Access: Those wishing to land (or join a work-party) should contact the National Trust, 0131-243-9300. There are a number of cruises to Hirta but weather conditions must be ideal for landing. Try Kilda Cruises, Tarbert, Harris, 01859-502060; Hebridean Whale Cruises, Gairloch, 01445-712458; Seatrek, Uig, Lewis, 01851-672464; or, on a different scale, the NTS' own cruise ship, 0131-243-9334; or *Hebridean Princess*, 01756-704704.

Anchorages:

1. Village Bay is the only relatively safe anchorage but can be untenable in winds NE–S. There is usually a swell. Squalls during gales can be violent. Anchor anywhere off the beach but best in 5–6m off pier below the church. Holding good, firm sand. The concrete pier has steps and

an iron ladder on its W side and a boat slip behind it. The pier is usually accessible but landing can be difficult due to the swell. (In 1993 most of Village Bay beach and part of the landing craft slip was reported to have been swept away in a storm).

2. Loch a' Ghlinne. (G. – glen bay). Temp. anchorage in SE gales. A valley and stream runs SE between the hills at head of bay. Landing possible beside the stream. Bay sheltered except from N, but too deep to anchor except very close to shore. Swell uncomfortable and there are strong winds off the cliffs.

9.2 Soay

[soa-ay] or [soy] (ON so-øy – sheep island).

OS Maps: 1:50000 Sheet 18 1:25000 Sheet 460
Admiralty Charts: 1:500000 No.2635 1:200000 No.2721
various scales No.2524 – the outliers

Area: 99ha (245 acres)
Height: 378m (1240 ft)

Owner: Together with the rest of the St Kilda group, Soay is owned by the National Trust

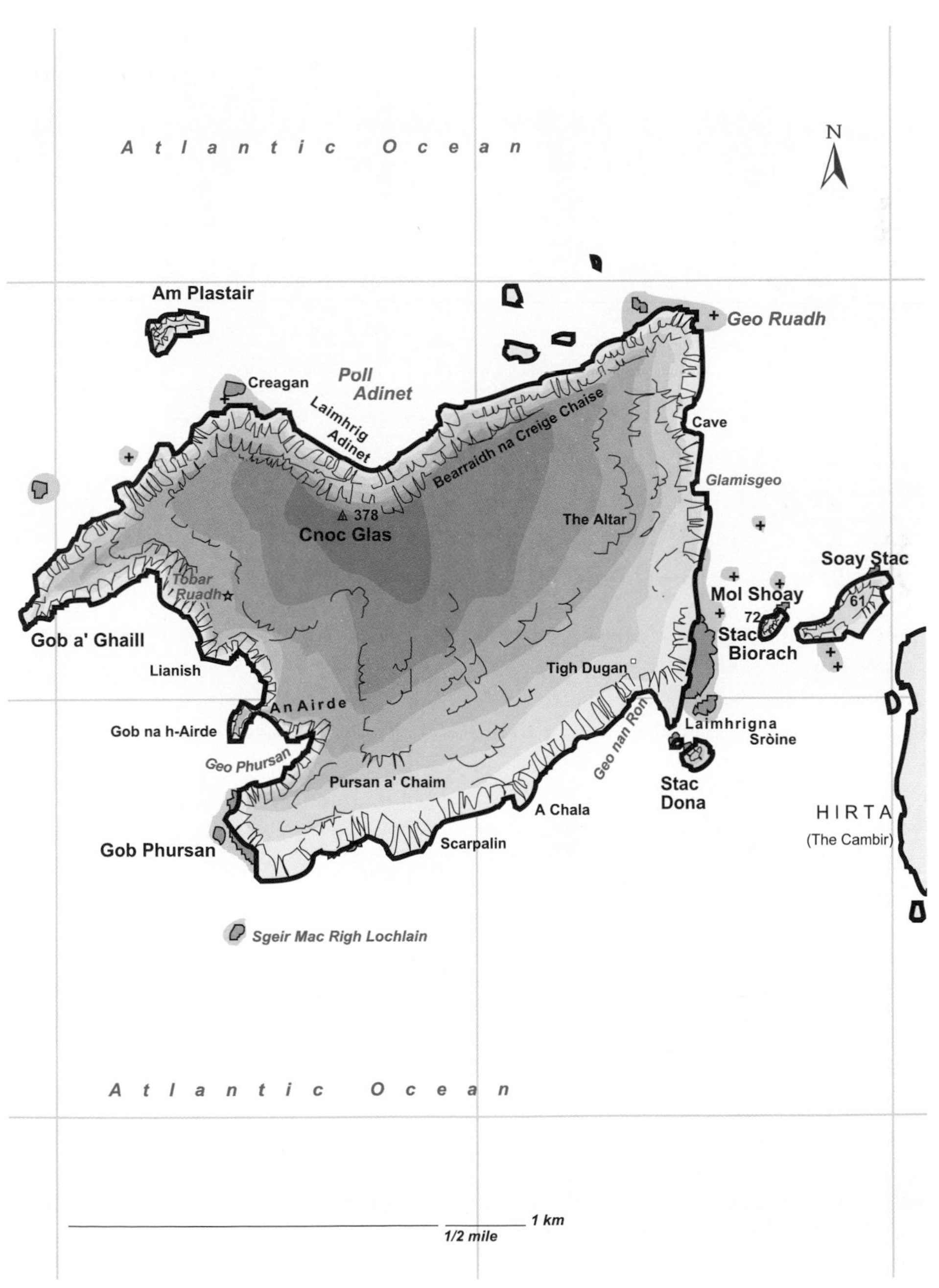

for Scotland and managed by Scottish Natural Heritage as a Nature Reserve.

Population: Uninhabited and has probably never been permanently inhabited.

Geology: Formed by a separate precipitous mountain peak rising straight from the same submarine mountain mass as Hirta it is composed mostly of a dark breccia of gabbros and dolerites, but with some granite. It has escaped any Ice Age erosion.

History: Although the St Kildans held everything in common ownership, the one exception was sheep. These could be personally owned, although there was communal interest in their well-being. Thus the Neolithic sheep on Soay belonged to a few St Kilda families. When these families emigrated to Australia in the 1850s the laird, MacLeod of MacLeod, paid them for their sheep to help defray their expenses.

After Hirta was evacuated in 1930 the Earl of Dumfries arranged for a balanced flock of 107 sheep to be collected from Soay by some St Kildans who had made a summer visit to their old home. The sheep were transported to, and released on, Hirta (No.9.1) and these form the basis of today's sheep population which is being studied by the Soay Sheep Research Team. All the islanders' domestic sheep were removed from Hirta at the time of the evacuation.

Wildlife: Soay is the home of the species of horned sheep, *Ovis aries*, which were first brought to the British Isles about 5000BC. They are like mountain goats in appearance, wild, but unconcerned with man so long as man is unconcerned with them. Until the 1930s the sheep were entirely confined to Soay and were not to be found anywhere else. When conditions permitted the St Kildans would climb the steep slopes of Soay to the lush grazing plateau and sometimes kill a beast for fresh meat. But mutton was considered a rare and special delicacy and the main interest was the wool. Soay sheep are never shorn. The fine soft wool is merely plucked when it is being shed naturally. The St Kildans used it to make tweed.

The soaring cliffs which surround Soay afford nest space for many thousands of gannet, fulmar, storm petrel, Manx shearwater, razorbill, great skua, and Leach's petrel although larger numbers of the latter bird nest on the Cambir on Hirta, opposite Soay Stac. Colonies of puffins inhabit the cliff-tops.

* * *

Ancient **SOAY** has no dinosaurs but it has primeval yellow-eyed sheep as compensation.

The inclined grassy, and boggy, plateau reaches a rounded summit, **Cnoc Glas**, (G. – grey eminence) 378m high where it falls away on the west coast in a nearly vertical black cliff, and it forms a very steep grassy incline to the east coast. The north and south have almost vertical cliffs but the cliff at the south-east end is less precipitous. The only objectional quality in this solid chunk of rock is that it overshadows the north end of Hirta at sunset.

The plateau is cut off abruptly at the Atlantic cliffs like a sliced piece of cheese at **Bearraidh na Creige Chaise** (G. – edge of the rocky precipice). On a level patch beneath a shallow escarpment on the west coast is **Tobar Ruadh** (G. – red well) [NA060015]. No doubt this provided water for the men from Hirta, when they spent some days on Soay wool-gathering. It is however quite a distance from the bothy site, **Tigh Dugan** (G. – Dugan's house), which is on the more sheltered south-eastern slope [NA068013]. To the north, below the **Altar** cliff lie the remains of a Wellington bomber which crashed in tyhe Second World War but was not investigated until 1978.

In the Sound of Soay at the end of rocky **Laimhrigna Sròine** (G. – nose of a landing place) stands a 15m-high rock called **Stac Dona**. There are two more rock stacks in the Sound, the awesome **Stac Biorach** [**peer**ich] and **Soay Stac**. Young St Kilda men were tested for their

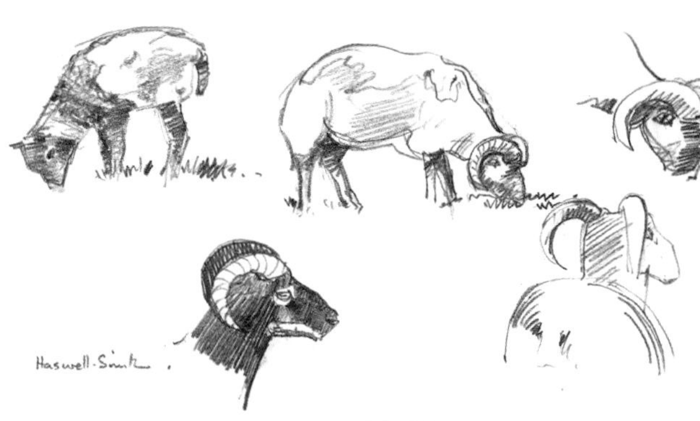

THE NEOLITHIC SHEEP OF SOAY

climbing ability on Stac Biorach (G. – sharply pointed stack) which at 72m (236ft) is certainly not the highest stack in the St Kilda group but is regarded as the most difficult and dangerous to climb. It was nicknamed the 'Thumb Stack' because the only hold on the rock was no bigger than a thumb. An interesting description was written by Sir Robert Murray in 1698: '... after they landed, a man having room for but one of his feet, he must climb up 12 or 16 fathoms high. Then he comes to a place where having but room for his left foot and left hand, he must leap from thence to another place before him, which if hit right the rest of the ascent is easy, and with a small cord which he carries with him he hales up a rope where by all the rest come up. But if he misseth that footstep (as often times they do) he falls into the sea and the (boat's) company takes him in and he sits still until he is a little refreshed and then he tries it again, for everyone there is not able for that sport.' The first recorded outsider to climb both this stack and Stac Lee was Charles Barrington in 1883 (he also made the first ascent of the Eiger).

It is reckoned that only three days in a summer month on average are suitable for landing on Soay and there is always the danger that a rapid change in the weather may leave you marooned.

Sailing through the deep but narrow channel between Soay Stac (61m) and Hirta is possible in good weather.

* * *

Access: Try Kilda Cruises, Tarbert, Harris, 01859-502060 or Seatrek, Uig, Lewis, 01851-672464.

Anchorages: There are no anchorages. The usual landing place at Laimhrigna Sròine near the SE corner, or Mol Shoay, a boulder beach, can only be used in very settled weather due to the swell. The Poll Adinet landing place, Laimhrig Adinet, entails mountaineering. The NTS warden from Hirta should be present during any landing.

9.3 Boreray

[baw-rĕ-ray or -rĕ] (ON borv-øy – fort island or island like a castle).

OS Maps. 1:50000 Sheet 18 1:25000 Sheet 460
Admiralty Charts: 1:500000 No.2635 1:200000 No.2721
various scales No.2524 – the outliers

Area: 77ha (190 acres)
Height: 384m (1260 ft)

Owner: The National Trust for Scotland.

Population: No Census records and uninhabited.

Geology: Boreray is almost entirely gabbro and there has been no Ice Age erosion.

History: Inextricably linked with Hirta and used as another food source by the St Kildans. The traces of lazybeds near the summit ridge may indicate a bygone settlement, but by the end of the 19th century the St Kildans were only visiting Boreray three or four times a year for fowling and tending the sheep.

Wildlife: In spite of its remote position and barren, rocky appearance there are at least 130 types of flowering plant on Boreray including some alpines which probably relish the cool climate and absence of disturbance.

The St Kildans kept some crossed black-face/Cheviot sheep on Boreray which had originally been introduced to Hirta from the mainland. Although the domestic sheep on Hirta were cleared in 1930 Boreray was fairly inaccessible and the sheep were abandoned when the islanders were evacuated. They have now reverted to a wild state.

A count in 1959 showed 45,000 pairs of gannets on Boreray and its two adjoining stacks, nearly half the British population and nearly 40% of the world population. On the relatively level top of Stac Lee alone there was a solid concentration of 6000 nests in 1971.

Many other seabirds also nest on Boreray in great numbers.

* * *

BORERAY is a quite remarkable, jagged heap of black volcanic rock rearing 386m (1260ft) above the sea. It is an unforgettable sight, particularly when the cloud swirls around its summit and the gannets plunge from breathtaking heights. It is an island of superlative emotions that change with the weather. In the words of the yachtsman, R A Smith, who sailed there in *Nyanza* in 1879: 'Had it been a land of demons it could not have appeared more dreadful.' But he probably saw it on a wild, grey day. It lies about 3½ miles to the north-east of Hirta and it has two enormous stacks standing guard beside it, Stac an Armin,

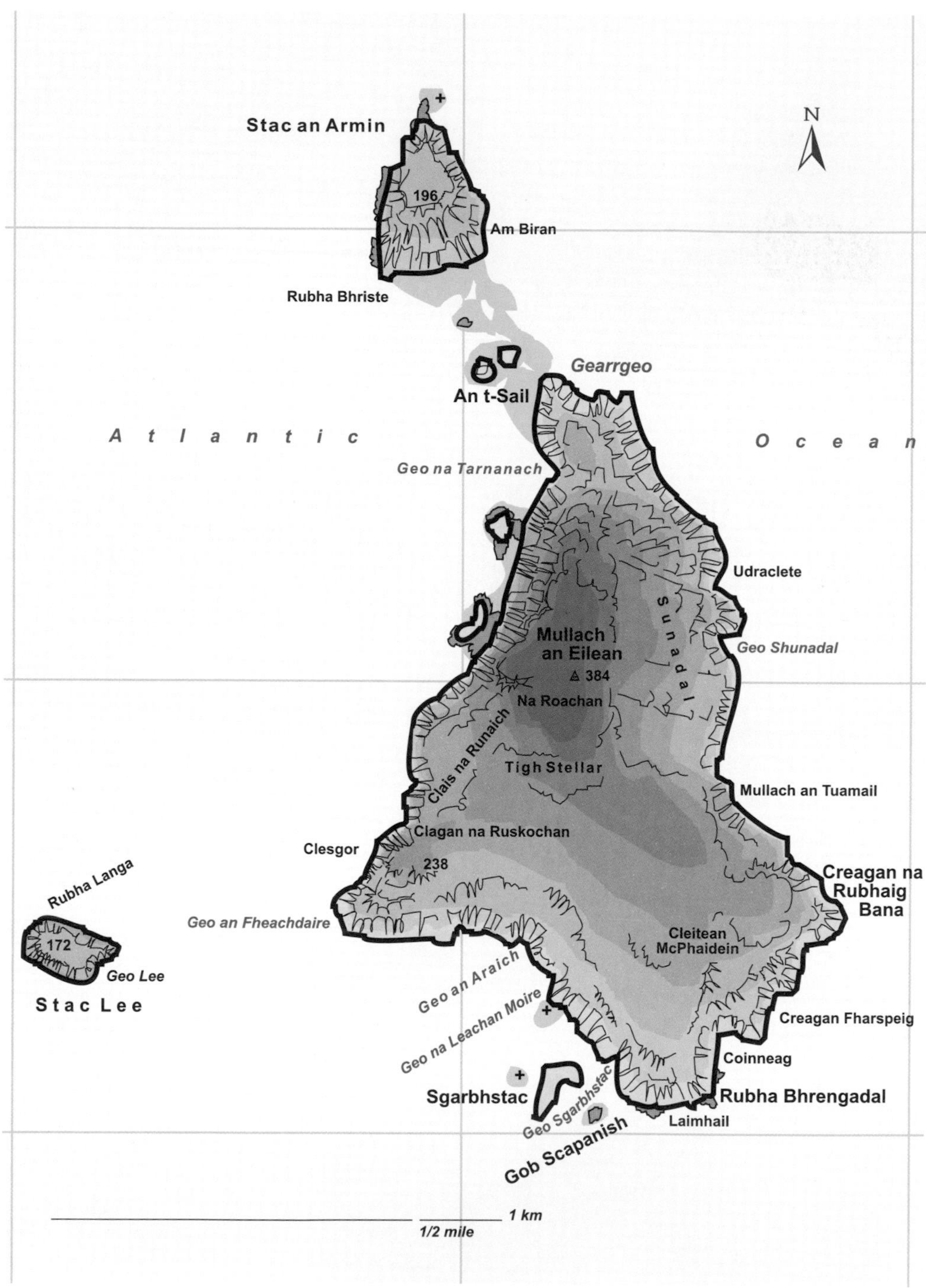

and Stac Lee. It is possible to sail between Boreray and Stac Lee – quite an experience – but the channel between Boreray and Stac an Armin is littered with rocks and should not be attempted.

Landing can be dangerous and considerable skill is required. The mountaineers, Williamson and Boyd, reported that a short distance above where they landed near **Sgarbhstac** (G. – cormorant stack) they came to a chasm in the southern crags. It is nearly two metres wide at the narrowest point and they had to jump across with the sea surging 30m below them.

A party from the University of Durham succeeded in landing on the island in July 1980

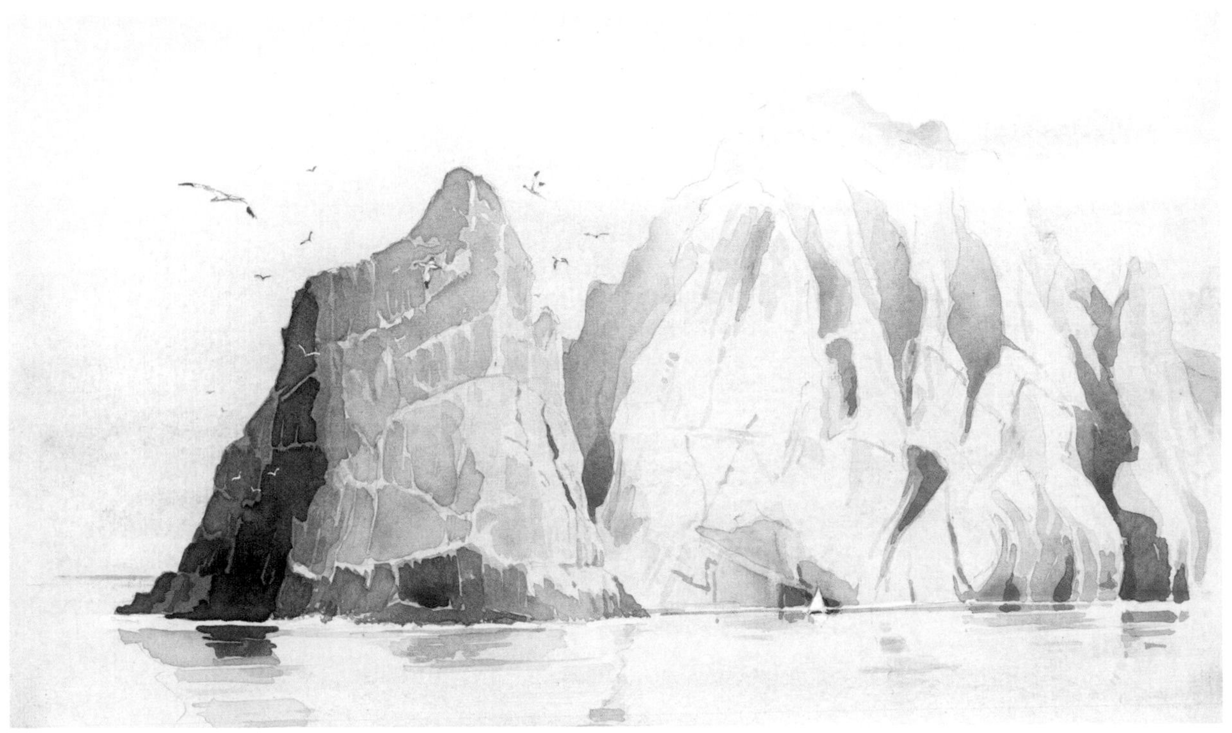

STAC AN ARMIN AND BORERAY

with Army assistance. They stayed on the island for about a fortnight studying the ecology and wildlife. They were helped by the presence of an old bothy which was used by the St Kildans for shelter and which may date from the Iron Age. There may be other undiscovered archaeological remains.

In spite of its exposed situation the skewed summit of Boreray is covered in lush grass. There are still traces of lazybeds and one can only marvel at the thought of carrying loads of seaweed up these high cliffs to manure the potato beds. Understandably, by 1889, sheep had replaced the lazybed culture and the St Kildans only made occasional visits each year.

The most dangerous annual visit took place in September. The gannets, or guga (G. *guga* – a young solan goose, or a fat silly fellow), had to be killed at night when they were on their nests. Normally, about seven men would land, wearing woollen socks at this stage to avoid slipping on the slimy rock. The boat would then stand off with a crew of five and drift around all night. Gannets always post a 'sentry' and this bird had to be killed silently first. Then the sleeping birds were quietly clubbed to death or strangled with fowling rods – which sounds easy until one remembers that the gannet is a big bird, ferocious when disturbed, and the rocky ledges are narrow and treacherous in the dark. Some birds would be gutted and left stored in the cleits on Boreray, but several hundred would be loaded aboard the Hirta boat at daybreak. Despite this annual massacre nature kept an equilibrium. Birds still survive on St Kilda, it is the human beings who have gone.

In April or May the St Kildans visited Boreray to collect eggs and count the sheep. In June they returned to collect the wool. These were not Soay sheep and had to be partly sheared but this was done with a penknife. Dogs were carried up the cliff to help gather the flock. After several days, the men would cut out an area of turf. This could be seen from Hirta and was the signal to send a boat – weather, of course, permitting. In earlier times women accompanied the men and while the men tended the sheep the women would catch and kill puffins.

Stac an Armin (G. or ON – stack of the warrior or steward) at 196m (643ft) is the highest monolith in the British Isles and yet it was regularly climbed by the St Kildans to collect eggs and birds. Sadly, it was on Stac an Armin that the last great auk seen in Britain was killed by two St Kildans who beat it to death in July 1840. They thought it was a witch.

Stac Lee (Martin called it Stac-Ly) is certainly

not in the lee of Boreray so far as the prevailing wind direction is concerned so the name probably derives from the Norse (ON *ly* – shelter) in a more general sense; a small, ancient bothy or shelter sits on top of Stac Lee, dry inside, and able to accommodate two people. When it was climbed by mountaineers in 1969 the south-east corner was considered the best landing point but best is a relative term – even on a calm day the Atlantic swell will move a boat up or down by five metres or more. Apparently the St Kildans lassoed an iron peg when landing. As the boat reached the top of the swell they would jump, find slippery hand and footholds, and start to climb.

* * *

Access: Try Kilda Cruises, Leverburgh, Harris, 01859-502060.

Anchorage: There are no anchorages but there is one place at the south end, close to Sgarbhstac, a rock lying close off the SW side of Boreray, it is possible to land when conditions are unusually calm. Landing on the E side at Sunadal must not be attempted during April–August, the bird breeding season. The NTS warden from Hirta should be present during any landing.

9.4 Rona

Probably (ON hraun-øy – rough island) but, maybe, (G. ròn, N -øy – seal island), or named after St Ronan to whom the island chapel is dedicated.

OS Maps: 1:50000 Sheet 8 1:25000 Sheet 460
Admiralty Charts: 1:200000 No.1954 1:25000 No.2524

Area: 109ha (269 acres)
Height: 108m (354 ft)

Owner: Barvas Estates Ltd

Population: 1796– 1 family. 1841–3 (last inhabitant evacuated in 1844). Uninhabited since, apart from one brief interlude (see below).

Geology: Gneiss and hornblende schist with pegmatite intrusions.

History: Dean Monro comments: 'Towards the north northeist from Lewis, three score myles of sea, lyes and little ile callit Roney, laiche maine land, inhabit and manurit be simple people, scant of ony religione.'

Monro found a people which had continuously inhabited North Rona for at least 700 years. The first inhabitant was supposed to have been St Ronan, who built a hermitage there during the 8th century, but the island may well have been occupied from earlier times. In 1680 Martin recorded the report of the Rev Donald Morison who had visited Rona that there were five families living in their own stone and thatched houses, each with a barn, storehouse, cattle-shed and 'a porch on each side to keep off the rain or snow'. He said they were simple and contented people who took their surname 'from the colour of the sky, rainbow and clouds'. Their only interest in the outside world was in the north part of Lewis which they very occasionally visited. They had no interest in money or wealth, using barter if necessary as they had enough food and raiment for all their needs. They restricted their population to 'thirty souls', by sending their 'supernumerary' people to Lewis.

Martin reported that soon after this came tragedy. Rats from a ship invaded the island and ate all the food. Then some seamen landed and killed the only bull. Within the space of a year 'all that ancient race of people' were dead.

The disaster was discovered by a party from St Kilda (100 miles away!) who were shipwrecked on Rona after being blown there by a storm. They lived for seven months on the island while they built a boat out of driftwood which they then sailed to Stornoway.

The minister of Barvas on Lewis had the island resettled. But by 1796 there was only one family left on Rona, that of a shepherd, as the rest had apparently drowned in a fishing accident. The island was rented by a Ness tacksman for £4 sterling per annum paid to the owner, MacLeod of MacLeod, and he in turn received produce from the islanders in the form of corn, butter, cheese, wild fowl and feathers, a few sheep and sometimes a cow.

When Dr MacCulloch landed on Rona in 1815, the shepherd, Kenneth MacCagie, with his wife, three children, and old deaf mother, ran away and hid. They had 'seen no face' for seven years and had taken MacCulloch's party for 'pirates or Americans'. MacCulloch managed to persuade them that he meant no harm. There was plenty of food and six or seven acres planted with potatoes and cereals. The shepherd was indentured for eight years at an annual wage of £2 worth of clothing. He had no boat in case he deserted but he caught fish without difficulty with a rod. His house was mostly underground. The MacCagies left Rona about 1820.

About this time, with the herring industry booming, it was seriously suggested that six fishermen from Great Bernera on Lewis should be settled on Rona to form a fishing 'station' at a rent of £30 per year but there were no volunteers. So in 1829 John MacDonald, known as Iain Buidhe, took over as shepherd on Rona accompanied by his wife Cirstina and daughter Catherine. Three more children were born on the island. The family returned to Lewis about 1834 and their recorded experiences are a valuable record of life on the island.

In 1844 Rona's single inhabitant, Donald MacLeod, the 'King of Rona', was evacuated after

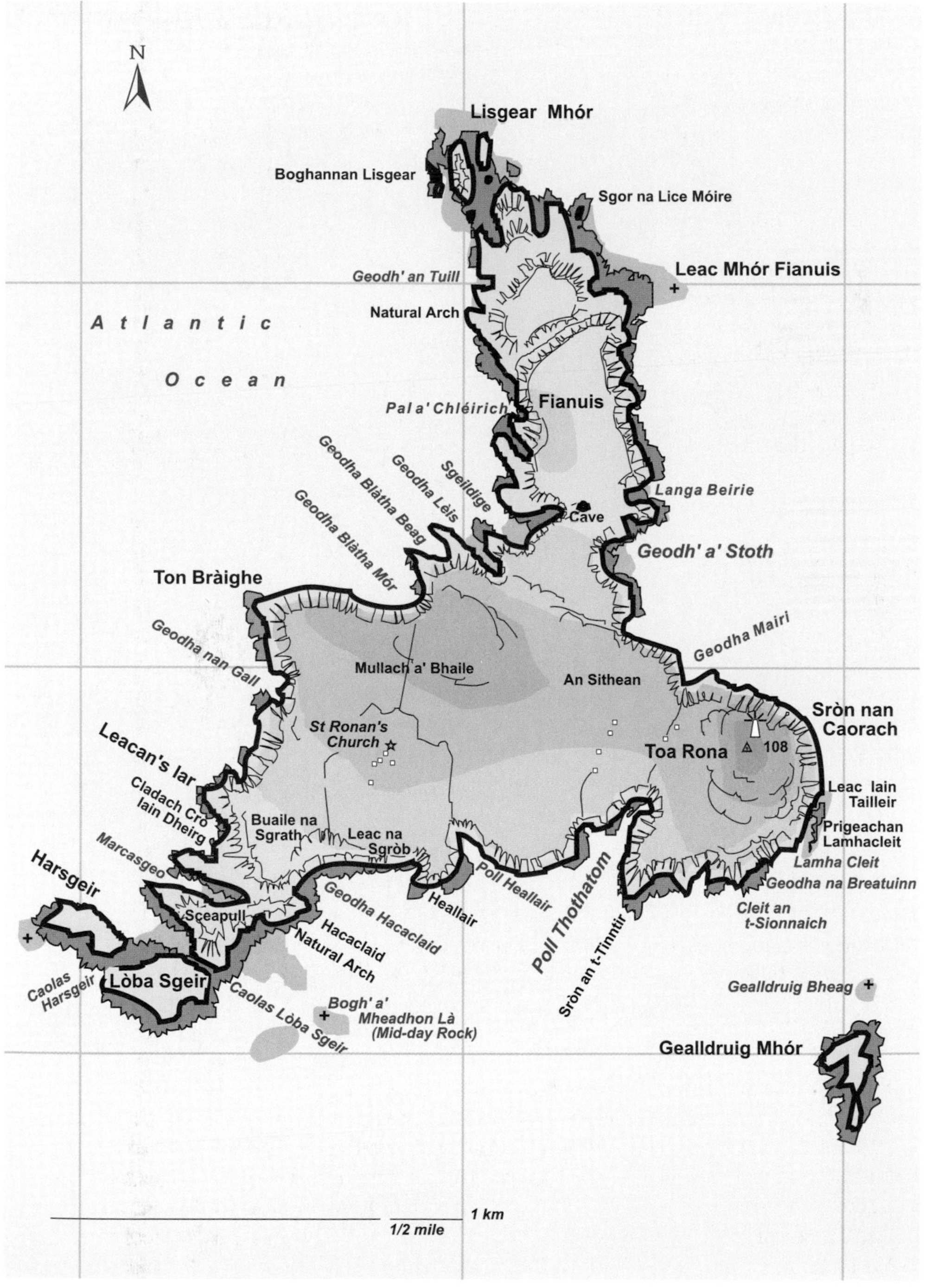

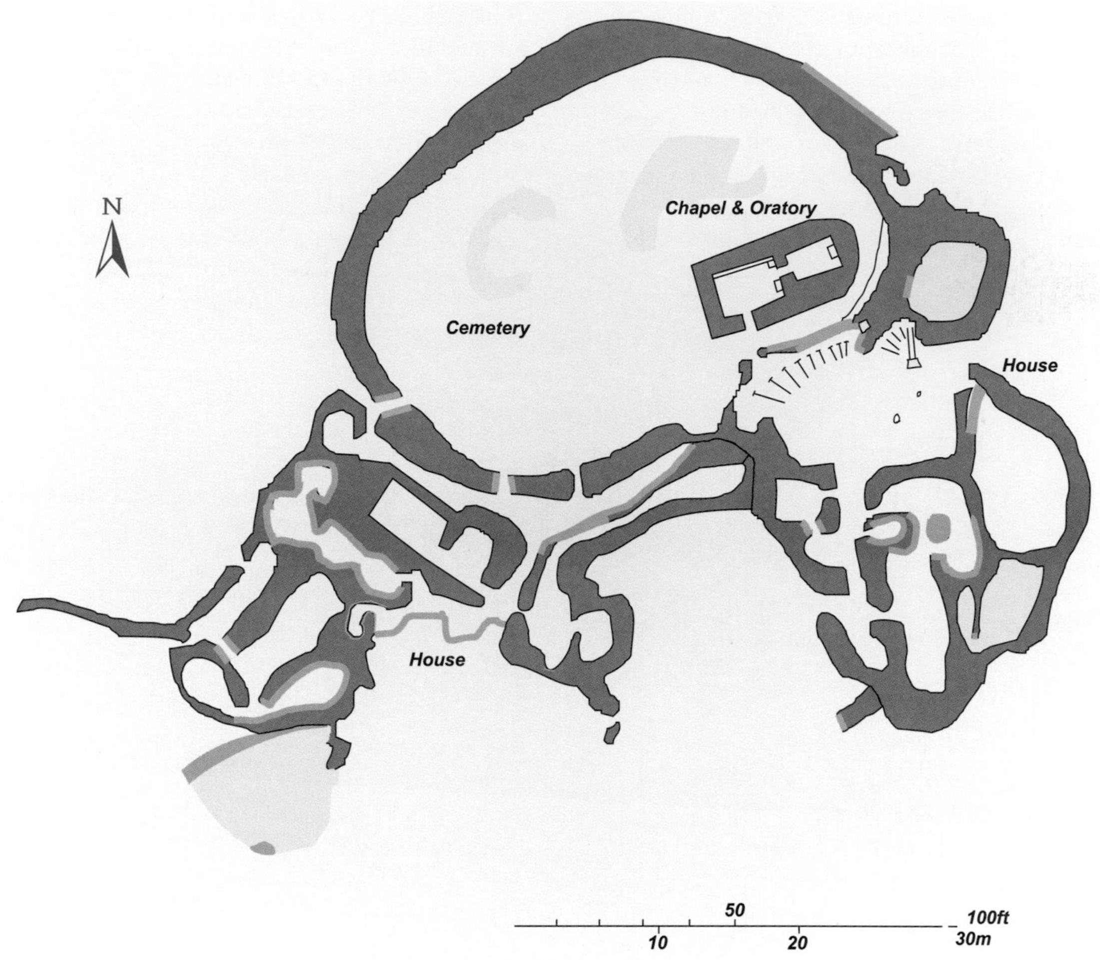

PLAN OF ST RONAN'S CHAPEL AND CEMETERY

spending a year there and in 1850 the island was offered free to the Government for use as a penal settlement. This was not accepted.

Rona lay deserted until 1884–5 when two men from Ness went there in a fit of pique after an argument with their minister. They vowed never to return to the parish. In February 1885 a relief boat called and found them both dead, one from natural causes, the other from 'exhaustion after nursing his friend.'

Wildlife: Harvie-Brown, a Victorian yachtsman, reported seeing whimbrel on Rona in June 1885. He was excited by the extensive bird life and also listed the island plants – about forty-three different species in all.

Rona (including Sula Sgeir) was declared a National Nature Reserve in 1956 because of its importance as a breeding ground for guillemot, puffin, kittiwake and fulmar. There are also large numbers of petrel, both Leach's and stormy, which breed in burrows.

Another reason for the importance of this wildlife station is that it is one of Britain's largest breeding grounds for the grey seal. More than 7500 of them breed here every autumn resulting in the birth of at least 2500 calves annually.

There are no rabbits.

* * *

RONA is an uninhabited island situated about ten miles east of Sula Sgeir and forty-four miles from the Butt of Lewis. It is roughly triangular in shape and covered with undulating turfy moorland but on the south-east corner there is a steep hill, **Toa Rona**, 108m high with a vertical cliff on its south side. Along the north-west coast the ocean storms have piled up an embankment of boulders over 20m (66ft) high. In spite of this protection sheets of seawater come splashing over the embankment during gales and the water has eroded deep channels in the turf which go right down to the bedrock.

During the many centuries of human habitation this remote little island was not only self-sufficient but even produced a surplus. Dean Monro said that there was an abundance of corn grown on the island and clover-grass for sheep. (The name of the hill, Toa Rona, may come from the Norse for a patch of grass.) A fine bere-meal (ground barley) was stuffed into the skins of sheep and sent with mutton and fowls to MacLeod each year as rent.

Nowadays the land supports only sheep which are shorn and tended by a party of Lewis shepherds on an annual visit.

St Ronan's Chapel is possibly the oldest relatively unaltered Christian building in Britain [HW809323]. Certainly the Royal Commission on Ancient Monuments lists it as one of the three oldest known structures of the Celtic Church but it is worth noting with some concern that Frank Fraser Darling claimed to have 'rebuilt' part of it. (*A Naturalist on Rona – Essays of a Biologist in Isolation. 1939*). The other two ancient structures are Annait in Skye and the nunnery on Canna (No.4.4). The ruin, which is near the remains of some houses, stands in pasture sloping down between the south-western and eastern promontories. The 'village' was possibly founded by Norse settlers in the 8th century.

In the burial ground beside the chapel there once stood a stone cross with three holes through it and the much-eroded figure of a naked man carved on it, possibly as a fertility symbol. This cross was removed in the 1930s and placed in Teampull Mholuaidh at Europie on Lewis (No.8.14). It is reputed to be 6th–7th century work and may have marked St Ronan's grave.

No one is very sure who St Ronan was. There were twelve saints of that name in Donegal, and two were recorded in Scotland. There are dedications to St Ronan on both North Uist (No.7.15) and Islay (No.2.4). Whether the island was named after this particular St Ronan or the saint was named after the island is a moot point.

Sula Sgeir, eleven miles south-west of Rona, is a narrow goose-neck shaped islet which is appropriately named gannet skerry (ON *sula skeri*). It is a small rocky island almost surrounded by cliffs and with a sea-cave running right through it. Although this is now a Nature Reserve the men of Ness in Lewis have special permission to harvest the young gannets (G. *guga*) once a year in September as this is an ancient tradition. The oily flesh of guga is considered a great delicacy but it is definitely an acquired taste.

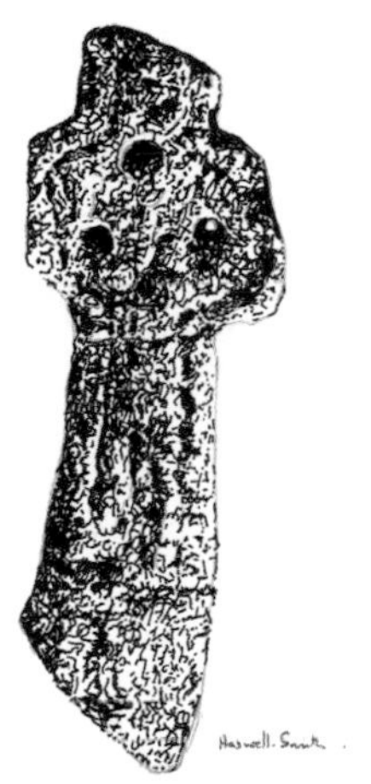

THE RONA CROSS

The Lewismen used to row the forty-one miles to Sula Sgeir in an open six-oared boat without a compass and yet accidents were very rare. A ring is fixed to the rocks at the only landing place, Geodha a' Phuill Bhàin, as there is no anchorage or beach. Nor is there any soil or fresh water on the islet but there are five stone bothies which the guga-hunters live in for a few days during their annual expedition.

* * *

Access: Permission to land is required from Barvas Estates Ltd, North Lewis and from Scottish Natural Heritage, Inverness, 01463-239431. Ness (Lewis) shepherds generally visit during July or August. Try Kilda Cruises, Leverburgh, Harris, 01859-502060, or Beyond the Blue Horizon, Stornoway, 07920-067774.

Anchorages: Approach Rona carefully, especially from the SW.

1. There is no recommended anchorage but Geodh' a' Stoth is usually favoured. Landing is generally difficult, but the best places, depending on wind direction and sea state, are a) Geodh' a' Stoth, b) Poll Thothatom or Poll Heallair, c) Sgeildige (requiring a climb up a cliff), or d) W side of Sceapull.

9–Appendix Flannan Isles

Named after St Flannan, St Ronan's half-brother.

Eilean Mór

(G – big island)

OS Maps: 1:50000 Sheet 13. 1:25000 Sheet 460. 1:10000 NA7146
Admiralty Charts: 1:500000 No.2635. 1:200000 No.2721.

1:15000 No.2524.

Area: 17.5ha (43 acres)
Height: 88m (289ft)

Population: Uninhabited.

Geology: Dark breccia of gabbros and dolerites intruding through Archaean gneiss.

History: St Flannan was St Ronan's half-brother by repute (see Rona. No.9.4): and there was St Flannan, an Irish prince, who became Abbot of Killaloe in County Clare and died in 778; and there again there was Flann, the son of Maol-duine, Abbot of Iona, who died in 890. Take your choice.

Wildlife: A good selection of sea-birds.

* * *

The **FLANNAN ISLES** can be seen on a fine day twenty-one miles west of Lewis (58° 17N 07° 35W). This group of islets consists of three small clusters. The main group has two islands, **EILEAN MOR** (G. – big island) and **Eilean Tighe** (G. – house island), two small islets in between, and some rocks scattered about. Eilean Tighe still has a ruined stone 'house' on it although it is a very tiny construction near the edge of a cliff. East of Eilean Mór are two small outliers, **Gealtaire Mór** and **Gealtaire Beag** (G – the big and little cowards). The smaller southerly cluster consists of **Soray**, **Sgeir Toman** and **Sgeir Righinn** (G. – princess skerry). The most westerly cluster, one-and-a-half nautical miles away, is **Eilean a' Ghobha** (G. – isle of the blacksmith), **Roareim** with a natural rock arch, **Bròna Cleit** (G. – sad sunk rock) and a plethora of rocks in between. These tiny islands are sometimes called the Seven Hunters but Dean Munro in 1549 called them the Seven Haley (Holy) Isles. He said they were uninhabited but with 'infinit wyld sheipe' which 'cannot be eaten be honest men' but make good tallow. People living in Uig on Lewis made an annual pilgrimage to worship in St Flannan's Chapel but *at* St Flannan's Chapel would be more appropriate. The chapel is so small that the lighthouse-keepers used to refer to it as the 'dog kennel'.

In Martin Martin's time (1695), landing on Eilean Mór was subject to strict conventions and newcomers had to be accompanied by someone who knew the rules. For instance, it was forbidden to relieve oneself near the mooring-place, to kill a bird after evening prayers – or at any time with a stone, to eat anything in private, or to take sheep suet back home. On reaching the plateau of the island it was essential to take one's hat off and

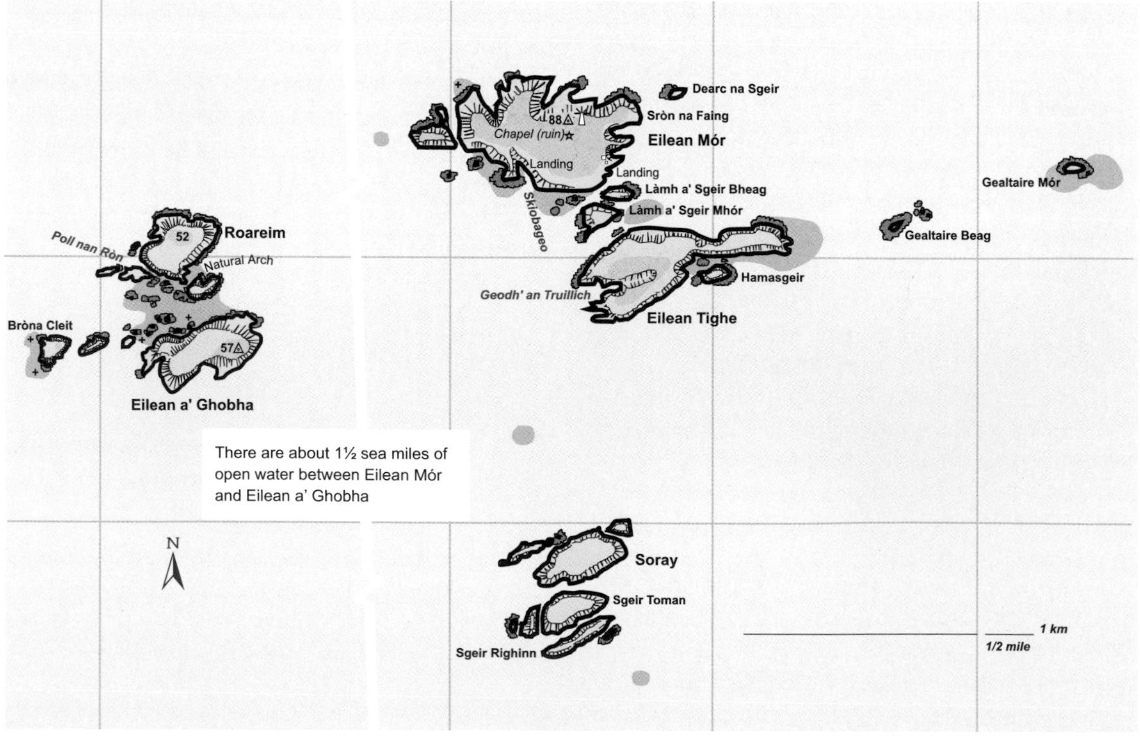

make a *deiseil* – a sunwise turn – giving thanks to God, and when twenty paces from the altar to strip off outer garments and place them on a stone. It was also important always to refer to the Flannans as 'the country', water as 'the burn' and rock as 'the hard'.

Grazing on the Flannans is of very high quality and sheep are still grazed there by the Bernera crofters. Landing can be a challenge as there is often a heavy swell. There is an expanse of slippery concrete reached by a rusty ladder and then a climb up a staircase of 195 steps partly cut from the cliff face with only the remains of a rusty guard-rail for protection.

The lighthouse, which was built by David Stevenson in 1899, is on the largest island in the group – Eilean Mór – where there are also the ruins of the tiny corbelled 6th(?) century St Flannan's Chapel and the Bothain Chlann 'ic Phail (G. – Macphail bothies) used by visiting shepherds. The light is 101m above sea-level and the stubby lighthouse which has been automatic since 1971 stands on high ground at the top of 88m (289ft) cliffs. This was the lighthouse which was the scene of a remarkable unsolved mystery.

On the night of 15 December 1900 it was noted in the log of a passing steamer that the light was not working. Before receiving this information at Oban, however, the lighthouse relief tender *Hesperus* had sailed for the Flannan Isles. She had to battle through an Atlantic gale and did not arrive until Boxing Day. The crew was surprised that there was no response to the ship's whistle and when the men landed they could find no trace of the keepers. The logbook was complete up to 13 December and notes for the log were recorded until 9am on the 15th. A meal of cold meat, pickles and potatoes was untouched on the kitchen table and, apart from one kitchen chair being knocked over, there was nothing amiss. The island was searched from end to end but nothing was found to explain the disappearance. It was however noted that equipment normally stored 110 feet above the West Landing was scattered about, the iron railings round the crane were badly twisted, and a boulder weighing about one ton was lying on the access steps.

A report by Superintendent Muirhead of the Commissioners of Northern Lights after a detailed examination decided that the men had gone to the West landing 'and that a large body of water going up higher than where they were, and coming down upon them, had swept them away with resistless force.' But this explanation is not entirely convincing. For instance, only two sets of oilskins were missing. If the third man had to rush out in his shirt-sleeves to help, how did he know there was an emergency in the first place? The landings are too far away from the lighthouse to hear a cry for help. And if he was in such a hurry, why did he close the doors and the gate?

> . . . Aye though we hunted high and low and
> hunted everywhere,
> Of the three men's fate we found no trace
> Of any kind in any place.
> But a door ajar and an untouched meal
> And an overtopped chair . . .
>
> *Wilfred Wilson Gibson (1878–1962)*

Walter Aldebert, who was a keeper of the Flannan light from 1953 to 1957, whiled away many hours trying to find a solution. The west landing is in a narrow inlet, Skiobageo, which ends in a cave. Aldebert photographed waves to show that occasionally a giant wave would thunder into the inlet causing air pressure in the cave to explode and throw tons of water across the cliffs. His conclusion was that such a wave washed one man into the sea. The second rushed back to the lighthouse for help then as the two reached the west landing a second wave carried them away. This is plausible but the records show that such explosive waves are very rare and for two to occur so close together would be an extraordinary coincidence.

Suffice it to say that when the news from Eilean Mór was first published the press had a heyday, with sea monsters, the ghost of St Flannan, and murder by the Secret Service all put forward as plausible explanations. The mystery has exercised lively imaginations ever since but, like the Marie Celeste, it is probably a better story left unsolved.

* * *

Access: Excursions by Kilda Cruises, Leverburgh, Harris, 01859-502060 or Seatrek, Uig, Lewis, 01851-672464..

Anchorage: There are two landing places, but these are no longer maintained and may be unsafe. Temporary anchorage is possible close to either landing place and there are rusty mooring rings, but the bottom is rock.

SECTION 10

Stroma and the Orkney Islands

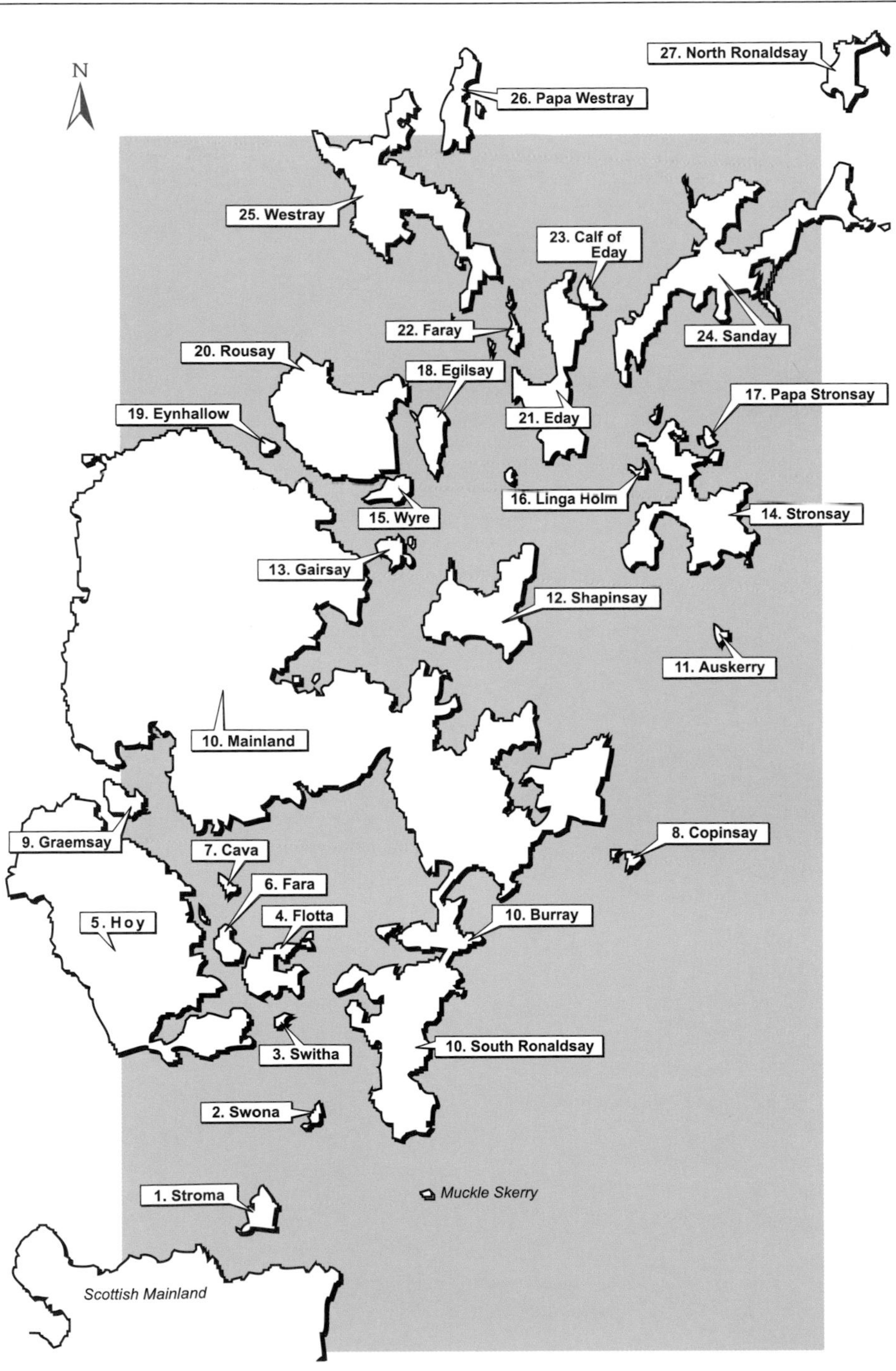

SECTION 10, Table 1: Arranged according to geographical position

No.	Name	Latitude	Longitude	Table 2* No.	Table 3** No.	Area in Acres		Area in Hectares
10.1	Stroma	58° 41N	03° 07W	59	114	927		375
10.2	Swona	58° 45N	03° 03W	114	130	227		92
10.3	Switha	58° 48N	03° 06W	158	151	101		41
10.4	Flotta	58° 50N	03° 07W	45	106	2165		876
10.5	Hoy	58° 51N	03° 18W	10	8	35380		14318
10.6	Fara	58° 51N	03° 10W	69	127	729		295
10.7	Cava	58° 53N	03° 10W	109	136	264		107
10.8	Copinsay	58° 54N	02° 41W	128	99	180		73
10.9	Graemsay	58° 56N	03° 17W	56	101	1011		409
10.10	Mainland (Orkney)	59° 00N	03° 05W	6	26	129295	52325	
	South Ronaldsay	*58° 47N*	*02° 57W*			12306	4980	
	Burray	*58° 51N*	*02° 54W*			2231	903	
	Hunda	*58° 51N*	*02° 59W*			247	100	
	Glimps Holm	*58° 53N*	*02° 55W*			136	55	
	Lamb Holm	*58 53N*	*02 53W*			99	40	58308
10.11	Auskerry	59° 02N	02° 34W	117	160	210		85
10.12	Shapinsay	59° 02N	02° 52W	25	100	7285		2948
10.13	Gairsay	59° 05N	02° 58W	78	67	593		240
10.14	Stronsay	59° 07N	02° 36W	23	124	8093		3275
10.15	Wyre	59° 07N	02° 58W	65	143	768		311
10.16	Linga Holm	59° 08N	02° 40W	141	162	141		57
10.17	Papa Stronsay	59° 09N	02° 35W	127	161	183		74
10.18	Egilsay	59° 09N	02° 56W	51	138	1606		650
10.19	Eynhallow	59° 09N	03° 07W	126	147	185		75
10.20	Rousay	59° 10N	03° 02W	19	28	12009		4860
10.21	Eday	59° 12N	02° 46W	27	68	6783		2745
10.22	Faray	59° 13N	02° 49W	89	145	445		180
10.23	Calf of Eday	59° 14N	02° 44W	77	116	600		243
10.24	Sanday	59° 15N	02° 34W	18	96	12461		5043
10.25	Westray	59° 18N	02° 57W	20	40	11646		4713
10.26	Papa Westray	59° 21N	02° 53W	43	122	2268		918
10.27	North Ronaldsay	59 22N	02 25W	49	158	1705		690

*Table 2: The islands arranged in order of magnitude
**Table 3: The islands arranged in order of size

Introduction

The islands to the north of Scotland are not easily confused with those of the west. Not only is the geology very different from that of, say, the Hebrides, but the entire social structure and language is distinctive. Both areas came under Norse influence in the first millennium but whereas within a few centuries Celtic civilisation had gained control in the west, the north remained a Norse dominion until comparatively recent times. Gaelic has never been a natural language in the north. When Norn (partly Old Norse, partly Icelandic) died out it was replaced by English or Lowland Scots.

Apart from a very few outliers, the islands in this region form two archipelagoes and just as the northern isles as a group are very different from the western isles so too does each archipelago have its own distinctive characteristics. The Orkney archipelago is agriculturally rich thanks to its base of Old Red Sandstone, while the Shetland archipelago, 50 miles further north, has poorer soil and its economy therefore depends on the wealth of the sea. Hence the well-known saying that 'an Orcadian is a farmer with a boat while a Shetlander is a fisherman with a croft.' The richness of the Orkney soil has always made fishing a secondary occupation. The sea is all around, but it is primarily for transport or recreation rather than for sustenance, whereas in Shetland it is a life-giving force.

Between Duncansby Head (beside John o' Groats) on the Scottish mainland and Brough Ness at the southern tip of South Ronaldsay is only a matter of six miles, or a mere ten kilometres. But this narrow strip of water contains the treacherous Pentland Firth in parts of which the spring tides run faster than almost anywhere else in coastal Britain. The western end of the Firth has a notorious tidal race called the Merry Men of Mey which forms on the ebb and which is so turbulent that a small vessel can be put in severe danger.

The eastern end also has its troublesome areas, such as near the Pentland Skerries in mid-firth. There are heavy breaking seas in this area which are particularly lethal when the wind is against the tide. **Muckle Skerry**, the largest of the Pentland Skerries, is a sizeable islet with a lighthouse (built in 1794) and a roadway up from the landing point in Scartan Bay. It has three tiny lochans and a table-shaped northern promontory called 'Tenniscourt'. In 1841 this islet had a population of eleven persons which by 1881 had increased to seventeen people living in four houses. After that the population declined, and in recent years it only consisted of the lighthouse-keepers; that is, until 1994, when the light was automated. Now, after 200 years, the lighthouse-keepers have left for good and the isle is deserted.

It would be a pity to discuss Orkney without mentioning the strange story of Henry Sinclair.

When the wealthy Order of the Knights Templar was branded heretical by the Vatican in 1307 many Knights fled to Scotland and set up their headquarters in Midlothian on the lands of the St Clair family. The St Clairs, or Sinclairs, were descended from Vikings and held powerful earldoms in Caithness and Orkney. Their connection with the Templars brought enormous additional wealth.

Henry Sinclair was born in 1345. Tall and strong, he could speak fluent Latin, Norse and Lowland Scots, and he hunted, crusaded, fathered thirteen children, and dreamed of conquest. He became a Knight Templar – a defender of the Holy Grail – and he wanted a kingdom so much that he was nicknamed 'Prince'.

Prince Henry had heard all the Norse tales of a land far west of Greenland so he persuaded two of his Venetian friends, Nicolo and Antonio Zeno, who had made vast profits from ship-building, to come to Orkney and join his venture. Nicolo died after an initial exploratory voyage to Greenland, but Antonio carried on and described events in long detailed letters to his family in Venice. These became known as the Zeno Narratives when they were eventually published in 1558.

According to these letters the adventurers fitted out a small fleet and Antonio armed it with Pietro cannons which he brought from Venice. In 1398 Prince Henry, Antonio Zeno and 300 colonists set sail for the west in twelve ships. They eventually reached Newfoundland and spent their first winter in Nova Scotia.

The Mi'Kmaq Indians' tribal history tells of the arrival centuries ago of a bird with a broken wing, and a prophet called 'Kluskap' and it was about this time that the Mi'Kmaqs started fishing with European-style nets. A couple of hilltop castle ruins in Nova Scotia have been dated to this period by Canadian archaeologists and a ship's cannon dredged from Digby Harbour in Nova Scotia in 1849 has been identified as a 14thC Pietro cannon. Hardly conclusive evidence but interesting nevertheless.

The following spring (1399), the colonists sailed down the coast to look for land on which to settle. Once again there is circumstantial evidence. A recently discovered boulder at Lake Memphremagog on the Canadian/US border near Montreal has been carved with an outline of the Sinclair coat-of-arms next to a fairly accurate map of the North American coastline while across the Lake a stone carving was found in a stream-bed which resembles the Rosslyn Apprentice Pillar.

In Rhode Island an ancient round stone tower, called the Newport Tower, has a striking resemblance to Orkney Mainland's church at Ophir (No. 10.10) and rock carvings in Westford, Massachusetts, accurately depict a medieval Scottish knight in full regalia.

It is known that Prince Henry sailed back to Orkney in 1400, possibly to collect more prospective colonists or essential provisions, but according to the Narratives he was killed by the English. (Henry IV of England invaded Orkney at that time.)

No one knows what became of the settlement but modern genetic testing of native Americans might have a story to reveal.

Some years later – in 1446 – the Sinclair family built Rosslyn Chapel on their land near Edinburgh with its famous Apprentice Pillar and stone carvings of Indian maize and aloe cacti. (And in 1537 the Dutch globe, Frisius-Mercator, shows the area west of Greenland as 'the land discovered by Britons').

So can one really be certain that it was Christopher Columbus who 'discovered' America in 1492?

10.1 Stroma

(ON straum-øy – island in the tidal stream).

OS Maps: 1:50000 Sheet 7 1:25000 Sheet 461
Admiralty Charts: 1:200000 Nos.1942 or 1954 1:50000 No.2162 1:26000 No.2581

Area: 375ha (927 acres)
Height: 53m (174 ft)

Owner: James Simpson, a Stroma man by birth and a former haulage contractor, has owned Stroma since 1960.

Population:1841–186 (42 houses). 1881–341. 1891–327 (66 houses). 1931–193. 1961–12. Uninhabited since 1950s except for lighthouse keepers and their families. 1971–8. 1981–0. 1991–0. 2001–0.

Geology: Weathered Middle Old Red Sandstone in flat layers known as Rousay flags. There is a fault line running north to south through the centre of the island – almost on the line of the road.

History: Svein Asleifsson (see Gairsay No.10.13) had to spend a night on Stroma sheltering from a gale according to the Orkneyinga Saga. The sagas make no other mention of Stroma.

It is usually true to say that the survival of an island population in the present day depends on the availability of good education and good communications. Well, Stroma is the exception that proves the rule.

Although there was an active and viable population of eighty people living there in the early 1950s with a good primary school to serve the children (and even with their own issue of postage stamps), tide-wracked Stroma lacked adequate harbour facilities. So officialdom rose to the occasion and in 1955 a new harbour was constructed at great expense and the contractors were pleased to employ the local people to carry out the work. Wages were so good that by the time the harbour was completed many of the islanders had made sufficient money to leave and establish themselves on the mainland. Too few were then left to maintain a viable population and within a few years the island was deserted except for the lighthouse-keepers; and they too left in 1996 when the lighthouse was automated.

Wildlife: Always a popular breeding ground for seals, the numbers have dramatically increased since the island became uninhabited.

STROMA is officially part of Caithness and not one of the Orkney isles. The powerful ocean tides, deflected by the British mainland, funnel into the Pentland Firth – the gap between Caithness and Orkney. Stroma obstructs their flow and turbulent seas are the result. Only a short distance west is the wide and dangerous tidal race known as the Merry Men of Mey and off Swilkie Point at Stroma's northern shore the sea can be equally violent.

The Picts are thought to have first settled in Orkney and the name of the Pentland Firth is a corruption of Pictland Firth. Stroma lies in the southern part of the Firth with the Inner Sound separating it from the mainland. The west side of the island is mainly cliffs but the east side is fairly low and flat. The Norse ruin of **Castle Mestag** [ND340764] caps Mell Head in the south-west and in the far north, beside the lighthouse which was automated in 1996, there is a chambered cairn [ND353791].

The evidence of Stroma's recent depopulation is there to be seen. A roadway runs down the centre of the island from the lighthouse in the north to the harbour in the south connecting what were the two main settlements, **Nethertown** in the north and **Uppertown** in the south. The main island farmhouse, **Mains of Stroma**, is central. **Cairn Hill** (53m), the highest point, is in the south-east.

The church and school, and the old croft houses, stand derelict. Only the sheep find shelter in them now.

A deep rocky pit in the north-west, known as **The Gloup** (ON *glup* – hollow, ravine), is filled with sea-water which feeds in through a subterranean passage under the cliffs. This is a particularly fine example of this type of feature of which there are many in the Northern Isles. Just north of the gloup are the remains of an Iron Age fort [ND350785].

* * *

Access: The owner who lives in Gills near John o' Groats runs boat trips to Stroma most weekends.

Anchorages:
1. Small harbour on S coast most of which dries. Good shelter and easy entrance at slack water but rock bottom and slight swell in outer basin. Inner basin recommended, sandy bottom. Tie up in SE corner just inside pierhead.
2. Comfortable anchorage out of tide midway between harbour and Mell Head off the sandy beach, 3m, sand with weed patches.

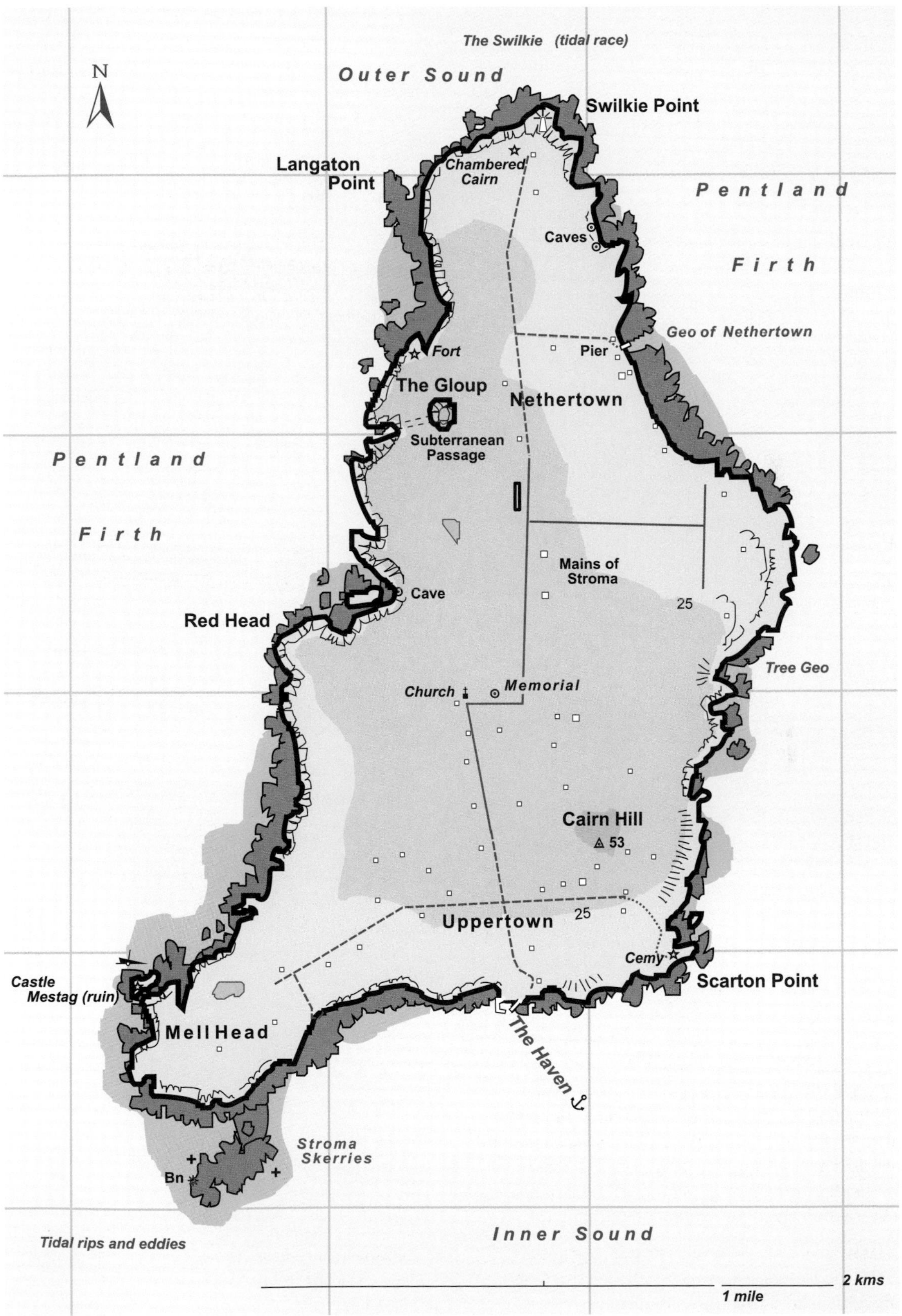
The Swilkie (tidal race)
Outer Sound
N
Swilkie Point
Langaton Point
Chambered Cairn
Pentland
Caves
Firth
Geo of Nethertown
Fort
Pier
The Gloup
Nethertown
Subterranean Passage
Pentland
Firth
Mains of Stroma
Cave
25
Red Head
Tree Geo
Church
Memorial
Cairn Hill
53
25
Uppertown
Cemy
Scarton Point
Castle Mestag (ruin)
Mell Head
The Haven
Stroma Skerries
Bn
Inner Sound
Tidal rips and eddies
2 kms
1 mile

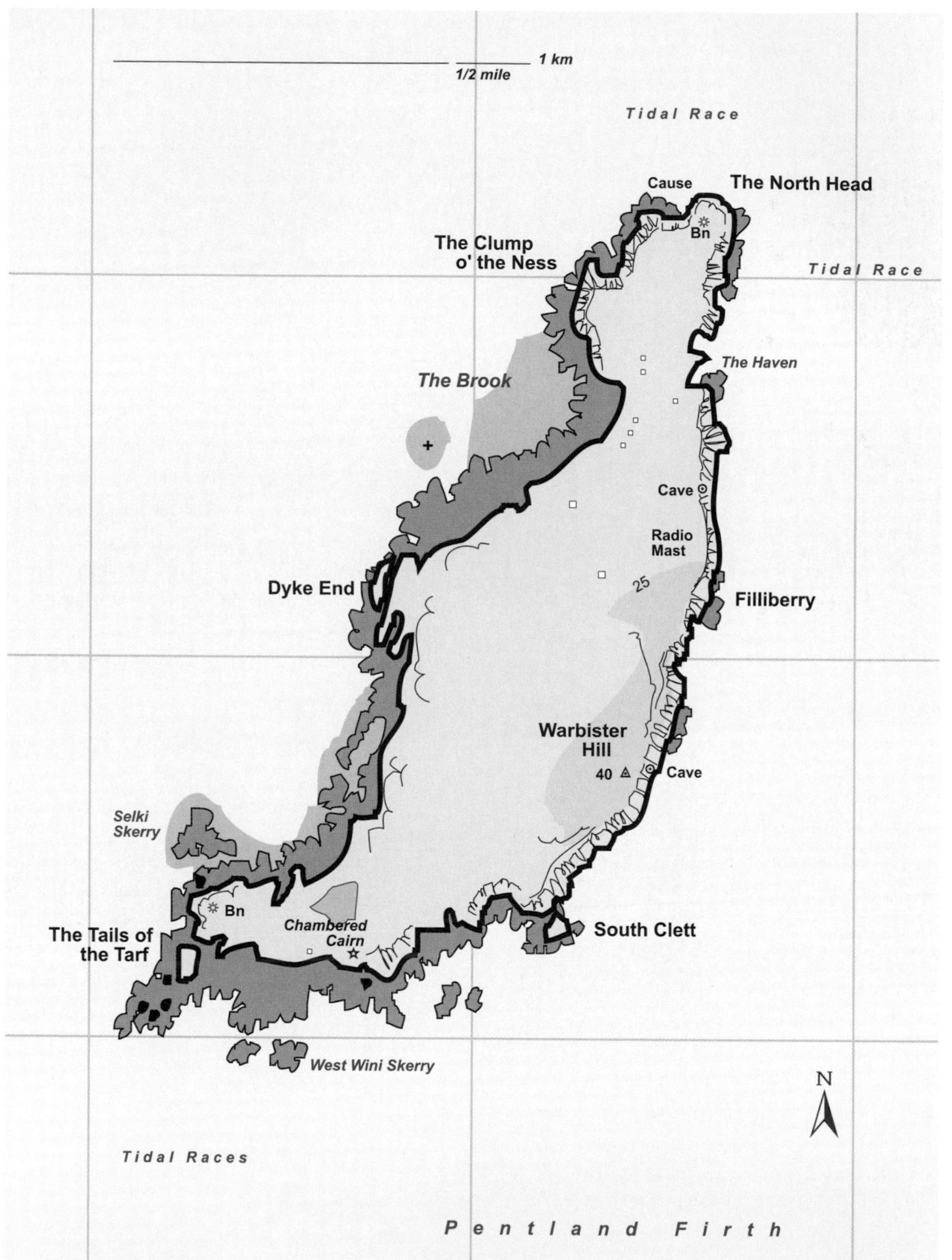

10.2 Swona

(ON svín-øy – pig island) or possibly (ON – Sveinn's island). Old records call it 'Swinna'. The Norse was sometimes used perjoratively – 'a swine of an island'.

OS Maps: 1:50000 Sheet 7 1:25000 Sheet 461
Admiralty Charts: 1:50000 No.2162 1:26000 No.2581

Area: 92ha (227 acres)
Height: 41m (134 ft)

Owner: Cyril Annal. His family has owned Swona since 1910.

Population: 1841–54 (8 houses). 1881–47. 1891–42 (7 houses). 1931–6. 1961–3. 1971–3. Abandoned 1974 and uninhabited since.

Geology: Weathered Middle Old Red Sandstone.

History: In spite of the difficulty of access,

archaeological evidence would suggest that Swona was probably first occupied 5000 years ago.

In the 12th century this was the home of Grim, father of two of Sweyn Asleifsson's close friends.

Wildlife: A small herd of feral cattle still survive. The original herd, which was abandoned in 1974, consisted of a mixture of black Aberdeen Angus and brown Shorthorns. The cattle eat seaweed during the grassless winter months, shelter from the cold in derelict buildings, and the young bulls fight for dominance in the spring. Such herds of feral cattle are very rare and this herd is being studied with interest by scientists. It is now officially recognised as a separate breed.

Thousands of rabbits breed unchecked, crop the grass which the cattle need and provide an occasional meal for the seagulls.

There is such a wealth of birdlife that the RSPB would like to have Swona declared a site of scientific interest (SSI).

* * *

SWONA lies in the south approach to Scapa Flow. The Tails of the Tarf (?N – the end of the seaweed) is the most southerly point marked by the small white tower of **Swona Light**. The east side of Swona is mainly cliff with the rounded green summit of **Warbister Hill** (41m) rising close above the cliffs midway along the east coast and a cave further to the north.

The settlement on Swona was in the lowest-lying part near the north end of the island. On the east side is a little cove called the **Haven**, Swona's best attempt at a harbour and on the west side is the **Brook**, an indentation with a wide stretch of shallow, treacherous rock and reef.

Associations with the distant past include a prehistoric chambered cairn [ND384837] in the extreme south of the island, an early Christian burial ground, and Viking remains.

In the 19th century the islanders' main occupation was line-fishing for cod. This was supplemented on occasion by piloting ships through the treacherous waters of the Pentland Firth – waters which they knew so well. Crofting was a marginal existence and by 1932 only one family remained on the island. The last inhabitant in 1974 was Jim Rosie. He was unmarried and had to leave when he developed Parkinson's disease. Now the solid stone and slated buildings have fallen into disrepair and old agricultural machinery rusts among the nettles.

Throughout history Swona has been the scene of many shipping disasters mostly on the west side during the east-going tidal stream. The tide is deceptive and can carry a boat on to the northern skerries with accelerating speed. By the time the danger is recognised it can be too late.

Martin Martin's (1695) solution should not be taken too seriously: '... Swinna isle, remarkable only for a part of Pentland Firth lying to the west of it, called the Wells of Swinna. They are two whirpools in the sea, which run about with such violence, that any vessel or boat coming within their reach, go always round until they sink. These wells are dangerous only when there is a dead calm; for if a boat be under sail with any wind, it is easy to go over them. If any boat be forced into these wells by the violence of the tide, the boat-men cast a barrel or an oar into the wells; and while it is swallowing it up, the sea continues calm, and gives the boat an opportunity to pass over.'

* * *

Access: No normal access but, weather and tides permitting, try Explorer Fast Sea Charter, Kirkwall, 01856-871225.

Anchorage: Swona is surrounded with very tricky tides and it is often impracticable to approach the island. There are tidal races at both N and S ends of the island and the west coast is particularly dangerous.

1. The Haven, a small cove on the NE side of the island, 2c S of North Head is the best landing place on Swona when an approach can be made.

10.3 Switha

Derivation uncertain but may be (ON sviv-øy – island that appears to be floating or swinging).

OS Maps: 1:50000 Sheet 7 1:25000 Sheets 461 or 462
Admiralty Charts: 1:50000 No.2162 1:26000 No.2581

Area: 41ha (101 acres)
Height: 29m (95 ft)

Population: No record of any habitation.

Geology: Well-weathered Old Red Sandstone of the Middle period.

Wildlife: There are many storm-petrel burrows in the light soil.

There is no written record of **SWITHA** ever having been inhabited in historic times and the Norse sagas make no mention of this little island. But Neolithic man lived here or, at least, visited the island for religious purposes, because he left two standing stones as evidence. The remarkable seamanship of these men in their flimsy craft never fails to astonish!

Sheep are grazed on Switha and probably have been for centuries. Every June, for at least a few days, the island echoes to the sound of human voices when shepherds, and occasionally members of their families, land on the island to clip the sheep.

Switha lies on the west side of the Sound of Hoxa amid tidal races beside the southern approach to Scapa Flow. Its most southerly point is called **The Ool** and between it and **The Kiln**, a

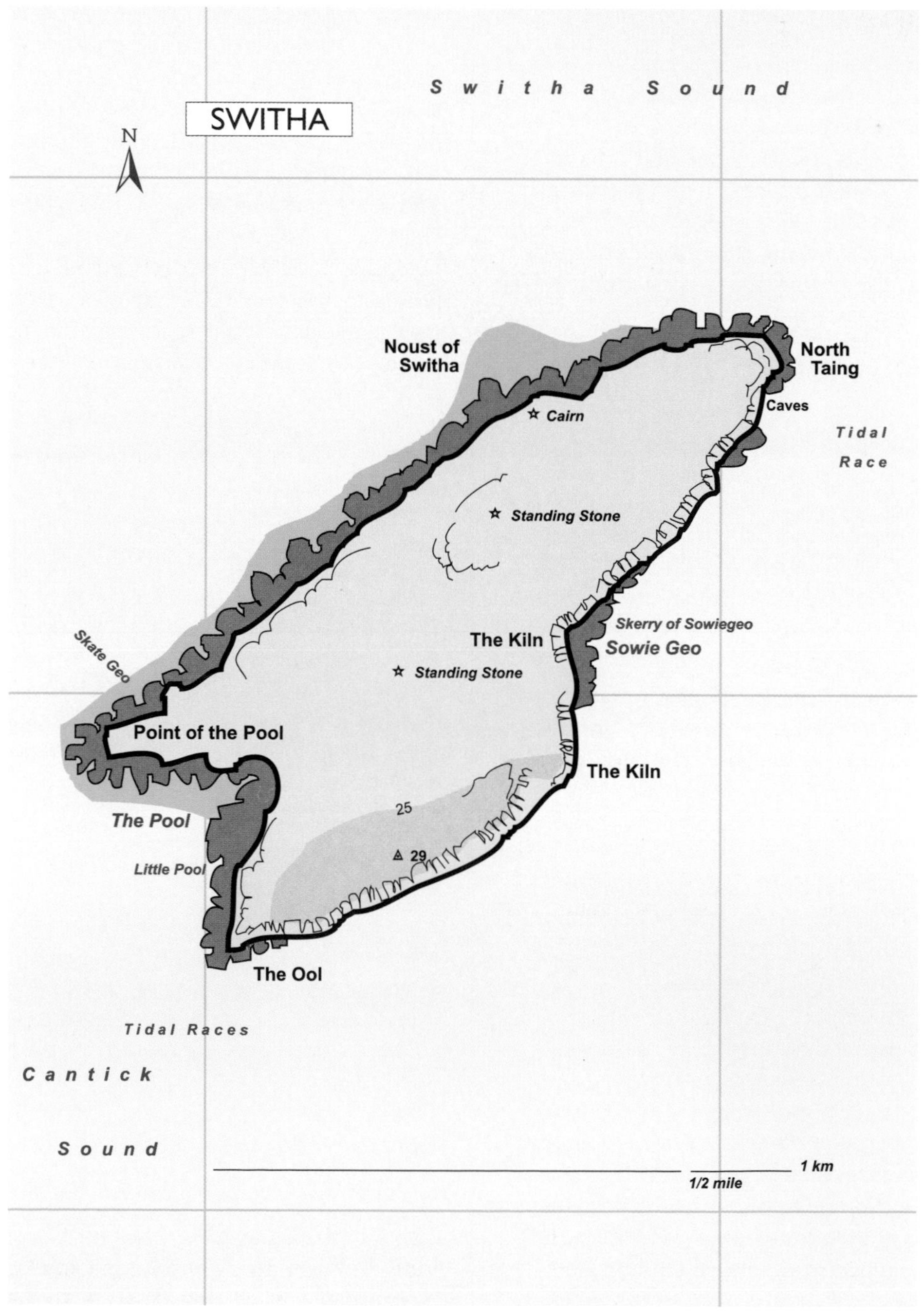

point halfway along the south-east side, the cliffs reach a height of 29m. This is the highest part of the island and the ground falls away behind the cliffs except for a small hill (24m) to the north with one of the standing stones on its summit. A shallow cove in the south-west, **The Pool**, lies between the Ool and a low promontory, Point of the Pool.

* * *

Access: No normal access but, weather and tides permitting, try Explorer Fast Sea Charter, Kirkwall, 01856-871225.

Anchorage: Approach from N if possible to avoid dangerous tides at SE entrance to Cantick Sound, or time the passage carefully.

1. Temp. anchorage in the Pool, at SW end of Switha off Cantick Sound, in suitable conditions.

10.4 Flotta

(ON flott-øy – flat grassy island).

O S Maps: 1:50000 Sheet 7 1:25000 Sheets 461 or 462
Admiralty Charts: 1:200000 Nos.1942 or 1954 1:50000 No.2162 1:30000 No.35 1:26000 No.2581 1:12500 No.2568 oil terminal

Area: 876ha (2165 acres)
Height: 58m (190 ft)

Population: 1841–405 (82 houses). 1881–425. 1891–423 (88 houses). 1931–282. 1961–123. 1971–73. (1975– introduction of oil industry) 1981–178. 1991–126. 2001–81.

Geology: The whole island is Middle Old Red Sandstone but the larger south-west portion is of Rousay Beds weathered into low hills, whereas the Golta peninsula and Quoy Ness are of Eday Beds – flagstones and sandstone of building quality.

History: An interesting sculptured stone slab from Flotta, thought to date from the 10th century, is in the Museum of Scotland in Edinburgh.

During the First World War Flotta became a naval base but after the war it returned to its former happy rural state. there were fields to be ploughed and lobsters to be caught in the rocky pools. Then the Second World War turned the island into an armed camp festooned with so many barrage balloons that it almost took off – the aim being to protect the southern entrance to Scapa Flow. Two new concrete piers were built with excellent access, and communication with Kirkwall and Stromness was improved. After the war the island once again slowly recovered from the shock, but, as with so many of the small islands, the population was decreasing and becoming more elderly. Improvement work was carried out, such as the laying of a water pipe in 1970 to bring fresh water from Hoy, but even so, the outlook was rather bleak.

Then Flotta, for the third time, was thrown irrevocably into the modern age because this flat little island, balanced near the edge of extinction, had the best-protected deep-water facilities in all of Orkney.

In 1974 the Occidental Group started construction of an oil terminal and linked it to the Piper and Claymore fields in the North Sea by 230km of pipeline. It became operational in December 1976. Many of the islanders were given employment but, inevitably, the work brought newcomers to the island and their assimilation was not always without problems. However, Flotta now has a thriving community with many young families and children, and, although the oil industry has passed its peak, there are still reasonable prospects for the foreseeable future.

The oil-terminal facilities are second only in size to those of Sullom Voe in Shetland but, unlike Shetland, practically all of the oil-related development, which copes with about 10% of all Britain's oil production, is confined to this one small island and has relatively little impact on the Mainland community.

Wildlife: Large number of Arctic tern, goodly population of Arctic skua and a compact seabird colony at Stanger Head.

* * *

Scapa Flow is no longer filled with men-of-war, iron-clads, or even sleek grey frigates of the modern fleet. The only continual signs of life and industry are the gas-flares of the huge oil terminal on **FLOTTA** sparkling on the water.

The island is almost rectangular except for the gaping mouth of **Pan Hope** in the east (the site of 17th-century salt pans). This wide bay cuts deep into the island with a northwards twist at Sands Taing. It then dries out in **Curries Firth**. Unfortunately all the inner part of the bay is too

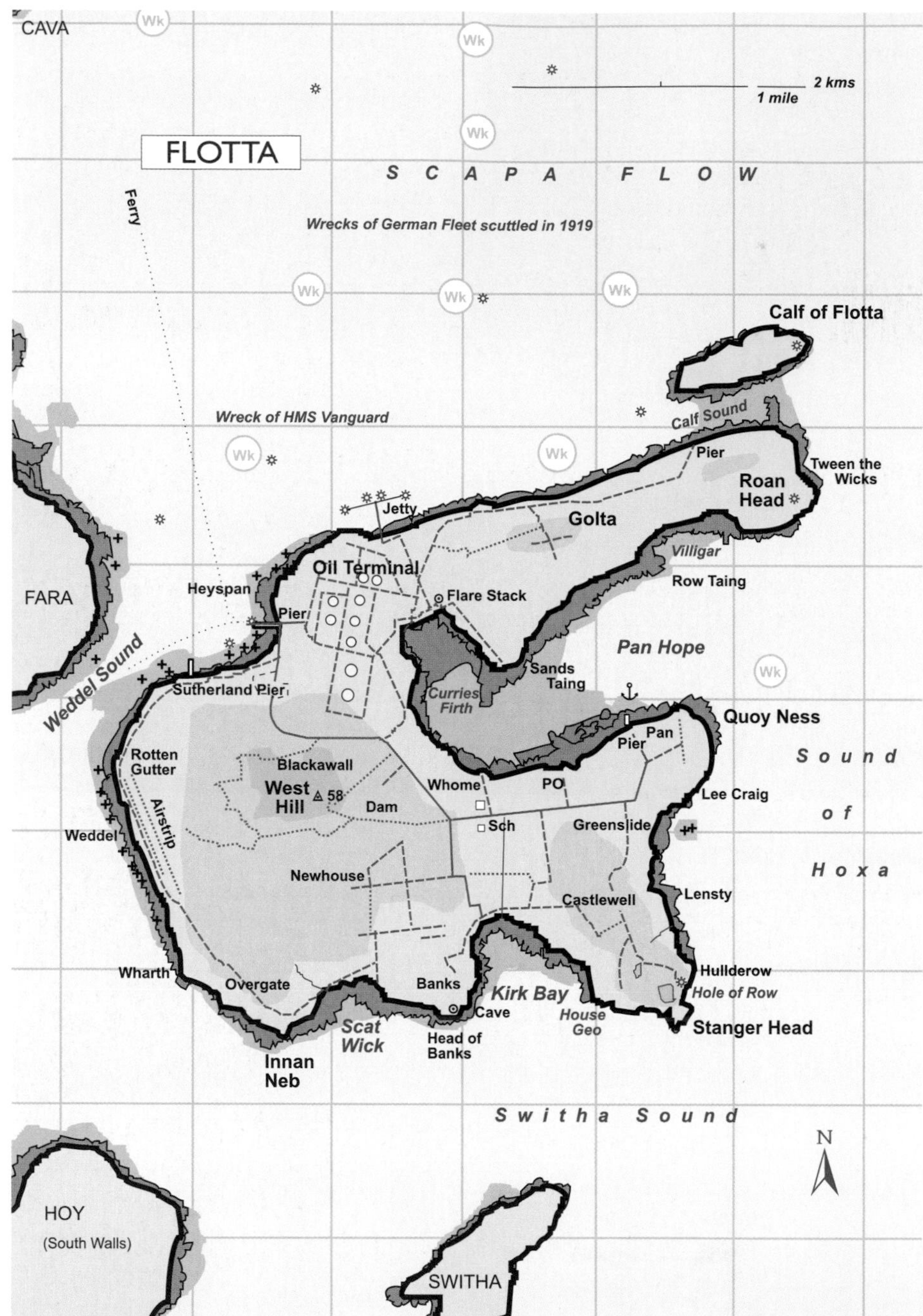

shallow to be of any use as an anchorage – but the waders don't mind.

In the pre-oil-terminal days the island was mostly moorland with some grazing and cultivated land and most of the farms were small. Lobster fishing was needed to augment the meagre return from farming, yet there was always an air of vitality despite the number of old people. Now more than half the total land area is covered with all the paraphernalia of industry and houses. **West Hill** (58m), Flotta's highest point, is relatively clear but the airstrip lies below it by Rotten Gutter on the west coast. North-west of the terminal the **Golta** (ON – barren, sterile) peninsula is more open, but that is all there is now to be seen of the old Flotta. The south-east corner at **Stanger Head** is covered with the remaining derelict military installations of the

Second World War – fascinating, or a suitable set for a disaster movie, depending on one's viewpoint. Most of the stone used came from the local quarry.

Calf of Flotta is a tiny island off Roan Head in the north. It nearly rates as a drying island because the water in Calf Sound which separates it from Flotta is very shallow. There is a narrow navigable channel between the rock-like obstructions there which are, in fact, large piles of anti-submarine cable discarded after the Second World War.

* * *

Access: Frequent ro-ro service by Orkney Ferries, 01856-811397, from Houton, 17km SW of Kirkwall, and Longhope or Lyness on Hoy. Bus service, Kirkwall/Houton and Stromness/Houton, 01856-870555.

Anchorages:

1. Pan Hope, large bay on E side of Flotta. Good fair weather anchorage in 4–5m N of pier and clear of underwater cable.
2. Kirk Bay, on S side. Temp. anchorage but rocky and exposed in S winds.
3. West Weddel Sound, bay in NW of Flotta. Shallow and rocky but good anchorage in settled weather. Gibraltar Pier on E side and Sutherland Pier on S side (0.6m at head).

10.5 Hoy

(ON há-øy – high island)

O S Maps: 1:50000 Sheet 7 1:25000 Sheet 462
Admiralty Charts: 1:200000 No.1954 1:75000 No.2249 north Hoy 1:50000 No.2162 south Hoy 1:30000 No.35 east coast

Area: 14318ha (35380 acres)
Height: 479m (1571 ft)

Owner: Sold in 1973 by the owner, Malcolm Stewart, to The Hoy Trust. After the passing of the Crofting Reform Act many crofters purchased their own land-holdings from the Trust which also sold 3237ha to the Royal Society for the Protection of Birds (including the Old Man of Hoy). The Trust hopes to encourage resettlement on the parts of Hoy which it still owns.

Population: 1841–1486 (294 houses). 1881–1380. 1891–1320 (271 houses). 1931–955. 1961–511. 1981–461. 1991–450. 2001–392.

Geology: Hoy is unique in being almost entirely composed of Upper Old Red Sandstone although there are a few small volcanic intrusive dykes in the north-west and some small areas of exposed basalt. This particular type of sandstone – massive, hard, and red or orange-coloured – is to be found nowhere else in Orkney. Its mode of weathering has resulted in the fantastic precipices of the west coast.

The sandstone lies above a basalt lava layer which is about 120m thick. This has been exposed by erosion at, for instance, the foot of the Old Man of Hoy where it forms a pedestal. The south-east of the island is of Middle Old Red Sandstone. In the extreme north there is a small area of Lower Stromness Flags – a finely laminated Middle Old Red Sandstone which weathers to a good soil.

History: It was on South Walls, according to the sagas, that Olaf Tryggvason, King of Norway from 995 to 1000, forced Sigurd Hlodvisson the Stout,

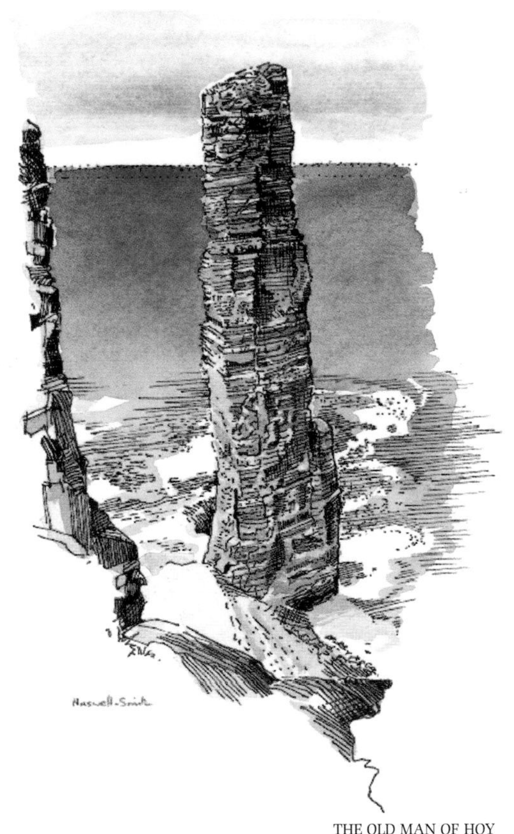

THE OLD MAN OF HOY

Earl of Orkney and a fearless warrior, to submit to baptism on pain of death. The Earl duly became a Christian – but in name only.

Wildlife: Hoy is a treasure-house of plant life – by far the best in Orkney and including a number of rare alpines but there is also deep heather covering many of the hill-slopes. The only remaining fragment of native woodland is at Berriedale west of the Old Man of Hoy with willow, birch, aspen and rowan, and a few indigenous trees still growing in the clefts of Ward Hill and Cuilags – rowan, hazel (only three survive) – *Corylus avellana*, aspen, birch – *Betula pubescens*, and sallow – *Salix atrocinerea*. Strangely, although it is common in the Highlands, there

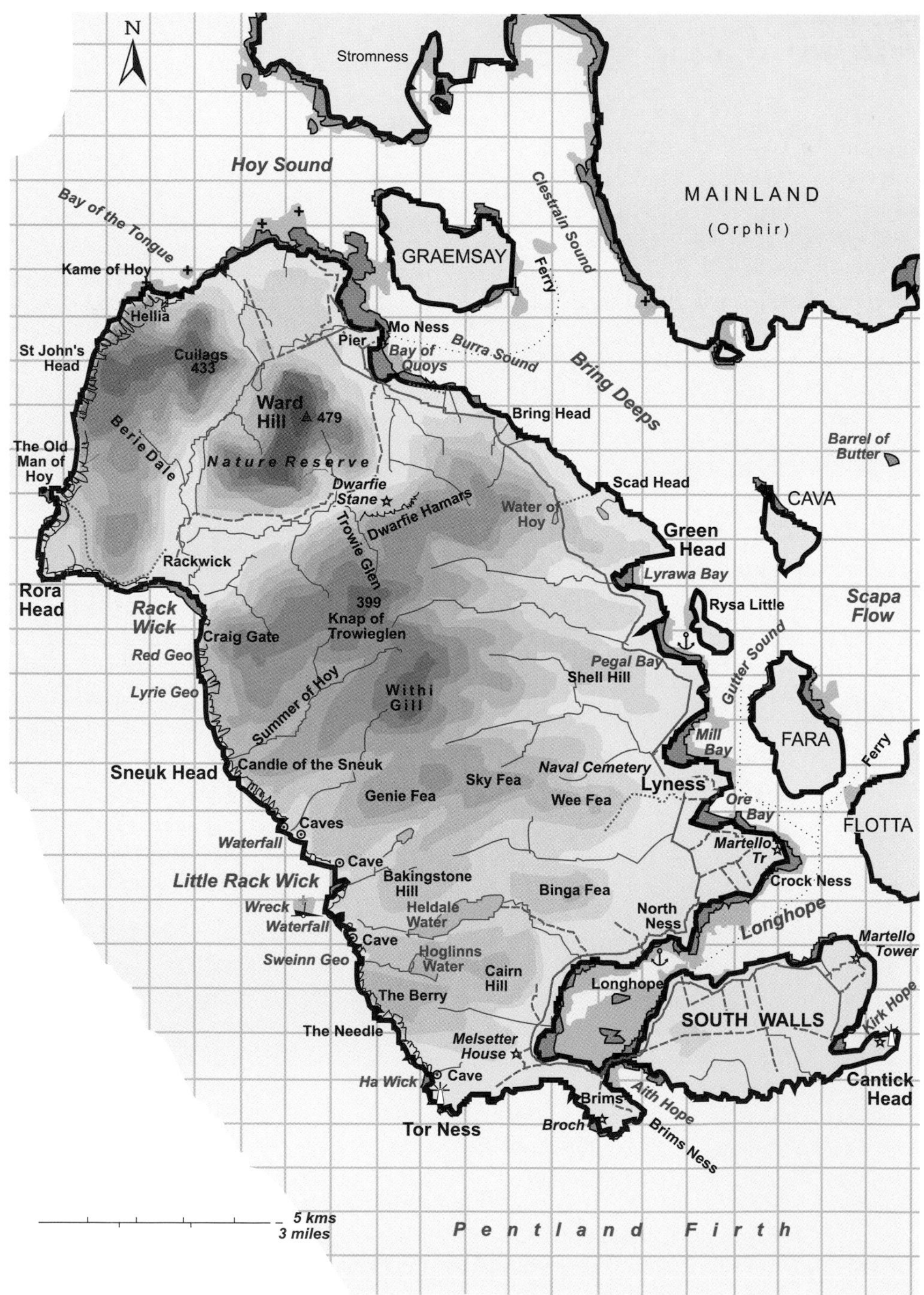

is no bog myrtle on Hoy. Mountain hares are to be found in the north of Hoy and nowhere else in Orkney although the brown hare is quite common. This area is also said to support Orkney's only grasshoppers.

North Hoy is an RSPB Nature Reserve. Breeding species of bird to be seen – if you can survive the midges – are red grouse, golden plover, dunlin, snipe and curlew, with some hen harrier, merlin and short-eared owl. There is an important skua population – over 400 pairs of Arctic and 1500 great skuas (bonxies) were recorded in 1982 and the lochans support half the 110 pairs of red-throated divers recorded on Orkney. Stonechat, wheatear, some ring ousel and many twite are in evidence. On the cliffs there are huge numbers of fulmar, shag, kittiwake, guillemot, razorbill, puffin, black guillemot, and rock dove. There are also buzzard, peregrine and raven, and barnacle geese appear in late winter at South Walls.

May to July are the best bird-watching months.

* * *

HOY is the highest and wildest and wettest (1500mm of rain) of all the Orkney islands. The high ground rises in three rugged masses, divided by 300m deep gaps, with **Ward Hill** in the middle. Ward Hill is the highest peak in Orkney (479m). Legend has it that on the steep north side of Ward Hill, where it hangs above the Hoy Outdoor Centre, there used to be a great carbuncle which gleamed ruddy red in the dark but which disappeared whenever you approached it. There has never been an explanation for this.

The outstanding view of the Hoy cliffs from the Scrabster ferry gives newcomers a very misleading impression of Orkney. As can be seen from Table III, most of the Northern Isles are low-lying. Yet **St John's Head** on the NW coast is, at nearly 350m, one of the highest sea-cliffs in Britain with the world-famous rock pinnacle, the **Old Man of Hoy** (137m), to the south and the remarkable echoing valley of the **Kame** in the far north. In 1970, mountaineers spent two days descending St John's Head as it was almost impossible to abseil in the vicious sea-wind, and the subsequent hair-raising ascent took five days.

Many legends attach to the **Dwarfie Stane**, – a huge block of red sandstone (8.5m long x 4.3m wide x 1.8m high) lying within a natural amphitheatre – the Dwarfie Hamars (ON *hamars* – crags), south-east of Ward Hill [HY243004]. This is the only example in Northern Europe of a rock tomb similar to the rock-cut chamber tombs of the Mediterranean region. The tomb, which was probably cut in Neolithic or Early Bronze Age times c.2000-1600BC, consists of a passage and two chambers hollowed out of the stone. Martin Martin thought there was a domestic purpose – 'at one of the ends... there is cut out a bed and pillow capable of two persons to lie in, at the other end there is a void space cut out resembling a bed, and above both these there is a large hole which is supposed was a vent for smoke'. Martin said that the 'common tradition is that a giant and his wife made this their place of retreat'. Sir Walter Scott said that 'the necromantic owner may sometimes still be seen sitting by the Dwarfie Stone.'. He considered the owner to be a troll, rather than a giant. Certainly the mysterious **Trowie Glen** (ON *troll* – evil monster, ogre or goblin) is beside the Dwarfie Hamars.

Even the **Dwarfie Hamars** have their legend. They are named after the dwarfs who, as everyone knows, are excellent smiths and who were responsible for forging Thor's famous hammer.

The track of roadway running through this legendary valley and past the Dwarfie Stane comes from **Moaness Pier** and the village of Hoy and ends up on the Atlantic coast at **Rackwick**, west of Rora Head. This picturesque old fishing village, stretching up the glen from a pebble beach, is Orkney's most isolated spot. The school closed in 1954 and the population has faded away although some of the cottages are reinhabited by visitors in the summer months and the famous composer, Sir Peter Maxwell Davies, used to live and compose in a converted croft in the hills above the village. Many years ago the men of Rackwick were known as fine fishermen and even finer country dancers. They cheerfully walked 6km over the ghostly hills to Hoy village, danced the night through, and then walked back home again.

Most of the north of Hoy is now sadly depopulated. The main road runs down the east coast overlooking Scapa Flow, to **Lyness** opposite the island of Fara (No.10.7). During the Second World War Lyness was home to about 30,000 men when it was the headquarters for the Scapa Flow naval base. The village has never recovered from this invasion and the Navy left behind a desolate landscape of abandoned structures.

The secluded natural harbour of **Longhope**

(ON – long bay) is south of Lyness. On each ness, guarding the harbour entrance like a Pictish broch, is a **Martello Tower** [ND324935 and 338913]. These were built for protection against U.S. privateers during the Napoleonic War (1813–15). As this was an assembly point for convoys, the Towers were each equipped with a 24-pounder canon on top, quarters for the gunners in the middle, and ammunition stores at ground level. A century later, they were armed once again for the First World War.

Melsetter House at the head of Longhope is one of Orkney's finest historic buildings [ND269893] set in a beautiful garden. It was a laird's house for the Moodie family until the late 19th century when it was bought by a wealthy Englishman, J G M Heddle, whose architect, W R Lethaby, enlarged it in the tradition of William Morris with furniture designed by Ford Maddox Brown and Dante Gabriel Rossetti. It can be visited by appointment.

The renowned **Longhope Lifeboat Station** is at Brims, in Aith Hope [ND291887]. This station has a remarkable record of daring rescues and will always be remembered for the loss of its entire crew when it went to the assistance of the Liberian cargo ship *Irene* in 1969. A force nine gale had raged for three days and the sea state was appalling. Eight men died including the coxswain and his two sons and the second coxswain and both his sons.

The south of Hoy is more green and mellow than the northern part and there is an active farming community on **South Walls**. South Walls was a tidal island until a narrow causeway – **The Ayre** – was constructed over the sandbank. The lighthouse on Cantick Head was built by David Stevenson in 1858.

* * *

Access: Orkney Ferries: every day passenger (and bike) service, Stromness/Graemsay/ Moaness, 01856-850624; ro-ro service Houton, Mainland/ Lyness (some via Flotta), 01856-872044; bus service, Kirkwall/ Houton; 01856-870555. No bus service on Hoy but car, taxi, mini-bus and cycle-hire available. Tourist information, 01856-872856.

Anchorages:

1. Mo Ness and Bay of Quoys. Temp. anchorage in 3m, SE of ferry pier. The bay is mostly shoal.
2. Aith Hope, between Brims Ness and South Walls on the S coast. Reasonable anchorage in 4–11m, sand, off the former Longhope Lifeboat Station. Useful while waiting for a favourable tide.
3. Kirk Hope. Temp. anchorage in 7m in centre of bay beyond fish-farm. Exposed N and E.
4. Longhope, between S Walls and Hoy. Visitors' moorings E of pier. Anchor in 4–6m E of pier on S Ness avoiding fish-farm. There is 4m depth at outer end of pier but avoid obstructing ferry. Heavy squalls can occur with NW winds and use plenty of cable because of the weed. Snug anchorage in 7–10m about 2½c NW of South Ness beyond submarine cables.
5. Ore Bay and Mill Bay, opposite Fara, are not recommended as the bottom is foul with old hawsers and there are fish-cages. Temp. berth alongside concrete jetty but keep clear of ro-ro jetty *(for access to Museum)*.
6. Pegal Bay, in Rysa Sound. Attractive anchorage with good holding but part obstructed by fish-cages and in W gales there can be violent squalls. Bottom shelves steeply.
7. Lyrawa Bay, S of Green Head is generally too deep and exposed for comfortable anchorage but excellent holding. Head of bay is shoal.

10.6 Fara

Possibly (ON vaer-øy – ram island). Previously called South Pharay.

OS Maps: 1:50000 Sheet 7 1:25000 Sheet 462
Admiralty Charts: 1:200000 Nos.1942 or 1954 1:50000 No.2162 1:30000 No.35 1:26000 No.2581 large scale No.2568

Area: 295ha (729 acres)
Height: 43m (141 ft)

Population: 1841–55 (10 houses). 1881–68. 1891–76 (15 houses). 1931–28. 1961–5. 1971–0. 1981–0. Uninhabited.

Geology: Rousay Flags of Middle Old Red Sandstone.

History: In the 19th century both Fara and Rysa Little were part of the Melsetter estate (Hoy and Walls) belonging to the Moodie family.

* * *

FARA has always had a good reputation for its rich pastures but, as with so many little islands which have a viable economic potential, it was abandoned because of poor communications. Without an adequate pier more and more of the inhabitants were attracted to secure centres of population. It became uneconomic to employ a teacher for the few remaining children and as numbers decreased further the pressure on the remainder increased. Eventually the number dropped below the critical minimum capable of manning a boat and carrying out similar communal tasks and the population collapsed. For Fara this point was reached in the 1960s yet the island lies close to the east side of Hoy and almost a stone's throw from Flotta, both populated areas. Today the ferry routes almost circumnavigate it, and neighbouring Flotta prospers. There is always hope that one day the island will be reinhabited.

The cultivated area was mainly on the north-east side and most of the abandoned houses are in the north. The summit, **Thomson's Hill** (43m), is in the centre of the island.

There is a small pier with a windmill close behind it on the west coast south-west of Thomson's Hill. A track runs up the hill from the pier to Upper Quoy (ON *koie* – hut or shelter).

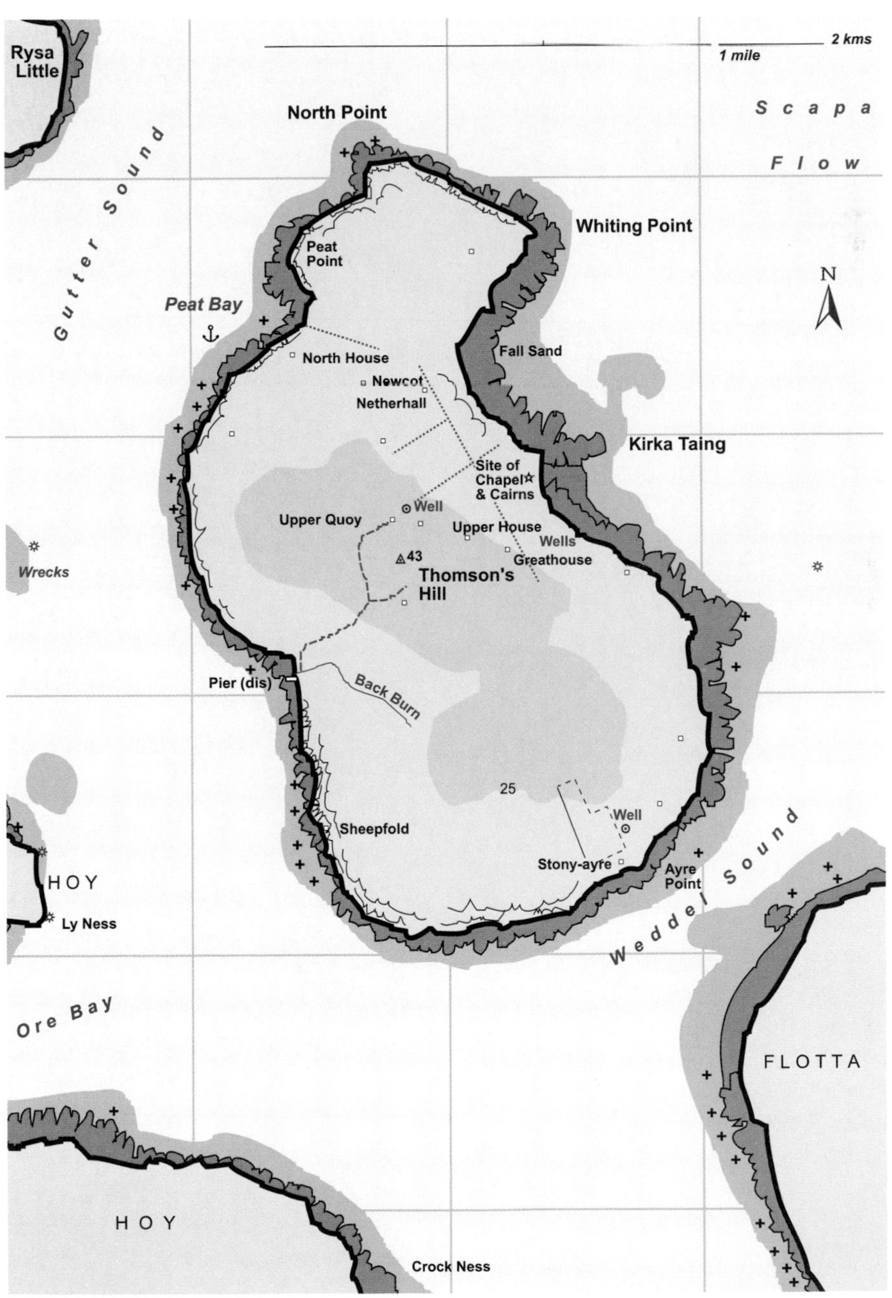

Peat Bay on the north-west coast is small and shallow with a stony beach, and **Kirka Taing** in the centre of the east coast means 'church point' – but there is little now to be seen of the chapel [ND331961].

* * *

Access: Try a Hoy or Flotta boatowner or Explorer Fast Sea Charter, Kirkwall, 01856-871225.

Anchorages: Most areas foul with old tackle so tripping line essential.

1. SW of Peat Point in Gutter Sound. Occasional anchorage in 4–6m, sand and shingle. Peat Bay is foul but suitable for landing by dinghy.
2. SW of Thomson's Hill. Temp. anchorage S of small pier. Beware rocks close in-shore further S.
3. West Weddel Sound opposite Sutherland Pier on Flotta. Settled weather anchorage in 3–4m, 1½c offshore.

10.7 Cava

(ON kálf-øy – calf island).

OS Maps: 1:50000 Sheet 6 or 7 1:25000 Sheet 462
Admiralty Charts: 1:200000 Nos.1942 or 1954 1:75000 No.2249 1:30000 No.35

Area: 107ha (264 acres)
Height: 36m (118 ft)

Population: 1841–23 (4 houses). 1881–25. 1891–13 (3 houses). 1931–14. 1961–0. 1981–2. 1991–2. 2001–0.

Geology: The underlying rock forms layers of flagstones and firm sandstones known as the Eday Beds of Middle Old Red Sandstone.

History: A notorious Orkney sailor, John Gow, who had become a pirate, returned to home waters in 1725. Having unsuccessfully tried to rob Clestrain House opposite Stromness, he visited Cava and kidnapped two or three girls which he took aboard his ship. A few days later they returned home. One story claims that they were laden with riches while the other declares that they were badly beaten and that one later died.

Gow went on to raid Graemsay (No.10.9) and Eday (No.10.21) but he was caught, tried, and sentenced to death by hanging. In life, Gow bungled every action and in death he was equally maladroit – or unlucky. The rope broke and he had to be hanged a second time. His total career in piracy lasted only six months.

A low grassy island with a stony shoreline, **CAVA** nowadays is mainly used for grazing.

Any small island lying off a larger island was often called Calf Island by the early settlers. Cava is distinct in being a Calf Island which has in turn its own Calf Island lying to the north – **Calf of Cava**. This is really a small peninsula which is joined to the north of Cava by a stony ridge. A small octagonal lighthouse stands on it.

A modest half-knot tide runs through the channel between Cava and **Rysa Little** (ON and E. – little heap of stones), an islet which does rise a little – 17m, to be precise. A small wrecked ship on this side of Cava lies to the north-west of a windmill standing near the shore. This is not exceptional as Scapa Flow is littered with wrecks.

After the German Fleet had surrendered to Admiral Beatty at the Firth of Forth on 21 November 1918, all the ships were transferred to Scapa Flow and held under the terms of the armistice. Most of the sailors were sent home and only skeleton German crews stayed aboard while the Allies argued about division of the spoils. The armistice was due to expire on 19 June 1919, with a return to hostilities so on the 17 June Admiral Von Reuter sent orders from his flagship *Emden* to make 'preparations for scuttling'. He was unaware that the armistice had been extended and the terms of a German surrender agreed.

On the 21 June 1919 – a quiet clear Saturday morning with the British Fleet away on exercise – all the mighty ships, some of the most modern fighting machines in the world, sank slowly beneath the waves. The entire fleet of more than 200 vessels was fully dressed with flags and the crews were in full dress uniform.

'Where they were sunk, they will rest and rust,' said the Admiralty in disgust. But in the following years many of the ships were salvaged or stripped of their valuable metal. The wrecks that remain are now a great tourist attraction and seen by thousands of divers.

The wrecks lying nearest to Cava, taken clockwise from the north-west, are the light cruiser *Karlsrühe*, the 25,000-ton battleships *Bayern*, *Kronprinz Wilhelm* and *Markgraf*, the light cruisers *Köln* and *Dresden* and the battleship *König*.

Cava Lodge, which is a conspicuous white house standing in the middle of the north part of the island, is an interesting example of a traditional old Orkney house. Only a very few examples still survive in fair condition.

Barrel of Butter to the north-east of the collection of wrecks is a small rock showing just above sea-level but marked by a beacon. Its quaint name comes from early times when the people of Orphir paid an annual rent of a barrel of butter to the local laird in return for permission to kill seals on the rock.

Access: Try Explorer, Kirkwall, 01856-871225 or Roving Eye Enterprises, Stromness, 01856-811309 which has an ROV to study the wrecks.

Anchorage: No recommended anchorages.

1. Point of the Ward, S extremity of Cava. Temp. anchorage in settled weather on sand-spit about 1½c S of Ward Point, 3–6m, sand and shingle. Tides are weak in this area.

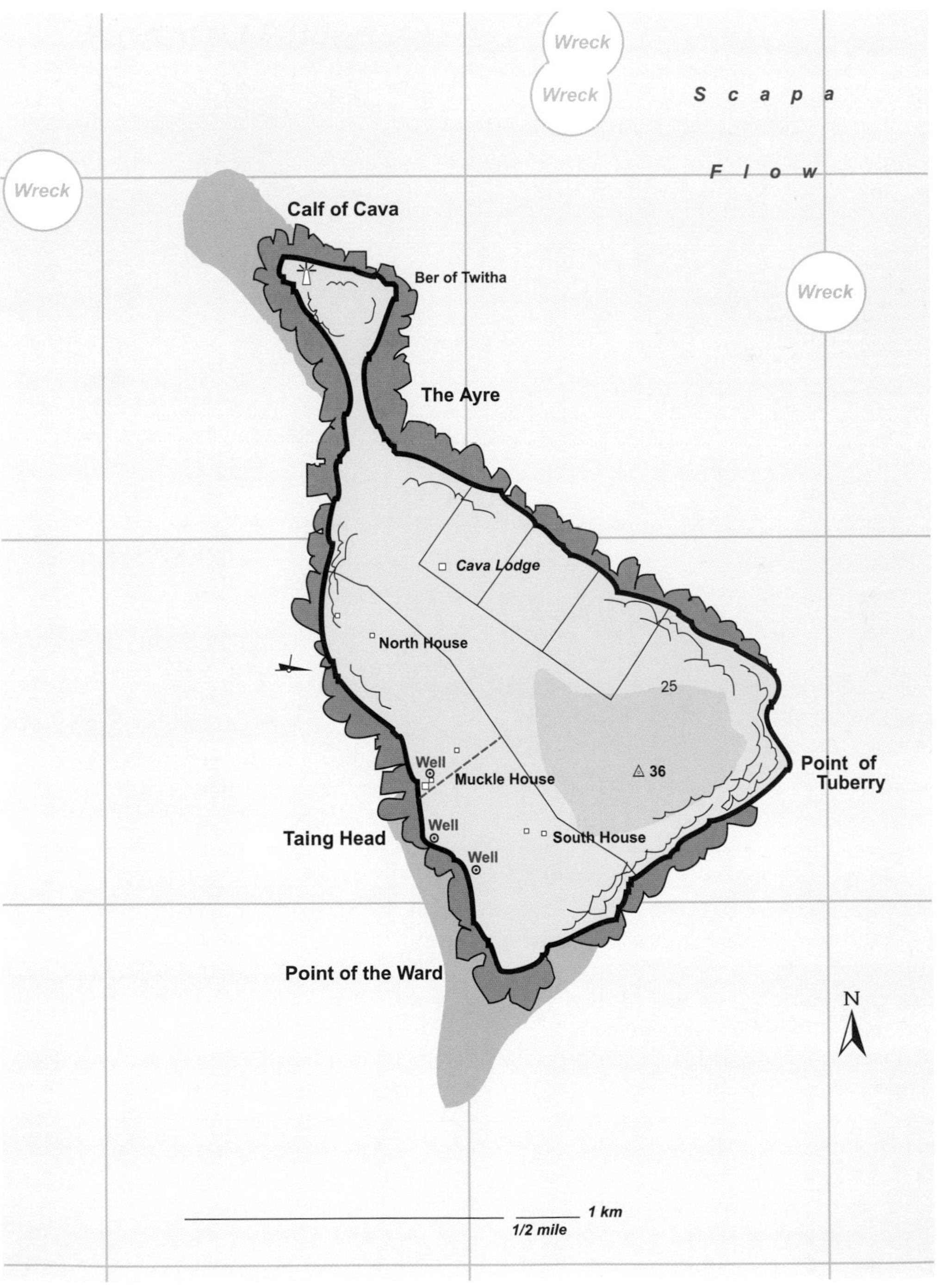

10.8 Copinsay

(ON kobbunge-øy – seal-pup island).

OS Maps: 1:50000 Sheet 6 1:25000 Sheet 461
Admiralty Charts: 1:200000 Nos.1942 or 1954
1:75000 No.2250

Area: 73ha (180 acres)
Height: 64m (210 ft)

Owner: Administered by the Royal Society for the Protection of Birds since 1972. Former lighthouse-keeper's cottage bought in 1991 by Paul Craig of Burston, Staffordshire as a holiday home. In 1993 he was very upset when Scottish Hydroelectric quoted nearly £1m to connect his house to the electricity mains.

Population: 1841–13 (1 house). 1881–5. 1891–9 (1 house). 1931–25. 1961–3 (lighthouse-keepers). 1981–0. 1991–0. 2001–0.

Geology: Tilted and eroded Rousay flags of Middle Old Red Sandstone with a top-skin of reasonable turf.

History: According to the sagas a great sea-battle was fought north of Copinsay, off the Mainland coast of Deerness. King Karl (there is some uncertainty who King Karl was but he might be King Duncan of Scotland, father of Macbeth) fought a battle with Thorfinn the Mighty. The ships were laid side by side and Earl Thorfinn leapt off his poop into the King's ship and struck out boldly. The King had eleven ships while Thorfinn only had five but his attack was so merciless that the King fled.

Wildlife: Copinsay has its fair share of seals but it is best known nowadays for its bird life. The most interesting time for bird-watching is from May to July but there is also much to be seen in the autumn. Copinsay is a Nature Reserve which has been administered by the Royal Society for the Protection of Birds since 1972 as the James Fisher Memorial Island. There are about 10,000 pairs of kittiwake, 30,000 guillemot, 1,000 razorbill, and many fulmar, eider, ringed plover, rock dove, raven and twite breeding here and even a few corncrake. No gannets have nested here since 1860. The adjacent Holms – which are accessible at low tide – also have arctic tern, puffin and black guillemot, plus a few common tern. The Horse rock-stack is covered with birds including a small colony of cormorant.

THE CLIFFS OF COPINSAY – GUILLEMOTS AND KITTIWAKES SPRINKLED LIKE CONFETTI

* * *

COPINSAY is a steeply-tilted green island which reaches a height of 64m right at the edge of the cliffs on its south-east side as though it had been abruptly sliced with a giant knife. From this high point the ground slopes steadily down to the west. The cliff summit is dominated by the lighthouse, a white tower standing 16m above the cliff-top and in summer the rock ledges are heavily populated with gulls, guillemots, razorbills, kittiwakes and shags.

A track runs down the hill from the lighthouse to the old farmhouse. This was still a working farm after the Second World War and although its isolation caused problems it was considered quite a good productive farm.

The **Giant Stone** is a huge boulder which according to legend was thrown at the island by a giant who lived on the farm of Stembister in Deerness on Mainland. The name Stembister means stone farm.

Apart from the south-eastern cliff-face the

island is surrounded by reefs, holms and skerries. The farmhouse stands on a small peninsula with a long rock saddle, Isle Rough, connecting Copinsay to **Corn Holm** in the west. This divides North Bay from South Bay and can be walked across at low water. There was once a little chapel on Corn Holm but the difficulty of access must have been a problem for the islanders intending to worship in it.

Corn Holm is linked by drying reefs to **Ward Holm** in the south and **Black Holm** in the west. Ward Holm has a prehistoric cairn on it.

Horse Sound which is about half a mile wide separates the **Horse of Copinsay**, a grass-topped rectangular stack 18m high, from North Nevi (ON *nøv* – fist), the north-east extremity of Copinsay. As with so many small islands the demand for grazing was so great that the islanders would

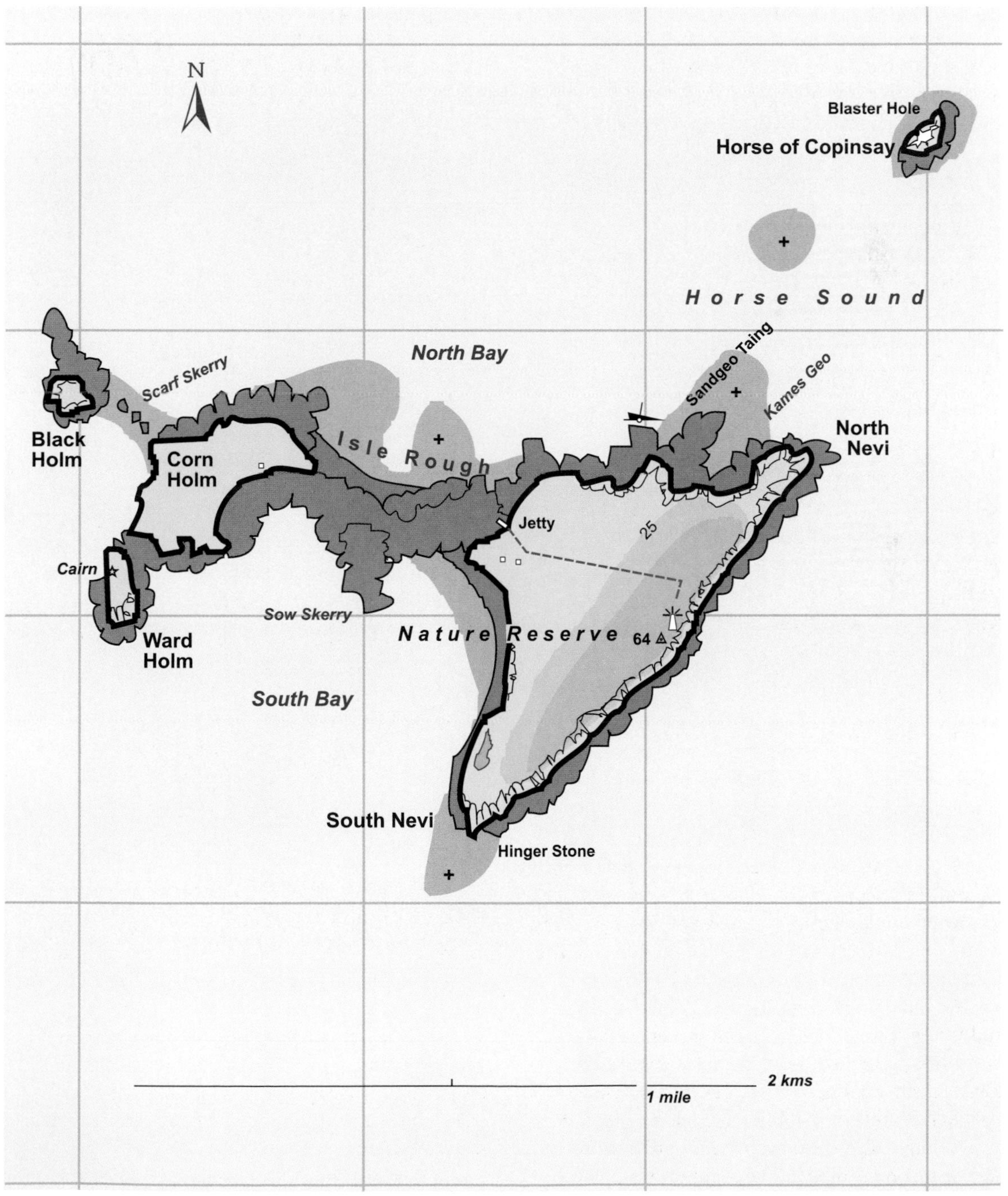

carry sheep to the top of the Horse, but it was said that it could fatten one sheep and feed two, but that three would starve. In the spring pigs were also hoisted to the top to fatten on the huge 'crop' of sea-birds' eggs. The pigs' coarse hair was used to make the strong rope needed for fowling. 'Lee-running' was the local name for the organised collection of seabirds' eggs which was still practised on Copinsay until the 1940s.

A hole through the Horse is called **Blaster Hole** because of the power of the water-jet which is forced through it and 60m into the sky by easterly gales.

* * *

Access: Boat trips by arrangement: *Verona*, Deerness, 01856-741252; or Explorer Charter, Kirkwall, 01856-871225.

Anchorage: No recommended anchorages but there is a landing jetty.
1. Horse Sound. Temp. anchorage in 6–8m slightly E of the line of the W coast of Copinsay (main island) and about 1½c offshore to avoid in-shore rocks.

10.9 Graemsay

(ON Gríms-øy – Grim's island).

OS Maps: 1:50000 Sheet 6 or 7 1:25000 Sheets 462 or 463
Admiralty Charts: 1:200000 No.1954 1:30000 No.35 large scale No.2568

Area: 409ha (1011 acres)
Height: 62m (203 ft)

Owner: Arthur Ritch, a crofter at Fillets, bought the 360-acre Sandside estate in 1996 for £55,000. A. D. Johnston of Stromness is another owner.

Population: 1841–214 (48 houses). 1881–236. 1891–223 (47 houses). 1931–114. 1961–51. 1981–21. 1991–27. 2001–21.

Geology: Mostly Lower Stromness Flags, a finely laminated Middle Old Red Sandstone, which has eroded on the surface to a fine soil. Two major volcanic faults on a north-south axis roughly divide the island into three equal sections. Apart from the outcrops of ancient granites and schists through the Old Red Sandstone there is a larger patch of granite-schist complex on the north coast – one of the few such outcrops to be found in Orkney.

History: Two early Celtic sites on Graemsay are dedicated respectively to St Bride and St Columba.

There are a number of crofts on the island but only one farm which is at Bu in Sandside. This was the original settlement of the natural son of Earl Robert Stewart when he was given the island by his father.

The 19th-century herring industry led to an increased interest in navigational safeguards and the construction of the two lighthouses, Hoy High and Hoy Low – both of which were built in 1851. Even so, on New Year's Day 1866, the *Albion*, en route to New York was wrecked off the Point of Oxan.

* * *

In Hoy Sound, off the comely island of **GRAEMSAY,** the tide can run so fast that the surface of the sea forms high ridges with whirlpools in the troughs. The ridges slowly but constantly move, like sand dunes during a sandstorm. These areas of violent turbulent water are called 'roosts' (ON *rost* – maelstrom) and Hoy Sound is a good example.

Graemsay is a green refuge with fertile soil encompassed by savage reefs, wrecks and shoals. It has two low hills, **East Hill** (49m) and **West Hill** (62m), the summit. The small lighthouse, **Hoy Low**, is on the north-western extremity, Point of Oxan, and a coastal battery was built beside it in the Second World War. The big lighthouse, **Hoy High** (33m), has an upper balcony supported on Gothic arches and keepers' houses built like Assyrian temples! It is in the north-east on the Taing of Sandside (ON – Sandside point) next to the island's only bay, the **Bay of Sandside.** This is also known as **The Hap** and it is shallow and rocky and guarded by the **Skerry of Cletts** and a dangerous reef called **The Lash.**

The small fishing pier and the ferry pier are east of Hoy High lighthouse. Further south a projection called **The Nevi** (ON *nøv* – promontory or fist) ends in the dangerous Sow Skerry.

A road runs across the island between the Bay of Sandside and a church at Kirk Geo on the south coast. Other roads feed off to the scattered dwellings and there is a small school beside West Hill. In 1996 Orkney Council decided to close the school as there was only one pupil. (This was sad news as the closing of any island school often spells eventual death for the community.)

The islanders own a number of boats. These are mainly used for lobster fishing but they are sometimes needed for last-minute shopping at Stromness as, although it has a post-office, Graemsay has no shop. The islanders are good innovative farmers and fishermen. It was Patrick Honeyman of Graemsay who first introduced the Scots plough to Orkney. He even risked buying two of them at a time when only single-stilted ploughs were in general use.

Access: Orkney Ferries every day passenger and cycle service (by request), Stromness/ Graemsay/ Hoy, 01856-850624. Stopover time to visit Graemsay is usually possible.

Anchorage: There is no recommended anchorage and there are many hazards. Temp lying alongside the pier must be timed to avoid causing obstruction.

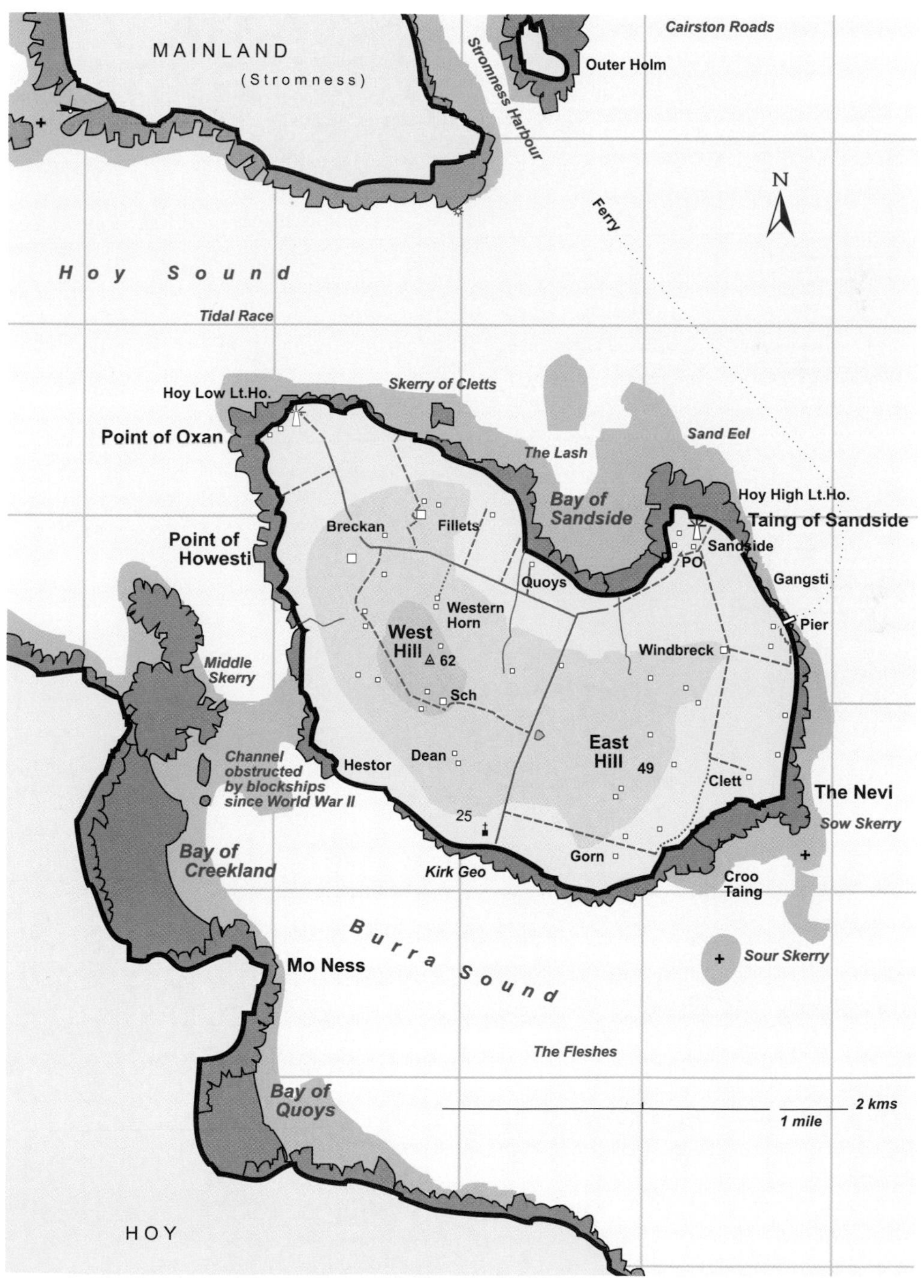

10.10 Mainland

(ON megenland – mainland) An alternative Norse name was 'Hrossey' – the island of horses. 16th century Latinist George Buchanan mistakenly called Mainland 'Pomona' and for a time the name was widely used but never by the islanders themselves. To Orcadians the Scottish mainland is simply 'Scotland'.

South Ronaldsay

(ON – Rognvald's island).

Burray

(ON borgr-øy – fort or broch island).

Hunda

(ON hund-øy – dog island).

O S Maps: 1:50000 Sheet 6 1:25000 Sheets 461 and 463. Admiralty Charts: 1:200000 No.1954 1:75000 Nos.2249 and 2250 1:30000 No.35 part S coast 1:25000 No.2584 part NE coast 1:12500 Kirkwall large scale No.2568 Stromness

Area: 58308ha (144079 acres)
Height: 271m (889 ft)

Owner: Multiple ownership.

Population:

	1841	1881	1891	1931	1961	1981	1991	2001
Mainland	16022	17165	16498	13352	13495	14000	15123	15315
S'th R'say	2331	2557	2315	1312	980	891	943	854
Burray	532	685	681	379	262	283	363	357
Hunda	6	8	7	0	0	0	0	0
G's Holm	0	0	0	0	0	0	0	0
L'b Holm	?	12	8	7	0	0	0	0
	18903	20423	19508	15043	14737	15174	16429	16526

Geology: As with all the Orkney islands, Mainland is sedimentary rock of Devonian (Old Red Sandstone) age except for some small patches of granite-schist complex. One of these is Brinkies Brae above Stromness which is the oldest place, geologically, in Orkney. The Dalradian foliated-granite rock was once an island in a great freshwater loch.

The sandstones in the west of Mainland are Upper and Lower Stromness Flags separated by a Fish Bed. These Stromness Beds are finely laminated and account for the dramatic cliff scenery in this area. The sandstones of the east are of the Rousay type although the Scapa Flow coastline, the Kirkwall area, Deerness and most of South Ronaldsay are Eday Beds, which are fine building stone. Deerness has some thick lava intrusions and the Gloup of Deerness on the east coast is a great rock hole connected to the sea by an underground fissure.

History: Mainland Orkney has so many notable relics dating from the late Stone Age that one must assume there was an advanced social structure on the island and considerable relative prosperity.

This age was followed by that of the broch-builders and the Picts (who may or may not have been the same people) but the Norsemen were not far behind them and some time in the 9th century the Earldom of Orkney was established. A dynasty followed which is well chronicled in the Norse Sagas and this reached its zenith in the 11th century under Earl Thorfinn the Mighty. Thereafter there was much infighting between rival descendants culminating in the death of Earl John in a drunken brawl in Thurso in 1231. He was the last of the Norse earls.

The succession passed to a son of the Earl of Angus, and various pale shadows followed him. King Haakon died in Kirkwall in 1263 and the Norse hold became ever more tenuous.

In 1379 Henry Sinclair of Roslin inherited the earldom and was formally invested by the King of Norway. He was a great sailor-adventurer and there is good evidence that he sailed to America and established settlements there long before Columbus.

In 1468 King Christian of Norway and Denmark included Orkney and Shetland as part of Margaret, Maid of Norway's, dowry but subject to a cash redemption. The total cash failed to be paid so Scotland wasted no time in annexing the islands in 1471.

Wildlife: Mainland has over 600 species of flowering plant, including wild lupins, daffodils and fourteen species of wild orchid. At places near the water's edge the rare Oyster Plant, *Mertensia maritima*, can be seen but the cliff-top home of the magenta-coloured Scottish Primrose, *Primula scotica*, is a secret.

Brown hares are very common on Mainland and so are rabbits. There are no frogs but there are toads. The otter is not nearly so common here as it is in Shetland, probably due to the amount of cultivation.

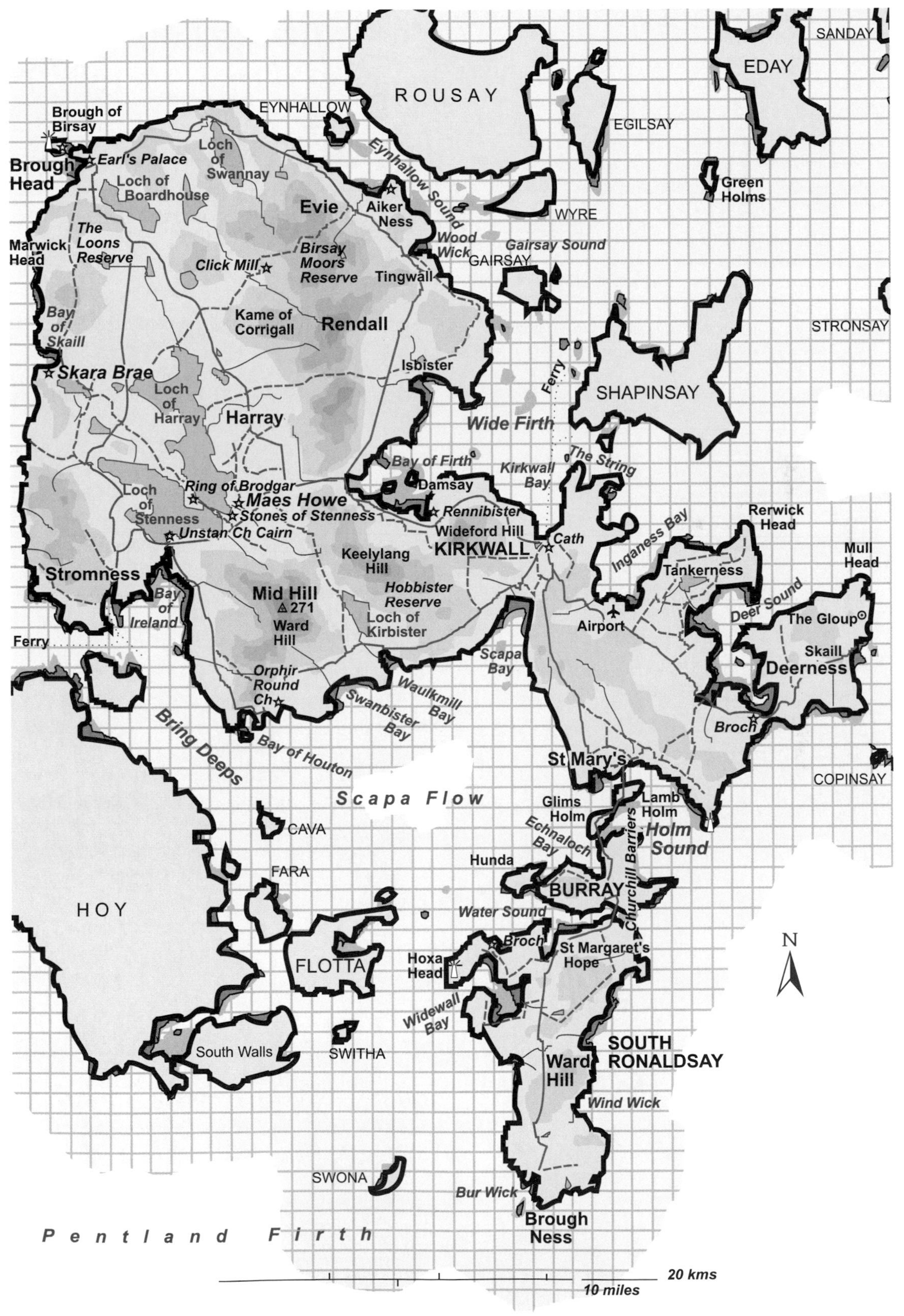
ROUSAY
EYNHALLOW
EDAY
SANDAY
EGILSAY
Brough of Birsay
Brough Head
Earl's Palace
Loch of Swannay
Loch of Boardhouse
Evie
Aiker Ness
Eynhallow Sound
Green Holms
WYRE
Marwick Head
The Loons Reserve
Birsay Moors Reserve
Click Mill
Wood Wick
GAIRSAY
Gairsay Sound
Tingwall
Bay of Skaill
Kame of Corrigall
Rendall
STRONSAY
Skara Brae
Isbister
Ferry
SHAPINSAY
Loch of Harray
Harray
Wide Firth
Bay of Firth
Kirkwall Bay
The String
Damsay
Ring of Brodgar
Maes Howe
Loch of Stenness
Stones of Stenness
Rennibister
Unstan Ch Cairn
Wideford Hill
Cath
KIRKWALL
Inganess Bay
Rerwick Head
Mull Head
Keelylang Hill
Tankerness
Stromness
Mid Hill
271
Hobbister Reserve
Bay of Ireland
Deer Sound
The Gloup
Airport
Ward Hill
Loch of Kirbister
Ferry
Skaill
Scapa Bay
Deerness
Orphir Round Ch
Waulkmill Bay
Swanbister Bay
Broch
Bring Deeps
Bay of Houton
St Mary's
COPINSAY
Scapa Flow
Glims Holm
Lamb Holm
CAVA
Echnaloch Bay
Holm Sound
Churchill Barriers
Hunda
FARA
BURRAY
HOY
Water Sound
Broch
St Margaret's Hope
N
FLOTTA
Hoxa Head
Widewall Bay
South Walls
SWITHA
SOUTH RONALDSAY
Ward Hill
Wind Wick
SWONA
Bur Wick
Brough Ness
Pentland Firth
20 kms
10 miles

West of Kirkwall there are three areas of heather moorland providing one of the finest moorland bird communities in Britain. Moor breeders include hen harrier, short-eared owl, red grouse, merlin, arctic and great skua, golden plover, dunlin, snipe, curlew, reed bunting, wheatear, stonechat, sedge warbler, twite, kestrel, woodpigeon and hooded crow. Lochan breeders are the red-throated diver, wigeon, teal, red-breasted merganser, eider and shelduck. On the lochs and wetlands are mallard, shelduck, wigeon, teal, pintail, shoveller, tufted duck, red-breasted merganser, dunlin, snipe, redshank, corncrake, sedge warbler and reed bunting. On the coasts there are kittiwake, guillemot, fulmar, razorbill and a few puffin. The Loch of Harray can sometimes hold 10,000 wintering duck and it is one of Britain's most important sites for pochard. Particular sites are: Birsay Moors and Cottascarth RSPB Reserve; Loch of Banks; The Loons RSPB Reserve; Loch of Boardhouse; Brough of Birsay; Marwick Head RSPB Reserve; Loch of Harray and Loch of Stenness; Binscarth Wood; Hobbister RSPB Reserve; and Stromness Harbour.

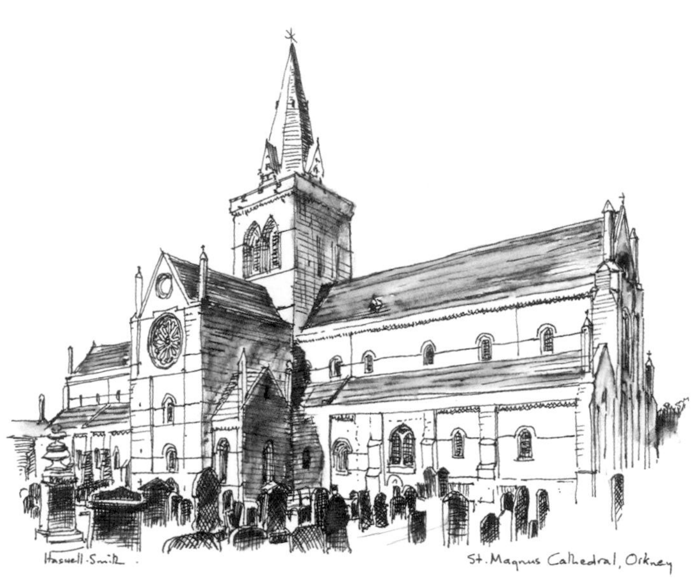

ST MAGNUS' CATHEDRAL

East of Kirkwall, Burray, and South Ronaldsay herring and lesser black-backed gulls predominate as breeders in the narrow band of moorland whereas the farmland is most noted for migrants rather than breeders and many rare ones have been recorded. Among coast breeders curlew predominate. Particular sites are: Graemeshall Loch; Deer Sound; Scapa Bay; Kirkwall Harbour; Loch of Tankerness; The Churchill Barriers; and Echnaloch Bay.

* * *

A narrow neck of land divides east and west **MAINLAND**. This is the strategic site of Orkney's 'capital' – Kirkwall.

Kirkwall (ON *kirkjuvagr* – church bay) was established by the Norse in the 11th century but reached prominence and city status in the 12th century thanks to its harbour and its new **Cathedral of St Magnus**. This massive edifice in early Norman style, founded in 1137 by Magnus's nephew, Rognvald III, contains the remains of both its founder and its saint built into the great piers in the central bay. The transepts, part of the choir and part of the nave with its interlacing wall-arcades are the oldest parts. It is almost surprising to find this magnificent Gothic structure in a town of less than 7000 inhabitants but, I suppose, this is a true picture of what a medieval cathedral city was really like. The small houses clustered like chickens round the mother-hen cathedral. The building was completed in the 15th century and was saved by the townsfolk from destruction during the Reformation but when Cromwell's men arrived they used it as a prison and for stabling their horses. After that only the choir continued to be used as a parish church and the neglected structure deteriorated. It was restored in 1913–1930 and again in the 1980s.

Close to the cathedral is the **Bishop's Palace** which is mostly a 16th-century reconstruction of the original 12th-century building. It was here that King Haakon died in 1263 after his defeat by the Scots at Largs. Across the road is the **Earl's Palace** which has been called the finest structure of 16th-century Scotland. This magnificent building was built with forced labour by Earl Patrick, known as 'Black Pate', a man who was so ignorant that his sentence of death was delayed for a week to allow him to 'better inform himself'.

When entering the harbour, after passing the

little islet called **Thieves Holm**, it is difficult to appreciate that much of the inner part of the bay, sheltered by The Ayre and called the **Peerie Sea**, was filled in during the 1800s to allow the town to expand to the west. Originally the cathedral and the Bishop's Palace would have dominated the harbour as well as the town. The shallow Peerie Sea must have provided excellent protection for Norse longboats.

For Orkney history it is worth visiting the Orkney Library in Laing Street and **Tankerness House Museum**, a well-restored example of a merchant's house.

Kirkwall is a charming town which was made a royal burgh by James III in 1486 when he also gifted the cathedral to the citizens. The main street, which used to run close to the seafront, is Albert Street, irregular and narrow, known simply as **The Street**.

East of Kirkwall and south of Inganess Bay is **Kirkwall Airport** set in an area of fertile fields and fat cattle. The road continues to the eastern extremity of Mainland – Deerness parish – the old Norse hunting ground where the

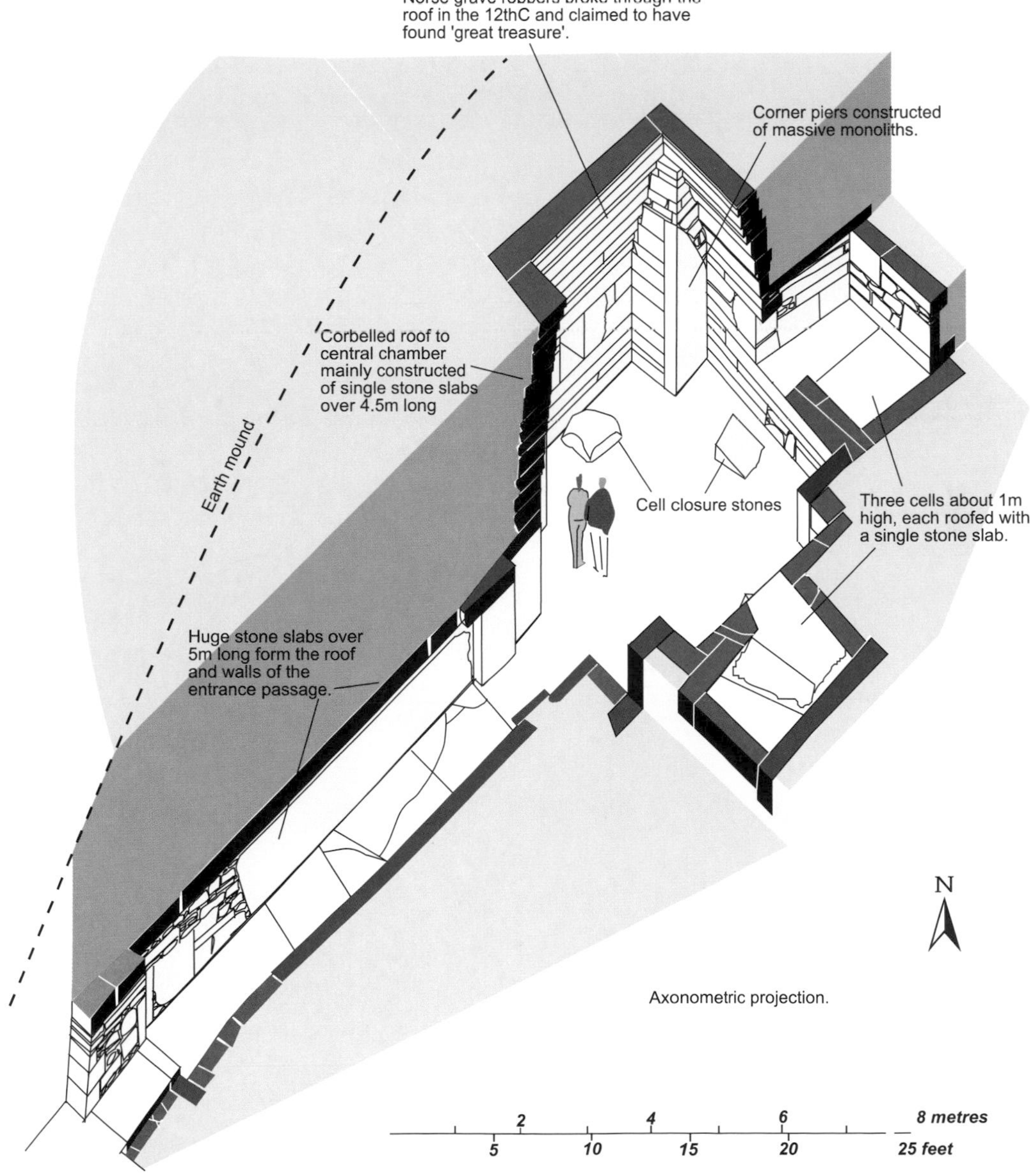
Norse grave robbers broke through the roof in the 12thC and claimed to have found 'great treasure'.
Corner piers constructed of massive monoliths.
Corbelled roof to central chamber mainly constructed of single stone slabs over 4.5m long
Earth mound
Cell closure stones
Three cells about 1m high, each roofed with a single stone slab.
Huge stone slabs over 5m long form the roof and walls of the entrance passage.
N
Axonometric projection.
2
4
6
8 metres
5
10
15
20
25 feet

MAGNIFICENT MAES HOWE

bones of red deer are still to be found in the peat bogs. Beside the road that crosses the narrow Deerness isthmus are the remains of the broch of Dingieshowe, and, to the north, the wide sands of St Peter's pool, covered with wading birds. At the **Brough of Deerness**, after passing The Gloup (ON *gljúfr* – hollow or ravine) [HY592079], a growling subterranean sea-vent caused by the sea breaking through the roof of a large cave, a rough walk of about 1km brings you to the remains of an ancient monastery which was a place of pilgrimage until the 17thC [HY595088]. Male pilgrims walked barefoot round and round the holy building chanting and scattering water and sharp stones behind them.

The road running due south from Kirkwall reaches the pleasant village of St Mary's in the parish of Holm [ham]. Here there is the first of the **Churchill Barriers**.

On 14 October 1939 a German submarine slipped past the blockships in the eastern approaches to Scapa Flow and torpedoed *HMS Royal Oak*. 833 men were lost. Britain had only been at war for one month and the disaster had a serious effect on morale. Churchill later ordered barriers to be built between the eastern islands and Italian prisoners-of-war provided the labour for this task. The Italians handled the engineering with skill and supported their faith by converting two Nissen huts into the delightful little **Italian Chapel** on Lamb Holm [HY488006]. This pious work was so appreciated by the Presbyterian Orcadians that in 1960 Signor Chiocchetti, and others who had done the original work, were invited to return to Orkney and restore the chapel paintings and interior to its wartime glory. Domenico Chiocchetti died in 1999.

Churchill Barrier No 2 crosses from **LAMB HOLM** to **GLIMS HOLM**, an islet which provides peat for local use, and the next Barrier reaches Burray. The old blockships can still be seen beside these causeways.

BURRAY has a great stretch of beach in its eastern bay, and the Reef linking it to **HUNDA**, which is particularly rich in birdlife, on its west coast. Burray is remembered for its colourful Jacobite laird, Sir James Stewart, who, in 1725, was involved in a murder in Kirkwall. He fled into exile and twenty years later joined the battle at Culloden. He survived the defeat and considered it safe after all these years to return home to Burray. But on arrival who should he meet but the son of his murder victim who promptly handed him over to the authorities. He died in a London prison.

Cross the 4th Barrier to **SOUTH RONALDSAY** and you are immediately greeted by a large windmill built for generating electricity [ND460938]. This was a trial to see if commercial electricity could be produced from Orkney's great power source – wind – but this early design was not particularly successful due to the high cost of maintenance. There has been talk of demolition of this obtrusive and noisy structure.

Nearby is **St Margaret's Hope** where there once was a chapel dedicated to Malcolm Canmore's Queen Margaret. It is sometimes wrongly claimed that the Hope is named after Margaret, Maid of Norway, who died in 1290. King Haakon's huge fleet of 120 ships anchored here at the start of August 1263 – the largest fleet in history ever to enter Scapa Flow before the 20th century. There was an eclipse of the sun that day which some would claim foretold the disaster that awaited him at Largs and his subsequent death in Kirkwall.

To the west is the Hoxa peninsula with a ruined broch where, according to the *Orkneyinga Saga*,

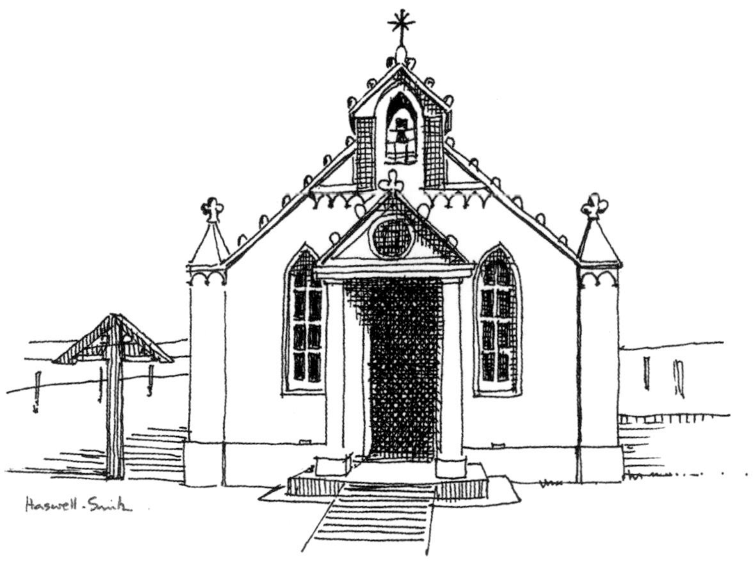

THE ITALIAN CHAPEL – A WARTIME WORK-OF-ART

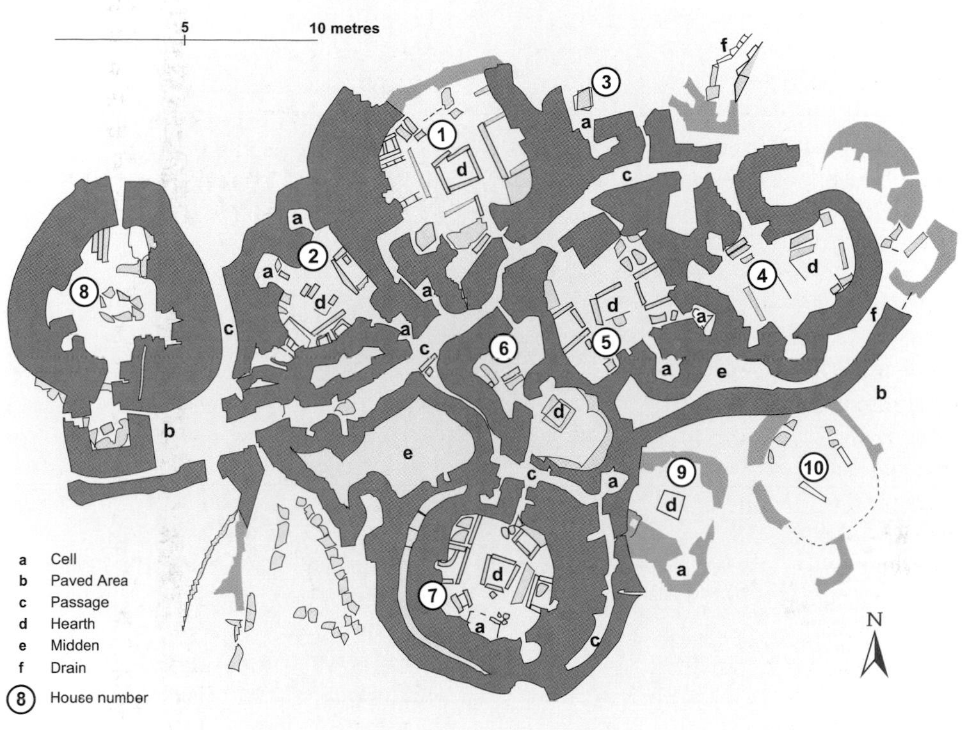

PLAN OF SKARA BRAE (*C.* 2800BC)

Thorfinn Skull-splitter is buried [ND425940].

Travelling southwards down the island the road passes **Ward Hill**, the summit of which is only 118m high but is a memorable viewpoint. From this distance tidal rips and treacherous seas fade into a vast expanse of untroubled ocean. But it was off this coast in 1969 that the Longhope lifeboat was lost with all on board while attempting to reach the wreck of the *Irene*.

In the south-west there is another 'Gloup' [ND472856] and a burned mound [ND465841]. These are both worth seeing, but they lie about a kilometre from the nearest road. Near here the 5000-year-old chambered cairn known as the **Tomb of the Eagles** was discovered in 1958. It contained around 16,000 human bones with their skulls lining the walls and the remains of at least eight sea eagles. It has an adjoining interpretative centre.

St Mary's Kirk at Burwick contains a penitent's stone, a block of whin with two foot-shaped hollows [ND439842]. One story claims that a man called Gallus prayed to the Virgin Mary for help when his ship sank. She sent a porpoise, who carried him ashore and then immortalised the poor beast by turning it into stone. Gallus built the church in gratitude.

The larger part of **MAINLAND** lies to the west of Kirkwall. The southern road from Kirkwall (A964) runs along the shores of Scapa Flow and through the **Hobbister Hill Nature Reserve**, where raptors can be seen while waders frequent the shores of Waukmill Bay. The next bay, Swanbister, was renowned in the 1830s for having a monster similar to the one which is reputed to inhabit Loch Ness (See also No.11.5).

Mainland's highest peak, **Mid Hill** (271m), is north of here and the last battle on Orkney soil was fought in the valley to the east of it. That was in 1529 when William Sinclair tried to wrest the earldom from his uncle, Sir William Sinclair. He raised an army with the support of the Earl of Caithness and sailed into Scapa Flow but his cousins raised a local army which defeated him.

This is the parish of Orphir (ON *or-fjara* – 'out of' low water) and beside **Orphir Bay** is a tiny church probably built by Earl Haakon Paulsson, the murderer of St Magnus [HY335044]. He must have done penance by a pilgrimage or crusade to the Holy Land, because the design echoes that of the Holy Sepulchre in Jerusalem. Only the apse now remains (the rest was demolished in 1757 for a Presbyterian preaching box) but the church is mentioned in the sagas as a 'magnificent church' facing the 'drinking-hall'. The Vikings had very clear priorities!

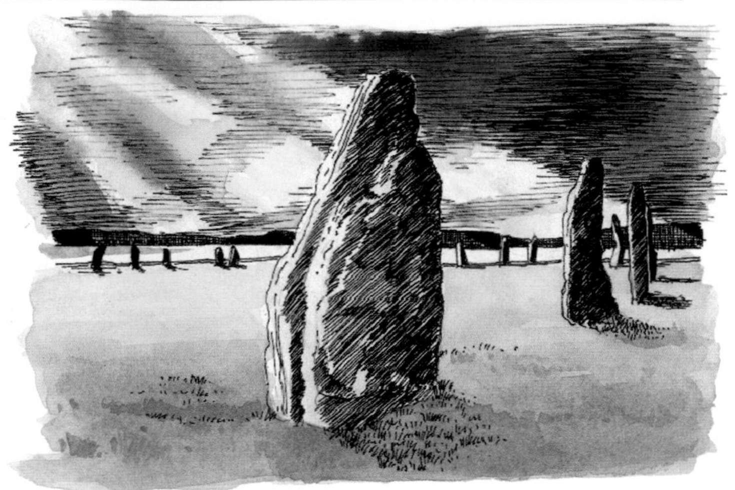

THE RING OF BRODGAR

The car ferry to Hoy sails from **Houton Bay** and the road then turns north up the coast of Clestrain Sound.

The northern road out of Kirkwall crosses a causeway and skirts **Wideford Hill** (225m) which is another marvellous view-point with a chambered cairn on its slopes [HY409121]. At **Rennibister** there is a good example of a souterrain or earth-house discovered in 1926 when a plough broke through the roof [HY397126]. The road continues along the south shore of Bay of Firth in which there are two small islands. The **Holm of Grimbister** is farmed, and **Damsay** (ON – pond island), which has several small pools on it, is mentioned in the sagas. It was in the days when Erlend and Sweyn were at war with Earls Rognvald and Harald. Erlend celebrated Christmas on Damsay with his men and then, dead-drunk, he returned to his ship to sleep. Although it was a full moon he and his men were taken by surprise and slaughtered. Tradition says that there was a nunnery on the island at one time and that no rats or mice are able to survive there.

This area of central Mainland is littered with prehistoric monuments but possibly the greatest concentration is around Lochs Harray and Stenness. By Tormiston Mill, a 19th century watermill, there is the green tumulus of **Maeshowe** (ON – great mound), Britain's largest chambered cairn and an example of truly breathtaking megalithic craftsmanship [HY318127]. A long, low, narrow passage leads into a large chamber with corbelled walls and smaller side chambers. The passage is accurately aligned to take advantage of the configuration of the hill silhouette on Hoy. This means that sunlight enters the chamber not only at the winter solstice but also with brief flashes of light on 11 November, 1 December, 11 January and 31 January. The work has a flavour of Egyptian design and constructional similarity to the Treasury of Atrius in Greece although the proportions are more modest. The smaller chambers are floored and roofed with single massive stones. Maeshowe was raided by the Vikings – howebreaking was a very popular pastime – and they also indulged in graffiti in the form of runic inscriptions. One comment refers to a great treasure but does not make it clear whether it was Norse or Neolithic treasure. The longest inscription has been translated as 'These runes were incised by the best runester in the west, using the axe that Gauk Thrandilsson once owned in south Iceland.' Other comments are timeless in character – 'Thorny was bedded; Helgi says so,' and 'Ingigerd is the best of them all.'

Close to Maeshowe are the **Standing Stones of Stenness** (ON *steine-nes* – promontory of the stones) [HY307125]. One of the remaining four stones is over 5m high and nearby is the, even higher, Watch Stone. Only 1½km north, on the narrow isthmus between Lochs Harray and Stenness, is the dramatic **Ring of Brodgar**, with twenty-seven of the original sixty stones still standing [HY294133]. And between these are freshly-excavated 5000-year-old structures and a monumental wall crossing the Ness of Brodgar. I remember visiting the Ring at dawn and seeing it washed with pale sunlight against an ominous dark sky surrounded by the grey lochs and windswept grassland.

Further west, where Loch Stenness spills into the Bay of Ireland is **Unstan Cairn** [HY283117], an important chambered cairn first excavated in 1844. It produced the largest collection of Stone Age pottery found in Scotland (now housed in the Royal Scottish Museum, Edinburgh) as well as two seated human skeletons.

Stromness was a prosperous port for many centuries. It has less than 2000 inhabitants but has a very long waterfront dating back to the time when it was overcrowded and busy with ships on the northern sailing routes. From 1670 to 1891 it was a base for the Hudson Bay Company, in the 18th and 19th centuries it was a supply base for the Davis Strait whaling fleet, and for a short time it was involved in the North American rice trade. The ships of Captain Cook were serviced here after his last ill-fated Pacific expedition as also were those of Sir John Franklin on the way to look for the North-West Passage. **Login's Well**, which provided the ships with fresh water, can still be seen, and the **Natural History Museum** has many interesting exhibits from Stromness's past. As for the future, a European Marine Energy Centre was opened here in 2004 making Orkney a world leader in the testing of wave power devices.

Stromness was also the home of the poet and writer, George Mackay Brown.

Some 10km north of Stromness on the west coast at the Bay of Skaill is possibly Orkney's most exciting archaeological site, **Skarabrae** [HY230187]. This astonishing prehistoric village dating from c.3100BC only came to light when it was exposed by a storm in 1850. A sandstorm buried the original village in about 2450BC, thus preserving a moment of time for posterity, and 5000 years later another storm revealed it. It was conscientiously excavated in 1928 and this has given us a marvellous chance to spy on the everyday domestic life of our ancient ancestors. The tiny individual 'houses' are closely linked by passages and each contains items of primitive Stone Age furniture – beds, dressers, lockers, hearth, fish-larder pools – and personal effects made of pottery, stone and whalebone. To the north of the Bay of Skaill a great Viking treasure was found in 1858 – the Skaill Hoard – enormous brooches, rings, ingots of silver, and coins. The Vikings were anything but parochial – some of the coins had been minted in Baghdad!

Further north the coast road passes between **The Loons**, an area of pools and swamps and breeding waders, and **Marwick Head**, whose cliffs support vast numbers of seabirds. Both are Nature Reserves.

Marwick Head is the site of the **Kitchener Memorial** [HY227251]. Field-Marshal the Earl Kitchener of Khartoum was invited by the Czar to visit Russia and discuss the progress of the First World War. He travelled to Thurso by night-train, crossed the Pentland Firth in a destroyer, lunched with Admiral Jellicoe on the *Iron Duke* in Scapa Flow and then boarded the cruiser *Hampshire*. It was 4 June 1916. In spite of a severe gale the *Hampshire* left by Hoy Sound and turned north. Then in very heavy seas off Marwick Head she struck a German mine and sank immediately with only twelve survivors. Local Orcadians were forbidden to assist in a rescue attempt or speak to the press and the official Government report was obscure. Naturally, this encouraged talk of a cover-up and many wild stories circulated that there was gold aboard, Kitchener was still alive, or even that he had been deliberately executed. This is still a war-grave and diving is forbidden.

The north-west corner of Mainland is Brough Head (ON *borg* – broch, or the island at the end of a tidal isthmus) in the parish of Birsay (ON – broch island). **Brough of Birsay** is a drying or tidal island with extensive remains of a Viking settlement and an early medieval chapel [HY240285]. The chapel is built on the remains of an earlier, 6th or 7th-century, chapel. The settlement may have been part of a well-garrisoned fortress. This island well repays a visit but avoid being trapped by the incoming tide covering the causeway.

Overlooking Brough of Birsay is **Earl Stewart's Palace** [HY248279]. The palace was rebuilt in 1574 but this is the site where the earls of Orkney had their palace before moving to Kirkwall in the 12th century. The present ruin shows little of the original splendour.

The north coast road passes Loch of Swannay (thought by some to be the best trout-fishing loch on Mainland), and skirts Eynhallow Sound in the parish of Evie (ON – swirling tide). Here, like a sentinel on windswept Aiker Ness, stands **Gurness Broch** [HY382268]. This is the best-preserved broch in Orkney but there is a great complex of ruins surrounding it which are also fascinating to explore.

About 6km south-west of Gurness Broch by an undulating minor road is Orkney's last surviving example of a **Click Mill** [HY325228]. These were old horizontal watermills, once common in Scandinavia and still to be found in North Pakistan. South of here is the parish of Harray (ON – hunting territory), the only land-locked parish in Orkney.

* * *

Access: NorthLink ro-ro, 0845-6000-449; Scrabster/ Stromness daily (2hrs): or Aberdeen/ Kirkwall (6hrs), Tue., Thu., Sat., Sun., return overnight (7hrs), Mon., Wed., Fri. Pentland Ferries ro-ro, 01856-831226, Gill's Bay/ St Margaret's Hope (1hr) daily. By air: scheduled flights most days to Kirkwall from Aberdeen, Edinburgh, Glasgow, Sumburgh, Inverness and Stornoway, 0870-850-9850 and 01856-872494. Kirkwall airport, 01856-886210. There is a good bus service on Mainland, 01856-870555 or 08457-740740. Tourist information, 01856-872856.

Anchorages: Considerable care and experience is needed due to the many erratic tidal conditions. Eynhallow Sound is particularly hazardous.

1. Stromness Harbour. Enter by buoyed channel using leading lights. New all-year marina beyond the harbour, excellent shelter. Anchorage between South Pier and Lighthouse Pier or centre W of Inner and Outer Holm.
2. Bay of Ireland. Anchorage 4c NE of Bu Point in 5–6m, sand. Exposed to S.
3. Bay of Houton. Enter E side of Holm of Houton (or Howton) and follow leading lights, depth 3.5m. Anchor in centre of bay, 4–5m, sand. Good shelter, good holding, but restricted space.
4. Swanbister Bay. Occasional anchorage in off-shore winds, NE of pier in 5–8m, sand and mud.
5. Waulkmill Bay, E of Ve Ness dries out 3c from head. Not recommended.
6. Scapa Bay (about 2km S of Kirkwall). Approach as sailing directions with buoyed wreck of *HMS Royal Oak (sunk by German sub in Oct 1939)* to starboard and Scapa Skerry buoy to port. Anchor mid-bay off the stone pier, clear of commercial traffic. Good anchorage, except in S'lies, which bring a swell. Untenable in SW gales.
7. Bay of Ayre (village of St Mary's on N shore with two piers). One visitors' buoy in centre. Good anchorage off village in 2–6m, or lie alongside pier. Keep well clear of Barrier and fish-farm.
8. Echnaloch Bay on NW side of Burray. Sandy beach at head with small pier on NE side. Temp. anchorage in S'lies.
9. Hunda Sound. Excellent in any weather but many fish cages. Best mid-sound, in 7–11m, sand over clay, very good holding. Head and sides are shoal.
10. Water Sound. Good anchorage just W of Barrier in 2–6m or end of Burray pier, 2m.
11. St Margarets Hope (bay on S side of Water Sound). Approach with care on leading line. Fairway only 2.7m depth. Anchor in centre in 6m avoiding fish-farm and ferry. 100m-long pier on W side has 3m at end. Head and shores are foul.
12. Widewall Bay. Bottom sandy and shelves gradually. Give Herston Head a 2c berth. Useful when awaiting slack water for passage S.
13. Sand Wick is shallow and exposed.
14. Bur Wick (SW tip of S Ronaldsay) is fringed with reefs but has a sandy beach at its head. Temp. anchorage off beach in 5–7m in quiet weather.
15. Wind Wick, between Hesta and Halcro Heads. Temp. anchorage in light W'lies, 5–10m.
16. Holm Sound. Temp. anchorage well off the sandy beach which heads the bay on the NE side of Burray, in 6–7m, sand, good holding but if wind is between NE and SE leave at once.
17. E Weddel Sound, SW Holm Sound. Excellent anchorage in centre of Bay, E of blockship, E of Barrier and clear of fish-farm, 2–4m, sand. Best anchorage in this area.
18. Kirk Sound. Anchorage in Mainland bay N of E end of Lamb Holm, close in-shore, avoiding fish-farm, 3–6m, sand and rock. Exposed SE. *(Visit Italian Chapel, Lamb Holm.)*
19. Deer Sound. Take care when entering and give shores a reasonable offing. Good shelter, good holding and very few squalls. Anchor off the stone pier on NW side of the Sound, below Hall of Tankerness, or off Mirkady Point, mid-channel in 4–5m. St Peter's Bay is not recommended.
20. Inganess Bay (Shapinsay Sound). Good anchorage with shelter from W and S and good holding in 6–8m, sand and shells. There are reefs and shallows off both entrance points.
21. Bay of Meil, W of Head of Holland. Visitors moorings. Good anchorage in centre of S part of bay clear of fish farm, 6–8m, sand.
22. Bay of Carness. Fringed with reefs but good anchorage in centre. Avoid fish-farm.
23. Bay of Kirkwall. Approach on leading line and anchor between Hatston Boat Slip and the CG lookout near W side of bay. SW side of bay is shoal. Exposed to N winds but these do not raise a heavy sea. Good holding but bottom foul. Harbourmaster's permission required to berth alongside the quays. New all-year marina within the harbour, excellent shelter.
24. Bay of Firth, shallow and many hazards. With care and local knowledge can offer good anchorage.

25. Bay of Isbister. Anchor 3½c ENE of Wald Taing in 8–10m, mud.
26. Wood Wick (Eynhallow Sound) dries out 3c from head. Temp. anchorage in suitable conditions 1½c S of Scara Taing, 6–8m.
27. Aiker Ness (Eynhallow Sound). Temp anchorage in bay SE of Aiker Ness, SE of Aikerness House, 1c off-shore in 5–6m, mud. Beware extensive shoal in centre and S of bay.
28. Sands of Evie (Eynhallow Sound). Rocky bottom, poor holding and not recommended.
29. Bay of Skaill. Centre of west coast of Mainland. Approach with caution. Temp. anchorage in calm conditions with no swell *(to visit Skarabrae)*. Exposed to W.

10.11 Auskerry

(ON østr sker – east skerry)

OS Maps: 1:50000 Sheet 5 1:25000 Sheets 461 or 465
Admiralty Charts: 1:200000 Nos.1942 and 1954 1:75000 No.2250

Area: 85ha (210 acres)
Height: 18m (59 ft)

Owner: Bought in 1973/4 by Michael Holgate, an oil industry consultant, and Simon Brogan. They are both resident at times with their respective families.

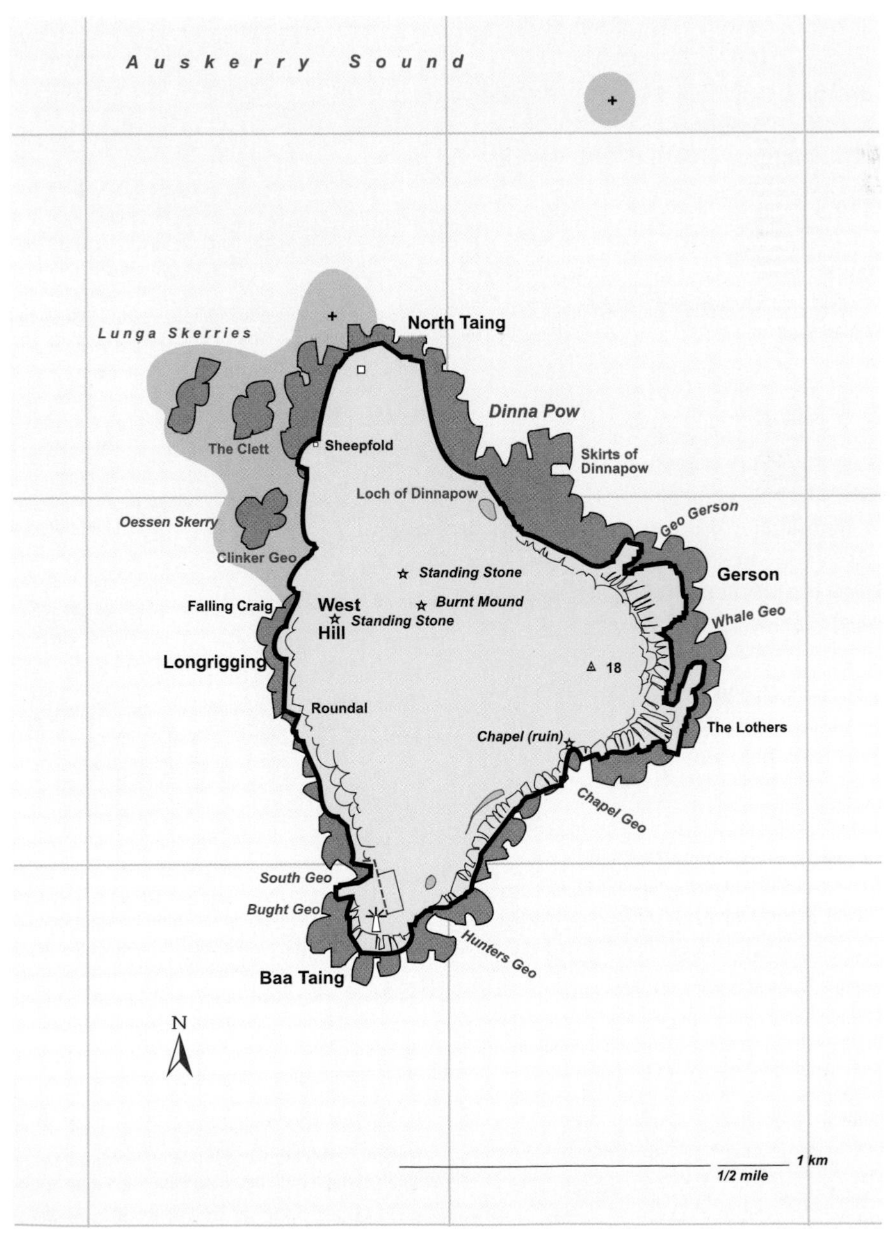

Population: 1881–8. 1891–7 (2 houses). 1931–4 (lighthouse-keepers). 1961–3. 1971–0. 1981–0. 1991 one, or two, families for most of each year. 2001–5.

Geology: Middle Old Red Sandstone in the form of weathered Rousay Flags.

History: This small island was more-or-less uninhabited for several decades (the lighthouse was made automatic in the 1960s) but it has an ancient history with standing stones making an abrupt statement on the wind-blown landscape, a burned mound, and the ruins of a medieval chapel [HY677160]. This is just the type of lonely outpost sought by the early Celtic Christians in their search for peace. It is a place to forget the passage of time. With only the sheep for company, the solitude is accentuated by the crashing of the surf and the screaming of the wind and seagulls.

Wildlife: A commercial flock of 300 North Ronaldsay seaweed-eating sheep. This is a Special Protection Area with a large colony of storm petrel, and a breeding site for puffin, arctic tern, and black guillemot.

* * *

AUSKERRY is a flattish grassy islet with a rocky shoreline and a conspicuous white lighthouse at **Baa Taing** (ON – tongue or promontory at the sea-rock). To sailors it could be easily confused with Muckle Skerry in the Pentland Firth which is very similar in appearance except that Muckle Skerry has two light towers.

Auskerry is about three miles south of Stronsay (No.10.14) and is separated from it by Auskerry Sound – a turbulent reef-rimmed stretch of sea. The food and mail at one time were delivered by a local fishing boat from Whitehall village on Stronsay but in the last years of lighthouse occupation the keepers provisions came from Kirkwall.

The inlet called **Hunters Geo** (ON *gja* – gully, creek) beneath the lighthouse on Baa Taing dates from the time when this was a favourite spot for seal-hunters. It is still a favourite spot for the grey seal, *Halichoerus grypus*, with its Roman nose, sad eyes (and halitosis) – known throughout the islands as the 'selkie'. In the late autumn many congregate on the skerries to pup and sing together.

Simon Brogan, Teresa Probert and their two home-taught sons lived here in comparative isolation for several years. There is a wind-generator and peat and driftwood provide heating but there is no plumbing. Mr Brogan, who tends the sheep, first moved to Auskerry in 1974 after travelling with a rock band. More recently the co-owner Michael Holgate, his wife Fiona – a former television presenter, and their son Adam have been in residence.

* * *

Access: Try Explorer Fast Sea Charter, Kirkwall, 01856-871225 or Groat's Charters, Shapinsay, 01856-711254.

Anchorage: No safe anchorage. Many hazards and strong tides. Landing place in South Geo.

10.12 Shapinsay

Possibly (ON hjalpandis-øy – helpful island) – because of a good harbour?

O S Maps: 1:50000 Sheet 6 1:25000 Sheet 462
Admiralty Charts: 1:200000 Nos.1942 or 1954 1:75000 Nos.2249 or 2250 1:25000 No.2584

Area: 2948ha (7285 acres)
Height: 64m (210 ft)

Owner: Multiple ownership. The Balfour family owned the entire island until the early 20th century, when they sold the freehold to their tenant farmers.

Population: 1798–730 (and about eighty boats). 1841–935 (199 houses). 1881–974. 1891–903 (179 houses). 1931–584. 1961–421. 1981–329. 1991–322. 2001–300.

Geology: This is a fertile island due to the breakdown of the Rousay Beds sandstone which covers all of it except the south-east corner. Here is extruded basaltic lava and Eday Beds of Middle Old Red Sandstone, which is a much better building stone than the Rousay Beds variety.

History: In 1263 King Haakon assembled his large fleet of galleys in Elwick before sailing south to Largs but the island itself was never mentioned in the sagas.

Always agriculturally fertile and reasonably prosperous, Shapinsay also enjoyed the kelp boom in the 18th century. The island produced over 3000 tons of burned kelp every year, which brought in about £20,000 of income for the inhabitants.

Wildlife: In 1805 the minister on Shapinsay first noted that the Orkney vole was a unique sub-species of the European vole, *Microtus arvalis*. This little creature is a puzzle as it is found nowhere else in the British Isles, including Shetland. It is of Spanish origin but did not come from an Armada wreck because its DNA shows that it reached Orkney about 6000 years ago. And anyway, unlike rats, voles hate ships!

The best time for bird-watching on Shapinsay is in the winter. Oystercatcher, lapwing and curlew nest on the farmland, and there are a few skua, gulls and terns in the south-east moorland. Inland is generally disappointing. In winter there are shelduck on The Ouse, an inlet on the north coast, and whooper swan on the Mill Dam, which is an RSPB Nature Reserve. Breeding waders such

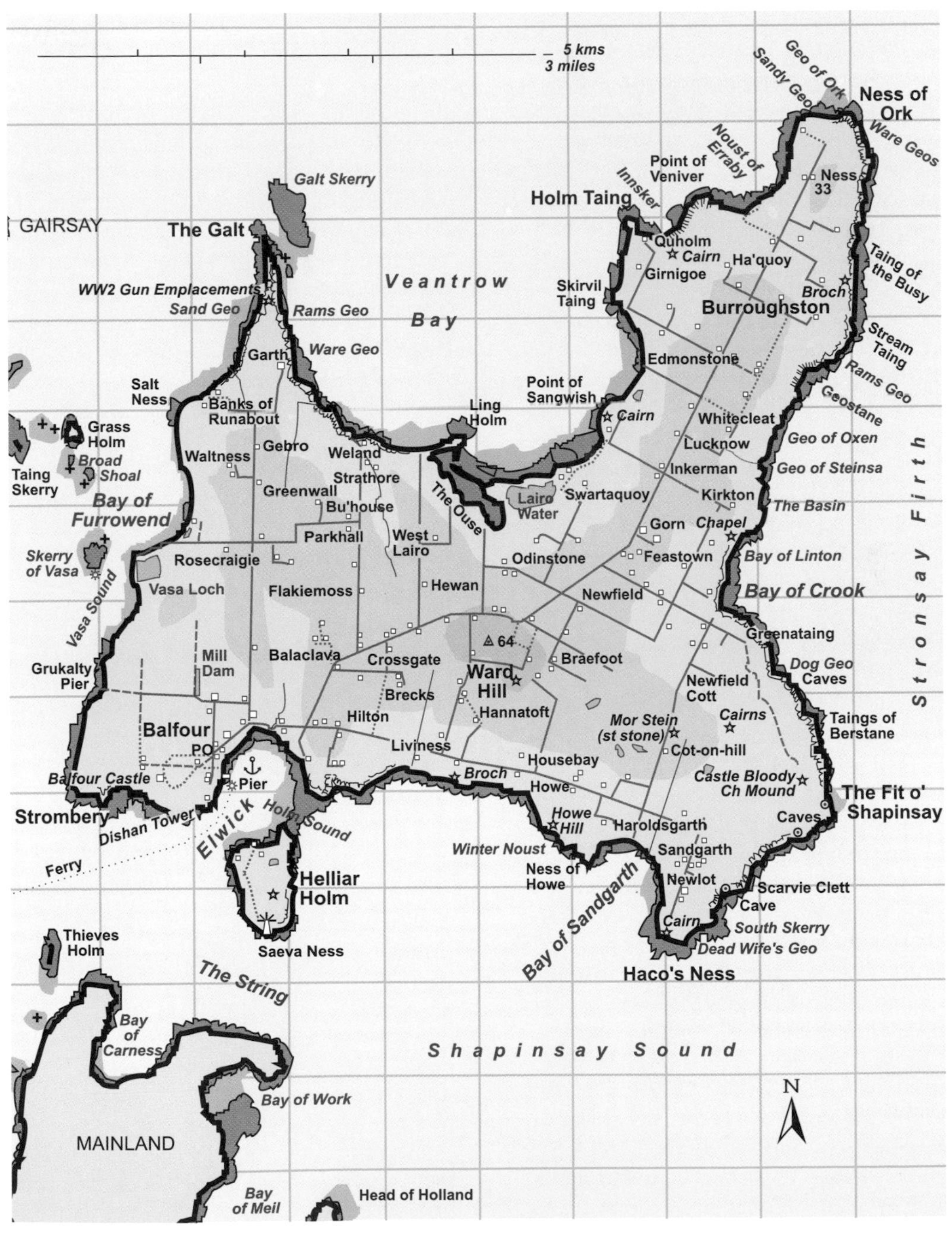

as redshank and snipe can be seen in spring and also various duck species. Balfour Castle woodland has many breeding birds and a variety of migrant species although the trees are generally small and stunted by the wind.

* * *

Intensively cultivated and close to Kirkwall, **SHAPINSAY** is a suburban sort of island. It is relatively low-lying with centrally situated **Ward Hill** (64m), its highest point flanked by two hummocks. The east coast has modest cave-riddled cliffs between **The Fit O'Shapinsay** in the south-east and **Ness of Ork** (pre-Norse – *orc* – boar) in the north-east. There is another minor escarpment flanking the north-west peninsula called **The Galt** (ON – boar) or Galt Ness. The rest of the coastline has little in the way of distinctive features with the exception of **Helliar Holm** (ON – holy island), a green tidal island with a lighthouse protecting the entrance to Elwick, and the remains of a broch, a chapel and a cairn.

Elwick (ON – holy bay) is another of the long line of famous anchorages used by King Haakon's fleet in 1263. As a harbour it was described by Rev Cruttwell's Gazetteer in 1798 as 'excellent for its extent as almost any one in this country. On the west side of it is a fine beach, with abundance of excellent fresh water'. The west side now has a ferry pier and a village with shops and a post-office. Cruttwell, incidentally, made an interesting claim: 'In this harbour it is high water at three quarters of an hour after nine o'clock, when the moon is new and full.'

Beside Elwick is the Victorian extravaganza of **Balfour Castle** [HY475164], with the only patch of woodland on Shapinsay. The building was completed in Scottish Baronial style in 1848 and is now run as a hotel.

The family of Balfour of Trenabie on Westray (No10.25) has a long association with Shapinsay. In the 18th century John Balfour made a fortune in India and then married the widow of a certain Colonel Mackennan. The Colonel had lent money to the Rajah of Tanjore and a number of other British expatriates were also caught in the same trap. The Rajah failed, or refused, to repay the loans so the lenders appealed for help from the British Government. They eventually received compensation, but only after John Balfour, by then (1790) MP for Orkney and Shetland, actively promoted their claim. Of course his wife, being Colonel Mackennan's widow, gained a substantial benefit from the settlement which contributed handsomely to John Balfour's fortune. Balfour bought estates on Shapinsay and several neighbouring islands and started building Balfour Castle.

But it fell to his son, Colonel Balfour, to complete most of the present structure with David Bryce as his architect. Colonel Balfour had raised a troop of volunteers and promoted himself to the status of colonel. The kelp industry had collapsed so he set about reforming the island's agriculture – squaring the fields into 10-acre units separated by open drains. He also built the attractive little village of **Balfour** populated with imported craftsmen such as joiners and weavers and the watermill which can be seen 1km north of the castle. A natural marsh beside it was dammed in the 1880s to provide the water. This is the **Mill Dam**. Balfour's improvements were generally of great benefit to the island but he himself is remembered as a petty tyrant. This is perhaps unfortunate as it was an age when many other landlords were clearing their islands for sheep.

Soon after the Second World War an expatriate officer of the Polish Lancers who had escaped the Katyn massacre, Tadeus Zawadski, bought Balfour Castle and the Balfour estate on Shapinsay. Like Balfour, he farmed it successfully, and he was a popular laird and resident of the island. He died in 1979.

Quholm in the north-east of Shapinsay [HY521218] was the family home of the parents of the American author, William Washington Irving. He was famous in his time and has been called the 'father of American literature' but is now often only remembered for his story of Rip Van Winkle. His father emigrated to the States in 1783 and set up shop as a hardware merchant in New York and his son was christened in honour of the first President.

* * *

Access: Ro-ro service by Orkney Ferries from Kirkwall, several sailings every day, 01856-872044. Balfour Castle Tour and cruise round Hellier Holm, 01856-711282. Tourist Office, 01856-872856.

Anchorages: There are turbulent tides in The String off Helliar Holm.

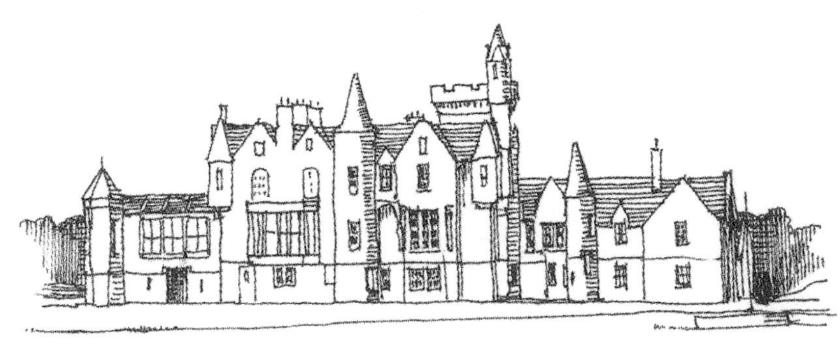

COLONEL BALFOUR'S CASTLE

1. Elwick Bay. Visitors morrings on W side. Anchor anywhere suitable in the bay, but note that shores are fringed by a shallow bank. Bottom sand. Pier on W side at village. Avoid obstructing ferry. Good shelter.
2. Veantrow Bay. Exposed to N and uncomfortable. Best on E side, 6–9m, sand and coral, avoid fish farm.
3. Helliar Holm. Temp. anchorage E of Helliar Holm and clear of prohibited area, sand.

10.13 Gairsay

(ON Gáreksøy – Gárekr's island). Gárekr is a man's name.

OS Maps: 1:50000 Sheet 6 1:25000 Sheet 461
Admiralty Charts: 1:200000 Nos.1942 or 1954 1:75000 Nos.2249 or 2250 1:25000 No.2584

Area: 240ha (593 acres)
Height: 102m (335 ft)

Owner: Bought in 1971 by Val and David McGill of Cornwall, who are resident on the island and farm it.

Population: 1841–71 (15 houses). 1881–33. 1891–33 (5 houses). 1931–5. 1961–0. 1971–7. 1981–6. 1991–3. 2001–3.

Geology: Fertile soil over Rousay type Middle Old Red Sandstone.

History: Gairsay will always be remembered as the home of the boisterous Sweyn Asleifsson, one of the last of the great Vikings. (His story would make a great opera but there is only space here for a 'potted' version.)

In the 12th century, Sweyn's father, Olaf Rolfsson of Gairsay, had supported Earl Paul of Orkney in a sea-battle off Deerness against Olvir Rosta in which Olvir was defeated. Seeking revenge Olvir set fire to Olaf's home and Olaf and five of his men were burned to death. Sweyn was fishing in the Pentland Firth at the time but when the young man returned and saw the carnage, he crossed to Orphir on Mainland to tell Earl Paul what had happened.

It was the night of the Yule feast. A big surly man called Sweyn Breastrope, the Earl's favourite and foremost fighter, was belligerent with drink. After the Earl had gone to bed there was a quarrel and in the ensuing fight Sweyn Asleifsson killed him. Fearing Earl Paul's anger Sweyn ran for cover and appealed to Bishop William of Egilsay for help and advice. The Bishop was sympathetic and suggested that he lie low for a while. He sent him to stay with friends on the island of Tiree (No3.10).

The following spring Sweyn visited Earl Maddad in Atholl and there learned that Earl Paul had declared him an outlaw. Maddad was married to Margaret, the beautiful but scheming sister of Earl Paul. She reckoned that both her son Harald, and her nephew Erlend, had a justifiable claim to the Orkney Earldom. Sweyn promised to support Harald's claim and in return he was paid compensation for the death of his father and given a merchant-ship with a crew of thirty men. Sweyn promptly sailed to Orkney, kidnapped Earl Paul (see Rousay No.10.20), and delivered him unharmed to Atholl. The Earl was never seen again and Margaret is reputed to have had her brother blinded and murdered.

Sweyn sailed back to Orkney and went openly to the assembled Parliament at Kirkwall. In a meeting with Bishop William, Kol, and Kol's son Rognvald – the good-natured earl-presumptive – he explained what had happened. His explanation was accepted and after the meeting Parliament acknowledged Rognvald's authority as Earl of Orkney.

Sweyn inherited his father's lands including Gairsay and persuaded Earl Rognvald to lend him two ships. He then sailed to Scotland and landed at Helmsdale. He failed to capture Olvir Rosta, which was his intention, so he plundered and burned Rosta's homestead. Turning south, Sweyn then spent two years fighting and pillaging in the Irish Sea and followed this by marrying Ingrid, the rich widow of the chieftain of the Isle of Man.

Back in Orkney, after a further successful cruise,

the volatile Sweyn fell out with Earl Rognvald, and after a nominal revolt, slipped away to Edinburgh and the court of David I, King of Scots. There he persuaded David to intercede on his behalf with Earl Rognvald. Rognvald duly forgave him and Sweyn returned to Gairsay.

Earl Rognvald meanwhile went on a crusade to the Holy Land and was absent for over two years leaving Harald in charge. Earl Maddad of Atholl had died and Harald was furious to discover that his widowed mother Margaret was having a child by Gunni, a brother of Sweyn Asleifsson. Harald outlawed Gunni but this enraged Sweyn. However Margaret by this time had already tired of Gunni and fallen instead for a handsome young Shetlander who carried her off to Mousa (No.11.2).

When Rognvald returned home he found Harald absent in Norway raising a force, possibly to usurp him. Sweyn and Erlend were jointly running his earldom. He sent Sweyn and Erlend north to defend Shetland against Harald and they captured three of Harald's ships. Taking advantage of Sweyn's absence in the north Harald approached Rognvald and asked for reconciliation. He explained that Rognvald had put him in charge during his absence but that Sweyn had turned against him. The easy-going Rognvald accepted this so he and Harald joined forces with a fleet of ships and lay in wait for Sweyn. As Rognvald and Harald had fourteen ships while Sweyn and Erlend had only seven Sweyn did not try to gain access to Mainland Orkney for supplies and assistance but chose instead to wait. Winter approached and Rognvald's fleet sheltered in Scapa Bay. It was a cold, dark, night with storm-force winds, poor visibility and gusts of sleet. Suddenly out of the spray Sweyn's ships appeared and his men leapt aboard the anchored ships. Rognvald was ashore and Harald escaped, but nearly everyone else was caught off-guard and slaughtered.

Strangely, in spite of all this bloodshed, Rognvald the peacemaker eventually arranged a reconciliation between Harald and Sweyn who, thereafter, became close friends.

Sweyn returned to his buccaneering exploits which included a raid on Port St Mary in the Scillies but a few years later, in 1158, Rognvald, the good-hearted warrior-poet, died in a skirmish in Caithness and Earl Harald succeeded him.

Sweyn continued to live on Gairsay. He farmed in the summer, drank away the winter in his drinking hall with his eighty men-at-arms, and went a-viking every spring and autumn. In one exploit, about 1171, with a fleet of five ships off Dublin he captured two English ships with a cargo of wine and cloth. They let the sailors go, stitched the brightly coloured cloth to their sails for show, and drank so much that they could not remember how they sailed home to Orkney. They called it their Cloth Cruise.

Eventually Sweyn decided to have one last cruise before retirement. He sailed south again to Dublin which was then held by the English. Fearless as ever, he stormed the city, captured it and held it to ransom. But the next day on his way to collect the ransom he was ambushed and killed.

One translation of the saga says: '... it is the judgement of men that he has been the greatest man in every way in the lands of the west, both in days present and days past, among men who were not of higher rank than he.'

Wildlife: Arctic and great skuas breed on the heather-covered moorland and arctic terns, sandwich terns and cormorants frequent the surrounding skerries.

* * *

Although **GAIRSAY** is much the same size as Wyre, its neighbour to the north, it has a distinctive summit (102m) with a cairn on top whereas Wyre is low-lying. The south-east corner of Gairsay, which is over 20m high and is called **Hen of Gairsay**, is only attached to the rest of the island by a narrow neck of land. It shelters a small cove on its west side which is the island's only anchorage. The sea south of Gairsay has many deceptive rock patches and skerries, and there are three tiny islets – **Holm of Boray**, **Grass Holm**, and **Holm of Rendall**. North of Hen of Gairsay is a more substantial islet – **Sweyn Holm** (ON – Sveinn's or servant islet) – is probably named after Sweyn Asliefsson.

Near the end of the 17th century Gairsay was bought by Sir William Craigie, a wealthy merchant who had been a tacksman of the Earl. There was an existing house on a prominent site opposite the shores of Rendall and he developed this into the imposing small mansion of **Langskaill**. Langskaill or Skaill is a name given to a Viking drinking-hall although in Norway it usually refers to a farmhouse or store. This particular Langskaill is sited on top of the remains of Sweyn's drinking-hall.

The front of the mansion courtyard has a curtain wall with a walkway along the parapet and there is an arched doorway with an armorial shield above it. A bowling green used to be between the house and the sea with access to a solid stone pier. After Craigie's death the house was deserted and eventually part of the decaying building was used as a farm steading. New owners renovated and occupied the building but after the Second World War it was once more abandoned and neglected for a period until it was again renovated by the present owners.

Gairsay provides good pasturage for sheep under a tenancy agreement but this may not help the economics of running an island farm.

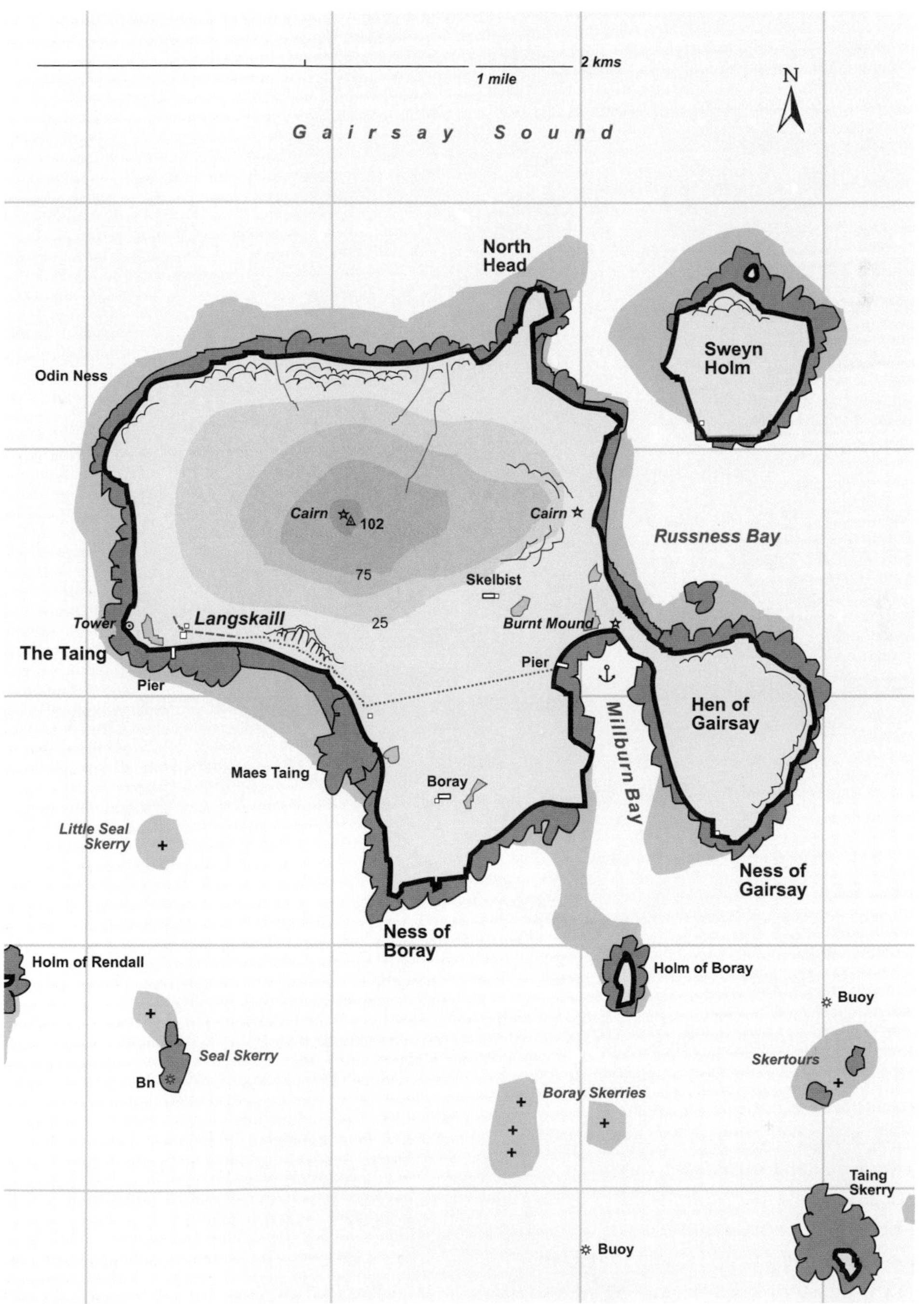

Access: Arrangements may be made at Tingwall or try Explorer, Kirkwall, 01856-871225.

Anchorages:

1. Milburn Bay, on S coast beside Hen of Gairsay. A submerged ridge (1.5m) joins W side of Milburn Bay to Holm of Boray. Shores are shoal. Anchor in centre, 6m mud.
2. Langskaill, by The Taing. Stone pier for owner's use.

10.14 Stronsay

Possibly (ON strjóns-øy – good fishing and farming island) – the inference being 'profitable property'.

O S Maps: 1:50000 Sheet 5 1:25000 Sheet 465
Admiralty Charts: 1:200000 Nos.1942 or 1954 1:75000 No.2250 1:25000 No.2622 Papa Sound

Area: 3275ha (8093 acres)
Height: 44m (144 ft)

Owner: Multiple ownership.

Population: 1798–887. 1841–1234 (250 houses). 1881–1274. 1891–1275 (269 houses). 1931–953. 1961–497. 1981–420. 1991–382. 2001–343.

Geology: Most of the island is the Rousay type of Middle Old Red Sandstone weathered into good soil and low hills but the south-west side of the Bay of Holland and a patch at Links Ness in the north-west is of the Eday variety of sandstone.

History: From the early 17th century to 1914 Stronsay was a fishing centre of constant importance. It was first exploited by the Dutch and built up to such an extent that by 1900 it had become the capital of the herring industry. This then declined but was revived for a time in the 1920s and 1930s. At one stage Whitehall had fifteen fish-curing stations (and forty pubs!) operating during the season, with a constant traffic of ships delivering the catch and exporting the cured and salted herring, mainly to Baltic markets. About 1960 there was an attempt to revive the industry with the formation of a co-operative to process white fish for export to the USA, but the great days are over.

Wildlife: In common with most of the Orkney islands this is a treeless landscape but the rich pastures have many wildflowers in spring and summer and examples of the rare blue-flowered oysterplant can be found near the shoreline at Lea Shun and on the shingle on the south side of St Catherine's Bay. A large area of naturalised Patagonian Ragwort (from south Chile) grows beside the path to The Pow, while Frog Orchids and Adder's Tongue can be found west of the beautiful Sand of Rothiesholm.

There is an enormous winter population of wildfowl including whooper swan and Greenland white-fronted geese, plus dabbling and diving duck and visiting shore-birds.

This is an excellent place for spotting rare migrant birds. American golden plover, tawny pipit, pied wheatear, Radde's, marsh and sub-alpine warblers, rustic bunting, Arctic redpoll and scarlet rosefinch have all been recorded. The lochs and wetlands are breeding haunts for redshank, snipe, shoveller and pintail and there are still a few corncrake and corn bunting nests and the occasional quail. Fairly large seabird colonies occupy the area between Odness and Lamb Head on the west coast.

Recommended bird-watching sites are: the Rothiesholm Peninsula, where there are breeding skua, gull, tern and various wildfowl and waders on the moorland, and also red-throated diver and twite. This is one of the best moorland sites in the Northern Isles. The cliffs are tenanted by shag, guillemot, razorbill, fulmar and black guillemot and there are also many rare and interesting shells to be found on the beautiful beach.

Mill Bay and Meikle Water, which are good for observing migrant passerines, sea-duck, divers, and waders. White-fronted and greylag geese frequent the area in the winter together with whooper swan, many duck and waders.

* * *

STRONSAY is a low-lying island of rich green pastures and wide beaches. **Burgh Hill** (44m) in the south-east is the highest of several rounded hills scattered across the island, all of similar height. Many typical maritime heath plants grow on its slopes.

Whitehall is the main settlement and ferry port. Its name comes from a house built in the 1670s by Patrick Fea, a retired privateer. For over two centuries, up to the outbreak of the Second World War, this was the most active herring port in the northern Orkney Isles and the large two-storeyed houses are a reminder of days of

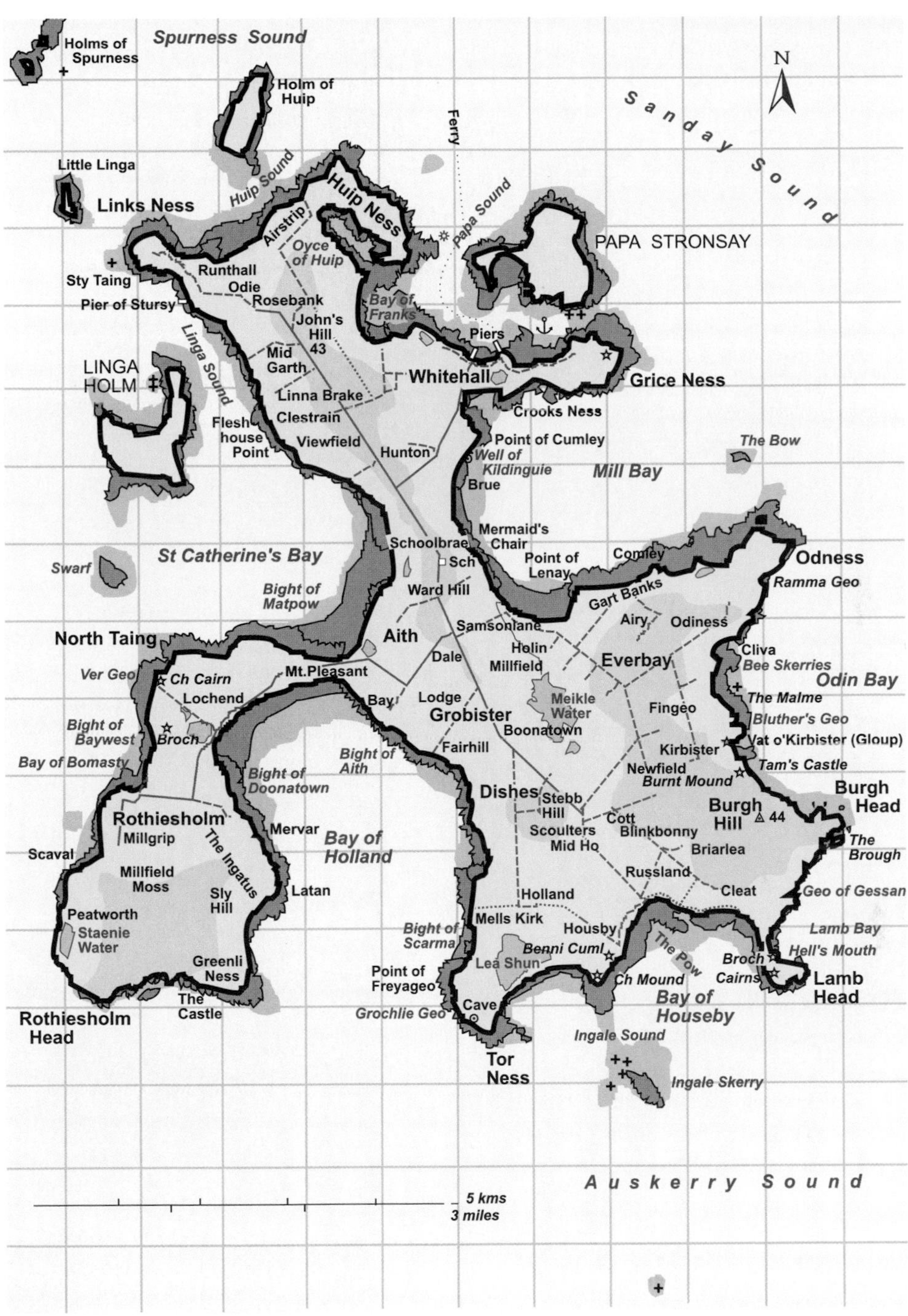

prosperous fishing, large families, and many lodgers. Today, Whitehall is a modest little place, with a fish factory, post-office, and hotel, and a few fishing boats in the harbour. At one time there was a fleet of 300 boats in Papa Sound, fifteen fish-curing stations, and 1500 'fishwives'. Occasional whaling occurred when there was the opportunity. A school of fifty whales was driven into Mill Bay in 1834 and slaughtered, yielding £100 worth of whale oil.

The road from Whitehall joins a road which runs north and south down the spine of the island, with a separate branch across the neck of land between St Catherine's Bay and Bay of Holland to the **Rothiesholm** [**row**sum] peninsula.

The airstrip is in the far north beyond John's Hill near the tidal wetland of **Oyce of Huip**, and across Huip Sound is **Holm of Huip** with five cairns on it, a tiny lochan and many Atlantic grey seals. It was up for sale in 2002 for £110,000. To the north-west is rocky Links Ness and the islet of **Little Linga** (ON – heather isle).

Wardhill with its village and school is in the geometric centre of the island and immediately west of **Mill Bay**. There is a long beach round Mill Bay with a rock seat in the middle called the **Mermaid's Chair** [HY655262]. Scota Bess, one of Orkney's storm witches, would sit here casting evil spells until finally the fisherfolk could stand no more of it. They beat her to death and buried her body but in the morning the corpse was found lying on the ground beside the grave. This happened several times so, in desperation, the islanders flung the body into **Meikle Water** (S. – little water), the loch south of Wardhill and it was never seen again. But it is said that any girl who sits in the Mermaid's Chair will be able to foretell the future.

Stronsay has long been a place of progressive farming and relatively large landholdings although there has been a natural change of character of the farming through the years. The kelp industry also played its part in the 18th century and circular, stone-lined kilns for burning the kelp can be seen dotted about the shores. James Fea of Whitehall started the industry in 1722 but the islanders feared the vengeance of *Nuckelavee*, a sea monster who hated smoke. Even forty years later they blamed the kelp industry for bad harvests and poor fishing and brought a case against James Fea, which they won. However, the next generation had a different attitude and the smoke from Stronsay's kelp kilns could be seen for miles.

The waters of Stronsay's **Well of Kildinguie** [HY654273] have long held the reputation for curing everything except the black death provided they are mixed with dulse from the adjoining sea-shore. However, close examination of the water may persuade one that the sickness is better than the cure.

Balanced on top of each of three rock-stacks in Odin Bay, – **The Malme**, **Tam's Castle**, and **Burgh Head**, – are the precarious ruins of anchorite cells. Here too is **Vat of Kirbister**, a dramatic 'gloup', boasting the finest natural rock arch in Orkney [HY686239].

The southern cliffs of Stronsay, on each side of the **Bay of Holland** (probably derived from the Old Norse for 'high land'), are rich in birdlife. It was from here that the islanders would collect the seabirds and eggs which were once an essential part of their normal diet. The Norse considered the area important because the adjoining Bay of Houseby indicates a farm which was an administrative and tax-collecting centre (ON *husabyr* – royal administrative farm). This also appears to have been a favoured area in prehistoric times as there are a number of tumuli, and on **Lamb Head**, the southern extremity, there are cairns and a small broch with a stone construction beside it which may be a Pictish or Norse pier [HY690214]. Here too is Hell's Mouth, a narrow, rocky, chasm in which breaking seas make a frightening sound.

* * *

Access: Orkney Ferries run daily ro-ro ferry services Kirkwall/ Eday/ Stronsay, 01856-872044. Scheduled daily air service Kirkwall, Sanday and Westray, 01856-872494 and 0345-222111. Tourist information 01856-872856.

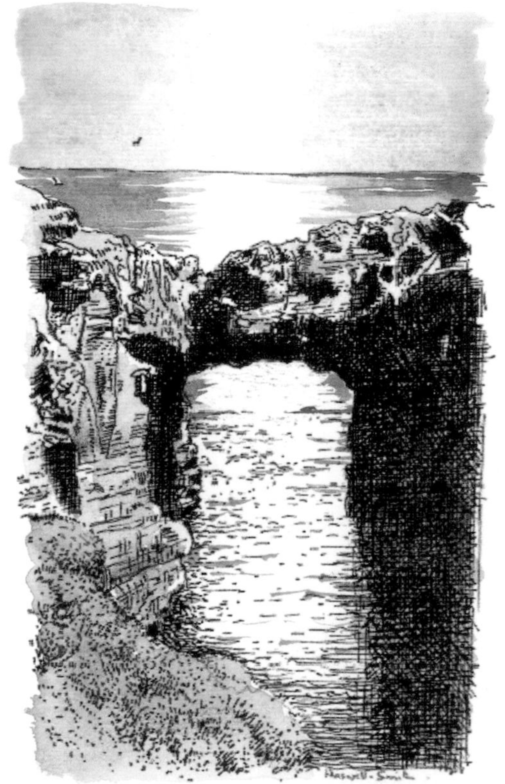

VAT OF KIRBISTER

Anchorages:

1. Whitehall Harbour. Good anchorage but many reefs and shoals. Use N entrance and anchor where space and depth available S of Papa Stronsay. There is water both sides of both piers but avoid obstructing ferry. E side of W pier recommended. Alternatively anchor about 1c W of red can buoy in Jack's Hole.
2. Linga Holm (St Catherine's Bay). Occasional anchorage out of tide E of SE extremity in 6–10m. In E winds temp anchorage off W side of Linga Holm in 9–10m. Midchannel rock reported, LD 0.4, in Linga Sound.
3. Bay of Holland. Good anchorage in 3–8m, sand. W side best. Well sheltered except from S.
4. Mill Bay. Fringed by shoals and bottom foul, not recommended, but temp. shelter in N'lies.

10.15 Wyre

Or Weir [wYr] (ON vigr – spear head) – derived from shape of island? There is a Norwegian island with a similar name and shape – and another off Iceland.

OS Maps: 1:50000 Sheet 5 or 6 1:25000 Sheet 464
Admiralty Charts: 1:200000 Nos.1942 or 1954 1:75000 No.2249 or 2250 various No.2562 plans

Area: 311ha (768 acres)
Height: 32m (105 ft)

Population: 1841–96 (20 houses). 1881–80. 1891–67 (14 houses). 1931–44. 1961–47. 1981–21. 1991–28. 2001–18.

Geology: Middle Old Red Sandstone of the same variety as neighbouring Rousay which weathers to a good fertile soil.

History: Wyre is noted for what is possibly the earliest stone castle to have survived in Scotland. This was built by Kolbein Hruga, remembered affectionately as 'Cubbie Roo', a mid-12th-century chief and descendant of Earl Paul I. He was born in Sunnfjord, Norway, and was established by Thorfinn the Mighty as a *gøding*, or best man.

Cubbie Roo's son was Bjarni (1188–1223). He became Bishop of the See of Orkney in about 1190 and he probably prevailed upon his father to build the delightful little Romanesque chapel on Wyre. Bjarni was also a poet who composed a lay about the legend of the Jomsvikings which is the only contribution to Norse literature to have come from the Scottish islands.

Cubbie Roo's castle is where Snaekoll Gunnason and fellow rebels sought refuge after killing Earl John, the last of the Viking earls, in 1232.

Wildlife: A large number of divers and sea-duck winter in the shelter of the adjoining sounds.

* * *

The flat little island of **WYRE** with its famous castle ruin is mentioned in the Norse Sagas. The *Orkneyinga Saga* speaks of 'Kolbein Hruga – the most haughty of men... He had a good stone castle built there that was a safe stronghold.' And *King Haakon's Saga*, eight years later, refers to the last Norse earl, Earl John, being slain in a Thurso cellar and how his murderers took refuge in Wyre castle. They were besieged, but as the castle was easily defended a truce was arranged.

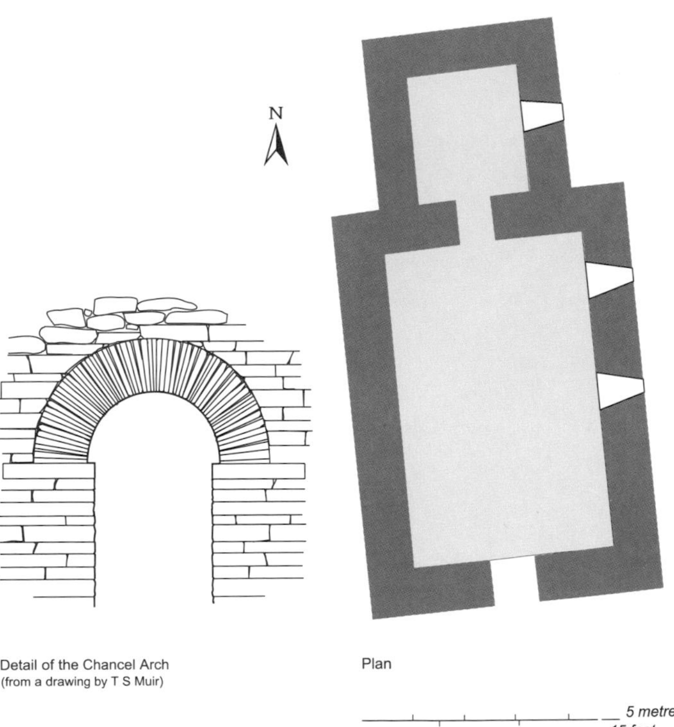

Detail of the Chancel Arch
(from a drawing by T S Muir)

Plan

THE 12TH-CENTURY CHAPEL ON WYRE

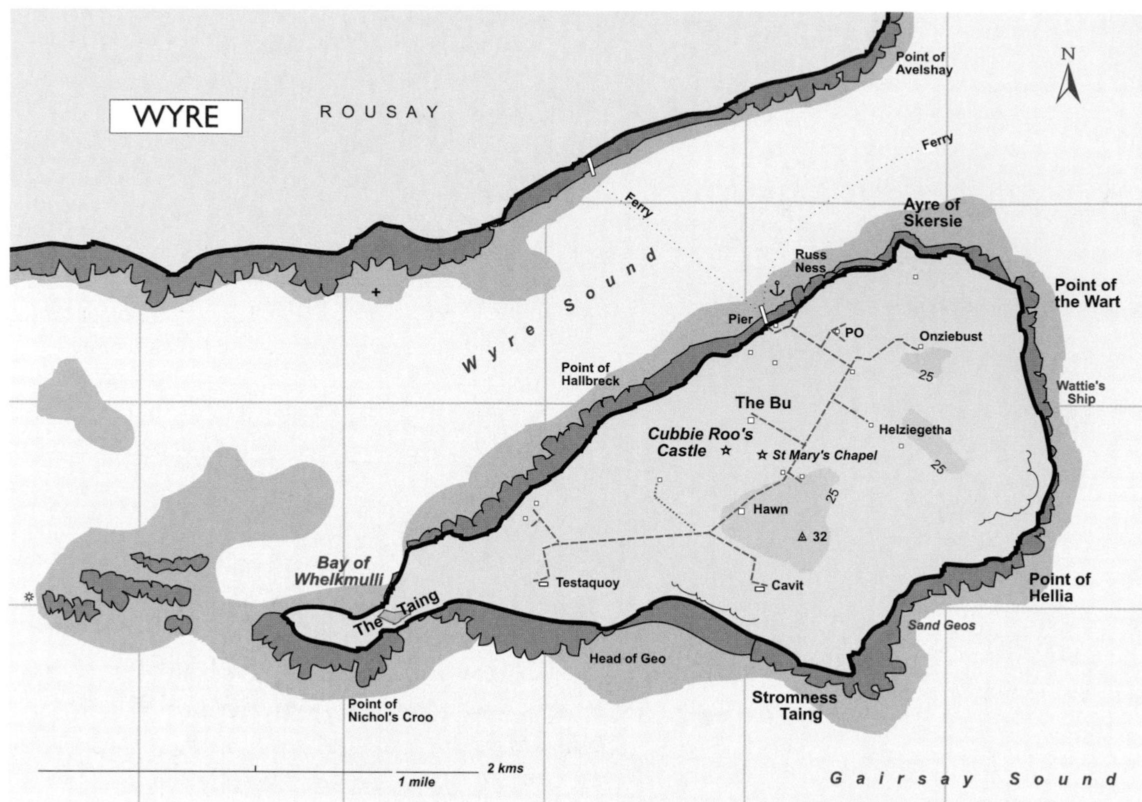

Cubbie Roo's castle ruin is in the centre of the island just north of the only hillock (32m) [HY442263]. The castle is a stone keep about 7½m square surrounded by a deep stone-faced ditch. The stonework is of high standard and there is evidence of at least one upper floor. A water tank is cut into the stone floor at ground level. The entrance was from the east with a door at upper level so that a ladder could be lowered for visitors. There are other ruins just visible around the castle but their purpose is uncertain.

North-east of the castle is the home farm, **The Bu of Wyre** [HY443264]. The farm buildings may have been built on top of Cubbie Roo's original farmhouse where Bishop Bjarni spent his boyhood.

Close to the castle ruin and farm buildings is a rectangular roofless chapel standing in a burial ground [HY443263]. The chapel dates from the late 12th century and was dedicated to either St Mary or St Peter. It has been partially restored and is of Romanesque design showing the influence of architectural ideas introduced to Orkney by Kol and Rognvald. The Vikings travelled widely and absorbed a remarkable amount of culture when they were not engaged in piracy.

In the centuries after the demise of 'haughty' Kolbein Hruga island folklore ascribed to him the character of a lumbering, well-meaning giant who could step from island to island. It was said that he tried to build bridges and causeways between the islands but the stones kept breaking his kishie (a straw basket normally used for carrying peat) which is why there are now so many rocks and skerries.

The renowned Orcadian poet, Edwin Muir, who was a contemporary and friend of the Orcadian painter, Stanley Cursiter, was born on Wyre in the late 1880s, and lived for a time in The Bu. 'I'm an Orkneyman, a good Scandinavian,' he said. In his autobiography he recalls his happy childhood on the island.

* * *

Access: Orkney Ferries ro-ro several sailings daily, Tingwall/ Rousay/ Egilsay/ Wyre, 01856-872044. Kirkwall/ Tingwall bus, 01856-870555.

Anchorage: Negotiate S end of Wyre Sound with care.

1. Wyre Sound. Reasonable anchorage and shelter E of the pier and close in-shore out of the tide.

10.16 Linga Holm

(ON lyng-øy, OE holm – heather island islet). Locally, sometimes called Midgarth Holm after the adjoining farm on Stronsay.

OS Maps: 1:50000 Sheet 5 1:25000 Sheet 465
Admiralty Charts: 1:200000 Nos.1942 or 1954 1:75000 No.2250

Area: 57ha (141 acres)
Height: 10m (33 ft)

Owner: Bought by the Scottish Wildlife Trust (SWT) in 1999 for £37,000 as a nature reserve.

Population: 1841–6 (1 house) 1891–0. Uninhabited.

Geology: Middle Old Red Sandstone of the Rousay type.

Wildlife: More than 2300 grey seal pups are born here annually – about 7% of the total world population. Bird life is prolific with red-throated diver, skylark, several colonies of endangered

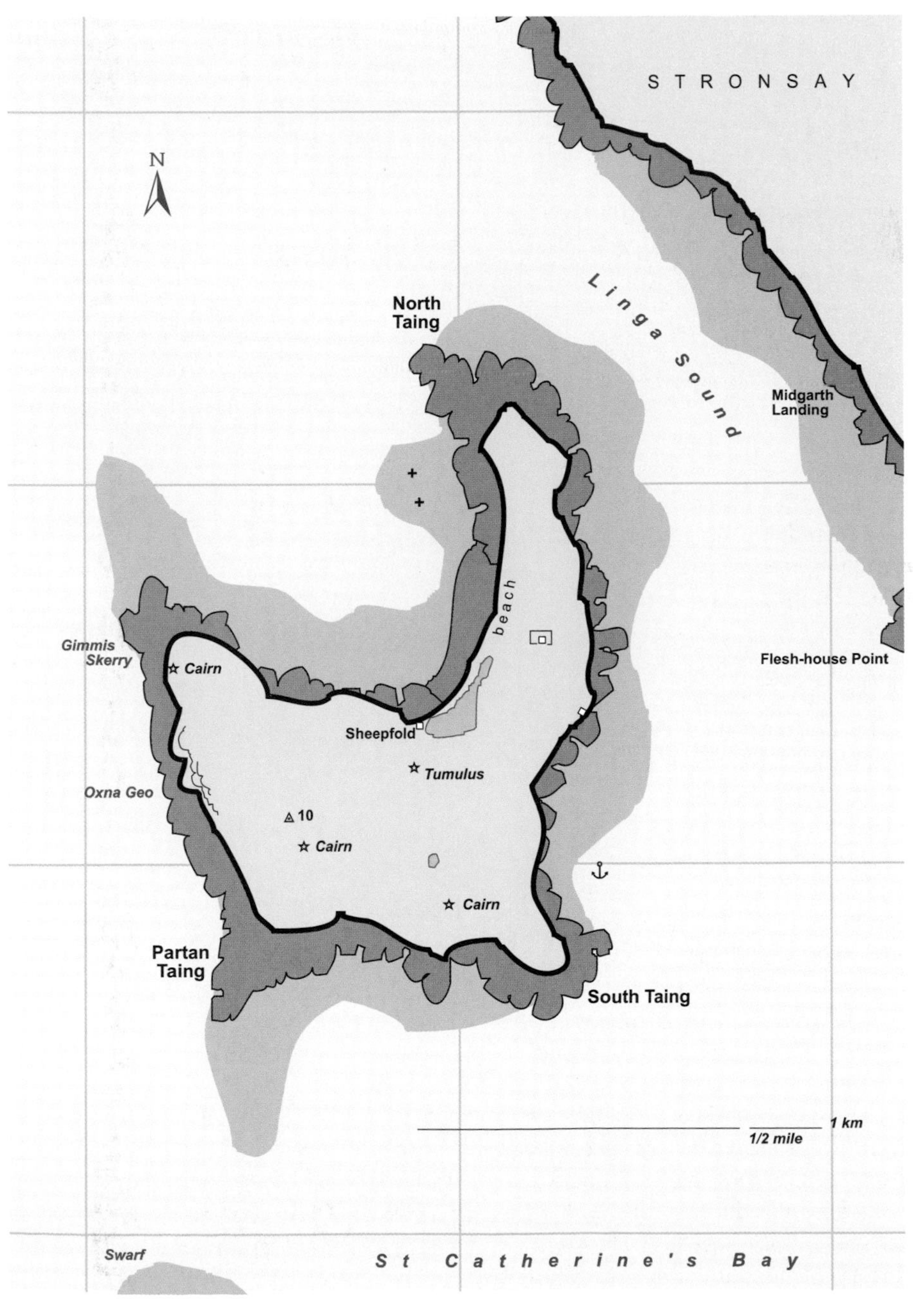

ground-nesting birds, and Greenland white-fronted geese in winter.

The last owner's North Ronaldsay sheep have gone but the SWT use some sheep as 'woolly lawnmowers' to maintain an open habitat for rare wildflowers such as adder's tongue fern.

* * *

Stretching open its arms to try to block the north-west winds which blow at intervals into St Catherine's Bay, **LINGA HOLM** is rather unsuccessful as this small island is only 10m high at its highest point. It has had a long association with Mid Garth on Stronsay which is only separated from it by narrow Linga Sound. The Sound can look deceptively peaceful but can suddenly become turbulent with very little warning.

The eastern arm of the island which stretches in a narrow tongue up the side of Linga Sound to North Taing has a building on it which has been in use as a boathouse. West of it is an extensive shallow pond beside a beach. The rest of the island is mainly open grassland rising gradually to its highest level in the south-west where there are the walls of a ruined house. Sometimes Shetland ponies have been seen grazing here. Prehistoric cairns in this area are evidence of the presence of early man but the most noteworthy archaeological item is the excellently preserved Pictish House.

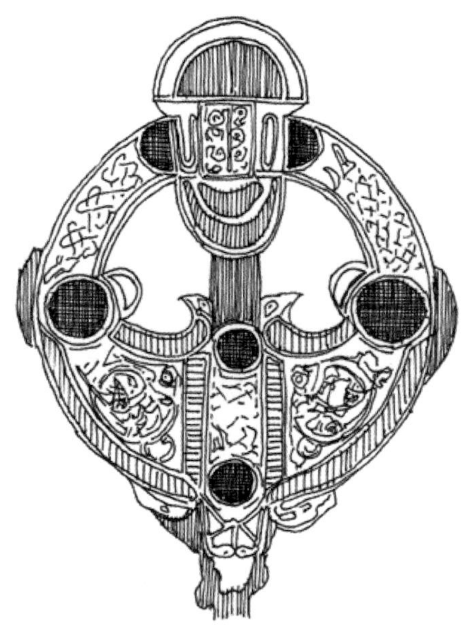

THE WESTNESS BROOCH OF ROUSAY

Partan Taing (G. – edible crab, ON *taing* – point) is a reef on the south-west side which runs out towards the **Swarf** (ON *svarf* – grit), a dangerous skerry in the middle of the entrance to St Catherine's Bay.

* * *

Access: Enquire at Whitehall, Stronsay. The SWT (0131-312-7765) may run controlled tours to the island or try Explorer, Kirkwall, 01856-871225.

Anchorage: Midchannel submerged rock reported in Linga Sound and beware Swarf south of Linga Holm.
1. St Catherine's Bay. Occasional anchorage E or NE of South Taing (SE extremity) in 6m out of tidal stream. In light E winds temp. anchorage off W side of Linga Holm beach in 9–10m.

10.17 Papa Stronsay

(ON – priest's island of Stronsay.) The Norse called it Little Papey (ON papøy hin litli) and to the local people it is just 'Papy.'

OS Maps: 1:50000 Sheet 5 1:25000 Sheet 465
Admiralty Charts: 1:200000 Nos.1942 or 1954 1:75000 No.2250 1:25000 No.2622

Area: 74ha (183 acres)
Height: 13m (43 ft)

Owner: Bought in 1999 for a reputed £250,000 by a Catholic community of priests, the Transalpine Redemptorists, from Charles Smith who had been the owner and resident since buying the island in 1988.

Population: 1841–28 (5 houses). 1881–23. 1891–27 (4 houses). 1931–18. 1961–4. 1971–3. 1981–0. 1991–0. 2001–10.

Geology: Middle Old Red Sandstone of the Rousay Flags variety.

History: Following the occupation of the island by prehistoric man, Papa Stronsay became a hermitage for Culdee monks.

In the early years of the 11th century fair-haired Earl Rognvald Brusason – gallant but unprincipled – arrived from Norway to take his share of the Orkney earldom granted to him by King Magnus of Norway. This Rognvald should not to be confused with the later Earl Rognvald of St Magnus cathedral fame. The incumbent Earl Thorfinn of Orkney accepted the position and

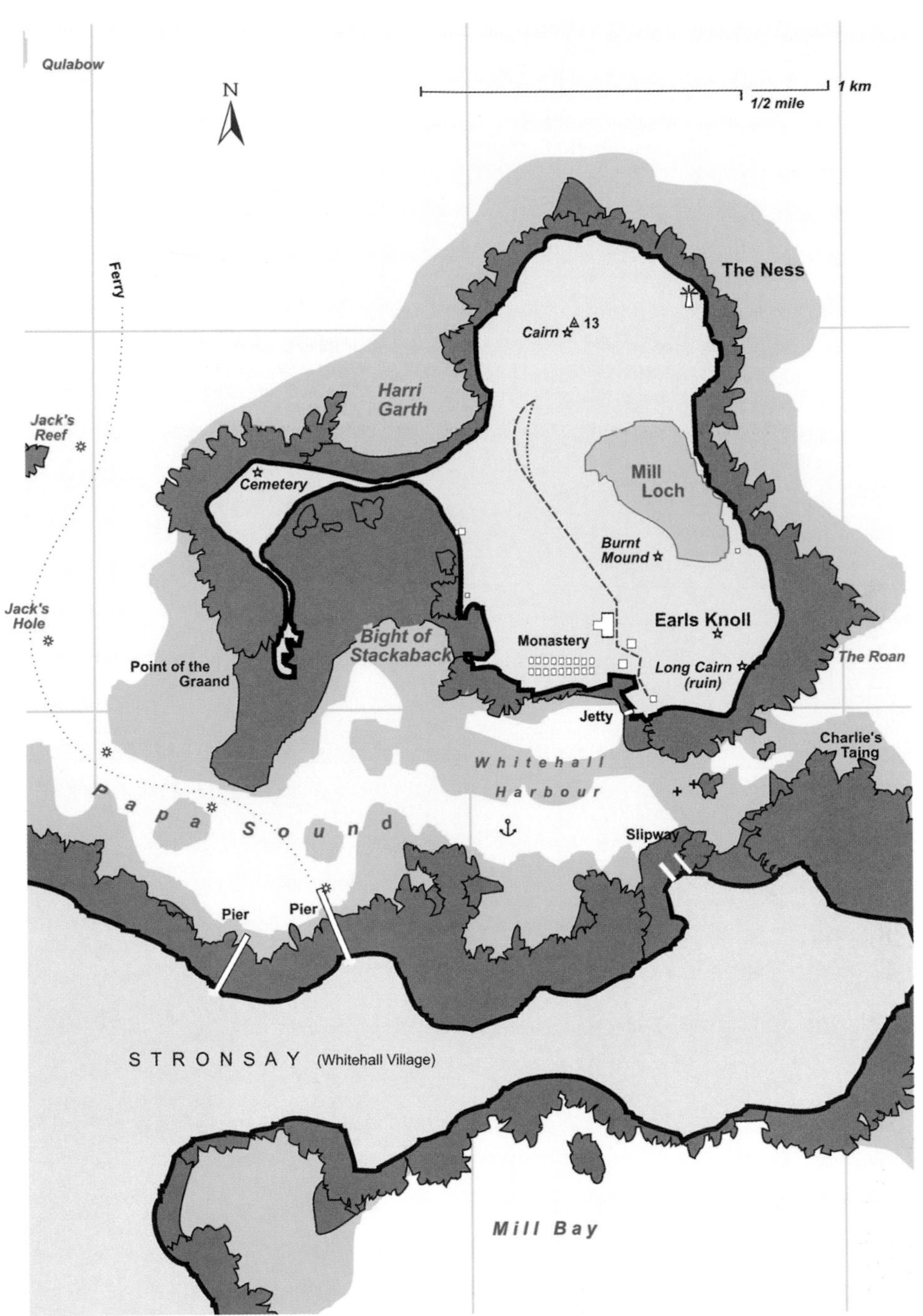

agreed that two-thirds of the revenue should go to Rognvald but asked, in return, for Rognvald's support and friendship. Rognvald agreed.

For several years Thorfinn and Rognvald enjoyed themselves rampaging up and down the west coast of Scotland, fighting and laying waste parts of the Hebrides, Ireland, Galloway and the north-west of England.

Then Kalf Arnison, a relative-in-law of Thorfinn who had fallen out with King Magnus, asked for refuge and hospitality in Orkney for himself and his men. Thorfinn agreed but Rognvald would not and a quarrel ensued. The two Earls prepared for battle and their fleets eventually met in combat off the west coast of Hoy. Only when Kalf's six ships joined the fray was the issue decided and the defeated Rognvald fled to Norway. But later, in mid-winter, Rognvald returned in a single ship and caught Thorfinn unprepared in a house in Orphir and set fire to it. Thorfinn escaped by leaping through the flames carrying his wife Ingibjorg and disappeared into the night. In a tiny skiff he then rowed across the Pentland Firth to safety.

Rognvald went to Papa Stronsay to obtain malt barley, which was grown on the island, probably by the Culdee monks, as he planned to brew ale for Christmas and hold a victory celebration, but while he and his men huddled by the fire in bitter December weather Thorfinn suddenly encircled them in flames. It was now Rognvald's turn to leap through the flames like Thorfinn, but he was carrying a lap-dog instead of a wife. He hid among the rocks and seaweed on the shore but the dog yapped and he was caught and slain by Thorkel Fosterer, one of Thorfinn's men.

And so Papa Stronsay played an important part in the history of Orkney for this episode led to a long period of peace and prosperity under the magnanimous rule of Thorfinn the Mighty.

Wildlife: Whooper swans winter on Mill Loch. The previous owner banned shooting and there are now many birds including breeding arctic terns and visitors such as snow bunting.

* * *

For many centuries **PAPA STRONSAY** was known for its fertility and its luxuriant crops of grain. And from the early 17th century until 1914 it also prospered from the fishing industry as, in spite of limited acreage, it had no less than five fish-curing stations. These worked in co-operation with the fifteen stations at Whitehall, just across the harbour on Stronsay and much of the produce went for sale to the Baltic ports. In the 1950s the farm was producing excellent crops of oats, turnips and potatoes.

Papa Stronsay is low and flat, only reaching 13m above sea-level but it has an ample water supply from the marshy Mill Loch which covers about 5% of the surface area. Most of the buildings are in the south of the island overlooking Whitehall Harbour and close to a mound (8m high) known as **Earls Knoll** [HY668292] which contains a Neolithic chamber tomb and a local tradition that the 'skeely skipper' Sir Patrick Spens is buried there. Two noteworthy cairns and a burnt mound are in the centre of the island and the excavated 12th century remains of St Nicholas Chapel have been found on the site of an 8th century Pictish church by the sea. Reminders of Papa Stronsay's popularity in the heady days of the herring boom are everywhere. A stone quay and a number of old piers are south of the house but only one curer's hut remains.

The original laird's house, now the Golgotha Monastery, is rambling and comfortable and the monks are building cells, a library, a small church and a cloister. They have a milking herd of cows and a further herd on Housebay farm (bought 2003) on Stronsay. In the words of Father Michael Mary: 'Commercial cheese production creates local jobs and gives us a financial infrastructure – after all, we can't just survive on prayers'.

A thin tongue of land curls out to the west and then southwards to **Point of the Graand** (ON *graand* – spit or sand bar). The whole area is very shallow and tidal and encloses the **Bight of Stackaback**. The light beacon at **The Ness** in the north-east is a white tower which is automatic and only 8m high.

It is well known in Orkney that when there is a

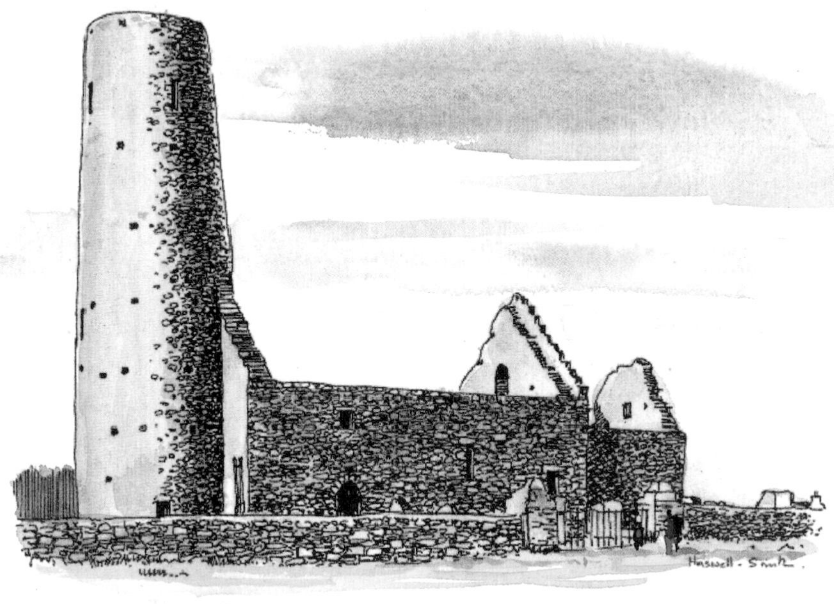

FAMOUS EGILSAY LANDMARK – THE 12TH-CENTURY CHURCH OF ST MAGNUS

spring tide on a Midsummer Night the grey seal or 'selkie' strips off his skin and becomes human and dances for sheer joy. A Papa Stronsay woman once fell in love with a selkie. The proof? Her children had thick horny skin on their hands and feet and always smelled of fish.

* * *

Access: No regular access but visits can be arranged with prior agreement from the owners. Enquire at Stronsay Hotel Hotel, 01857-616473.

Anchorage:

1. Whitehall Harbour. Good anchorage but many reefs and shoals. Use N entrance and anchor where space and depth available S of Papa Stronsay. Tidal stream slight.

10.18 Egilsay

(G. eaglais or EI ecclais, ON -øy – church island) or possibly (ON – Egil's island). In 1529 described as 'insularum ecclesia'. The possible Celtic derivation, very unusual in Orkney, is supported by the drying island at the north extremity being called Kili Holm which could be (G. cille – chapel or cell islet).

OS Maps: 1:50000 Sheet 5 or 6 1:25000 Sheet 464
Admiralty Charts: 1:200000 Nos.1942 or 1954 1:75000 Nos.2249 or 2250 various No.2562 plans

Area: 650ha (1606 acres)
Height: 35m (115 ft)

Population: 1795–210. 1841–190 (35 houses). 1881–165. 1891–147 (33 houses). 1931–85. 1961–54 (15 houses). 1981–23. 1991–46. 2001–37.

Geology: Middle Old Red Sandstone similar to that on Rousay.

History: Erlend's son, Magnus, reluctantly accompanied King Magnus of Norway when he plundered Wales in 1098 but he refused to fight, although to prove he was no coward he stood on the poop-deck singing psalms during the battle. Needless to say this was not a popular gesture and soon after the battle was won young Magnus had to make a quick exit. He took refuge for a number of years at the court of Edgar, King of Scots (the son of Malcolm Canmore) avoiding all contact with King Magnus. The Norwegian King was by then known as Magnus Barelegs presumably because he chose to wear a kilt. In 1103 Magnus Barelegs was killed in Ireland so young Magnus returned to Orkney in 1106 and claimed his earldom and half the Orkney revenues. The other half belonged to Earl Haakon, his cousin.

In spite of his piety Magnus was a fairly unpredictable character but nevertheless he had the popular support of many Orcadians. He married a girl called Ingigerd but never consummated the marriage. Apparently cold water helped him to maintain a state of chastity. After some years he lost interest in marital life and travelled south to stay at the court of King Henry I of England. Henry was married to King Edgar of Scotland's sister.

Haakon took advantage of Magnus's absence to assert his complete authority in Orkney when suddenly Magnus reappeared with five warships. Haakon rushed to arms but the Althing, or Parliament, counselled peace and arranged a parley on the island of Egilsay during Easter week, 1117. Both parties were to take no more than two ships and equal numbers of men. Magnus landed first, but then saw Haakon approaching with eight ships and many men.

Magnus refused to let his men defend him and spent the night praying in a small chapel while Haakon camped on the shore. With Magnus was a Celt called Holdbodi who recorded what then happened.

In the morning Magnus came out of the chapel, met Haakon on the shore and offered, for the sake of peace, to go into exile – to Rome or the Holy Land – but Haakon dismissed the idea.

Magnus then said he would accept imprisonment, but this too was rejected. He next offered to be maimed or blinded and to this Haakon agreed, but Haakon's men objected as they did not wish Orkney to continue to be divided between two earls. They said they would prefer to kill either cousin outright – no matter which. Haakon is then reported to have said: 'I like my Earldom better than death, so kill him.' But no one was keen to strike the fatal blow in such a cold-blooded fashion.

Magnus said nothing, knelt, prayed, and then commanded Lifolf, (who was Haakon's cook), to use his axe to hew a great wound in his head. This Lifolf did, and also struck a second time.

Holdbodi's account has since been supported by the discovery in 1919 of what is almost certainly Magnus' skeleton entombed in St Magnus' cathedral in Kirkwall. The skull has been pierced with an axe and the upper jaw severed.

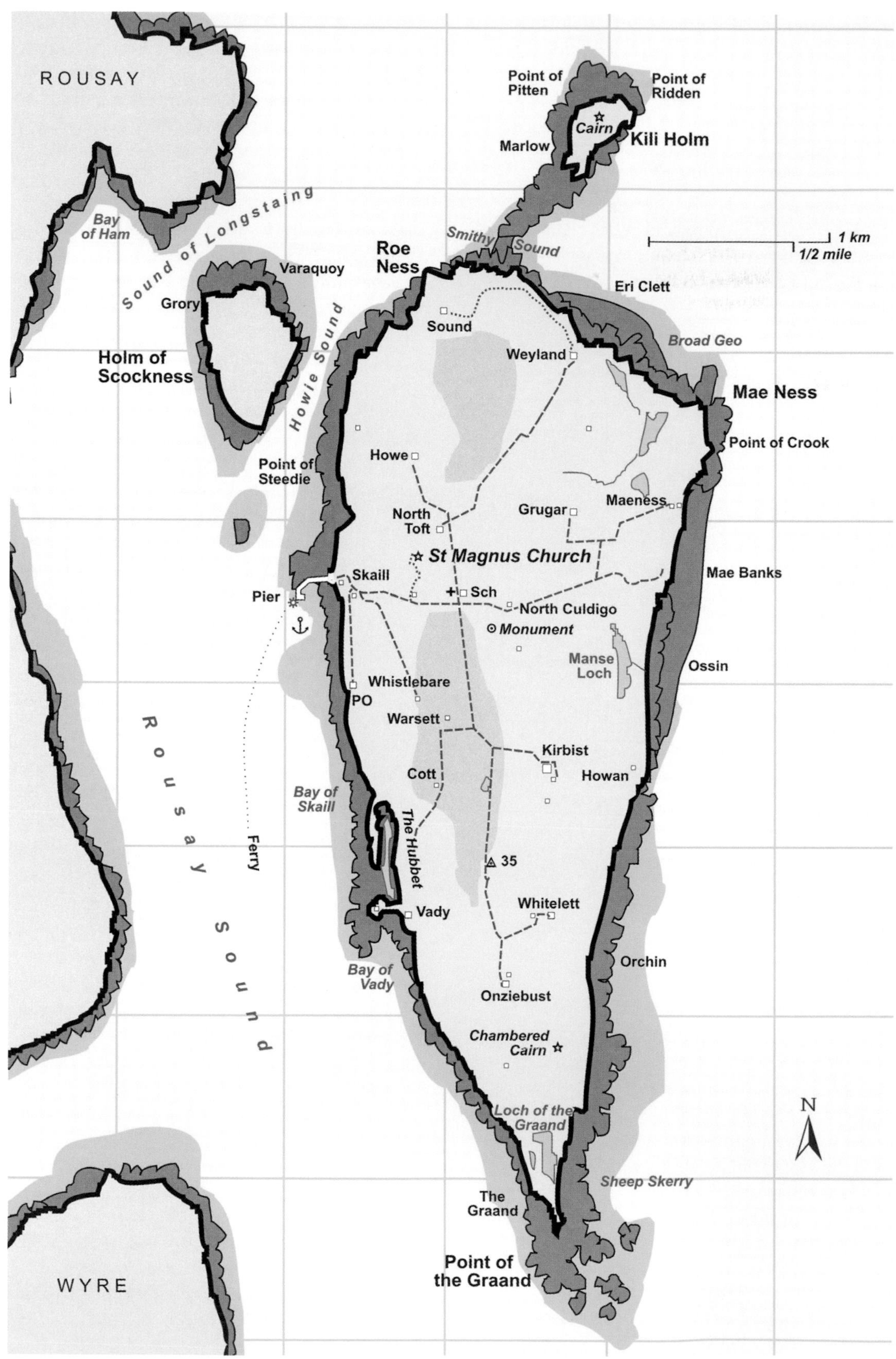
ROUSAY
Point of Pitten
Point of Ridden
Cairn
Kili Holm
Marlow
Bay of Ham
Sound of Longstaing
Smithy Sound
1 km
1/2 mile
Roe Ness
Varaquoy
Grory
Eri Clett
Sound
Holm of Scockness
Howie Sound
Weyland
Broad Geo
Mae Ness
Point of Crook
Howe
Point of Steedie
Maeness
Grugar
North Toft
St Magnus Church
Mae Banks
Skaill
Pier
Sch
North Culdigo
Monument
Manse Loch
Ossin
Whistlebare
PO
Warsett
Rousay Sound
Kirbist
Howan
Cott
Bay of Skaill
Ferry
The Hubbet
35
Vady
Whitelett
Orchin
Bay of Vady
Onziebust
Chambered Cairn
N
Loch of the Graand
Sheep Skerry
The Graand
Point of the Graand
WYRE

Wildlife: Breeding ducks, waders and black-headed gulls frequent the small lochs. In winter the coastline supports many waders, purple sandpiper and turnstone with numerous divers and sea-duck in the sounds. But rats have become a serious and growing problem.

* * *

EGILSAY is a spearhead-shaped island with a low central ridge rising to 35m. Conspicuous on the ridge is the great round tower of **St Magnus' Church** [HY466304]. From the distance it could, unromantically, be a factory chimney or grain silo but closer inspection reveals the beautiful masonry of this well-preserved 12th-century tower. The style is unique in Orkney and follows an Irish ecclesiastical style of the 11th century. Even on mainland Scotland there are only a limited number of examples. The tower was reduced in height in the 19th century to improve its stability but it is still nearly 15m high. Originally, it was probably about 20m high and included several storeys. Its internal diameter at ground level is about 3m and the walls are over 1m thick.

The church nave, originally covered with Orcadian stone slabs,is now roofless but the church was in use until well into the 19th century. The walls are almost complete but they are dotted with 'put-log' holes, possibly for scaffolding, and there used to be a second storey above the chancel, roofed with a barrel vault.

This is not the church where St Magnus kept vigil before his death although it is dedicated to him and quite probably stands on the site of the earlier chapel. The place where the saint was murdered is not far away and marked by a stone cenotaph which was erected in 1938.

The name of this island with its probable Celtic connections, the design of the church and even the presence of a Celt as witness to the death of St Magnus leads one to wonder whether this may have been the site of an early Celtic monastery set in the heart of Norse territory?

There is a good little road running from the pier at **Skaill** (ON *skáli* – hall), on the west side of Egilsay, up to the schoolhouse near St Magnus' Church. Here a road runs along the spine of the island serving the dozen or so small farms. Apart from a chambered cairn [HY474278] near the southernmost tip, **Point of the Graand** (ON – spit or sandbank), there are few other known prehistoric relics.

At the north of Rousay Sound which separates Egilsay from Rousay there is a small island like a stepping stone, **Holm of Scockness** (ON – islet of the crooked headland). **Kili Holm**, the islet to the north of Egilsay, is tidal. Both are used as rough grazing for sheep.

* * *

Access: Orkney Ferries daily ro-ro service, Tingwall/ Rousay/ Egilsay/ Wyre, 01856-872044. Kirkwall/ Tingwall bus, 01856-870555.

Anchorage:

1. Skaill. Anchor in Rousay Sound off the Skaill pier, 3–6m, sand. Avoid obstructing ferry. Shelter from W but subject to swell in S'lies and NE'lies.

10.19 Eynhallow

*[**Yn**-hal-oa] (ON øyin helga – holy island)*

OS Maps: 1:50000 Sheet 6 1:25000 Sheets 463 or 464
Admiralty Charts: 1:200000 Nos.1942 or 1954 1:75000 No.2249

Area: 75ha (185 acres)
Height: 30m (98 ft)

Owner: Owned by Duncan Robertson (an ornithologist) and subsequently by his daughter, Jean Robertson. She died in 1979 and Eynhallow was then bought from her estate by Orkney Islands Council for £60,000.

Population: 1841–26 (4 houses). 1891–0. 1931–0. 1981–0. Uninhabited.

Geology: Middle Old Red Sandstone of the Rousay variety.

History: This was probably the site of one of the earliest monastic settlements in Orkney and may only have been preceded by Christ Church on the Brough of Birsay. Although it was established after Earl Thorfinn's period of rule at the height of Norse dominance, it almost certainly had Celtic antecedents.

The *Orkneyinga Saga* records that Sweyn Asleifsson and his men once hid in the sea-cave (at Cave Geo?) on Eynhallow when being pursued by Earl Harald. The tide rose above the cave entrance, concealing it and leaving Earl Harald mystified by their disappearance, but the fugitives survived in the pocket of air trapped at the back of the cave.

Eynhallow is another of the small group of

islands which is allowed to issue its own postage stamps.

Wildlife: It used to be claimed that rats and mice could not live on this enchanted isle but rats, in fact, prospered so well that they had to be eradicated. Not so the many common seals as these may be Fin Folk. Their enchanted summer home is called Hildaland and some think Hildaland is really Eynhallow.

On a more practical note this is a sea-bird sanctuary run as a Nature Reserve by Orkney Islands Council. Thirty-three species nest regularly on the island, including the fulmar (the 'malliemak'), whilst many others come as visitors. The fulmar, many of which live for over 40 years, is now quite common but was unknown in Orkney before 1900.

* * *

With the exception of the exposed west side **EYNHALLOW** is surrounded by reefs, shoals and dangerous tides which must have required expert seamanship by the early Christians when they chose to settle there. The island has a compact

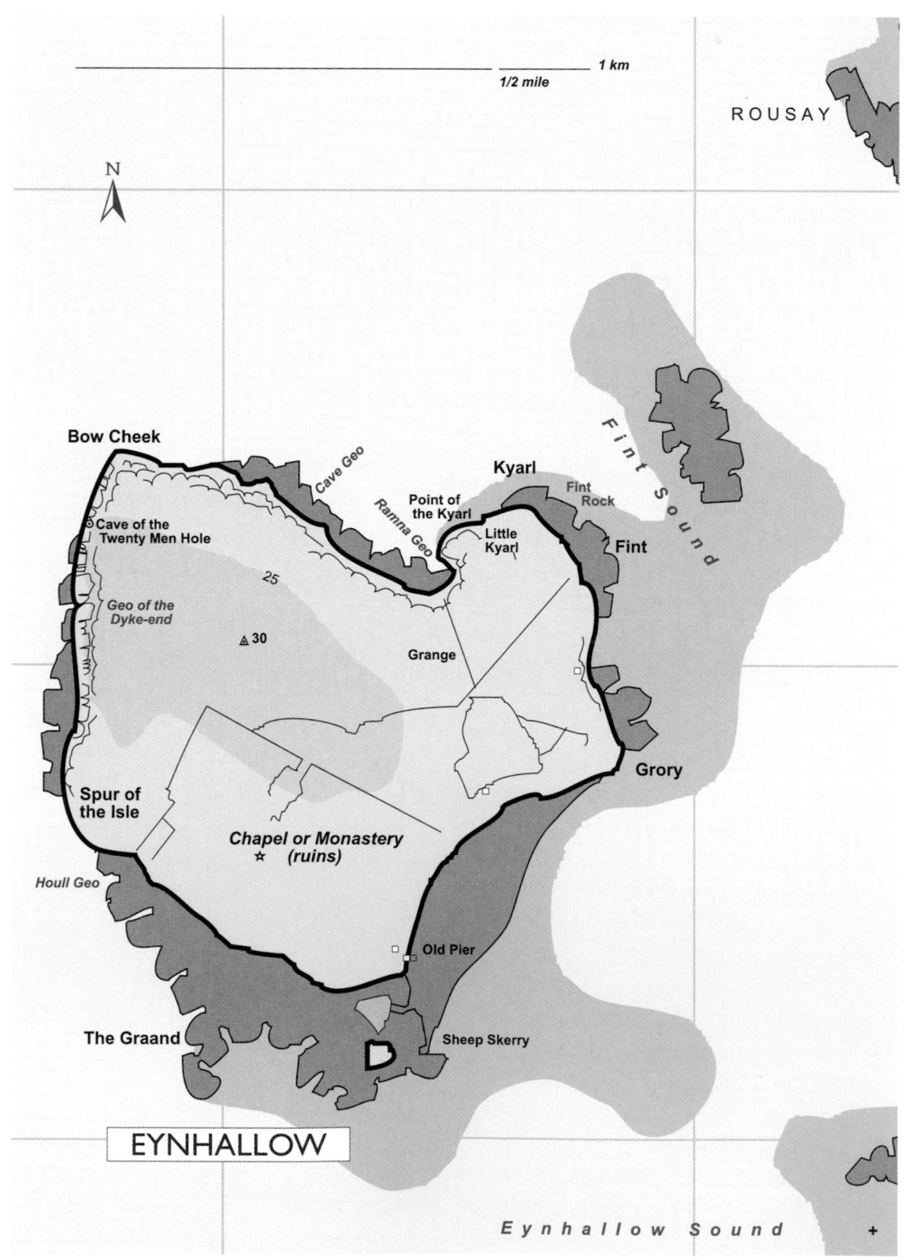

shape with the highest ground (30m) being just north-west of the centre and a gently sloping valley called the **Grange** divides the island. The ruins of a small medieval church in what may be a Cistercian monastery site can be seen facing across Eynhallow Sound to the parish of Evie on Mainland [HY359288]. Evie means 'swirl' and the Reef of Burgar opposite the church creates the dangerous Burgar Rost, a vicious tidal rip that has to be treated with great respect. On the other side of the island is the even more turbulent Cutlar Rost.

The relatively recent history of the ruined church is of interest because it was only rediscovered by David Balfour, the island's owner, in 1851. The owner cleared the island when a virulent disease – possibly typhoid from a contaminated well – killed several of the crofters living in the small interconnected settlement of houses. When the tenants had gone the houses were set alight as a safety-precaution and it was only when the thatched roofs and timber partitions had burned away that it was seen that the stone walls formed parts of old monastic buildings – church, cloisters, refectory and dormitories. It is probable that the domestic occupation occurred at the time of the Reformation.

The church itself is thought to be early 12th-century and is almost certainly part of the Orkney monastery to which Abbot Lawrence was appointed in 1117 according to the records of Melrose.

The ruined bothy by the south shore is in fact the old 19th century schoolhouse and 'The Lodge', a summer residence clad with corrugated-iron sheet, was built near the landing beach by the then owner in the late 1800s. It is now used as a research centre by Aberdeen University, mainly for the study of fulmars.

The west coast is steep with cliffs of piled up sandstone slabs and its **Cave of the Twenty Men Hole** recalls the days when it was imperative for all the able-bodied men to hide from the naval press-gangs.

Eynhallow is an island rich in tradition and mystery and in the past was known as the enchanted island. It has, for instance, been known to vanish as one's boat approaches it. The only way to avoid this navigational disaster (so they say) is for the helmsman to keep his eyes resolutely fixed on the island while clasping an iron object.

* * *

Access: Excursions may be arranged at Tingwall or try Explorer Charter, Kirkwall, 01856-871225.

Anchorage: Local knowledge is essential. The tidal stream (Burgar Rost) S of island is very strong, unpredictable, and conditions can change suddenly. Tidal stream on NE side is dangerous. Temp. anchorage off beach in SE bay only when conditions are favourable.

10.20 Rousay

(ON Hrólfs-øy – Hrolf's island).

O S Maps: 1:50000 Sheet 6 1:25000 Sheet 464
Admiralty Charts: 1:200000 Nos.1942 or 1954 1:75000 No.2249

Area: 4860ha (12009 acres)
Height: 250m (820 ft)

Owner: Multiple ownership.

Population: 1841–982 (225 houses). 1881–873. 1891–774 (187 houses). 1931–468. 1961–237. 1981–209. 1991–217. 2001–212.

Geology: The Middle Old Red Sandstone of which Rousay is almost entirely composed has been adopted as a standard for its particular type – it yields greyish-coloured flagstones. These underlie the peat-covered uplands.

History: In the on-going struggle for control of Orkney, Earl Rognvald had landed and mustered his forces on Westray (No.10.25) and Earl Paul, known as Paul the Silent, who was effectively in control, had established his defences on Mainland. Battle seemed imminent until Rognvald asked Bishop William to mediate. The Bishop agreed, and a fortnight's truce was declared.

Paul decided that a few days' holiday would do him good so he sailed over to Rousay to stay with his friend Sigurd of Westness and early in the morning he, and a group of his men, went down to the shore to hunt otters.

The wild card in this idyllic scenario, however, was young Sweyn of Gairsay (No.10.13) – Sweyn Asliefsson – who had been rather unjustly outlawed a year before by Earl Paul. Sweyn had stayed on the Scottish mainland with Earl Maddad of Atholl and his wife, Margaret, whose son Harald also had claims to the Orkney title. He promised to support Harald's claim and

Margaret's uncle provided him with a merchant ship and a crew of thirty men.

When Paul failed to return to the house for his morning ale, Sigurd sent out a search party, which found the bodies of Paul's men and six strangers. There had obviously been a fight but no trace of Paul could be found. It was only discovered later that Sweyn had sailed his new ship through Scapa Flow, up the Atlantic coast of Mainland, and into Eynhallow Sound – waters which he knew well from his life on Gairsay. There he had surprised and kidnapped Paul and slain his followers.

Paul was taken to Atholl and given a friendly reception although held as a prisoner but later, when Sweyn had returned to Orkney, the ruthless Margaret had him blinded and then murdered.

* * *

Wildlife: There is a lot of angelica to be seen on Rousay – the plant which the Norsemen are said to have introduced. It looks something like hogweed.

The brown hare is fairly common but the enormous population of rabbits is most in evidence. There are more families of otters on these coasts than elsewhere in Orkney.

Bird-watching on Rousay is good at any time but probably best from May to July. Inland, there are many breeding species such as the red-throated diver, hen harrier, merlin, curlew, golden plover, short-eared owl and five gull species. The common sandpiper can be seen here although it is generally uncommon in Orkney.

The best sites are: Brings Heath and Quendale in the north-west where there are some 4000 pairs of arctic tern, 100 pairs of arctic skua and some great skua. Many fulmar, kittiwake, guillemot and razorbill are to be found on the cliffs.

Trumland RSPB Reserve in the south-east; here the red-throated diver, hen harrier, and golden plover breed, while merlin, arctic and great skua and short-eared owl can be seen.

Great northern diver, eider, long-tailed duck, velvet scoter and red-breasted merganser winter in Eynhallow Sound.

* * *

ROUSAY is a hilly island and the sandstone strata have given the hills a terraced appearance. From the summit of **Blotchnie Fiold** (250m) in the south-east it is possible to see Foula (No.11.6) on a clear day nearly 100km distant on the Atlantic horizon.

This is possibly the most interesting of all the Orkney Islands and one of the best of the Northern Isles for anyone interested in prehistory. It has the added advantage that some of the best sites are quite near the ferry pier on the south coast. West of the pier are three remarkable burial cairns: **Taversoe Tuick** [HY426276] has two storeys and separate entrance passages, **Blackhammer** [HY414276] has seven divisions in the chamber (in 1936 two skeletons were found in it), and **Knowe of Yarso** [HY405280], a stalled cairn with four compartments. When this latter cairn, which is about 3km from the pier, was excavated in 1934 a large collection of mixed bones were discovered including the remains of twenty-one humans, several sheep, thirty deer, and a dog.

The pier and village settlement were built in the 1870s by General Traill Burroughs who is sometimes given the dubious distinction of being Orkney's most-detested 19th-century landowner. His home, **Trumland House,** was designed in a truly Victorian Scottish Baronial style by David Bryce in 1873 [HY428278]. The General made his money in India and married the heiress to the Traills of Rousay. She took an interest in the landscaping around the house – which has resulted in a pleasant patch of woodland – and chose a knoll for a viewpoint and on which to place a seat. This led to the discovery that the knoll was a 5000-year-old burial cairn with an adjacent earth-house (Taversoe Tuick).

The Traill family home was at **Westness** [HY383289], a couple of kilometres beyond Knowe of Yarso. It was burned down when John Traill, a Jacobite supporter, was hiding in the Gentleman's Cave on Westray (No.10.25) but was rebuilt later in the 18th century.

Excavations were started in 1978 on a number of Viking buildings beyond Westness. According to the *Orkneyinga Saga* this was the home of Sigurd where Earl Paul was kidnapped while hunting otters although there is some dubiety because not far away, at **Skaill** (ON *skáli* – hall), a farmer in 1963 started digging a hole to bury a cow and broke into a Norse grave. A young woman was buried in it with three magnificent silver brooches dating from about the 9th and 10th centuries. There is an old church at Skaill

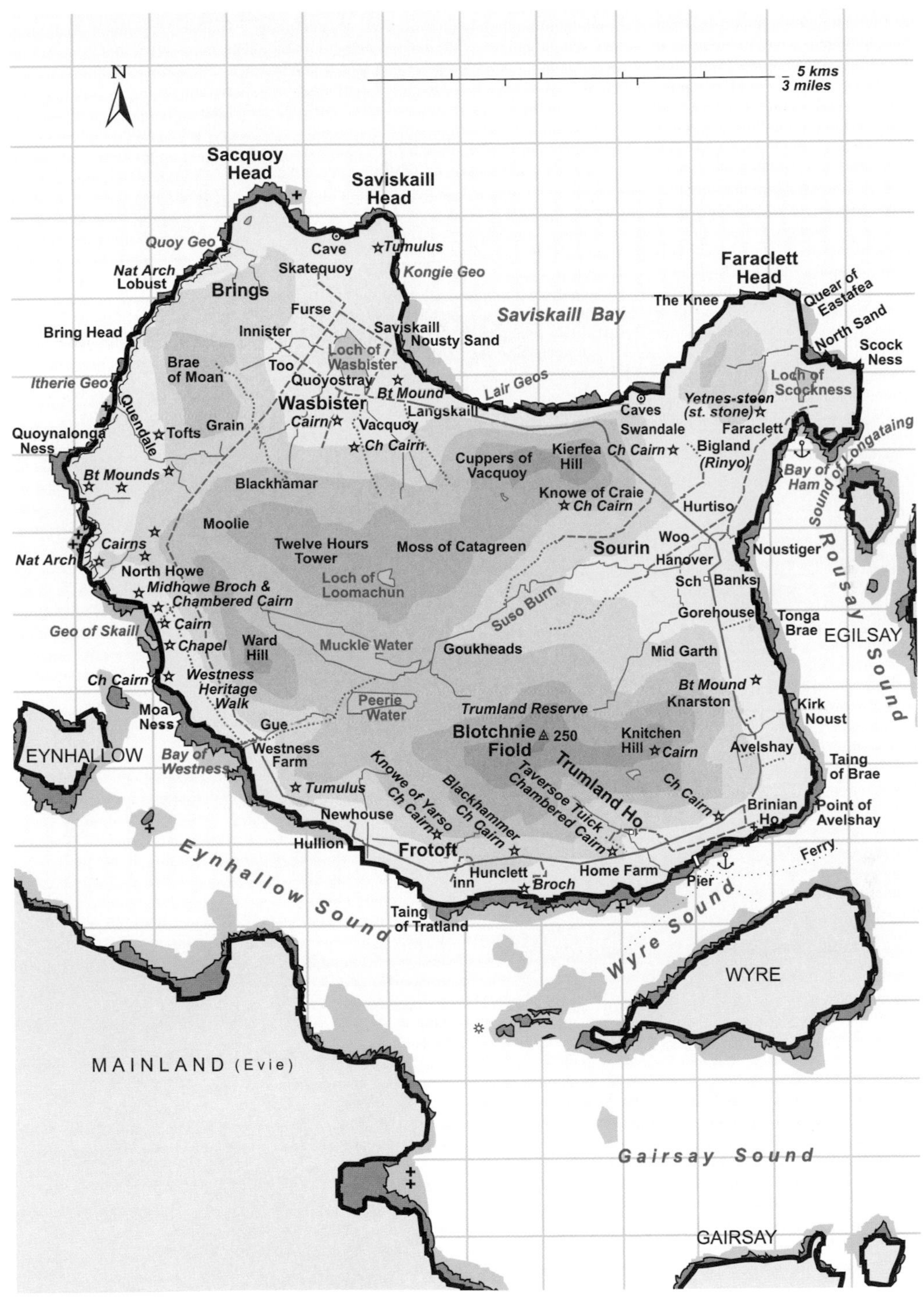

which may be pre-Reformation [HY374302].

Without doubt, the most significant archaeological site on Rousay is **Midhowe** [HY372306] which is just beyond Skaill and opposite Eynhallow (No.10.19). Here there is an enormous chambered cairn which predates Maeshowe on Mainland. The Midhowe chamber is 23m long and over 2m wide with 12 burial stalls arranged along each side. Unstan type pottery was found here and the remains of twenty-five individuals. There were also the remains of cattle, deer, sheep and even an Orkney vole. The original chamber height would have been about 2½m. Midhowe was excavated in the 1930s having been discovered, and the work paid for, by W G Grant who had bought Trumland House and much of the south-west of the island. It was Grant's forebears who founded the Highland Park whisky distillery at Kirkwall.

Near the tomb is an Iron Age broch [HY370307] which is over 9m in diameter and with walls over 4m high and clustered by it are the remains of later buildings like a small village. During excavation many domestic implements were revealed, some of which were of Roman origin.

Rousay is littered with the relics of prehistory. There are two more brochs in the immediate vicinity of Westness, at least fifteen brochs on the shores of Eynhallow Sound, and any number of cairns and burned mounds.

After the road turns northwards it crosses Quendale where the old mansion of **Tofts** stands – said to be the oldest two-storeyed domestic house in Orkney. The site is south of Brae of Moan [HY373326]. There is interesting cliff scenery all along this coastline due to the regular rock strata, with caves, geos, and a natural rock arch.

The place names by Saviskaill Bay on the north coast confirm associations with the Norse period, **Wasbister** (ON – west farm), Langskaill (ON – longhouse drinking-hall) and a number of 'quoy' suffixes (ON *koie* – shelter or enclosure), often applied to hillcrofts.

The north-east corner of the island forms a protuberance ending at Faraclett Head. Here, on the farm of Bigland, there is a fine example of a Stone Age village of the Skarabrae type called **Rinyo** [HY438321]. This has been dated to about 3700BC from pottery shards discovered at foundation level and this, in turn, has assisted the dating of Skarabrae. It also shows that these dwellings were contemporary with the chambered cairns.

On Faraclett Farm nearby there is an enormous standing stone called **Yetnes-steen** (ON *jötna-steinn* – the male giant's stone) [HY447327]. To prove there is no discrimination, at Swandale to the west, some rock-outcrops are called the **Gyro-stones** (ON *gyger* – a female giant).

There are a number of lochs on Rousay all rich in birdlife, such as **Loch of Wasbister** in the north-west, and in the desolate centre of the island where there is marvellous hill-walking, **Muckle Water** (big), **Peerie Water** (little) and **Loomachun** (ON – lochan of the red-throated diver or loon).

Although Rousay supported about 1000 people at the start of the 19th century it has always been restricted by its lack of agricultural land. Only the coastal strip can be profitably worked.

Access: Orkney Ferries daily ro-ro service, Tingwall/ Rousay/ Egilsay/ Wyre, 01856-872044. Kirkwall/ Tingwall bus, 01856-870555. Rousay History Tour by mini-bus, 01856-821234. Tourist Office, 01856-872856.

Anchorages:

1. Bay of Ham, N of Rousay Sound, good shelter from N and W. Anchor in 3½-6m. Avoid fish-farm. *(Access to the Stone Age village of Rinyo).*
2. Saviskaill Bay. Not recommended. Rocky bottom and exposed.
3. Wyre Sound. Anchor E of Rousay ferry pier. Close inshore out of the tide gives reasonable shelter from all directions. *(Access to Taversoe Tuick, etc.)*

10.21 Eday

*[**ee**-day] (ON eid-øy – isthmus island.) Eday has a narrow waist.*

O S Maps: 1:50000 Sheet 5 1:25000 Sheet 465
Admiralty Charts: 1:200000 Nos.1942 or 1954 1:75000 No.2250

Area: 2745ha (6783 acres)
Height: 101m (331 ft)

Owner: Multiple ownership since 1925. Previously owned by the Hebden family. Most small farms are owner-occupied.

Population: 1841–944 (193 houses). 1881–730. 1891–647 (138 houses). 1931–430. 1961–198. 1981–147. 1991–166. 2001–121.

Geology: Most of Eday is of an eponymous type of Middle Old Red Sandstone which is an excellent and attractive building stone. The fine yellow sandstone used in St Magnus Cathedral was quarried here. This is a true sandstone which is stratified in distinct slabs that are easily fashioned into blocks. It over-lies the Rousay type of sandstone except in a small patch at Backaland where Rousay Beds reach the surface.

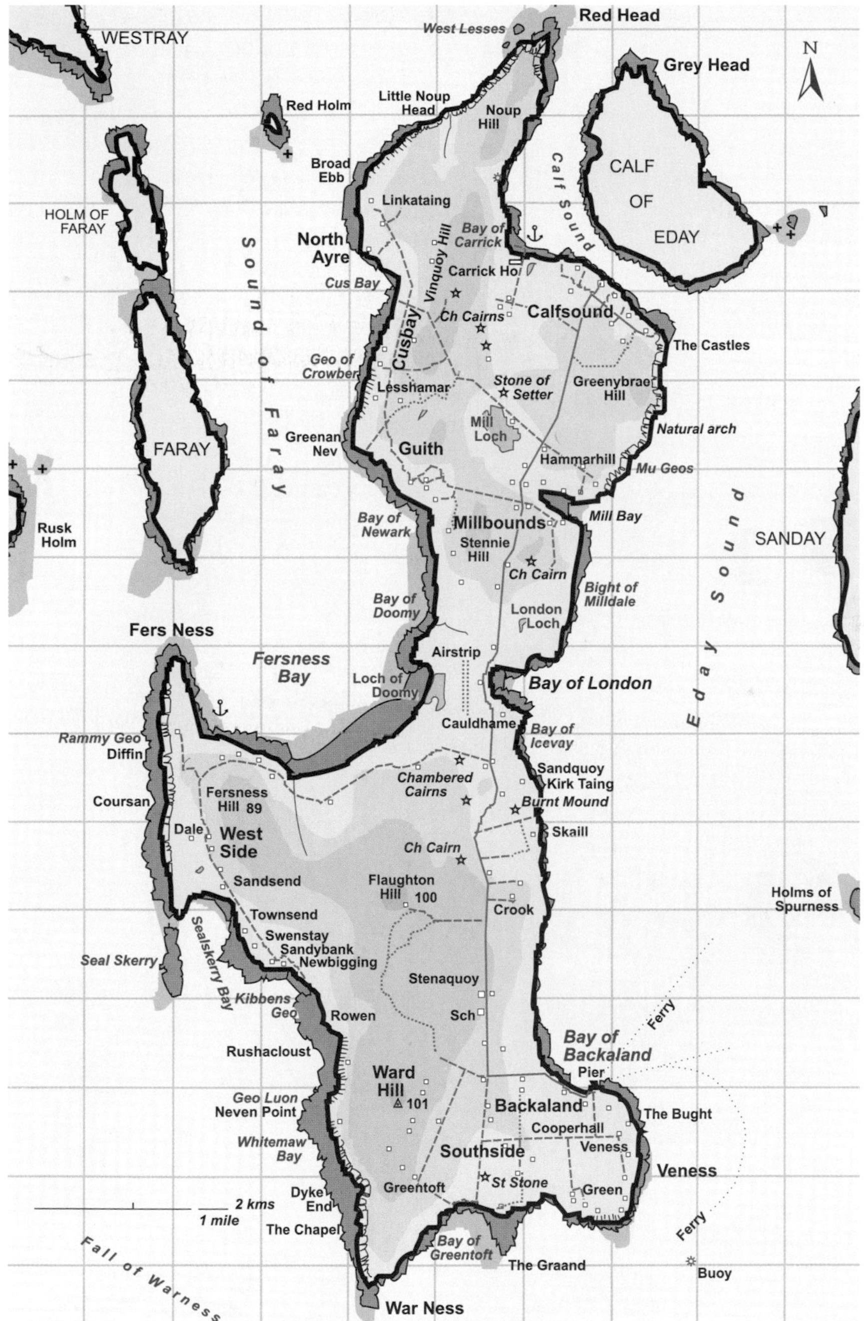

The ridge of hills running down the spine of Eday is covered with peat. Only the narrow coastal strip is suitable for cultivation. The islands of Sanday (No.10.24) and North Ronaldsay (No.10.27) obtained most of their fuel requirements from Eday and the peat was also exported to a number of whisky distilleries throughout Scotland.

History: Near the start of the 17th century the youthful John Stewart, second son of the Earl of Orkney, was accused of poisoning his brother Patrick. It was claimed that he had colluded with a witch called Alysoun Balfour. Alysoun was tortured but John was acquitted and in 1628 was created Earl of Carrick. In 1632 he was granted the island of Eday and immediately set about building a home in the pleasant Bay of Carrick overlooking Calf

Sound. The date 1633 is still to be seen inscribed over the courtyard gateway at Carrick House.

The notoriously inept pirate, John Gow, after raiding Cava (No.10.7) and Graemsay (No.10.9) decided to raid Carrick House on Eday. He sailed into Calf Sound but was unaware that the fast tides could set him onto the Calf of Eday shore. His ship *Revenge* got into difficulties and ran aground. He spent some time in full view of the House struggling for control and by the time he came ashore his old schoolmate James Fea, the owner of Carrick House, was waiting for him. He was arrested and handed over to the authorities. His ship's bell is still in Carrick House.

Wildlife: This is the only Orkney island on which bog myrtle, *Myrica gale*, can be found. The hills are used for rough grazing for sheep and are regularly burned to encourage the growth of young heather.

A number of otters, fairly uncommon in Orkney, frequent these coasts, particularly in the south-west between West Side and War Ness. There are lots of rabbits but no hares.

Eday has some special treats for bird-watchers, particularly from May to July. On Mill Loch there are several pairs of red-throated divers, probably representing the densest concentration of these fine birds in Britain (a bird hide is provided), and a few pairs of whimbrel nest on the moors which is a rare sight on Orkney. The moors also harbour arctic and great skua, curlew, snipe and golden plover. Fulmar and herring gull breed on Red Head in the extreme north and black guillemot can be seen on the shore. There are many migrants in the woodland at Carrick House particularly in spring and autumn.

* * *

EDAY can be dark and bleak with hills clothed in a deep layer of peat moorland. Only the southern part is cultivated and although there are many farms they are mostly very small and owner-occupied. This is a long island with a low narrow waist where the airstrip is sited beside the shallow Loch of Doomy.

The north extremity is called **Red Ness**, or **Red Head**, and the islet beside it in the Sound of Faray is **Red Holm**. These names are explicit – the red rock colour is distinctive, and because Red Ness is so much higher (70m) than its surroundings it is a useful landmark clearly indicating the entrance to Calf Sound. **Carrick House** [HY567385] was built in 1633 by the Earl of Carrick, younger son of the unpopular Earl Robert Stewart. Carrick Farm and the village of Calfsound look north across the narrow tide-rippled sound to Calf of Eday (No.10.23). The Bay of Carrick is sheltered by the western ridge of Noup Hill (ON *gnupr* – headland crag), Muckle Hill of Linkertaing, and Vinquoy Hill. The remains of chambered cairns in these hills can be seen but the best example, although little remains, is at **Huntersquoy** (ON *koie* – shelter or enclosure) [HY563377]. This, like Taversoe Tuick on Rousay (No.10.20), has two storeys with separate entrances. **The Stone of Setter**, almost 5m high, stands proudly between Huntersquoy and Mill Loch, where red-throated divers can be seen among the reeds [HY564372].

A road runs southwards for the entire length of the island, from Calfsound to the standing stone at Southside. There are more chambered cairns and other evidence of early man, particularly among the moorland hills – Fersness, Whitemaw, Flaughton, Leeniesdale, and **Ward Hill** (101m), the highest on the island. Although the ferry route leads through Calf Sound in the north the ferry pier is at **Backaland** in the south-east.

The thick layers of peat on Eday were its salvation in the 18th and 19th centuries as it provided much-needed fuel for the other islands and prosperity also came from its quarries which supplied Kirkwall with slate. But increasing imports of coal destroyed the peat trade in the 1860s and the island has not yet fully recovered its self-esteem.

South-west of Warness, across the Fall of Warness where North Sea gales stir up fierce tidal rips, are **Muckle Green Holm** and **Little Green Holm**. They are occupied by a small cormorant colony and a number of nesting shags while Otter Pool on Muckle Green Holm still shelters a family of otters. The islet was called Hellisay (cave island) by the Norse and it was another hiding place used by Sweyn Asliefsson.

Access: Orkney Ferries ro-ro service every day from/to Kirkwall and most days from/to Stronsay/ Sanday, 01856-872044. Scheduled air service from Kirkwall, usually Weds. only, 01856-872494 or -873457. Tourist information, 01857-622248 or -622260.

Anchorages:

1. Bay of Carrick, Calf Sound. Follow the white sectored light identifying the fairways in the Sound. Bay of Carrick is SE of Calf Sound Light-tower. Good shelter. Anchor below Carrick House off the stone jetty close in-shore out

of the tide in 3–4m sand. Avoid lobster boat moorings.

2. Fersness Bay. Shelter from all S'lies. Anchor off S shore in 3½–7m, sand and weed. Good holding.

3. Bay of Backaland, an indentation on the E coast ½M N of Veness. Temp. anchorage in suitable conditions 2c NW of pier, bottom stony, or possibly lie alongside pier but keeping a constant watch.

4. Bay of London, small inlet at centre of E coast. Temp. anchorage at entrance to bay.

5. Mill Bay, small inlet on the E coast ¾M SSW of Greeny Brae. Temp. anchorage at entrance to bay.

10.22 Faray

(ON vaer-øy – ram island). Previously called North Pharay.

OS Maps: 1:50000 Sheet 5 1:25000 Sheets 464 or 465
Admiralty Charts: 1:200000 No.1942 or 1954 1:75000 No.2249 or 2250

Area: 180ha (445 acres)
Height: 32m (105 ft)

Population: 1841–67 (14 houses). 1871–83. 1881–72. 1891–58 (8 houses). 1931–40.

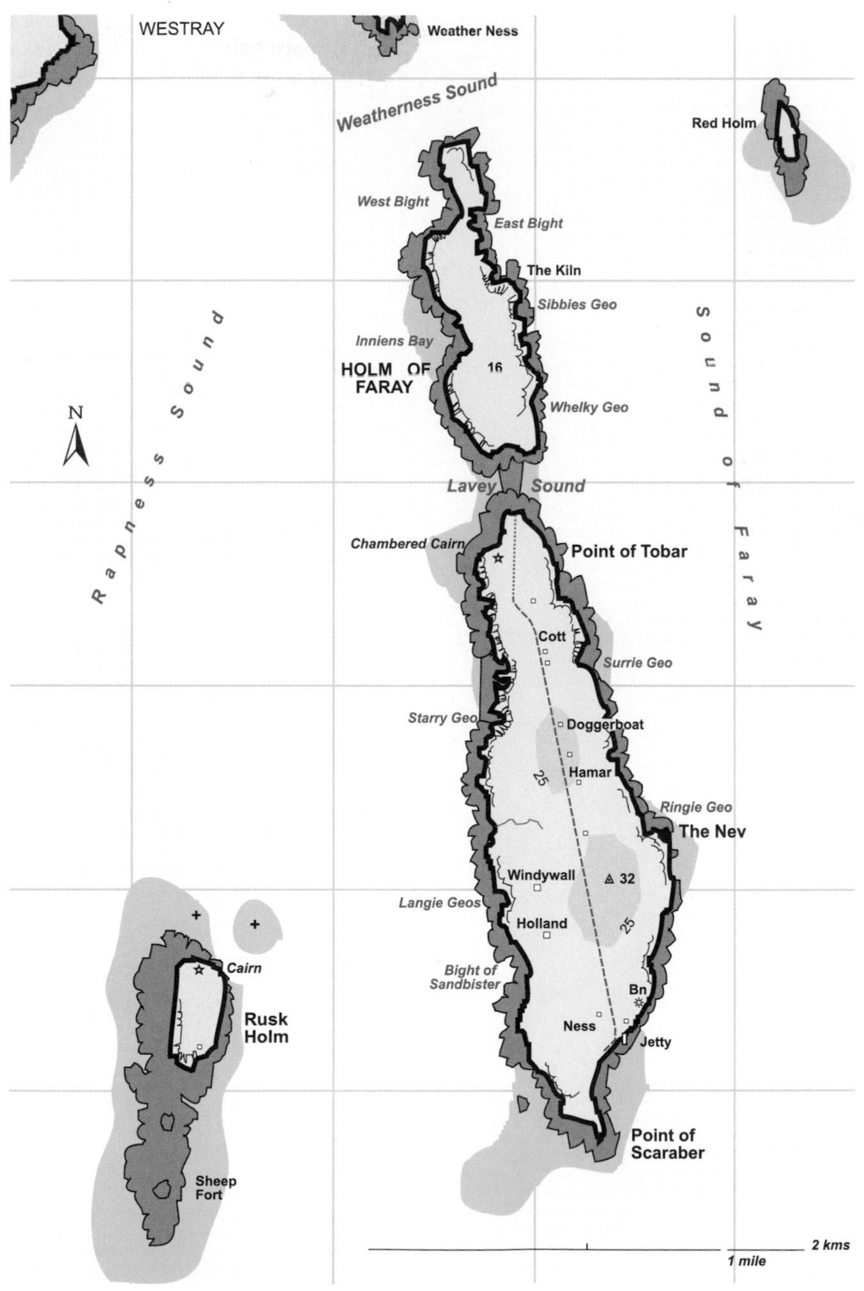

1961–0. 1971–0. 1981–0. 1991–0. No permanent habitation.

Geology: Middle Old Red Sandstone of the Rousay type with the exception of a small area of Eday type sandstone on the south-east coast.

History: A lone chambered cairn near Lavey Sound is the only apparent historic artefact on the island.

Wildlife: Holm of Faray and the islet due west of Faray, Rusk Holm, is a favourite breeding ground for grey seals which can often be seen lying in great numbers on the wet rocks like well-cooked giant sausages. Rusk Holm also has its own flock of wild native sheep.

* * *

FARAY is part of a ridge which almost connects Fers Ness on Eday to Weather Ness on Westray. There is a wider gap to the south through which the Kirkwall Ferry sails into the Sound of Faray and a narrower gap at the north forming Weatherness Sound. In the middle, Faray is separated from Holm of Faray by Lavey Sound which dries out at low water but through which it is possible to sail after half-tide.

Faray rises to a height of 32m near the centre of the island.

A road still runs up the central axis serving the scattered empty houses. It was reported that during the General Election of 1992 three voters on Faray were unable to deliver their votes because the rudder of their boat was broken. Democracy was saved by the use of a pet homing skua which carried their voting papers to Mainland.

One of the crofts on the ridge is called 'Holland' – a name which is quite common throughout Orkney. Although the Dutch were well-known to the Orcadians the name is, in most cases, actually derived from (ON *há-land* – high land).

In the late 1930s there were eight families living on the island. They had crofts and supplemented their income by a spot of lobster-fishing. Then the Second World War intruded and a new world opened up. Comparisons were drawn and the simple but strenuous island life seemed less than perfect. By 1947 the last hard-working family had left and the island was deserted except for occasional summer occupation.

The only man-made relic of note is the chambered cairn beside Lavey Sound but it has been proposed that the rich peat bogs of both Faray and Holm of Faray should be made Special Areas of Conservation (SACs).

* * *

Access: Try Pierowall Charters, Westray, 01857-677493 or Eday Tourist Information, 01857-622248.

Anchorage: There are no recommended anchorages but temp. anchorage may be found using the chart. In S'lies anchor in Fersness Bay, Eday and in N'lies anchor by Weatherness, Westray to await suitable conditions for an approach to Faray. Avoid shoal area SW of Faray, and Lavey Sound which dries.

10.23 Calf of Eday

See Eday (No.10.21.) 'Calf' refers to a satellite of a larger island.

OS Maps: 1:50000 Sheet 5 1:25000 Sheet 465
Admiralty Charts: 1:200000 No.1942 or 1954 1:75000 No.2250

Area: 243ha (600 acres)
Height: 50m (164 ft)

Population: 1841–0. 1891–0. 1931–0. 1981–0. 1991–0. Uninhabited.

Geology: The island is composed of Middle Old Red Sandstone, mostly of the Eday variety but there is a thin intersection of Rousay flags on the north-south axis.

History: In the 18th and 19th centuries most of Orkney's salt came from the salt pans on this small island.

Wildlife: On Grey Head and the eastern cliffs there are large colonies of guillemot, razorbill and kittiwake, with black guillemot around the shores and moorland-nesting black-backed gulls on the heather top. A large cormorant colony thrives on the south side of the island.

* * *

Narrow Calf Sound between Eday and **CALF OF EDAY** is scenically attractive. The approach by sea from the north lies between the imposing **Red Head** of Eday and **Grey Head** of the Calf. The stone colours are subtle and dramatic.

The savage spring tide runs through the sound at six knots at both flood and ebb and in gales is whipped up into a turbulent race but at slack water in fine weather the sea becomes idyllic.

Among the group of chambered cairns on the heather slopes opposite Calfsound village, one is of particular interest as it has been built above an even earlier stone structure – whether a tiny dwelling or a tomb it is hard to say [HY579386].

Nearby [HY575390] is one of the finest examples of ancient saltworks in Britain.

Access: Try Pierowall Charters, Westray, 01857-677493, or ask Eday Tourist Information, 01857-622316.

Anchorage:

1. Bay of Carrick, Calf Sound. Follow the white sectored light identifying the fairways in the Sound. Bay of Carrick is SE of Calf Sound Light-tower on Eday. Good shelter. Anchor below Carrick House off the stone jetty close in-shore out of the tide in 5m sand. Avoid lobster boat moorings. Cross the sound *only* at slack water for dinghy landing.

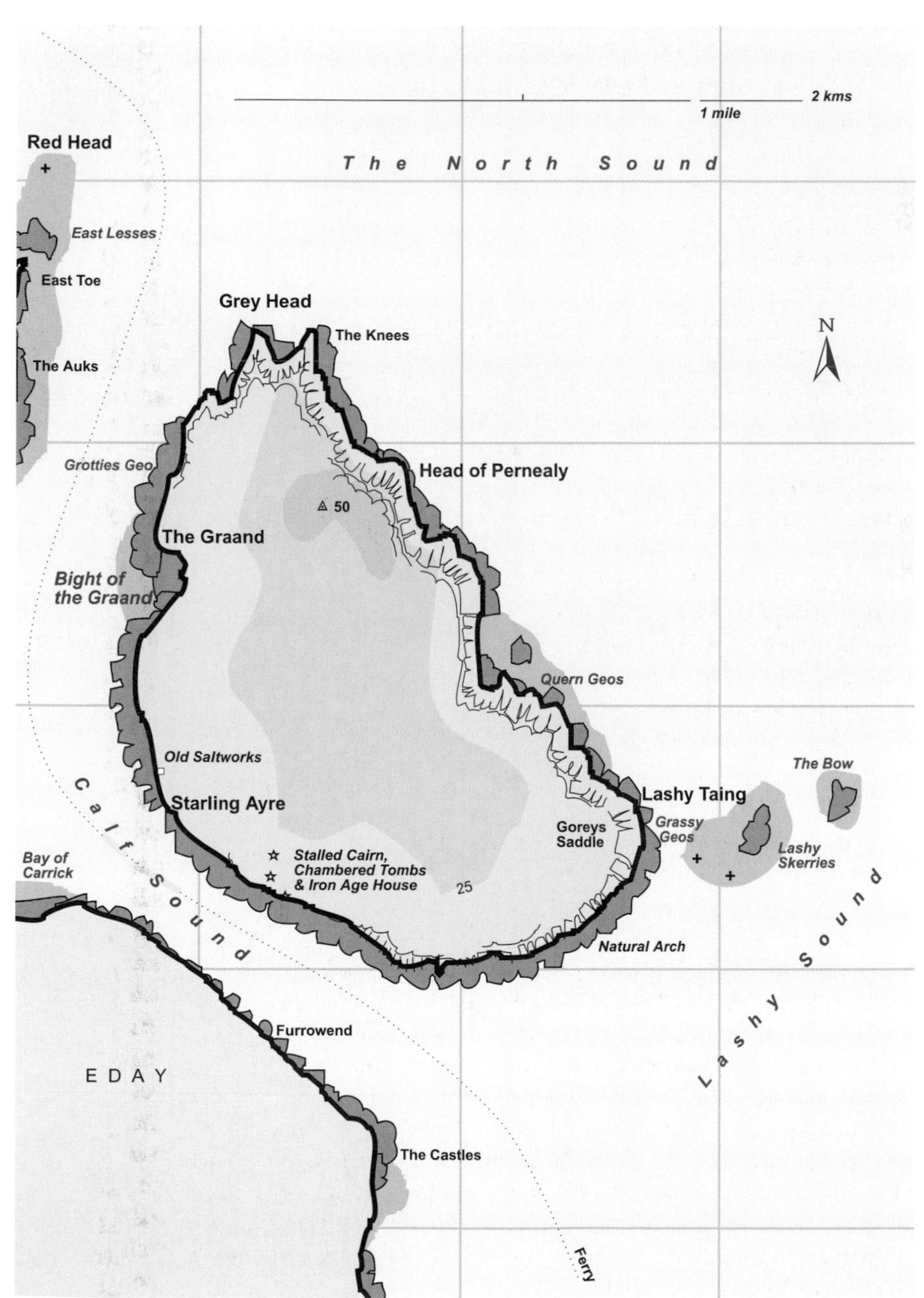

10.24 Sanday

(ON sand-øy – sand island).

O S Maps: 1:50000 Sheet 5 1:25000 Sheet 465
Admiralty Charts: 1:200000 Nos.1942 or 1954 1:75000 No.2250

Area: 5043ha (12461 acres)
Height: 65m (213 ft)

Owner: Multiple ownership. Most of the farms are owner-occupied.

Population: 1798–1772. 1841–1892 (372 houses). 1881–2082. 1891–1929 (402 houses). 1931–1160. 1961–670. 1981–525. 1991–533. 2001–478.

Geology: Well-weathered Middle Old Red Sandstone with a greyish colour. This is mostly of the Rousay type which accounts for the good soil but the south-western extremity is of the firmer Eday type of sandstone. A fault crosses the island from Ness of Brough to Tresness.

Wildlife: The Site of Scientific Interest (SSI) at North Loch includes Early March and Frog Orchids. Seaweed is plentiful around the coasts and *Laminaria digitata, L. cloustonii* and wracks such as *Fucus nodosus* and *F. serratus* are collected for alginate processing.

Sanday has prolific birdlife with colonies of Arctic tern, large numbers of ringed plover, and some corncrake and corn bunting. Many waders settle on the shoreline in winter including grey and golden plovers, bar-tailed godwit, dunlin, and turnstone. Rats have been a problem but were, hopefully, eradicated in 2007.

Lady Parish has many spring and autumn migrants and breeding wildfowl such as teal, widgeon, shoveller, tufted duck, red-breasted merganser, eider and some breeding waders. At Gump of Spurness there are Arctic skua and short-eared owl.

* * *

Eric Linklater thought that, from the air,

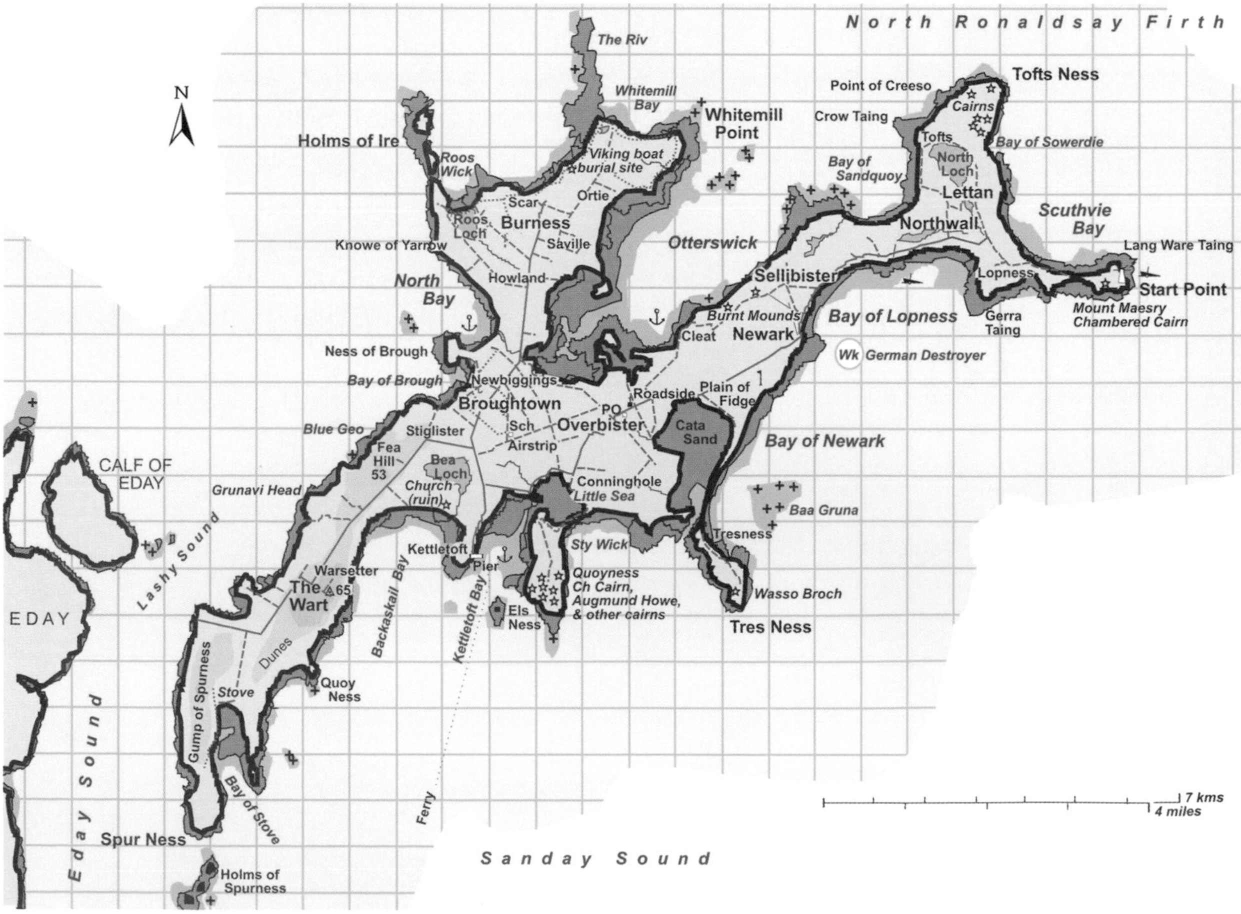

SANDAY looked like a fossilised, gigantic bat but we can be sure that the Norsemen never saw it from this angle. There are three peninsulas projecting from a common central base. The island is low-lying, the highest point being **The Wart** (65m) (The Ward or lookout point) and the peninsulas divide the long coastline into a large number of fairly shallow and exposed bays with beautiful wide white sandy beaches. These are usually deserted except for multitudes of wading birds. From a comparison with old maps it is possible that the sand-banks are slowly being extended by the sea and that the island is growing although in Otterswick the remains of a submerged willow forest dating from 5000BC show that the sea-level has risen by three metres.

In dark misty weather this low sprawling island is virtually invisible from the sea. Consequently, as there is no peat on the island, wrecks of wooden ships were very welcome and it is even said that prayers in church asked for the Lord's assistance in this respect.

The light, sandy soil is very fertile. It is tied in at the coasts by the roots of marram grass although thousands of rabbits do their best to disturb this delicate balance. A golf course spreads across the dunes of the Plain of Fidge at Newark. Kelp was the major industry in the 18th century with one quarter of Orkney's total production coming from Sanday. When the kelp boom died it was of little concern as during the 19th century the farms here were the most prosperous in Orkney. It is still productive but nowadays the farming is possibly more relaxed and supplemented by lobster-fishing and seaweed-gathering for alginate.

Although there are a few small lochs, the sandy soil is not good at retaining moisture, and as the rainfall is sometimes low water shortage can be a problem.

For many centuries agriculture took precedence over the preservation of ancient monuments on Sanday so there are few visible ruins although almost every ness has the faint trace of a broch. **Els Ness**, which at one time would have been a separate island but is now connected by an ayre, is on the south coast overlooking Sanday Sound. It has escaped the plough and is spattered with cairns like convex craters on the surface of the moon. Here there is a very interesting chambered cairn (central chamber and six cells) at **Quoyness** (ON – hut or shelter headland) which is the largest such cairn yet excavated in Orkney (key available at Lady post-office). Bones found in it were radiocarbon dated to about 2900BC [HY676378].

Stone Age burial mounds were treated with fear by the old crofters. This was because every mound had a resident hogboon. The hogboon was bad-tempered and untrustworthy and could cause a lot of trouble. At Hellihowe on Sanday one hogboon created so much trouble that the desperate farmer sold the croft and moved out. But as he carried his possessions into his new crofthouse the hogboon stuck its head out of a kirn and said: 'We're gettan a fine day tae flit on, guidman.'

Maybe the most interesting relic yet found is that of a Viking ship-burial north-east of **Scar** (ON – cleft) on the north-central peninsula of Burness [HY678458]. This was discovered in 1991 when about half the boat (6.5m long) had already been washed away by the sea. But the remaining – lengthwise – half contained a compartment with the skeletal remains of a man, a woman and a child. Beside the man was a sword, a quiver of arrows and some bone gaming pieces. Beside the woman were two spindle whorls, a pair of shears and some iron objects which might be parts of a wooden box. There was also a decorated whalebone plaque, a sickle, a brooch and some other remains possibly of textiles.

Scar itself is the site of the **Saville Stone**, a 20-ton block of Scandinavian gneiss – an obvious glacial erratic. It is said that this was thrown by a furious witch on Eday at a man on Sanday with whom her daughter had eloped. She missed, and the couple lived happily ever after.

At the eastern extremity of Sanday, the lighthouse stands above Tobacco Rock on the tidal island of **Start Point**. First built in 1802 it was fitted by Robert Stevenson in 1806 with the first revolving light in Scotland. The tower was rebuilt in 1870.

* * *

Access: Orkney Ferries daily ro-ro service, Kirkwall/Eday/Sanday, 01856-872044. Scheduled air service from Kirkwall, 01856-872494 or -873457.

Anchorages:

1. Kettletoft Bay, on S coast. Possible to lie alongside ferry pier on W side of bay, 3.5m depth at head, or anchor in

bay in 4m. Approach bay using leading line. Very exposed. SE and S'lies bring in a swell.

2. Otterswick, on N coast. Large shallow bay. Care needed on entering and give shores a wide berth. Good shelter but quite uncomfortable in N and E winds. Anchor to suit wind direction.

3. North Bay, on W coast, S of Holms of Ire. Enter from NW. Anchor in 3–5m. Exposed to W'lies.

10.25 Westray

(ON vestr-øy – western island).

O S Maps: 1:50000 Sheet 5 1:25000 Sheet 464
Admiralty Charts: 1:200000 No.1942 or 1954 1:75000 No.2249 1:37500 No.2622 NW coast

Area: 4713ha (11646 acres)
Height: 169m (554 ft)

Owner: Multiple ownership. Most of the larger farms are owner-occupied. Westray has a policy of giving local Orcadians first refusal when farms are for sale.

Population: 1841–1791 (387 houses). 1881–2200. 1891–2108 (433 houses). 1911–1668. 1931–1269. 1961–872. 1981–701. 1991–704. 1998–600. 2001–563.

Geology: Westray is entirely composed of Middle Old Red Sandstone of the Rousay Beds variety. The harder bedrock has a bluish colour, but most of the rock is a greystone flag which used to be used for building and slating. There is only a limited quantity of poor-grade peat and most of the island is fertile soil.

History: Earl Rognvald landed on Westray in 1136 on his second expedition to Orkney and gained the submission of the two local chieftains, Kugi of Rapness and Helgi of Hofn (Hofn – 'haven' – was the old name for Pierowall).

During the Reformation, in the mid-16th century, the last Catholic Bishop of Orkney, Adam Bothwell, followed the example of many of his brethren at the time and bestowed part of the Church lands, the island of Westray, on his sister Margaret and her husband. Margaret was married to Gilbert Balfour, scion of an ancient Fife family and one who, as Master of the Household to Mary Queen of Scots, had been involved in the murder of Mary's husband, Darnley, in 1567. (He had previously been implicated in the murder of Cardinal Beaton in 1546.) Gilbert, who was also Sheriff of Orkney and Captain of Kirkwall Castle, immediately set about building a magnificent castle in his new domain. It is possible that the ground-work was already there in the form of an unfinished castle started by Bishop Thomas Tulloch a century earlier. However, in due course Noltland Castle was completed and after Mary had married the Earl of Bothwell she instructed Gilbert to make it ready for the reception of

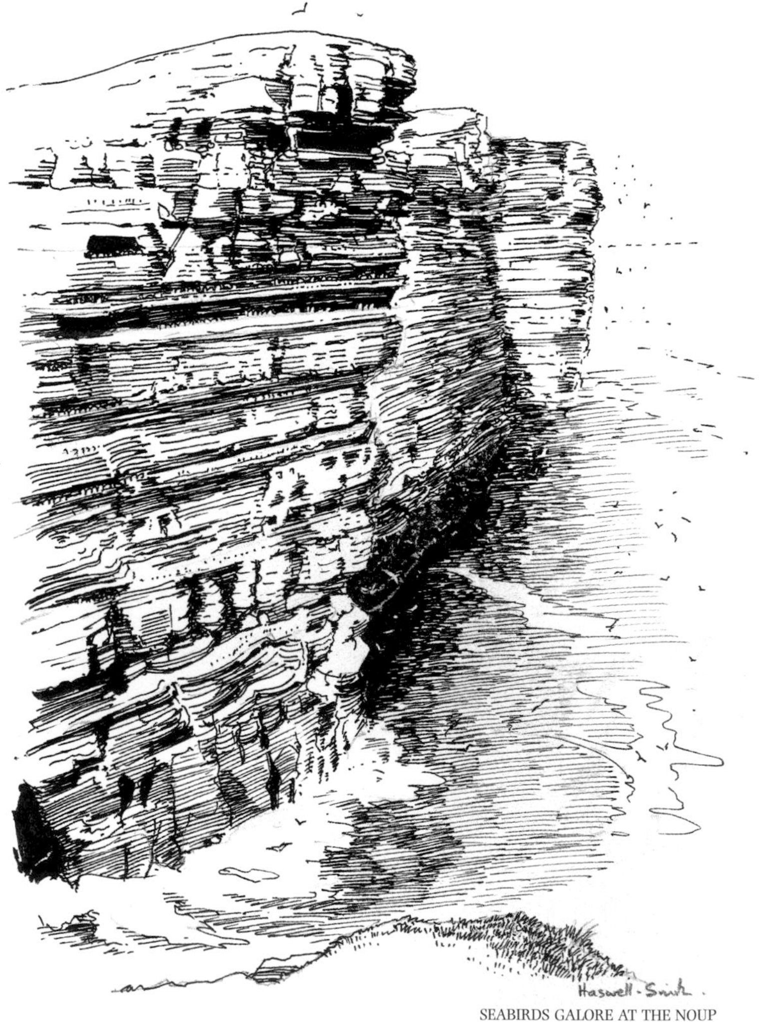

SEABIRDS GALORE AT THE NOUP

herself and her new husband. At the same time she created him Duke of Orkney.

Mary was deposed before her visit could take place but Bothwell fled north to Orkney hoping for refuge. Gilbert, though, refused to let him stay and as he also failed to find shelter in Shetland, he had to sail on to Bergen, where he was arrested and given a life sentence in a Danish prison.

Gilbert Balfour meanwhile joined an uprising in favour of the exiled Queen but it was defeated and he was found guilty of treason. He fled to Sweden but could not resist being involved in a plot against the Swedish King for which he was arrested and executed.

In spite of all Gilbert's unfortunate conspiracies and Lord Robert Stewart's occupation of Noltland

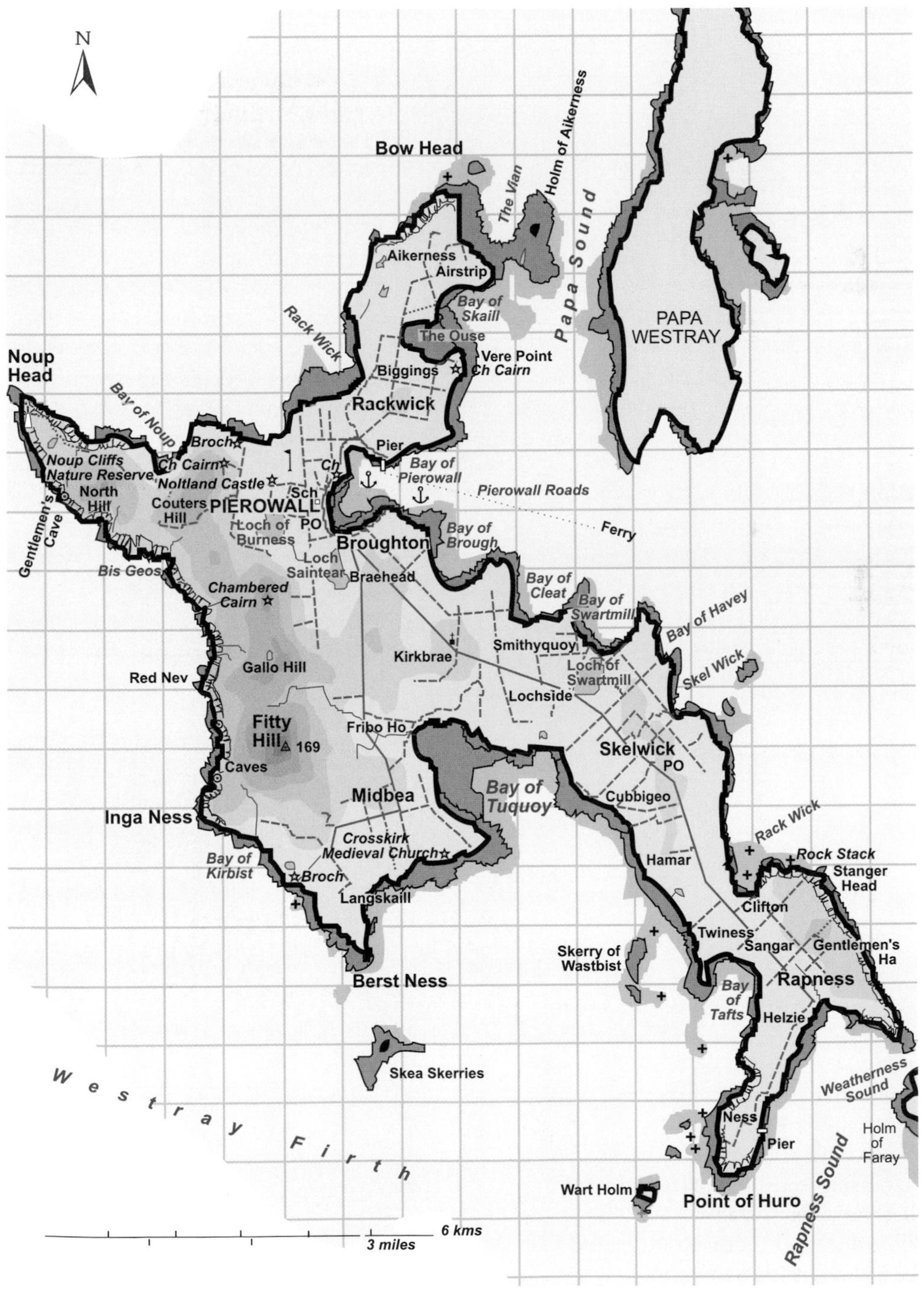

Castle for a time, the Balfour family held on to Westray and their ownership of the island continued for many generations. This might be attributed to the fact that Bishop Bothwell after his deposition as a Catholic Bishop suddenly chose to become a staunch Protestant.

Wildlife: Common plant species are bird's-foot trefoil, lady's smock, bog orchis, grass of parnassus, butterwort, eyebright and scabious. In the spring there are primroses everywhere including examples of the rare *Primula scotica*.

Mice, and the Orkney vole, are common but otters are only occasionally to be seen. The first rats only appeared on the island during the Second World War after an enemy grain ship ran onto the rocks.

The seabird colonies on the west coast are probably the main interest for bird-watchers. The cliffs between Noup Head RSPB Reserve and Inga Ness are packed with birds including some 60,000 guillemot, 3000 razorbill, and 30,000 pairs of kittiwake, as well as shag, puffin, black guillemot and occasional continental migrants. On the inland heath near the cliffs there are about 2000 pairs of arctic tern, fifty pairs of arctic skua, and eider, oystercatcher, ringed plover and four species of gull. On the lochs and wetland areas there are breeding wildfowl and waders many of which over-winter here. A few corncrake can be heard. In winter, purple sandpiper and turnstone can be seen on the rocky foreshore, with sanderling in the sandy bays. The most interesting time is possibly mid-May to mid-July.

Other sites of interest are Stanger Head for puffin, Aikerness Peninsula for black guillemot and Loch of Burness near Pierowall which is the northernmost habitat of the little grebe. Here also are mute swan, teal, shoveller, tufted duck, moorhen, coot, snipe and redshank.

Although the hills and sea-cliffs of **WESTRAY** are not as high as others in the Orkneys, they are very impressive and beautiful. In fact there is such a diversity of scenery that this is often called the 'Queen of the North Isles'. The inhabitants are also noted for their own distinctive brand of 'bloody-Mary' humour.

In the south-west are three cairn-pimpled hills, Knucker Hill, Gallo Hill and **Fitty Hill** which is the highest point on the island at 169m. South of Fitty Hill on the road to Inga Ness is the deserted village of Netherhouse, a favourite of artists and photographers; and beyond it, at the Bay of Kirbist, is a stimulating cliff-top walk all the way to **Noup Head** (ON *gnupr* – craggy headland) which projects into the Atlantic and towers above the swell – when it can be seen through the clouds of wheeling seabirds. (Allow 3½hrs walking time.)

To the east is Bay of Noup and Rack Wick culminating at **Bow Head**, the northern extremity of a dangerous but dramatic coastline. Near Bow Head are **The Querns of Aikerness** which is a huge cauldron surrounded by rock pillars and arches.

South of the airstrip at Aikerness and overlooking the tidal race in Papa Sound is **Bay of Skaill** (ON *skáli* – hall).

The cliffs in this region and on the west coast in particular are riddled with caves. One of the most famous of these is **Gentlemen's Cave** on the south side of Noup Head [HY398486]. The Westray islanders are said to have been the only Orcadians who supported the Jacobite cause and after the defeat at Culloden in 1746 a number of the local lairds are thought to have hidden in this cave throughout the winter to avoid Hanoverian vengeance. Among them was one of the Balfours of Trenabie whose descendant John Balfour became landowner of a large part of Shapinsay (No.10.12) in the 18th century. For many years after the uprising supporters would meet in the cave to drink the health of the 'King over the Water'. For the inexperienced it is a fairly risky climb down to the cave.

The principal village is **Pierowall** tucked in to the sheltered Bay of Pierowall. Viking graves dating back to 800 have been found here and there are the remains of an ancient church, **Lady Kirk**. Another church ruin, **Cross Kirk**, also of the Norse period, is about 6km to the west, at Tuquoy.

On the slope of a hill west of the village is mysterious **Noltland Castle** [HY429487]. Mysterious, because it is unclear why such a mammoth structure was ever built by Gilbert Balfour. It stands alone like a man-of-war, a great stone fort with walls 2m thick pierced with tiers of gun-loops. It could have withstood a massive siege – but who would want to attack it? Gilbert Balfour, of course, had the character of a robber-baron so possibly he and his brother-in-law, the Bishop-about-to-be-deposed, had dreams of starting up their own mini-kingdom in Orkney using the combined fortresses of Noltland and

Kirkwall.

Inside the forbidding bulk of the castle is a large staircase installed later by Earl Patrick Stewart, son of Queen Mary's bastard brother, Robert Stewart. It is elegant but quite out-of-keeping with the original design. More to the point is the inscription over the arched doorway – 'When I see the blood I will pass over you in the night.'

On a lighter note, the length of festivity following a wedding in the Northern Isles is renowned. The longest party on record was held at Noltland Castle. It continued from Martinmas to Candlemas without a break – three months!

Another Skarabrae-type Stone Age village was partly excavated, then reburied, on the shore near the golf course at Links of Noltland and further south, at **Knowe of Skea** near Inga Ness, the discovery of a large well-preserved 5,000-year-old Stone Age tomb similar to Maes Howe (see No.10.10) is proving of great interest.

A road runs the length of Westray from the airstrip in the north to near the southern extremity of **Point of Huro**, where the tiny islet of **Wart Holm** lies near Rull Rost, a frenetic tidal rip in the middle of the Westray Firth.

Westray plans to go entirely 'green' and use nothing but energy from wind, wave, tide, solar panels, methane from waste and, possibly, fuel made from rapeseed and sugar beet.

* * *

Access: Orkney Ferries daily ro-ro services Kirkwall/ Westray, 01856-872044. Scheduled air service Kirkwall/ Westray and Papa Westray, 01856-872494 or -873457.

Anchorages:

1. Bay of Swartmill, Papa Sound. Occasional anchorage in off-shore winds but holding unreliable.
2. Bay of Cleat. As above.
3. Bay of Brough. As above but sheltered from SE'lies if Pierowall uncomfortable.
4. Pierowall Harbour. Easy access, well-sheltered except from SE. Serviced visitor pontoon facility. Anchorage possible clear of the pier, but very restricted space. Also anchorage SE of pier off S shore in 5m, sand and weed.
5. Bay of Skaill. Shallow and not recommended.
6. Bay of Tuquoy on S coast. Temp. anchorage in settled weather, sand, 3–6m. Exposed, but negligible tidal stream.
7. Rapness Sound, SE side of Westray (Weather Ness). Useful anchorage in N'lies. Exposed S and heavy swell in bad weather. Good holding.
8. Rack Wick too deep and Skel Wick has rocky bottom. Neither is suitable.

10.26 Papa Westray

(ON papøy meiri – big Papay or priest's island.) Known as 'Papay' to the Orcadians.

O S Maps: 1:50000 Sheet 5 1:25000 Sheet 464
Admiralty Charts: 1:200000 No.1942 or 1954 1:75000 No.2249 or 2250 1:37500 No.2622

Area: 918ha (2268 acres)
Height: 48m (157 ft)

Owner: Belonged to the Traill family for three centuries but now in multiple ownership.

Population: 1841–340 (69 houses). 1881–345. 1891–337 (76 houses). 1931–237. 1961–139. 1981–92. 1991–85. 2001–65.

Geology: The geology of Papa Westray is similar to that of Westray – Middle Old Red Sandstone of Rousay Beds with a fertile soil.

History: According to the *Orkneyinga Saga*, after Earl Rognvald Brusasson was murdered by his uncle in 1046 he was buried on Papay, but the location of his grave is a mystery. It is thought by some to be in the vicinity of Munkerhoose because an ornate cross with a gilt finish was found there in the St Boniface churchyard.

In 1567 Gilbert Balfour, Master of the Queen's Household, Captain of Kirkwall Castle and Sheriff of Orkney, and Margaret, his wife, were granted both Papa Westray and Westray by Margaret's brother, Adam Bothwell, Bishop of Orkney. The Westrays belonged to the Catholic church but with the Reformation came a rapid disposal of church lands. Gilbert (together with his two brothers) had been implicated in the murder of Cardinal Beaton in 1546 and also the later murder of Darnley, Mary Queen of Scots' husband.

Wildlife: The dwarf shrub-heath in the north of the island is rich in herbs and specialised plants which will only grow on Old Red Sandstone. Among them is the Scottish primrose, *Primula scotica*, which has a purple flower with a yellow eye.

The low cliffs on the east coast were possibly one of the last breeding sites of the great auk before its extinction. Early in the 19th century a pair nested here, but the female died or was killed and the male bird was shot in 1813.

Some rare migrants have been recorded on Papa Westray particularly during easterlies in spring and autumn.

The best sites are: North Hill RSPB Reserve. This is the largest ternery in Europe with

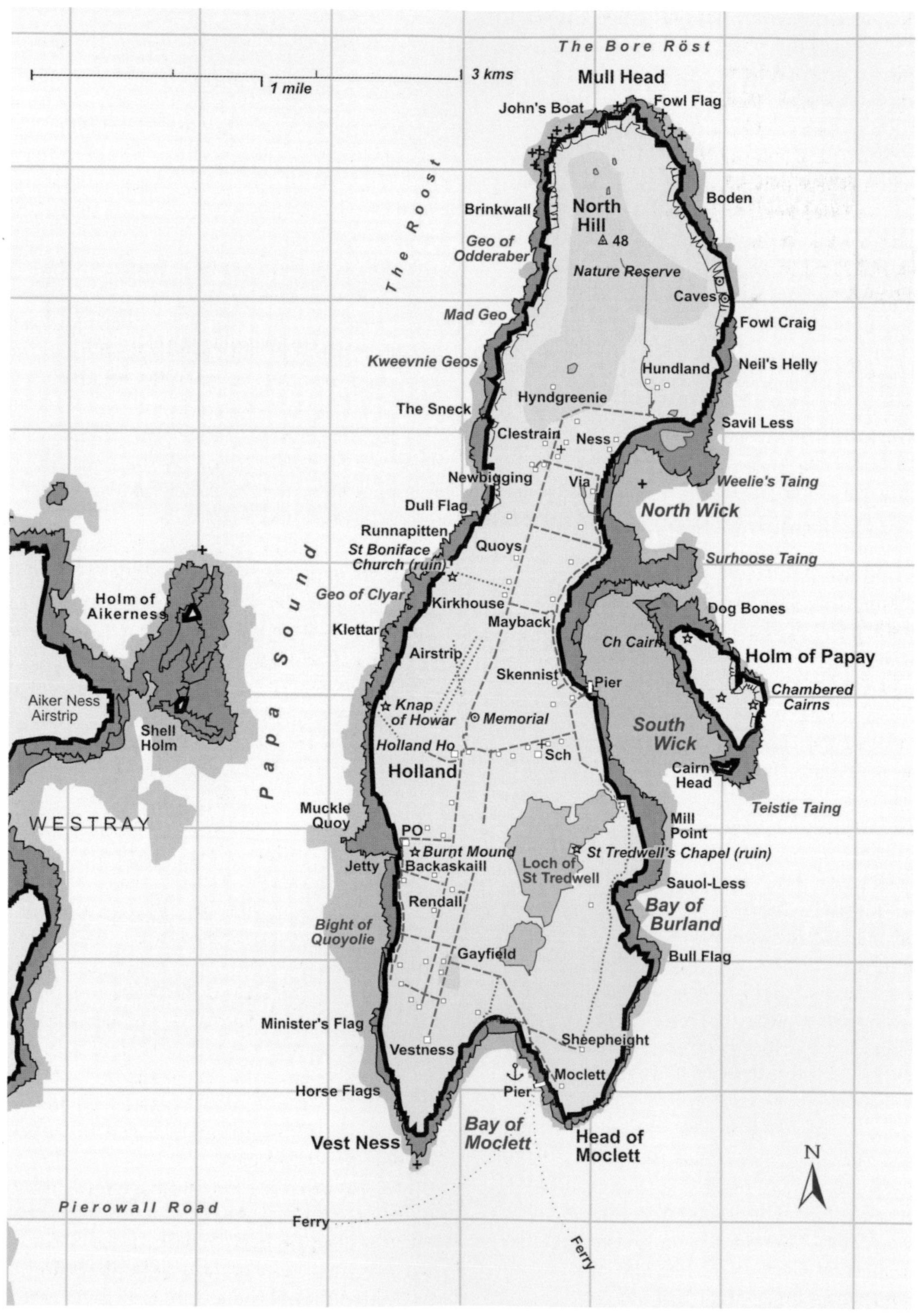

about 100,000 Arctic tern and some common and sandwich tern. There are also arctic skua (constantly nagging the terns), eider, four gull species, several wader species, and colonies of guillemot, kittiwake, razorbill, puffin and some black guillemot. Sooty shearwater and long-tailed skua can be seen at sea.

Holm of Papa: here there is, possibly, the largest breeding colony of black guillemot in Britain – some 130 pairs at the last count. There are also gulls, terns and some storm petrel.

Loch of St Tredwell: this was a former breeding site of the red-necked phalarope and many varieties of wildfowl and waders breed here.

Mid-May to July, and August to mid-October, are the best bird-watching times.

* * *

The attractive 'priest' island of **PAPA WESTRAY** has a long association with early Christianity. In fact it is claimed that this was the fountainhead of Christianity in Orkney.

But it has a much longer association with early man. The **Knap of Howar** on the west coast is a settlement that has been dated to about 3700BC [HY483518]. Two solidly built stone houses, which are thought to be the oldest preserved domestic dwellings in northern Europe, stand side by side, facing the turbulent 'Rôst' of Papa Sound. They are near the airstrip and the **House of Holland** (ON *há-land* – high land), former home of the Traills of Holland, past owners of the entire island [HY488515]. **Beltane House** is a nearby group of cottages which has been converted to a Youth Hostel, guest accommodation and a shop.

The flight across Papa Sound from Westray is the shortest scheduled air-flight in the world according to the *Guinness Book of Records*. It normally takes two minutes but was once accomplished in fifty-eight seconds; the distance between the two airstrips is less than the length of Heathrow's longest runway.

North of the airfield is Munkerhoose religious site where the early Christian anchorites probably set up camp. The beautifully-restored pre-Reformation **Church of St Boniface** is built on the site of a much earlier building [HY488527]. Boniface was known as the 'German Apostle' for as a missionary bishop he converted much of Germany to Christianity. Several stone Celtic crosses from the graveyard can now be seen in the Tankerness Museum at Kirkwall and the Royal Scottish Museum at Edinburgh. A Viking grave remains on the site with a carved hog-backed gravestone of Red Sandstone. Nearby, a roundhouse (c.900BC) has recently been excavated where the cliffs are being eroded by the sea.

Papa Westray's fertile soil supports a number of active smallholdings, although some are now owned by absentee Westray farmers. The islanders are fighting to maintain their community in spite of a dwindling population. The shop closed in the 1980s and the resident doctor left but they formed a co-operative to run a community shop and hostel.

The north of the island is devoted to the RSPB's famous **North Hill Nature Reserve**, a wonderland for bird-watchers. **North Hill** is the island's highest point at 48m. Beneath the low cliffs of the northern tip, Mull Head, there is a notoriously dangerous tidal race called 'The Bore'. During gales even the sea bottom 40m below the surface is savagely scoured by the cross-currents, and erosion is almost continuous.

The large expanse of the Loch of St Tredwell, with many wildfowl nesting on its shallow shores, is at the opposite end of the island. On a small peninsula on its east bank is a tiny ruined chapel, the **Chapel of St Tredwell** [HY496509]. Triduana or Tredwell was a devout 8th-century Celtic girl who is said to have lived alone on this little peninsula. Nechtan, King of the Picts, told her that he was aroused to passion by her beautiful eyes and attempted to rape her but his ardour was quickly dampened when she plucked out her eyes and handed them to him. It is said that this proves that spiritual attributes are more important to a true Christian than physical ones. The blind girl was later rewarded by being made abbess of a nunnery at Restalrig in Midlothian and in due course she was canonised.

The chapel, which is dedicated to her, became by the 12th century a place of pilgrimage for anyone with eye troubles. There used to be a spring beside it at which pilgrims would bathe their eyes. Bishop John of Caithness claimed to have regained his sight here in 1201 after being blinded by Earl Harald.

The east coast has two large bays, North and South Wick, which are separated by an islet, **Holm of Papay**. Even this tiny piece of Orkney has its remnants of prehistory for there are several cairns and the largest is a chambered cairn, 20m long [HY509518]. The walls are as thick as those of Midhowe (See Rousay No.10-20). There is a narrow central chamber with compartments at each end and small cells opening off it – ten single and two double cells. On the walls are unusual 'eyebrow' decorations. The cairn was first opened in 1849 but no human remains were found in it. However, it is contemporary with the houses at Knap of Howar – older than Maeshowe on Mainland – and may have been the place where these people buried their dead.

* * *

Access: Orkney Ferries ro-ro service from Kirkwall and Westray, Tues., Fri., 01856-872044. Several daily passenger ferry crossings, 01857-677216. Scheduled air services Kirkwall/ Westray/ Papa Westray, 01856-872494. Papay car hire, 01857-644202. Tourist Information 01856-872856.

Anchorages:

1. Bay of Moclett, between Head of Moclett and Vest Ness, the S extremity. Excellent anchorage, sand. Avoid submarine cable and ferry approach. Good holding but exposed S.
2. South Wick, on E coast, W of Holm of Papa. Very shallow, sandy bay, 2m and less in depth. Anchor off pier on E side or off Holm of Papa ESE of the pier. Exposed SE.
3. North Wick. Occasional anchorage, sand and stones, 4–5m. Best approach at LW to avoid reefs. Beware rock and shoal in NW area.

10.27 North Ronaldsay

The name is of uncertain derivation. The Norse name was Rinansøy (?Ringa's isle) so it is almost certainly not derived from (ON Ragnvalds-øy – Ronald's island).

OS Maps: 1:50000 Sheet 5 1:25000 Sheet 465
Admiralty Charts: 1:200000 No.1942 or 1954 1:75000 No.2250

Area: 690ha (1705 acres)
Height: 20m (66 ft)

Owner: Multiple ownership. Bought by James Traill, an Edinburgh lawyer, for £2222 in 1727 and held by the Traill family until quite recently when some of the tenants purchased their properties and became owner-occupiers.

Population: 1841–481 (92 houses). 1881–547. 1891–501 (86 houses). 1931–298. 1961–161. 1981–109. 1991–92. 2001–70.

Geology: Old Red Sandstone of Rousay Flags mainly greyish or bluish in colour. The south and east coasts have wide sandy beaches, north and west is more rocky. There is no peat and a shortage of fuel has always been a problem.

History: In spite of its remote location the island has been continuously occupied since prehistoric times.

King Harfagar of Norway had a son called Halfdan Highlegs who fought a sea-battle against Earl Einar (Torf Einar – 'the first man to cut peat for fuel') in North Ronaldsay Firth. Halfdan lost the battle and swam ashore but Einar followed and slew him.

Rinansøy (North Ronaldsay) is mentioned on a number of other occasions in the Norse sagas.

In November 1983 North Ronaldsay was connected to the national grid and received electricity for the first time.

Wildlife: The range of habitat and lack of human interference encourages a wide selection of wildlife – everything from breeding seals to a wealth of botanical varieties.

Apart from the usual Orkney plant life there are rare examples of the Arctic sandwort, *Arenaria norvegica*, and skull-cap, *Scutellaria galericubata*.

The island is noted for its primitive, and intelligent, sheep which exist on a diet of seaweed except when lambing. They are small, goat-like in shape, and variously coloured, and they produce very fine wool and delicious dark mutton. They are descendants of the original Orkney sheep, well adapted to the environment and producing their best mutton in mid-winter just when it is most needed. The flock is maintained at around 4000 head with each family having an agreed allocation according to an elected committee – The Sheep Court. Because of their diet of seaweed an oil-spill could have disastrous consequences so a small flock is now kept in England as a safeguard.

This remote island also has wonderful birdlife – in many ways equal to Fair Isle (No.11.1) and a bird observatory was therefore established here in 1987. There are records of fifty-one breeding species of which thirty-four are regular and there

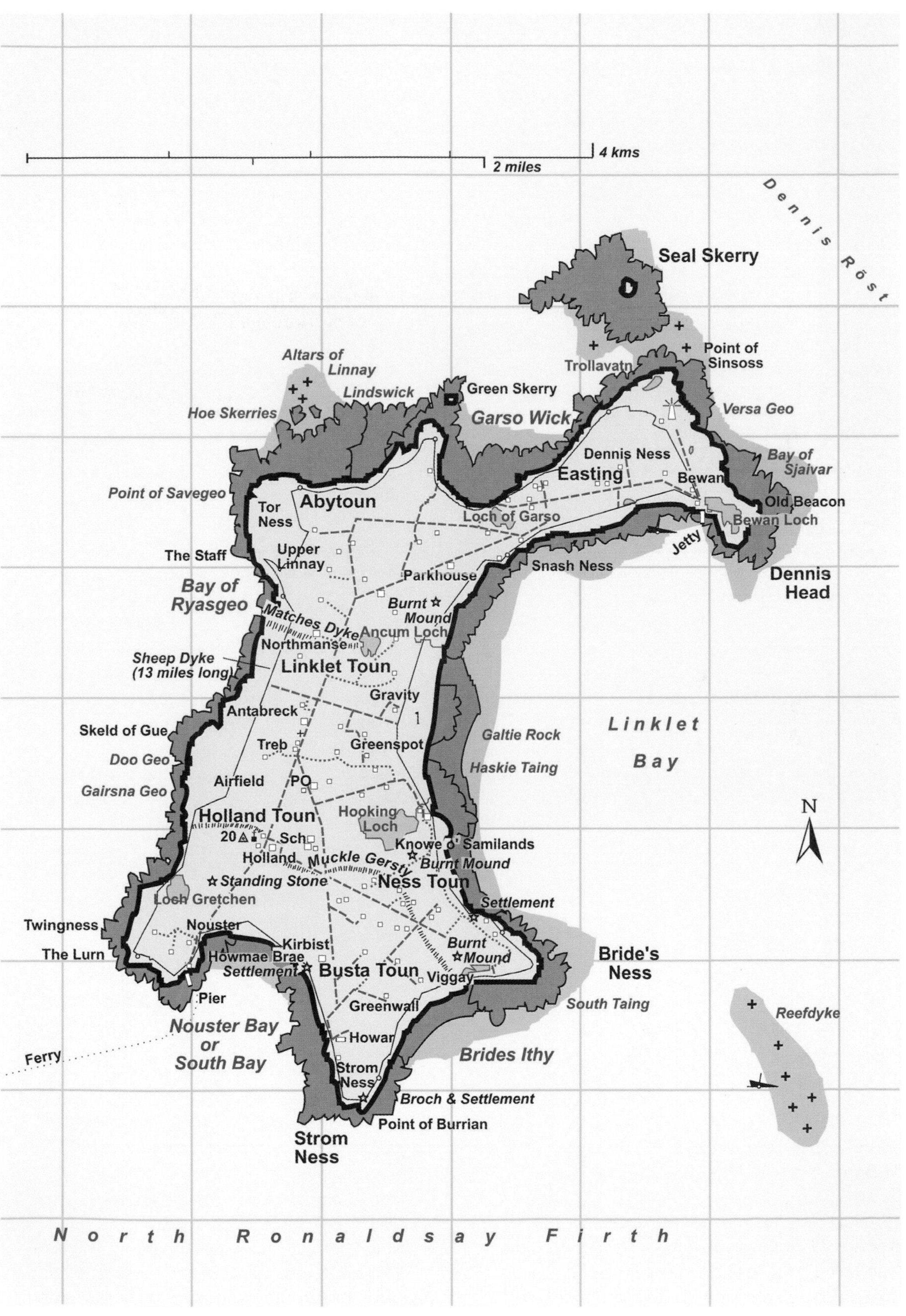
4 kms
2 miles
Dennis Röst
Seal Skerry
Point of Sinsoss
Trollavatn
Altars of Linnay
Lindswick
Green Skerry
Hoe Skerries
Garso Wick
Versa Geo
Dennis Ness
Bay of Sjaivar
Easting
Bewan
Point of Savegeo
Abytoun
Tor Ness
Old Beacon
Loch of Garso
Bewan Loch
Upper Linnay
Jetty
The Staff
Snash Ness
Parkhouse
Dennis Head
Bay of Ryasgeo
Burnt Mound
Matches Dyke
Ancum Loch
Northmanse
Sheep Dyke (13 miles long)
Linklet Toun
Gravity
Antabreck
Skeld of Gue
Galtie Rock
Linklet Bay
Treb
Greenspot
Doo Geo
Haskie Taing
Airfield
PO
Gairsna Geo
Hooking Loch
N
Holland Toun
20
Sch
Knowe o' Samilands
Holland
Muckle Gersty
Burnt Mound
Standing Stone
Ness Toun
Loch Gretchen
Settlement
Twingness
Nouster
Kirbist
Burnt Mound
The Lurn
Howmae Brae
Bride's Ness
Settlement
Busta Toun
Viggay
Pier
Greenwall
South Taing
Reefdyke
Nouster Bay or South Bay
Ferry
Howar
Brides Ithy
Strom Ness
Broch & Settlement
Point of Burrian
Strom Ness
North Ronaldsay Firth

is a colony of about fifty pairs of cormorant on Seal Skerry. Mute swan, shelduck, teal, gadwall, pintail, mallard, eider, shoveller, coot, moorhen, water rail, oystercatcher, ringed plover, lapwing, snipe, curlew, redshank, common and herring gulls, rock dove, sandwich tern, skylark, meadow and rock pipits, pied wagtail, wren, blackbird, hooded crow, starling, house sparrow, reed bunting, twite, raven, and the rare corncrake are all in evidence.

Hedgehogs were thoughtlessly introduced in 1972 (although fortunately there are still no rats) with a consequent loss of many ground nests but a scheme to remove them was introduced. Many migrant birds can be seen including continental passerine migrants. Rarities which have been recorded are the olive-backed pipit, Spanish sparrow, Pallas's rosefinch, snowy owl and the pine bunting. At sea, Sabine's gull, long-tailed skua, Leach's petrel and sooty shearwater may be seen.

Apart from birds, Seal Skerry – Orkney's most northern rock – supports large colonies of both grey and common seals during the breeding season.

* * *

NORTH RONALDSAY has many similarities with Papa Westray (No.10.26), in size, population and land use, but its situation is even more remote. It is low-lying – nowhere is the ground higher than 20m above sea-level – extensively cultivated and studded with cottages. The inhabitants make up a closely-knit and competent community, well able to cope with their isolated situation. The County Library apparently has a full-time job keeping them supplied with books, while even the average Orcadian has quite a struggle understanding the local dialect. This contains many similarities to the traditional Norn dialect which was at one time the language of Orkney.

Because of its unique, primitive, seaweed-eating sheep the entire island is surrounded by the **Sheep Dyke**, a wall about 2m high. This great construction which was completed in the mid-19th century ensures that the sheep stay on the seashore because, although they survive well on seaweed, they would eat the local agricultural produce for choice. It is only when they are lambing that they are allowed to vary their diet.

Normally the dyke is maintained by the islanders as a matter of course, but in 1993 the worst storms in fifty years knocked down more than 3km of the 20km of wall allowing the scruffy little sheep to wander all over the farmland. The island community was much too small to undertake such a massive repair by itself so the Royal Navy, financially assisted by Prince Charles's Prince's Trust, came to the rescue and helped to rebuild the wall and save the crops.

The meat of these sheep has a unique flavour which is a delicacy much sought after by some of the top London restaurants. The wool also has special qualities and the islanders now spin their own fleeces in a mini-mill set up in the redundant lighthouse buildings in 2004.

The New Lighthouse in the north, overlooking Seal Skerry and now automatic, is the tallest land-based lighthouse in the British Isles. It is 33m (109ft) high and was built in 1854 to replace the Dennis Head Old Beacon built in 1788 and abandoned in 1809. Yet at Dennis Head on 11th March 1926, three German ships ran aground one after another!

In the past, communal farms or groups of smallholdings in Orkney were defined by boundary walls which have, in general, long since disappeared. But this is not so on North Ronaldsay, where many farming traditions can still be identified and two old boundary dykes, **Matches Dyke** and **Muckle Gersty** stretch right across the island in the form of raised mounds, dividing the island into three roughly equal portions. They are thought to be over 3000 years old.

Another old tradition is the use of 'plantiecruives', miniature walled gardens outside the sheep-dyke by the seashore. These are used as cold frames to bring on the young kale plants, wind-proof and relatively frost-free.

North Ronaldsay was first occupied in the remote past and the first settlers have left much evidence of their activities. There is a standing stone near **Loch Gretchen** which is about 4m high and pierced by a hole [HY752529]. Two hundred years ago the islanders still danced round this stone on the night of the New Year but the meaning of the ritual has been forgotten.

The remains of a settlement at **Kirbist** [HY758523] may be another Skarabrae (see No.10.10) and there is also an unusual ruin near Hooking Loch which could be a primitive house.

At **Strom Ness**, the southern tip of the island, **Burrian Broch** has walls 4½m thick and four concentric ramparts on the side facing the land [HY762514]. Objects inscribed with Pictish symbols have been found in it and there are the remains of a settlement alongside. Unfortunately this site is now in some danger of being washed away by the sea.

A hazardous patch of rocks called **Reef Dyke** lies off Bride's Ness in the south-west. Many ships have been wrecked here including, the wreck of an armed merchant ship of the Swedish East India Company, the *Svecia*, which went down in 1740 with two-thirds of its crew and a valuable cargo of silks and spices. It was investigated by marine archaeologists in 1975.

* * *

Access: Car-ferry return service Tues. and Fri. by Orkney Ferries, 01856-872044. Scheduled daily air service from Kirkwall, 01856-872494. Accommodation at N. Ronaldsay Bird Observatory, 01857-633200.

Anchorages:

1. Linklet Bay, S of Dennis Head. Occasional anchorage in 7m–9m, sand. Best W of jetty at N of bay. Exposed to E.
2. South Bay between Twinyess and Strom Ness. Temp. anchorage in middle of bay, 7m, sand. Exposed S to W and liable to swell. Sufficient depth to lie alongside pier but also subject to swell. There is one visitor's mooring.

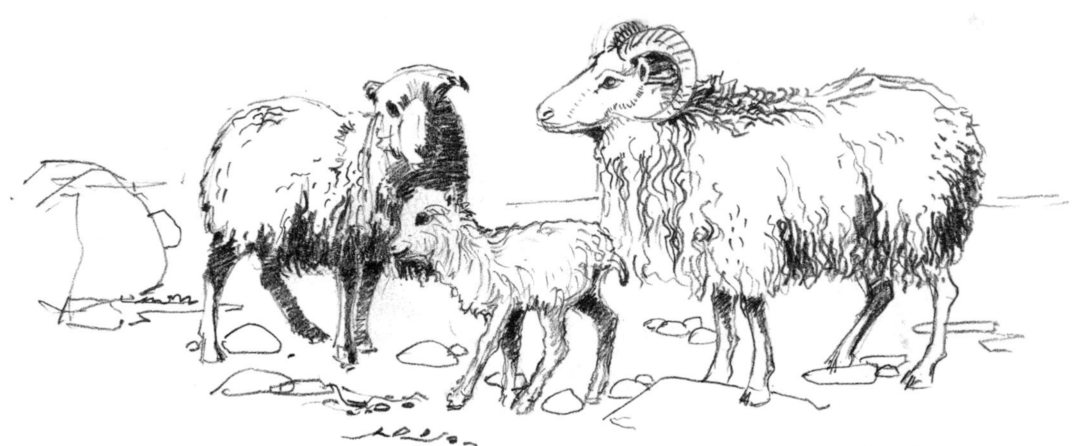

THE SEAWEED-EATING SHEEP OF NORTH RONALDSAY

SECTION 11

Fair Isle and the Shetland Islands

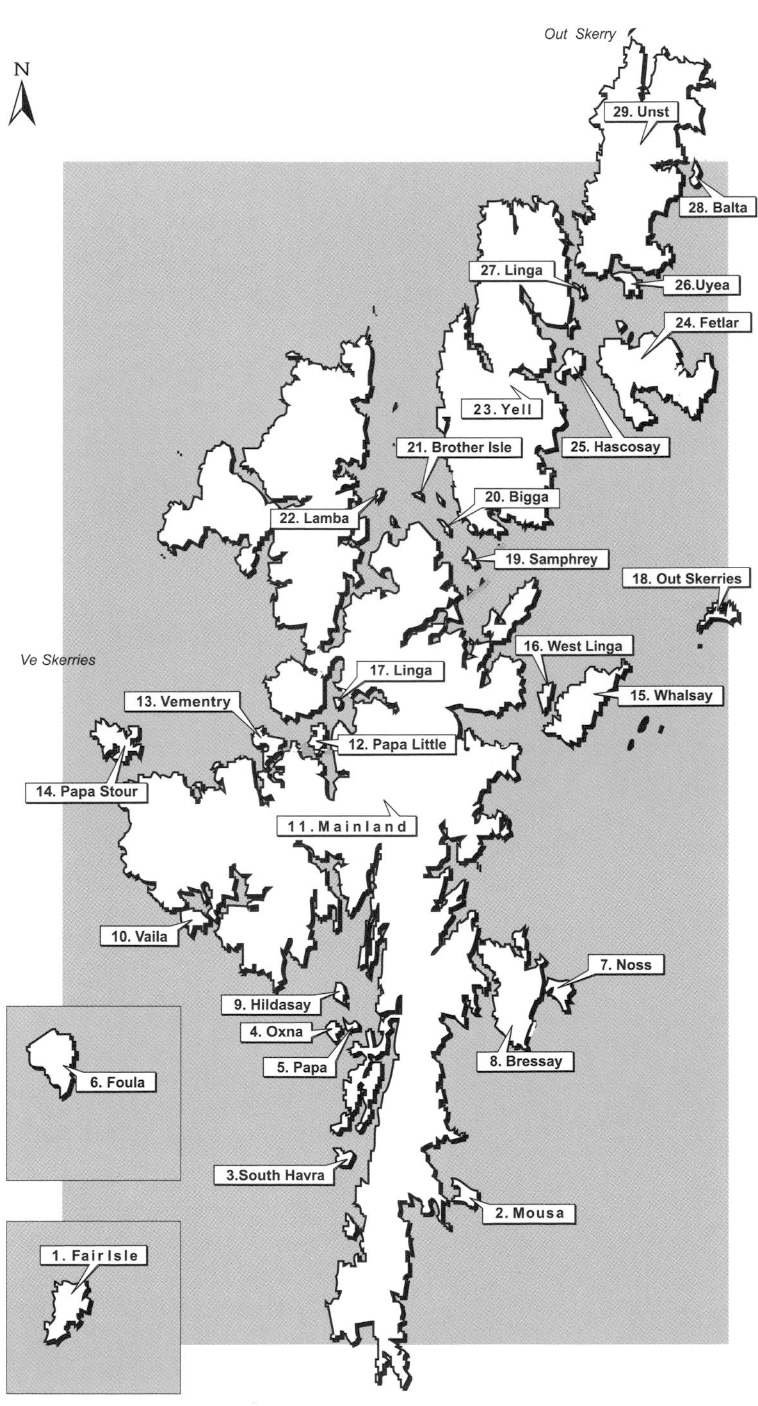

SECTION 11, Table 1: Arranged according to geographical position

No.	Name	Latitude	Longitude	Table 2* No.	Table 3** No.	Area in Acres	Area in Hectares	
11.1	Fair Isle	59° 32N	01° 38W	48	30	1898		768
11.2	Mousa	60° 00N	01° 10W	88	110	445		180
11.3	South Havra	60° 02N	01° 21W	138	129	146		59
11.4	Oxna	60° 07N	01° 22W	132	133	168		68
11.5	Papa	60° 07N	01° 21W	139	144	146		59
11.6	Foula	60° 08N	02° 04W	37	13	3126		1265
11.7	Noss	60° 09N	01° 01W	62	38	848		343
11.8	Bressay	60° 09N	01° 05W	26	29	6931		2805
11.9	Hildasay	60° 09N	01° 21W	108	146	267		108
11.10	Vaila	60° 12N	01° 36W	63	73	808		327
11.11	Mainland	60° 15N	01° 20W	2	9	239388	96879	
	Muckle Roe	*60° 22N*	*01° 25W*			4381	1773	
	West Burra	*60° 05N*	*01° 20W*			1836	743	
	East Burra	*60° 04N*	*01° 19W*			1273	515	
	Trondra	*60° 07N*	*01° 17W*			680	275	
	Uyea	*60° 37N*	*01° 25W*			111	45	100230
11.12	Papa Little	60° 20N	01° 23W	80	81	558		226
11.13	Vementry	60° 20N	01° 28W	60	76	914		370
11.14	Papa Stour	60° 20N	01° 42W	46	79	2046		828
11.15	Whalsay	60 21N	00° 58W	31	57	4868		1970
11.16	West Linga	60° 22N	01° 02W	101	115	309		125
11.17	Linga (Olna Firth)	60° 22N	01° 22W	130	92	173		70
11.18	Housay (Out Skerries)	60° 25N	00° 46W	81	113	403	163	
	Bruray	*60° 25N*	*00° 45W*			136	55	218
11.19	Samphrey	60° 28N	01° 09W	135	150	163		66
11.20	Bigga	60° 30N	01° 11W	123	142	193		78
11.21	Brother Isle	60° 31N	01° 13W	162	156	99		40
11.22	Lamba	60° 31N	01° 17W	157	140	106		43
11.23	Yell	60° 35N	01° 05W	9	34	52412		21211
11.24	Fetlar	60° 36N	00° 52W	22	43	10077		4078
11.25	Hascosay	60° 37N	00° 59W	70	149	680		275
11.26	Uyea	60° 40N	00° 54W	83	117	507		205
11.27	Linga (Bluemull Sd)	60° 40N	00° 59W	156	155	111		45
11.28	Balta	60° 45N	00° 47W	121	125	198		80
11.29	Unst	60° 46N	00° 52W	12	23	29820		12068

*Table 2: The islands arranged in order of magnitude
**Table 3: The islands arranged in order of height

Introduction

It is extremely rare to find a map of the British Isles in which the Shetland archipelago is shown in its true position. Almost invariably it is squeezed into a small inset. The result is that nearly everyone on mainland Britain fails to appreciate that Shetland, as the northern outpost of the British Isles, is closer to Bergen than to Aberdeen – and that Muckle Flugga is further from the Scottish/English border than Lands End.

Shetland was to the Norsemen what Gibraltar was to the British – a key naval base conveniently situated where world sea-routes converged. When the North Atlantic is seen from the correct viewpoint it is clear why the Vikings used Shetland as their first landfall, whether to raid Ireland, trade with the Isle of Man, or cross the Atlantic to Greenland.

Although they had no magnetic compasses these remarkable navigators could not only use a crude sextant and gnomonic (sun/shadow) compass by day, and follow the stars at night, but they also knew how to read the Atlantic swell – a method still known to the Polynesians – and follow natural indicators such as the drift of seaweed and the flight of seabirds.

Take the story of 'Raven' Flokki and his two beautiful daughters. There was said to be a Land of Ice and Volcanoes beyond the Faeroes and Flokki wanted to find it and make it his home. So he set sail from Norway but when he had reached Shetland one of his daughters, Geirhild, died and he buried her beside the loch which still bears her name, Loch of Girlsta. Flokki then sailed on to the Faeroes where his second daughter met and married an islander and would travel no further. Flokki was determined to continue although no one could tell him how to reach the land of Ice – only that they thought it was in the direction of the setting sun. So Flokki captured three ravens and sailed west. After a few days he released the first raven and saw it fly back the way he had come. The next day he released the second raven, but it flew ever higher and was lost to sight. The following day he released his last raven which flew high, but then set course to the north-west. He followed it and reached his chosen land, and that is how Flokki became the first Icelander.

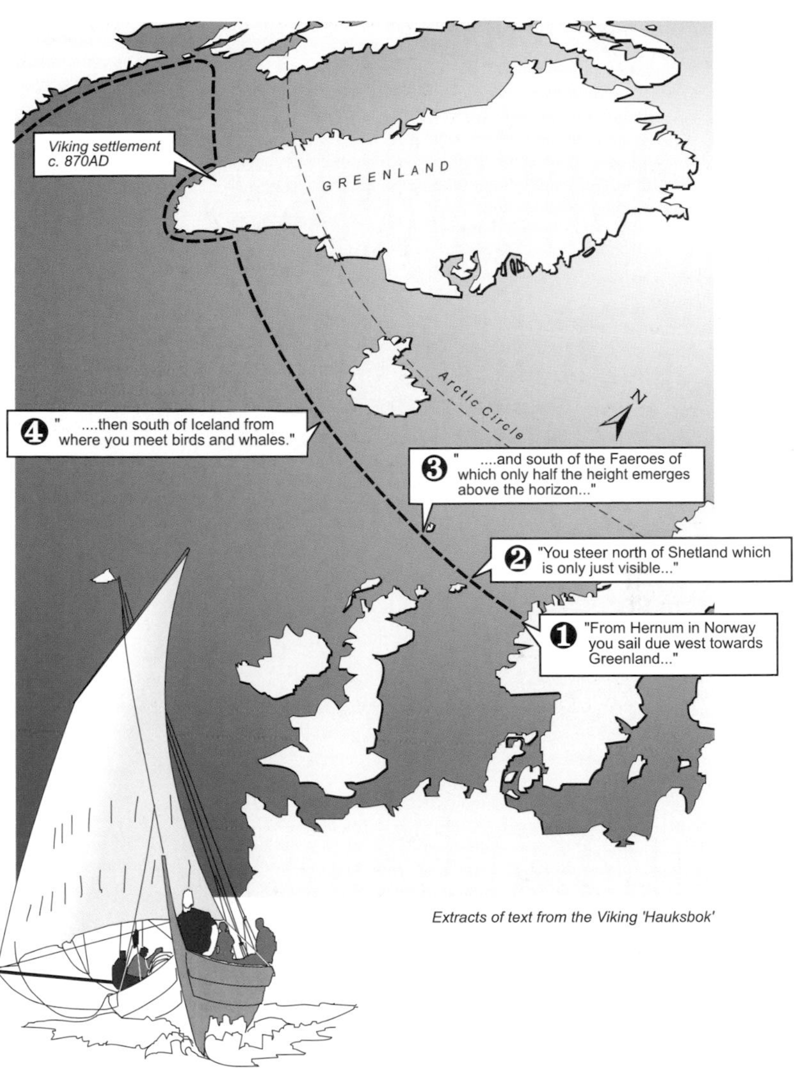
Viking settlement c. 870AD
GREENLAND
Arctic Circle
N
4 " ....then south of Iceland from where you meet birds and whales."
3 " ....and south of the Faeroes of which only half the height emerges above the horizon..."
2 "You steer north of Shetland which is only just visible..."
1 "From Hernum in Norway you sail due west towards Greenland..."
Extracts of text from the Viking 'Hauksbok'

THE VIKING ROUTE TO GREENLAND AND BEYOND

In the Icelandic sagas, which were put in writing in the 13th century, Shetland is consistently called *Hjaltland* and that is still the Icelandic name. This has led to all sorts of scholarly assumptions regarding the derivation of the Norse name although in the Faeroe Islands and West Norway it was known as *Hetland*. In 1221 one of Henry III's clerks at Westminster called Shetland *Heclandensis* and the pope's clerk in 1226 called it *Ihatlandensis*. But in 1289 the Norwegian king in a letter to the English king called it plain *Shetland* although in 1299 in Shetland itself it was written as *Hiatlandi*.

The pre-Norse name for Shetland was *Inse Catt* according to early Irish documents, i.e. the islands of the Catt tribe, whose totem was a cat. This was the same tribe that gave its name to Caithness – Catt Cape. The equivalent name for Orkney was Inse Orc – islands of the tribe of Orc, whose totem was an *orc* or boar.

The Icelandic, and assumed early Norse, name of *Hjaltland* has been variously interpreted by the experts as meaning 'high land', 'land shaped like the hilt of a sword', or 'Hjalti's land' (– whoever Hjalti may have been). I am sure these are all carefully considered and learned interpretations but the Norwegian historian, A W Brøgger, has suggested that the Norsemen were merely talking of the land of Catt, or Cattland. As they would have pronounced Catt as 'chat', i.e. chatland – this seems to me to be an absolutely brilliant piece of common sense. It is the hardest task in the world to reach a simple solution!

In spite of its northern situation Shetland's winter climate is only marginally colder than that of mainland Britain thanks to the North Atlantic Drift. This is an extension of the Gulf Stream. Summers are certainly cooler but the very long hours of daylight tend to compensate. In fact in midsummer the Simmer Dim (the summer gloaming) is an unforgettable experience. Wind speeds can be high, and sometimes very high, but rainfall is not excessive and less than that of many areas of the British mainland.

Shetland's geology is very different from that of Orkney, although there are some large areas of Orkney's ubiquitous Old Red Sandstone. Generally, though, the rocks are Precambrian and of the Dalradian group giving an undulating rather than a slab-shaped profile. These rocks do not decompose into fertile soil. Consequently, there are large areas of blanket peat and few rock outcrops. The coastlines have been eroded to form high cliffs and whereas Orkney's cliffs are mainly limited to its Atlantic coast – Shetlands intrude everywhere.

Shetland, like the south of England, and the Outer Hebrides to a lesser degree, is sinking and at a rate sufficient to make a marked difference in the last few centuries. A mere century ago one could walk from Muckle Roe to Mainland at low water.

The geology and poor soil combine to create a landscape which is more primitively picturesque than that of Orkney but in spite of the poverty of much of the soil there is a feeling of affluence which is not entirely due to the oil industry. Perhaps it can be attributed to the rich character and open generosity of the Shetland Islanders themselves.

11.1 Fair Isle

Referred to in the sagas as (ON frioar-øy – fair isle) but a derivation from (ON feoer-øy – far off isle) seems more plausible.

O S Maps: 1:50000 Sheet 4 1:25000 Sheet 466
Admiralty Charts: 1:200000 No.1942 or 1119 1:25000 No.2622

Area: 768ha (1898 acres)
Height: 217m (712 ft)

Owner: Acquired by the National Trust for Scotland (NTS) in 1954 from Mr George Waterston with the help of Lord Bruntisfield.

Population: In 1701 the population was decimated by smallpox but it recovered and in 1790 was 220. 1841–232 (35 houses). 1861–380. 134 emigrated to Nova Scotia in 1862. 1881–214. 1891–223 (34 houses). 1931–108. 1955–about 50. There was talk of evacuation but the NTS improved amenities and encouraged repopulation. 1961–64. 1981–58. 1991–67. 2001–69 2005/6 – many applications for four vacant houses.

Geology: Red sandstone cliffs and natural sandstone arches and stacks surround the island. The highest cliffs are in the north but Sheep Rock in the south-east has some of the finest arches. There is copper ore on Fair Isle at Copper Geo.

History: In the Norse saga of *Burnt Njal*, Kari the viking came from Iceland and landed on Fair Isle. He spent the winter there, staying with his good friend David the White. And in the *Orkneyinga Saga* Earl Rognvald sent Uni to Fair Isle in preparation for his invasion of Orkney. When the time was due, Uni soaked a warning beacon with water so that it could not be lit and the Earl was able to pass Fair Isle and land on Westray (No.10.25) unopposed.

In 1588 the 38-gun *El Gran Grifon*, a Spanish fleet auxiliary flagship was wrecked at Fair Isle. After the Armada's defeat she had withstood an attack in the English Channel by Sir Francis Drake's *Revenge* but managed to escape northwards. Then on a night in late summer there was a severe squall and she ran onto the rocks in Sivars Geo, on the south-east side of Fair Isle. About 200 men survived the catastrophe and struggled ashore. They had already been without food for days and were weak and starving. The islanders supplied what little food they had but found it difficult to support such a large number of extra mouths. As the rations were small the men set about raiding the winter stocks, killing poultry and slaughtering the few precious cattle and sheep until, in desperation, the islanders managed to round them up and ship them off to Shetland. There they were well fed and well treated until they were repatriated. In 1984 a Spanish delegation dressed as conquistadors dedicated an iron cross in the island's kirkyard to those who had died.

This was just one wreck out of many. A survey has shown that, up to the advent of radar, there was a major shipwreck on the rocks of Fair Isle every four to five years on average.

In 1630 Fair Isle became part of the Shetland estates of Sinclair of Quendale and it was held by his family until 1750. They obtained rent

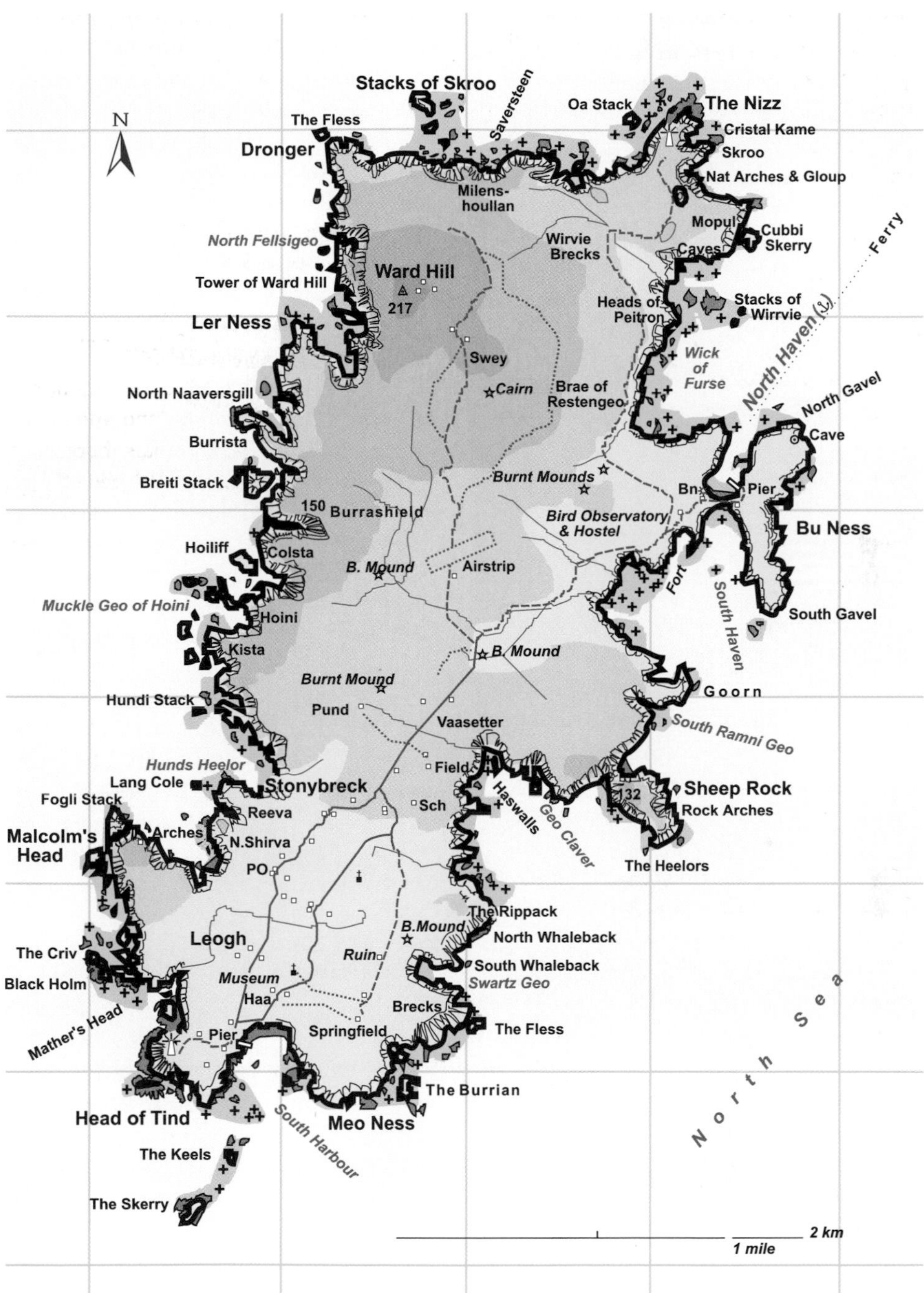

from twenty-four households in four townships and a 'Hamburg Merchant's' booth by the south harbour.

For several centuries the Dutch had turned herring fishing into a very profitable industry. Their fishing boats or 'busses' crowded the waters of Orkney and Shetland protected by naval men-of-war and the catches were exported to Europe, the Mediterranean, and even South America. The French cast covetous eyes on this wealth and in a famous sea-battle in 1702 their navy attacked Dutch men-of-war off Fair Isle with some success.

In 1770 Fair Isle was purchased by Stewart of Brough in Sanday, Orkney, and in 1866 was sold to J. Bruce of Sumburgh.

Wildlife: About 240 different species of flowering plant have been recorded, including juniper, which is rarely found elsewhere in Shetland. White campion and reed grass are widespread with swathes of blue spring squill and thrift. There are also examples of the rarer orchids. Heather and cranberry are common, and dwarf willow and alpine bistort can be found in the hilly moorland.

Like Hirta (No.9.1), Fair Isle has its own distinctive sub-species – the Fair Isle wren *(Troglodytes troglodytes fridarienis)* and the Fair Isle fieldmouse *(Apodemus sylvaticus fridarienis)*. The rabbits are so multi-coloured that some could be wearing Fair Isle jerseys, but they have not yet achieved the status of a separate sub-species.

The Bird Observatory was founded in 1948 by George Waterston, a well-known ornithologist, who bought the island because of its exceptionally interesting birdlife. Over 345 species of bird have been recorded, which is more than anywhere else in Britain, and well over 220,000 birds of about eighty different species have been ringed such as puffin, pipit, wheatear, brambling, fieldfare, redwing, crossbill, siskin and sometimes, Lapland bunting, barred warbler and pied woodpecker.

There are large colonies of seabirds including great and arctic skua. Other breeding species are eider, oystercatcher, ringed plover, lapwing, and snipe. Curlew, whimbrel and dunlin occasionally breed here and breeding passerines include raven, wren, starling, house sparrow, twite, wheatear, white and pied wagtail, skylark, and rock and meadow pipit.

The best all-round months for bird-watching are April, late June to early September, and late October. The best time to spot rare migrants is between mid-September and late October when the wind is from the east.

* * *

FAIR ISLE lies twenty-four miles south-west of Shetland's Sumburgh Head which is roughly half-way between the two northern archipelagoes. It has a distinctive outline with high red sandstone cliffs in the north sloping down to a low, bare southern coastline. **Ward Hill** (217m) in the north-west is the highest part of the island. The Hill Dyke and the ancient Feelie Dyke separate the northern hill-grazing land from the southern fields.

The majority of the inhabitants live in the south where there is a limited amount of ground suitable for cultivation. Here, the scattered settlement of **Stonybreck** (ON *brekke* – hillside) includes a post-office, general store, school, museum, Church of Scotland kirk, and Methodist chapel (each used on alternate Sundays).

The airstrip is centrally situated and to the east of it is the **Bird Observatory and Hostel**. East again, **Bu Ness** (ON – home headland) is only joined to the island by a very narrow isthmus dividing two relatively sheltered bays, North and South Haven. **North Haven** is the port for the passenger ferry, *The Good Shepherd*. Rough roads continue north from the airstrip and the Bird Observatory (roads south of the airstrip are macadamed). One road leads to the radio mast by Ward Hill, and the other serves the lighthouse on **The Nizz** (ON *nes* – the headland). Both the island lighthouses were built by Stevenson in 1892. In this area, known as **Skroo** (ON – stack of oats built to withstand winter gales), the cliffs have been savagely bent by primeval forces and perforated with caves and natural arches by the sea. But this is in keeping with the whole north of the island which is generally wild and barren. In summer the Ward Hill area becomes a test of nerve as the great skua, or 'bonxies', dive-bomb all intruders.

Once again long sea crossings obviously did not deter early man for there are a number of tumuli which date back to about 3500BC (Houlalie is the largest) and an Iron Age fort is at Landberg near the Observatory [HZ226722].

The population decline was halted thanks to the timely intervention of the ornithologist George

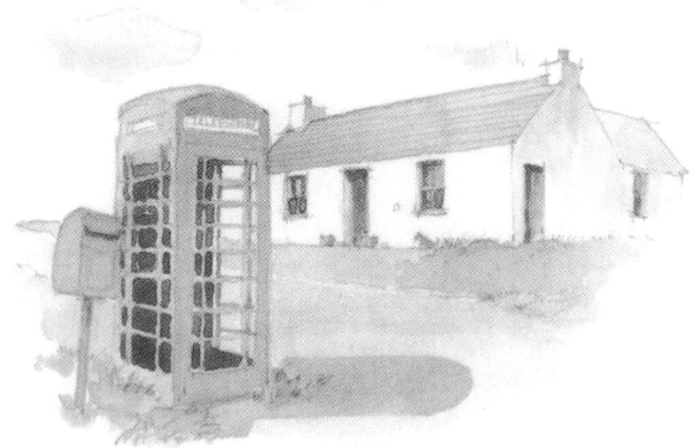

FAIR ISLE POST OFFICE, SHIRVA. A POST OFFICE WAS OPENED AT SOUTH HARBOUR IN 1877. IT MOVED HERE IN 1948.

Waterston who gained international recognition for the island by publicising its varied birdlife. He had visited it regularly since 1935 but while a prisoner-of-war in Germany he dreamed of purchasing the island and setting up a bird observatory. After the war he realised his dream and in due course he also enabled the National Trust for Scotland to continue the good work. The Trust improved the mail-boat pier, good communications being the essential ingredient for a viable island community, and also improved much of the property. The Bird Observatory and Hostel was rebuilt in 1969 with accommodation for twenty-four visitors.

All the buildings are connected to a mutually owned electricity generating station. The electricity previously came solely from diesel generators but for the last twenty years or so two wind turbines have contributed 80% of the power.

The school has probably the highest pupil-to-staff ratio in Britain with – in 2007 – eight staff (some part-time) for eight pupils. As so often with small island schools the results are exceptional. At the age of twelve pupils go to a boarding school in Lerwick for their secondary education. The school hall, built in 1980, is a popular community hall in the evenings.

Apart from those directly involved with the Nature Reserve or in community service, the main occupation is crofting, supplemented by some fishing, and the knitting of traditional jerseys. The distinctive, brightly-coloured and non-repetitive geometric patterns of Fair Isle knitwear are sometimes said to have been introduced by the shipwrecked Spanish sailors from *El Gran Grifon* but it is almost certain that they were an insular development from traditional Nordic designs.

Although this rocky island would seem to be a climber's paradise, with the semi-detached headland of **Sheep Rock** south of Bu Ness considered a prime test of climbing ability, the stone is reported to be of poor quality and unreliable. However as the top of Sheep Rock provided four hectares of valuable pasture the islanders used to climb it with chains and then used ropes to raise and lower the sheep.

A few examples of the traditional Shetland boat – the 'yoal' – can still be found at Fair Isle. She is a lightweight craft with a raked stem and stern, clinker-built, and very similar to the Danish Gokstad ship of 1000 years ago. The islanders used their yoals to trade with passing ships but the construction of the lighthouses stopped this practice as ships then gave the island a wide berth.

The Thief's Hole in the cliff-face of **Malcolm's Head**, behind Fogli Stack, was the traditional smugglers' or press-gang hideout. Another feature of interest is an 80m subterranean passage, the **Kirn of Scroo**, at the North Light which ends in a 'gloup' or borehole.

* * *

Access: Passenger ferry: Grutness (by Sumburgh), (booking essential); three times a week; Lerwick alternate Thurs. in summer, 01595-760222. Air service from Tingwall, Shetland: Mon.,Wed., and Fri., 01595-840246. Air service from Kirkwall, Orkney: Thur. and Sun., 01856-872494. Bird Observatory Lodge, 01595-760258. There are NTS volunteer work parties in the summer to restore buildings, etc., 0131-243-9300.

Anchorages:

1. North Haven, Bu Ness. Small secure harbour (built 1992) but limited space for lying alongside. Anchorage possible but occasional swell and very restricted space, sand and weed. Follow leading marks for entry. Mail-boat pier was built 1958 and slipway 1981.
2. South Haven, Bu Ness. Temp. anchorage in N'lies but poor holding due to rocky bottom. Anchor in 4m. Careful entry required.
3. South Harbour, a small bay at the S end between Meo Ness and Head of Tind. Recognised anchorage and landing place but many dangers.

11.2 Mousa

[moo-së] (ON mós-øy – moor or mossy island).

OS Maps: 1:50000 Sheet 4 1:25000 Sheet 466
Admiralty Charts: 1:200000 No.1119 1:75000 No.3283

Area: 180ha (445 acres)
Height: 55m (180 ft)

Owner: George Bell

Population: 1774–11 families. 1841–12. 1861–0 and uninhabited since.

Geology: The old quarry on Mousa was the source of many of the flagstones used for the streets of Lerwick.

Copper ore is to be found at Sand Lodge on Mainland, just opposite Mousa.

History: Mousa, and its famous broch, are best remembered for their part in the sagas.

According to the Icelandic *Egil's Saga* about 900AD a young man in Norway, Bjorn, fell in love with a girl called Thora Jewel-hand. They eloped from her family home and he took her to his mother's house on the Sogne fjord where she stayed throughout the winter, virtue intact. In the spring Bjorn's father gave him a trading-ship and suggested that he make for Dublin where business was good. His parents wanted Thora to remain with them until his return but the couple would not be separated and Thora sailed with him. A violent storm blew up and they were in grave danger but they managed with difficulty to run the ship aground on Mousa. The young lovers married and made the ancient broch into their honeymoon home for the winter. Meanwhile the crew set about repairing the ship.

The following spring news came that Thora's family had persuaded King Harald of Norway to outlaw Bjorn. As his ship was now ready for sea Bjorn and Thora sought refuge in Iceland. It was another stormy voyage but they were given a very friendly welcome on arrival. Not long after, Thora produced a daughter called Asgerd and they all lived happily ever after.

In the Norse *Orkneyinga Saga* the story is told of Margaret, wife of Earl Maddad of Atholl, daughter of Earl Haakon and mother of Earl Harald. After the death of her husband, the mature but beautiful Margaret, wasted no time in moving in with Gunni, brother of the buccaneering Sweyn Asleifsson of Gairsay (see No.10.13). She soon became pregnant but Margaret was mercurial, oversexed and not really made for motherhood. She gave birth to the child in 1153 but, growing tired of Gunni, she turned her attention to a handsome young man from Shetland, Earl Erland Ungi son of Harald the Fair-spoken. She was of course only too delighted to be carried off to Shetland by Erland and taken to the broch on Mousa. There the couple established their love nest and, although the broch does not look particularly cosy by present-day standards, no doubt love overcame all discomforts. At least the chosen spot was private and defensible, which was important as it was not long before Margaret's twenty-year-old son, Earl Harald Maddadson, besieged it. He was enraged by his mother's behaviour but her hide-out proved 'an unhandy place to get at'. So, in the end, after a long siege he agreed to forgive her provided she married Erland. This she did and after the

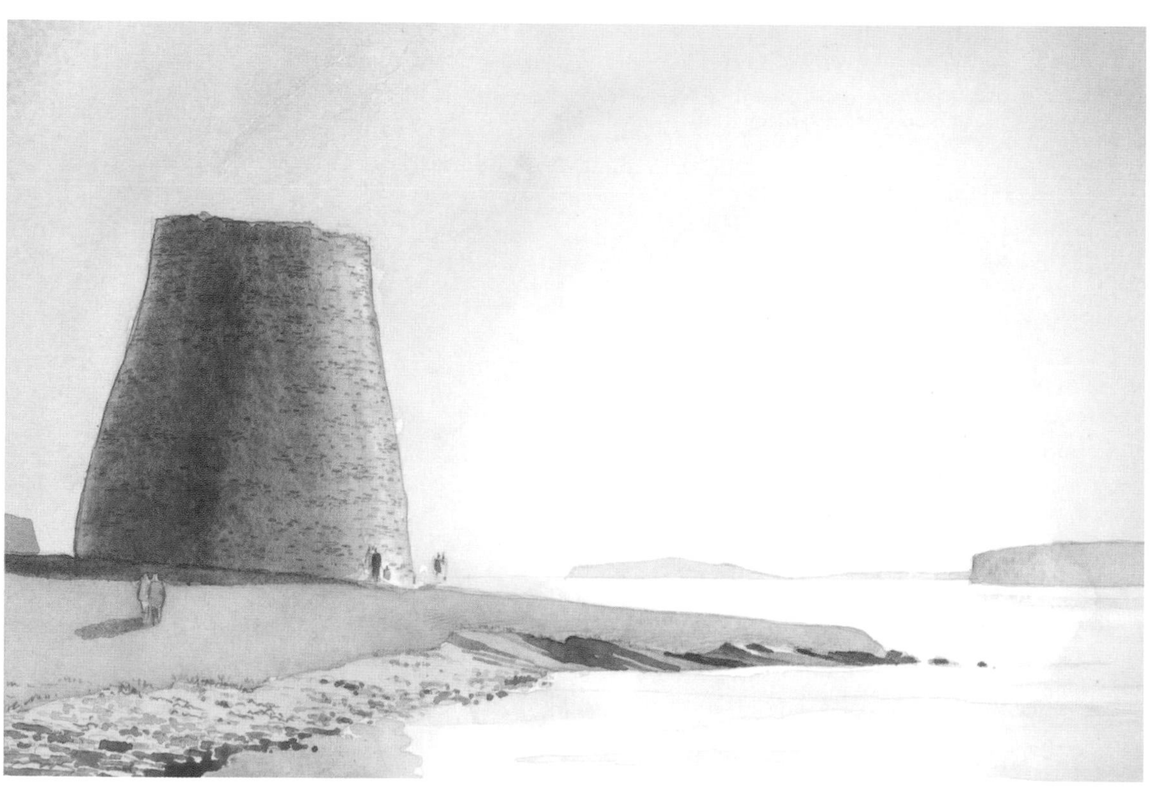

THE BROCH OF MOUSA

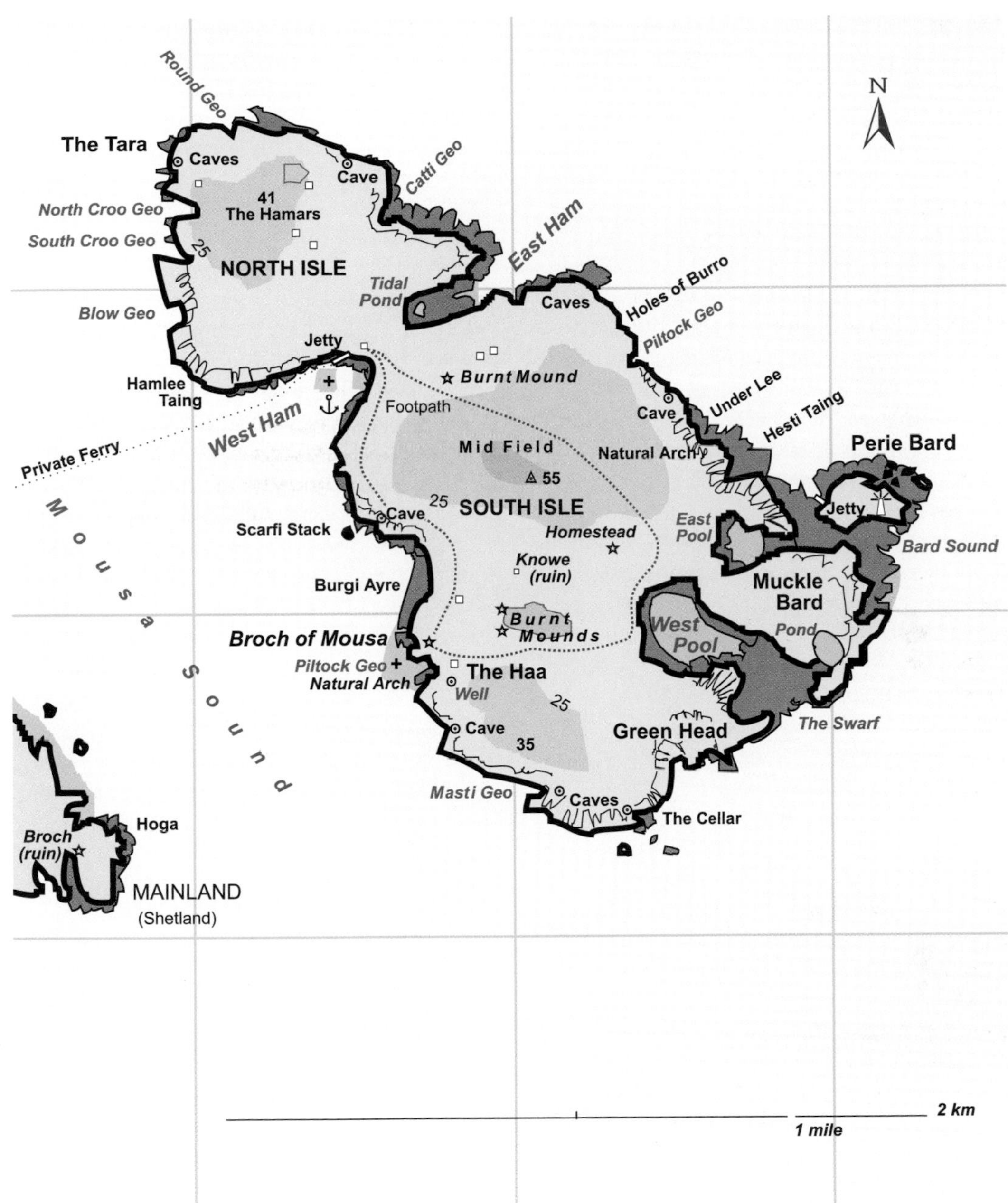

ceremony Harald sailed them over to Norway for a legitimate honeymoon.

Wildlife: The most noticeable life-forms are sheep, seals and sea-birds. The seals, both common and grey, particularly favour East and West Ham.

Botanically the island has an interesting mixture of moorland and salt-water plants.

This is an RSPB reserve. Breeding species of birds include great and arctic skuas, eider, storm petrel, fulmar, many arctic tern and black guillemot. A colony of storm petrel and a few rock doves nest in the broch's dry-stone walls and migrant waders frequent the lochans.

* * *

Two men fishing in a small boat off **MOUSA** in September 1779 were surprised when a strange ship approached from the south and asked for help. They climbed aboard only to discover that it was a French warship wanting to be piloted into Lerwick harbour. They immediately lied to the French saying that two powerful British warships were waiting in Lerwick. They were able to describe the ships because they had seen them sailing south some months before. This persuaded the French not to attack Lerwick but they refused to release the two fishermen. Months later the French man-of-war – still with its two prisoners aboard – was captured by a British ship, and strangely enough it turned out to be one of the actual British ships which the men had lied about! So nearly a year after their abortive fishing trip the two well-travelled fishermen returned home.

To the Vikings an island was a piece of land which a boat could circumnavigate but the term 'circumnavigation' included transporting a boat across dry land. It was for this reason that the Mull of Kintyre was judged to be an island. Similarly little Mousa counted as two islands, **North Isle** and **South Isle**, because it has a narrow waist or isthmus which a boat could be carried across.

North Isle is the smaller part and rises to a height of 41m. It is divided from South Isle by two bays, **West Ham** (ON *ham* – harbour) and East Ham. South Isle's highest point is **Mid Field** at 55m and there is a further small hill in the south which rises to 35m. The south-east is indented to form what are almost two drying islands with saltwater pools separating them, **Muckle Bard** and **Perie Bard** (ON – big and subordinate sandbar or reef). A lighthouse stands on Perie Bard.

There are two tiny lochans on Mousa, one on each 'island', with ancient tumuli beside the southern loch. The remains of old farm-buildings are on an attractive site above this loch and nearer the east coast is a ruined water mill. There is also an old two-storeyed building known as **The Haa** [HU458236]. On the east coast itself the wreck of the first *St Sunniva* can be seen. She ran aground in 1930 in thick fog.

On the western shore, the world's finest, best-preserved and most complete broch can be clearly seen from Mainland across the Mousa Sound. The **Broch of Mousa**, dating from the Iron Age, has lost its upper courses but is still some 13m tall. It is a very fine example of the craft of the ancient builders. Unlike many other brochs there is no sign of a surrounding settlement – the broch of Mousa appears to stand alone. The external diameter at ground level is about 15m with the walls gracefully curved inwards so that the upper diameter is about 12m. The circular internal courtyard is approximately 6m in diameter and contains a wheelhouse which was probably added in the 2nd or 3rd century. The stairs between the double walls lead upwards through six galleries.

Many brochs have been built in tandem facing each other over a stretch of water, and this broch is no exception as on a headland projecting into Mousa Sound there are the remains of its sister Broch of Burraland. The real purpose of these structures, probably built before the Roman invasion of British waters, is still a mystery.

Mousa's broch is built of small stones of a local schistose slate meticulously laid dry to give a smooth exterior. The workmanship is quite remarkable when one remembers that timber was an exceptionally scarce commodity and the curved walls were probably built without templates and to a line depending on the eye of the stonemason. This skill and accuracy has resulted in a building, possibly 1000 years old at the time of the Vikings and now 1000 years older still, appearing today as though the builders had just laid the last stone and gone home for the night.

* * *

Access: Regular summer boat trips from Leebitton pier, Sandwick. No dogs. Weather permitting so check first. (Jamieson, 01950-431367). Also late night storm petrel trips in season (booking essential).

Anchorage: Near the broch the bottom is rock and unsuitable for anchoring.

1. West Ham, Mousa Sound – a bay ½M N of the broch. There is a cottage and boat slip. Anchor in 4m, sand. Sheltered from NW through N to E. Fresh S'lies cause a swell.

11.3 South Havra

(ON hafr-øy – ewe island.) Less probable alternatives are (ON havari-øy – shipwreck island) or (ON – Halvor's island). Formerly written as Halvera and Hevera.

OS Maps: 1:50000 Sheet 4 1:25000 Sheet 466
Admiralty Charts: 1:75000 No.3283 1:25000 No.3294

Area: 59ha (146 acres)
Height: 42m (138 ft)
Population: 1841–37. 1881–35. 1891–24 (4 houses). Uninhabited since 1923.

Geology: Soil with no peat deposits over an area of epidotic syenite, undifferentiated schist and gneiss.

History: South Havra was the home of the Foud (Magistrate) of all Shetland, Olaf Sinclair, in the 16th century. He was also laird of the great odal estate of Brew.

South Shetland occasionally suffered raids by men from Lewis (No.8.16). There was one such raid which ended in a pitched battle at Sumburgh in which sixty men died. It is said that Olaf Sinclair only escaped death by diving off the high cliffs at Sumburgh Head.

* * *

SOUTH HAVRA could easily be called the island of shipwrecks as it lies directly across the southern approach to the comparatively sheltered waters of Clift Sound and the Burras. The east

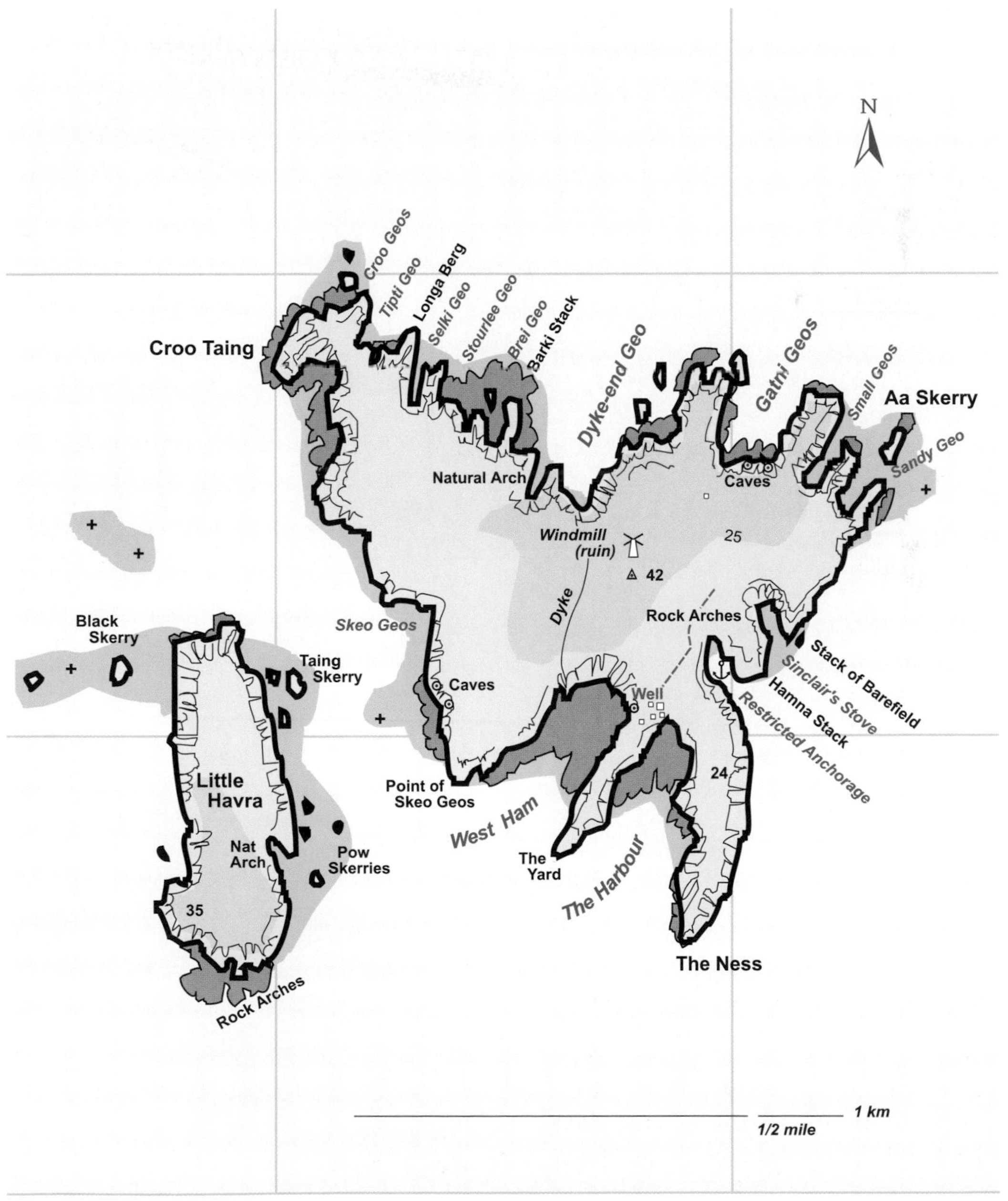

side is steep-to but elsewhere there are reefs and skerries galore particularly in the channel between South Havra and Little Havra and also stretching north from Little Havra to the west of Croo Taing. The cliffs and broken shoreline of both islands are made up of a tumble of interesting rock formations perforated with caves and arches.

Eight families were living on the island until May 1923 when they all decided to leave. Up to that time it seems to have been a viable small community with a full-time schoolteacher and eight pupils. The ground was fertile and productive and, although there was no peat for fuel, this could be found at Deepdale on the Mainland shore. However, the operation was not easy as the peat had to be brought down the hillside on a sledge, controlled by ropes to stop it falling over the cliff and into the sea. It then had to be manhandled across the slippery rocks and into a heaving boat. It must have been difficulties such as these which persuaded the islanders to abandon their homes.

The island's summit is 42m high and on top of it stands the conspicuous ruin of a **windmill** which itself is nearly 8m high. This was, strangely, the only corn-grinding windmill in Shetland, a land of wind-whipped islands with a long association with the Dutch. This windmill was built by the islanders in the middle of the 19th century to grind their corn as there was no stream to operate a water mill. The ruin is worth visiting and the island is an exciting place to explore.

The two larger coves on the south coast are optimistically called the Harbour and West Ham (ON *ham* – harbour). Both bays are exposed and partly filled with drying rocks.

The Havra rock formations are repeated on the adjacent Mainland with a tiny rocky islet, **Holm of Maywick**, in the centre of the separating channel.

* * *

Access: By arrangement: MV Cycharters, Scalloway, 01595-696598. Tourist Office, 01595-693434.

Anchorage:

1. In the S inlet on the E coast. (There are two narrow inlets close together but the N inlet is foul with rocks). Anchor in middle of pool in 2m with warps ashore.

11.4 Oxna

(ON yxn-øy – ox island).

OS Maps: 1:50000 Sheet 4 1:25000 Sheet 466
Admiralty Charts: 1:75000 No.3283 1:25000 No.3294

Area: 68ha (168 acres)
Height: 38m (125 ft)

Population: 1841–19 (2 houses). 1871–29. 1881–30. 1891–31 (5 houses). 1901–36. 1931–0. Uninhabited since.

Geology: Much of the rock is epidotic syenite, which is like a dark granite.

History: At the end of the 19th century a young Oxna boy was playing with his friends near a skarf's (cormorant's) nest. The surrounding turf had been scalped away by the islanders to improve the soil in the arable areas and consequently the ground was bare. Something glinted in the sunlight and with some difficulty the boy prised the object from the roots and took it proudly home. A visiting schoolteacher from Burra was shown the find and he informed the museum authorities in Edinburgh. I hope the bright-eyed lad or his family were paid 'treasure trove'. They deserved it because he had unearthed an exquisite example of Norse jewellery – a solid gold armlet about 7cm (3 inches) in diameter, plaited from four heavy gold wires.

* * *

OXNA has a compact shape, uneven surface and a number of small lochans. Its summit to the south of the centre is 38m high. Extending for a considerable distance to the north is a broken line of islets and skerries. Joined to Oxna by a drying reef are the **Hoggs of Oxna** with a narrow channel, Bulta Sound, separating them from the next group called the **Cheynies**. Bulta Sound is navigable, but only 100m wide.

The Cheynies are a group of three drying islets forming a single unit and to their south-east is a further little islet called **Spoose Holm**.

When Oxna was inhabited the main settlement was beside the narrow inlet called **Sandy Voe**, facing the island of Papa (No.11.5). It seems that the First World War was the beginning of the end for Oxna. With the menfolk away it was virtually impossible for the women and children to maintain a viable community in such a

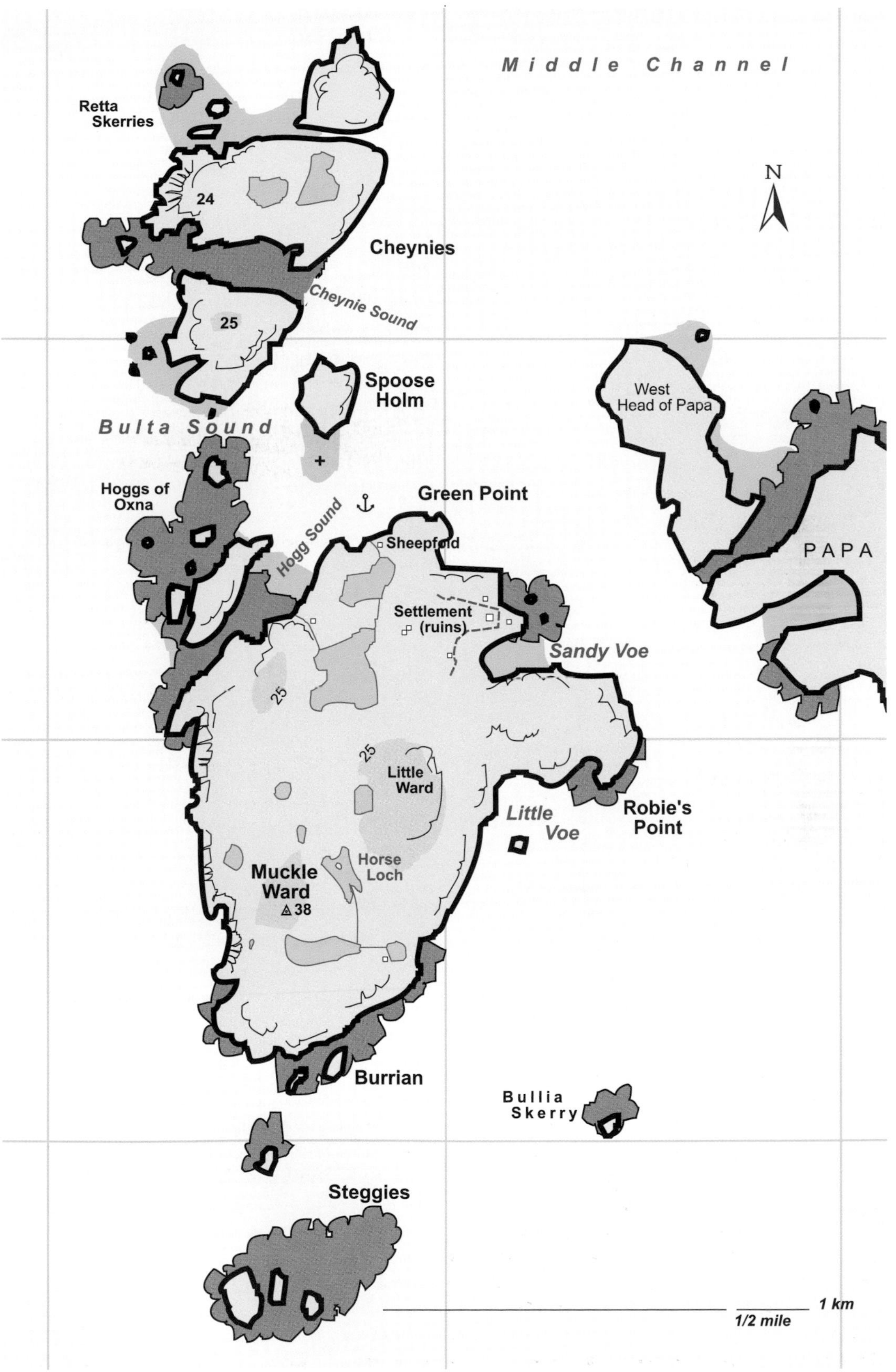
Middle Channel
Retta Skerries
24
Cheynies
Cheynie Sound
25
Spoose Holm
Bulta Sound
Hoggs of Oxna
Green Point
Hogg Sound
Sheepfold
Settlement (ruins)
Sandy Voe
25
25
Little Ward
Little Voe
Robie's Point
Muckle Ward
38
Horse Loch
Burrian
Bullia Skerry
Steggies
West Head of Papa
PAPA
N
1 km
1/2 mile

demanding environment. Difficulties of transport and communication, fishing and subsistence crofting, hard enough at the best of times, must have become insurmountable. And even when the war was over many of the islanders never returned – mere statistics among the losses on the Somme or at sea.

* * *

Access: By arrangement: MV Cycharters, Scalloway, 01595-696598. Tourist Office, 01595-693434.

Anchorage:
1. Anchor NNE or SSE of Spoose Holm, 6–9m, sand over rock. Area partly obstructed by fish-cages. Beware reef close S of Spoose Holm. Reasonably sheltered except from the N.

11.5 Papa

(ON pap-øy – priest or hermit island).

OS maps: 1:50000 Sheet 4 1:25000 Sheet 466
Admiralty Charts: 1:75000 No.3283 1:25000 No.3294

Area: 59ha (146 acres)
Height: 32m (105 ft)

Population: 1841–21. 1881–14. 1891–23 (2 houses). 1931–0. Uninhabited since.

Geology: Much of the bedrock is epidotic syenite, which is similar to a coarse granite.

Wildlife: The island is said to be infested with rats but if so, they are well concealed.

* * *

All Shetland's holy islands are clustered in the south-west of the archipelago and it has been suggested that by the time the early Irish Christians had sailed in their currachs all the way to Shetland they were only too content to settle down where they had landed and go no further.

Why the first missionary chose **PAPA** and not Oxna or Langa (an islet to the north) will never be known but maybe Oxna was already inhabited and the poor chap was just too tired to sail over to Langa. Certainly Papa has a lot to commend it. It has some pools of fresh water, enough land to cultivate for food, and reasonable proximity to Mainland.

Before the island was vacated in the 1920s it supported three or four crofts.

There is a deep and narrow channel separating Papa from Oxna and the coast of Papa is indented with a series of small inlets. Off the north-east headland is the **Hogg of Papa** – to balance the Hoggs of Oxna at the opposite side of the group – and the west side of the island has a tidal channel joining it to a fair-sized islet called **West Head of Papa**. This tidal islet alone is actually larger than the aforementioned **Langa** (ON – long island) and yet Langa supported one croft and a population of nine souls in 1841 and thirteen in 1881 although it was deserted by the 1890s. Papa has a goodly stock of peat and the Trondra (Mainland) islanders have the right to cut it as they have none of their own.

Even smaller islets lie to the east of Papa in the centre of the shipping route into the port of Scalloway – **Green Holm** with **Merry Holm** and a scattered group of skerries beside it. To the north is **Burwick Holm** by the Ness of Burwick.

In May 1903 the crew of *Adelong* fishing near Papa reported that a sea-monster, known locally as a 'sifan', had ruined ten of their nets.

A similar report from the other side of Shetland was given in a sworn account by six men crewing the *Bertie* in June 1882. They had been fishing south-east of Fetlar for two days. Their holds were full of fish and they were hauling in their lines to return home when they saw a sifan heading for their boat. It was 150 feet long with a huge head covered with barnacles, a square mouth with bright green whiskers – 'probably of seaweed' – and it had humps and a long neck. They fired at it at close range and threw ballast stones at it but that only infuriated it and it followed the boat for three hours.

Access: By arrangement: MV Cycharters, Scalloway, 01595-696598. Tourist Office, 01595-693434.

Anchorages: A tripping line is advised.
1. North Voe. Temp. anchorage in 6m in centre of gut.
2. West Head of Papa. Temp. anchorage in 5m in bay between Papa and West Head of Papa. Beware rocks on Papa shore and keep nearer the West Head of Papa shore. Head of bay is shoal.
3. NNE of Spoose Holm. (See Oxna, No.11.4). Safest anchorage except in N'lies but a considerable dinghy distance from Papa.
4. Temp anchorage in South Voe in centre of gut, 6m.

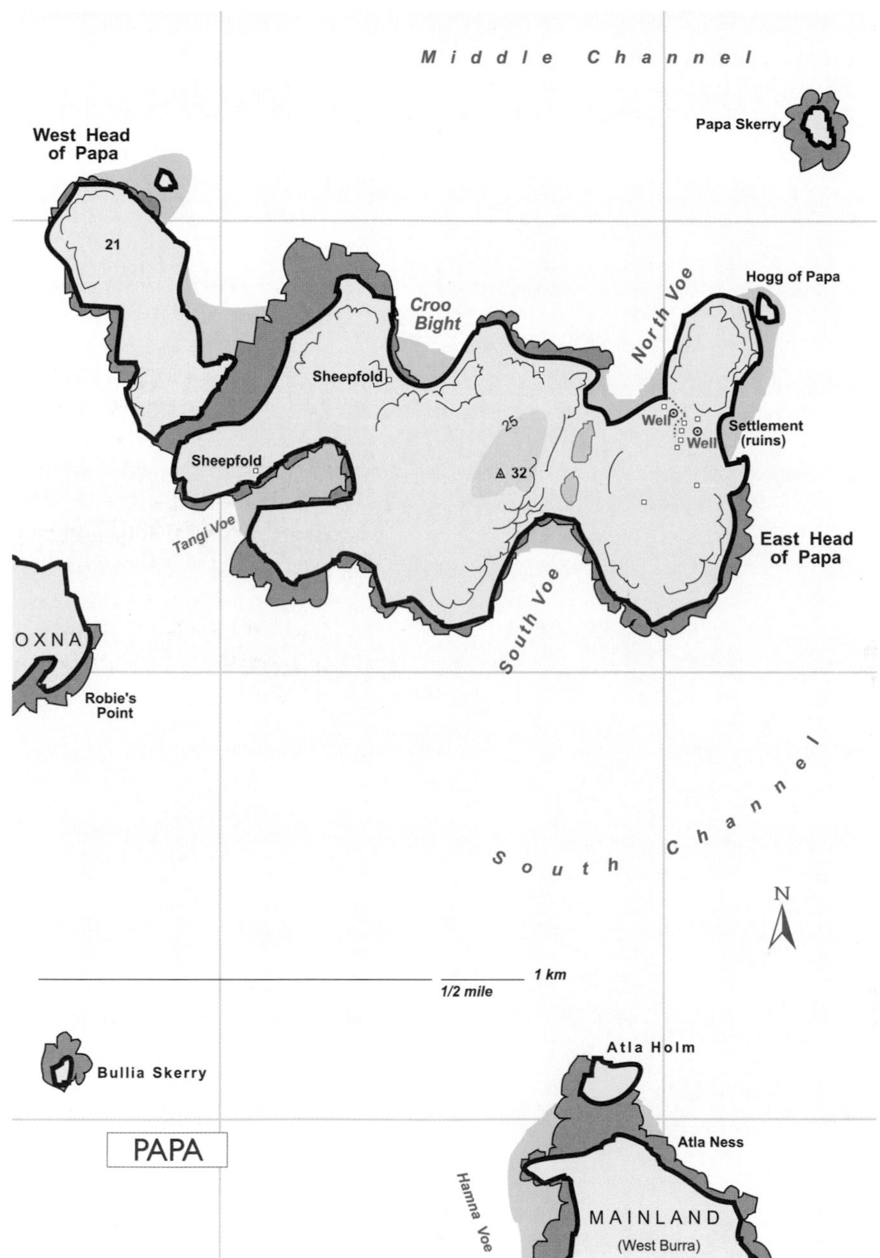

11.6 Foula

[foo-lë] (ON fugl-øy – bird or fowl island.) Sometimes called Uttrie – the outer isle.

O S Maps: 1:50000 Sheet 4 1:25000 Sheet 467
Admiralty Charts: 1:75000 No.3283 1:75000 No.3281 NE part only.

Area: 1265ha (3126 acres)
Height: 418m (1371 ft)

Owner: South Foula has been owned by the family of P R H S Holbourn of Pendre, Brecon, Wales since 1900.

Population: In the early 18th century the 'Mortal Pox', or smallpox, almost depopulated the island but it was replenished from Mainland. 1841–215. 1881–267 (and 7 fishing boats or 'sixareens'). 1891–239 (47 houses). 1901–222. 1931–118. 1951–70. 1961–54. 1971–33. 1981–39 (15 occupied houses). 1991–40. 2001–31. 2006–26.

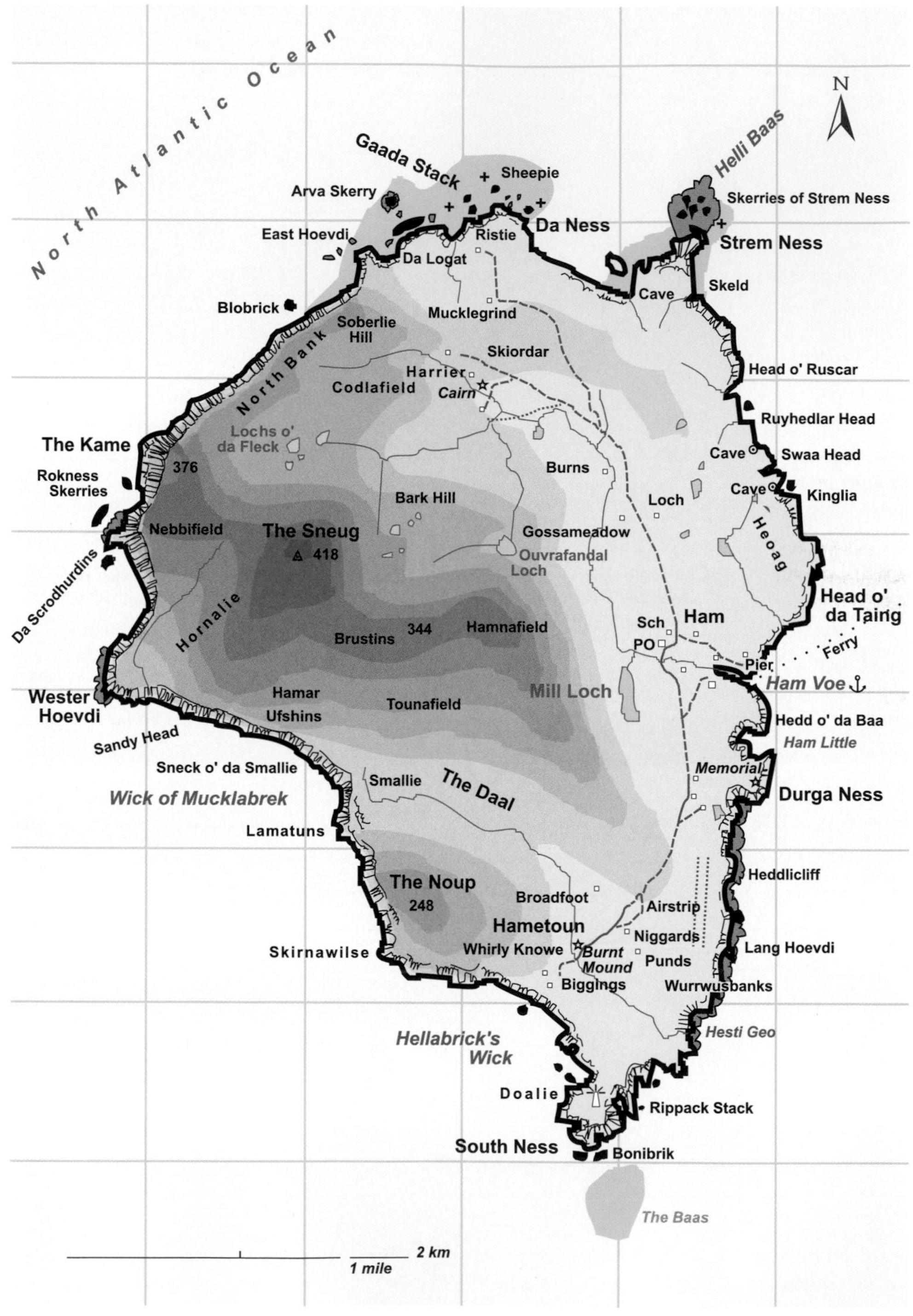

Geology: The west and centre is sedimentary (Old Red Sandstone) and the land terminates abruptly with high sandstone cliffs of variegated colours. The north-east side is metamorphic, consisting mainly of schists and gneiss. Foula has some of Shetland's best arable land.

History: In 1490 Foula became the possession of Alv Knutsson. Previously it had belonged to the Norwegian family of Ciske. When the last Queen of Foula, Katherine Asmunder, died in the late 17th century Norse udal law was still recognised by the islanders who were unaware of the advent of Scots Law in the rest of Shetland.

About this time, according to island tradition, a ship's surgeon named Scott visited the island and gained the trust of the islanders. He persuaded them to hand over their old Norse title-deeds on the pretext that they needed to be registered in Edinburgh. They never saw them again and the family of Scotts of Melby, owners of Vaila (No.11.10) and various estates on Shetland Mainland, thereby acquired possession of the island. This was merely another reputed case of the theft of land by 'carpetbaggers' from the south which had become widespread throughout the Northern Isles during the previous two centuries. As a result crofters lost their udal rights, under which they were freemen land-owners. Instead they became tenants and virtual bondsmen subject to the whims of their landlords. Luckily, as fishermen, the islanders were more rent-productive than those depending solely on crofting and this saved them from clearance for sheep-farming. But their insecurity continued until 1882, when they gained some protection under the Crofting Acts.

Until 1800 Norn was still the normal tongue of this isolated community although it was no longer spoken anywhere else in Britain. Even in 1894, Jacobsen, the Faeroese linguist, was surprised at the similarities with Faeroese.

Foula still uses the old Julian calendar which most of the rest of Britain (see Jura No.2.5) discarded in 1753 and Christmas on the island is therefore still celebrated on the 6th of January. And New Year's Day, or 'Nuerday', is on 13 January. According to the islanders this is neither old-fashioned nor heathen, but just downright independent.

Wildlife: Foula is yet another island with its own variety of sheep although they are not as distinctive as the Soay (No.9.2) sheep of the St Kilda group or even the seaweed-eating sheep of North Ronaldsay (No.10.27). They are known as 'hardback' sheep and, in common with all primitive sheep, they have exceptionally hairy fleeces. They were possibly introduced by the Vikings. Recently the sheep have been found to have a carnivorous streak – they bite the heads off young arctic tern and skua nestlings. Red deer on Rum (No.4.3) have a similar habit. The RSPB has suggested that the sheep should be given minerals as they are probably trying to compensate for a deficiency in the vegetation. On the other hand they may have just discovered a new gastronomic treat.

Foula, like Fair Isle (No.11.1), has its own sub-species of field mouse, *Apodemus sylvaticus thuloe* – a charming little creature with big feet. It also has rabbits, hedgehogs and house mice.

The Viking name of Foula is still apt for this is an internationally recognised seabird station with over 125,000 breeding birds (twelve species) including the rare Leach's petrel. It is the most prolific breeding site in the North Atlantic for that ponderous pirate, the great skua or 'bonxie'. In the 19th century bonxies bred nowhere else in Britain except Foula and Unst (No.11.29) but, thanks to the attention of egg-collectors, only about fifteen pairs were left by the late 19th century and only *three* pairs by 1920. However, with protection, it has made a remarkable recovery and there are about 3000 breeding pairs on Foula's cliffs and boulder fields. The great skua – large, dark brown and heavily built – will attack even a gannet or black-backed gull forcing it to vomit up its catch. During the nesting season it will fearlessly attack men or dogs yet, strangely, the smaller arctic skua, or 'scootie-allan', shows no fear of it.

Parts of the sheer northern cliffs provide no foothold for nesting birds but elsewhere the narrow ledges are packed with noisy activity. The south-east of the island, which is almost bare of peat, has high densities of nesting oystercatcher, ringed plover, arctic skua and arctic tern. Unfortunately, there are now greatly reduced numbers of puffin (or 'Tammy Norie'). This may be due to a reduction in sand-eels caused by over-fishing or it may be a result of the increased numbers of bonxies. After all, a bonxie will even take an occasional lamb so, puffins are an easy meal.

* * *

FOULA is the most isolated inhabited island in the British Isles and the most westerly of the Shetland group, lying fourteen miles out in the Atlantic. Bad weather can cut off the island for up to six weeks at a time so the difficulty for a visitor is not merely the matter of getting there, but the twin problem of getting there *and* getting back. Be sure to carry ample provisions in case of an enforced stay and if you are visiting in your own boat remember to keep a very close watch on the weather as there is no adequate harbour.

The land rises from east to west with low, broken cliffs and some small coves on the east coast, but a west coast of precipitous cliffs rising to a height of 150–365m. There are five distinct peaks all leaning to the north; the **Sneug**, which is the highest at 418m, just west of centre; **Hamnafield** or Hamnafjeld (344m) at the centre; the **Noup** (248m)(ON – precipitous crag) on the south-west coast; the **Kame** (376m) on the west coast; and **Soberlie Hill** (221m) on the north-west coast. The Noup is separated from the other peaks by a glacial valley called the **Daal** (ON *dal* – valley).

At one time the menfolk of Foula were almost entirely engaged in fishing but nowadays crofting has had to take precedence. All the crofts are on the east side with about half the population settled in **Hametoun** (S. – home town) in the south-east and the remainder living at **Ham** near Ham Voe (ON – harbour inlet). Here there is a post-office, a school (rebuilt at considerable expense), a church and a chapel. The 'smiddy' sells items made by the islanders like colley lamps, ram's head knives, sheepskin rugs and items made from copper salvaged from the *Oceanic*, sister ship to the *Titanic*. She was wrecked off Foula in 1914.

Ham Voe is the best that Foula can provide in the way of harbour facilities. The island's only 'beach' is at the head of the narrow little voe and the fishing boats have to be drawn well up to clear the big waves which tumble in, particularly when the wind is in the east. Even the small mailboat/ferry, after it has had all the goods and equipment off-loaded by the islanders, has to be power-hoisted onto a concrete pad at the pier for security. A monthly mailboat service began in 1879, when the local minister wrote to Queen Victoria and received a reply from Disraeli. But 'monthly' was an optimistic term as there was no harbour and passengers and goods had to be landed on the rocks. It was not until 1914, after thirty years of petitioning, that a tiny concrete pier was built using local labour and shingle from the back of Smell Geo. It included a step for a gun because of the advent of the First World War. The officials chose to site the pier alongside the only skerry in the Voe so consequently one side of the pier is inaccessible. Many years later a power-driven crane and winch was fitted to allow the mailboat to be lifted out instead of being manhandled. The winter service from Walls is entirely dependent on the weather but there have been many problems since 1990 as a new ferry was built which was found to be unable to cope with the severe conditions.

The strong sense of community in this gaunt and beautiful outpost is very evident. For about a century the population was slowly disintegrating and in 1965 Eric Linklater claimed that this 'old folks' home remote in the pitiless Atlantic will not survive much longer as a human habitation'. Yet today the population has stabilised, shows signs of increasing, and new houses and a school for the next generation have been built. There is no doubt that this is the result of better communications; access to an airstrip, a telephone, and a radio transmitter. But a different attitude by mainlanders is also helping to save the last few populated islands from complete desolation. Local authorities have at last realised that island schools may be uneconomic but that they are an essential element in maintaining a population, and that this also applies to improved harbours and services.

Foula has many physical similarities to Hirta, St Kilda (No.9.1). Both these Atlantic islands have high mountains, skyscraping cliffs and little land suitable for cultivation. In both cases an essential source of food was seabirds and eggs collected from the terrifying cliffs. But there the similarity ends because the St Kildans were basically crofters who had virtually no concept of private property. All decision-making had to be communal following the tenet that the community is more important than the individual.

On Foula, on the other hand, the islanders were fishermen rather than crofters and like all sailors they were intensely independent and self-assured. They believed in private enterprise and standing on their own feet. The community was important, but only as a collection of individuals. Even the houses on Foula stand apart whereas on St Kilda they cling together.

Is there a lesson to be learned? The St Kildans have gone, but Foula is still a thriving community.

Foula's stacks are not as high as those of Hirta but they are just as interesting. For instance, near **Hellibaas** (ON – flagstone rocks on which the sea breaks in bad weather) on the north coast there is a high square-topped stack with a natural arch at its base which looks like a ruined castle. But Foula's cliffs are unequalled in dramatic impact even if they just fail by 2m to match the height of the awesome St Kildan cliffs. There is a narrow chimney on top of **Hamnafjeld** (ON – harbour mountain) which is so deep it is said to go straight down to Hell; and at the head of the Daal in the **Wick of Mucklabrek** is the Sneck of the Smallie, another secret chimney which plunges down between the sea-cliffs in a narrow slit until only the sky is visible 60m above.

Relics of the quaint Norn language still linger in the dialect on Foula, noticeable in place names such as Hedd o' da Baa (head of the underwater rock) and Wester Hoevdi (western height). Linklater recalled how when the menfolk had finished fishing they would dance the Foula Reel to the tune of *The Shaalds of Foula* (shaald – shoal) – 'Up wi' da lines and link it awa, awa, ta da shaalds o Foula.'

One of these famous, but dangerous, shoals – **Hoevdi Grund** (ON – high ground) – which were once rich in cod, haddock, mackerel, halibut, saithe and ling, lies only three miles east of South Ness.

* * *

Access: Mail boat/ passenger ferry, May to Sept. weather permitting, from Walls, 2 or 3 times per week, 07881-823732, or 01595-743976 for information. Advance booking essential. Scheduled flights from Tingwall, weather permitting, Mon., Tue., Wed., and Fri. 01595-840246.

Anchorage: There is no adequate harbour. Local boats are hauled out and even the mailboat/ferry is lifted out by crane each trip.

1. Ham Voe. Very restricted. Beware rocks on N and S sides of Ham Voe and on E side of pier. Approach with care on a WNW course to just off the SW corner of the pier. The stone pier is 27m long with steps halfway along its NW side and a depth of 1.8m at its head and on its west side. Anchor in corner of Voe with warp to hold stern off. No turning room for boats of over 36'. Best to leave promptly if bad weather likely.

11.7 Noss

(ON nos – nose, or high rocky promontory) or (ON nes – headland.)

OS Maps: 1:50000 Sheet 4 1:25000 Sheet 466
Admiralty Charts: 1:75000 No.3283 1:17500 No.3291 excludes E coast.

Area: 343ha (847 acres)
Height: 181m (594 ft)

Owner: John Hamilton Scott of Garth and Wendy Scott. Noss is part of the Garth Estate.

Population: 1841–24 (3 houses). After 1871 partly cleared by Walker, the owner's factor. 1881–3. 1891–3 (1 house). 1931–4. Only summer habitation since. 1961–0. 1971–3. 1981–0. 1991–0. 2001–0.

Geology: Old Red Sandstone cliffs stratified and eroded in horizontal slabs which provide perfect shelves for nesting birds with occasional traces of volcanic vents.

History: A small chapel existed in front of the old homestead at Gungstie (now the SNH visitor centre) in 1633, built by 'shipwrakt' persons. The walls were still standing in 1774 and the burial ground beside the Sound was used until the middle of the 19th century. There is good reason to believe that the chapel site was originally Celtic and pre-Norse but, unfortunately, the burial ground is now being eroded by the sea. In 1969 the tenant found an underground passage beside the house.

The homestead was built some 400 years ago and for a time was the only inhabited house on Noss. In the early 19th century the farm was reputed to produce the best butter and milk in Shetland. The tenant farmer at the time was the father of Dr James Copland who published the *Dictionary of Medicine* in 1832.

In 1869 the Marquis of Londonderry leased the island and turned it over to pasture for his prize breed of Shetland stallions. These were used in his Durham coal mine as a substitute for child labour. The mares were kept on Bressay to allow controlled breeding.

Since 1900 Noss has been used for sheep-farming providing pasturage for about 420 Shetland ewes.

Wildlife: The island, which has been a National Nature Reserve since 1955, is managed by Scottish Natural Heritage. Explanatory leaflets are available at the visitors' centre. Visitors are required to keep to the cliff-top path and no camping is permitted.

There are 150 species of flowering plants here including the semi-parasitic Lousewort or 'Sookie Flooer', but Noss is best known for its seabirds,

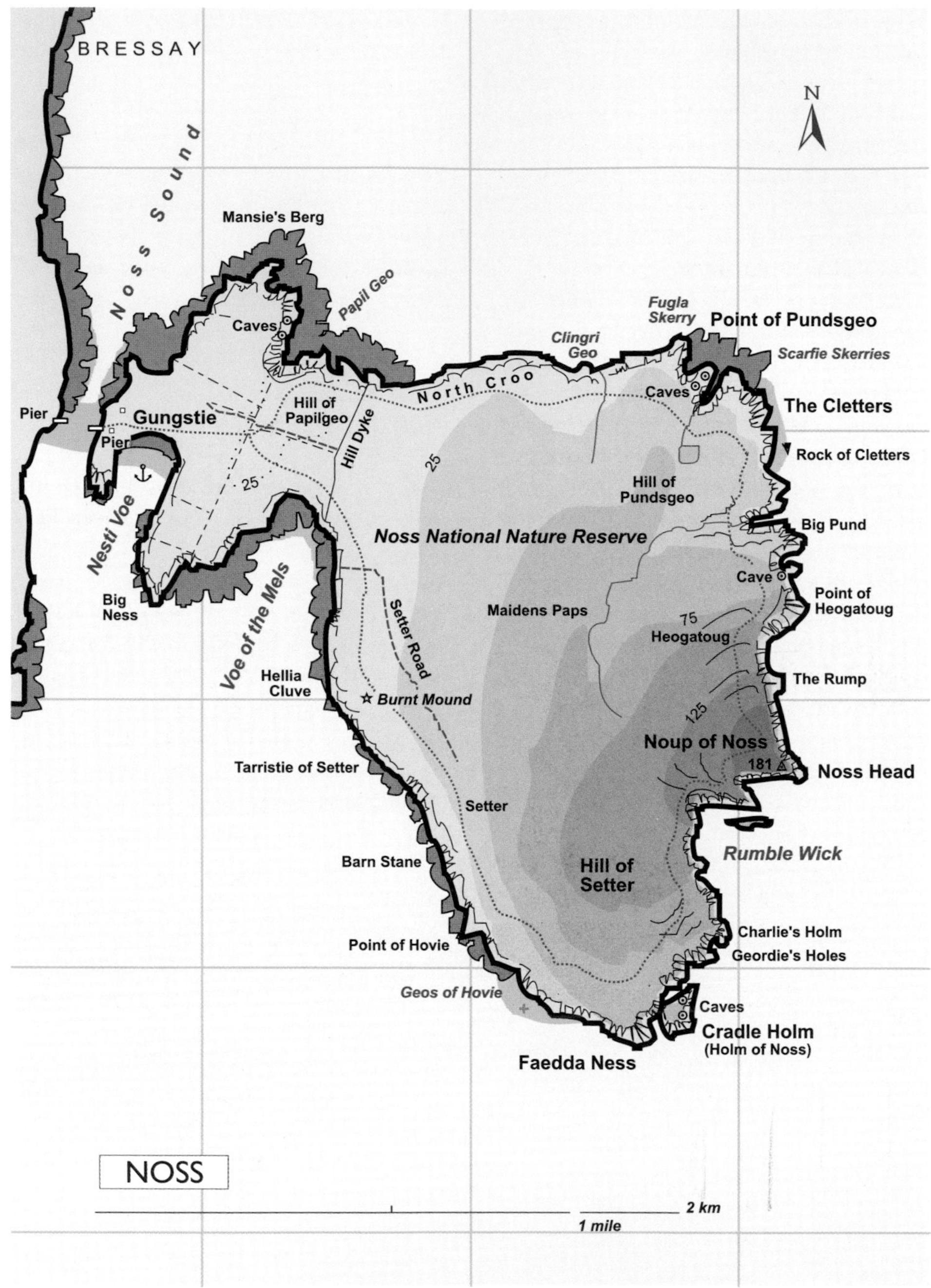

more than 160,000 of them. The first gannet colony only became established on Noss in 1911. Now there are over 5,000 pairs nesting on the headland with over 10,000 pairs of kittiwake and 65,000 pairs of guillemot. Twenty pairs of arctic skua and 300 pairs of great skua (bonxie) nest inland. There are also many fulmar, eider (dunter), great black-backed gull, razorbill, puffin, shag and black guillemot (tystie).

The best bird-watching period is mid-May to July.

* * *

The isle of **NOSS** is a veritable metropolis of seabirds and the cacophony of sound from their cries is so loud that it can sometimes be heard far to seaward when even the island itself is out of sight. The cliffs of Noss are made up of narrow horizontal beds of sandstone which the sea has carved into thousands of attractive ledges. These are ideal sites for seabirds' dream-houses and competition is intense in Bird City.

The **Noup of Noss**, towering 180m above the waves, is the highest point on Noss and the 'city centre'. Every precipitous dormitory suburb has a suitable name which rolls off the tongue delightfully: to the north – the Cletters, Whiggie Geo, Point of Heogatoug, and the Rump; and southwards – Rumble Wick, Geordie's Holes, Feadda Ness and Holm of Noss. The best viewpoint is from the sea.

Holm of Noss, also known as Cradle Holm, is a stack standing 48m high and considered now to be almost impossible to climb. It is separated by a 20m gap from the cave-riddled cliffs of Feadda Ness. This used to provide a handy anchorage for small boats until a rockfall blocked it. In the 17th century a crofter was wagered a cow that he could not reach the top of the Holm and he won the wager, reputedly by climbing a ship's mast for part of the way. While on the top he fixed stakes in the turf and constructed a replaceable rope railway which could support a box cradle large enough to carry a man and a sheep. Unfortunately, after completing the work he slipped and fell to his death. It was of little consolation to him that his engineering was faultless and that his famous 'Cradle of Noss' was used every summer for over 200 years to graze sheep on the top of the Holm. It was dismantled in 1864 by Mr Walker, the laird's factor, who considered it unsafe. He had a safety wall built along the cliff-head.

Noss Sound is shallow, rocky and narrow (less than 200m) and wind and tide can funnel through, making it decidedly unpleasant at times. It has been the scene of many shipwrecks. An old track along the south shore ends at **Setter** where there are still the ruins of a settlement. In Norse times there were five settlements along this south coast according to the records. The visitors' path continues from here and circumnavigates the island.

The old house at Gungstie was restored as staff accommodation in 1986 and includes a visitor information room. The Pony Pund – the stables building built by the Marquis of Londonderry in 1870 – was converted at the same time and contains an interpretative display.

The name of **Papil Geo** (G. – priest's inlet) on the north coast below the **North Croo** might be a reminder that an early Christian hermit once lived on Noss – possibly in the caves which open on to the Geo, or it may be related to the chapel site at Hametoun.

From the landing place at Gungstie the ground climbs towards the west, gently at first and then quite steeply. The 'Hill Dyke' crosses the island's neck and during the lambing season this separates the lambs from the nesting bonxies. The ground cover is mostly heather and coarse grass but the grazing was once fine grass pasture for the Marquis of Londonderry's ponies. In the nesting season when climbing up the slopes to the cliff-head the bonxies dive-bomb with determination. This is rarely dangerous but is certainly intimidating. On the cliff-top path expect also to have your senses assaulted. The sight of prolific birdlife is unbelievable, the noise is deafening, and the smell overpowering.

* * *

Access: Lerwick to Bressay (See No.11.8) then car, bus, taxi or walk (5km) to Noss Sound. For crossing to Noss by inflatable from Bressay (summer only, and no dogs) hail the Scottish Natural Heritage warden at Gungstie on Noss, 01595-693345. For wildlife trips round Bressay and Noss try Alluvion Trips, 01595-693434 or contact Tourist Office, 01595-693434.

Anchorages: Noss Sound is shallow, rocky and has a strong tidal current. Passage requires a shallow-draught and local knowledge.

1. Nesti Voe, at S end of Noss Sound. Occasional anchorage. Enter mid-channel and anchor in the middle, sand. Exposed S.
2. Voe of the Mels, W of Nesti Voe. Occasional anchorage. Approach E of mid-channel and anchor near head of voe in 4m sand. Exposed S.
3. Noup of Noss, steep-to. There are mooring rings on the rocks below the Noup for use in quiet weather to watch the birds.

11.8 Bressay

In 1490 called (ON Brús-øy – Brusi's island) from a proper name, but in 1263 was possibly referred to as (ON breid-øy – broad island).

O S Maps: 1:50000 Sheet 4 1:25000 Sheet 466
Admiralty Charts: 1:75000 No.3283 1:17500 No.3291
Area: 2805ha (6931 acres)
Height: 226m (741 ft)

Owner: Mr John Hamilton Scott of Garth, who farms Maryfield Farm, is the principal landowner. He inherited the Bressay estate from his uncle, Mr Norman Ogilvie Mouat Cameron of Garth.

Population: 1841–904 (167 houses). 1881–847. 1891–799 (166 houses). 1931–448. 1961–269. 1981–334. 1991–352. 2001–384.

Geology: Almost entirely composed of Middle and Upper Old Red Sandstone with a few volcanic outcrops and some thin bands of tuff between the flagstones on the east coast. Much of Shetland is roofed with 'slates' – thin flagstone slabs – from Bressay, and building stone was quarried at Aith.

History: A selection of prehistoric remains are scattered across Bressay but the best-known early historical artefact is probably the Bressay Stone which was found near Culbinsbrough churchyard and which can be seen in the Scottish National Museum of Antiquities in Edinburgh. It is a Pictish cross-slab with an ogam inscription which includes two Gaelic words and one Norse word which could indicate that the early inhabitants were co-operating peacefully. It is exquisitely carved with a Celtic cross, representations of priests, a horseman, some animals and, possibly, Jonah and two whales.

In the 11th century Harald Hardrada's ships lay in Bressay Sound (ON *Breideyjarsund*) before sailing south to a Viking defeat by Harold Godwinsson at Stamford Bridge. In the 13th century King Haakon's fleet also sheltered in the Sound before meeting a similar fate at Largs.

From the 15th to the mid-17th century most of Bressay was owned by Sigurd Jonsson, a Norwegian nobleman. John Neven the Younger of Unst became owner of the estate in 1660 and then it passed to the Hendersons, who were also of Norwegian origin. Most of the remainder of the island belonged to the Bolts of Cruister, Magnus Bult being 'Foude' of Bressay in 1612. The Bolts lived in the Haa of Cruister but the building was abandoned – it is now a ruin – when the Mouats of Garth acquired the Bolts' estate in the early 19th century.

In 1640 ten Spanish men-of-war sailed into the Sound and attacked four Dutchmen, two of which were sunk. Later, an English fleet of ninety-four ships commanded by Admiral George Monk anchored here for several days in 1653 while searching for Van Tromp and the Dutch fleet.

In the early 18th century French privateers sailed through and 'pillaged like gentlemen' and a French fleet in a fishing war with the Dutch burned 150 busses anchored in the Sound. The area was a favourite fishing ground for the Dutch and in 1774, for instance, over 400 busses – mostly Dutch – anchored in the Sound. It was said that Amsterdam was built 'oot o' da back o' Bressa'.

During the Peninsular War, naval press-gangs raided the area and removed numerous young Shetlanders, magnificent seamen whom the islands could ill-afford to lose, for service with Nelson's fleet.

1871 was 'da year 'at Walker made da uproar'. The laird at that time was Miss Mouat and her factor, Walker, cleared many of the crofts for sheep. He built Maryfield House for himself and named it after his wife. The site, opposite Lerwick, was previously a croft called Troubletoon.

The German High Seas Fleet visited the Sound in the early years of the 20th century and Bressay boasted gun emplacements in both World Wars.

Wildlife: Many migrant birds reach the crofts in the west of the island. Waders and whooper swans can be seen at the Loch of Grimsetter on the east coast. Further south, bonxies nest near Sand Vatn, seabirds nest on the cliffs and a colony of arctic skua nests near Bard Head.

* * *

Lerwick and **BRESSAY** are symbiotic. Lerwick could not exist if it were not for the protection which the island gives to its excellent harbour; Bressay owes much of its livelihood to close proximity to Lerwick.

The merits of an anchorage in Bressay Sound were known by the Vikings but it was the Dutch fishermen in the 15th century who turned it into a port. The Dutch busses – two-masted craft of over 80 tons – and their accompanying men-of-war which would now be called 'fishery protection vessels' would crowd into the Sound in vast numbers. At times it was said one could cross from Mainland to Bressay by stepping from boat to boat. For the Dutch this was a great government-protected industry with more than 2000 busses exporting their catch of Scottish herring to countries throughout the western

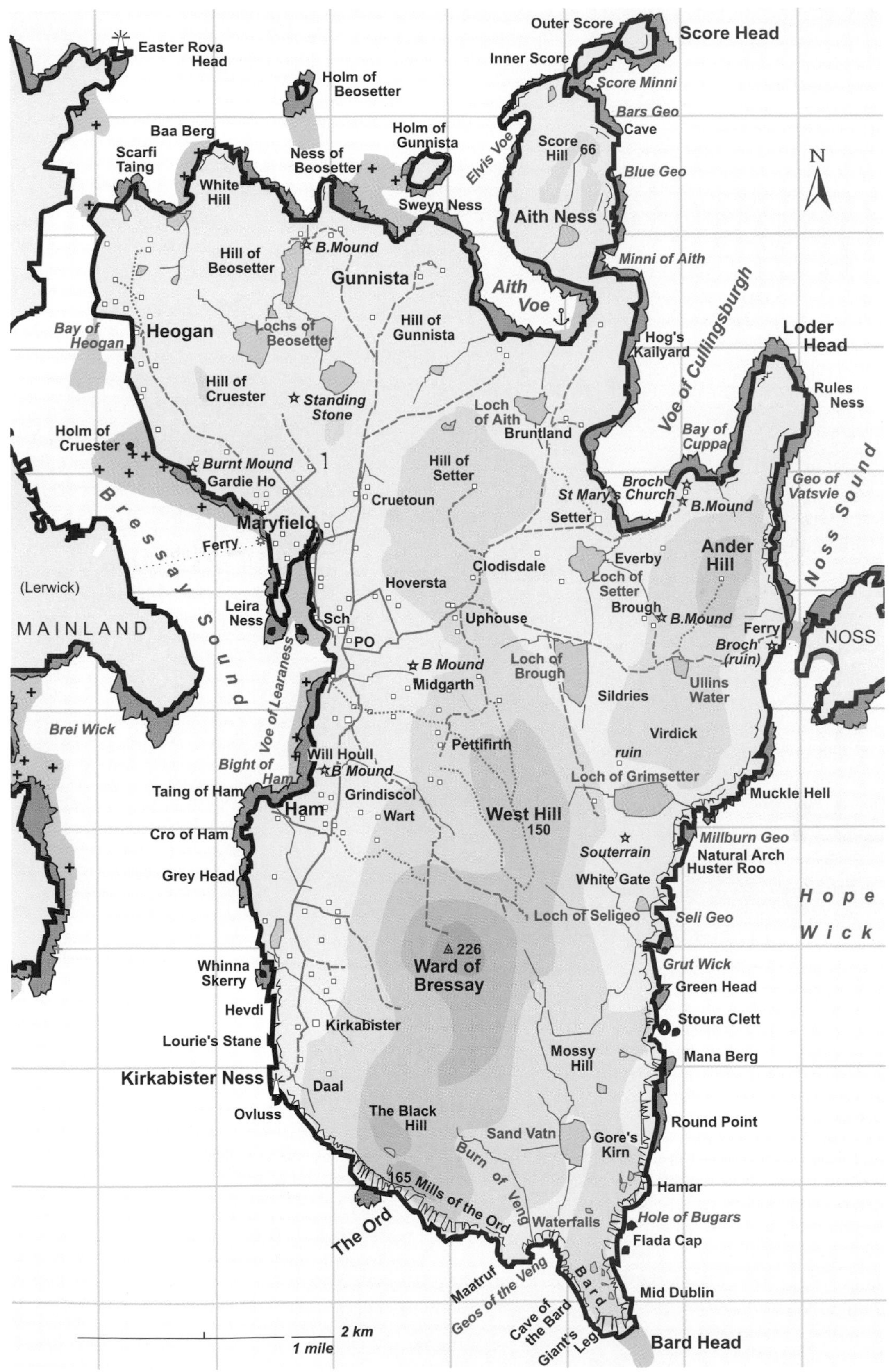
Outer Score
Score Head
Inner Score
Easter Rova Head
Holm of Beosetter
Score Minni
Bars Geo
Cave
Baa Berg
Holm of Gunnista
Score Hill
66
Scarfi Taing
Ness of Beosetter
Elvis Voe
Blue Geo
N
White Hill
Sweyn Ness
Aith Ness
B.Mound
Hill of Beosetter
Gunnista
Minni of Aith
Aith Voe
Voe of Cullingsburgh
Bay of Heogan
Heogan
Lochs of Beosetter
Hill of Gunnista
Loder Head
Hog's Kailyard
Hill of Cruester
Standing Stone
Rules Ness
Loch of Aith
Bruntland
Bay of Cuppa
Holm of Cruester
Burnt Mound
Hill of Setter
Gardie Ho
Broch
Geo of Vatsvie
St Mary's Church
B.Mound
Cruetoun
Bressay Sound
Noss Sound
Maryfield
Setter
Ferry
Ander Hill
Everby
Clodisdale
(Lerwick)
Loch of Setter
Hoversta
Leira Ness
Brough
B.Mound
Uphouse
Sch
MAINLAND
Ferry
NOSS
PO
Broch (ruin)
Voe of Leraness
B Mound
Loch of Brough
Midgarth
Ullins Water
Sildries
Brei Wick
Pettifirth
Virdick
Will Houll
ruin
Bight of Ham
B Mound
Loch of Grimsetter
Taing of Ham
Grindiscol
Muckle Hell
Ham
Wart
West Hill
150
Cro of Ham
Millburn Geo
Souterrain
Natural Arch
Huster Roo
Grey Head
White Gate
Hope Wick
Loch of Seligeo
Seli Geo
226
Ward of Bressay
Grut Wick
Whinna Skerry
Green Head
Hevdi
Stoura Clett
Kirkabister
Lourie's Stane
Mana Berg
Mossy Hill
Kirkabister Ness
Daal
Ovluss
The Black Hill
Round Point
Sand Vatn
Gore's Kirn
Burn of Veng
Hamar
165
Mills of the Ord
Hole of Bugars
The Ord
Waterfalls
Flada Cap
Maatruf
Geos of the Veng
Bard
Mid Dublin
Cave of the Bard
2 km
1 mile
Giant's Leg
Bard Head

world. James VI (James I of England) tried to introduce a licensing system to control them but it was ignored. Later Charles I enlisted the help of the Navy and after an exchange of fire the Dutch agreed to pay an annual fee and obey the rules. One such rule was that fishing could not begin before the Feast of St John the Baptist (Johnsmas – 24 June). By mid-June the Sound would fill with boats preparing for the start and the Shetlanders meanwhile would make what profit they could from the event by setting up booths and bars on the shore.

By 1798 a few Shetland boats had succeeded in joining the bonanza. According to the Rev. Cruttwell: 'The inhabitants of Bressay fit out about twenty-six large fishing boats.'

It is a sad historical fact that the social structure in the Scottish islands denied most of the inhabitants the chance to own an ocean-going fishing boat with the result that the vast wealth of the northern seas was largely exploited by foreigners. It is only in very recent times that Scottish fishermen have had the opportunity to participate.

The south and east coasts are high, barren and precipitous whereas the north and west coasts are lower with rocky foreshores and productive crofts. **Ward of Bressay** – 'Da Wart' – is a pyramid-shaped hill in the centre of the southern part of the island. It is the highest point on the island at 226m but its interesting silhouette is not appreciated by the inhabitants of Lerwick as on sunny winter mornings it casts a shadow across the town.

On the south coast above the cliffs there is another hill called **The Ord** which reaches a height of 165m. East of here is the bleak expanse of **Sand Vatn** and the most southerly point of Bressay, **Bard Head**. The sandstone cliffs which stretch round this point and up the west coast are composed of interesting rock formations. Beside the aptly-named **Giant's Leg** is the Cave of the Bard, better known as **Orkneyman's Cave** [HU514360]. No one is certain now who the Orkneyman was: he might have been a Jacobite, or a fugitive from the naval press-gangs, or the name might come from an earlier age. The cave is only accessible by boat but is well worth the trouble. The entrance is a symmetrical archway which is wide enough for several boats to enter abreast and the water within is clear and deep with extraordinarily beautiful variegated colours on the roof and walls. The cave then narrows but opens up again into a spacious hall with stalactites. It is possible to go in by dinghy for a considerable distance.

Bressay has had its brochs but only traces of these remain. In Culbingsbrough Voe (ON Kolbeinsborg) in the north-east, called Cullingsburgh by the Ordnance Survey, there is one on a small promontory [HU521423]. Beside it is the ruined wall of a chapel, **St Mary's Church**, which is claimed to have been the only cruciform church in Shetland and which may date back to the Norse era. In the burial ground is a stone commemorating a Dutch captain, Claes Bruyn, who was master of a merchantman *Amboina*. In 1636 after a foray with Portuguese ships off Mozambique, he took on a cargo of Persian silk at Surat in India, was delayed by violent gales off the Cape of Good Hope, lost twenty-nine of his crew from disease, and then at last, months later, reached Bressay Sound. He dropped anchor thankfully and promptly dropped dead.

St Mary's is overlooked by **Ander Hill** which has a derelict lookout tower on top of it built by the Admiralty before the First World War. Ander Hill has a similar profile when viewed from every point of the compass.

Gunnista was also the site of an early church dedicated to St Ola or Olaf and the parish church until 1722. It was demolished by the laird, William Henderson of Gardie, despite the minister's protests, to use the materials for a new church to be built nearer Gardie House. **Aith Voe**, between Gunnista and twisted Aith Ness, is a fair anchorage with its entrance guarded by two islets, **Holm of Beosetter** and **Holm of Gunnista**.

A third early church existed at **Kirkabister** in the south-west dedicated to St John, but it has long since disappeared. **Bressay Lighthouse** is close by, at Kirkabister Ness, marking the southern entrance to Bressay Sound. It was built in 1858 and is now automatic.

The ferry docks by **Maryfield**, the main house for Maryfield Farm (452ha). To the north is the charming little mansion, **Gardie House**, the laird's house, which was built in 1724 but had its facade remodelled about 1900.

* * *

Access: Frequent daily ro-ro ferry from Lerwick, (voicebank) 01595-743974. Tourist Office, 01595-693434.

Anchorages:
1. Visitor berth in marina (2m least depth) at Voe of Leiraness.
2. Lerwick Harbour, (Mainland). Berth in Small Boat Harbour or Albert docks subject to HM's agreement or temp. anchorage S of Small Boat Hr.
3. Bard Head. Mooring rings for use while visiting the Cave of the Bard (Orkneyman's cave) by dinghy in settled conditions.
4. Aith Voe, N coast. Enter E of Gunnista Holm. Anchor in 5½–7m. Good shelter but fish cage obstruction.

11.9 Hildasay

Possibly (ON hildis-øy – battle island). Hild was the battle goddess of Norse mythology. The Vikings liked to settle a quarrel by single combat on an uninhabited island in order to avoid interference by spectators. The island name is sometimes spelt Hildesay. Alternatively (ON Hildis-øy – Hildir's island). Hildir is a man's name.

OS Maps: 1:50000 Sheet 4 1:25000 Sheet 466
Admiralty Charts: 1:75000 No.3283 1:17500 No.3294

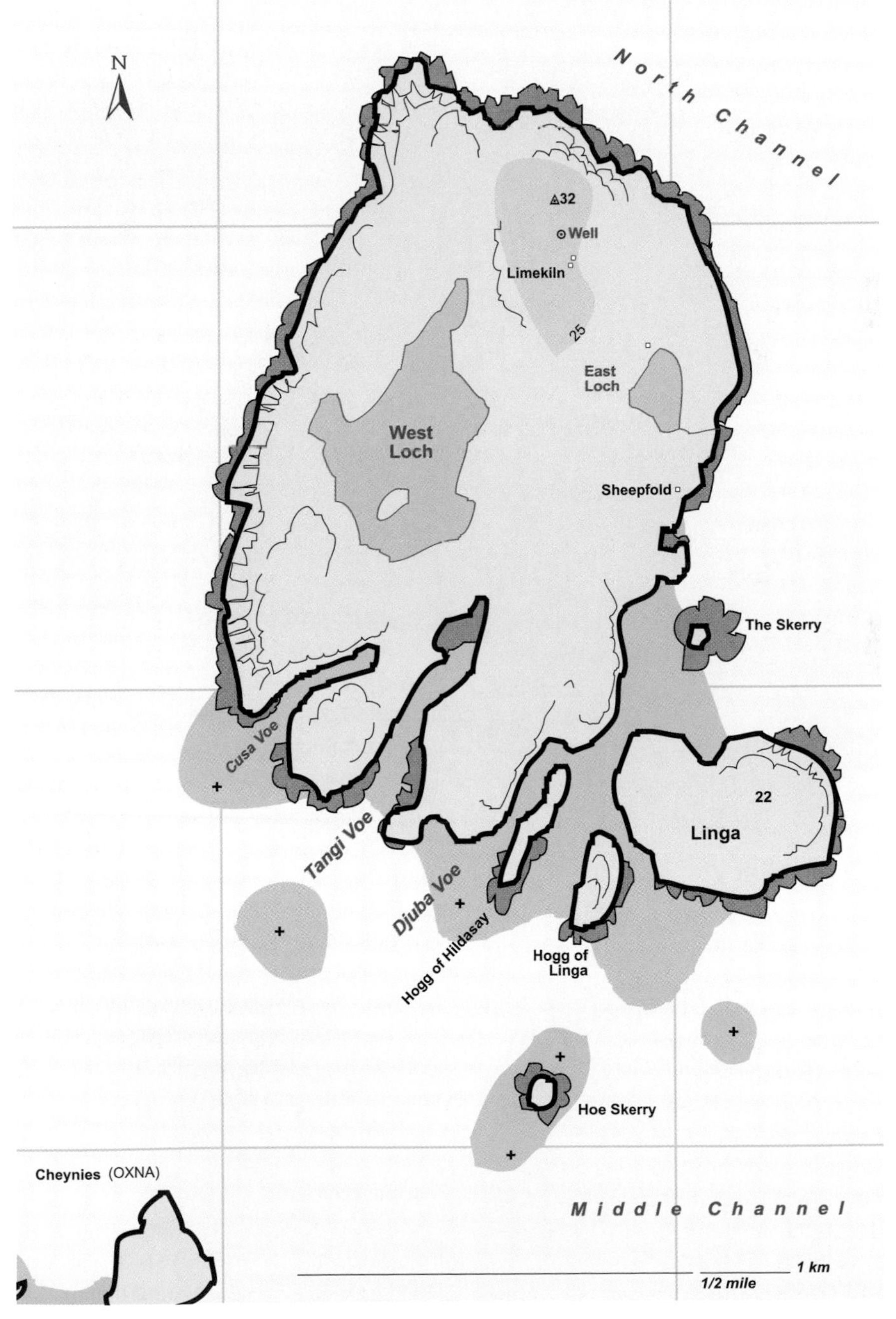

Area: 108ha (267 acres)
Height: 32m (105 ft)

Owner: Hildasay was for sale in 1996.

Population: 1881–7. 1891–30 (5 houses). 1901–0. Uninhabited since.

Geology: The high-quality red-green 'granite' on Hildasay – actually an epidotic syenite – was quarried for many years and was even said to have been exported to Australia but with the advent of concrete the quarry became uneconomic and closed down.

History: Hildasay was bought by an American with Shetland family connections in 1897.

* * *

HILDASAY is an oval island, shaped like a yeti's footprint. It reaches a height of 32m near its north end. There are rocky escarpments on the west and north coasts and the south coast has three 'toes' formed by two narrow inlets, Cusa Voe and Tangi Voe (ON – seaweed inlet). A large loch, **West Loch**, with a lone islet covers a considerable part of the west side of the island.

Hildasay has a satellite island – the yeti's big toe – called **Linga** (ON – heather island). It is close to the south-east coast and it was a separate croft in the 19th century.

To the north-west, but separated by a deep navigable channel, is a long reef of skerries and holms including **North Score Holm**, **Easter Score Holm** and **Sanda Little**. It culminates in **Sanda Stour** (ON – big sandy island) at its south end. This little islet is 19m high and the sea has carved its rocks into a natural arch.

The ruins of Hildasay's small settlement, which reached its maximum size of five houses towards the end of the 19th century, is on the hillside in the north. At that time the island was going through a relatively prosperous stage. Apart from three or four crofts there was a curing-station for herring and a granite quarry. The quarry had a small railway track to carry the cut stone down to the landing place – the only such railway track in Shetland. The owner allowed islanders from Burra and Trondra to cut peat on the island as they had none on their own islands. The peat on Hildasay was of particularly good quality and the peat-cutting visits were always a good excuse for a social occasion.

Unfortunately, the good times came to an end. The quarry closed down when the sale of its stone became uneconomic and almost simultaneously the curing-station was closed because of the decline in the herring industry. Only sheep remained. The island was abandoned about 1900 but it was determined not to be forgotten and in the latter years of the last century issued its own postage stamps.

* * *

Access: By arrangement: MV Cycharters, Scalloway, 01595-696598. Tourist Office, 01595-693434.

Anchorage: There is no recommended anchorage and temp. anchorage by The Skerry (N of Linga) is risky owing to the proximity of fish-cages but there is an old pier for a landing place.

11.10 Vaila

Probably (ON val-øy – falcon island) but could also be horse island, battlefield island or round island.

OS Maps: 1:50000 Sheets 3 and 4 1:25000 Sheet 467
Admiralty Charts: 1:75000 Nos.3283 or 3281 1:25000 No.3295

Area: 327ha (808 acres)
Height: 95m (312 ft)

Owner: Dorota Rychlik and Richard Rowland, of London. Purchased in 1993 from Mr Henry Anderton. The new owners have restored Vaila Hall.

Population: 1841–29 (4 houses). 1881–9. 1891–19 (2 houses). 1901–30. 1931–5. 1961–9. 1971–5. 1981–0. 1991–1. 2001–2.

Geology: Fine, dark-grey sandstone typical of the Walls region. It was deposited about 400 million years ago but has since been folded and metamorphosed and subsequently glaciated. The south-east corner has an intrusion of complex Sandsting granite seen in the red cliffs by the Gaada Stacks.

History: A Neolithic house site has been discovered and there are Bronze Age burned mounds in the fertile north-west of the island.

In 1490 the estates of the Norwegian family of Ciske were divided and Vaila and Foula (No.11.6) became the possession of Alv Knutsson. Gorvel Fadersdatter 'of Geskie' succeeded to the title in 1537 and she leased Vaila, and Walls, to Robert Cheyne of Ury (later to become Commissioner of Zetland) in 1576 with permission to build a fortress for safety from 'Heland men, perattis and utheris invasionis'. There was some confusion concerning national ownership of all the Northern Isles at this time as they had been mortgaged to Scotland for Princess Margaret of Norway's dowry in 1468 and Scotland had later foreclosed on the unpaid debt and annexed them. Consequently, Andrew Hawich of Scatsa contested Cheyne's claim to Vaila but Cheyne was

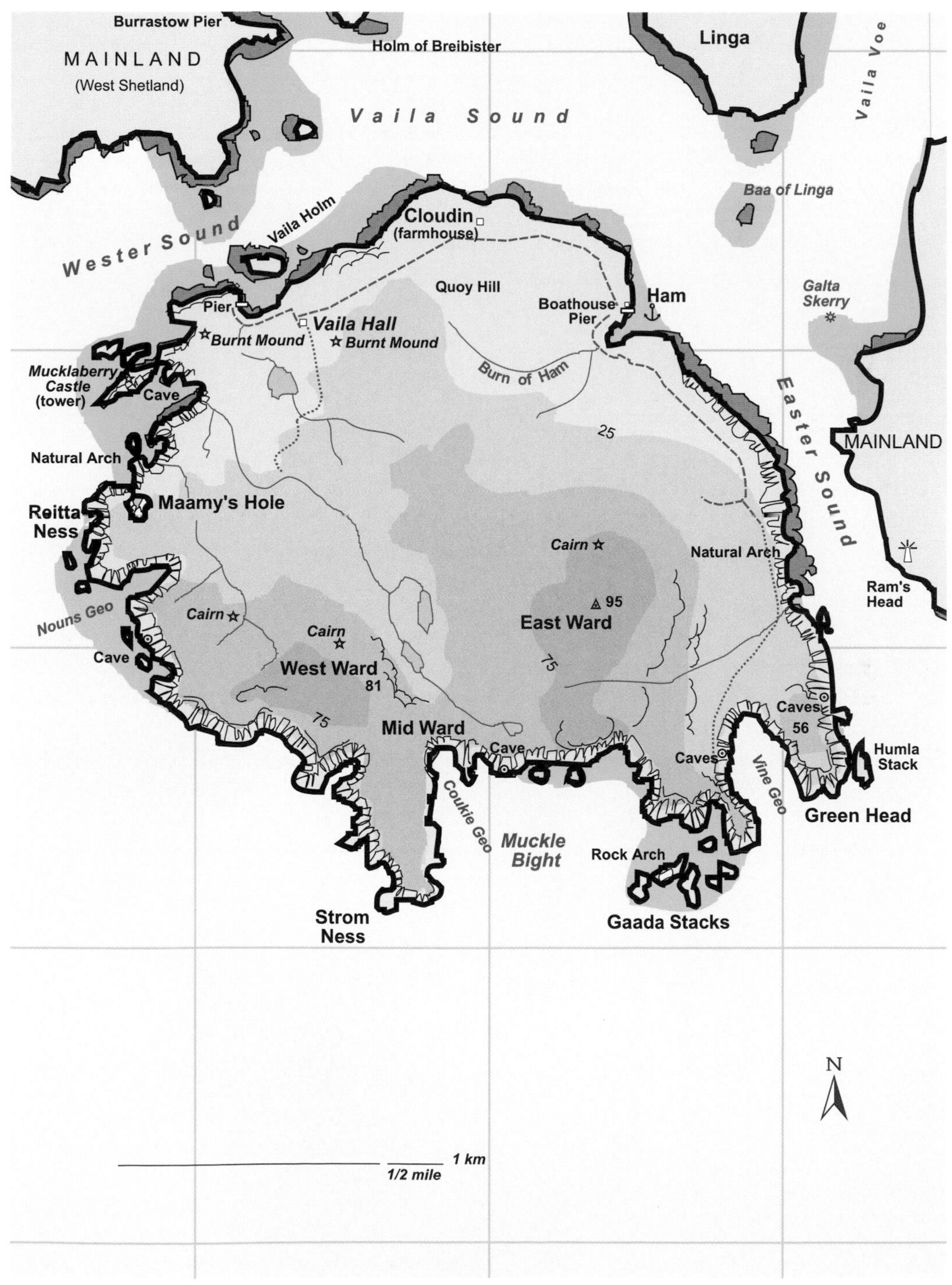

able to produce proof of title from the Scottish king. Two years later (1582) Gorvel transferred all her estates to the King of Denmark but he too confirmed Cheyne's right to lease the property for 66 'good dollars' a year.

The Scandinavian claim became more and more tenuous and by 1661 the Danes were complaining that the rent was seldom received.

In 1696 the Cheyne's sold Vaila to James Mitchell, a Scalloway merchant and he built a house on the island which now forms part of the south wing of Vaila Hall. In 1736 the island was inherited by James Scott of Melby (see also No.11.6) and it was the Scott family who leased it to that notable Shetlander, Arthur Anderson.

Arthur Anderson was born in Shetland in 1792. He was a beach-boy (fish-drier), who acquired some education and volunteered to join the Navy. He became a midshipman and, in due course, a Captain's clerk. He then left the Navy and obtained employment with a London shipowner, Willcox, who eventually offered him a partnership. This gave him time to travel during which he intervened successfully in a civil war in Portugal and founded a Liberal newspaper in Shetland. In 1837 he and Willcox started the Peninsular Steam Company which, three years later, became the Peninsular and Oriental (P & O), running regular mail services to India and China with a strict discipline that almost matched the Royal Navy.

Meanwhile Anderson continued to take a great interest in Shetland's welfare. He presented Queen Victoria with a fine knitted Shetland shawl which made these shawls instantly popular in fashion-conscious London society and created a new cottage industry. Also in 1837 he leased Vaila and established the Shetland Fishery Company – breaking the existing feudal system by which all catches, and most of the boats, belonged to the laird. And in the following year he started a regular steamship mail-service to Shetland, which existed until recently in the form of the P & O Ferries serving the Northern Isles.

This untiring and benevolent man was Member of Parliament for Orkney and Shetland for several years – establishing a Liberal tradition which has remained part of the philosophy of the islands. But his outlook was far from insular: for instance, he suggested the cutting of a Suez Canal long before de Lesseps. He was philanthropic, founding the Widows' Homes in Lerwick for widows of seamen and fishermen, never priggish, and always retained a great sense of humour.

Arthur Anderson, who died aged seventy-seven, may have had only a passing connection with the island of Vaila but the island gains much by association with one of the truly great Shetlanders.

In 1893 Herbert Anderton, a rich Yorkshire mill-owner on a wool-buying business trip to Shetland, fell in love with Vaila and bought it. He immediately carried out a massive building programme with similarities to the Bullough developments on Rum (No.4.3). Anderton used Vaila Hall as a summer residence and accommodated large house parties. His brother, Francis Swithin, a Royal Academician, assisted with other developments on the island and his brother-in-law and fellow mill-owner, Colonel Foster, bought nearby Burrastow House on Mainland.

During the slump Mr Anderton's fortune largely disappeared as he tried to maintain full employment for his mill-workers. He retired to the island in 1933 and lived there in virtual isolation until he died in 1937. Colonel and Mrs Foster then inherited Vaila but they had both died by 1953 and their daughter was confined to the deteriorating building with multiple sclerosis. Meanwhile, the farm also fell into disrepair so that when, on Miss Foster's death in 1969, Herbert Anderton's great-nephew inherited the island, it was almost too late for him to take remedial measures to stop further serious deterioration of the property. To assist in the cost of maintenance he ran banquets in the Hall, and opened a hostel for bird-watchers and sea anglers. He sold Vaila to the present owners in 1993. Burrastow House (built 1759) on Mainland is a hotel with a well-regarded restaurant and can usually organise a boat to Vaila.

Wildlife: Over 100 different species of wildflower have been recorded on Vaila.

The blue (mountain) hare was introduced in the 20th century and the peat and heather moorland and cliff fringe provide nesting sites for many seabirds.

* * *

Green fertile ground on the north of **VAILA** slopes upwards to moorland in the south. Here there are two cairn-topped rounded hills, West Ward (81m) and **East Ward** (95m), the island summit. The moor has some scattered pools and lochans and on the south-east coast it falls abruptly to the sea in red granite cliffs which rear up again in arches and rocky stacks like Dracula's teeth where they are split by narrow geos.

On the west coast the cliffs are of more modest height but they also have a natural arch and the explosive **Maamy's Hole**, where the waves are forced under pressure through a fissure into a 'gloup' [HU221464].

Vaila is separated from Mainland by Wester Sound and Easter Sound, which form entrances to **Vaila Sound** with its good natural harbour of Walls. This used to be a port of call for ships from Aberdeen and Leith, and for the Shetland deep-sea fishing fleet, and is still the terminus for the Foula passenger ferry (No.11.6). The islet of **Linga** (ON – heather isle) which lies in the middle of Vaila Sound had a population of nine in 1841. This increased to thirteen in 1881 and there were still two inhabitants in 1931.

Derelict cottages by Vaila's west beach were probably built in the early 17th century. Near them, on the narrow peninsula running parallel with Wester Sound, is **Mucklabery Castle** [HU221468], an ancient two-storey watch tower of unknown origin but which may have been of use to smugglers watching for excisemen. The tower was restored by Herbert Anderton with added crenellations and an angle turret.

West Pier is sheltered by **Vaila Holm** at this north-west corner. It is the landing point for the boat from Burrastow House on Mainland which crosses the narrows of Wester Sound, passing the **Holms of Breibister** and **Burrastow**.

There is another pier at **Ham** (ON – harbour) in the north-east – the **East Pier**. The boat-house with studio above was possibly the first reconstruction project undertaken by Anderton. Both he and his wife were keen artists and his brother was a member of the Royal Academy. Anderton's work had often taken him abroad and among the many artefacts he brought back was a Buddha from Japan. With true Victorian abandon he constructed a small Buddhist temple beside the studio. (This is quite unique for Shetland but not for Scottish islands in general. Both Eilean Righ (No.2.8) and Holy Island (No.1.3) also have Buddhist connections). Unfortunately, the temple and studio later fell into serious disrepair but the gardens at Ham, which Herbert Anderton created, still shelter his tomb.

The fertile ground in the north supported a productive farm and **Cloudin Farmhouse** was built in 1894. When Lord Londonderry's famous stud of Shetland ponies on Bressay (No.11.8) was sold Anderton bought foundation stock and built up a large herd. He also had sheep, Clydesdale horses and a small herd of dairy cows.

Work started on **Vaila Hall**, which is the largest house of its kind in Shetland, in 1895. The south wing incorporates James Mitchell's laird's house as well as the original entrance doorway with the Mitchell coat-of-arms above it inscribed with the date 1696. The north wing of the hall was reconstructed from various outbuildings with a central courtyard which became the hall itself. Some of the stone and skilled labour for the work was imported from England and many of the ornaments and contents came from further afield. The stone griffons flanking the entrance steps, for instance, are thought to have come from Germany.

As befitted an island laird, a brass cannon made in Yorkshire was ceremoniously fired from the terrace whenever the Andertons arrived on Vaila.

* * *

Access: Crossing from Burrastow pier only by prior arrangement, 01595-809307.

Anchorages:

1. Ham (Boathouse Pier). Reasonable shelter in all winds. Anchor off pier but beware old moorings.
2. Burrastow Pier (on Mainland). Anchor off pier. Sheltered W–N.

11.11 Mainland

(ON megenland – mainland).

Muckle Roe

(S. and ON – big red island).

West *and* East Burra

(E. and ON – west and east broch island).

Trondra

Probably (ON – boar island) but may be from the man's name (ON – Þrondr's isle) or, improbably, the Norse tribe's name (ON – Praendir island), from which Trondheim in Norway derives.

O S Maps: 1:50000 Sheets 1, 3 and 4 1:25000 Sheets 466 to 470 inclusive.
Admiralty Charts: 1:500000 No.219 1:200000 Nos.1119 and 1233 1:75000 Nos.3281, 3282 and 3283 1:30000 No.3298 Yell Sound 1:17500 No.3291 approaches to Lerwick various scales: No.3294 Clift Sound, Scalloway, Sand and Hos Wick, Seli, Sandsound and Weisdale Voes: No.3295 Vaila Sound, Gruting, Dales and Ronas Voes, Bay of Quendale, Swarbacks Minn, Olna and Ura Firths 1:12500 No.3297 Sullom Voe

Area: 100230ha (247668 acres)
Height: 450m (1476 ft)

Owners: Multiple ownership. Shetland Council owns a large area in the north.

Population:

	1841	1881	1891	1931	1961	1981	1991	2001
M'land	20572	20821	19741	15172	13282	17722	17562	17550
E/W B'a	586	642	695	767	653	884	889	819
M'e Roe	214	230	213	154	103	99	115	104
Trondra	244	133	154	91	20	93	117	133
	21616	21826	20803	16184	14058	18798	18683	18606

Geology: Mainland is formed from a ridge of very old rocks made up of granite, schist, and gneiss. The southern leg or promontory is mainly of dark blue and grey slates and mica-schists but with a band of Old Red Sandstone on the east coast. North of here the ridge of stratified metamorphic rocks continues in more crystalline forms of schist and gneiss interrupted by long bands of limestone as far north as Laxfirth. West Mainland is generally of Old Red Sandstone but North Mainland is a very complex structure with granites and diorites predominating and basaltic lavas and tuffs on the west side.

On top of the ancient core of igneous and metamorphic rocks great beds of sediment (Old Red Sandstone) were laid down in geologically recent times. There were occasional volcanic intrusions of lava forming layers of igneous rock.

During the last Ice Age the Scandinavian ice sheet spread across Shetland and scoured the surface, removing much of the 'new' Old Red Sandstone from the central spine and smoothing the topography into rounded hills, wide valleys and many small lochs. The ice brought debris with it. There is a two-ton boulder of laurvikite in the roadside wall of Dalsetter croft in Boddam (near Sumburgh), which was deposited there by the ice. It has come from just south of Oslo.

INSIDE AN IRON AGE WHEEL-HOUSE AT JARLSHOF

History: There are none of the Orkney-style chambered cairns on Shetland which could lead one to

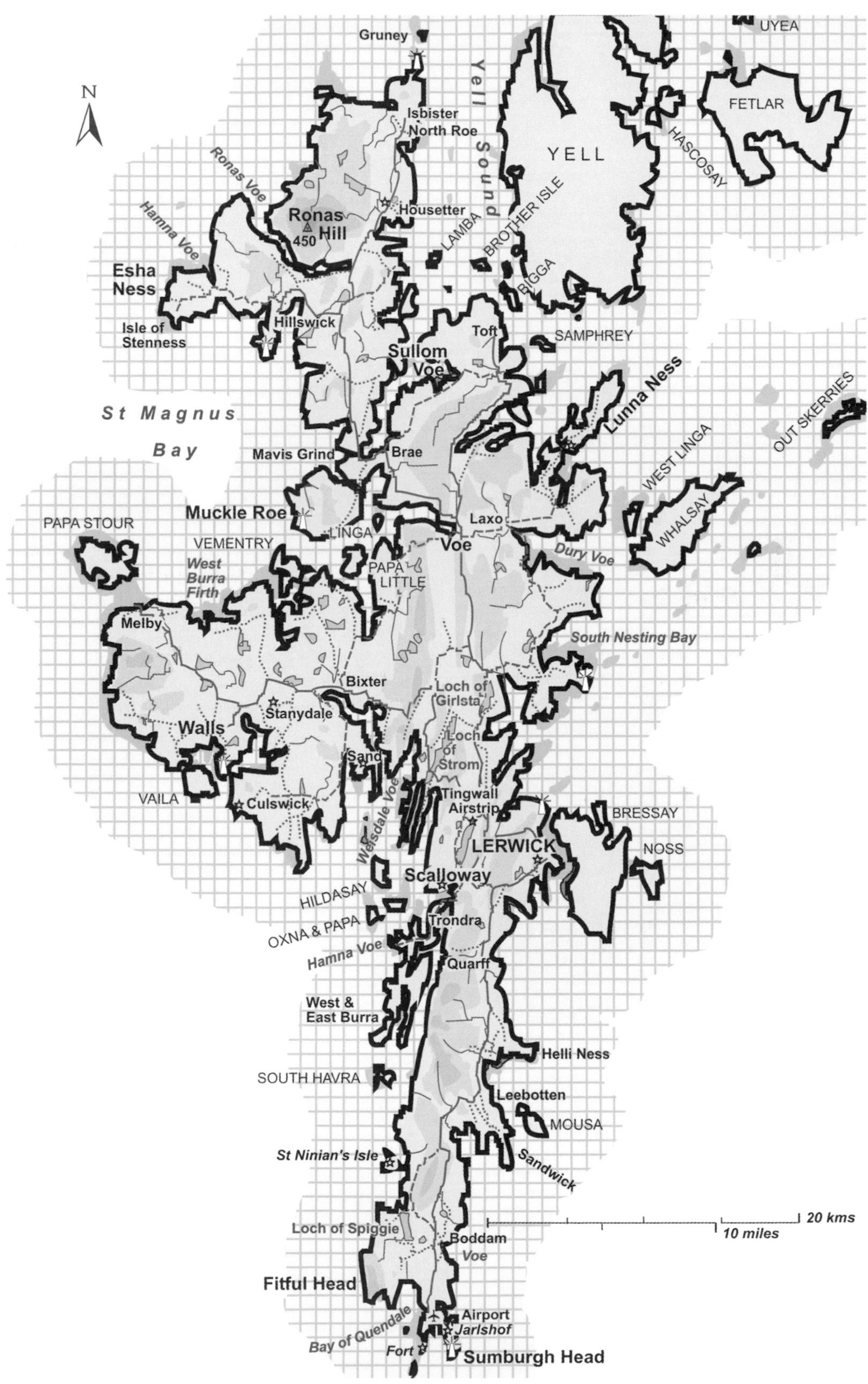
N
Gruney
UYEA
Isbister
North Roe
Yell Sound
FETLAR
YELL
HASCOSAY
Ronas Voe
Hamna Voe
Ronas Hill
450
Housetter
LAMBA
BROTHER ISLE
Esha Ness
BIGGA
Isle of Stenness
Hillswick
Toft
SAMPHREY
Sullom Voe
Lunna Ness
OUT SKERRIES
St Magnus Bay
WEST LINGA
Mavis Grind
Brae
PAPA STOUR
Muckle Roe
Laxo
WHALSAY
VEMENTRY
LINGA
Voe
Dury Voe
West Burra Firth
PAPA LITTLE
Melby
South Nesting Bay
Bixter
Loch of Girlsta
Stanydale
Walls
Loch of Strom
Sand
VAILA
Culswick
Tingwall Airstrip
BRESSAY
Weisdale Voe
LERWICK
NOSS
Scalloway
HILDASAY
OXNA & PAPA
Trondra
Hamna Voe
Quarff
West & East Burra
Helli Ness
SOUTH HAVRA
Leebotten
MOUSA
St Ninian's Isle
Sandwick
20 kms
10 miles
Loch of Spiggie
Boddam
Voe
Fitful Head
Airport
Jarlshof
Bay of Quendale
Fort
Sumburgh Head

suppose that these islands were inhabited by a different prehistoric race or, at least, a people with its own distinctive social and religious code.

Christianity filtered north into Shetland slightly later than to Orkney which is understandable and the islands played a lesser part in Norse history. This is possibly due to their geographical position as a staging post on the route to the Faeroes, Iceland, Greenland, western Scotland and Ireland. In general terms, however, the history of Shetland in the Norse period was similar to that outlined for Mainland Orkney (No.10.10).

In 1468 King Christian of Norway and Denmark mortgaged both Shetland and Orkney to the Scottish Crown as part of Margaret of Norway's marriage dowry. As the cash redemption was not forthcoming, Scotland foreclosed and annexed the islands in 1471.

Apart from a few churchmen there were virtually no Scots living in Shetland at that time but the next one hundred years saw a considerable influx of land-hungry Scots. It was in this period also that the Lowland Scots dialect started to mingle with the native tongue. The Sinclair family was there before 1469 and by 1600 Sinclair was the commonest surname among the one-third of the population which used Scottish surnames. The native Shetlanders still used patronymics.

In 1564 Mary, Queen of Scots, granted the feu of Orkney and Shetland in perpetuity to her half-brother, Lord Robert Stewart. By 1568 Lord Robert had forced the Bishop to resign, gained the right to all crown, church and earldom property together with the right to claim revenue from every islander, and had made himself the chief magistrate. No Norse earl had ever held such power.

By 1571, Lord Robert had installed his half-brother, Laurence Bruce, as foud (chief magistrate) and Bruce used and abused this position to confiscate land on every excuse. He soon lost his position as chief magistrate but, nevertheless, by 1638 the Bruce family held one-eighth of all the lands of Shetland.

In 1581 Lord Robert was made Earl of Orkney and in 1591 his son, Earl Patrick Stewart, succeeded him. He built the castle at Scalloway, and the house at 'Jarlshof' and as chief magistrate he nominally supported the Norse legal forms, but would confiscate land readily. However, his main interest was in reducing the land-holdings of the entrenched landowners such as the Bruce family of Muness and this made him many powerful enemies. He was imprisoned in 1609 and executed in Edinburgh in 1615 by James VI. Norse law was superseded by Scots law; udal was replaced by feudal. The landowning families had now gained enormous power and fought among themselves to divide the spoils.

A very few items of udal law have survived to the present day in Shetland and Orkney such as the right of a crofter to own the foreshore down to the low-water mark. In the rest of Scotland the foreshore, with a very few exceptions, belongs to the Crown Estates. Understandably, the islanders insist that there should be no further erosion of their few remaining udal rights.

Wildlife: There are very few trees to be found, but the largest plantation in Shetland is at Kergord, north of Weisdale. Many interesting alpine plants grow on Ronas Hill including dwarf specimens of willow, *Salix herbacea*. Shrubs generally are heather and juniper as much of the landscape consists of upland peat bog, grass, and moorland, with many small lochs, but about 680 flowering plants and ferns, and nearly 1000 varieties of fungi, have been recorded. The Alpine Mouse-Ear Chickweed, *Cerastium arcticum edmondstonii*, can be found nowhere else in the world but the Shetland Isles and there are also a number of unique microspecies of Hieracium, or Hawkweed. White water lilies, *Nymphaea alba*, flourish in some of the lochans.

Native domestic mammal species are the small, hardy, Shetland ponies (about 1m high) and the distinctive black and brown Shetland sheep which are thought to be identical to Siberian wild sheep. Arctic hares, introduced for sport about 200 years ago, are common.

There is good fishing in many of the lochs but in Loch of Spiggie the fish are said to be 'dour'.

Mainland Shetland is of ornithological interest throughout the year with the great asset of nineteen hours of summer daylight. East and south-east winds bring in migrants with May, September and October being best for unusual sightings. The red-necked phalarope and the Slavonian grebe are scarce and the black-throated diver can probably not be found.

Sites: Sumburgh and Fitful Head for breeding seabirds. About 2500 moulting eider off-shore in autumn and long-tailed skua occasionally seen.

Pool of Virkie, north of Sumburgh has intertidal sand and mud flats for wintering and migrant shore-birds.

Quendale Bay, sand-dunes and machair. Wintering divers and sea-duck with Loch of Hillwell to the north an important breeding site for wildfowl. Corncrake sometimes heard here.

Loch of Spiggie RSPB Reserve is the most important winter wildfowl site in Shetland. Shelduck, teal, oystercatcher and curlew nest here. Great and arctic skuas, kittiwake and arctic tern are often present, and whooper swan, sometimes, in autumn. Greylag geese, wigeon, tufted duck, pochard, goldeneye and long-tailed duck in spring.

At Boddam Voe, on east coast opposite Loch of Spiggie there are wintering divers, grebe, sea-duck, gulls and waders. Great skua and raven are attracted by the nearby slaughter-house.

Scalloway and Lerwick Harbours, gulls and black guillemot. Migrant passerines in town gardens. Loch of Clickhimin on west side of Lerwick is a wintering wildfowl site.

Lochs of Asta and Tingwall, pochard, tufted duck, and possibly the only mute swans in Shetland.

Weisdale, Sandsound, and Tresta Voes for goldeneye, sea-duck, grebes and wintering divers.

Kergord woodland, north of Weisdale, gives cover for nesting birds, rook, tree sparrow, goldcrest, and migrant species.

Sandness, west extremity of Mainland, wintering wildfowl and sea-birds.

Lunna Ness, red-throated diver on the lochans, migrants in the sycamore trees.

Sullom Voe, wintering great northern diver, Slavonian grebe, eider, long-tailed duck and velvet scoter. Also ravens, waders and gulls.

Esha Ness, guillemot and kittiwake colonies in Old Red Sandstone cliffs. Nearby breeding terns, whimbrel and skuas.

* * *

MAINLAND, the principal island of the Shetland group, lies at about the same latitude as the south of Greenland. It has a landscape of hills which are mostly smooth, low and covered with rough grass, heather and upland peat bog. The highest point is the massive barren crest of **Ronas Hill**, or Rønies Hill, at 450m (1476ft). This is also the highest point in all Shetland.

The long leg of land stretching from **Sumburgh** in the south to Lerwick in the north is undulating peat moorland with a border of neat meadows. The great tilted wedge of Sumburgh Head is set between Grutness Voe and West Voe of Sumburgh with busy **Sumburgh Airport** straddling the connecting isthmus.

Grutness Pier on the east is the departure point for *The Good Shepherd* on its trips to Fair Isle (No.11.1) and south-west, facing **Horse Island** and Scat Ness with its substantial ruined Iron Age Fort on **Ness of Burgi**, are the world-famous ruins of Jarlshof.

Jarlshof [HU397096] was given its fanciful Viking name by Sir Walter Scott in his novel *The Pirate* but it is rather misleading because the site covers at least five distinct archaeological periods over a span of some 3000 years. The ruins are complex and fascinating. There are Bronze Age huts and farm buildings, earth-houses from the Iron Age with a broch and wheel-houses (1st–8th century), a variety of Norse long-house remains (9th–14th centuries), the foundations of a medieval farmhouse (14th–16th centuries), and the walls of the house belonging to Earls Robert and Patrick Stewart (16th century). In 1997

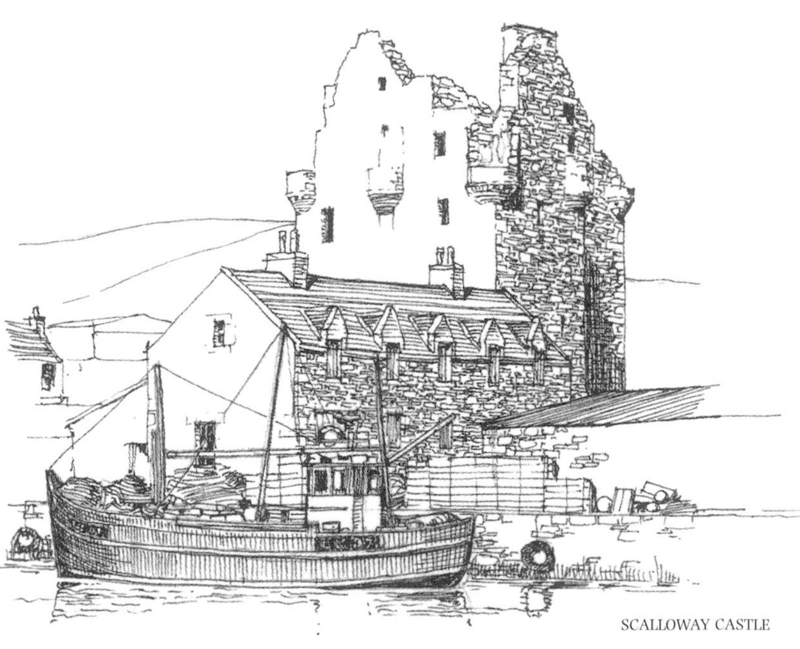

SCALLOWAY CASTLE

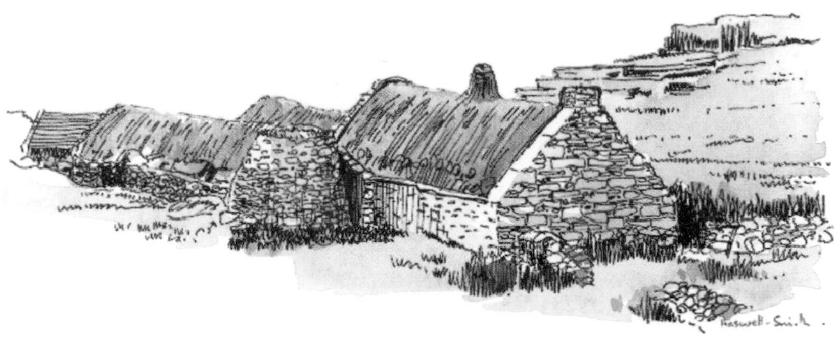

BODDAM CROFT MUSEUM. THE SMOKESTACK OF THATCH AND TIMBER IS CALLED A 'TEØFI'.

some equally remarkable ruins were discovered by chance at **Scatness**, only one mile from Jarlshof. These are also now open to the public and well worth seeing.

The land stretches west to the awesome heights of **Fitful Head** (ON – *hvitfugla* – white birds). It encloses the wide sandy sweep of Bay of Quendale, scene of the 1993 *Braer* tanker disaster. South of the bay are two islets, **Lady's Holm** and **Little Holm**.

East of the main road by Gallow Hill and south of the village of **Boddam** is the **Croft House Museum** which portrays croft life in the 19th century beside a working horizontal water-mill of original Norse design [HU399147].

Although the main road continues north to Channer Wick, a more interesting secondary route branches west at Boddam by the eutrophic **Loch of Spiggie** (Sc *spigg* – stickleback), rich in water-plants, fish and wildfowl. Beyond, the bleak Bay of Scousburgh shelters behind the island of **Colsay** with its prehistoric cairn.

St Ninians Isle is Shetland's answer to Mont St Michel but most of the remains of the early-Christian monastic settlement have now disappeared. Only the lower courses of a 12th-century chapel [HU367209] can be seen amid the bare sheep-grazed downs where a sandy isthmus crosses to the island. But in 1958 excavation revealed the remains of an earlier (pre-Norse) church, and a hoard of 8th-century Celtic silver was found under a stone slab in a box made of Norwegian larch. This may have been hidden by the monks before a Viking raid. South of the chapel is a Holy Well – a spring of crystal-clear water.

North of St Ninians Isle the tiny islet of **Griskerry** lies close to the Ness of Ireland with a road running up the Ness to Maywick.

Back on the east coast after rejoining the main road a number of scattered settlements surround Sand Wick and the pier at **Leebotten** where the boat leaves for Mousa (No.11.2) on pre-arranged visits.

Hollanders Knowe is where a secondary road cuts off to the west through the hills to Scalloway while the main road continues to Lerwick. This was once a Dutch trading post.

Scalloway [skalaway or -awa] (ON *skallivaagr* – voe of the booths) is on the west coast and only 8km from Lerwick. It was the capital of Shetland until Lerwick claimed that title about two centuries ago but it is still an important little village port and a centre for the fish-processing industry. The pier was built in the 1830s for the export of salt cod to Spain and it was extended in 1896. The most prominent feature is **Earl Patrick's Castle**, built with forced labour in 1600 to a medieval design which was already out-of-date. It was abandoned only fifteen years later when its owner was executed. A resident told me that the lime mortar was mixed with 'the hair of maidens'.

In 1942 Prince Olaf, later, King of Norway, visited Scalloway in recognition of the many Norwegians who were carrying out clandestine wartime operations. Fascinating information on these operations (and the 'Shetland Bus') can be found in Scalloway Museum on the waterfront.

* * *

Mainland is now connected by bridges with the long, narrow islands of **TRONDRA**, **WEST BURRA** and **EAST BURRA**. The busy fishing port of **Hamna Voe** is on West Burra.

The main road to Lerwick passes Sandy Loch Reservoir and as it enters the town, the Loch of Clickimin is on the left – unfortunately now surrounded by new housing. In it, but connected to the shore by a causeway, is possibly Lerwick's most memorable feature [HU464408], the massive structure of **Clickimin Broch** [klich-imin]. The broch is 20m in diameter, has walls 5½m thick and 4½m high, and the entire structure stands on a great stone platform with a gateway leading into an enclosure. The site is thought to have been occupied from the 6th century BC up to possibly the 7th century AD and to have been in turn a dun, a broch and, latterly, a wheelhouse. There are a number of inexplicable features and the ruin is so tidy that one must wonder whether the Victorian lady who carried out the excavation was occasionally overcome by idealism. (Such questions, however, should not be allowed to spoil your appreciation.)

LERWICK (ON *leir vik* – mud creek) is a cosmopolitan town built round a lively waterfront and harbour. Nowadays visiting Dutch sailors have been largely replaced by Russians but a close association with Scandinavia continues. Although Norsemen probably founded the town and appreciated the safe anchorage in Bressay Sound, it was the Dutch who developed it in the early 17th century by using Lerwick as a base for their fishing activities. The Shetlanders were glad to sell their wares to the visiting sailors and consequently a shanty town of booths, shacks, bars and brothels grew up leading to 'great abominatioun and wickednes'. In 1640 ten Spanish warships sailed into Bressay Sound and sank two of the four Dutch men-of-war who were there to protect the fishing 'busses'. In 1653 Cromwell, instead of knocking Lerwick about, tried to impose an English claim to the fishing grounds by sending Admiral George Monk with ninety-four ships to search for Van Tromp. He landed an army of troops to build what is now **Fort Charlotte**, possibly Lerwick's first permanent building. But twenty years later the Dutch returned, set fire to it and carried on fishing. Then the French took an interest and in 1702 their privateers attacked the Dutch and sailed around the Shetlands which they 'pillaged like gentlemen'. They burned 150 busses off Lerwick.

Strangely, neither Shetland, nor for that matter, Scotland, seem to have had much to say in these Continental battles over the local fishing grounds. In 1798 the Rev Cruttwell reported that: 'The herring fishery is carried on almost wholly by foreigners, 200 busses from Holland, 50 from Denmark, 40 from Prussia, 20 from Dunkirk and about the same from the Netherlands.'

Flagstoned **Commercial Street**, Lerwick's main street, meanders behind the waterfront buildings, attractively irregular and criss-crossed with narrow alleys and dark wynds. **Fort Charlotte** at its north-west end was first repaired after the Dutch attack and then it was thoroughly renovated and a barrack block added in 1781. It is, today, the only Cromwellian military structure which survives intact in Scotland.

The district of Hillhead, a chaotic composition of old stone gables and slated roofs, is above Commercial Street. It contains the **Town Hall**, 1882 Scottish baronial with fine stained glass windows and a Victorian interpretation of a Viking drinking hall. Nearby is the interesting and comprehensive **Shetland Museum**. Both of these are certainly worth visiting. The Fort is rather uninspiring but provides commanding views from its ramparts. The town itself has intriguing corners to explore and a replica Viking longship which makes trips around the bay (information at the Tourist Office) provides a very different view of Lerwick.

A winter visit to Lerwick should be timed for the last Tuesday of January when the nostalgic Viking fire festival of Up-Helly-aa is celebrated with great gusto by the locals. There are 'guisers', lighted torches, songs, revelry and a burning longship.

North of Lerwick Harbour the town fades away into rough land round the Bight of Vatsland. A small group of rocks called the **Holms of Vatsland** lie in the bay. The road runs to the head of Dales Voe and then turns north to the scattered community of Veensgarth and **Tingwall Airfield** where a route strikes off to Weisdale and the west Mainland. Near the **Tingwall Agricultural Museum** a secondary road runs south to Scalloway and passes Loch of Tingwall. This is an interesting diversion as the Viking parliament and law court, the Althing, used to meet here in the valley. The actual site is thought to be **Law Ting Holm** [HU418434], a small promontory at the north end of the loch which was an island in Norse times. There is a standing stone at the foot of the loch and, on **Gallow Hill** to the west, a mother and daughter were burned as witches in the early 18th century.

North of Tingwall the road runs alongside the **Loch of Girlsta** named after a Norse maiden, Geirhilda, who is said to be buried on the island in the loch. The districts of North and South Nesting, a remote area of low hills skirted by the loop of a secondary road, lie to the east. Off their indented coastline are the **North** and **South Isles of Gletness** with **Green Holm** far to the south, **Hoo Stack**, **Eswick Holm**, **Cunning**

Holm, **Holm of Skellister**, **Hog Island** and **Green Isle**. A line of skerries called the **Stepping Stones** runs far out to sea punctuated by **Muckla Billan** and **Muckle Fladdicap**.

Near the head of Dury Voe (South Voe) at **Laxo** (ON *lax* – salmon) is the pier of the car ferry to Whalsay (No.11.15). A secondary road skirts the Voe and becomes unclassified as it turns north. Halfway up the Ness is **Lunna Kirk** which was built in 1753 [HU486691].

West Lunna Voe is remembered as the anchorage for the 'Shetland Bus', small fishing boats which courageously dodged the Germans to assist the Norwegian resistance during the Second World War. This was a lifeline for supplies, rescuing refugees and transferring agents, but in the end, fuel shortages in Norway so reduced the local fishing fleet that the Shetland boats became more and more conspicuous. German patrols also became more efficient with the result that many brave men and their ships were lost. **Lunna House** (1660), now a summer hotel, was the headquarters for the operation. For cover, most of the trips had to be undertaken in the long, dark, sub-Arctic nights of winter when the weather was at its worst. Lt-Com David Howarth (in *The Shetland Bus*) recalled five days of November storm with winds of over 100mph. 'At Lunna the salt water snatched from the wave crests in Vidlin Voe streamed over the isthmus and over the house to a height of a hundred and fifty feet. From the upper windows the spray looked as solid as streamers of grey silk...'

Just beyond Lunna, at Grut Wick, the Ninian oil pipeline to Sullom Voe makes its first landfall after 103 miles on the seabed. **Lunna Holm** marks the extreme end of Lunna Ness.

The main road divides again at **Voe**. One branch leads north up Dales Voe to **Booth of Toft**, where the car ferry leaves for Yell (No.11.23). The other takes a north-westerly direction along the shore of the Olna Firth, scene of the last whaling station in Shetland, and up to the uninspiring village of **Brae** (ON *breio eio* – broad neck) on Busta Voe. Here, a road turns off for the oil terminal at **Sullom Voe**. These sheltered waters supported an active flying-boat base during the Second World War and they are now the setting for giant tankers visiting Europe's largest oil terminal. Part of the area is reclaimed land where excavated material was dumped in Orka Voe. The Ninian and Brent pipelines – both of nearly one metre diameter – discharge their oil here.

Beyond Brae, a road crossing a bridge to the south-west links the round, hilly island of **MUCKLE ROE** with Mainland. Almost completely encircled with high cliffs of red granite there are some crofts in the south-east but the rest of the island is of broken high moorland – wild walking country.

At **Mavis Grind** (ON *maev eids grind* – gate of the narrow isthmus) Mainland almost splits into two islands [HU340684]. To the right of the road are the head waters of Sullom Voe, to the left is a small sea-loch and the waters of St Magnus Bay. **Egilsay**, a group of drying islets, lies off-shore, and further north, **Isle of Gunnister** and **Isle of Nibon** with **Oe Stack** and a rock arch. This is the district of Northmavine, an area of scenic beauty. After about 8km the road divides with the left fork heading for **Hillswick** (ON *hildiswik* – battle bay) on the shores of the Ura Firth. The Ness of Hillswick is a peninsula with many multi-coloured rock formations. Off its west coast is **Isle of Westerhouse**, **Isle of Niddister** and **The Drongs** – spiky stacks and grotesque shapes carved by the sea out of the Old Red Sandstone with one huge perpendicular column over 30m high. Hillswick was developed in the 18th century as a haaf fishing station by Thomas Gifford of Busta. A haaf (ON *haf* – sea) is a deep-sea fishing ground in the Northern Isles. Gifford provided all the equipment and the fishermen provided all the fish – a somewhat inequitable arrangement, but normal practice at that time.

A secondary road continues westwards into the forbidding landscape of **Esha Ness** eventually reaching Stenness (ON – stone headland) where there was also a small haaf fishing-station partly sheltered by **Isle of Stenness** which has a natural arch on it. In 1933 Joan Grigsby camped on the isle and wrote a successful book about the experience called *An Island Rooin*. Nearby stack-shaped **Dore Holm** (ON – doorway islet) has a flying buttress on its north-west side making a natural arch 21m high and the islet is completely perforated by a cavernous passage which looks like a giant doorway. The Esha Ness area has many prehistoric relics and interesting walks. Moorland lochans sprinkle the ground above the western cliffs which are broken into fantastic shapes, weathered and tilted and a home for many seabirds. There are arches, caves and subterranean passages and the precipitous view north from the lighthouse track to **Grind of the Navir** (ON – gateway of the giants) is particularly dramatic.

The north side of Esha Ness is indented by **Hamna Voe** (ON – harbour bay), an anchorage and one-time whaling station with a narrow rocky entrance which is difficult to identify from the sea. Luckily three islets lie to the north, **Muckle Ossa**, **Little Ossa** and **Fladda**, and Muckle Ossa has a hole right through it. A line of sight through the hole leads directly to the voe entrance.

A certain John Williamson who was born here in 1740 became known as Johnny Notions. He was a blacksmith, clock repairer, weaver, joiner and bonesetter at different times in his life but he became renowned for protecting people from smallpox when the disease was rife and the medical profession could only advocate leeches. He is said to have collected vesicles from victims of the disease, dried them by a peat fire and buried them for several years. These were then inoculated under his patients' skin and the wound was dressed with a cabbage leaf.

An unclassified road near Hillswick leads to the headwaters of lovely **Ronas Voe**. Beside the voe is a knowe called **Hollanders' Grave** where Dutch seamen were buried in 1674 [HU299804]. They were on a crippled Dutch East-Indiaman, the *Wapen van Rotterdam*, which sheltered here during the war with the English. She was discovered by the frigate *Newcastle* and taken after a fight.

Another Dutch East-Indiaman, the *Wapen van Alkmaar* carrying ivory from Ceylon foundered in a Shetland storm in 1689. (These ships took the long route past Shetland in order to avoid the English Channel.) In the early 1930s a fishing boat dredged up two tusks thirty miles north-east of Shetland which were sent to Aberdeen University for identification. The University claimed they had come from a Shetland mammoth and this myth was not dispelled until they were radio carbon-dated in 1993.

Across Ronas Voe is Shetland's highest hill, **Ronas Hill** (450m), with a chambered cairn at the summit. An invigorating hill-walk to the top is rewarded by a striking panoramic view stretching from the Atlantic, with the little islets of **The Cleiver** and **Gruna Stacks** beyond the entrance to the cutlass-shaped Ronas Voe, Foula (No.11.6) on the horizon, Sullom Voe to the south-east, Yell Sound to the east with the **Holms of Burravoe**, and **Muckle** and **Little Holm**. Beyond the northern tip of Mainland lies **Gruney**, **Outer Stack**, **Scordar**, **Turla**, **Fladda**, and assorted skerries collectively known as **Ramna Stacks** – a group designated as a 'Special Protection Area' on account of its prolific birdlife. The district of North Roe lying at the foot of Ronas Hill and west of the road is a huge expanse of trackless wilderness peppered with lochs and bog pools. Heading north the road skirts Colla Firth and passes the **Loch of Housetter**. Beside the road are two standing stones [HU361855] and chambered cairns. The road ends at Isbister by Sand Voe. Mainland tapers away at **Point of Fethaland**, 4km to the north, while to the north-west is the drying island of **Uyea** [oe-yë]. Climbers consider the cliffs and stacks in this region offer a worthwhile challenge but, whether climbing or not, it is a place of extraordinary beauty.

Taking the left fork where the road divides at Veensgarth and passing west of the Tingwall Airstrip the road climbs **Wormadale Hill** with its magnificent view down **Whiteness Voe**. There is a workshop here (called Hjaltasteyn) making,

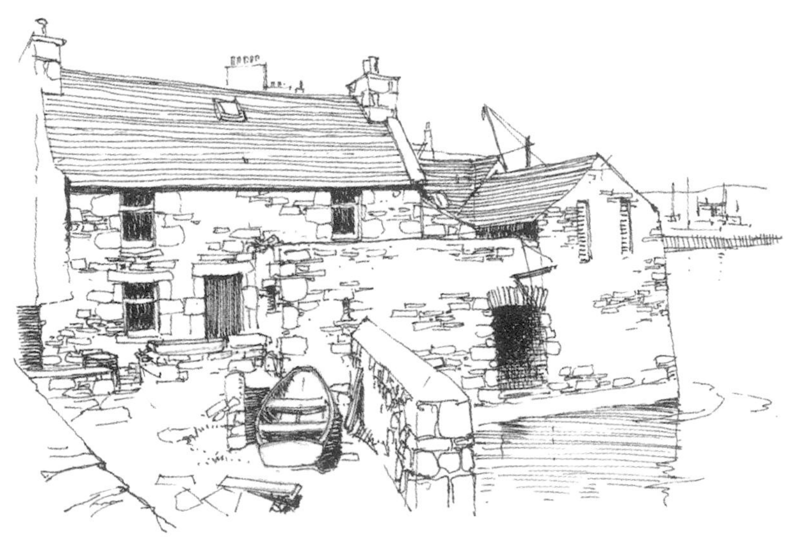

OLD LODBERRIES SOUTH OF LERWICK HARBOUR

and selling, handmade jewellery from Shetland's own gemstones. **Loch of Strom** has the ruin of a medieval castle on a crannog-like islet [HU396475]. This may have been a residence of the Sinclairs before the castle at Scalloway was completed.

Weisdale Voe has a strange claim to fame. It was the birthplace in 1786 of John Clunie Ross who was recognised by Queen Victoria as 'King' of the Cocos Islands. Far down the voe, off the shores of Strom Ness are the islands of **Flotta** (ON – flat island) and **Hoy** (ON – high island).

The road crosses the hills and runs along the shore of Tresta Voe and **The Firth** to **Bixter**. Here a secondary road meanders northwards for 16km eventually meeting the main north road at Voe on the Olna Firth. At the head of Bixter Voe another minor road runs south to Sand, where there are the arched remains of **St Mary's Chapel**, which is said to have been built by the crew of a wrecked Spanish Armada galleon but is actually of Norse origin [HU346472]. At the entrance to the voe are two tiny islets, **Fore Holm** and **Kirk Holm** with the latter, surprisingly, having the remains of an ancient settlement on it. This road continues through Easter Skeld to the south coast at Culswick where, 2kms away beside a cave, are some remnants of the **Broch of Culswick** [HU254448]. The islet of **Giltarump** lies to the south and **Muckle Flaes** is near the broch. A hermit is reputed to have lived at one time on the storm-lashed **Burgi Stack**.

A more interesting archaeological site, well sign-posted, is to the north at **Stanydale** – a large heel-shaped cairn on the open moors. It dates from about 1600BC and is thought to have been a Neolithic temple or meeting place of religious significance. The nearest known similar structure is in Malta. The walls are nearly 4m thick and they enclose an oval chamber with stalls. The floor has post holes in which are traces of spruce. Live spruce was almost certainly only introduced to Scotland in the 16th century so driftwood is the most likely explanation. There are many settlement remains round about indicating that this windswept moorland once supported a sizeable community.

An abandoned village at **West Houland** is reminiscent of the cleared settlements in the Western Isles – thankfully a rather uncommon sight in this part of the world.

Near here an unclassified road runs north to West Burra Firth where the ferry sails to Papa Stour (No.11.14). **Galta Stack** is in the middle of the firth and at the entrance are **The Heag** and **Isle of West Burrafirth**.

Walls (ON – voes) is a little township with a snug harbour which once knew a certain prosperity providing barrels of salted fish for export to Aberdeen and Leith. The Foula ferry (No.11.6) sails from here. The mapmakers thought the Shetlanders' pronunciation, which sounded like Wa's, was a Scottish form of 'walls' so they anglicised the name accordingly. It actually comes from the Norse *vágar*, or *voes*, the 'v' being pronounced as a 'w'.

Unclassified roads from Walls service a fairly large area of crofts but to the north the landscape is wild and barren. The road ends at Melby which looks past the **Holm of Melby** in the Sound of Papa to Papa Stour (No.11.14) and the North Atlantic.

* * *

Access: Ro-ro service by NorthLink Ferries daily between Aberdeen and Lerwick (via Kirkwall, Orkney), 0845-6000-449.

Sumburgh Airport, 01950-461000, scheduled air services daily to/from: Aberdeen, 08700-400006; Edinburgh, 08700-400007; Glasgow, 08700-400008; Inverness, 01667-462280; Kirkwall (Orkney), 01856-886210. Also scheduled flights, Bergen, Norway.

Ro-ro weekly ferry service (summer) by Smyril Line between Lerwick, Faroe Islands, Norway, Iceland and Denmark, 08704201267.

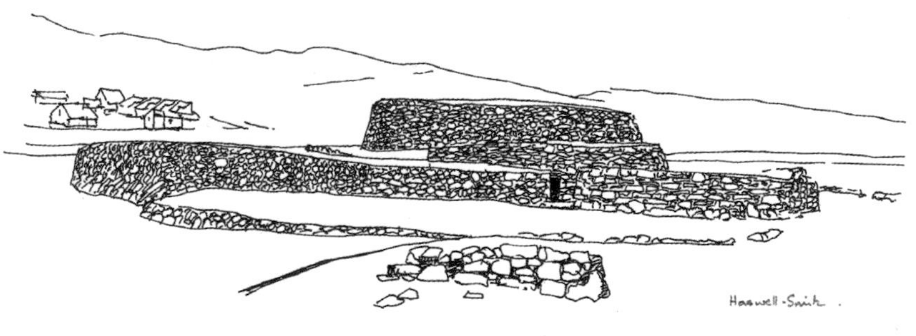

CLICKIMIN FORT, BLOCKHOUSE AND BROCH

Shetland Islands Tourist Information publish an Inter-Shetland Transport Timetable, 01595-693434.

Anchorages:

1. Grutness Voe, 1½M N of Sumburgh Head. Well sheltered except that NE'lies and E'lies bring a swell. Beware shallows in S half of entrance. Noisy due to airport *(but convenient for Jarlshof visit)*. Concrete pier has depth of 2.7m alongside but avoid obstructing it. Anchor off pier in 6m A small boat marina is in Pool of Virkie, behind breakwater.
2. Voe Bay. Reasonable shelter in NE'lies. Head and N shore are shoal and also avoid S headland. Anchor off SW shore in 6m sand and heavy weed.
3. Leven Wick. Good shelter from S and W. Anchor in SE corner ¾c off beach in 6m sand.
4. Hos Wick. Good shelter from N and W. Anchor at NW corner but beware rocky patches. Head is shoal. Alternative anchorage in bight N of Broonies Taing south of derelict pier. *(Sea-cave with blowhole to explore on Ness of Cumliewick.)*
5. Sand Wick. Anchoring not advised due to abandoned submarine cables.
6. Wick of Sandsyre (N Mousa Sound). Rocky ridge extending 1c from SE side affords some shelter for occasional anchorage. Anchor mid-bay off small stone pier on S side.
7. Aith Voe is shallow, narrow and partially obstructed with rocks. Temp. anchorage when conditions allow.
8. Gulber Wick. Holding good but exposed SE. Anchor near head.
9. Voe of Sound. Foul ground and submarine cables restrict anchorage. Best avoided.
10. Brei Wick. Anchor in NW where depth permits. Avoid rocks in SE.
11. Lerwick Small Boat Harbour with 70m pontoon *(easy access to town centre)*. For a berth contact HM (Ch.12. Office opposite Victoria Pier). Berthing alongside breakwater not recommended.
12. Lerwick Harbour. For berth in Albert Dock contact HM on Ch.12.
13. Gremista Marina. Possible but first contact Port Control Ch 12 for details.
14. Dales Voe. Reasonable shelter except from NE. Beware entrance dangers, keep mid-channel, and avoid fish-farm. Anchor just beyond Muckle Ayre promontory in centre, 6m mud.
15. Lax Firth. Good shelter. Enter on W side. Anchor at head in 6m off stone pier. Anchor at head beyond the ayre on E shore in 5–6m.
16. Wadbister Voe. Excellent shelter in SW winds. Beware centre rock at entrance.
17. Cat Firth. Excellent shelter but holding unreliable. Anchor N of Little Holm in 6m between the burns and W of mid-channel. Beware two wrecks which cover.
18. Vassa Voe. Excellent shelter but little room. Follow sailing instructions closely.
19. South Voe of Gletness. Temp. anchorage in fair weather off W side of South Isle of Gletness in 4m sand. Many dangers.
20. North Voe of Gletness. Exposed N and E. Approach with care. Anchor near head of voe in 4m sand.
21. Dock of Ling Ness (South Nesting Bay). Good anchorage for yachts drawing less than 1½m. Numerous rocks to be avoided.
22. Grunna Voe, S side of head of Dury Voe. Excellent anchorage in 5–10m, black mud, good holding. Approach keeping towards N shore of Dury Voe and turn into Grunna Voe when fully open. Keep 1c off both shores.
23. Vidlin Voe. Sheltered anchorage in pool off pier in 4m, mud. If insufficient room anchor S of Vidlin Ness clear of fish-cages in 6–10m, mud but in NE and E gales a swell sets in to this area. Careful attention to charts needed. Avoid ro-ro terminal. Visitors' berths at marina have depth at LWS of 1.7m.
24. Boatsroom Voe, at head of Hamna Voe, W side of Lunna Ness. Excellent anchorage in SW or NE corner but partly obstructed by fish cages. Good holding. On approach keep over 1c off Lunna Ness.
25. West Lunna Voe *(Shetland Bus anchorage)*. Excellent anchorage about ½c off-shore below the tower, 10-12m or in N centre of pool 4-8m. There are several rocks to avoid. Follow sailing instructions carefully for approach.
26. Swining Voe. Good anchorage but most parts too deep for small craft, mud and shingle.
27. Dales Voe, beyond Colla Firth. Excellent holding and free of swell but subject to violent gusts in W'lies. Keep ¾c off when passing Scarvar Ayre and anchor in 5–15m, mud.
28. Firths Voe. Temp. anchorage in summer weather. Both sides clear beyond ½c and head dries 2c.
29. Garths Voe, off Sullom Voe. Tug and boat harbour for oil terminal. Avoid.
30. Sullom Voe. Excellent anchorage anywhere above the Ness of Haggrister narrows in depth to suit. For approach through Yell Sound to Sullom Voe it is essential to contact Harbour Control (Ch.14) and follow sailing instructions. The head of Voxter Voe is shoal.
31. Gluss Voe. Good sheltered anchorage in pool at head of voe in 4–12m, sand. W end of pool dries. Easy approach up centre of voe.
32. Bay of Ollaberry. Occasional anchorage with good shelter from W. Anchor at head of bay in 5m.
33. Quey Firth. Temp. day anchorage only.

34. Colla Firth. Good shelter from W. Best anchorage off pier in Voe of the Brig or anywhere on W shore. On approach keep 1c off shores. Pier is 32m long with 4m at its head. It is used by trawlers. SW arm pleasant but weedy.
35. Burra Voe (North Roe). Drying rocks at middle of entrance. Keep less than ½c from Burgo Taing when entering. Good anchorage centrally off N shore in 4–6m, sand. Temp anchorage in SW opposite the houses but holding poor.
36. Easter Wick of Fethaland. Temp. anchorage in good weather.
37. Sand Voe on N coast. 60 36.2N 01 20.0W. Good sheltered anchorage close to W side of inner part of Sand Voe in 4–5m but difficult to get out in NW'lies. Good anchorage in outer voe in depths over 7m but exposed to NW.
38. Ronas Voe, NW Mainland. Subject to violent squalls. Secure anchorage at head of voe in 4–10m but winds fitful. Enter mid-channel till S of Burries Ness then tend towards the NE shore, moving into mid-channel once above the narrows. Dramatic scenery. *(Access to climb Ronas Hill.)*
39. Hamna Voe. Tricky entrance only 65m wide needs careful attention to sailing instructions. Reasonably sheltered anchorage in E of the voe where it shoals rapidly or in S. Temp. anchorage off the beaches on SE side. Good holding but bottom may be foul.
40. Brae Wick and Sand Wick. Coast foul but with local knowledge temp. anchorage possible.
41. Hills Wick, Ura Firth. Good shelter except from S, 4–10m, sand, holding unreliable.
42. Ura Firth, at head N of Cro Taing. Good shelter in 4–10m sand, but holding unreliable.
43. Hamar Voe, Ura Firth. Excellent shelter and holding good. The head of the pool at the head of the voe is shoal but has no hidden dangers. Anchor where depth suitable.
44. Mangaster Voe. Good anchorage near the head in 4–6m but north of the moorings. Partly obstructed by fish cages.
45. Roe Sound. Approach with care and avoid in W'lies. Good anchorage just W of islet, Crog Holm, but exposed W.
46. Busta Voe, Swarbacks Minn. Fair anchorage off Brae in 6m but bottom mainly seaweed. Visitors' berths available at 52-berth marina. 2m at MLWS.
47. Olna Firth, Swarbacks Minn. Excellent shelter. Anchor in 4–8m above the narrows. Centre of firth clear for approach. Small marina behind pier/breakwater. Visitors welcome.
48. Gon Firth. Well-sheltered anchorage in bight at SE corner but weedy.
49. Sound of Houbansetter. Good shelter in N'lies. Anchor at any suitable depth.
50. Aith Voe. Well sheltered. Anchor anywhere to suit but if strong N'lies tuck into entrance to East Burra Firth or in Bight of Warwick E of Papa Little.
51. Uyea Sound, S side of Swarbacks Minn. Good shelter and holding in bay on N side, 4–8m, but fish cages and many weedy patches. Approach with care. Landing possible at pier in tiny harbour on S side. Passage through to Cribba Sound best tackled at near HW. MLWS depth 1m.
52. Vementry Sound. Many sheltered anchorages but the entrance to the sound is not well defined and there are many dangers. Interesting area to explore but not for the faint-hearted.
53. West Burra Firth, St Magnus Bay. Occasional anchorage subject to a heavy swell. Anchor about 2c beyond narrows towards W shore in 9–12m sand. Approach needs care. New pier for Papa Stour ferry (built 1992) affords shelter but avoid ferry berth.
54. Voe of Snarraness, St Magnus Bay. 60 17.7N 01 34.7W. Clear of dangers beyond ½c off-shore. Excellent holding, and more sheltered than West Burra Firth. Anchor in 9–14m in pool centre (fish cages), mud, or in shallow bay on E side, sand.
55. Lera Voe, Vaila Sound. Approach through Easter Sound. Anchor N of pier on S side of voe. Several hazards and fish-farm.
56. Walls. Anchorage, and Marina (built 1995).
57. Vaila Voe. Many moorings N of Saltness in 4–5m, mud. Good holding and more room off Skeo Taing. Better anchorage than Lera Voe. Beware Baa of Linga NW of Galta Skerry beacon, otherwise approach is relatively simple.
58. Gruting Voe. Well-sheltered anchorages in any of the voes leading off Gruting Voe: Browland Voe, Scutta Voe, or Seli Voe. Olas Voe is shallow. Keep mid-channel but at entrances to Browland Voe and Scutta Voe keep N of mid-channel. Anchor anywhere suitable, mud generally.
59. Skelda Voe, The Deeps (W of Hildasay). 60° 09N 01° 27W. Marina with 8 visitors' berths in depths up to 2.5m. Secure anchorage in pool S of marina in 5.5m but can be subject to swell in S'lies.
60. Rea Wick, Seli Voe and Sand Voe. Best visited at LW. Temp. anchorages in quiet off-shore winds.
61. Sandsound Voe. Pier at Omunsgarth suitable for boats at all times. Anchor in bight N of Omunsgarth or wherever suitable in The Firth, Bixter Voe or Tresta Voe. Beware Billy Baa off Fora Ness on first approach and there are several reefs and shoals to be avoided at Salt Ness and the upper reaches. Holding good.
62. Weisdale Voe. Good anchorage N of narrows at Hellister Ness sheltered except for S'lies. Head of voe is shoal. In S'lies use Bay of Haggersta.
63. Stromness Voe. Restricted entrance with rocks and strong tide but attractive anchorage in 8m on E side after the narrows.

64. Whiteness Voe. Temp. anchorages in quiet off-shore winds.
65. Scalloway harbour. Approach with care. Well sheltered. Anchor off the town on a line between Blacks Ness and Gallow Hill, 6–10m, soft mud. Below the castle there is a quay with depths exceeding 3m alongside, contact HM. Also for pontoon berthing next to marina.
66. Scalloway Bay. Anchor off W side of bay, 8m, soft mud. Use anchor buoy. Better shelter in East Voe in SW'lies, 4m, well NE of fish quay.
67. West Burra Firth, S of Scalloway entrance. Good shelter and holding. Approach mid-firth and anchor in centre N of bridge in 10–12m sand.
68. Hamna Voe, NW extremity of West Burra. Good shelter and fairly easy approach but restricted room, and bottom can be foul with moorings. There is a 75m long jetty at the head of the voe with 3.4m depth alongside its head.
69. West Voe leading to South Voe. Small marina behind breakwater at Bridge End but shallow and bottom foul.
70. Clift Sound. Good shelter except from strong S'lies in entrances to Voe of North House and Stream Sound and West Voe of Quarff avoiding submarine cables in Clift Sound and crossing the S part of W Voe of Quarff to Stream Sound.
71. May Wick. Occasional anchorage off pleasant sandy beach in 3m, sand. Extensive shoal.
72. Bigton Wick, St Ninians Isle. Good shelter except from N. Anchor on W side as near the isthmus as possible, sand. Some swell possible. *(Visit St Ninian's Isle.)*
73. St Ninians Bay. Good shelter except from S. Anchor on W side as near the isthmus as possible, sand. Some swell possible. *(Visit St Ninian's Isle.)*
74. Bay of Scousburgh. Temp. anchorage in quiet conditions.
75. Bay of Quendale not safe except as temp. anchorage in very settled weather.

11.12 Papa Little

(ON pap-øy litla – little island of the priest.) Shetlanders call it Papa Litla.

OS Maps: 1:50000 Sheet 3 1:25000 Sheet 469
Admiralty Charts: 1:75000 Nos.3281 and 3282 1:25000 No.3295

Area: 226ha (558 acres)
Height: 82m (269 ft)

Population: 1841 – 11 (1 house). Uninhabited since.

Geology: Papa Little lies at the junction of two faults: the Walls Boundary Fault (which may be an extension of the Great Glen Fault), and a lesser fault running westwards to Sandness Hill. Most of the island is Old Red Sandstone but the west is peat-covered metamorphic schists and phyllite.

History: Although this was obviously recognised by the Norsemen as a 'papar' island it is not known whether it was associated with any specific religious figure. It is, in fact, possible that at that time it was part of the religious lands of Papa Stour. It was inhabited, possibly for centuries, by some farmers and fisherfolk, but abandoned or cleared in the mid-19th century. The islanders of Papa Stour (No.11.14) have a traditional right to cut peat on Papa Little and this became essential in the 1870s when their own stocks ran out.

* * *

The south-west side of **PAPA LITTLE** is steep with low cliffs surrounding the projection of Moo Ness (ON – ness like a heap of stones). These dwindle to Green Banks in the south. There are several small hills with the highest being **North Ward** (82m), and South Ward (also 82m) topped with a cairn.

The large deep bay on the west coast is defined by two projecting entrance points. The southerly of these is called **Point of Hamna-ayre** (E. and ON – point of the shingle-spit of the harbour), where boats were once drawn up on the shingle beach when the island was inhabited. There are vivid patches of sea pinks in the grass round the shore – a plant known locally as 'banksflooer.'

Papa Little no doubt served its early inhabitants well with its bare but pleasant slopes, generous stock of peat for fuel, relatively sheltered position, and two little lochans, one in the north and one in the south, to provide fresh water.

The advantage of having peat on one's doorstep cannot be overestimated. To collect it from the mainland or another island required an enormous amount of toil and trouble and even an element of danger. After the peat blocks had been cut and dried they were loaded into each individual's 'kishie' – a large basket slung on the back – to bring them to the shore, or to a steep-sided rock which a boat could approach. There they were stacked up in preparation for the loading, which often had to be carried out fairly promptly because of weather and tide. If the boat

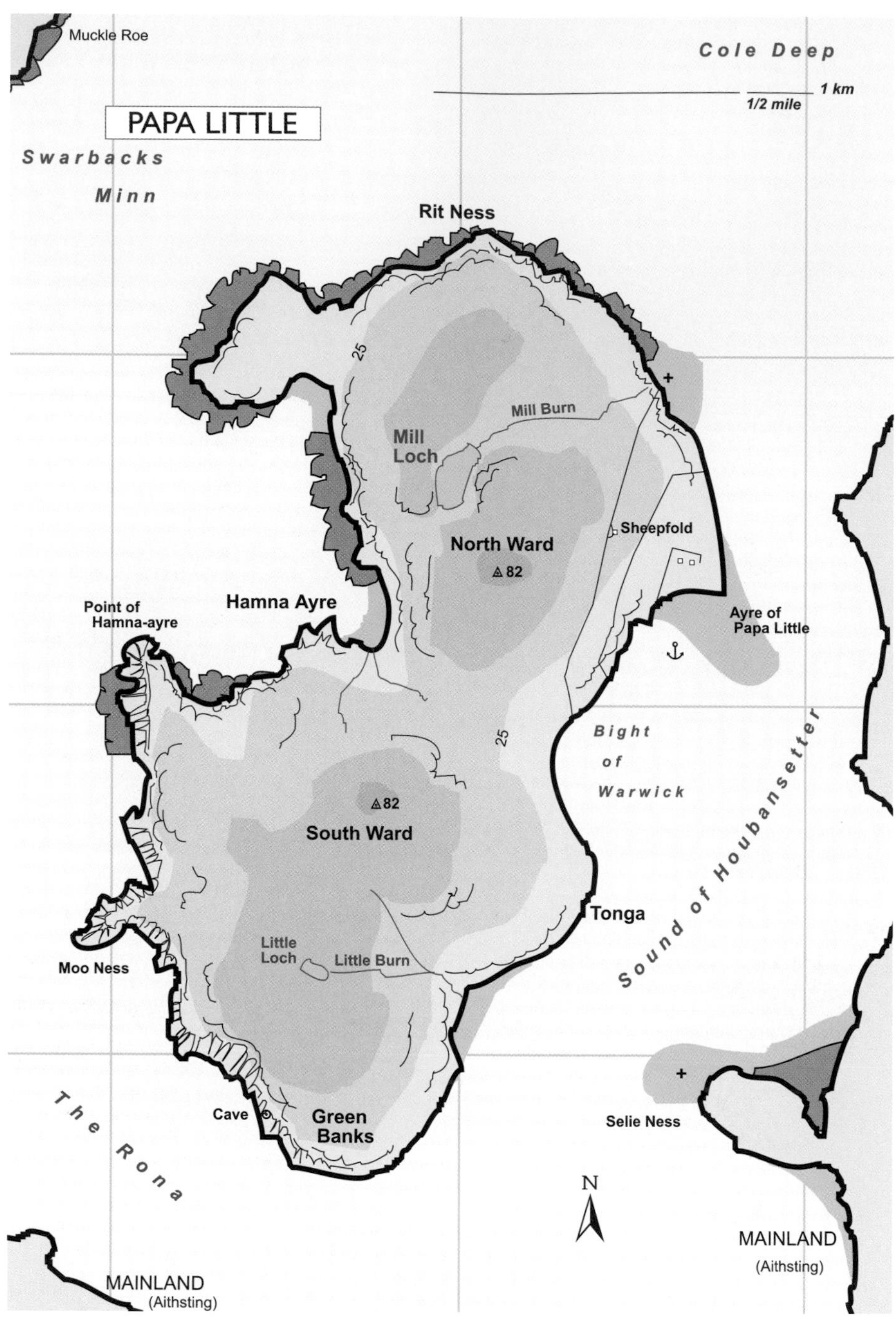

lay off a beach the people would wade out to it while the skipper or one of the crew stowed the peats neatly. As the boatload increased the boat had to be moved further out into deeper water making access more difficult.

If the boat could come alongside a rocky shore distance was less but the work was just as back-breaking and unpleasant. Controlling the boat in a swell, or if the weather was poor while the peats were being emptied into it and stowed, required skilful seamanship. And carrying a full kishie over slippery seaweed-covered rocks could be difficult and dangerous.

After the heavily laden boat had arrived at its destination the whole procedure began all over again but in reverse, and even when the peats were finally delivered to each croft door the work was not over, for they still had to be stacked

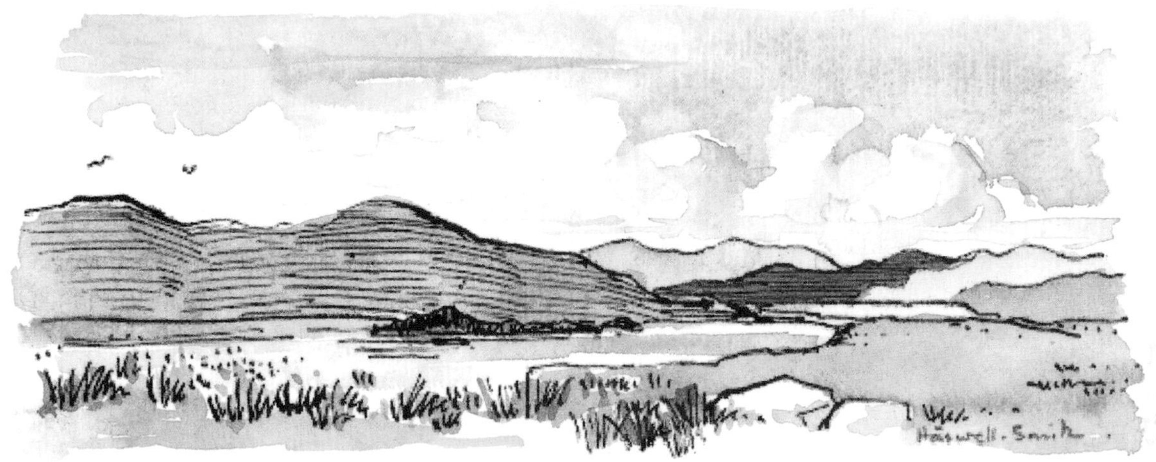

MAA LOCH, VEMENTRY

expertly to keep each precious particle dry and safe from winter storms. It is little wonder that some said there was more heat generated by the peat-gatherers than by the peat itself.

* * *

Access: No regular access but try St Magnus Bay Charters, West Mainland, 01595-810378.

Anchorage:

1. Bight of Warwick, Sound of Houbansetter. Anchor off E shore of Papa Little in the bight S of the drying sand-spit in 7–10m. Good holding and well sheltered except, possibly, from N–NE.

11.13 Vementry

(ON Vémundar-øy – Vémundr's island) Vémundr is a man's name.

OS Maps: 1:50000 Sheet 3 1:25000 Sheet 467
Admiralty Charts: 1:75000 No.3281 1:25000 No.3295

Area: 370ha (914 ft)
Height: 90m (295 ft)

Population: 1841 – 2 (1 house). No permanent habitation since.

Geology: Although the area is predominantly of undifferentiated schist and gneiss, Vementry has a large intrusive sheet of coarse granite on the north-west side composed mainly of pink orthoclase, felspar, and quartz – but with very little mica. Across the Cribba Sound near Clousta there are volcanic rocks and Old Red Sandstone.

History: Swarbacks Minn was an important naval anchorage during the First World War and Vementry was fortified with two six-inch guns to protect it.

* * *

VEMENTRY, in the parish of Aithsting, is a good example of a typical small Shetland island with a broken landscape of lochs, voes, rocky shoreline, windy heath, and some relics of man's ancient past. Old records mention a chapel on Vementry but its site is uncertain.

Swarbacks Head (ON and E. – headland of the black-backed gull) in the north, guards the entrance to the large irregular area of sheltered water called Swarbacks Minn. Above its rocky bluff and skerry there is an emplacement of two six-inch guns from the 1914–18 war [HU290619]. **Northra Voe** (ON – northern creek), the small inlet beside Swarbacks Head has a chambered cairn on its west side beside a small burn [HU290612].

There are several small hills on Vementry. The highest, **Muckle Ward** (90m), has a magnificent, circular (8m diam.), stone-faced cairn on its summit [HU295609]. It stands on a heel-shaped platform made of big stone blocks with an 11m-wide facade. A passage with some of its lintels still in position leads to a trefoil-shaped chamber. This type of tomb is to be found only in Shetland and has its chambers laid out like the heel of a shoe. These cairns are usually built in a prominent position, such as at the top of a hill, but the size varies and may depend on the importance of the interred individuals. This tomb on Muckle Ward is a large one and the best preserved in Shetland – probably because its situation is not readily accessible. It is also unusual because it has no entrance and was presumably closed after the last burial.

The west coast is divided by shallow, rocky, Suthra Voe (ON – southern creek), which penetrates into the heart of the island. Two islets almost obstruct the entrance, **The Heag** and **Gruna** (ON – green island), while **Linga** to the south spreads halfway across the sound. Only a shallow, narrow channel separates Vementry from Mainland as a neck of land projecting out of Mainland divides Cribba Sound from Uyea Sound. Vementry House stands, white-walled, at the root of this peninsula with its snug little harbour beside it.

* * *

Access: A boat-owner in Vementry harbour (Mainland) may take you across or try St Magnus Bay Charters, West Mainland, 01595-810378.

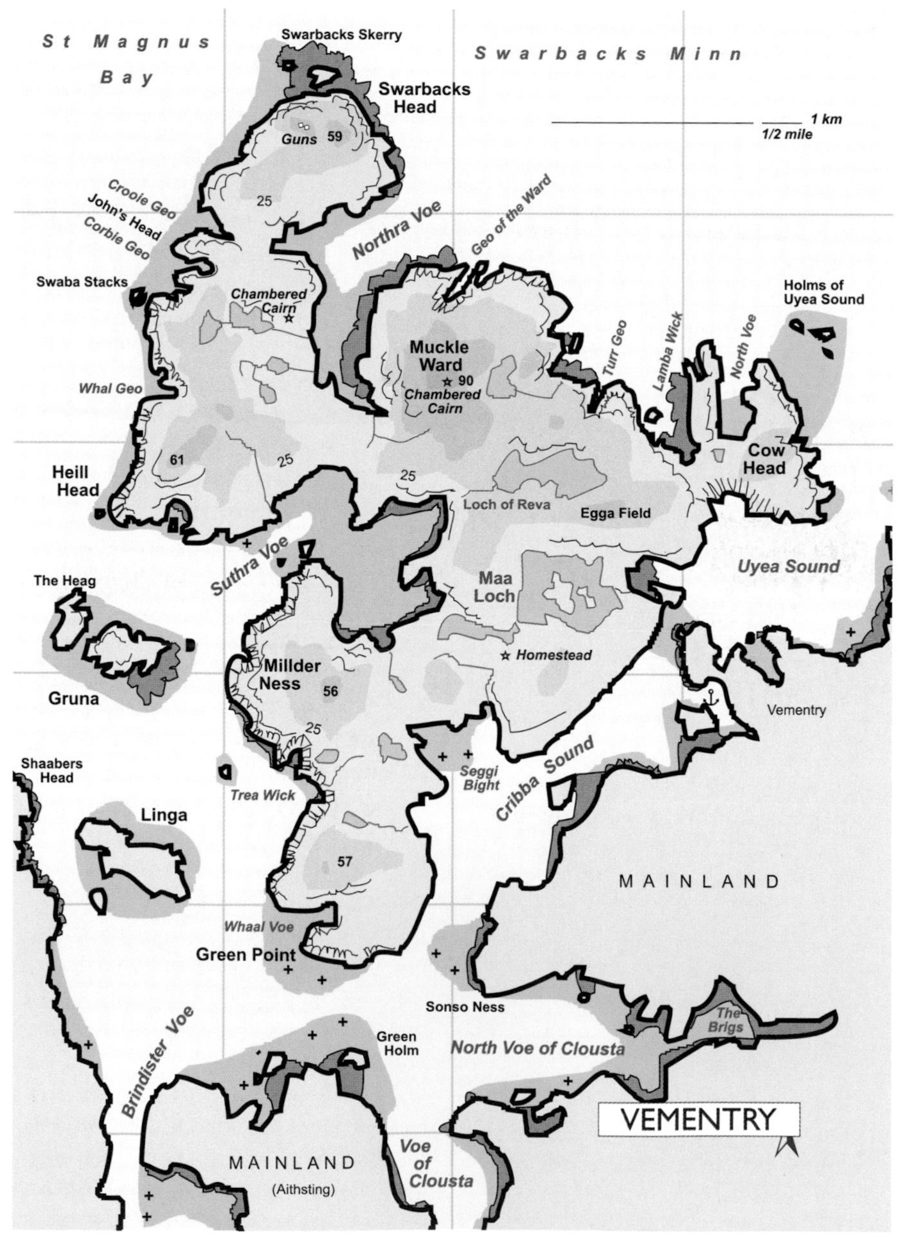

Anchorages: Vementry Sound has a number of suitable anchorages but passage is difficult with many rocks and dangerous reefs. Proceed with great care using large-scale chart and sailing instructions.
1. Uyea Sound. Reasonable shelter. Anchor in bay on N side in 4–8m, good holding when not in weed, but restricted by fish cages. Narrow passage through to Cribba Sound has minimum depth of 1m.
2. Cribba Sound. Good shelter in NW half. Fish cages.
3. Suthra Voe. Approach with great care as both sides foul with rocks. Well-sheltered anchorage in centre of NE bay, 8m.

11.14 Papa Stour

(ON papøy stóra – big island of the priests).

O S Maps: 1:50000 Sheet 3 1:25000 Sheet 467
Admiralty Charts: 1:75000 No.3281

Area: 828ha (2046 acres)
Height: 87m (285 ft)

Owner: Multiple ownership.

Population: 1841–382 (66 houses). 1871–351. 1881–254. 1891–244 (44 houses). 1931–100. 1961–55. 1981–33. 1991–33. 2001–23.

Geology: Formed from volcanic lava and ash and then sculpted by the sea resulting in some of the finest sea caves in Britain. These, however, are only accessible in fine weather. There are also many interesting skerries, stacks and voes.

History: Papa Stour, with its fertile soil, is thought to have been first settled about 3000BC. When the Norsemen came they presumably found monks or hermits in residence but they settled here themselves nevertheless. A fascinating piece of archaeological detective work by Dr Barbara Crawford of St Andrews in the early 1980s has revealed what is almost certainly the 13th-century residence of Duke Haakon, later King of Norway, who had a farm on the island beside Housa Voe.

In the early 16th century merchants from Hamburg and Bremen considered the island of sufficient importance to build a summer trading booth to buy fish and fish oil from the islanders and exchange various commodities. But the haaf (ON deep-sea) fishing decreased and herring fishing had taken its place by the mid-19th century. A herring station was constructed at Hamna Voe and curers and gutters came from far afield, even from Ireland. Fuel was so scarce and the fishermen so busy that the islanders started burning the turf and even today large areas lie scalped and bare. By the 1870s the situation was so bad that people started to leave.

In 1970 the school closed because there were no more young children. In fact the total population by then was only sixteen fairly elderly people. Although the Sound of Papa is relatively narrow, tides rage through it and the island can be isolated for days at a time. But after an advertisement was placed in *Exchange and Mart* mentioning that crofts would be granted free together with five sheep each, young people started to flood in from all over Britain. It was a refuge from the rat-race – a place for 'human values' and flower-power. Shetlanders started calling it the 'Hippy Isle'. Most of the incomers gave up quickly when they discovered the rigours of island existence but a few remained and they gave the island new life. The population rose to about thirty. By 1992, however, numbers were once again falling and a new search was on.

As a result the Primary School was able to reopen in 2003 with pupils enjoying the undivided attention of the teacher who had previously taught the three pupils on Foula (No.11.6). But peace was short-lived for in 2005 a serious dispute between families again threatened the stability of the island.

Wildlife: This is a fertile island and it is said that fishermen can locate the island in a summer haar by the pungent smell of the wild flowers – 'Fir da scent o flooers in Papa leds wis aa da wye.'

Papa Stour and Foula (No.11.6) were the last refuges of the primitive and goat-like Shetland sheep. These were classified as an endangered species.

The stacks and inlets support many sea-birds and there are quite large colonies of cormorant and Manx shearwater. It is interesting to learn that although the fulmar is relatively widespread now, in 1890 an ornithologist visiting Papa Stour noted with delight that he had seen one.

Common seals breed on the skerries.

* * *

Each volcanic island being formed today off the coast of Iceland will become a **PAPA STOUR** tomorrow. Already their soft ash is being eaten away by the sea from its hard volcanic base leaving tunnels and arches and weird, grotesque,

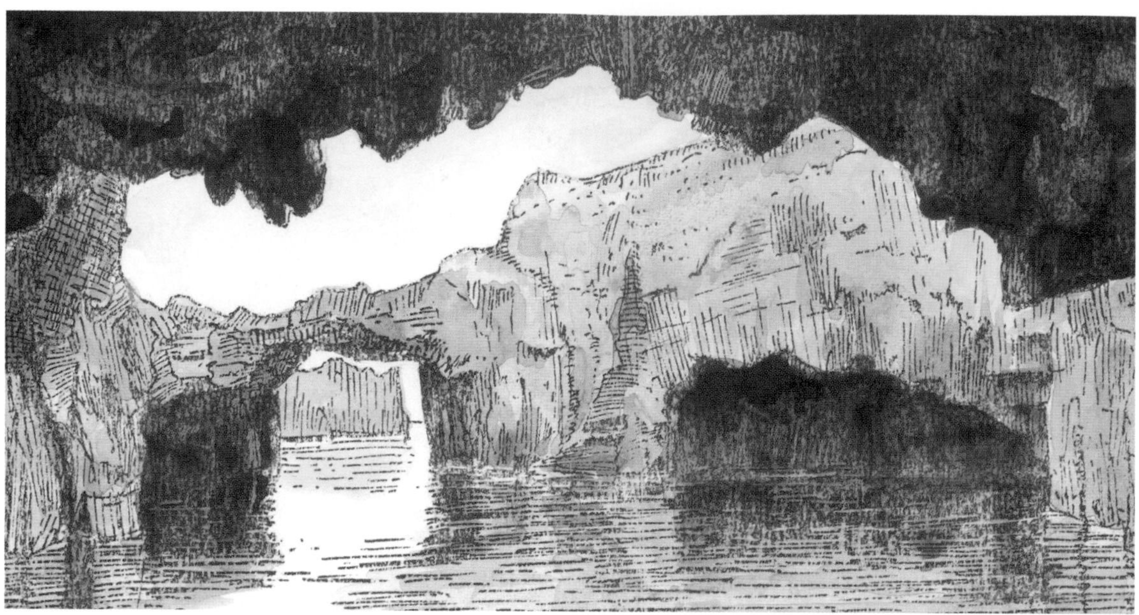

VOLCANIC SEA-CAVES BY BREI HOLM, PAPA STOUR

tortuous shapes. On the surface, where the sea cannot wash it away, seeds dropped by the seabirds take root and the ash is converted into fertile soil, rich in essential nutrients.

Papa Stour is one of the most fertile of the Shetland Islands, its only failing being a total lack of fuel in the form of peat. It has exciting volcanic forms and a precipitous coastline, indented and eroded, above a tumble of detached rocks, stacks and skerries – a wonderland for climbers and potholers. In the north-west there is an immense cliff with a natural tunnel, the **Hole of Bordie**, penetrating it for nearly 1km (½M)! **Virda Field**, the highest hill (87m), sits above it. Beyond the narrow cleft of Akers Geo are the **Fogla** (ON *fugl* – bird) and **Lyra** (ON *lyrie* – Manx shearwater) **Skerries**. They also have subterranean passages through which the tide surges. Here too a great column of rock, the **Stack of Snalda**, reaches skywards, and far out to sea the **Ve Skerries** (ON – suffering skerries), a favourite seal-hunting ground in days gone by, lie low and menacing among the Atlantic waves.

Probably Britain's finest sea-cave, **Kirstan's** (or Christie's) **Hole**, is on the south-west side of the island [HU152606]. It is at the head of a narrow creek and confined between vertical rock faces about 30m high. A columnar stack stands like a sentry beside the 27m-wide natural arch forming the cave entrance. Within there is an enclosed space with glistening walls standing open to the sky. The cave then continues for about another 70m, ending at a beach.

John Tudor, a Victorian traveller, raved about the caves of Papa Stour. His favourite was **Francie's Hole** nearer Hamna Voe. This is smaller than Christie's Hole, but in his view more beautiful. The entrance is perfectly arched and inside you are 'in fairyland, so exquisite is the colouring of the roof and sides, and so pellucid is the water'. Caves branch off on one side and at the back is a small pink beach above which 'are alcoves or recesses like stalls in a church'.

Hamna Voe (ON – haven or harbour creek) is an almost land-locked lagoon. Red cliffs on the east side by the entrance conceal the modest island airstrip and the school. There is a natural rock arch in these cliffs with the remnants of two chambered cairns above it. The church is above a small beached cove known as **Kirk Sand** and there are more cairns and burned mounds nearby. The odds are that the church, which looks across the Sound of Papa to Melby on Mainland, was built on the most sacred pagan site. **Forewick Holm** lies off-shore.

All the habitation is in the east, mainly around **Housa Voe** (ON – voe of the houses). Although more exposed than Hamna Voe, Housa Voe has a pier for the small ferry-boat from West Burra Firth on Mainland. Off the headland between Kirk Sand and Housa Voe there are many interesting rock formations and a small islet, **Brei Holm**,

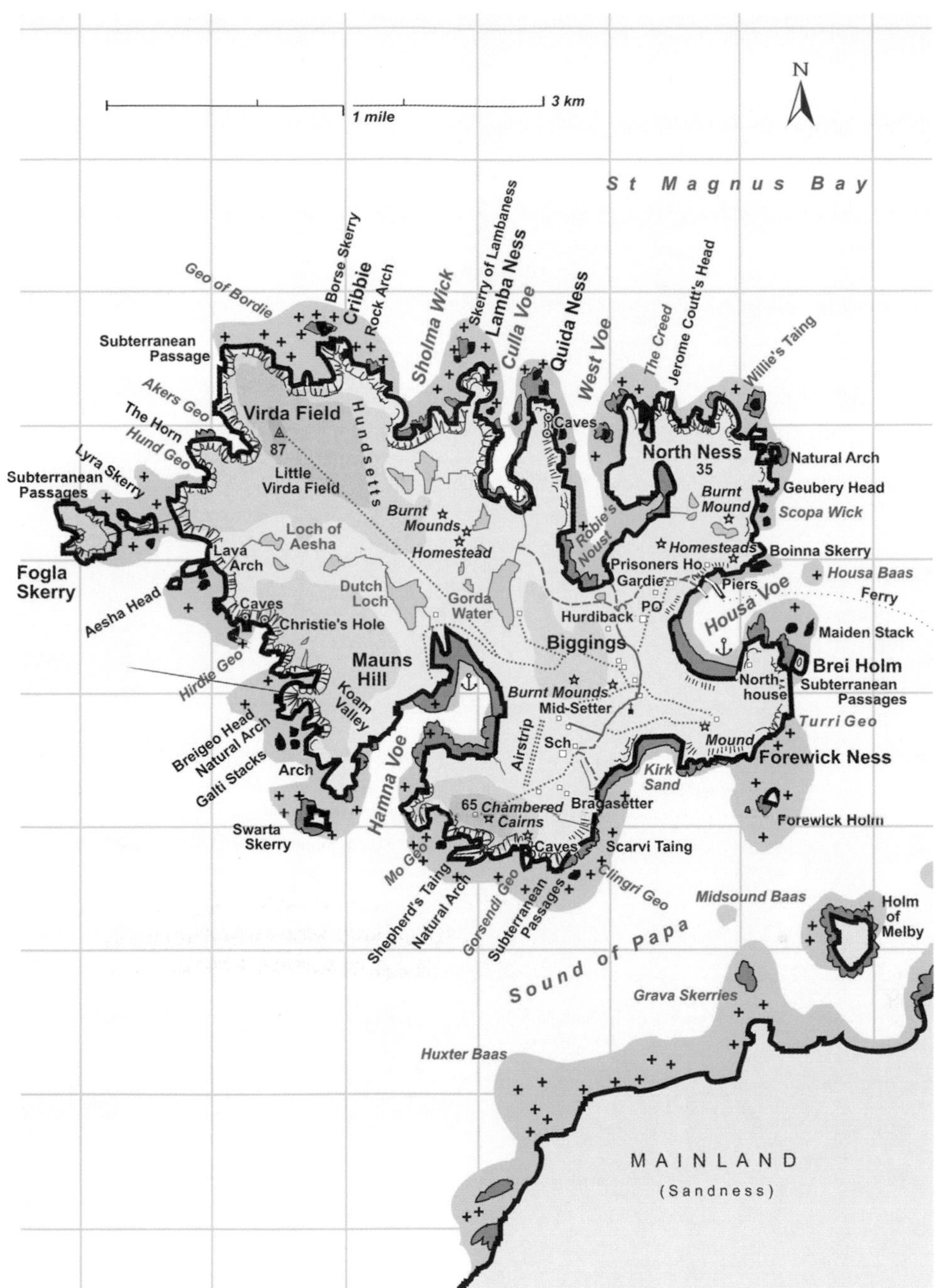

joined to the ness by a drying reef. Said to have been the precarious site of a leper colony in the 18th century recent excavations have shown that it might first have been an early Norse monastic community.

Near Brei Holm is an isolated stack with the vestige of a stone house to be seen on its narrow top. This is the **Maiden Stack**, or Frau Stack. In the early 14th century Lord Thorvald Thoresson is said to have built this for his daughter to live in to ensure that she would not be in the company of men. But it was all to no avail for when he released her she was found to be pregnant.

The group of houses which cluster behind the post office at Housa Voe is known as **Biggins** (ON *byggja* – buildings) and is probably the island's earliest settlement. At the start of the 19th century the Hon Edwin Lindsay was sent here in disgrace by his family for refusing to fight a duel. They had him declared insane and he was kept under guard on the island for twenty-six years. It was a Quaker preacher, Catherine Watson, who arranged his escape and he was then able to claim his inheritance. There is a spring at the south of the island called Lindsay's Well, where he was allowed to bathe.

Papa Stour's mood changes with the weather and at times it has either a magical or a sinister quality. This is particularly noticeable on the north coast when a haar creeps in and blankets the wicks and geos. But even Housa Voe is not immune. The islanders tell of a strange ship that sailed into the voe on a sunny day long ago. The crew were seen to be preparing to attack the village so the local witch, Minna Baaba, immediately created a storm, which blew the ship far out to sea.

* * *

Access: Ro-ro ferry from West Burrafirth, daily except Tues. and Thur., 40 minutes, 01957-722259, weather permitting and prior booking essential. Scheduled air service from Tingwall, Tues. only, 01595-840246.

Anchorages: Passage in the Sound of Papa requires great care as there are strong tides and many off-shore dangers. There are severe overfalls off the NW coast.

1. Hamna Voe. Shelter from all weather but entry impossible in strong S'lies. At the narrows there is only 2m depth at LWS, and 20m width. Follow instructions for entry, which requires care. Anchor N or S in 4–6m.
2. Housa Voe. Reasonable shelter in 4–6m, sand. There is a new pier/breakwater with alongside depth of 2.5m. Enter from N 1c off and parallel to NW shore to avoid Housa Baa.
3. West Voe. In E bay which dries at head, 4–6m, sand. No shelter from N'lies.
4. Culla Voe. Good holding and shelter from all weather. Approach mid-channel to avoid sunken rocks at entrance. Anchor near head of Voe in 3m.

11.15 Whalsay

(ON hvals-øy – whale island).

O S Maps: 1:50000 Sheet 2 1:25000 Sheet 468
Admiralty Charts: 1:75000 No.3282

Area: 1970ha (4868 acres)
Height: 119m (390 ft)

Owner: Multiple ownership.

Population: 1841–628 (112 houses). 1881–870. 1891–927 (167 houses). 1931–900. 1961–764. 1981–1031. 1991–1041. 2001–1034.

Geology: The bedrock is almost entirely of gneiss with granite veins. There are good stocks of peat which the Out Skerries islanders are entitled to cut.

History: The Bruces of Muness in Unst gained possession of Whalsay from its crofter-owners and brought in a period of harsh rule. In the 19th century the punishment for any small misdemeanour was exile from the island.

Naval press-gangs valued the sailing ability of Whalsay men and would sometimes remove them from their 'sixerns' when they were out fishing. The families were not informed.

The recent history of Whalsay is the 'boom and bust' history of fishing for this is an island of fishermen. In 1832 many lost their lives when there was a great storm at sea but fishing continued and 1834 was the peak year for herring catches. Second-hand 'half-deckers' were bought on the Scottish mainland to replace the native sixerns and improve the Whalsay fleet. But this optimism was followed in 1839 by a slump in the herring market followed in 1840 by another violent storm in which many men were drowned. Bankruptcy and poverty were rife.

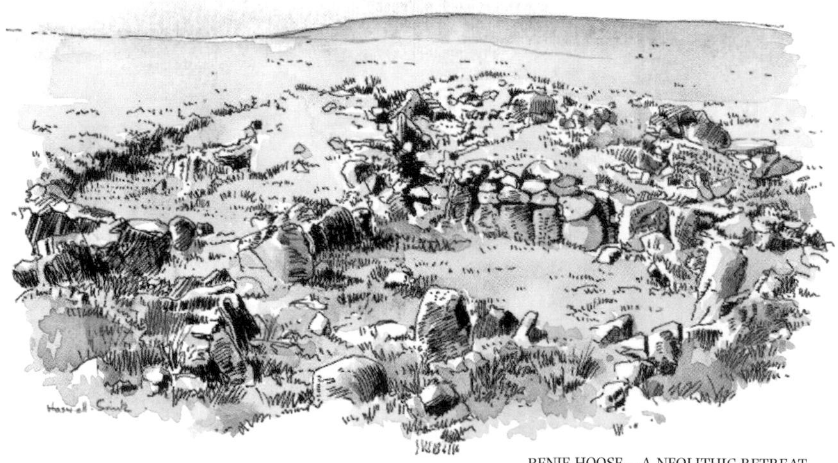

BENIE HOOSE – A NEOLITHIC RETREAT

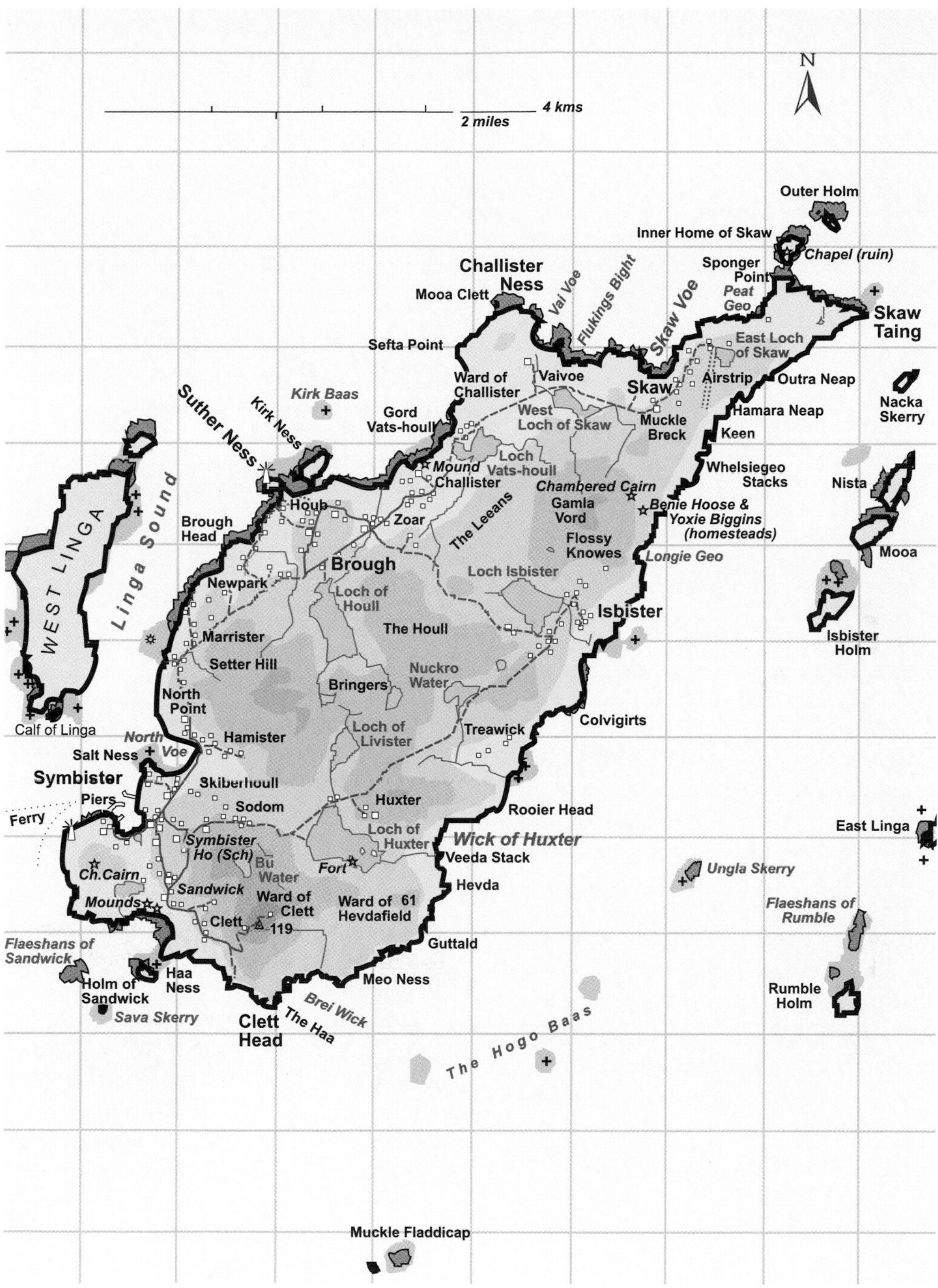

By the late 19th century, however, the industry had recovered and bigger boats were introduced. For a time all was well, and then steam drifters created new problems as the Whalsay men lacked capital to compete.

Between the two World Wars Whalsay fishermen survived by catching what herring they could in the summer and supplementing this with in-shore haddock-fishing in the winter, but after the Second World War conditions improved when Government grants and loans assisted the purchase of superior dual-purpose vessels.

This 'mini-boom' continued until 1965 when 200 Norwegian ships appeared fitted with power tackle and sonar and swept the seas of fish. The Shetlanders tried to follow the Norwegian example and for a few years there were huge catches but by 1977 the stocks had disappeared and herring-fishing was banned. Since 1983 there has been limited intermittent fishing, complicated by the predation of foreign fleets and the requirements of the European Union.

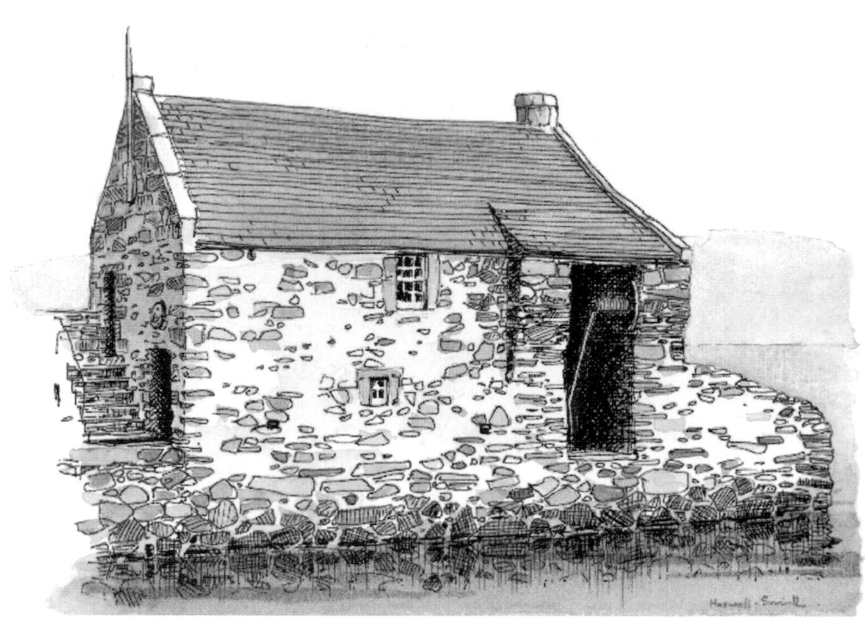

BREMEN BÖD – A 17TH CENTURY HANSEATIC TRADING POST

Wildlife: The Shetland record brown trout – 9lb 4oz – was caught in Whalsay's Loch of Huxter.

Small colonies of kittiwake and puffin nest at the south end of the island and whimbrel, arctic tern and arctic skua nest on the moors and by the lochans. A few red-throated diver, known as 'rain geese' in Shetland, may also be seen. This is an important staging-post for migrant birds; unusual species such as the red-rumped swallow, hoopoe, and Pallas' warbler, have been recorded.

* * *

WHALSAY is the 'Bonny Isle'. Pleasant green pastures could easily support livestock but few do, for the islanders are fishers not farmers and the economy revolves round fish. Off-shore there are rocks, reefs and skerries with fascinating names like the **Hogo Baas** and **Rumble Holm** which give shelter to lobsters, prawns, and a surprising number of white fish. It takes a local to know all these sand-banks and crevices. Furthermore, Whalsay's millionaires – and it is said there are more than twenty of them – now own some supertrawlers which search the distant oceans for fish. As a result, there is an expanding and relatively prosperous population, a fish-processing plant, and a desire by every young man to get to sea in his own boat. Why waste time milking cows when there are fish in the sea? Lerwick can supply all the milk required. Recently, however, the European Union has cast a dark shadow over this idyllic scenario and the future is uncertain.

Ward of Clett, a well-defined hill in the south of the island, is the highest point at 119m. It rises south-west of the **Loch of Huxter** (ON – prehistoric-mound farm) with its Iron Age holm fort [HU559620]. This is thought to be one of the earliest versions of a broch – the idea from which the later versions evolved. Unfortunately, many of the stones were removed to build cabbage enclosures or 'plantiecruives', but sufficient remains to be of interest.

Generally, the island has an attractive rolling landscape of low hills and small lochs, with activity mainly centred around the small port at **Symbister** in the south. The airstrip is at the other end, at **Skaw** (ON – point) in the north. There are two islets off Skaw Taing, **Outer** and **Inner Holm of Skaw**, with a ruined chapel on Inner Holm.

The lighthouse on **Symbister Ness** in the south-west is close to the busy little harbour, which is in the most southerly of two small voes. **Bremen Böd**, near the Symbister pier, has an old wooden windlass beside it. This is a Hanseatic store set up by German merchants in the 17th century to trade brandy, tobacco, linen, muslin, fruit, and salt for haddock, fish oil, cod and other fishy delicacies. It is the only complete surviving example in Scotland of such a building. It was rescued from dereliction and is now used as a visitors' interpretative centre.

Symbister House is an extravagant solid-granite Georgian mansion sited east of the harbour, which has served as a Junior High School since 1940 [HU543622]. It was built in

1823 by the head of the distinguished Shetland family of Bruce at great cost (£30,000), not because he needed a second home – he already had a fine house on Mainland – but for the rather petty reason that he did not wish to leave the money for his heirs to enjoy. The grounds, incidentally, are reputed to be haunted by an old sailor who was murdered by the gardener for winning a game of cards.

Between Symbister and Loch of Huxter is the ruined cottage where the poet Christopher Grieve (Hugh MacDiarmid) lived from 1933 to 1942. The place name is **Sudheim** (ON – south home) but the Ordnance Survey had anglicised this to **Sodom**! – much to MacDiarmid's amusement.

A shallow bay on the south coast, Sand Wick, has Bronze Age burned mounds beside it. Several skerries and an islet, **Holm of Sandwick**, obstruct entrance to the bay.

Halfway up the north-west coast the village of **Brough** (ON – stronghold) is beside Kirk Ness with a narrow isthmus leading to a church [HU555655] and at Suther Ness there is another lighthouse. Directly across on the other side of the island is **Isbister** (ON – east farm), a settlement of houses clustered beside a loch and looking south-east over two strings of islets. Nearby are the delightfully named **Nista** (ON – northmost isle), **Mooa** (ON – narrow isle), and **Isbister Holm** with **Nacka Skerry** to the north, and further out are **East Linga** and the **Grif**, **Swarta**, **Longa** and **Rumble Skerries** (ON – beside the deep sea, black, long and round-rocks skerries respectively). The Grif Skerry was a haaf fishing station where the boats could be beached in bad weather while the men sheltered in primitive huts.

Some of these names can be very confusing. For instance, the Admiralty Chart attaches names to the rocks south of Whalsay which are incorrect according to the Whalsay fishermen. They say that a sailor should read **Muckla Fladdacap** as Muckle Fladdacap, **Muckla Billan** as Peerie Fladdacap, **Litla Billan** as Haerie, and **Haerie** as Ooter Vooder!

Midway between Loch Isbister and Loch of Huxter is pewter-coloured **Nuckro Water** (ON *nøkk* – water monster). This is the home of a vicious water demon, known in Shetland as the 'njuggle', which usually appears in the form of a beautiful, friendly, horse. But once seated on its back the human victim is carried into the water and drowned. The njuggle can also appear in other forms and it is most dangerous after sunset. Another njuggle lives in Njugals Water near Tingwall on Mainland.

Between Isbister and Skaw the **Yoxie Biggins** may date from about 3000BC. This is a heel-shaped structure somewhat like Staneydale on Mainland. It was first assumed to have religious significance but now it is thought more likely to have been a Neolithic farmhouse. A ruin from the same period, **Bunzie** (or **Benie**) **Hoose**, is adjacent and it has a clover-leaf layout [HU587652].

Access: Frequent daily ro-ro ferry service from Laxo, Mainland, (½hr), 01806-566259. Scheduled flights Tingwall/Out Skerries, Mon., Wed., Thurs., lands at Whalsay on request, 01595-840246. Tourist Information, 01595-693434.

Anchorages:

1. Symbister Harbour. Sheltered but busy fishing-boat harbour on W coast. Tie alongside S breakwater/jetty, 102m–long, provided those already berthed are agreeable or try the marina which has depths of 2m.
2. North Voe. Only use as a last resort. Bottom foul with old moorings.

11.16 West Linga

(E. and ON – west heather-island).

OS Maps: 1:50000 Sheet 2 1:25000 Sheet 468
Admiralty Charts: 1:75000 No.3282

Area: 125ha (309 acres)
Height: 52m (171 ft)
Population: Uninhabited.

Geology: Coarse micaceous and hornblendic gneiss with granite veins. There is a raised beach above Croo Wick (ON – sheep-pen bay) at the south extremity.

History: Liv Schei in her fascinating book, *The Shetland Story*, notes that on the 7 August 1485 at Korskirken in Bergen a meeting was held to discuss an illegal purchase of various lands in Shetland. The most important piece of land listed was ten merks on 'Liungøuo i Hwalsøyo.'

WEST LINGA is a long narrow island covered in rough heath with its highest point (52m) almost in the exact geometrical centre. There is a further minor hill in the southern part with a cairn on it and two small lochans in the northern half. It is somewhat surprising that an island of this size with a supply of drinkable, if brackish, water has so little sign of human habitation but this is probably due to the lack of an anchorage. There is not even a suitable place to beach a boat easily for any length of time. However, in spite of such difficulties the island seems to have been inhabited intermittently until, possibly, the end of the 18th century.

It is said that while the Bruce family were 'acquiring' Whalsay the udaller of West Linga went out fishing. While he was absent his young son got his head stuck in a large jar and

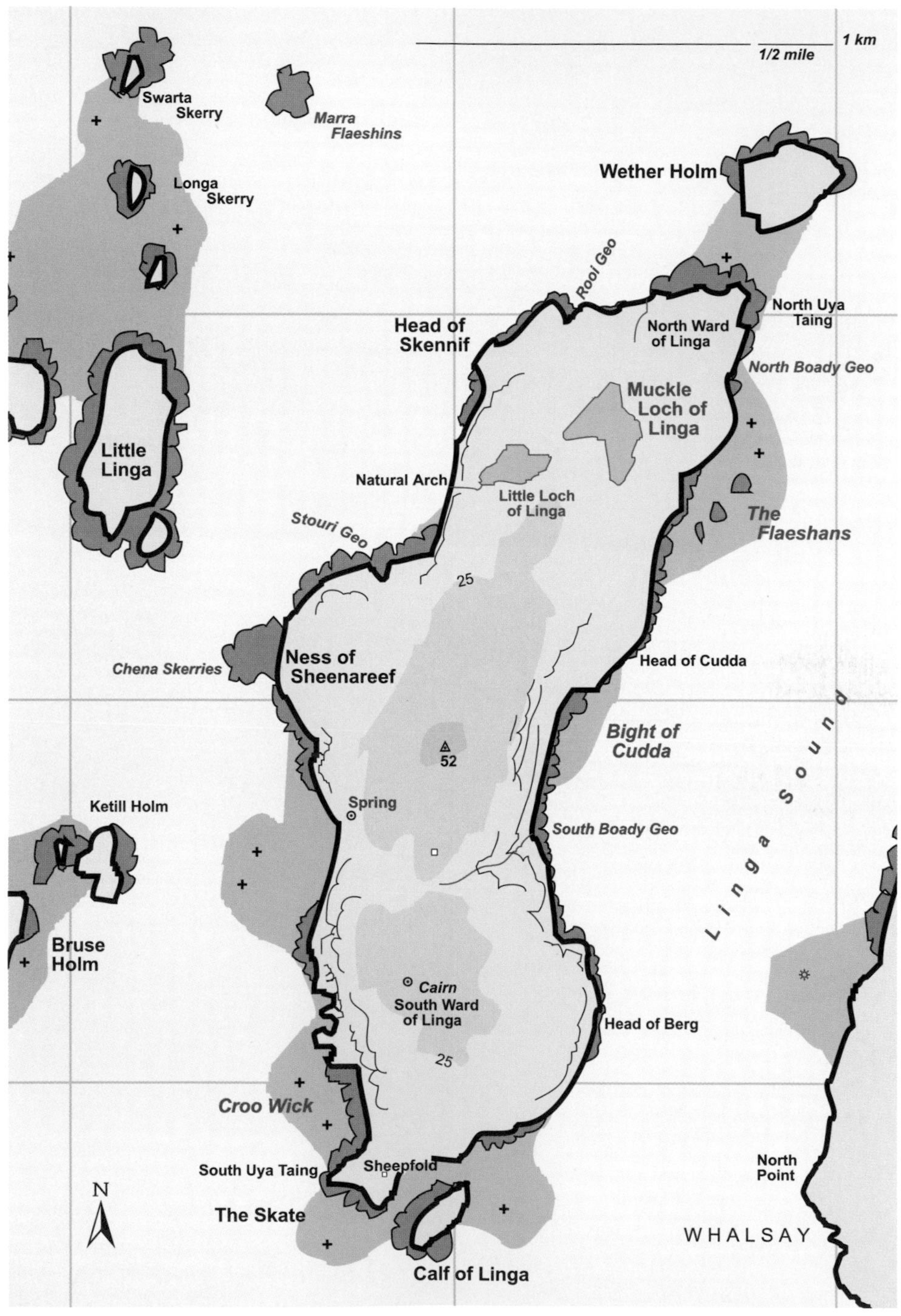

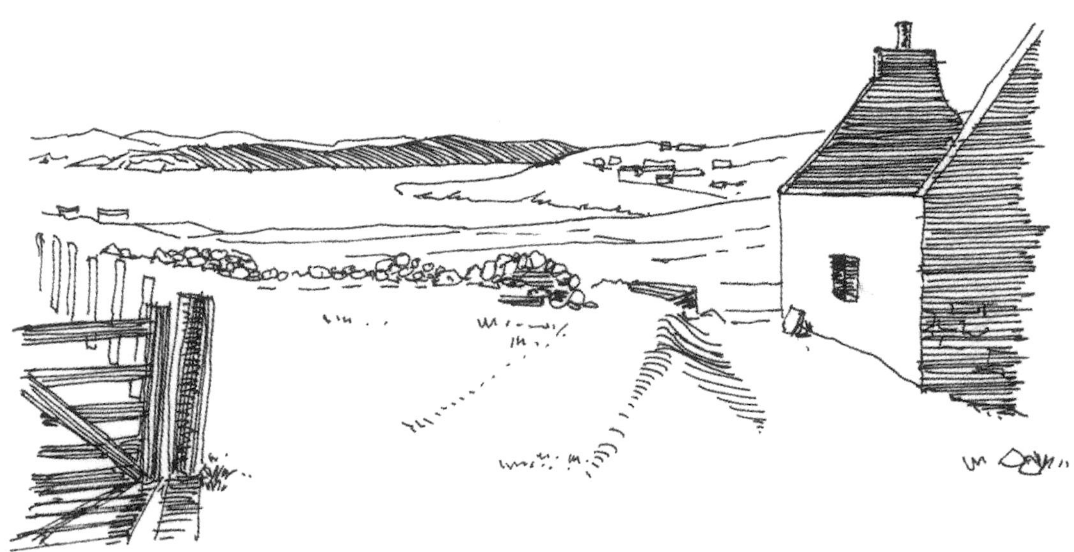

WEST LINGA SEEN FROM SODOM (HUGH MACDIARMID'S COTTAGE) ON WHALSAY

his mother was frantic with worry. The Bruce representative happened to land on the island during this incident and the mother appealed to him for help. He refused until the mother signed over the land, whereupon he calmly broke the pot. This story may have grown with the telling but it no doubt had some basis in fact.

The **Calf of Linga** is a drying islet off the Skate (ON – a rock or sand-shelf) at the southern extremity. At the opposite extreme in the north there is another islet called **Wether Holm**. This is separated from West Linga by a narrow 3m-deep channel.

West Linga divides the sea area between Whalsay and Mainland into two Sounds, Linga and Lunning. Both have fierce tides but Lunning Sound is broken up with many islets and skerries which create swirls and eddies understood only by the Whalsay fishermen. The islets are **Hunder Holm** according to the Ordnance Survey but known locally as 'Unerim' (ON – Arnorr's holm), **Bruse Holm** or 'Brusim' (ON – Brusi's holm), **Ketill Holm** or 'Kettlim' (ON – Ketill's holm), **Score Holm** or 'Skurim' (ON – Skori's holm) and **Little Linga**.

The poet and author, Hugh MacDiarmid, who lived in a Whalsay cottage which overlooked West Linga, claimed in *The Uncanny Scot* to have spent three days on the island. He said that he asked a boatman to leave him there and not to look for him for three days and that he had with him only a good stock of matches, some thick black tobacco, and two books. He slept in a cave in the rocks and caught four sillocks with a bent pin on a string. It transpired later that the story was entirely imaginary – although he had spent part of a day on the island with the man who grazed his sheep there.

* * *

Access: No regular access. Try the Tourist Office, 01595-693434 or ask at Symbister on Whalsay.

Anchorage: No recommended anchorages.

11.17 Linga

(ON lyng-øy – heather island).

OS Maps: 1:50000 Sheet 3 1:25000 Sheet 469
Admiralty Charts: 1:75000 Nos.3281 or 3282 1:25000 No.3295

Area: 70ha (173 acres)
Height: 69m (226 ft)

Population: Uninhabited and no Census records.

Geology: Gneiss, schists and some quartzite and pelite.

* * *

A circumnavigation of **LINGA** reveals all. From every viewpoint its rounded surface of rough grass and heather resembles a well-cooked pudding in a rock-encrusted pie-dish. There are no coves or

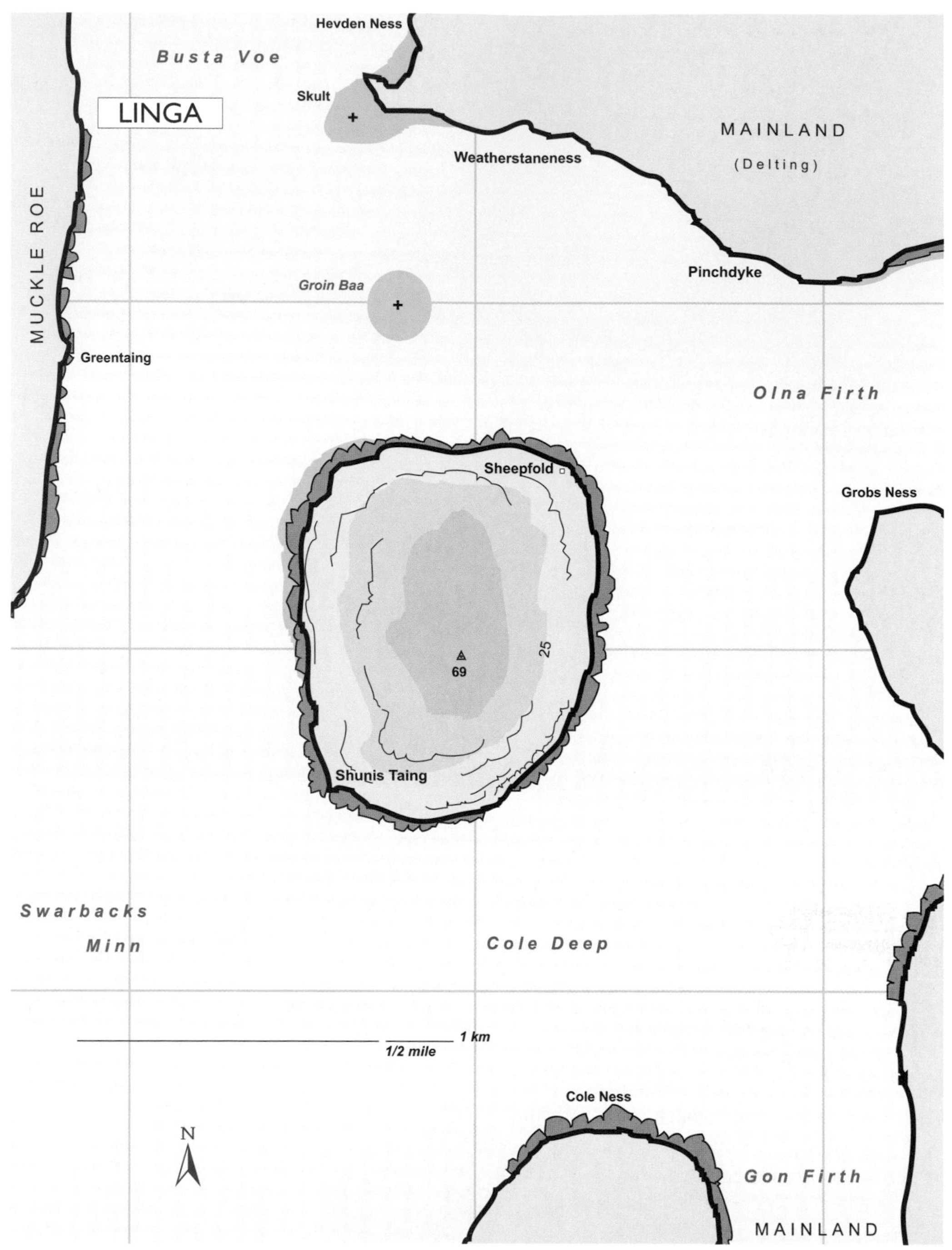

caves or crags, no hidden secrets, no ancient ruins. To its credit the view from the top of the dumpling (69m) is striking and worth the effort of achieving a landing, and to be fair, Linga is not unwelcoming to visitors – merely indifferent.

Access: No regular access but try St Magnus Bay Charters, West Mainland, 01595-810378.

Anchorage: No recommended anchorages. Beware Groin Baa in the north channel.

1. Possible temp. anchorage, if conditions are suitable, off NE side in 12–15m but use tripping line.

11.18 Housay

or West Isle (ON hús-øy – house island).

Bruray

or East Isle (ON brúar-øy- island forming a bridge) – together with

Grunay

(ON – green island). These are known as the Out Skerries (ON út-skeri – outer skerries) or just 'The Skerries' (ON austrskeri – eastern skerries).

OS Maps: 1:50000 Sheet 2 1:25000 Sheet 468
Admiralty Charts: 1:75000 No.3282
Area: 218ha (539 acres)
Height: 53m (174 ft)

Owner: Housay, Bruray and the nearby stacks and skerries are owned by Cussons Estate. They were bought by A S Cussons (of Imperial Leather fame) in 1967. The only exception to this is Laurence Anderson who owns his own property of 'Sunnyside' beside Da Stripe.

Grunay changed hands many times in the 20th century. The present owner, Torquil Johnson-Ferguson of Dumfriesshire also owns Lunga (No.2.11). He put Grunay up for sale in 1993, but is still the owner.

Population:

	1841	1881	1891	1931	1961	1981	1991	2001
Housay		71	86	68	71	49	58	50
Bruray		59	54	34	34	33	27	26
Grunay		25	25	6	0	0	0	0
Total	122	155	165	114	105	82	85	76

Geology: The Mio Ness peninsula (joined to Housay by The Steig which is a collapsed cave) is granite. Apart from a strip of fragmented limestone which stretches from the southern coast of Housay through the centre of Housay and Bruray the rest of the islands are of gneiss and schist. Grunay has granite bedrock.

History: The extent of settlement by early man still awaits scientific investigation. Norse habitation is much more clearly recorded by the hundreds of Norse place-names. These could never have arisen from a few transitory visits and point to continuous settlement over a long period of time.

But the real history of the Skerries is the history of the sea that surrounds them because through the centuries many ships have foundered on these treacherous rocks and the people of the Skerries have had to live with, and understand, the sea in all its moods. One of the earliest recorded wrecks was a Spanish Armada horse-carrier which was said to have sunk in the narrow channel called The Rett.

With the outbreak of the second Anglo-Dutch war in 1664 Dutch East-Indiamen, being merchant ships, avoided the English Channel and preferred to take the longer route ('Achter Om') round the north of Scotland. Although, following the accession of a Scottish King to the English throne in 1603, Scotland and England had a shared monarchy, both countries still had independent Parliaments and the Scots were not at war with the Dutch. On the night of the 11 December 1664 the *Kennermerland*, bound for the Cape of Good Hope ran hard on to Stoura Stack and broke up in the South Mouth. The foremast fell ashore and three men in the rigging survived. The rest were swept out to sea and drowned. The only body washed ashore, a drummer-boy, is buried near the old fish factory. The Earl of Morton, who owned the islands at that time, recovered about 120,000 guilders by promptly setting up a primitive salvage operation but King Charles II stepped in and claimed ownership. There was a court case in Edinburgh which the King won and the Earl lost both the guilders and his Orkney and Shetland estates. The islanders also got nothing, but at least enough barrels of spirits came ashore to keep them inebriated for

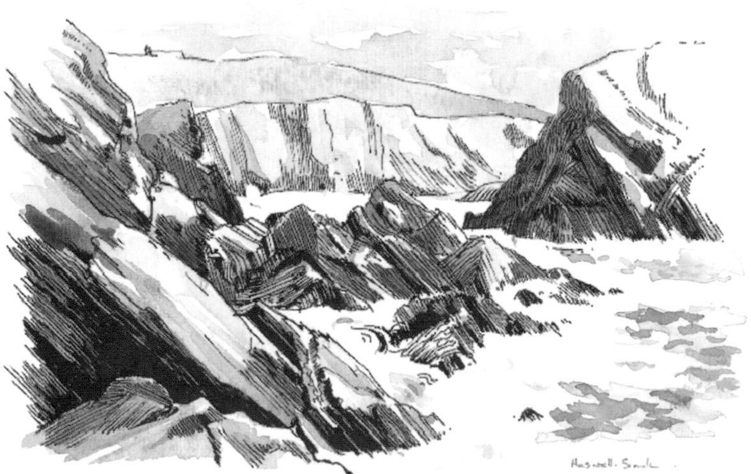

THE SKERRIES SHORELINE – A GRAVEYARD FOR SHIPS

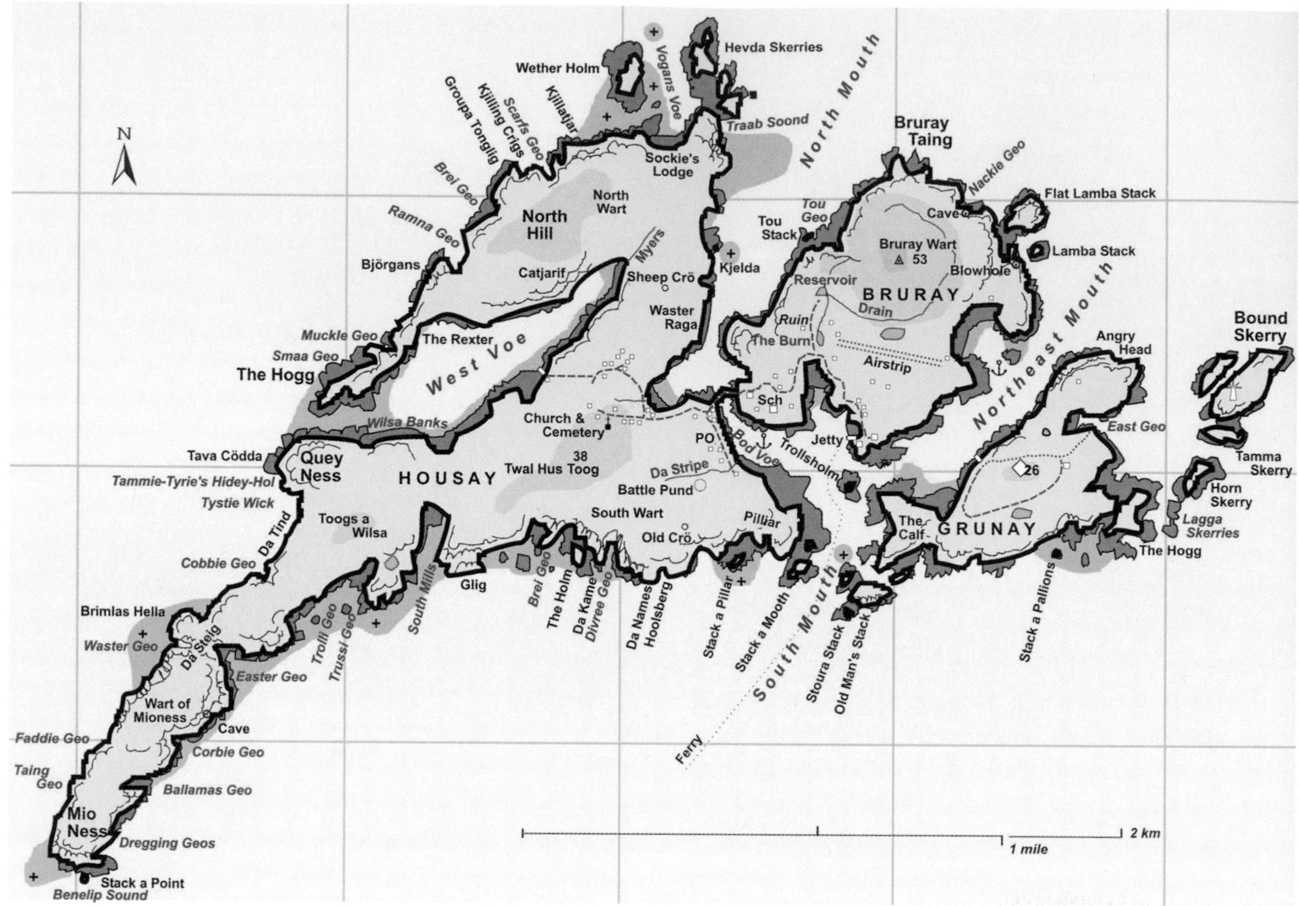

weeks and it is still said that a chest of gold was hidden on the seashore. It is also said that the first hens on Out Skerries came from this wreck.

The *De Liefde*, one of a convoy of ships laden with gold and silver coins to pay for exotic goods in Java, ran into Mio Ness on 8 November 1711 and was lost with all hands except for the look-out in the crow's-nest who was thrown onto the grassy top of the cliff. He reported that there were millions of guilders and several chests of gold coins on board. Most of the money may still be somewhere on the seabed. Occasional coins turn up and an official dive in 1967 recovered a chestful of silver coins and some gold ducats. Diving to these wrecks, however, without official permission is forbidden and strictly enforced.

More recently, in 1906, the wreck of the *North Wind* with a cargo of wood provided the islanders with wooden floors in every house – a great luxury.

But shipwrecks only brought occasional and limited prosperity. Fishing is the historic means of livelihood and in the 19th century Out Skerries provided a valuable haaf fishing station and intermittently throughout the 20th century it was a centre for the industry.

Wildlife: Very well placed to receive continental migrants when the wind is in the east so, apart from islanders' relatives, divers and island-hoppers, the majority of visitors are bird-watchers. The islands support small breeding colonies of gulls, terns, eider and black guillemot but, otherwise, there is only limited birdlife on the cliffs which are not high enough to provide attractive nesting sites.

HOUSAY and **BRURAY** are linked by a concrete bridge built in 1957, replacing the first bridge built in 1899 and a subsequent 'improvement', and they are nowadays the only inhabited islands in the Out Skerries group. Although this cluster of little islands and skerries, exposed and isolated, reach tentatively into the vast inhospitable wastes of the North Sea they are considered to be one of the happiest and most flourishing parts of

Shetland. On approach by sea the cliffs, which are not particularly high, still look forbidding and impregnable. But on a close approach a gap appears and once through the narrow 'mouth' a different picture presents itself. In between the three main islands of the archipelago, Housay, Bruray and Grunay, is a landlocked haven and a pier, completed in 1986, where the ferry docks. Neat, trim and colourful cottages scattered around deep-green miniature fjords create a Nordic flavour. Behind, low grassy hills are used for grazing. There is a little cultivation on a belt of relatively fertile soil but generally the people are fisherfolk, not farmers.

The Skerries is a world in miniature with about 1500 tiny geographical features, each of which is specifically named by the islanders. Housay has a long precipitous leg stretching south-westwards and ending at **Mio Ness** (ON – narrow headland). It humps up like a bent knuckle to a height of 48m near its south extremity. The island itself has a hill on each side of **West Voe**, a deep inlet on the west coast and a modest settlement with a post-office and a cemetery in the middle. At the northern extremity is **Wether Holm**.

North Hill is covered with mounds of stones like 2m-long upturned boats. These are said to be prehistoric graves. There is other evidence of early man – lengths of walls built of Cyclopean masonry, 'skeos' round West Voe (a 'skeo' is the Shetland equivalent of a St Kildan 'cleit', or stone larder), and a mysterious stone rectangle of large boulders called **Battle Pund**. This has some similarity to Hjaltadans on Fetlar (No.11.24). There are varying explanations for both it and its name.

Across the bridge, on Bruray there are more houses, a school overlooking the harbour, and the airstrip beyond. North of the airstrip is the highest point on the archipelago at 53m where a much-needed fresh-water collection system was installed in 1957. Even so, water sometimes has to be brought over by tanker from Mainland.

As ever in such small communities, the school is a vital requirement for stability and the islanders insisted that their children should be fully educated on the island. Consequently a new school was built in 1965. It has two teachers and provides both primary and secondary education – including a course in computer graphics! It is the smallest secondary school in Britain. The old school was converted into a church and a new Community Hall was built in 1981.

There is about a mile of surfaced road which can be quite busy as, since the introduction of the ro-ro ferry, there are about twenty cars. Every family owns a boat, and a fish-processing factory was built here in the productive early 1970s but fish is no longer such a prolific commodity and the factory is idle.

The small island of **Grunay** on the east side of the harbour is separated from the others by South Mouth and Northeast Mouth. The entrance to South Mouth is guarded by both **Stoura Stack** – cause of the *Kennermerland* (or *Carmelan*) disaster – and **Old Man's Stack**, while **Lamba Stack** stands by Northeast Mouth. East of Grunay is **Bound Skerry** with a lighthouse which is now automatic. It was twice bombed by the Germans in the Second World War as they thought it was a munitions factory! The lighthouse was built in 1857 for £21,000 and the keepers were housed on Grunay. Robert Louis Stevenson's signature is in the visitors' book. Since the war the house on Grunay has been in ruins and the island is reputed to be rat-infested.

On its route to Out Skerries the ferry passes a group of islets and skerries stretching south from Mio Ness – **Benelip**, consisting of linked islets – **North and South Benelip** and **Easter Skerries** – is the largest, while the ferry is named after **Filla**, which lies immediately to the south.

* * *

Access: Ro-ro ferry on prior booking from Vidlin, (90 mins), Fri., Sat., Sun., Mon., or Lerwick on Tues. and Thurs. (150 mins), 01806-515226. Flights from Tingwall, Mon., Wed., Thurs., 01595-840246. Tourist info., 01595-693434.

Anchorages:

1. Between Housay and Bruray. Berth at pier usually available (charge) with good facilities, or anchor in 6m towards bridge, abreast school, but many moorings. Use tripping line. Good shelter.
2. Between Bruray and Grunay. Anchor in 4m in entrance to bight on Bruray shore central between the rocks. Use tripping line. Reasonable shelter but NE'lies bring an uncomfortable swell.
3. North Mouth, pool N of bridge (Stringa Voe). Sheltered but not recommended as room very restricted.
4. West Voe on W side of Housay. Mouth obstructed by the Hogg, a rocky islet 2c long. The narrow difficult entrance is at S end of the Hogg where a bar restricts least depth to only 0.6m. Inside the depth increases and there is excellent shelter but the entrance at HW or in any swell is tricky.

11.19 Samphrey

(ON Sandfridar-øy – Sandfridr's island) Sandfridr is a woman's name.

OS Maps: 1:50000 Sheet 2 or 3 1:25000 Sheet 468
Admiralty Charts: 1:75000 No.3282 1:30000 Nos.3292 or 3298

Area: 66ha (163 acres)
Height: 29m (95 ft)
Population: 1841–36 (6 houses). 1881–0. Uninhabited since then.
Geology: Coarsely crystalline gneiss with occasional granite veins.

History: In late 1832 a terrible storm blew up unexpectedly and caught six Samphrey men out fishing on the haaf. Their sixern was blown through mountainous seas until it eventually ended up on a Norwegian beach. It suffered only minor damage and the men were given accommodation and treated very hospitably by the Norwegians. In the spring they returned home, none the worse for their holiday abroad, to a great welcome from their families who had

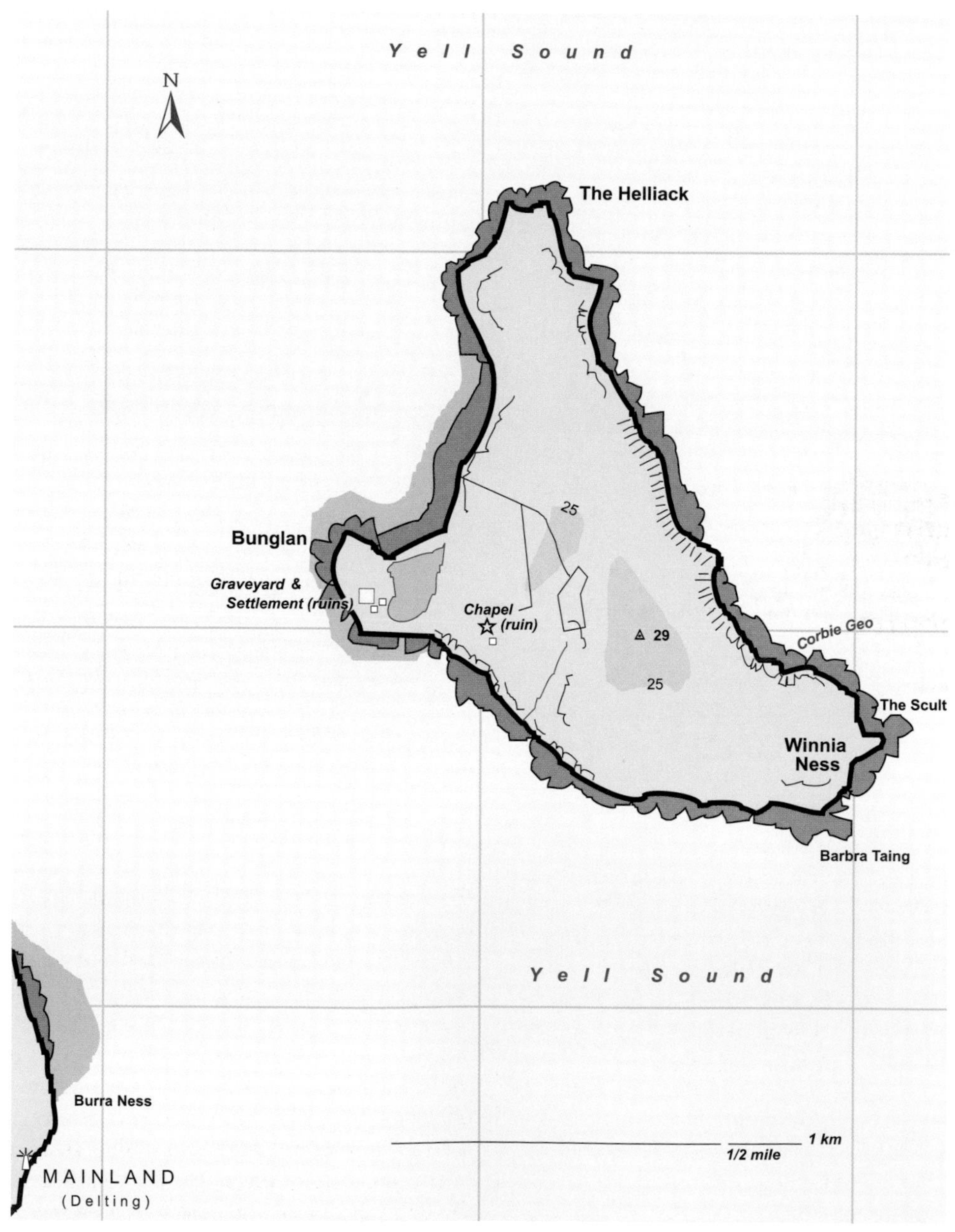

believed they were dead.

Wildlife: The grazing is reasonably good for sheep but wildflowers are scarce, not only because of the grazing but also, because the island is so flat, it catches the worst of the salt-spray.

A number of sea-birds breed here and both Samphrey and neighbouring Fish Holm are managed by the RSPB as a bird sanctuary.

* * *

SAMPHREY defensively straddles the southern entrance to Yell Sound. The tides can run fast past its shores. It is low-lying, shaped something like the jaw-bone of an ass, and the highest ground in the centre of the island is only 29m above sea-level.

Samphrey is relatively clear of rocks in the surrounding sea except for the shallow **Bunglan** promontory on the west side. A large pool or lochan on this headland is only cut off from the sea by narrow margins of land on two sides.

Many of the remnants of human occupation have already disappeared but there is a wee kirkyard. It is reputed to have very few men buried in it as according to tradition: 'Samphrey men are always taken by the sea.' Such certainty could only have arisen in a community dedicated to fishing and the sea which, in the end, may have taken too many, for slowly during the 19th century the number of fishermen and their families dwindled until the island was entirely depopulated. Samphrey is now merely habitation for seabirds and sheep.

On Hogmanay 1941 a Gloster Gladiator N5642 of 152 squadron flying over Yell Sound, had engine failure, made a forced landing in a bog on Samphrey and overturned. The pilot, Sgt. Makin, had done this once before and was unhurt.

South of Samphrey there is an island, **Linga** (ON – heather island) which only just fails to meet my target of forty hectares. South of it is yet another, **Wether Holm** (ON – islet of the castrated ram), and to the north is **Fish Holm**.

A rock outcrop, The **Rumble**, north-east of Samphrey is marked by a beacon. Orfasay (ON *orfyrisøy* – tidal island), is across the sound and linked to the south coast of Yell (No.11.23).

* * *

Access: Try Tourist Information, 01595-693434 for recommended boatmen.

Anchorage:
1. Temp. anchorage in suitable weather in the bight N of Bunglan, the W promontory. Approach with care and anchor in 5m. Use tripping line. Beware submarine cable which is on a line between the W extremities of the two headlands.

11.20 Bigga

(ON bygd-øy – island of the building).

OS Maps: 1:50000 Sheet 2 or 3 1:25000 Sheet 470
Admiralty Charts: 1:75000 No.3282 1:30000 No.3298
Area: 78ha (193 acres)
Height: 34m (112 ft)

Population: 1841, 1881 and 1891 – no separate Census records. 1931 – 1. Since uninhabited.

Geology: Moine bedrock of coarsely crystalline gneiss and quartzite.

Wildlife: Storm petrel and puffin occasionally breed here. Uynarey, to the north, is a nature reserve managed by the RSPB.

* * *

BIGGA is now a 'sheep isle' but it appears to have been inhabited until the 1930s. It is long and narrow with a head and torso. The neck is between two bays, Easter and Wester Hevda Wick (ON – east and west bays of seaweed or manure). The torso rises to a central height of 34m and there is a small hill at the north extremity or head with a prehistoric cairn on its eastern slope.

In the south of the island there is a house which is used as a shepherd's bothy. The local newspapers reported the story of two sailors from Yell (No.11.23), who were given home leave during the Second World War. They were home-sick and desperate to rejoin their families in time for Yule. The weather was very wild and the ferry from Mainland refused to sail so they borrowed a small open boat from a friend and set off. The snow-covered hills of Yell could just be seen through the spume over the wind-whipped open Sound and the tide was in full racing flood but they were accomplished sailors and knew the waters well. However, they could make no headway as the storm increased in strength and it was many hours later before they managed to struggle ashore on Bigga. They sheltered in the bothy but it was so cold that they spent the night playing the fiddle and dancing Shetland reels to keep warm. The next day they were given assistance by a passing drifter and arrived on Yell just in time to join their family celebrations.

There is a reef at the north end of Bigga which crosses the narrow sound separating Bigga from Uynarey. Uynarey (ON – venerated island) is slightly higher than Bigga with steeper sides.

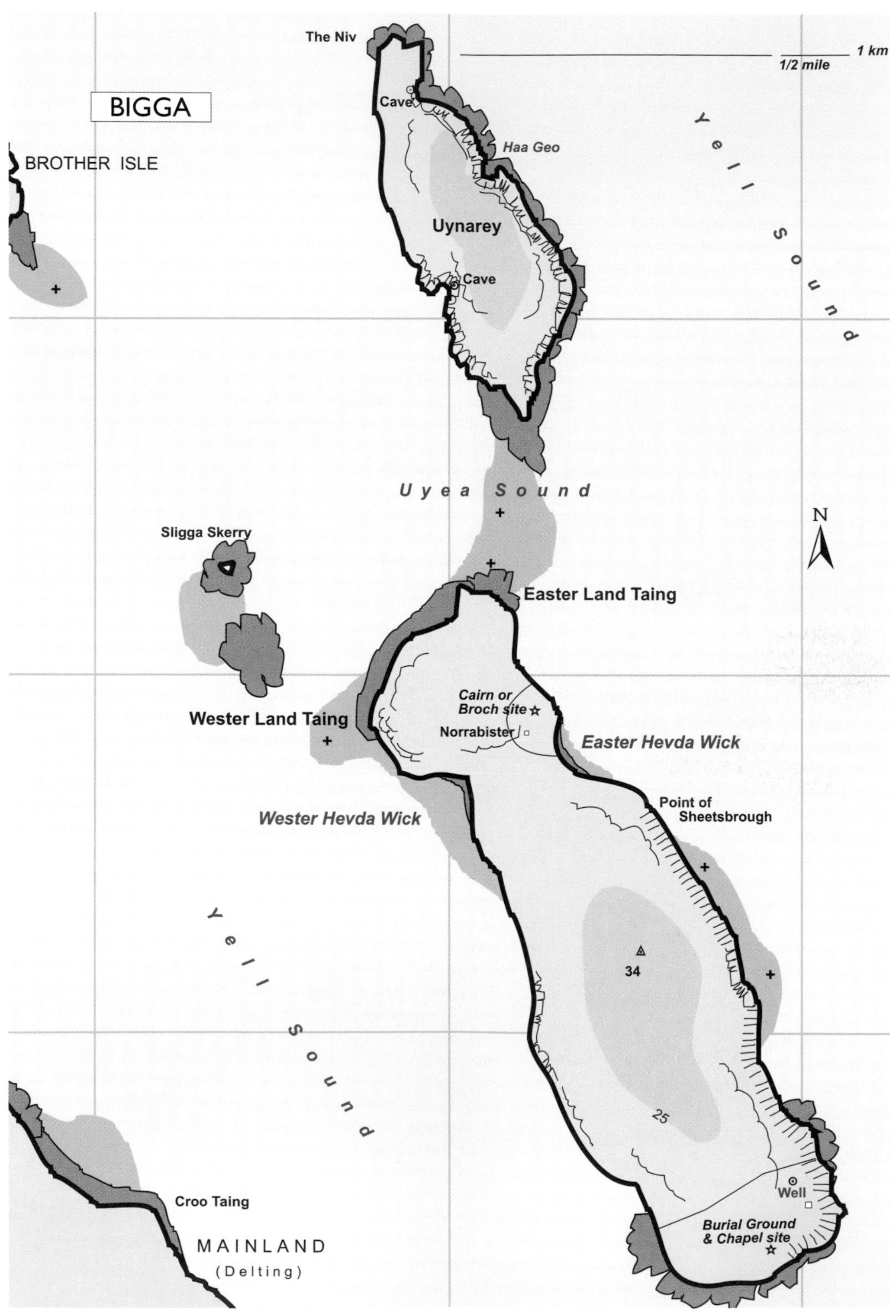

Access: Try Tourist Information, 01595-693434 for recommended boatmen or the Yell ferryman may advise.

Anchorage: Strong tides and a number of rocks make this area hazardous.

1. Temp. anchorage when conditions suitable in Wester Hevda Wick. Beware rock with less than 1.8m over it ½c off NW extremity.

11.21 Brother Isle

(ON breidare-øy – broad beach island.) The alternative (ON brodur-øy – brother island), is improbable.

OS Maps: 1:50000 Sheets 1, 2 or 3 1:25000 Sheet 469
Admiralty Charts: 1:75000 No.3282 1:30000 No.3298

Area: 40ha (99 acres)
Height: 25m (82 ft)

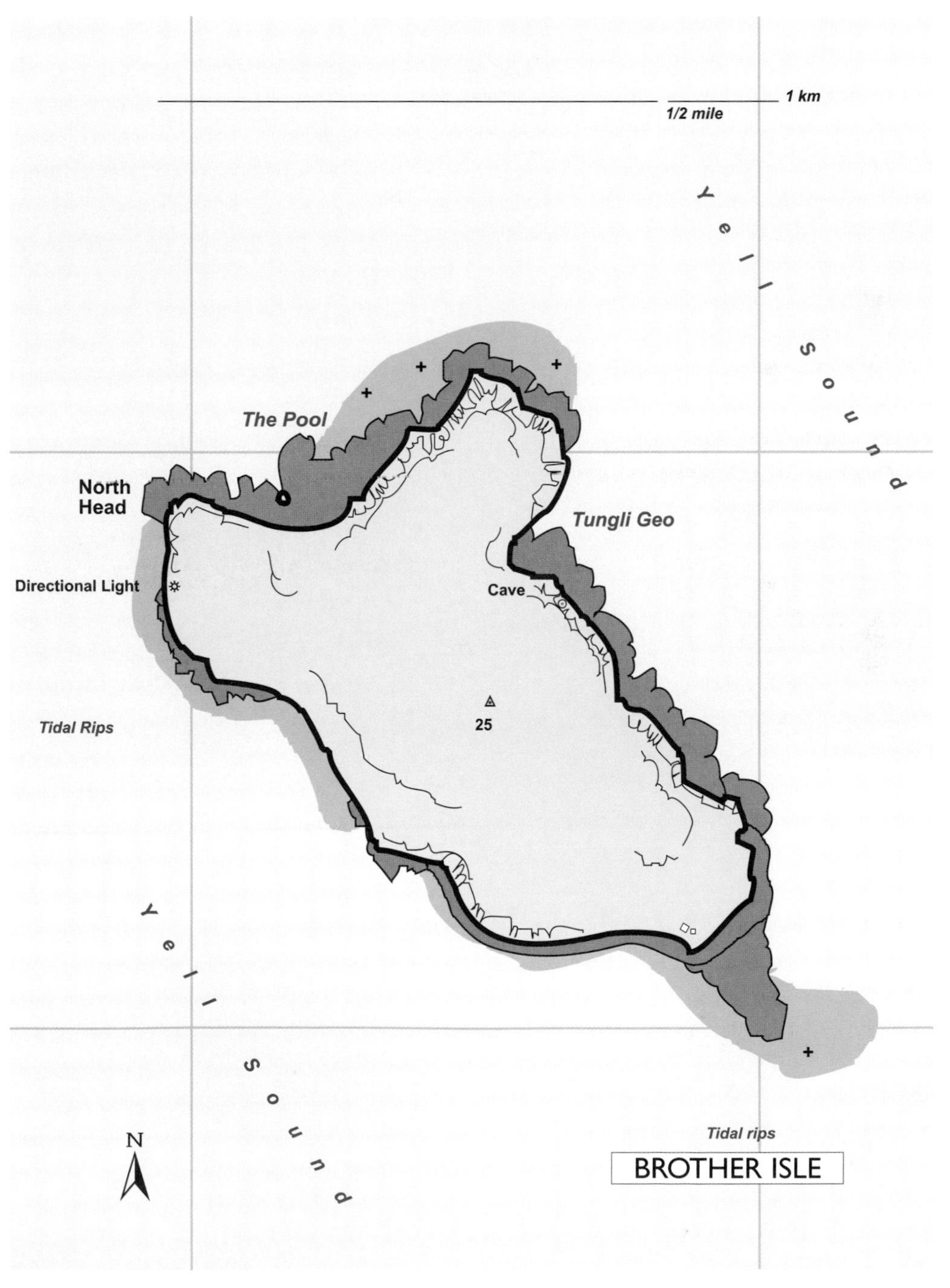

Population: Uninhabited and no Census records.

Geology: Undifferentiated Moine gneiss and quartzite.

Wildlife: Occasional site for breeding storm petrel.

* * *

BROTHER ISLE does not extend a welcome to visitors. If an anchorite or hermit monk ever did live on it, he must certainly have enjoyed solitude for Brother Isle like a pirate ship repels boarders on all sides. The shallow depression on the north side, known as **The Pool**, is full of hidden rocks and there is an evil drying rock called Stoura Baa lurking a short distance away. The southern tip has a long reef of rocks extending to the south-east amid vicious tidal rips. There are also tidal rips off the east and west coasts.

When gales are blowing against the tides in Yell Sound the surface of the sea is whipped into a demonic frenzy. It is then that the South Yell folk refer to the tides familiarly as 'bitin' grices' – or, in other words, swine.

The island itself (with an area of just under one hundred acres it is the smallest in my over-forty-hectares classification), is unremarkable. There is a central hillock of 25m height and a dent on the east side called **Tungli Geo** (ON – gloomy inlet). Nearby is a substantial cave, which could, I suppose, have provided some shelter for a hermit.

To the west of Brother Isle, the ugly head of **Tinga Skerry**, rears 5m above the dark waters of Yell Sound and, like an iceberg, conceals most of its body beneath the surface.

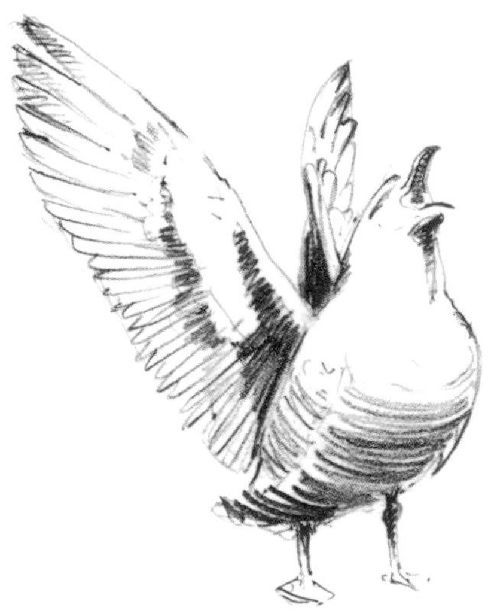

THE 'BONXIE', OR GREAT SKUA, LORD OF THE SKIES

* * *

Access: Try Tourist Information, 01595-693434 for recommended boatmen or the Yell ferryman may advise.

Anchorages: No recommended anchorages.

11.22 Lamba

(ON – lamb island).

OS Maps: 1:50000 Sheets 1, 2 or 3 1:25000 Sheet 469
Admiralty Charts: 1:75000 Nos.3281 or 3282 1:30000 No.3298

Area: 43ha (106 acres)
Height: 35m (115 ft)

Population: Uninhabited.

Geology: Intrusive igneous rocks – mainly granite and syenite.

Wildlife: A family of otters is to be seen quite often in the cleft on the north-east side beside the eponymous Otter Had.

Storm petrel and puffin usually take up residence in the nesting season.

* * *

LAMBA's main claim to distinction is the tall (27m) light tower at its southern extremity, **South Head**. This helps to define the entrance to busy Sullom Voe oil terminal.

There are caves in the steep bluff beside the light tower and a cleft called **Hesti Geo** (ON – horse inlet). On the east coast a wider indentation called the **Wick of Lamba** (ON – Lamba Bay) is at least partly sheltered from the tidal currents in this area. These are clearly seen in the turbulence which builds up off both South Head and North Point. There is another bay on the north-west side but it is full of rocks and dries out at low water.

Lamba is surrounded by low escarpments which means that access can be something of a scramble but once above the shore the ground rises more gradually to a height of about 35m at the centre.

An interesting wreck of a Norwegian steamer – the *SS Robert Lee* – lies near Lamba in a depth of only 10 metres but divers should be very wary

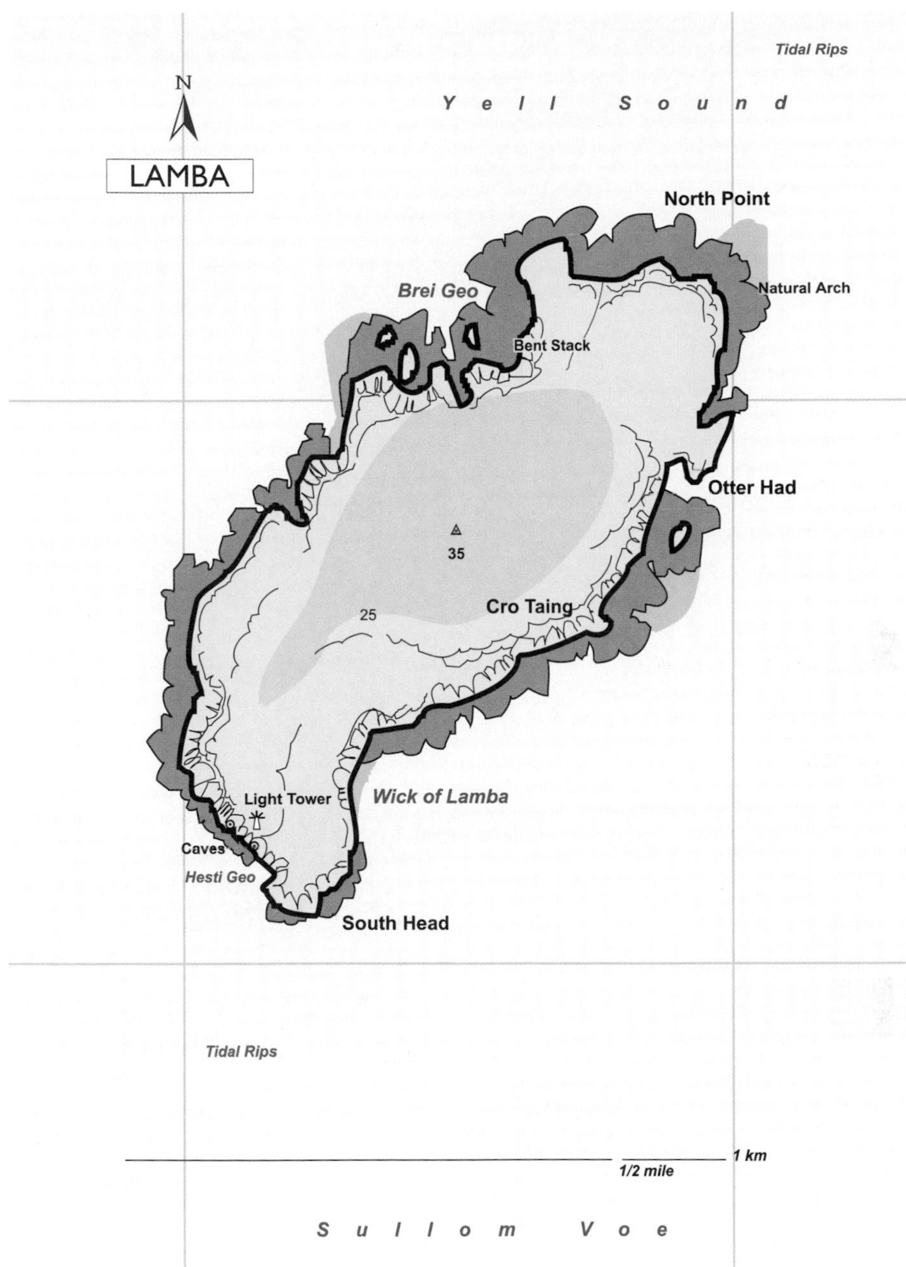

of the strong currents.

Near the entrance to Sullom Voe is another, smaller, island with a light beacon. This is **Little Roe,** which in 1841 was inhabited by eleven people sharing a single house.

* * *

Access: Try Tourist Information, 01595-693434 for recommended boatmen or the Yell ferryman may advise.

Anchorages: No recommended anchorages.

1. Temp. anchorage in suitable weather conditions in Wick of Lamba, 7–10m.

11.23 Yell

(ON gjall – barren) but some think the name may be Pictish. The early Norse name was 'Jala' or 'Jela' which might mean white island (i.e. sandy beaches).

O S Maps: 1:50000 Sheets 1 and 2, or 1 and 3 1:25000 Sheet 470.

Admiralty Charts: 1:75000 No.3282 1:30000 Nos.3292 and 3298 1:12500 No.3293 Basta Voe

Area: 21211ha (52412 acres)
Height: 205m (672 ft)
Owner: Multiple ownership, including the RSPB, A Cunningham-Brown, J Ballantyne, Wilson, and L H Johnson.

Population: 1841–2611 (550 houses). 1881–2529. 1891–2511 (525 houses). 1931–1883. 1961–1155. 1981–1191. 1991–1075. 2001–957.

Geology: Pre-Cambrian rocks under a thick blanket of peat. Most of the island is of garnetiferous mica plagioclase gneiss but the north-eastern coast and the south-east corner have an underlay of striped granulitic oligoclase gneiss and some bands of calc-silicate rock. The central highland is thick lenticular quartzite and the western cliffs are muscovite biotite gneiss with some silvery mica schists.

History: Early prehistoric remains are scattered around the coasts of Yell with hardly any to be found inland and there are a number of Iron Age structures such as the important broch at Ness of Burraness, overlooking Fetlar. About twelve broch sites have been identified and at least fifteen sites of ancient chapels.

Yell moorland was possibly of less interest to the past landowners because it was never formed into really large estates and has always had multiple ownership. The largest landowners in the 19th century were Mouat in the north, Leask in the west and MacQueen in the Burravoe district.

Wildlife: The moors and heaths of Yell provide a habitat for most of Shetland's eight species of orchid with the heath spotted orchid by far the most common.

The coasts are otter territory and the lochans are well-stocked with brown trout. The west coast in particular is favoured by grey seals but a bearded seal, a stray from the Arctic drift ice, was recorded here in 1977.

At the Lumbister RSPB Reserve in the north-west near Whale Firth there are typical breeding species for the Shetlands – red-throated diver, red-breasted merganser, golden plover, eider, merlin, curlew, snipe, lapwing, arctic and great skuas, dunlin, great black-backed gull, raven, twite and wheatear. Oystercatcher, black guillemot, puffin and ringed plover breed on the coast.

Generally speaking, the waters of Yell Sound offer an important wintering area for divers, eider, and long-tailed duck.

The ferry to **YELL** docks at Ulsta. As you cross the Sound, what appears to be a reef at the southern extremity of the island turns out to be the lonely remains of a broch built precariously on a skerry. Yell itself has a gloomy appearance – low-lying hills blanketed in peat bog – yet for many this is the real Shetland. The peat of course has its merits as the Rev. Cruttwell pointed out in the 18th century: 'The inhabitants have plenty of fuel, catch immense quantities of small fish and live comfortably.' On the other hand, Buchanan in the 16th century claimed that Yell was 'so uncouth a place that no creature can live therein, except such as are born there'. By the 1960s Yell's danger of serious depopulation became a matter of grave concern. Some said that part of the problem was the islanders' 'social egalitarianism,' which denied anyone the opportunity to be a leader or entrepreneur. This is unlikely but airing the matter seems to have helped because the numbers now appear to have more or less stabilised. Yell is quite a large island – half the size of Arran – but it has such a bleak landscape that human settlement, and attitudes, tend to cling to the edges.

Two roads run north from **Ulsta**, the main road on the west coast and a secondary, more scenic and interesting, road following the south and east coasts.

This secondary road skirts Hamna Voe (ON – harbour voe) and runs into **Burravoe** (ON – broch voe) in the extreme south-east. The whitewashed crow-stepped **Old Haa of Burravoe**, built in 1637, is the oldest surviving building on the island [HU522796]. It is used as a local museum and craft centre. Burravoe has a tiny well-protected harbour which discourages visitors by its welter of skerries surrounding the islet, **Green Holm**, at its entrance.

The east coast has pleasant hamlets and crofts and touches of cultivation to relieve the dark peat mosses on the slopes of Yell's highest hill, **Ward of Otterswick** (205m). Beyond the cliffs the expanse of steel-blue sea is broken by Fetlar (No.11.24) and when the weather is favourable Out Skerries (No.11.18) can be seen on the horizon.

In 1924 a German 3-masted barque, *Bohus*,

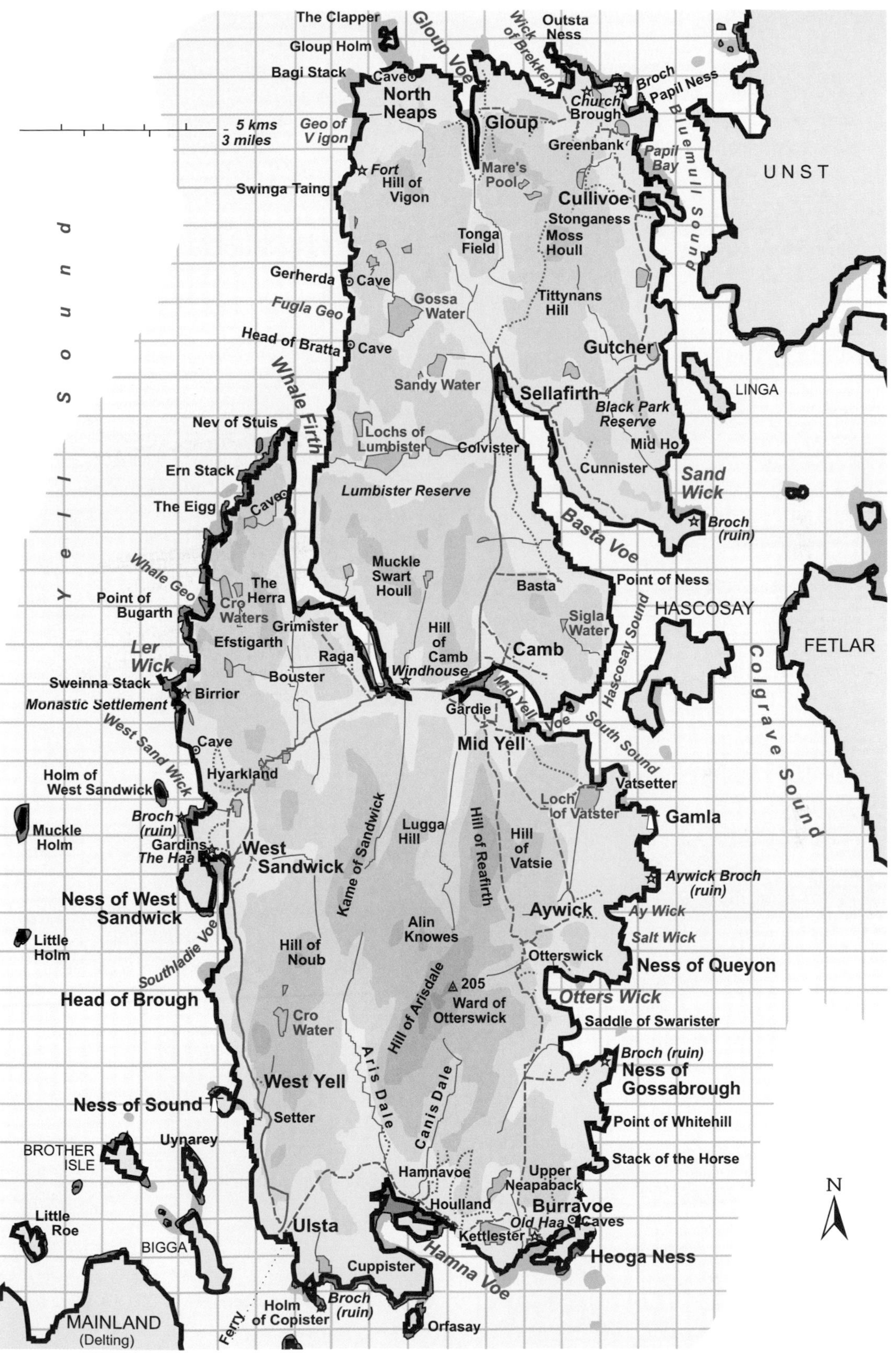

The Clapper
Gloup Holm
Bagi Stack
Cave
North Neaps
Gloup Voe
Wick of Brekken
Outsta Ness
Broch
Papil Ness
Church
Brough
Gloup
Greenbank
Papil Bay
Bluemull Sound
UNST
5 kms
3 miles
Geo of Vigon
Fort
Hill of Vigon
Swinga Taing
Mare's Pool
Cullivoe
Stonganess
Moss Houll
Tonga Field
Gerherda
Cave
Gossa Water
Fugla Geo
Tittynans Hill
Head of Bratta
Cave
Gutcher
Whale Firth
Sandy Water
Sellafirth
LINGA
Black Park Reserve
Nev of Stuis
Lochs of Lumbister
Colvister
Mid Ho
Ern Stack
Cunnister
Sand Wick
Lumbister Reserve
The Eigg
Cave
Broch (ruin)
Basta Voe
Yell Sound
Whale Geo
Muckle Swart Houll
Point of Ness
Point of Bugarth
The Herra
Cro Waters
Basta
HASCOSAY
Sigla Water
Grimister
Hill of Camb
FETLAR
Ler Wick
Efstigarth
Camb
Raga
Hascosay Sound
Colgrave Sound
Sweinna Stack
Bouster
Windhouse
Birrior
Monastic Settlement
Mid Yell Voe
Gardie
West Sand Wick
Cave
Mid Yell
South Sound
Hyarkland
Vatsetter
Holm of West Sandwick
Loch of Vatster
Gamla
Broch (ruin)
Kame of Sandwick
Lugga Hill
Hill of Reafirth
Hill of Vatsie
Muckle Holm
Gardins
The Haa
West Sandwick
Aywick Broch (ruin)
Ness of West Sandwick
Aywick
Ay Wick
Alin Knowes
Salt Wick
Little Holm
Hill of Noub
Otterswick
Ness of Queyon
Southladie Voe
205
Ward of Otterswick
Otters Wick
Head of Brough
Cro Water
Hill of Arisdale
Saddle of Swarister
Aris Dale
Broch (ruin)
Ness of Gossabrough
West Yell
Canis Dale
Ness of Sound
Setter
Point of Whitehill
Uynarey
BROTHER ISLE
Stack of the Horse
Hamnavoe
Upper Neapaback
N
Little Roe
Houlland
Burravoe
Old Haa
Caves
Ulsta
Kettlester
BIGGA
Heoga Ness
Cuppister
Hamna Voe
Broch (ruin)
Holm of Copister
MAINLAND (Delting)
Ferry
Orfasay

ran aground and broke up here with the loss of two of its crew. The figurehead lay for many years on the shore until it eventually rotted and disintegrated but not before a fibreglass reproduction had been made and set up on the shore as a monument. This is known as the '**White Wife of Queyon**' [HU529853].

The only settlement of note on the main road up the west coast is **West Sandwick**, a pretty spot with houses clustered round the sandy beaches of Southladie Voe [HU440887]. The remains of a broch on a drying islet on the coast look across to the **Holm of West Sandwick** which has a rock arch through which the sea breaks. A challenging walk along these west coast cliffs past the prehistoric settlement at **Birrier** [HU438913] beside **Sweinna Stack**, and **Ern Stack** (which was the last recorded nesting-place of the sea-eagle in Shetland) leads to Stuis of Graveland at the entrance to **Whale Firth.**

Yell is almost bisected where the west- and east-coast roads rejoin at **Mid Yell**, the island's main settlement. It is here that the narrow twisted Whale Firth nearly meets the sheltered anchorage of **Mid Yell Voe**, a suitable venue for many sailing regattas. The lonely haunted **Windhouse** at the head of Whale Firth is on a site which has been occupied since Neolithic times.

The ruined herring curing station halfway up Whale Firth at **Grimister** closed shortly after the Second World War – and apart from a few crofts the firth is deserted. The Germans claimed that their U-boats often sheltered here during the First World War and one could hardly imagine a better hiding-place! The whole west-coast area beyond Whale Firth to North Neaps at the remote northern extremity of Yell is an untouched wilderness of peaty heath and mire with many small lochans rippled by the continual wind. Yet this desolate expanse containing the **Lumbister RSPB Reserve** has some of the most interesting scenery and hill-walks on the island. The coast is wildly indented with green hollows, great rock arches, caves and tumbled cliffs.

The main road continues beyond Mid Yell – with its islet of **Kay Holm** hidden by a headland – round the length of Basta Voe, and ends at **Gutcher**, which is the ferry terminal for Fetlar (No.11.24) and Unst (No.11.29). But before jumping aboard at this point remember that the best of Yell lies north where a secondary road continues up the shores of attractive Bluemull Sound through the rural village of **Cullivoe.**

As the road passes the priests' loch on Papil Ness, and turns along the north coast at **Brough**, the roofless **Kirk of Ness** [HP532049] can be seen by the west shore of Kirk Loch. This medieval parish church was dedicated to St Olaf but has been deserted since 1750. There is no historical proof but legend claims that it is from here that Leif the Lucky set off on his expedition to America. The rough wilderness is, incomprehensibly, covered with the remains of ancient settlements which have never yet been adequately investigated. To the west on the cliff top is the broch which has given the area its name [HP540051]. There is a delightful walk along these cliffs and the views are stunning but it is important to keep clear of the edge which is brittle and crumbles easily.

Skeletons have been found in the sands of the **Wick of Brekken** which may once have had a settlement like Jarlshof.

The road ends at **Gloup Voe** (ON – ravine creek), although there is a track continuing round the head of the voe to West-a-Firth on the far side. The **Fishermen's Memorial** [HP507044] here on the hillside above the voe commemorates yet another devastating island disaster. The entire male community in this remote northern haven (ten sixerns with fifty-eight fishermen on board) was lost in a savage storm on 20 July 1881.

A track leading north from Gloup connects with the Coastguard Lookout Station which is set on the cliffs between two wicks. To the west is **Gloup Holm** with jagged **Eagle Stack**, **Whilkie Stack** and **The Clapper**. To the east, Muckle Flugga lighthouse is on the horizon – convincing proof that this is the end of the road.

* * *

Access: Daily ro-ro ferry from Toft, Mainland to Ulsta, Yell, (20mins), approx. half-hourly, 01957-722259. Also daily frequent ro-ro from Belmont, Unst to Gutcher, Yell (10mins). and from Hamars Ness, Fetlar to Gutcher, Yell, (20mins), 01957-722259. Tourist Information, 01595-693434.

Anchorages:

1. Hamna Voe on S coast. Exposed SE–S. Anchor W of Ness of Galtagarth in 8–10m, good holding. Head is shoal. Approach on central course and beware Burga Skerry 3c S of Green Holm.
2. Burra Voe at SE extremity of Yell. Approach from S and

enter with great care following directions. There are many dangers in the approach. Anchor anywhere inside in 4-6m but bottom foul with old moorings; N of the bay is best.

3. Wick of Gossabrough on E coast. Small stone pier on S side. Easy access but beware Wick Skerry at entrance. Exposed N to E. Anchor off beach in SW bay. Holding unreliable.

4. Otters Wick has many rocks and careful use of chart required. Exposed E to SE.

5. Mid Yell Voe, mid E coast, good secure anchorage. Head dries for ½M. Approach on mid-channel course and anchor anywhere in wide part of voe in 2½–10m, mud and sand. Gusty in N winds. Pier has depth of 3m. Small marina for shallow draught boats.

6 Basta Voe. Good shelter. Both sides clear to ¾c from shore. Shingle bank off point on NE shore. Anchor beyond the shingle bank in 5–15m, clay, good holding mostly.

7. Wick of Gutcher, small bay in Bluemull Sound with ferry terminal. Berthing reserved exclusively for ferry.

8. Culli Voe, in Bluemull Sound, is shallow but concrete pier at entrance to voe projects 42m from shore and has 3.5m depth at head. Fair anchorage as far into the voe as depth permits or temp. anchorage south of pier in 5m, holding good, sand and shells. Small marina for shallow draught boats at head of voe.

9. Wick of Breckin (Breakon) on N coast. Temp. anchorage in S or E winds, holding poor (Lunda Wick on Unst is better).

10. Gloup Voe, not recommended. Mostly too deep, heavy sea with N–NW winds, and voe dries out halfway to head.

11. Whale Firth on W coast. Quiet, secluded anchorage. Beware sunken rock 2c NE of Nev of Stuis at entrance and rocks off S shore at Grimister. Otherwise clear of dangers.

12. Southladie Voe, close E of Ness of West Sandwick. Good anchorage except in S'lies. Limited anchorage in the pool at head, 1½m, soft mud. Keep to W side at narrow passage off Urabug ayre where there is only 1m depth.

11.24 Fetlar

(ON – fat/prosperous land). Intriguing suggested alternative derivation (ON fetill – a strap or tie) with (ON -ar) as the plural form. See below.

O S Maps: 1:50000 Sheet 1 or 2 1:25000 Sheet 470
Admiralty Charts: 1:75000 No.3282 1:30000 No.3292 west part

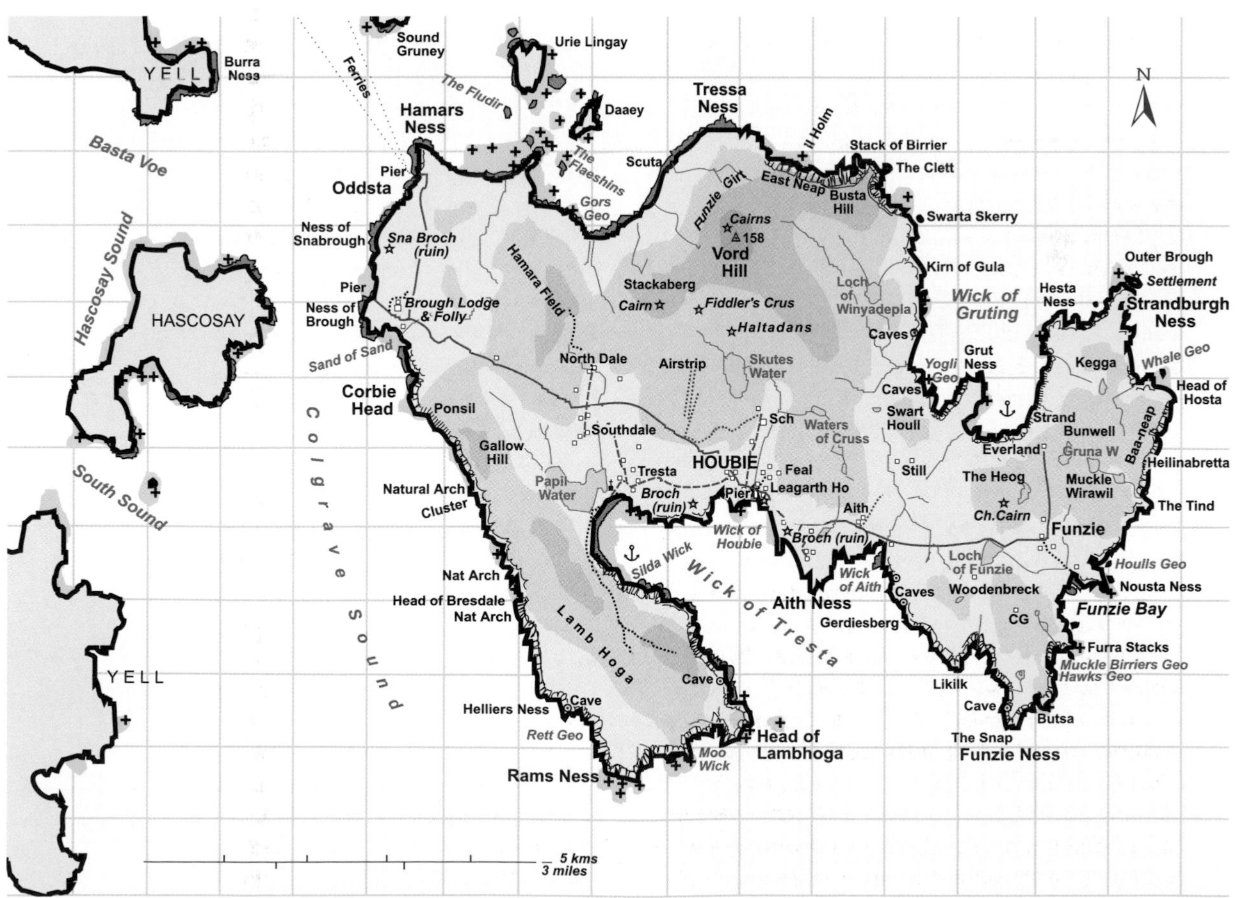

Area: 4078ha (10077 acres)
Height: 158m (518 ft)
Owner: Most of the island was inherited by Mrs Borland, Edinburgh, on the death of her aunt, Lady Nicolson (c.1980). Fetlar has been owned by Nicolsons since the early 1800s but the recent owners were not direct descendants of Sir Arthur Nicolson.

Population: 1841–761 (137 houses). 1881–431. 1891–363 (70 houses). 1931–217. 1961–127. 1981–101. 1991–90. 2001–86. 2007–60.

Geology: There is gneiss in the west including Lambhoga. East of a fault line there are magnificent serpentine outcrops which are only equalled by those of Cornwall and which account for the interesting cliff formations. There is also metagabbro and phyllite. The sand in the Wick of Houbie is magnetic and at Moo Wick at the tip of Lambhoga there is a residual deposit of kaolin. At Hesta Ness in the north-east the serpentine has been altered to antigorite and steatite. Here too there are bands of pure talc, which was mined at one time.

History: The story of Fetlar goes back a long way. Yet Fetlar, in spite of its great contrast to its neighbour, the rather desolate Yell, has never achieved a distinctive place in Shetland history, probably due to its lack of a safe harbour. The first Norse settlers are thought to have landed here, and swashbuckling King Harald the Fair-haired landed on Fetlar during his pursuit of 'Vikings' in the 9th century but he swiftly moved on to a secure anchorage at Unst.

The first large-scale clearances in Shetland started here on the Lambhoga peninsula in 1822 when the landowner, Sir Arthur Nicolson, evicted the crofters to make room for sheep. By 1858 he had emptied the whole of the north and west part of the island and cleared nearly 30 townships. He built himself the three-storey tower folly at Grutin using stone from the crofters' houses.

A serious drop in population during the 1980s led to the local community council advertising for settlers. The two biggest drawbacks are that older children have to travel to Yell for schooling and there is no adequate harbour. The Shetland Council are trying to improve this situation as the population is again decreasing.

Like so many Shetland islands, Fetlar has a history of shipwrecks. An incomplete list illustrates this:
1601– a Danish vessel. 1699– a packet, wrecked at Hamars Ness. 1710– a vessel from Emden. 1737– *Wendela*, Danish. 1765– a vessel at Whale Geo. 1773– *James*. 1794– a vessel at Aith. 1799– *Good Intent*. 1811– *Stadt Memel*. 1847– *Clarenden*. 1848– *Neptune*. 1870– *Johan Caesar*, Hamburg. 1882– *Lizzie*. 1897– *Flosta*. 1897– *Anna*. 1900– *Hedevig*, Norway. 1962– *Maia*, Russian trawler.

Wildlife: More than 200 different species of wildflower have been recorded on this verdant isle. Rarer species include frog orchid and northern gentian, but the rarest are members of the sedge family. In the sheltered area at Leagarth House there used to be a number of quite exotic trees.

There are many grey and common seals around the coasts and otters can often be seen, particularly between Brough Lodge and Urie.

The lochs, some with restricted access, offer fly fishing for brown trout.

Fetlar is an outstanding bird sanctuary, especially for breeding waders of which there is the highest density in Britain. All visitors should first contact the RSPB warden. Lapwing, oystercatcher and ringed plover breed on the crofts, and golden plover, dunlin, curlew, and many whimbrel nest on the moorland. Snipe, redshank and red-necked phalarope breed on the lochans and wetlands. There are also breeding seabirds. Manx shearwater, storm petrel, shag, kittiwake, guillemot and puffin are to be seen on the cliffs, particularly on the Lamb Hoga peninsula which has Britain's largest colony of storm petrels. There are common tern and about 4500 pairs of arctic tern.

Fetlar is probably most renowned for the snowy owls, which were found nesting at Stakkaberg in 1967. This is the extreme southern limit of their breeding range. Unfortunately the old male, having driven off all competitors, died of old age in 1975 leaving several morose females without a mate. Consequently, there are now no resident snowy owls although they still occasionally make an appearance.

Other breeders on the island are red-throated diver, eider, raven and twite and recorded migrants include two-barred crossbill and greenish warbler. In the autumn there are many fieldfare and redwing.

* * *

Let your imagination take over for a moment and think of **FETLAR** in the dark ages of prehistory – a fair and fertile land populated by Mesolithic farmers.

Now let us suppose that two tribes live on the island and because the grass is always greener next door they engage in intermittent feuding and fighting. The wars go on for years until at last someone decides to call a truce. There is a meeting at which, after argument, they agree to a division of land, and so that there can be no further dispute whatsoever, they join forces and build a big wall right across the centre of the island. With their territories now clearly defined, they live happily ever after.

This idyllic state continues until the 7th or 8th century AD and then the unexpected happens. Land-hungry Norwegian settlers, following in the wake of the first marauding Vikings, come to Shetland. Their first landfall is Fetlar, which is about as near to Norway as you can get and here they see a land of milk and honey. History does not record the viewpoint of the original islanders but we can be sure the land was acquired while they were slaughtered, enslaved or merely absorbed.

The Norsemen would be surprised to find Fetlar divided by a huge wall and, as they lacked a scientific definition for an island, they thought of it as two islands. This is much the same as their view that a mountain barrier divided Lewis and Harris into two separate islands or a narrow isthmus turned the Mull of Kintyre into an island. At this point an element of fact creeps into our reconstruction because early Norse records always spoke of Fetlar as Est Isle and Wast Isle. Fetlar, as a name for the whole island, is first found in a document dated 1558 although an earlier document in 1490 talks of Foetilør. As 'fetill' means a strap or a tie in Norse one might guess that they thought of Fetlar as two islands tied together.

Meanwhile, the ancient wall itself took on an aura of mystery. 'Who had built it?' the settlers wondered. And as time passed their descendants attributed its creation to the Finns, magical figures in Norse folklore, who might have been Laplanders, or giants, or trolls, or all three rolled together. It was said that the Finns built the wall in a single night in exchange for a farmer's best cow.

Today, the one-metre wide wall, or what little is left of it, is still called **Funzie Girt** [fin-ee girt] which means the Finns' dyke and it cuts round the west side of Vord Hill but disappears near Whilsa Pund. It then reappears south of Skutes Water, crosses the Vallahamars and ends by the Stack of Billaclett where there is a cave in which the trolls lived. It divides Fetlar into two almost equal sections.

There are other mysteries too in this mid-island region. Between Vord Hill and Skutes Water, are the **Fiddler's Crus** [HU618927]. These are three mysterious stone circles set in a triangular pattern and almost touching each other. Each circle is about 13½ metres in diameter. Nearby, about 200 metres north of Skutes Water, there is another strange monument called **Haltadans** (or Hjaltadans) which means 'limping dance' [HU622924]. This is an outer circle of thirty-eight serpentine stones, about 11½ metres in diameter, with an internal, low and concentric earth bank. Two stones lie at the centre.
Both these structures seem to be related but archaeologists have no satisfactory explanation of their purpose. The local explanation is that a fiddler and his wife were dancing in the moonlight one night with trolls and all were enjoying it so much that they failed to notice the dawn. Everyone was instantly petrified by the light of the rising sun. The stone circles are the dancing trolls and the two prostrate central stones are the fiddler and his wife. This is a typical Norse legend with trolls as creatures of the night coupled with a Christian flavour of retribution for ungodly pleasures.

Fetlar is Shetland's most fertile island and it is still known as the Garden of Shetland although it is not quite as well tended as it once was. It is quite hilly with **Vord Hill** (ON – watch hill) at 158m being the highest point. Two Neolithic heel-shaped cairns on the hill are possibly 5000 years old. The shelter in the southern cairn was built during the First World War [HU622936].

It is a pity that such an attractive island has no secure anchorages, although it is usually possible to find shelter provided there is no sudden change of wind. The survival of any island's population today depends on reliable communications and on-site education. In Fetlar's case, the former criterion was satisfied in 1974, when a regular vehicle ferry service to a pier at Oddsta was inaugurated, but the island still lacks the facilities for secondary education, which Out Skerries,

(No.11.18) with a similar population, already has.

Fetlar's single road runs west to east across the island. To the south there is the great **Lamb Hoga** (ON – sheep pasture) peninsula with its steep gneiss cliffs. Shetland ponies sometimes graze here on the open moorland. The lairds of **Brough Lodge** [HU580926], the Nicolsons, crossed the native stock with Norwegian to achieve an improved breed. Beneath the stretch of **Papil Water** (ON – priests' water) is the magnificent sweep of beach at **Tresta**, well sheltered from the prevailing wind.

The adjoining cove at **Houbie** (ON *hopr* – light), with the airstrip to the north of it, also has a pleasant, but much smaller, beach. Prominent **Leagarth House**, by the small pier, was built by Sir William Watson Cheyne in 1900. He was a Houbie lad who became a famous surgeon after assisting Joseph Lister in his development of antiseptic surgery in 1867. Sir William died in 1932. The **Fetlar Interpretive Centre**, almost opposite Leagarth House, should not be missed. It is a treasure trove of island history.

The road continues through pleasant green valleys to the east coast settlement, and old haaf station, of **Funzie** [fin-ee], a picturesque collection of cottages, many of which are unfortunately deserted. As the name suggests, it was here that the very first Vikings are said to have settled. The land in summer is swathed in wildflowers and on almost every rocky headland there is a lichen-covered ruined broch. The cliffs here are not as high as elsewhere but their rugged serpentine rock-faces are full of colour. **Funzie Bay** was the site of a haaf fishing station in the 19th century.

Under Baa-naap is a rocky point called **Heilinabretta** where the Danish ship, *Wendela*, ran aground and sank in 1737 [HU675911]. She was carrying a large quantity of unspecified silver currency, most of which was immediately salvaged by the islanders. A diving team in the 1970s investigated the wreck and collected a number of silver coins in the area. Unauthorised diving is forbidden.

Broken cairns top Vord Hill and, below, the landscape is dotted with ancient mounds. The view from here is magnificent. The whole island can be seen stretching from The Snap, a headland beneath the Coastguard Lookout-point in the south-east, to **Hamars Ness** near the ferry pier in the north-west; and from **Rams Ness** in the south to **Strandburgh Ness** in the east. The latter has a tiny islet, **Outer Brough**, beside it with the remains of a broch and ancient settlement. Great natural arches in the Wick of Gruting (ON – stony area) flank **Kirn of Gula**, a blowhole, where fishermen took refuge in the 18th century when the press-gangs called [HU645931]. Beneath the cliffs of East Neap are rock-stacks, including the remarkable shape of **The Clett** [HU641944] off Busta Pund with, believe it or not, a hermitage perched on it! The sea between Fetlar and Bluemull Sound is sprinkled with low-lying islets including **Daaey**, **Urie Lingey** and **Sund Gruney** (ON – south green island).

* * *

Access: Ro-ro ferry several times daily from Gutcher, Yell, or Belmont, Unst, 01957-722259. Tourist Information, 01595-693434.

Anchorages:

1. Vehicle-ferry terminal at Oddsta, Hamars Ness, in NW is reserved for ferry only.
2. Brough Lodge, W coast. Convenient temp. anchorage except in W'lies. Anchor off the pier and below the tower, N of Ness of Brough, in 4–6m. Good holding.
3. Wick of Tresta. Good shelter if wind W or N, but swell comes in with W gales. Open to SE. Head shoals. Anchor in 6–8m sand, good holding. Approach on central course and beware rock 2c E of Head of Lambhoga. Magnetic anomalies.
4. Wick of Gruting. Good shelter in S winds. Open N. Keep 1c off all shores. Anchor centre-bay E or W of Ness of Gruting in 10m sand, good holding.

11.25 Hascosay

[ha-skoa-say] (ON huskot-øy – cottage or cottages island) or (ON haf-skogen-øy – sea-wood or driftwood island).

OS Maps: 1:50000 Sheet 1 or 2 1:25000 Sheet 470
Admiralty Charts: 1:75000 No.3282 1:30000 No.3292

Area: 275ha (680 acres)
Height: 30m (98 ft)

Owner: Part of the Nicolson of Fetlar estate inherited in the 1980s by Mrs O Borland of Edinburgh, a niece of Lady Nicolson.

Population: 1841–42 (6 houses). 1851–13. 1861–0 Uninhabited since.

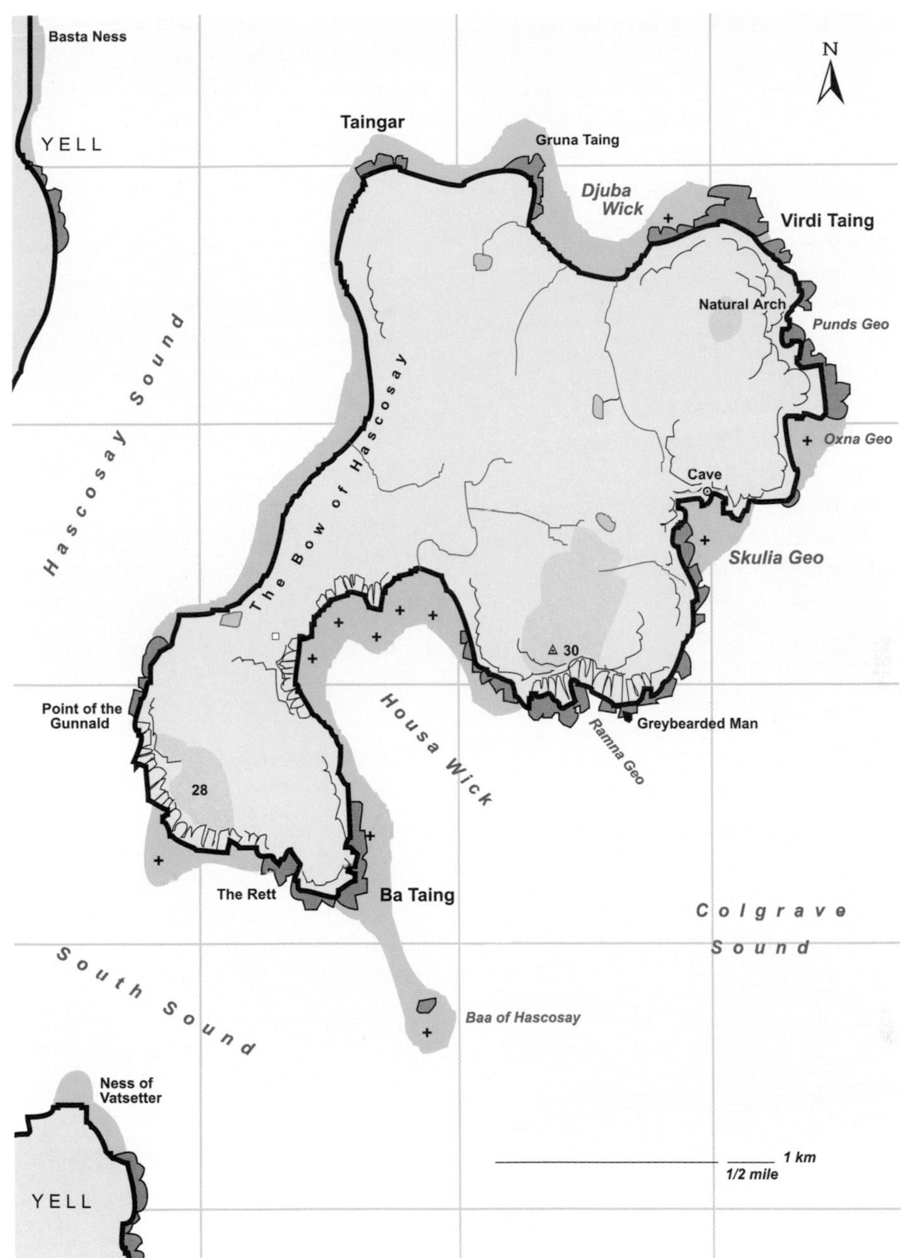

Geology: The bedrock is a coarse micaceous gneiss.

History: A branch of the Edmondston family once owned the island and a James Edmondston is named as laird of Hascosay in 1645.

Hascosay was home to a small but thriving community until it was bought by Sir Arthur Nicolson, the laird who cleared much of Fetlar for sheep in the mid-19th century. His house on Fetlar, Brough Lodge, overlooked Hascosay and this may have been why the islanders decided to leave before they were forcibly evicted. On the other hand, the trouble may merely have been lack of a good supply of fresh water and nothing to do with Sir Arthur.

Wildlife: Hascosay is an RSPB reserve and a Special Area of Conservation on account of its blanket bog. So, although it is reputed to have magic soil which keeps mice away, removing its soil would not be appreciated.

The BBC cameraman, Hugh Miles, visited Hascosay with the renowned Shetland ornithologist, Bobby Tulloch, in 1979, to make a BBC *Wildtrack* programme on otters. Hascosay is noted for its otters but on this occasion they failed to appear and the film was eventually shot on Fetlar and (Basta Voe) Yell. Nevertheless, Tulloch's books include many of his beautiful photographs of the Hascosay otters.

* * *

HASCOSAY has an undulating surface, the highest point being 30m above the south-west bluff. The island is criss-crossed with burns or rivulets fed by several small pools, none of which is large enough to merit the title of lochan and none of which provides a supply of good drinking water. Even when the pools are filled with rainwater they quickly turn brackish with the salt-spray and there is only one rather inadequate well. **Housa Wick** (ON – house bay) is an attractive rocky inlet which cuts deep into the island in the south-west. On a shallow isthmus behind it are the walls of the Edmondston's old hall which they vacated before 1800. There is also the site of a chapel but it is not known to whom it was dedicated.

A smaller bay on the north side is used for fish-farming. It is called **Djuba Wick** (ON – deep bay) but with a depth of less than 10m according to the Admiralty Chart the derivation of the name is open to conjecture.

The broken cliffs in the south fall away to **The Rett** (ON – the straight) and **Ba Taing** (ON – point of the underwater rock). On the opposite headland of Housa Wick there are more cliffs and an off-shore stack called **Greybearded Man**. Continuing up the west coast there is **Skulia Geo** (ON – hiding-hole inlet) with a submerged rock concealed in the middle of the geo and a fair-sized cave to explore on its shore. Nearby the rocks form a natural arch. There are a number of fine caverns on Hascosay.

* * *

Access: No regular access. Try Muckle Flugga Charters, 01806-522447, or Tourist Information, 01595-693434.

Anchorages: No recommended anchorages.

1. The Bow of Hascosay, Hascosay Sound. Temp. anchorage at N end of Bow in 5–10m.

2. Housa Wick. Temp. anchorage in centre of Wick, 8–10m. The head is foul. Beware Baa of Hascosay 3½c SSE of Ba Taing.

11.26 Uyea

[yoo-ay] Possibly (ON ve-øy – home island or island of the sacred place).

OS Maps: 1:50000 Sheet 1 1:25000 Sheet 470
Admiralty Charts: 1:75000 No.3282 1:30000 No.3292

Area: 205ha (507 acres)
Height: 50m (164 ft)

Owner: Sold by Jim Smith, a local farmer, in 1990 for about £100,000 including the livestock (320 sheep) and the islet of Wedder Holm. It was bought by Peter Hunter of Uyeasound on Unst, a crofter and salmon-farmer.

Population: 1841–23 (3 houses). 1881–5. 1891–8 (1 house). 1931–12. 1961–0. 1981–0. 1991–0. 2001–0.

Geology: Hornblende-schists in the west, mica-schists in the east.

History: Uyea Hall was the five-bedroom home of Basil Neven-Spence who was the Member of Parliament for Orkney and Shetland from 1935 until he was defeated in 1950 by Jo Grimond. Sir Basil is buried in the chapel cemetery.

Wildlife: Although mice are plentiful on Unst, there are none on Uyea we are told. Maybe some of Hascosay's magic soil is responsible (see No.11.25).

Otters can be seen by the shores, and many seals.

* * *

UYEA is only two-thirds the size of Vaila (No.11-10) but is similar in respect that it is dominated by a single large house originally built by the owner. On Uyea **The Hall** stands amid a group of structures on the central ridge near the middle of the island and is therefore fairly conspicuous. The highest point on the ridge is 50m.

Farm roads or tracks lead from a bay on the north coast with a rough jetty on the foreshore to the main house.

There are a number of antiquities which mirror those just across the sound on Unst. Part of the old chapel beside **Brei Wick** (ON – broad bay) dates from the 12th century [HU608985], while **Tur Ness**, just north of Brei Wick, is the site of an ancient settlement. At the northern end of the island there is a chambered cairn representing even earlier times.

Quite close to **Hawks Ness**, the southern extremity, is an islet called **Wedder Holm** (ON – ram islet) and further away to the east is the small island of **Haaf Gruney** (ON *hafgroenøy* – green island in the fishing grounds). This island is now classified as a national nature reserve on account of its colony of breeding storm petrel. The remains of a disused chromate mine are on it and its green pastures have for long been used for grazing.

In the early 18th century two young girls from Uyea rowed themselves over to Haaf Gruney to milk the cows. On their return a storm blew up and increased in fury. For several days they could do nothing but bail and hang on until they were at last cast ashore on the island of Karmøy off the south-west coast of Norway. The superstitious islanders at first took fright but when one of the girls made the sign of the Cross they helped them. In any case there was a severe shortage of women on Karmøy at the time so, needless to say, before long the girls were happily married and their descendants still live there today.

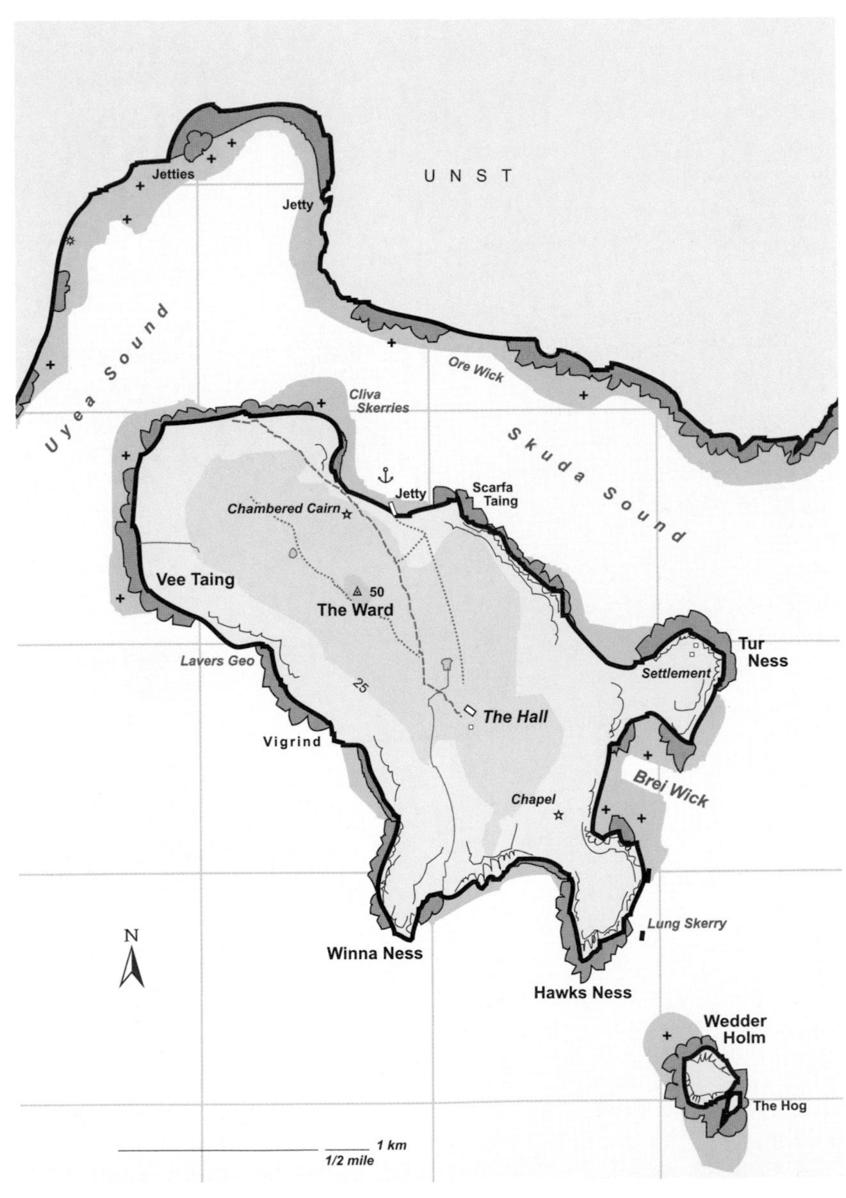

Access: No regular access. Try Muckle Flugga Charters, 01806-522447, a boat-owner in Uyeasound, or Tourist Information, 01595-693434.

Anchorages:

1. Skuda Sound, bay W of Scarfa Taing. Anchor off the jetty in 5–6m, mud and sand. Reasonable shelter and holding. Beware Cliva Skerries, W of the bay.
2. Bay on S side between Winna Ness and Hawks Ness. Temp. anchorage in suitable conditions. Approach and anchor centrally towards the head in 5–6m.
3. Brei Wick. Avoid. Shallow and foul.

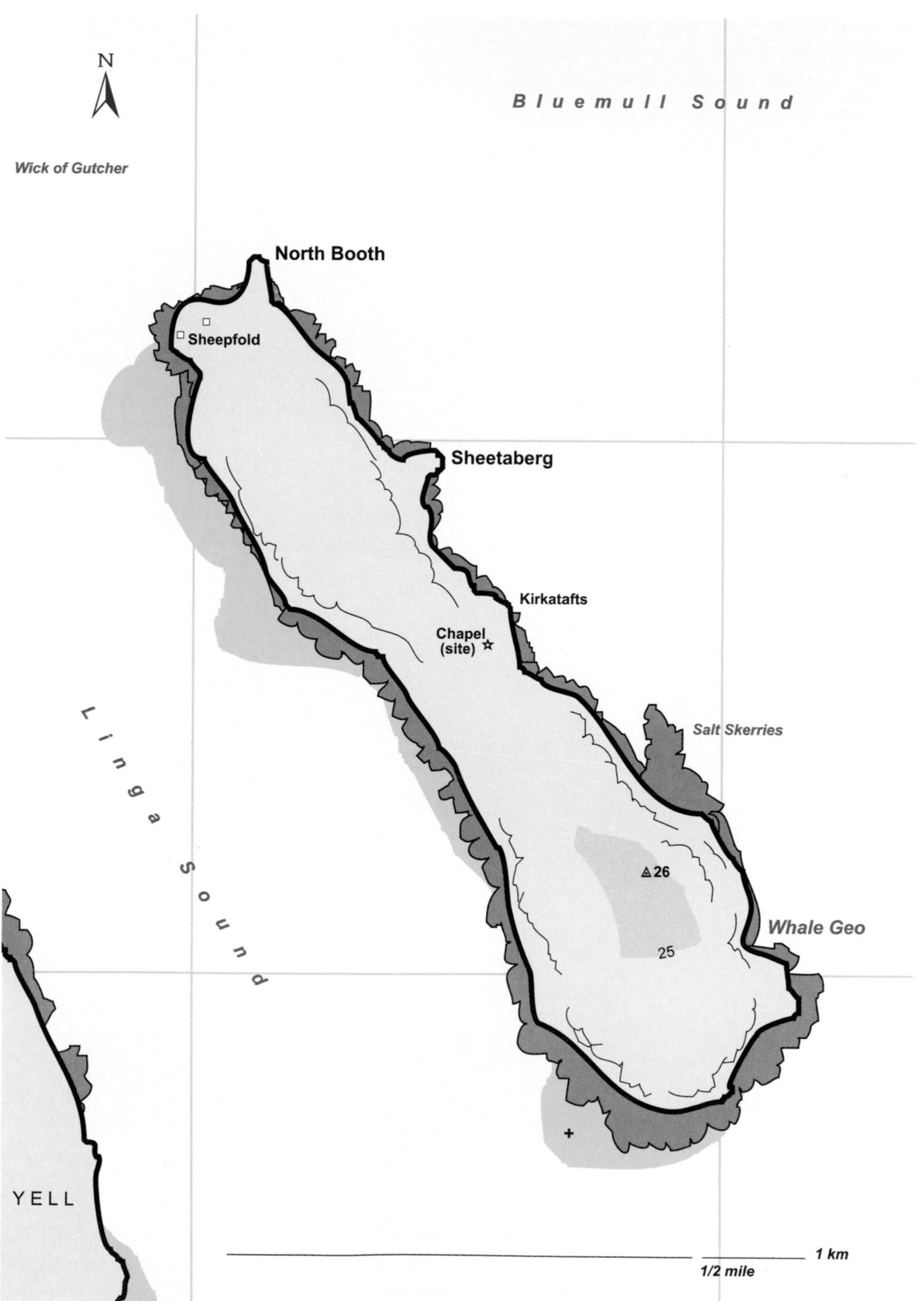

11.27 Linga

(ON lyng-øy – heather island).

OS Maps: 1:50000 Sheet 1 1:25000 Sheet 470
Admiralty Charts: 1:75000 No.3282 1:30000 No.3292

Area: 45ha (111 acres)
Height: 26m (85 ft)

Owner: The island was bought in the 1980s by a Mr Renwick who started building a pseudo-Norman castle at North Booth, but was refused planning permission. He abandoned the project (and many unused concrete blocks) and sold out to Charles Henderson of Yell. He, in turn, sold Linga to an American lady but kept the crofting rights and uses the land for grazing sheep.

Population: No Census records and uninhabited.

Geology: A bedrock of coarse mica-schist and gneiss.

Wildlife: In spite of its name, very little heather is to be found on Linga. Many seabirds breed here – particularly guillemot – and there are resident otters. Seals breed in the season.

* * *

LINGA is a long narrow island lying roughly parallel to the coast of Yell, and separated from it by Linga Sound. This is a fairly secluded corner of Shetland – if anywhere in this part of the world can truly be called secluded. Yell holds out two tentative arms, Head of Gutcher and Burra Ness (with a ruined broch on it) to shelter the waters of Linga Sound. There is often little in the way of activity in or near the Sound except for the ferry plying its path between Gutcher on Yell and Oddsta on Fetlar.

The long low ridge of Linga reaches a maximum height of 26m near its southern end. It has few known antiquities but there is the site of an old chapel [HU559986], which would indicate that it might have had a number of inhabitants at some time. The source of an adequate supply of fresh water is a puzzle although it may have been brought over by boat from neighbouring Yell. The island is now used for grazing sheep.

There is said to be a ring of green turf on the island (although its position is elusive!) called the **Bear's Bait**. An ancient Norse tale says that Jan Tait of Fetlar killed one of the King of Norway's men after an argument and the King had him brought to Norway to answer for the crime. After the King had spoken to Jan he was so impressed by his courage and candour that he promised to grant him his freedom provided he captured a giant bear that was causing trouble in the district. Jan put out a barrel of drugged butter for the bear to eat and had no trouble capturing it and taking it to the King. The King kept his promise and granted him his freedom but he was surprised that Jan had not killed the bear. He ordered him to do so and then to leave Norway forthwith. Jan, however, was proud of his capture and wanted to show it to his friends so he brought the bear back to Shetland and kept it tethered on Linga. The ring marks the spot where the poor old bear walked round and round its stake for the rest of its days.

Access: No regular access. Try Muckle Flugga Charters, 01806-522447, or Tourist Information, 01595-693434.

Anchorages: No recommended anchorages.
1. Linga Sound. Temp. anchorage in suitable conditions off the mid-point of the W coast in 3–6m. Approach with caution and use tripping line.

11.28 Balta

Perhaps (ON Balti-øy – Balti's island) from the man's name.

OS Maps: 1:50000 Sheet 1 1:25000 Sheet 470
Admiralty Charts: 1:75000 No.3282 1:12500 No.3293

Area: 80ha (198 acres)
Height: 44m (144 ft)

Population: No Census records and uninhabited now.

Geology: Metagabbros interspersed with some hornblende-schist.

History: The remains of a broch at South Sail at the top of the northern cliffs may once have had a 'brother' broch across the Sound on Swinna Ness – they often came in pairs – but there is no record of it. It does suggest, however, that Balta was inhabited at that time.

Wildlife: The eastern cliffs provide residential sites for nesting seabirds. A Glaucus gull nested for several years on nearby Huney during the 1980s.

* * *

BALTA is a long narrow island like Linga (No.11.27) but with a more complex shape. It has three hills spaced along its length, the central one at **Muckle Head** (S. – big head) being the highest (44m). The southern hill is 38m high.

The east coast, facing the stormy North Sea, consists of steep cliffs broken by fissures and rocky coves and with tumbled half-submerged rock-falls close to the foot where they have not slipped away down the steep submarine slopes. There is a shallower patch, **Salta Skerry**, at the southern extremity of the island. Heavy seas break over this area when the wind is in the south-east. The whole of this east coast is slowly being eroded by the sea which pounds against it relentlessly.

The rock strata tips the whole island up towards the east while the west side is low-lying with a short stretch of sandy beach extending up the slope at South Links. Balta has the best dune grassland in Shetland but it is steadily

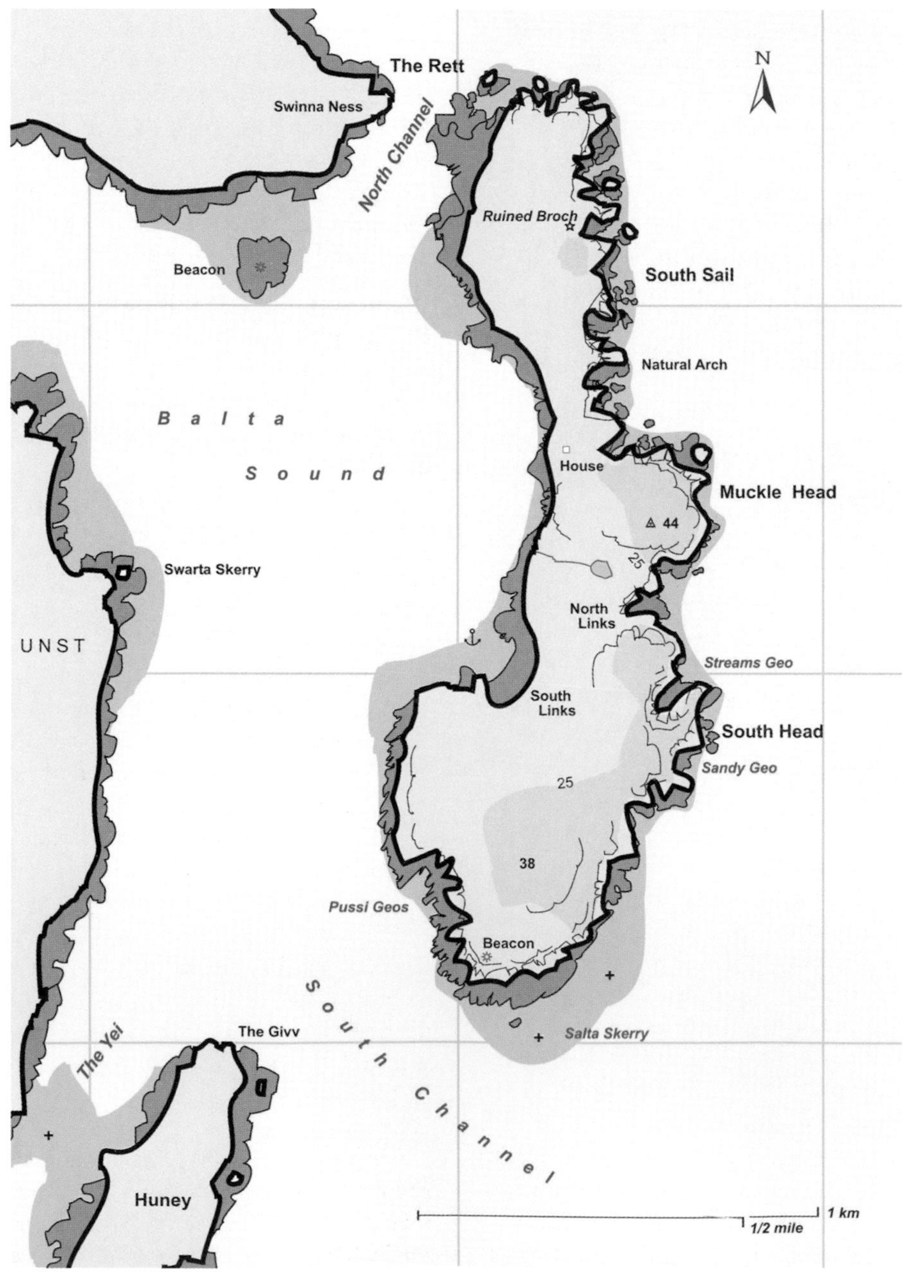

deteriorating due to wind erosion, rabbit damage and, possibly, overgrazing. The shallow western bay protects Shetland's most northerly fish farm.

Apart from the broch ruin at **South Sail** [HP660089], another site of archaeological interest is that of an ancient chapel dedicated to the popular Norse saint, St Sunniva.

Balta Sound was a busy and popular harbour in the early 1900s and the island must have seen a lot of activity as hundreds of brown-sailed luggers of the Scottish fishing fleet bustled in and out to off-load their herring catches.

In 1917 a Royal Navy submarine, *E49*, struck a mine and sank in Balta Sound. The wreck, which lies at a depth of thirty-five metres, is classed as a 'war grave' and permission to dive must be obtained from the Ministry of Defence.

On the west side of South Channel is the small uninhabited island of **Huney** which has a flat grassy top about 19m high. There is a narrow channel called the Yei between Huney and the coast of Unst which is full of rocks and sand-banks but which the local fishermen negotiate with ease (at the right state of the tide).

* * *

Access: Try Muckle Flugga Charters, 01806-522447, a boat owner at Baltasound or Tourist Information, 01595-693434.

Anchorages: Approach mid-channel by S Channel when entering Balta Sound. The N Channel is tricky and requires great care.

1. Mid E-side of Balta. Good anchorage and well sheltered except for S–SW in which case move to the Unst side. Best spot with Buness House, Unst, in line with Skeo Taing but may be obstructed by fish cages. Anchor as near Balta as depth permits, sand.

11.29 Unst

[unst – not oonst] Derivation obscure and may be of Pictish origin, but possibly (ON ørn-vist – home of the eagle or erne).

O S Maps: 1:50000 Sheet 1 1:25000 Sheet 470
Admiralty Charts: 1:75000 No.3282 1:30000 No.3292 southern part only 1:12500 No.3293 Balta Sound only

Area: 12068ha (29820 acres)
Height: 284m (932 ft)
Owner: Multiple ownership. Family descendants of Saxby (who wrote *Birds of Shetland*) and Edmonston (*A Flora of Shetland*) still have sizeable land-holdings, as do John and Wendy Scott of Garth.

Population: 1798–1688 (300 houses) approx. 1831–2730. 1841–2808 (517 houses). 1881–2173. 1891–2269 (470 houses). 1931–1326. 1961–1148. 1981–1140. 1991–1055. 2001 –720.

Geology: Unst has a complex but fascinating geology. The western side, defined by Loch of Cliff and the Loch of Watlee by Valla Field is coarse-grained gneiss, sometimes studded with tiny garnets, under peat moorland, which is very similar to that of adjacent Yell. The eastern side is composed of metagabbro and serpentine interspersed with schists. The serpentine has veins of iron chromate, and black and green jasper. A complex dislocation zone divides these two zones.

Limestone can be found in the south and talc at Haroldswick in the north-east. Unst has the only surviving talc mine in Britain.

History: Harolds Wick is named after King Harald Haarfagr (Fair-hair) who anchored here in 875 after first visiting Fetlar (No.11.24). Norway was being harassed by Viking, or pirate, raids from Shetland and Orkney so the king visited the islands and annexed them in the name of Norway. The pirates were, in any case, probably descendants of Scandinavian settlers.

Wildlife: This was the home of Thomas Edmonston, who published *A Flora of Shetland* in 1845, when he was still in his teens. He discovered the Norwegian Sandwort here in the Keen of Hamar which is found nowhere else in Britain but North Ronaldsay (No.10.27) and Rum (No.4.3), and protected by law since 1981, and the Shetland Mouse-ear Chickweed, which is unique to Unst. Edmondston was killed accidentally by a musket during an Amazon expedition when he was still a young man.

The Keen of Hamar is now a National Nature Reserve and the Warden's permission is needed to enter, 01463-239431. It is a remarkable site of broken serpentine scree. A number of other unusual and rare plants such as the fragrant and frog orchids can also be found here and occasionally elsewhere on Unst.

Small groups of Shetland ponies, whose numbers are in decline elsewhere, can still be seen on Unst. There are no bats, weasels, frogs, toads, hedgehogs or adders but there are plenty

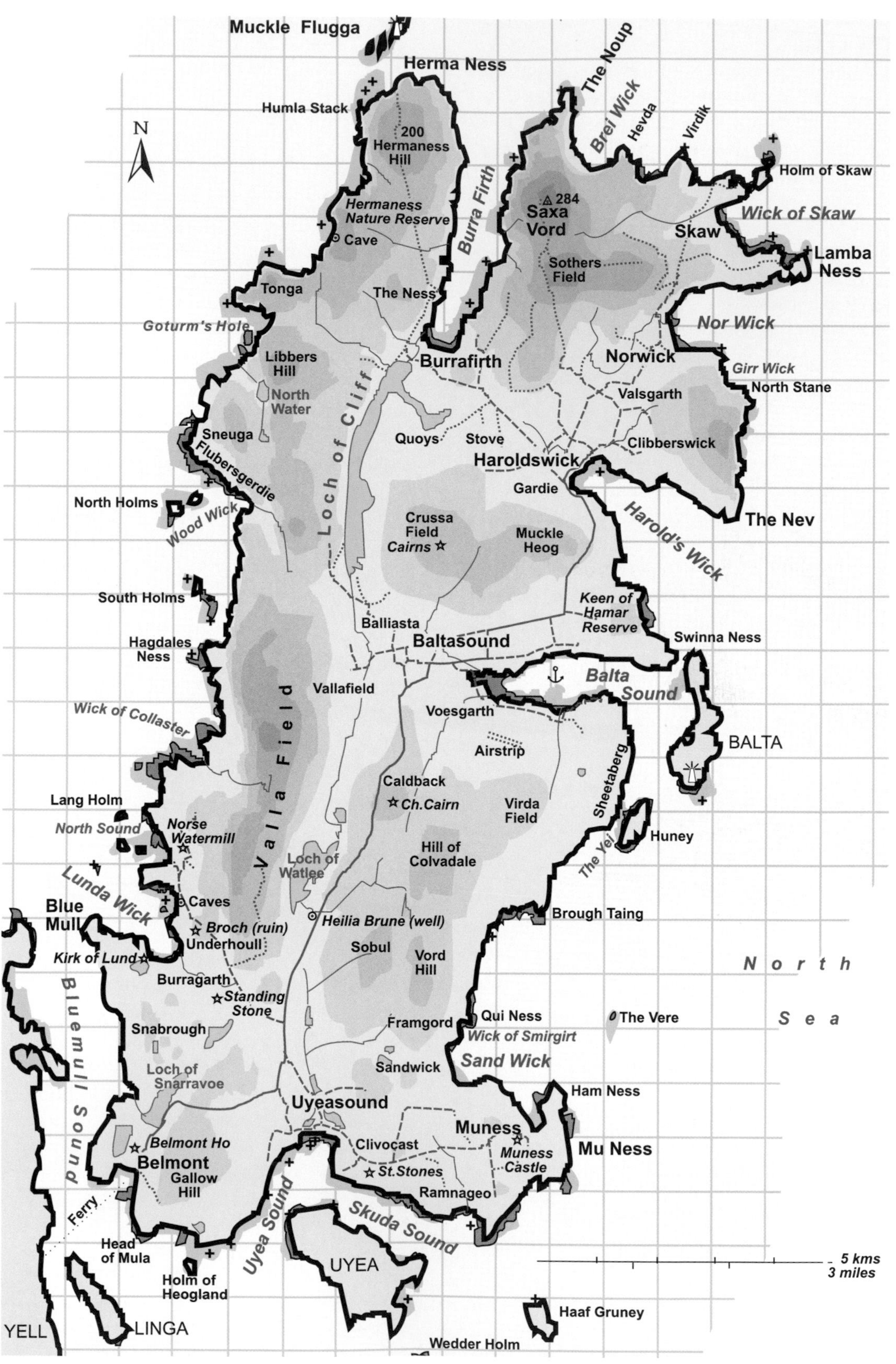
Muckle Flugga
Herma Ness
Humla Stack
N
200
Hermaness
Hill
Hermaness
Nature Reserve
Cave
Burra Firth
The Noup
Brei Wick
Hevda
Virdik
Holm of Skaw
284
Saxa
Vord
Wick of Skaw
Skaw
Lamba
Ness
Sothers
Field
Tonga
The Ness
Goturm's Hole
Nor Wick
Libbers
Hill
North
Water
Burrafirth
Norwick
Girr Wick
North Stane
Valsgarth
Loch of Cliff
Sneuga
Quoys
Stove
Clibberswick
Haroldswick
Flubersgerdie
Gardie
North Holms
Wood Wick
Crussa
Field
Cairns
Muckle
Heog
The Nev
Harold's Wick
South Holms
Keen of
Hamar
Reserve
Balliasta
Hagdales
Ness
Baltasound
Swinna Ness
Vallafield
Balta
Sound
Wick of Collaster
Voesgarth
Airstrip
BALTA
Valla Field
Caldback
Sheetaberg
Ch.Cairn
Lang Holm
Virda
Field
North Sound
Norse
Watermill
Huney
Hill of
Colvadale
Loch of
Watlee
The Yei
Lunda Wick
Caves
Blue
Mull
Heilia Brune (well)
Brough Taing
Broch (ruin)
Underhoull
Kirk of Lund
Sobul
Vord
Hill
North
Bluemull Sound
Burragarth
Standing
Stone
Snabrough
Qui Ness
The Vere
Sea
Framgord
Wick of Smirgirt
Sand Wick
Sandwick
Loch of
Snarravoe
Ham Ness
Uyeasound
Muness
Belmont Ho
Clivocast
Muness
Castle
Mu Ness
Belmont
Gallow
Hill
St.Stones
Ramnageo
Ferry
Uyea Sound
Skuda Sound
Head
of Mula
5 kms
3 miles
UYEA
Holm of
Heogland
Haaf Gruney
YELL
LINGA
Wedder Holm

of rabbits. Rats were first recorded in 1903, and otters are common.

Hermaness National Nature Reserve is one of the few breeding sites of a rare moth and the cliffs of this, Britain's most northerly peninsula, hold one of our largest seabird colonies. 10,000 pairs of fulmar, the same of gannet, 5000 pairs of kittiwake, 16,000 pairs of guillemot, 2000 pairs of razorbill, and some 25,000 pairs of puffin have been recorded. There are a small number of arctic skua and, this being with Foula the last stronghold of the bonxie (great skua) when it was nearing extinction, now boasts at least 800 pairs.

It is also at Hermaness that the famous black-browed albatross returned each spring from the early 1970s to the late 1990s. A vagrant from the South Seas and trapped in the northern hemisphere, it kept hoping to find a mate. It occasionally winked at a passing gannet but was always violently rebuffed.

Many seabirds visit Bluemull Sound, particularly in winter and early spring, when eider and tysties (black guillemot) breed here.

* * *

Britain's most northerly inhabited island, **UNST** is one of the most interesting in the Shetland group. It has its share of dreich peat moorland, particularly in the west, but the cliff scenery is spectacular.

The ferry from Yell (No.11.23) docks at the chunks of serpentine which make up Belmont pier. The shell of **Belmont House**, a Lowland-style mansion built in 1777, can be seen across the fields [HP565010]. The main road branches off to Uyeasound, past standing stones, and on to **Muness Castle** [HP629011]. This desolate ruin in a desolate landscape could have been devised by Edgar Allen Poe for *The Fall of the House of Usher*. It was built in 1598 by Lawrence Bruce of Cultmalindie in Perthshire, an evil man and a relative of the notorious tyrant Earl Patrick. Bruce also built the castle at Scalloway on Mainland (No.11.11). Muness is a handsome ruin, a high stone rectangle with circular towers and similarity of detail to the Earl's Palace in Kirkwall (No.10.10) built in the same period. Above the entrance is inscribed (the Shetland phonetics are unmistakable):

> 'List ze to knaw yis bulding quha began
> Laurence the Bruce he was that worthy
> man quha ernestly his airis and ofspring
> prayis to help and not to hurt this vark
> aluayis – the zeir of God 1598'

In spite of this urgent plea, the work at Muness Castle was soon destroyed, for the castle burned down in the 17th century. The history of the disaster is confused. One story in Norn verse claims it was a certain Hakki of Dikkeram, possibly in response to the abduction of a girl called Helga and the murder of her father by one of the Bruce family. Another story claims the castle was sacked and torched by French privateers.

Beside Mu Ness (ON – maiden headland) is the islet of **Hunts Holm** and to the north a Norse

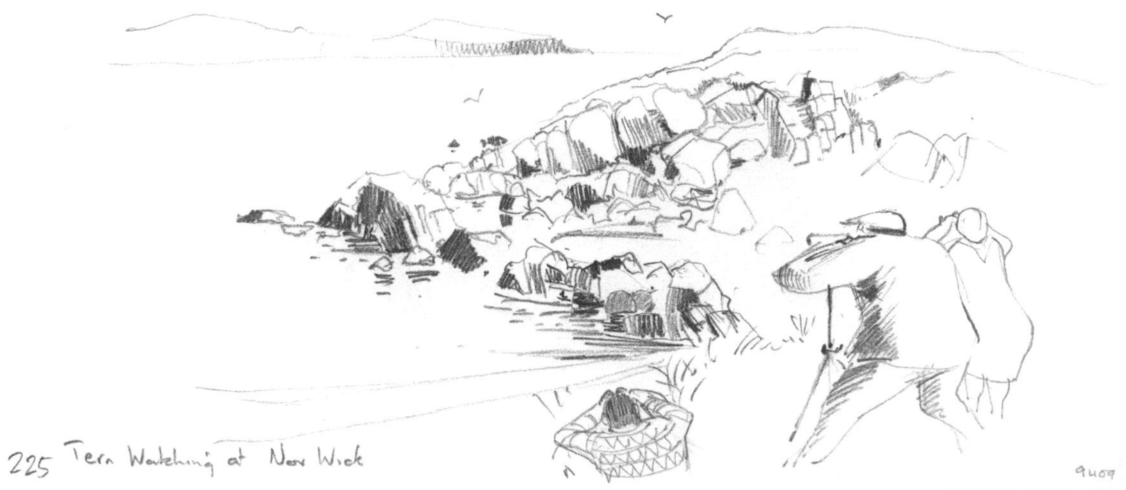

TERN WATCHERS AT NOR WICK

settlement has been excavated at **Sandwick**.

A branch to the west off the main spinal road leads to a track which passes **Bordastubble**, Shetland's largest standing stone [HP579034], and arrives at **Lunda Wick**. Here there is the ruin of the 12th-century **Lund Church**, last used for worship in 1785 [HP566041]. In the cemetery are the 16th-century graves of two Bremen merchants, probably representatives of the Hanseatic trade. (See Whalsay, No.11.15.) Lund Church – or St Olaf's Chapel – is built on **Blue Mull**, the headland which gives its name to Bluemull Sound. The mull is best admired from the sea, where it has a distinct blue colour when seen from the distance. On the opposite side of Lunda Wick at **Underhoull** are grass-covered earthworks surrounding the ruin of a broch [HP575044]. A 9th-century Viking longhouse, excavated in the 1960s, was built on an earlier Iron Age site. Further north, where the road crosses a burn, there is a restored Norse-type horizontal click mill.

Islets are scattered about North Sound, north of Lunda Wick, called **Lang Holm**, **Round Holm**, **The Vere** and **Brough Holm**. As expected, this latter islet has the remains of yet another broch on it. Further north up this dramatic coastline are two more groups, **North Holms** and **South Holms**, which has a subterranean passage.

The main road continues over a relatively featureless landscape with the ridge of **Valla Field** (ON – hill of mythological battle) to the west reflected in the brown waters of **Loch of Watlee**. The wishing well of **Helia Brune** [HP594046] is beside the loch and there are a few scattered chambered cairns. It is interesting, by the way, to note a resemblance between the map of Unst and Robert Louis Stevenson's map of Treasure Island. RLS visited Unst after his Uncle David had built Muckle Flugga lighthouse. Not long after the visit he began writing *Treasure Island*.

Baltasound is Unst's 'capital' with two hotels and an airstrip. The Swedish Church was built in 1910 and used by Scandinavian fishermen until the 1950s. The Sound used to be the centre of the northern herring industry and in its heyday had a seasonal population of 10,000, but its main use as a port today is for the export of talc. It is also a collection point for the oil industry – hence the busy little airfield.

To reach the large scattered settlement of **Haroldswick** the road skirts **Crussa Field** and **Muckle Heog**, hills which have clusters of ancient cairns on them. One is called Harald's Grave and is supposed to be the burial site for King Harald the Fair-haired. Haroldswick has the most northern post-office in Britain and is always happy to frank your letters accordingly.

Nor Wick, a bay with a glorious sweep of beach and weathered rocks, is an old haaf fishing station site. In 1700 a sea-eagle stole a baby girl, Mary Anderson, from the croft on the hill above the wick and carried her off to its eyrie on the cliffs of Fetlar. This was seen by a Fetlar islander and a young boy, Robert Nicolson, was lowered down to the nest by rope. He rescued the baby and she was returned unharmed to Unst and, according to the story which is sworn to be true, when Mary grew up, Robert married her and the happy couple settled in Yell and raised a family.

At **Wick of Skaw**, Britain's most northerly dwelling, a croft farmhouse, nestles among marsh marigolds in a small valley by the beach. One of the outhouses is made from an old upturned boat [HP658164], – normal island practice where nothing is wasted.

A visit to the summit of **Saxa Vord** (ON – Saxa's lookout), Unst's highest point at 284m is no 'big deal' as there is a road climbing the one thousand feet or so to the top. The view is breathtaking. The furthest outpost of the British Isles, **Out Stack** – or 'Oosta' – is only 3km further north. Lady Franklin landed on this bare rock in 1849 and prayed for her husband when he failed to return from his North West Passage expedition. Out Stack may be in the lead but **Muckle Flugga** with its lighthouse, built by David Stevenson in 1858 for £32,000 and surrounded by wheeling seabirds, is close behind. (It was automated in 1995.) Beneath one's feet are some of Shetland's most spectacular cliff-scenery and the deep, beautiful, but ominous, cleft of **Burra Firth**. At the entrance to Burra Firth there is a 100m-long natural tunnel through the rock at **Hol Hellier** through which a dinghy can sail on a calm day. Looking back, to the south, the firth almost meets the long and narrow Loch of Cliff, which in turn leads to a distant valley stretching the length of Unst, splitting the island longitudinally. Across the Burra Firth, the **Herma Ness** peninsula is a wild area almost uncontaminated by man. It is a Nature Reserve run by Scottish Natural Heritage.

The Ministry of Defence has had radar and other installations on and around Saxa Vord since the 1950s but these were closed in 2005 with devastating consequences for the island population. This is a windy place. In 1962 an unofficial all-British wind speed record of 177mph was recorded on top of Saxa Vord. It may have reached a higher speed but the anemometer blew away.

Saxa was a giant who lived on Saxa Vord and Herma was another giant who lived on Hermaness Hill and they were always quarrelling; or so the story goes. One day, Herma, using a ship's mast as a fishing rod, caught a whale for supper and asked Saxa to boil it for him in his kettle. (Saxa's Kettle is a huge rock-cup in Nor Wick in which the tide boils and gurgles.) Saxa agreed provided he could keep most for himself but Herma objected to this. The giants started throwing stones at each other and one of the stones which Herma threw can be seen on the west side of Saxa Vord and a stone which Saxa threw is a skerry on the west shore of Burra Firth called **Saxa's Baa**.

I suppose it is fitting that the end of the world should be a land of giants, for there is nothing beyond here but the icy wastes of the Arctic.

* * *

Access: Frequent daily ro-ro ferry service from Gutcher, Yell (10 mins), 01957-722259. Tourist Information, 01595-693434.

Anchorages:

1. Uyea Sound. Fairly good shelter except from S'lies.There is a pier on NW side at head of sound. Anchor NE side in suitable depth, mud and sand. If caught by S'lies try Skuda Sound. See Uyea (No.11.26).
2. Sand Wick, Ham of Muness. Exposed NW–N–E. Temp. anchorage towards head of bay in 3–6m. Head shoals to shingle beach. Approach needs care.
3. Balta Sound, only safe all-weather anchorage on Unst. Pontoon berth W of main pier (charge) is accessible at all states of the tide or anchor where suitable but best SW of pier,4-8m, mud. Good holding.
4. Harolds Wick. Exposed SE–E. Temp. anchorage near E side of head but holding uncertain. Approach mid-channel. *(Visit Unst Boat Haven marine museum.)*
5. Nor Wick, on NE coast. Unsafe in E'lies. Temp. anchorage near centre of head, 8–10m, good holding in stiff grey sand.
6. Wick of Skaw. Dangerous due to tidal roost. Best to avoid this area by at least 1M.
7. Burra Firth. Exposed N. Sides high and steep-to but wide sandy beach 2½M up firth at head. Easy access. Temp. anchorage off beach, holding good. *(Hermaness Visitor Centre.)*
8. Muckle Flugga. No anchorage and landing only possible in fine weather at steps cut in rock.
9. Lunda Wick, just E of Blue Mull. Sheltered S and E, otherwise exposed. Anchor in SE towards head, sand and mud, holding good. Approach with care S of mid-channel.
10. Wick of Belmont, off Bluemull Sound. Vehicle ferry terminal at head with berthing reserved exclusively for ferry. Rocky bottom.

SECTION 12

The East Coast

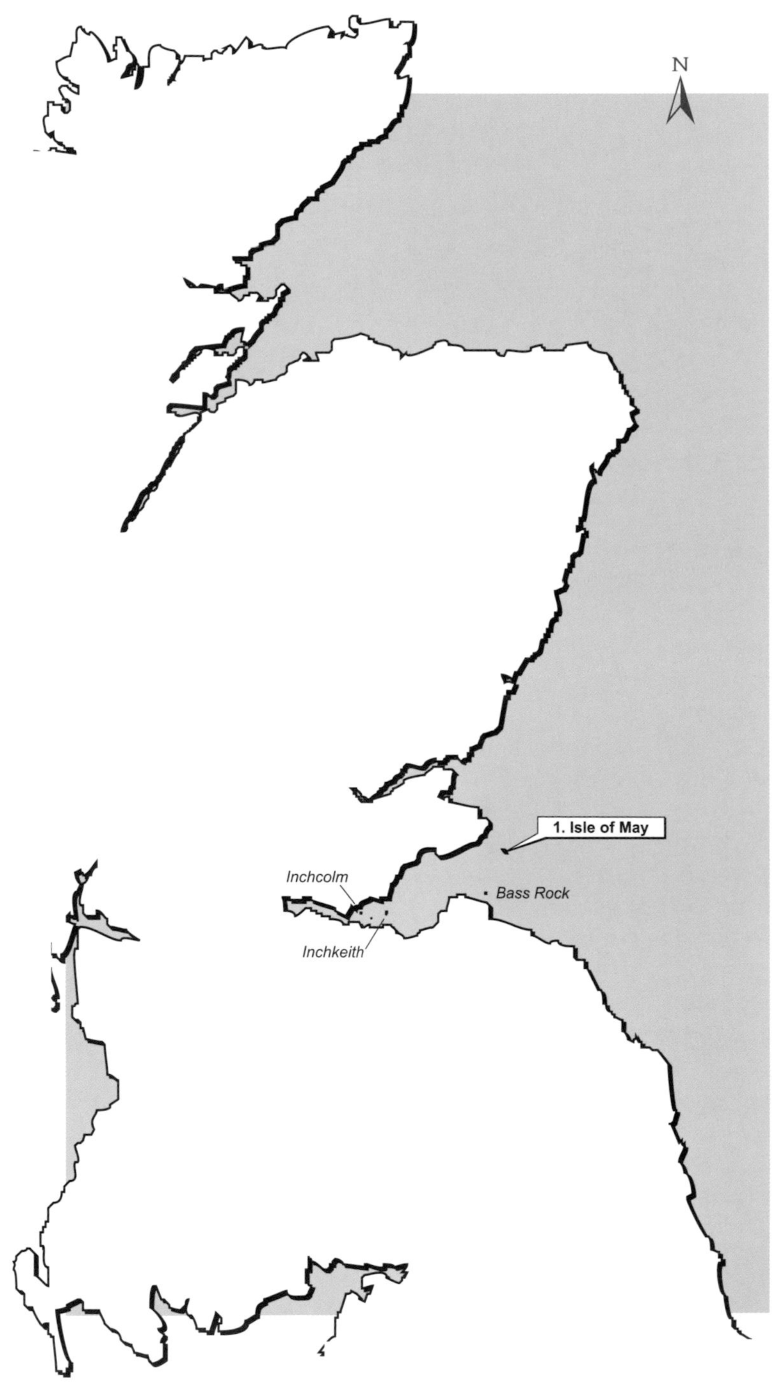

SECTION 12, Table 1: Arranged according to geographical position

No.	Name	Latitude	Longitude	Table 2* No.	Table 3** No.	Area in Acres	Area in Hectares
12.1	Isle of May	56° 11N	02° 33W	154	118	111	45
12.A	*Bass Rock*	*56° 05N*	*02° 38W*			*19*	*8*

*Table 2: The islands arranged accourding to magnitude
**Table 3: The islands arranged according to height

Introduction

It is remarkable that over the entire length of the east coast of mainland Scotland, from John o' Groats – or more accurately, Duncansby Head – to the border north of Berwick-upon-Tweed, there is only one island which comes within the terms of classification for this book by having an area of forty hectares or more. And even this single example – the Isle of May – only just meets the conditions as it is a mere forty-five hectares (111 acres) in area.

There are no islets really worth mentioning north of the Tay except, possibly, the **Halliman Skerries** off Branderburgh and Lossiemouth – a mere line of seaweed-covered rocks; a few broken shards of land at the extreme head of the Cromarty Firth; **Keith Inch** which is part of the docks at Peterhead; and **Inchbroach** which is part of Montrose.

In the Firth of Tay itself there is only the quaintly named **Mugdrum Island** (G. – hog-back island) while out in the open sea beyond the Firth is the lonely and infamous **Bell Rock**. During the 1980s, radio broadcasts had to drop Bell Rock readings from the inshore shipping forecasts when a fire gutted the interior of the lighthouse. The Bell Rock, incidentally, was originally known as **Inchcape** (G. – island stumbling-block), which is understandable as this tiny rock chip with some skerries around it is only just large enough to support a lighthouse and seems to be there for no logical reason. It was certainly the cause of many shipping tragedies (an average of six ships each year) before Robert Stevenson built the famous lighthouse which marked its position in 1811.

We have to look to the Firth of Forth to find every other islet on the east coast. The Isle of May has been mentioned. The Bass Rock, although below the classified size, is of such historic interest that it has been included as an appendix to this section. But the remaining little islands also have fascinating histories.

To the west of the Bass Rock is the rugged island of **Fidra** (ON – feathered arrow shape) with a broken reef, called the Briggs of Fidra, spanning between it and the shore. On the Briggs are the remains of a Cistercian Hermitage which belonged to a Nunnery founded at North Berwick in the 12th century. At the time of the Dissolution of the Monasteries in Scotland (1561) the North Berwick and Fidra sisterhood consisted of eleven nuns, each drawing an annual income of £20. Although this was a very comfortable income, and they came of good families, not one of them could sign her name. It is possible to anchor on the east, west or south sides of Fidra, although there is often an uncomfortable swell. On the east side there is a landing jetty for the lighthouse. The south anchorage is tricky because of the rocks and submarine cables.

Two smaller islets lie between Fidra and the Bass Rock – **Craigleith** and **Lamb**. The Lamb has a Dog guarding each side of it (they are skerries) while Craigleith's claim to fame is that it was used as a rabbit warren.

Further up the Forth, standing conspicuously foursquare in the middle of the seaway opposite the Port of Leith is **Inchkeith**. It is about half the size of the Isle of May but slightly higher and also has a lighthouse on the summit. It is now unkempt but it once supported a viable small farm with good pasturage and there are several springs providing drinking water. The geology, apart from a few beds of sandstone, is chiefly sheets of igneous rock separated by thin strata of sedimentary deposits – shale with many fossils, coal, and limestone.

The plant life is varied and I can vouch for the virility of the birdlife. During the nesting season the gulls strafe visitors relentlessly.

Some time between 679 and 704 St Adomnan, abbot of Iona, founded a 'school of the prophets' on the island and it was here that he met St Serf who had just arrived in Scotland from Rome. In 1010 Malcolm II rewarded Robert de Keth of the Catti (Chattan) clan from Caithness (Cattiness) for his assistance in repelling the Danes and gave him large estates which included Inchkeith and Dalkeith. This is the probable derivation of the name of the island although there are other possibilities. In 1497 the sufferers from a contagious disease called 'grandgore' were shipped from Edinburgh to a Hospital on Inchkeith. The crew of a plague-stricken ship was also quarantined here in 1580; more plague-victims were sent over in 1609; and in 1799 many Russian sailors who had died of an infectious disease were buried on the island.

In 1547 after the battle of Pinkie Cleugh, the victorious English general – the Duke of Somerset – landed marines on Inchkeith and ordered them to fortify the island. A large square fort with corner towers was accordingly built on the summit (site of the present lighthouse). Italian mercenaries held the fort for the English until 1549 when D'Essé, a French general, led a joint Scottish and French force in a brilliant manoeuvre which recaptured the island. The Queen Regent, Mary of Guise, landed on Inchkeith the following day to see the 'three and four hundred of her dead foes still unburied'. As the date of capture was June 29th – the day of *Fête Dieu* in France – she renamed the island *L'Ile de Dieu*. D'Essé demolished the fort and built a larger and stronger one on the same site with an outer surrounding wall and a moat crossed by a drawbridge. Mary, Queen of Scots inspected the French garrison of this fort in 1564 and the commemorative stone from the original gateway with the inscription 'M.R. 1564' can still be seen where it has been built into a wall beside the lighthouse.

After Mary's deposition the Castle of Inchkeith was ordered to be 'raisit' but ended up instead being used as a prison. However, it was refortified during the Cromwellian Wars and, even when the ubiquitous Dr Johnson visited Inchkeith with Boswell in 1773, Boswell noted that the fort was strongly built. It was not until 1808 that it was at last 'raisit' to make room for the lighthouse.

In 1878, after twenty years of deep thought, the Admiralty realised that Inchkeith had a commanding position in the Forth and decided to fortify it once again. They installed elaborate batteries at the three corners of the island designed by the Royal Engineers as three separate fortresses. Each battery is partly underground and these magnificent fortifications can still be explored today. In fact Inchkeith is an island so rich in history that it is surprising that it has not received more detailed archaeological study, particularly before all its valuable artefacts disappear. It also has, incidentally, Scotland's *lowest average rainfall* (21.75ins). Dr Johnson said: 'I'd have this island: I'd build a house... A rich man of an hospitable turn here, would have many visitors from Edinburgh'. When the lighthouse was made automatic, Inchkeith was purchased from the Lighthouse Commissioners by Sir Tom Farmer, a well-known Edinburgh businessman, but he has not yet followed Dr Johnson's advice.

Inchmickery (G. *innis na bhicaire* – isle of the vicar) is an insignificant islet lying between **Cramond Island** (which is a drying island, accessible at low water) and Inchcolm. It probably had some past connection with the abbey on Inchcolm. The story goes that James IV, who had an enquiring mind, wanted to discover the 'Original Language' of the human race. So he sent two newly born infants with a dumb nurse to live on uninhabited Inchmickery. After a year or two he and his courtiers seriously agreed that the children 'spak extremely guid Ebrew'.

The remnants of various Second World War fortifications make Inchmickery today an interesting piece of abstract sculpture.

Inchcolm (G. – island of St Columba) was named in the 12th century in memory of Columba's visit to it in about 567. Its old name was Aemonia or Emona. It is best known for the monastery which dominates its skyline and which was founded in 1123 by Alexander I. A century earlier when a Danish force under King Sueno entered the Firth of Forth and pillaged Fife with the support of an English force sent by Sueno's brother King Canute, Macbeth drove them off. In return for 'a great summe of gold' Macbeth agreed that the defeated invaders could bury their dead on St Colme's holy island (Shakespeare put the price at 'ten thousand dollars').

Naturally, as a well-endowed monastery, Inchcolm was fair game for plunder and an English ship first raided it in 1335 carrying off all the treasures including a famous image of St Columba. A storm almost wrecked the ship on Inchkeith so the sailors vowed to return the image if they survived. In due course they landed at Kinghorn, sent the image back to Inchcolm, and then sailed for home with the rest of the booty, a clear conscience, and a fair wind. There was another English raid in 1384 and this time the raiders tried to burn down the monastery, but St Columba sent a change of wind which put the fire out.

In 1547, after the battle of Pinkie Cleugh, the Monastery was fortified, and there were occasions when it was, like the Castles of Inchkeith and Inchgarvie, also used as a state prison. Euphemia, mother of Alexander, Lord of the Isles, was imprisoned here, as was Patrick Graham, Archbishop of St Andrews. But there were dark secrets too, as revealed in the 1880s, when a human skeleton, standing upright, was found built into one of the walls.

The various buildings on Inchcolm are too extensive to discuss in detail here but they form a most interesting group and some parts of the monastery are remarkably well preserved. The site is maintained by the Government and has a resident custodian. During the summer there are occasional boat excursions from South Queensferry and for yachtsmen the best anchorage is in the north bight.

The island beneath the Forth (Rail) Bridge – **Inchgarvie** (G. – rough island) – also has a long and interesting history but as the bridge has destroyed its insularity it is not a subject for this book. Like Inchkeith it had its castle fortification which was considered an important stronghold and was also used as a state prison on occasions, and even a hospital for the quarantine of infectious diseases. It was demolished by Cromwell but rebuilt in 1779 for protection against John Paul Jones. In the end stone from the castle was used to help build the bridge caissons in 1883.

For the defence of the bridge a gun emplacement was maintained on Inchgarvie during the Second World War.

12.1 Isle of May

(ON maa-øy – gull island). In 13th century recorded as 'Maeyar' leading to a comparison with (G. machair – level land) because of the island's plateau-like structure but this is not convincing.

OS Maps: 1:50000 Sheet 59 1:25000 Sheet 59
Admiralty Charts: 1:75000 Nos.175 or 190 1:25000 No.734

Area: 45ha (111 acres)
Height: 50m (164 ft)

Owner: The Commissioners of Northern Lights. Scottish Natural Heritage (SNH) manage it as a National Nature Reserve.

Population: 1881–22. 1891–27. 1931–10. 1961–7. 1971–10. 1981–2. 1991–0. 2001–0.

Geology: The rock is mainly hard fine-grained basalt of a dark-grey colour with tinges of green and greenstone. There are fewer sea-caves than there are on the Bass Rock as the rock here is harder.

History: The island became a celebrated place of pilgrimage after St Adrian, first Bishop of St Andrews, was discovered and murdered when attempting to shelter here from the Danes in about the year 870. He was buried on the island but half his stone coffin is supposed to have miraculously floated over to Anstruther and ended up in Anstruther Wester churchyard. Six thousand Fife Christians are said to have been slaughtered in this attack, including another saint – Monance.

David I (1124–53) gifted the May to the Benedictine Monastery of Reading in Berkshire on the promise that nine priests would say mass for his soul and that of

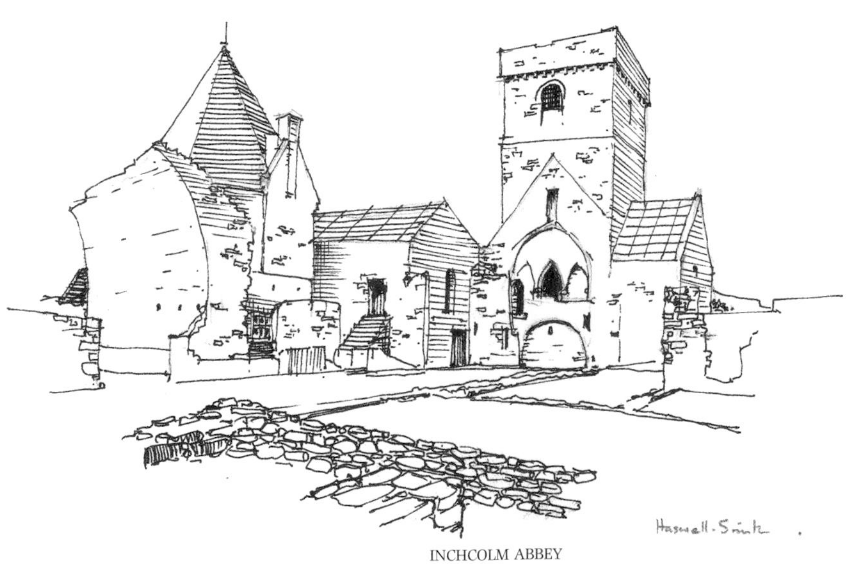

INCHCOLM ABBEY

his successors in perpetuity. He built a chapel on the island dedicated to St Adrian for the new Priory.

The May was sold by the abbot of Reading privately to William Wishart, archbishop of St Andrews c.1270. This may have been encouraged by Alexander III, who disliked the idea of the May being under English control, and certainly the brethren in Reading tried to rescind the deal when they learned of it.

When Edward I installed John Balliol on the throne of his 'vassal kingdom' of Scotland in 1292, the very first Parliament was asked to return the May to the Benedictines of Reading. Bishop Fraser of St Andrews, however, appealed to the Pope for a ruling and this delayed any settlement. The Battle of Bannockburn in 1314 eventually resolved the matter, although the Scottish monks had meanwhile deserted the island and established themselves in more comfort at Pittenweem. For the next two centuries the monks continued to till the island but live elsewhere while the English demolished the island Priory during many incursions. Later, however, a small Hermitage was built among the ruins.

In 1549 the Provost of St Andrews took a feu on the island which was described then as waste land providing no income, due to the rabbit warrens having been destroyed by the English. It was agreed that a chaplain should stay in the Hermitage and continue to conduct services in the chapel 'out of reverence to the relics and tombs of the saints buried in the island; and for the reception of pilgrims...' Two years later a feu charter was conferred on the Balfours of Montquhanny and in 1558 it passed to the family of Forret of Fyngask. Then sometime before 1636 the island was bought by the Cunynghames of Barnes and it was agreed that together with James Maxwell of Innerwick they could levy an 'impost' on ships for erecting and maintaining a Light on the Isle of May. Parliament ratified this in 1641 and again in 1645 for the 'true and thankeful service done to his hieness... Be his Majesty's Lovitt Johne Cunnynghame of Barnes In bigging and erecting upoun the yle of Maij belonging to him Lyand in the mouth of the firth Of ane Lighthous...'

In 1672 the Earl of Kellie is recorded as the owner but he sold it to the Scotts of Scotstarvet. The Marquis of Tichfield, 4th Duke of Portland, inherited it from the Scotts by marriage in 1795 and the Duchess eventually sold it to the Northern Lighthouse Commissioners for the sum of £60,000 in 1815. In the 20th century the island played an important part in anti-submarine defense during both world wars.

Wildlife: A number of interesting plant communities are to be found and over sixty varieties of seaweed have been recorded here.

The Scottish Seabird Centre in North Berwick has a direct video link to the Isle of May similar to its remote interactive cameras on the Bass Rock and Fidra. This allows visitors to watch the birds and other wildlife such as seals throughout the year without disturbing them. By individual control of the cameras they can pan the area and zoom in on points of interest.

Renowned for its birdlife, in early summer the Isle of May is a wonderful nesting place for many seabirds but, unlike the Bass Rock, there are no gannets. April/May and August/October are the most interesting periods for bird-watching. Breeders: Large numbers of shag, kittiwake,

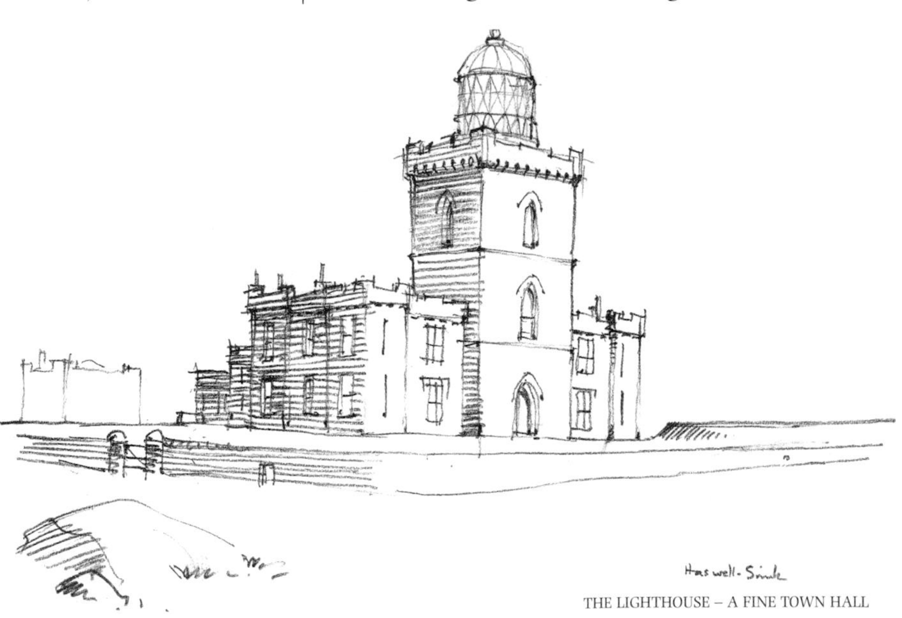

THE LIGHTHOUSE – A FINE TOWN HALL

guillemot, razorbill, puffin, and also, fulmar, herring gulls and lesser black-backed gulls, eider, oystercatcher and a few common and arctic terns, wheatear and rock pipit.

Over 240 bird species have been recorded and in autumn there are often enormous numbers of relatively common birds. Other species seen include wryneck, bluethroat, icterine, barred and yellow-browed warblers, great grey and red-backed shrikes, red-breasted flycatcher, Lapland

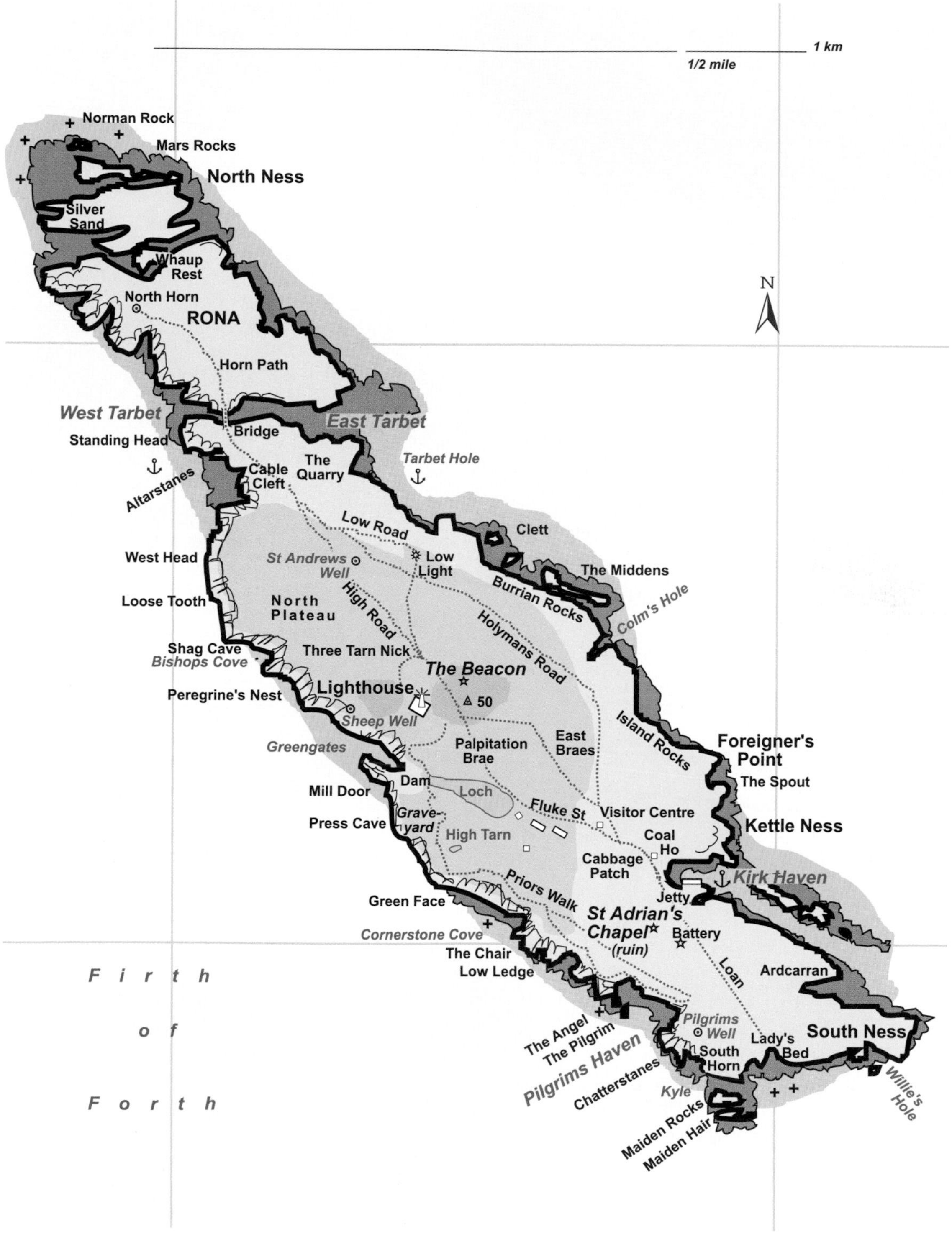

and ortolan buntings, and scarlet rosefinch. Rarities recorded include the red-footed falcon, spoonbill, Pallas's sandgrouse, Daurian redstart, Siberian thrush, pied wheatear, Pallas's-, paddyfield-, melodious-, olivaceous-, and subalpine warblers, red-throated pipit, yellow-breasted and rustic buntings, and pine grosbeak. At sea: divers, shearwaters, sea-duck, petrels and skuas.

* * *

The verdant islet May,
Whose fitful lights amid surrounding gloom,
. . . from danger warns the home-bound mariner.

Fergusson, 1772.

The **ISLE OF MAY** is well known for three diverse reasons – its archaeological interest, its historic lighthouse and its birdlife. The island itself is a long narrow slab of hard basalt with a grassy and reasonably fertile surface partly surrounded by cliffs. The highest point at 50m is near the centre with the lighthouse on it.

Most of the antiquities are at the southern end not far from **Kirkhaven**, where there is a jetty and crane built for the lighthouse keepers. The main ruin is of a rectangular building nearly 10m long with two Norman-style window openings in the west wall [NT658990]. The building is on a north-south access and has had several alterations such as the addition of a defensive tower. The north part of the structure, defined by a partition wall, may have been a chapel but about 1600 a small smithy and forge were constructed inside the ruins of the church which had probably been abandoned years before. Although this building was joined to **St Ethernan's Priory** (c.1140), the Priory itself was demolished in a succession of English invasions. However, during archaeological excavations in 1992, a monastic church was uncovered. The cloister garth and numerous graves were investigated in 1995 and excavation under the 13th-century Benedictine church has revealed signs of an earlier building. Large quantities of pottery included a 13th, or 14th, century decorated jug which probably came from Scarborough and shards of Iron Age and Beaker vessels.

David I was the son of the saintly Queen Margaret and he was determined to substitute the Roman faith for the Culdee faith of St Columba and the other early Christians. He spent money lavishly on abbeys, cathedrals, and churches, gave generous donations to Augustinians, Cistercians, and Benedictines and was profligate in his distribution of Crown lands to the Church. His friendship with the Benedictines of the House of Reading on the Thames came about through his marriage to Henry I of England's sister. His endowment made the Priory of May one of the kingdom's wealthiest establishments.

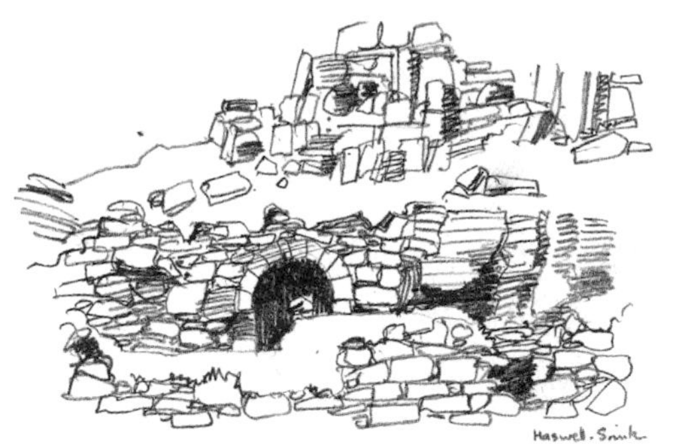

A CHAPEL IN THE CLIFFS NEAR ST ADRIAN'S PRIORY

There are records that shortly after David had founded the Priory Sweyn Asliefsson (See Gairsay, No.10.13), the likable buccaneering Orcadian, plundered it and then sailed up the Firth of Forth to Edinburgh to be received by King David with great honour. It seems that he proudly told David of his exploits and was severely reprimanded so he promptly sailed back down the Forth, restored all the plunder to the monastery, and then sent his greetings to David whereupon he was restored to his position of honour.

A creek at the south-west corner of the island is known as the **Pilgrims' Haven**. It has two outlying rock-stacks (one of these isolated pinnacles is 24m high and supposed to look like a bishop's mitre but I found that to be somewhat imaginative) and a shingle beach in the cove on which a small boat can rest. In the 14th and 15th centuries a steady stream of pilgrims landed here and flocked up the slope to pay their respects at St Adrian's shrine. On the way they would stop to drink brackish water from the **Pilgrim's Well** [NT659989], which was reputed to cure many ailments and bring about remarkable miracles. One of these pilgrims was Mary of Gueldres, *en route* from the Netherlands in 1449 to marry James II. Another was James IV who made the pilgrimage on a number of occasions – 1490, 1503, 1505 and 1513. James V may also have visited the May in 1540.

In the 17th century there was a small village

just south of the Priory and there is a tradition that the inhabitants lived by ship-wrecking and smuggling. Contraband was kept in the cave near the **South Ness** which the excisemen were told was inhabited by a colony of kelpies. The May caves were also used by Fife fishermen to avoid the press-gangs and one well-concealed cave is still called 'Press Cave'. Archaeologists are investigating the village remains.

In a hollow near the cliff-edge is a solitary tombstone for a John Wishart who died in 1730. This was probably the site of the village cemetery.

West of the lighthouse-keepers' cottages and outbuildings there is a deep gorge which has been dammed to provide a water supply. Prior to this there was no satisfactory source of fresh water as, although there are several wells, they are either brackish or dry out at intervals. The lighthouse is now automatic but on an earlier visit to the island a keeper proudly showed us his walled garden, well protected to keep out the rabbits and full of superb vegetables.

The lighthouse is a handsome structure which would make a fine town hall but is quite out-of-keeping with the landscape. It was started in 1816 and contains a square light-tower with mock battlements and a spacious two-storey building with accommodation for the superintendent keeper.

The track running past the lighthouse and on to **Altarstones Landing** in the north-west is called **Holyman's Road** because it was the path customarily taken by the Prior.

In the centre of the island and not far from the modern lighthouse is a platform-like structure which is all that remains of the original lighthouse or **Beacon** [NT657994]. When Alexander Cunningham had it built in 1635 it was the first and only lighthouse in Scotland – a mere platform 12m high with a burning beacon on it. When Cunningham's son, John, together with James Maxwell, obtained permission to charge ships an impost for the light, they improved the design by raising the beacon platform to 18m and constructing the tower like a Border keep. This was in 1656. The impost was four Scots shillings a ton for foreign ships and two shillings for home vessels collected by Customs officers on the Fife coast and bringing in about £280 sterling per year. The light came from burning a ton of coal each night in a grate or chauffer at the top of the tower. In gales, up to three tons of coal were consumed.

The architect for the beacon tower was drowned when his boat capsized while on a supervision visit. Several old ladies of Pittenweem were blamed for the tragedy and burned as witches.

The lighthouse was rather unsatisfactory, particularly as in a gale very little light could be seen on the dangerous windward side. In January 1791 the light was out for two nights during a severe storm. It was found that the lighthouse-keeper, his wife, and five children, had been asphyxiated by the fumes although a baby survived. There were many shipwrecks and complaints but nothing was done until two Royal Navy frigates, *Pallas* and *Nymph*, were wrecked on the rocks near Dunbar in 1810. The pilots said they thought a limekiln at Broxmouth was the May light, and that the May light was the Bell Rock. At last the Government acted. The Commissioners of Northern Lights bought the island in 1815 and started construction of the present lighthouse – using the latest design of oil lamps and reflectors.

Maiden Hair Rock, near the Pilgrims' Haven, is supposed to be named in honour of St Thenaw. King Loth of Lothian was reputed to have been gifted his kingdom by King Arthur of the Round Table. The legend claims that in the year 516, Princess Thenaw, Loth's young unmarried daughter, was found to be pregnant. The king was furious and ordered her to be cast headlong from Traprain Law (then known as Dunpender) as punishment for fornication. After praying for forgiveness the girl was thrown from the height, but she landed on soft ground and suffered no injury. King Loth was convinced that only a witch could have had such a remarkable escape and decreed that she be put to death by drowning. So she was rowed out from Aberlady and cast into the water near the Isle of May. She managed to clutch on to the seaweed on Maiden Hair Rock for a time but after crying for help from God she was swept away by the tide far up the Forth. She was at last washed ashore beside the Monastery at Culross and it was here, lying on the beach, that she gave birth to her son, Kentigern, later known as St Mungo, patron saint of Glasgow. Soon after, mother and son were discovered by a monk and St Serf, Abbot of Culross, looked after them.

Access: Information on boat trips from Anstruther and Crail, 01333-311073. Scottish Natural Heritage, Fife, 0334-54038.

Anchorages: Use plenty of chain as holding is poor.
1. Altarstones Landing, W side. Subject to surge and exposed to all W'lies. Occasional anchorage in 5m, opposite the steps. Moored dinghies subject to damage except in flat calm. Hoist inflatables clear of sea.
2. Kirkhaven, E of S Ness. Long, narrow gut entered from SE with jetty at head. Pleasant in calm weather but subject to surge in S–SW winds and dangerously exposed to E'lies and breaking seas. Depth only 1.2m but with space for small yacht to tie to rings. Very narrow, but mid-channel approach under power is straightforward.
3. East Tarbet or Tarbet Hole. Subject to swell and exposed to E. Awkward landing on rocks. Occasional anchorage in 4m.

12-Appendix Bass Rock

Derivation uncertain. Possibly named after a man named Bass mentioned in the Book of Lecain (Chronicles of Picts and Scots). In Old Norse 'Baa' is a sunken rock on which the sea breaks in bad weather – maybe this is an inaccurate application meaning 'a dangerous rock'; or (ON berserk – in a bear's shirt) meaning 'a wild warrior'.

O S Maps: 1:50000 Sheet 66 1:25000 Sheet 351
Admiralty Charts: 1:75000 No.175 1:50000 No.734

Area: 7½ha (19 acres)
Height: 107m (350 ft)

Owner: Sir Hew Hamilton-Dalrymple.

Population: (Lighthouse-keepers) 1961–5. 1971–3. 1981–0. 1991–0.

Geology: A volcanic plug of phonolite rock.

History: Most of the rock belonged to the Bishopric of St Andrews when Malcolm Canmore is said to have granted the remaining part of it to the Lauder family in 1056. The Lauders became known as the Lauders of the Bass and they held it until the mid-17th century. In 1706 it became the property of Sir Hew Dalrymple and it is still in the ownership of his family.

St Baldred, an Irish missionary may have been the first inhabitant. He died in 606.

In 1338, the siege of Dunbar Castle by the English was broken because the Bass Rock was able to provide Black Agnes, Countess of March and Dunbar, with provisions.

The date when the fortress was built, probably by the Lauders, is not on record. It is first mentioned in 1405 when Prince James, the twelve-year old son of Robert III, later to become James I, was sent here for safety by

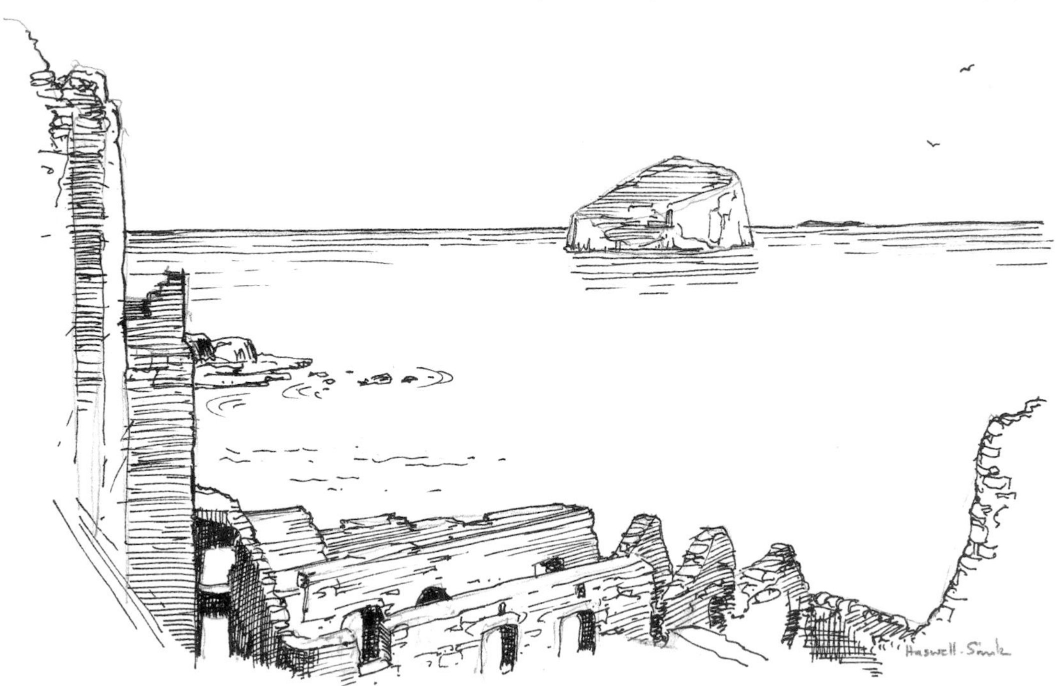

THE BASS ROCK FROM THE RAMPARTS OF TANTALLON CASTLE. THE ISLE OF MAY LIES ON THE HORIZON.

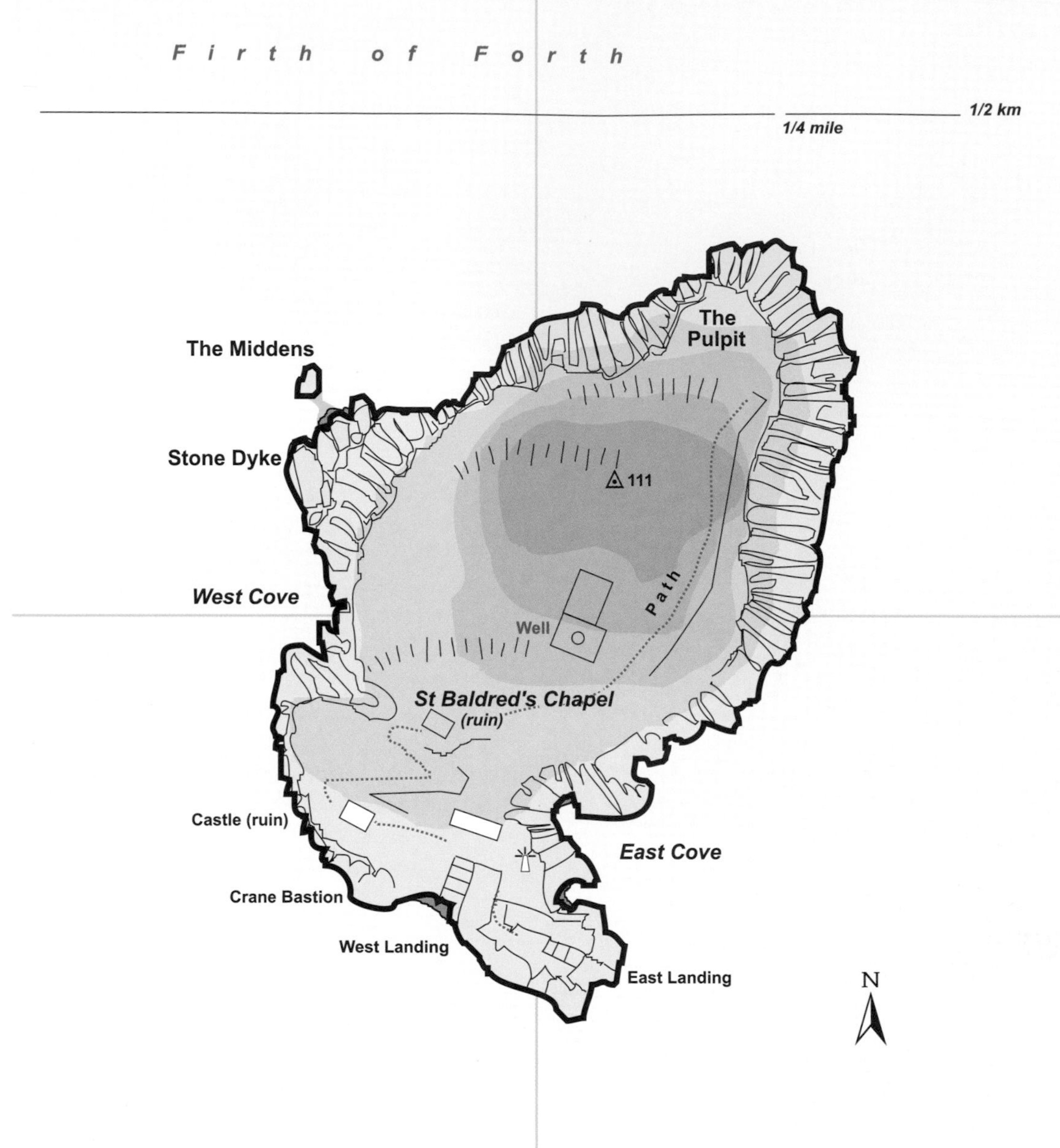

his father until a vessel could be found to take him to France, as the king's brother, the Duke of Albany, had designs on the throne. Albany tipped off the English who intercepted James' ship, and imprisoned the prince in the Round Tower at Windsor for nineteen years. When James was eventually ransomed for £400,000 he, understandably, decided to get his own back and imprisoned the son of the Duke of Albany in the fortress on the Bass Rock.

In 1542 the crude little chapel which had been built about 1491 was consecrated and dedicated to St Baldred.

When Cromwell stormed north and defeated the Presbyterians at Dunbar (they had offered allegiance to Charles II), there was an attempt to send the Church Records over to the Bass Rock for safe-keeping. But the Rock surrendered to Cromwell's forces in 1651, the Records were removed to London, and it is thought they were lost in the fire at the House of Commons in 1834.

When Charles II was restored as monarch in 1660 he set about destroying the Church of Scotland, but the Covenanters fought back with secret 'conventicles'. Many Presbyterians were arrested and in 1671, the Bass Rock was bought (for £4000) and used as a prison for the recalcitrant Covenanters. It was not until 1688 that many of these men were released when James VII was relieved of the Crown and William of Orange proclaimed king. Much of Scotland however remained faithful to James until the Battle of Killiecrankie after which the only remaining Jacobite stronghold was the Bass Rock. It held out for nearly two years under its Governor, Sir Charles Maitland, but was eventually starved into submission in 1690.

It was now the turn of four Jacobites to be held prisoner. But not for long, because while the new Governor, Fletcher of Saltoun, was away they captured the garrison and with only a gunner and sixteen friends from Lothian to help them they held the Bass Rock from 1691 until 1694. Even then they only surrendered because they were granted an amnesty.

In 1701, the fortress was dismantled and the island was sold to Sir Hew Dalrymple, whose family still own it. Its main use at this time was for grazing sheep and collecting gannets to eat.

In 1902 the lighthouse was constructed and the island was once again temporarily inhabited.

Wildlife: Forty-eight species of wildflower have been recorded here. This includes the tree mallow, *Lavatera arborea*, a tall biennial with attractive rose-coloured flowers. It was introduced to the Bass Rock by sheep farmers in the 17th century (its woolly leaves make good bandages). It is thriving in the milder winters and as its seeds can survive in water for more than three months it is invading surrounding islands and destroying the puffin burrows. Another unusual plant is the Pheasant's-eye Daffodil, *Narcissus poeticus*, which comes from central Europe. Examples can also be found of the native Sea Beet, *Beta vulgaris maritima*.

Birdlife is prolific. There are common inland species such as blackbird, hedge sparrow and rock pipit, while seabirds are packed onto every steep rock-ledge. The island is most famous for its huge gannet colony of over 40,000 pairs and the bird is even named after the island – *Morus bassanus*. There are also large numbers of kittiwake, razorbill, shag, fulmar, herring gull, guillemot and puffin. These, together with the birdlife on St Kilda and the Isle of May, can all be viewed live by remote video at the Scottish Seabird Centre in North Berwick.

* * *

The **BASS ROCK** can be thought of as the Ailsa Craig (No.1.1) of the East Coast but it is very much smaller. There was a fortress on it for centuries and most of the materials were brought over from the mainland. Considering the difficulty of landing in even comparatively quiet conditions, one marvels at the dogged determination of the builders.

There is a huge cave which cuts right through the base of the Bass Rock from east to west. The sea – and the seals – slip through, and it can be explored by dinghy in calm weather. Its least height is about 10m, length 170m, and there is a patch in the middle where there is a small gravel beach.

Sailing around the rock is an unforgettable experience. The view of the cave may be beautiful and fascinating but it is the assault on all the senses which is beyond belief. The eyes are dazzled by clouds of wheeling and diving birds set against rock formations draped in guano and deep shadows of caverns and overhanging ledges. The ears are deafened by the high-pitched cries of the seabirds as a descant to the surging bass tones of the sea growling in the rock clefts – what a subject for Mahler! And the nose really suffers. The smell is overpowering.

The rock itself appears from the mainland to slope gradually down to the sea but this slope is in fact divided into three rough terraces. The lowest terrace with the landing place has the remains of the fortress on it which was purchased by the Government in 1671 as a state prison. On the second terrace are the ruins of **St Baldred's Chapel**, probably built on the site of his original anchorite cell. The highest terrace has what was once a walled garden and a well – although this is no more than a catchment for surface water. There is a cairn at the summit (111m).

* * *

Access: There are boat trips from North Berwick in the summer months. The owner's permission is required for landing.

Anchorages: No anchorages.

1. Landing jetty on S side, below lighthouse. Unless flat calm (very rare), advisable to lie off and approach in dinghy. Even then, landing can be difficult due to the swell.

Table 2:

The islands arranged in order of magnitude

NO.	NAME	TABLE 1 NO.	AREA IN HECTARES
1	Lewis/Harris	8–14	220673
2	Mainland (Shetland)	11–11	100230
3	Mull	3–3	87794
4	Uists/Benbecula	7–15	74540
5	Islay	2–4	61956
6	Mainland (Orkney)	1010	58308
7	Arran	1–4	43201
8	Jura	2–5	36692
9	Yell	11–23	21211
10	Hoy	10–5	14318
11	Bute	1–8	12217
12	Unst	11–29	12068
13	Rum	4–3	10463
14	Tiree	3–10	7834
15	Coll	3–13	7685
16	Barra	7–6	6835
17	Raasay	5–7	6405
18	Sanday	10–24	5043
19	Rousay	10–20	4860
20	Westray	10–25	4713
21	Colonsay	2–6	4617
22	Fetlar	11–24	4078
23	Stronsay	10–14	3275
24	Eigg	4–2	3049
25	Shapinsay	10–12	2948
26	Bressay	11–8	2805
27	Eday	10–21	2745
28	Scalpay	5–3	2483
29	Ulva	3–7	2415
30	Lismore	3–9	2351
31	Whalsay	11–15	1970
32	Luing	2–13	1543
33	Taransay	8–9	1475
34	Scarba	2–9	1474
35	Gigha	2–3	1395
36	Canna	4–4	1314
37	Foula	11–6	1265
38	Kerrera	3–2	1214
39	Great Cumbrae	1–6	1168
40	Scarp	8–13	1045
41	Soay	5–1	1036
42	Rona	5–9	930
43	Papa Westray	10–26	918
44	Iona	3–1	877
45	Flotta	10–4	876
46	Papa Stour	11–14	828
47	Pabbay	8–4	820
48	Fair Isle	11–1	768
49	North Ronaldsay	10–27	690
50	Hirta (St Kilda)	9–1	670
51	Egilsay	10–18	650
52	Mingulay	7–2	640
53	Ronay	7–17	563
54	Muck	4–1	559
55	Shuna	2–10	451
56	Graemsay	10–9	409
57	Sandray	7–4	385
58	Wiay	7–16	375
59	Island of Stroma	10–1	375
60	Vementry	11–13	370
61	Ceann Ear (Monach Isles)	7–19	357
62	Noss	11–7	343
63	Vaila	11–10	327
64	Little Cumbrae Island	1–5	313
65	Wyre	10–15	311
66	Tanera Mór	6–7	310
67	Handa	6–9	309
68	Isle of Ewe	6–2	309
69	Fara	10–6	295
70	Hascosay	11–25	275
71	Seaforth Island	8–12	273
72	Eilean Mór (Crowlin Islands)	5–6	270
73	Inchmarnock	1–7	266
74	Lunga	2–11	254
75	Holy Island	1–3	253
76	Pabbay	7–3	250
77	Calf of Eday	10–23	243
78	Gairsay	10–13	240
79	Fuday	7–11	232
80	Papa Little	11–12	226
81	Housay (Out Skerries)	11–18	218
82	Carna	3–14	213
83	Uyea	11–26	205
84	Berneray	7–1	204
85	Boreray	8–1	198
86	Gruinard Island	6–3	196
87	Ensay	8–3	186
88	Mousa	11–2	180
89	Faray	10–22	180
90	Killegray	8–2	176
91	Isle Martin	6–4	157
92	Shuna	3–12	155
93	Sanda	1–2	151
94	Wiay	5–5	148
95	Garbh Eilean (Shiant Islands)	8–8	143
96	Hellisay	7–9	142
97	Garbh Eileach	2–15	142
98	Eilean nan Ron	6–10	138
99	Little Bernera	8–20	138
100	Longa	6–1	126
101	West Linga	11–16	125
102	Eilean Iubhard	8–11	125

NO.	NAME	TABLE I NO.	AREA IN HECTARES
103	Mealista Island	8–15	124
104	Pabay	5–2	122
105	Priest Island	6–5	122
106	Eorsa	3–6	122
107	Rona (North)	9–4	109
108	Hildasay	11–9	108
109	Cava	10–7	107
110	Pabay Mór	8–19	101
111	Ailsa Craig	1–1	99
112	Soay	9–2	99
113	Gighay	7–10	96
114	Swona	10–2	92
115	Little Colonsay	3–5	88
116	Eilean Righ	2– 8	86
117	Auskerry	10–11	85
118	Vuia Mór	8–17	84
119	Fuiay	7–8	84
120	Lunga	3–8	81
121	Balta	11–28	80
122	Muldoanich	7–5	78
123	Bigga	11–20	78
124	Boreray	9–3	77
125	Eilean Kearstay	8–16	77
126	Eynhallow	10–19	75
127	Papa Stronsay	10–17	74
128	Copinsay	10– 8	73
129	Hermetray	7–20	72
130	Linga (Olna Firth)	11–17	70
131	Gunna	3–11	69
132	Oxna	11–4	68
133	Tanera Beg	6–8	66
134	Cara	2–2	66
135	Samphrey	11–19	66
136	Eilean Dubh Mór	2–14	65
137	Isay	5–8	60
138	South Havra	11–3	59
139	Papa	11–5	59
140	Floddaymore	7–18	58
141	Linga Holm	10–16	57
142	Eileach an Naoimh	2–12	56
143	Inch Kenneth	3–4	55
144	Horse Island	6–6	53
145	Tahay	7–21	53
146	Longay	5–4	50
147	Eileanan Iasgaich	7–13	50
148	Eilean Macaskin	2–7	50
149	Scotasay	8–7	49
150	Stockinish Island	8–6	49
151	Texa	2–1	48
152	Shillay	8–5	47
153	Soay Mór	8–10	45
154	Isle of May	12–1	45
155	Stuley	7–14	45
156	Linga (Bluemull Sound)	11–27	45
157	Lamba	11–22	43
158	Switha	10–3	41
159	Fiaray	7–12	41
160	Vacsay	8–18	41
161	Flodday (E Barra)	7–7	40
162	Brother Isle	11–21	40

Table 3:

The islands arranged in order of height

NO.	NAME	TABLE 1 NO.	HEIGHT IN METRES
1	Mull	3–3	966
2	Arran	1–4	874
3	Rum	4–3	812
4	Lewis/Harris	8–14	799
5	Jura	2–5	785
6	Uists/Benbecula	7–15	620
7	Islay	2–4	491
8	Hoy	10–5	479
9	Mainland (Shetland)	11–11	450
10	Scarba	2–9	449
11	Raasay	5–7	443
12	Hirta	9–1	430
13	Foula	11–6	418
14	Eigg	4–2	393
15	Scalpay	5–3	392
16	Boreray	9–3	384
17	Barra/Vatersay	7–6	383
18	Soay	9–2	378
19	Ailsa Craig	1–1	338
20	Holy Island	1–3	314
21	Ulva/Gometra	3–7	313
22	Scarp	8–13	308
23	Unst	11–29	284
24	Bute	1–8	278
25	Mingulay	7–2	273
26	Mainland (Orkney)	10–10	271
27	Taransay	8–9	267
28	Rousay	10–20	250
29	Bressay	11–8	226
30	Fair Isle	11–1	217
31	Seaforth Island	8–12	217
32	Canna/Sanday	4–4	210
33	Sandray	7–4	207
34	Yell	11–23	205
35	Pabbay (Sound of Harris)	8–4	196
36	Berneray (Bishop's Isles)	7–1	193
37	Kerrera	3–2	189
38	Noss	11–7	181
39	Pabbay (Bishop's Isles)	7–3	171
40	Westray	10–25	169
41	Carna	3–14	169
42	Shiant Islands	8–8	160
43	Fetlar	11–24	158
44	Muldoanich	7–5	153
45	Colonsay/Oronsay	2–6	143
46	Tiree	3–10	141
47	Soay	5–1	141
48	Muck	4–1	137
49	Great Cumbrae	1–6	127
50	Lismore	3–9	127
51	Rona	5–9	125
52	Handa	6–9	123
53	Little Cumbrae	1–5	123
54	Sanda	1–2	123
55	Tanera Mór	6–7	122
56	Isle Martin	6–4	120
57	Whalsay	11–15	119
58	Ronay	7–17	115
59	Crowlin Islands	5–6	114
60	Garbh Eileach	2–15	110
61	Rona (North)	9–4	108
62	Fuiay	7–8	107
63	Gruinard Island	6–3	106
64	Coll	3–13	104
65	Lunga	3–8	103
66	Wiay	7–16	102
67	Gairsay	10–13	102
68	Eday	10–21	101
69	Gigha	2–3	100
70	Iona	3–1	100
71	Lunga	2–11	98
72	Eorsa	3–6	98
73	Vaila	11–10	95
74	Gighay	7–10	95
75	Luing	2–13	94
76	Vementry	11–13	90
77	Shuna	2–10	90
78	Fuday	7–11	89
79	Papa Stour	11–14	87
80	Tanera Beg	6–8	83
81	Papa Little	11–12	82
82	Eileach an Naoimh	2–12	80
83	Shillay	8–5	79
84	Hellisay	7–9	79
85	Priest Island	6–5	78
86	Mealista Island	8–15	77
87	Eilean nan Ron	6–10	76
88	Eilean Iubhard	8–11	76
89	Isle of Ewe	6–2	72
90	Shuna	3–12	71
91	Longa	6–1	70
92	Linga (Olna Firth)	11–17	69
93	Pabay Mór	8–19	68
94	Vuia Mór	8–17	67
95	Longay	5–4	67
96	Sanday	10–24	65
97	Eilean Macaskin	2–7	65
98	Tahay	7–21	65
99	Copinsay	10–8	64
100	Shapinsay	10–12	64
101	Graemsay	10–9	62
102	Little Colonsay	3–5	61

NO.	NAME	TABLE 1 NO.	HEIGHT IN METRES
103	Wiay	5–5	60
104	Inchmarnock	1–7	60
105	Horse Island	6–6	60
106	Flotta	10–4	58
107	Scotasay	8–7	57
108	Boreray	8–1	56
109	Cara	2–2	56
110	Mousa	11–2	55
111	Eilean Righ	2–8	55
112	Eilean Dubh Mór/Beag	2–14	53
113	Housay/Bruray	11–18	53
114	Stroma	10–1	53
115	West Linga	11–16	52
116	Calf of Eday	10–23	50
117	Uyea	11–26	50
118	Isle of May	12–1	50
119	Ensay	8–3	49
120	Inch Kenneth	3–4	49
121	Texa	2–1	48
122	Papa Westray	10–26	48
123	Killegray	8–2	45
124	Stronsay	10–14	44
125	Balta	11–28	44
126	Stockinish Island	8–6	44
127	Fara	10–6	43
128	Flodday (E Barra)	7–7	42
129	South Havra	11–3	42
130	Swona	10–2	41
131	Little Bernera	8–20	41
132	Stuley	7–14	40
133	Oxna	11–4	38
134	Eilean Kearstay	8–16	37
135	Soay Mór	8–10	37
136	Cava	10–7	36
137	Gunna	3–11	35
138	Egilsay	10–18	35
139	Hermetray	7–20	35
140	Lamba	11–22	35
141	Vacsay	8–18	34
142	Bigga	11–20	34
143	Wyre	10–15	32
144	Papa	11–5	32
145	Faray	10–22	32
146	Hildasay	11–9	32
147	Eynhallow	10–19	30
148	Fiaray	7–12	30
149	Hascosay	11–25	29
150	Samphrey	11–19	29
151	Switha	10–3	29
152	Isay	5–8	28
153	Floddaymore	7–18	28
154	Pabay	5–2	28
155	Linga (Bluemull Sound)	11–27	26
156	Brother Isle	11–21	25
157	Eileanan Iasgaich	7–13	23
158	North Ronaldsay	10–27	20
159	Ceann Ear/Iar	7–19	19
160	Auskerry	10–11	18
161	Papa Stronsay	10–17	13
162	Linga Holm	10–16	10

Appendices

Islands permitted to issue their own postage stamps

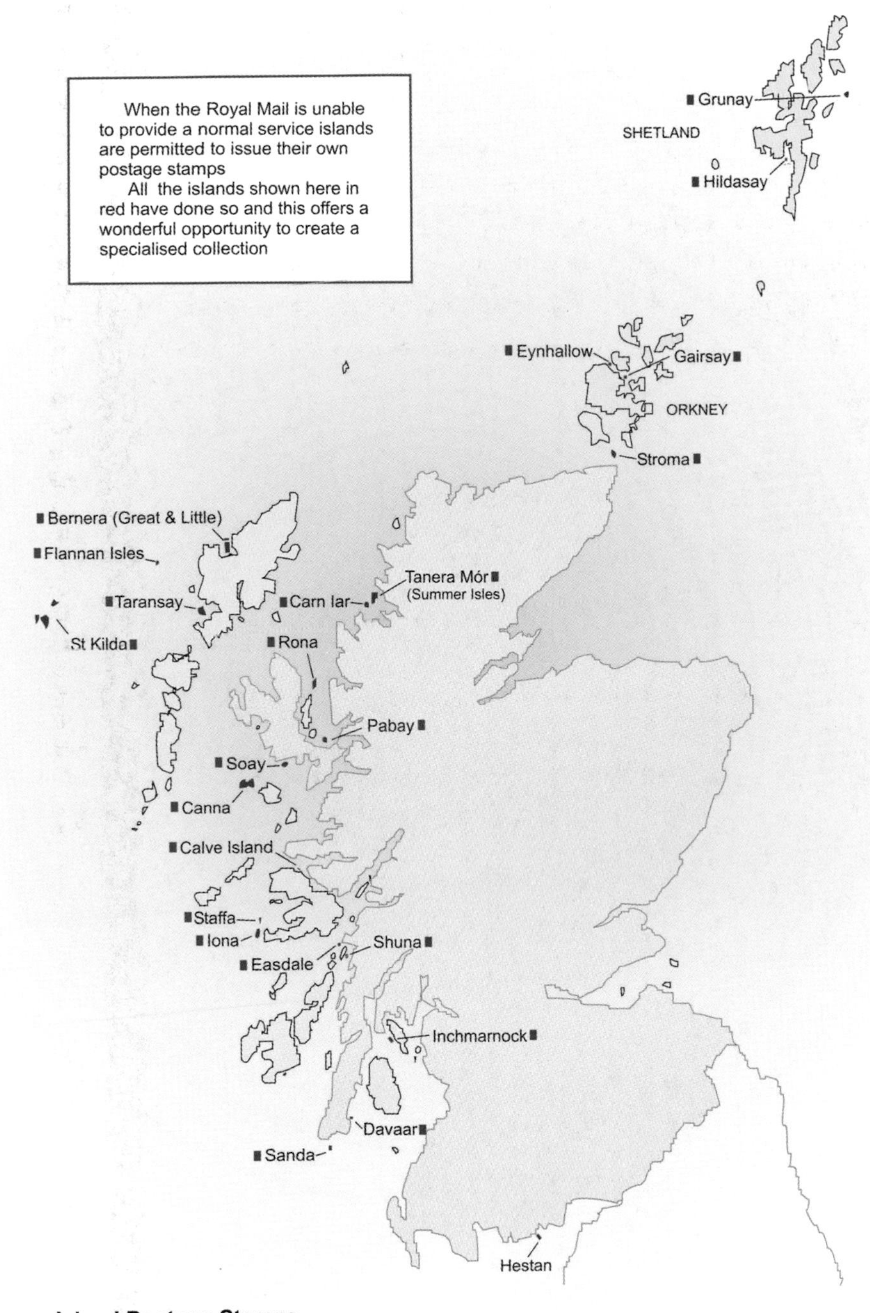

Island Postage Stamps

00x-stampC3

Island whisky distilleries

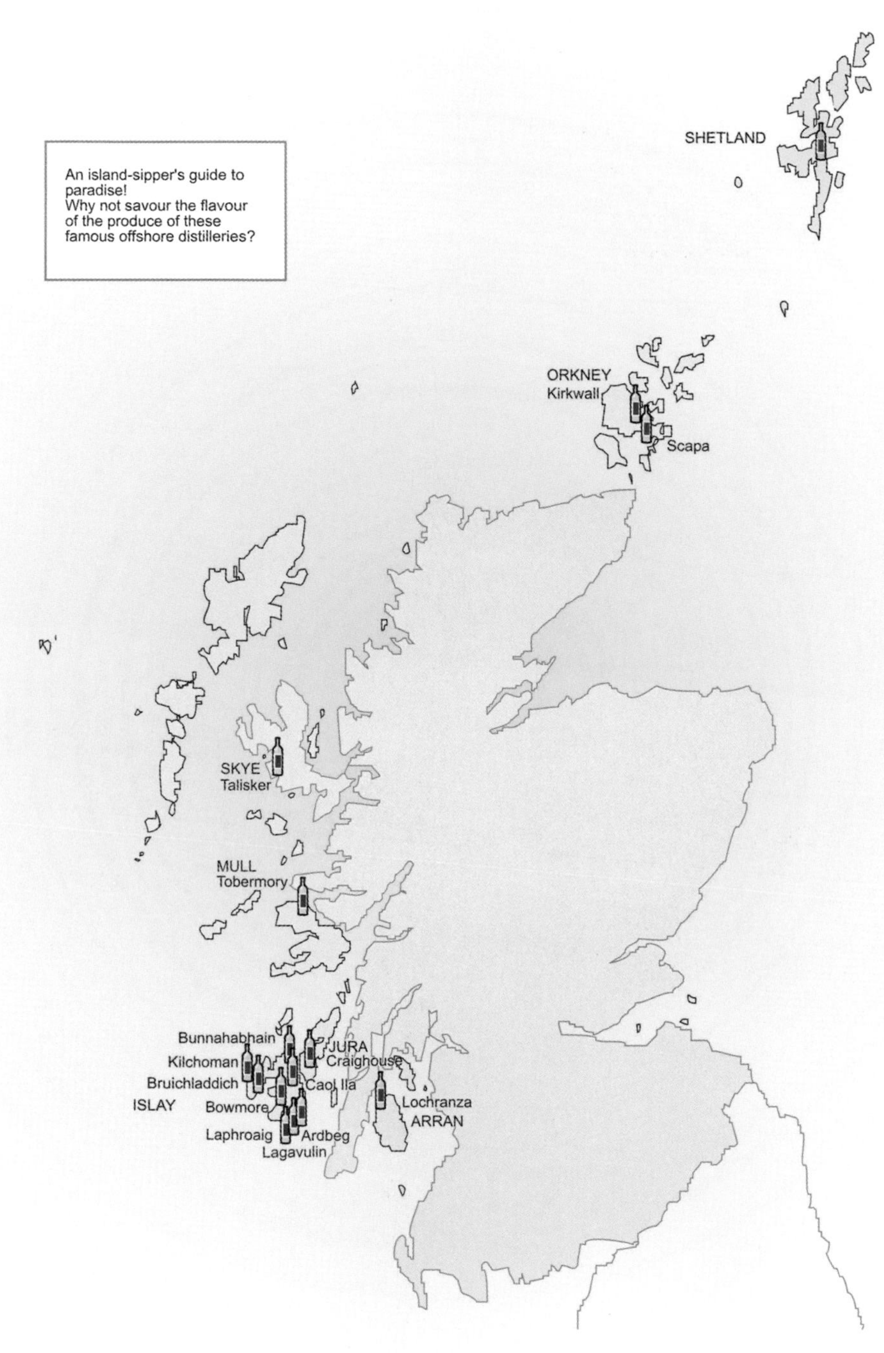

An island-sipper's guide to paradise!
Why not savour the flavour of the produce of these famous offshore distilleries?
SHETLAND
ORKNEY
Kirkwall
Scapa
SKYE
Talisker
MULL
Tobermory
Bunnahabhain
Kilchoman
Bruichladdich
ISLAY
Bowmore
Laphroaig
Lagavulin
Ardbeg
Caol Ila
JURA
Craighouse
Lochranza
ARRAN
Island Distilleries

Island golf courses

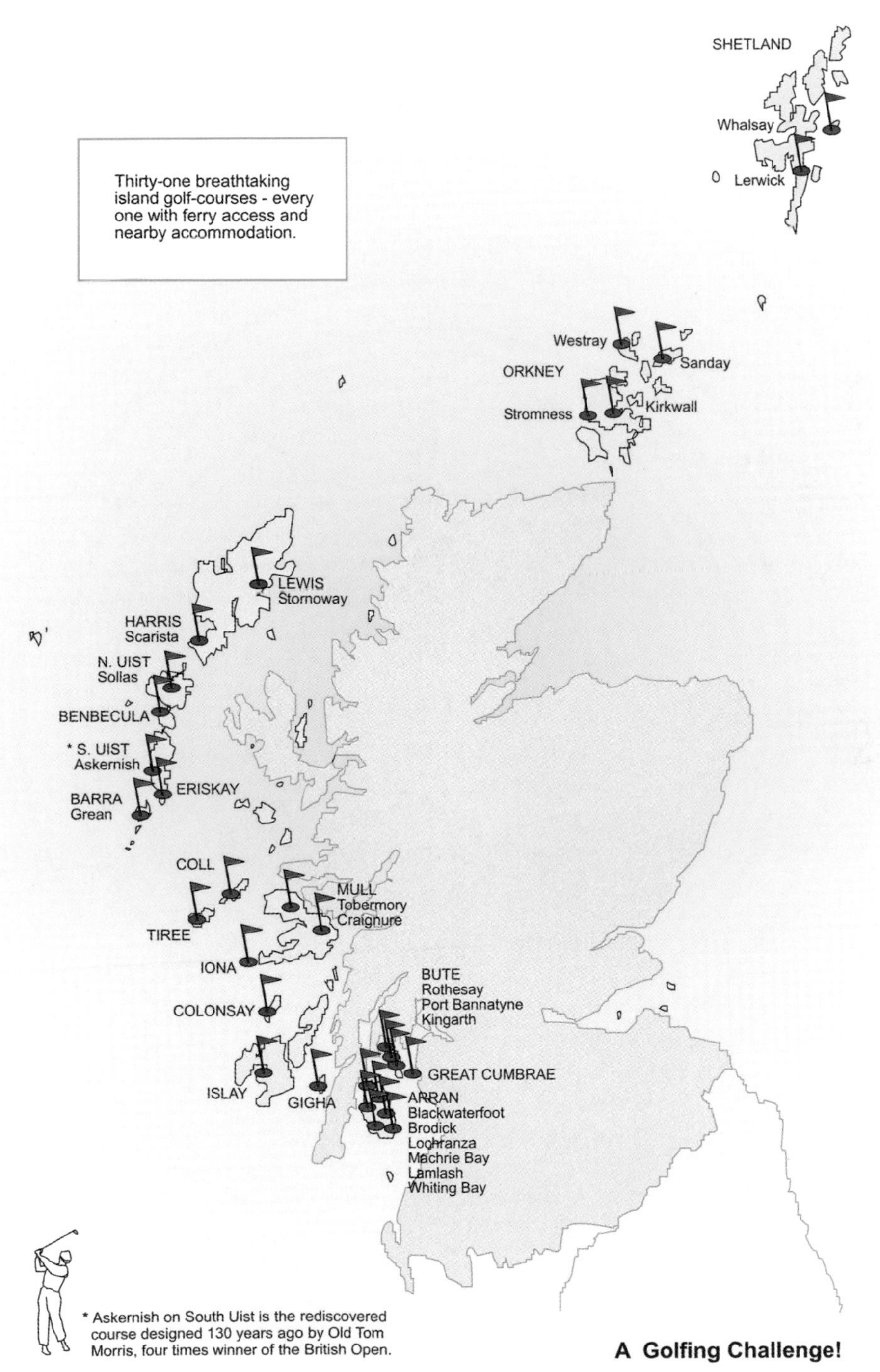
SHETLAND
Whalsay
Lerwick
Thirty-one breathtaking island golf-courses - every one with ferry access and nearby accommodation.
Westray
Sanday
ORKNEY
Stromness
Kirkwall
LEWIS
Stornoway
HARRIS
Scarista
N. UIST
Sollas
BENBECULA
* S. UIST
Askernish
ERISKAY
BARRA
Grean
COLL
TIREE
MULL
Tobermory
Craignure
IONA
COLONSAY
BUTE
Rothesay
Port Bannatyne
Kingarth
GREAT CUMBRAE
ISLAY
GIGHA
ARRAN
Blackwaterfoot
Brodick
Lochranza
Machrie Bay
Lamlash
Whiting Bay
* Askernish on South Uist is the rediscovered course designed 130 years ago by Old Tom Morris, four times winner of the British Open.
A Golfing Challenge!

Bibliography

The relevant section(s) are in square brackets after each entry. [G]= general

Admiralty Hydrographer. *North Coast of Scotland Pilot.* [G]
----------*West Coast of Scotland Pilot.* [G]
Allen, J Romilly, *The Early Christian Monuments of Scotland.* 1903. [G]
Anderson, A O, and M O, *Adomnan's Life of Columba.* 1961. [G]
Anderson, Joseph (ed), *The Orkneyinga Saga.* 1873. [10,11]
Anderson, R S G *The Antiquities of Gigha.* 1978. [2]
Arbman, H *The Vikings.* 1961. [G]
Atkinson, George Clayton, *Expeditions to the Hebrides in 1831 and 1833.* David A Quine (ed). 2001. [5,8,9]
Atkinson, Robert, *Island Going.* 1949. [G]
----------*Shillay and the Seals.* 1980. [7,8]
Bailey, Patrick, *Orkney.* 1971. [10]
Barclay, R S, *The Population of Orkney 1755–1961.* 1965. [10]
Barry, G, *History of the Orkney Islands.* 1805. [10]
Bathurst, Bella, *The Lighthouse Stevensons.* 1999. [G]
Blake, George, *The Firth of Clyde.* [1]
Booth, C Gordon, *A Guide to Islay and Jura.* 1984. [2]
Boswell, James, *The Journal of a Tour to the Hebrides. 1785.* [G]
Botanical Society of the British Isles. *Proceedings.* [G]
Bray, Elizabeth, *The Discovery of the Hebrides. Voyagers to the Western Isles 1745–1883.* 1986. [G]
Brøgger, A W, *A History of the Norse Settlements in Scotland.* 1929. [G]
Brown, G M, *An Orkney Tapestry.* 1969. [10]
Brown, P. Hume, *Early Travellers in Scotland.* 1891. [G]
Budge, Donald, *Jura, an Island of Argyll.* 1960. [2]
Butler, David, *Isle of Noss.* 1990. [11]
Buxton, Ben, *Mingulay. An Island and Its People.* 1995. [7]
Caldwell, David H., *Islay, Jura and Colonsay. A Historical Guide.* 2001 [2]
Campbell, A J, *Fifteen Centuries of the Church in Orkney.* 1938. [10]
Campbell, J F, *Popular Tales of the West Highlands.* 1860–2. [G]
Campbell, John Lorne, *Canna: the Story of a Hebridean Island.* 1984. [4]
Carmichael, Alasdair, *Kintyre.* [G]
Carmichael, Ian, *Lismore in Alba.* 1947. [3]
Childe, V Gordon, *Prehistory of Scotland.* 1935. [G]
----------*Skara Brae: A Pictish Village in Orkney.* 1931. [10]
Clouston, J Storer, *A History of Orkney.* 1932. [10]
Clouston, J Storer, *The Orkney Parishes.* 1927. [10]
Cluness, A T, *The Shetland Isles.* 1951. [11]
Clyde Cruising Club Publications Ltd.
-----------Sailing Directions (with annual updates):
Clyde Area. [1]
Kintyre to Ardnamurchan. [2,3]
Ardnamurchan to Cape Wrath. [4,5,6]
Outer Hebrides. [7,8,9]
North and North-East Coasts and Orkney. [6,10]
Shetland. [11]
Cooper, Derek, *Hebridian Connection.* 1977. [G]
----------*Skye.* [5]
----------*The Road to Mingulay.* 1985. [7,8]
Council for Scottish Archaeology,
Discovery and Excavation in Scotland. [G]
Scottish Archaeological News. [G]
Cowan, E J, McDonald, R A, et al, *Alba: Celtic Scotland in the Medieval Era.* [G]
Cruttwell, Clement, *The New Universal Gazetteer.* 1798. [G]
Craig, David, *On the Crofters' Trail.* 1990. [G]
Craig, G Y, *Geology of Scotland.* 1991. [G]
Cummins, W A, *The Age of the Picts.* 1995. [G]
Cursiter, J W, *List of Books relating to Orkney and Shetland.* 1894. [10,11]
Darling, Dr Frank Fraser, *Island Farm.* 1944. [6]
----------*Island Years.* 1942. [3,6,9]
----------*A Naturalist on Rona.* [9]
----------*West Highland Survey.* [G]
Darling, F Fraser and Boyd, J Morton, *The Highlands and Islands.* 1969. [G]
Dasent, G W, *The Orkneyingers' Saga.* 1894. [10]
Delaney, Frank, *The Celts.* 1989. [G]
Dey, Joan, *Out Skerries.* 1991. [11]
Dickson, John, *Emeralds Chased in Gold.* 1899. [12]
Donaldson, M E M, *Wanderings in the Western Highlands and Islands.* 1920 [G]
----------*Further Wanderings – Mainly in Argyll.* 1926. [G]
Drever, W P, *Udal Law in the Orkneys and Zetland.* 1914. [10,11]
Drummond, Maldwin, *West Highland Shores.* 1990. [G]
Duncan, Angus, *Hebridean Island: Memories of Scarp.* 1995. [8]

Edmonston, T, *Glossary of Shetland and Orkney Dialect.* 1866. [10,11]
Fabian, D J *et al. The Islands of Scotland including Skye.* [G]
Faux, Ronald, *The West.* 1982. [G]
Feacham, R, *A Guide to Prehistoric Scotland.* [1963]
Fenton, Alexander, *The Northern Isles: Orkney and Shetland.* 1978. [10,11]
Fenton, Alexander and Palsson, Hermann, *The Northern and Western Isles in the Viking World.* [G]
Forth Yacht Clubs' Association Pilot Handbook. *Berwick-on-Tweed to Peterhead.* 1974. [12]
Garms, Harry, *The Natural History of Europe.* 1967. [G]
Gear, Sheila, *Foula. Island West of the Sun.* 1983. [11]
Gordon, Seton, *Highways and Byways in the West Highlands.* 1935. [G]
----------*Afoot in Wild Places.* [G]
Gorrie, D, *Summers and Winters in the Orkneys.* 1868. [10]
Graham, Henry Grey, *The Social Life of Scotland in the Eighteenth Century.* 1899. [G]
Grant, I F, *The Lordship of the Isles.* 1982. [G]
Grant, James Shaw, *Discovering Lewis and Harris.* 1987. [8]
Gregory, D, *History of the Western Highlands and Islands.* 1881. [G]
Grieve, Symington, *The Book of Colonsay and Oronsay.* 1923. [2]
Grigsby, Joan, *An Island Rooin.* 1933. [11]
Grimble, Ian, *Highland Man.* 1980. [G]
----------*Scottish Islands.* 1985. [G]
Groome, F Hindes, *Ordnance Gazetteer.* 1900. [G]
Gunn, J, *The Orkney Book.* 1909. [10]
Harker, Alfred, *The West Highlands and the Hebrides.* 1941. [G]
Heddle, J G F M and Mainland, T., *Orkney and Shetland.* 1920. [10,11]
Henderson, Isabel, *The Picts.* 1967. [G]
Hewison, James King, *Bute in the Olden Time.* 1893. [1]
Hewitson, Jim., *Clinging to the Edge.* 1996. [10]
Higgins, L R, *A Tangle of Islands.* 1971. [G]
Hogg, Garry, *The Far Flung Isles.* 1961. [G]
Hossack, B H, *Kirkwall in the Orkneys.* 1900. [10]
Howarth, David, *The Shetland Bus.* 1953. [11]
Jakobsen, Jakob, *Old Shetland Dialect and Place-Names of Shetland.* [11]
----------*Etymological Dictionary of the Norn Language in Shetland.* [11]
Jamieson, Peter, *Letters on Shetland.* 1949. [11]
Johnson, Samuel, *Journey to the Western Isles of Scotland.* 1775. [G]
Knox, John, *Tour of the Highlands of Scotland and the Hebride Isles in 1787.* 1787. [G]
Lacaille, A, *The Stone Age in Scotland.* 1954. [G]
Lamont, W D, *The Early History of Islay.* 1966. [2]
Lawrence, Martin, *Clyde to Colonsay.* 2001. [1,2]
----------*Crinan to Canna.* 2004. [2,3,4]
----------*Skye and Northwest Scotland. 2002.* [5,6]
----------*Western Isles.* 2003. [7,8,9]
----------*North and East Scotland.* 2003. [6,10,12]
Lawson, Bill, *The Teampull on the Isle of Pabbay.* 1994. [8]
Linklater, Eric, revis. J R Nicolson. *Orkney and Shetland.* 1990. [10,11]
Linklater, Eric, *The Ultimate Viking.* 1955. [G]
Loder, J de V, *Colonsay and Oronsay in the Isles of Argyll.* 1935. [2]
Love, John A., *Rum. A Landscape Without Figures.* 2002 [4]
MacCaig, Norman, *Collected Poems.* 1988. [G]
MacCormack, John, *Island of Mull.* 1923. [3]
MacCulloch, J, *The Highlands and Western Isles of Scotland.* 1824. [G]
Macdonald, Donald, *Lewis. A History of the Island.* 1978. [8]
MacDonald, James, *General view of the agriculture of the Hebrides or Western Isles of Scotland: with observations on the means of their improvement, together with a separate account of the principal islands.* 1811. [G]
McEwen, John, *Who Owns Scotland.* 1981. [G]
MacGregor, Alasdair Alpin, *Searching the Hebrides with a Camera.* 1933 [7,8]
Mackenzie, Compton; Campbell, J L; Borgström, Carl, *The Book of Barra.* 1936. [7]
McKerral, Andrew, *Kintyre in the Seventeenth Century.* 1948. [1,2]
MacKillop, Donald, *Sea-Names of Berneray.* 1990. [7,8]
Mackintosh, W R, *Around the Orkney Peat Fires.* 1914. [10]
Maclean, Charles, *The Isle of Mull. Placenames, Meanings and Stories.* 1997. [3]
McLellan, Robert, *The Isle of Arran.* 1970. [1]
Maclennan, John, *Place-Names of Scarp.* 2001 [8]
Macnab, P A, *Mull & Iona.* 1982. [3]
McNeill, F Marion, *Iona.* 1959. [3]

Madders, Michael, and Welstead, Julia, *Where to Watch Birds in Scotland.* [G]
Marshall, David, *The Story of Inchkeith.* [12]
Martin, Martin, *A Description of the Western Isles of Scotland.* 1703. [G]
----------*A Late Voyage to St Kilda.* 1698. [8,9]
Marwick, H, *Ancient Monuments of Orkney. Official Guide.* 1952. [10]
----------*Orkney.* 1951. [10]
----------*Orkney Farm Names.* 1952. [10]
----------edit. Nicolaisen, W F H, *The Place-Names of Birsay.* 1970. [10]
----------*The Place-Names of Rousay.* 1947. [10]
Mercer, John, *Hebridean Islands: Colonsay, Gigha, Jura.* 1982. [2]
Millman, Lawrence, *Last Places.* 1992. [7]
Mitchison, Rosalind, *A History of Scotland.* 1982. [G]
Mooney, J, *Eynhallow. The Holy Isle of the Orkneys.* 1923. [10]
Morton, Tom, *Hell's Golfer – a good walk spoiled.* 1995. [7,8,10,11]
Muir, Edwin, *Autobiography.* [10]
Munro, Dean Sir Donald, *Description of the Western Isles of Scotland.* 1549. [G]
Munro, Neil, *Children of the Tempest.* [7]
----------*The Clyde River and Firth.* [1]
New Statistical Account of Scotland. 1845. [G]
Murray, Frances, *Summer in the Hebrides.* 1887. [G]
Murray, W H *The Islands of Western Scotland.* 1973. [G]
----------*The West Highlands of Scotland.* 1988. [G]
Newton, Norman S, *Colonsay and Oronsay.* 1990. [2]
----------*Islay.* 1988. [2]
Nicolaisen, W F H, *Scottish Place-Names.* 1976. [G]
Nicolson, A, *History of Skye.* 1930. [5]
Nicolson, Adam, *Sea Room. An Island Life.* 2001. [8]
Nicolson, James R, *Traditional Life in Shetland.* 1990. [11]
O'Dell, A C and Watson, Kenneth, *The Highlands and Islands of Scotland.* 1962. [G]
O'Dell, Andrew, *Historical Geography of the Shetland Isles.* [11]
Orkney Antiquarian Society.
Proceedings. [10]
Pennant, T, *A Tour in Scotland, and Voyage to the Hebrides.* 1776. [G]
Perrot, David, *Guide to the Western Isles.* 1986. [G]
Philip, Kathleen, *The Story of Gigha.* 1979. [2]
Rea F G, *A School in South Uist.* 1964 [7]
Reed, Laurence, *The Soay of Our Forefathers.* 2002 [5]
Rendall, R, *Orkney Shore.* 1960. [10]
Robson, Michael, *Rona, the Distant Island.* 1991. [9]
Royal Commission on the Ancient and Historical Monuments of Scotland.
Argyll. 1971–92. [1,2,3]
Orkney. 1946. [10]
Outer Hebrides, Skye and Small Isles. 1928. [4,5,6,7,8]
Sawyer, P H, *The Age of the Vikings.* 1962. [G]
Schei, Liv Kjørsvik and Moberg, Gunnie, *The Orkney Story.* 1985. [10]
----------*The Shetland Story.* 1988. [11]
Scott, M A, *Island Saga. The Story of North Ronaldsay.* 1968. [10]
Scottish Mountaineering Club. District Guide Books,
Islands of Scotland
Munro's Tables
Shaw, Frances J, *The Northern and Western Islands of Scotland: their Economy and Society in the Seventeenth Century.* 1980. [G]
Shaw, Margaret Fay, *From the Alleghenies to the Hebrides.* 1993. [G]
Sharpe, Richard, *Raasay: a Study in Island History.* 1982. [5]
Sheddon, Hugh, *The Story of Lorn.* [3]
Simpson, W Douglas, *The Ancient Stones of Scotland.* 1965. [G]
----------*The Celtic Church in Scotland.* 1935. [G]
Simpson, Sir James Y, *Inchcolm.* [12]
Sinclair, Andrew, *The Sword and the Grail.* 1993. [10]
Sissons, J B, *The Evolution of Scotland's Scenery.* 1967. [G]
Skene, W F, *Celtic Scotland.* 1876. [G]
Smout, T C, *A History of the Scottish People.* 1985. [G]
Smith, G Gregory, (ed.) *The Book of Islay: Documents Illustrating the History of the Island.* 1895. [2]
Society of Antiquaries of Scotland.
Proceedings. [G]
Steel, Tom, *The Life and Death of St Kilda.* 1975. [9]
Steven, Campbell, *The Island Hills.* 1955. [G]
Storrie, Margaret C, *Islay: Biography of an Island.* 1981. [2]
Teignmouth, Lord, *Sketches of the Coasts and Islands of Scotland.* 1836. [G]
Tennent, Norman, *The Islands of Scotland.* [G]

The Statistical Account of Scotland. 1791–99. 1800. [G]
The Third Statistical Account of Scotland. 1961. [G]
Thompson, Francis, *Harris and Lewis, Outer Hebrides.* 1968. [8]
----------*Northern Scotland & the Islands.* [G]
----------*The Uists and Barra.* 1976. [7]
Tranter, Nigel, *Argyll & Bute.* 1977. [1,2,3]
Tulloch, Bobby, *Bobby Tulloch's Shetland.* 1993. [11]
Tulloch, Vie, *The Isle of Gigha.* 1988. [2]
Wainwright, F T (ed.) *The Northern Isles.* 1962. [G]
----------*The Problem of the Picts.* 1955. [G]
Walker, John, edit. McKay, Margaret M., *The Rev Dr John Walker's Report on the Hebrides of 1764 and 1771.* 1980. [G]
Watson, W J, *The History of the Celtic Place-Names of Scotland.* 1926. [G]
West, R G, *Pleistocene Geology and Biology.* 1968. [G]
Westwood, Jennifer, *Albion. A Guide to Legendary Britain.* 1985. [G]
Whitehouse, G K, *The Wild Goats of Britain and Ireland.* 1972. [G]
Whittow, J B, *Geology and Scenery in Scotland.* 1979. [G]
Wightman, Andy, *Who Owns Scotland.* 1996. [G]
Williams, Ronald, *The Lords of the Isles: the Clan Donald and the Early Kingdom of the Scots. 1984.* [G]
Williamson, Kenneth and Boyd, J. Morton, *Mosaic of Islands.* 1963. [G]
----------*St. Kilda Summer.* 1960. [9]
Wilson, Neil, *Scotch and Water: an Illustrated Guide to the Hebridean Malt Whisky Distilleries.* 1985. [G]
Youngson, Peter, *The Long Road: a Driver's Guide to Jura.* 1987. [G]
----------*Jura. Island of Deer.* 2002 [2]

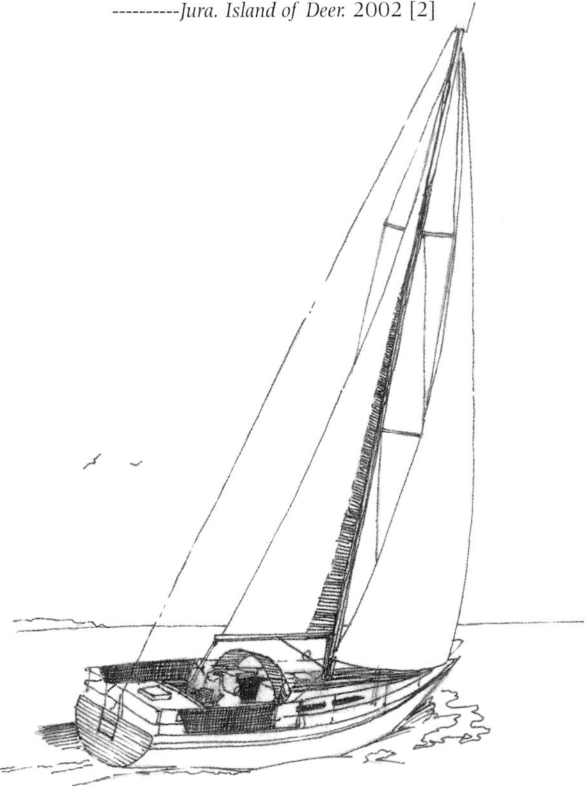

JANDARA

Index of Islands

The section and island reference number is given for each entry. Int = Introduction. Ap = Appendix